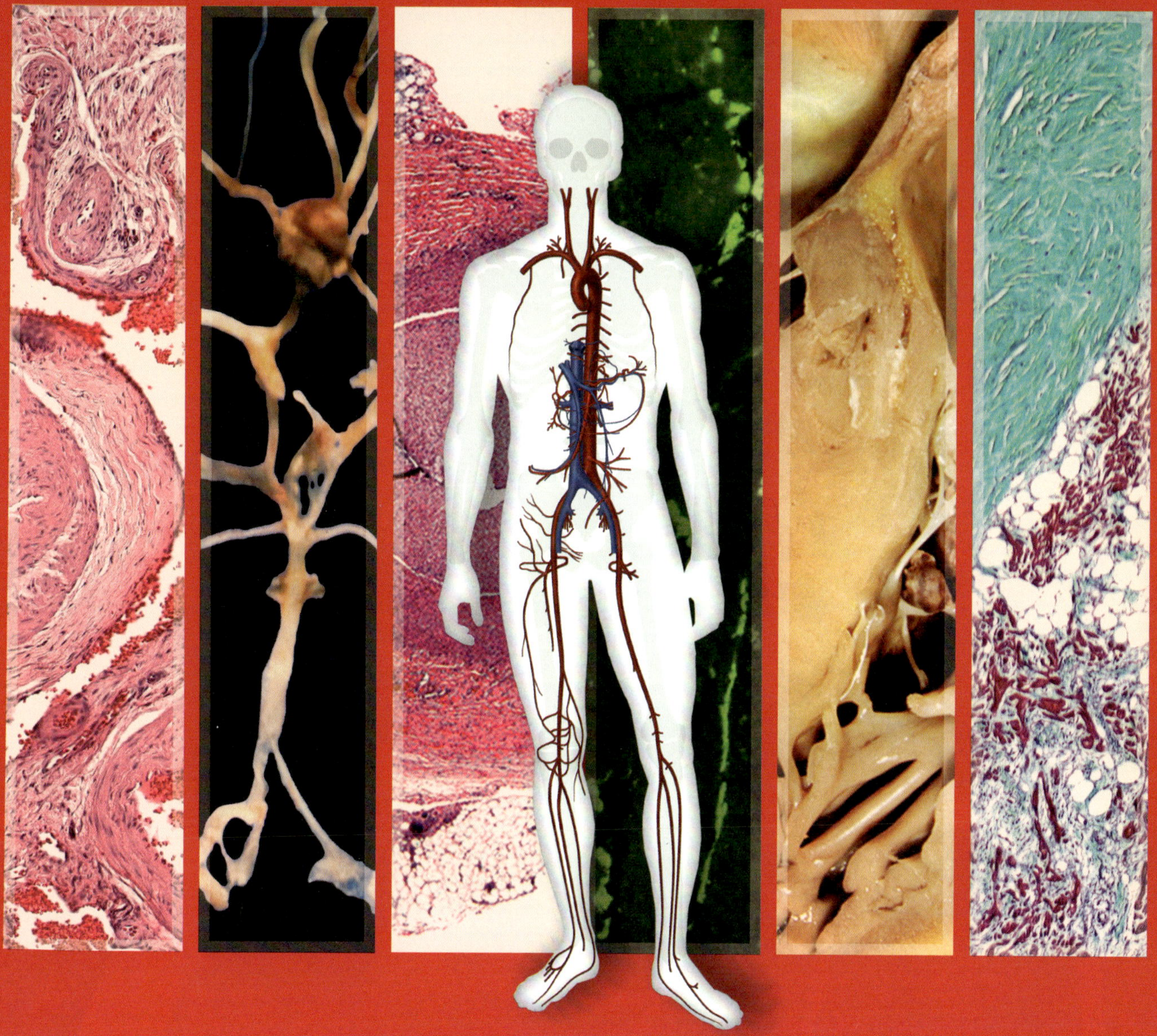

Diagnostic Pathology

Cardiovascular

Miller | Revelo

ELSEVIER

THIRD EDITION

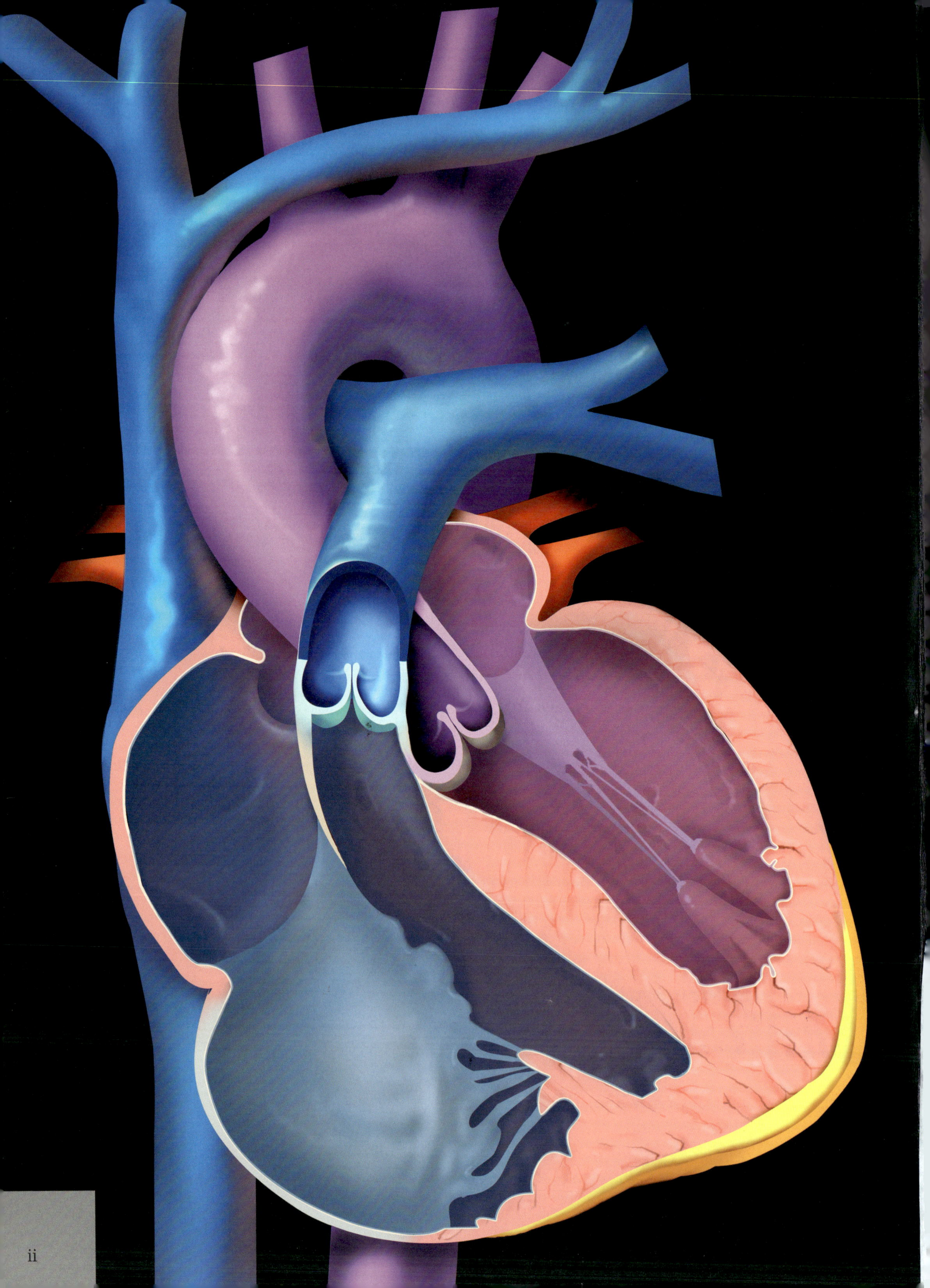

Diagnostic Pathology
Cardiovascular

Third Edition

Dylan V. Miller, MD
Professor (Clinical)
Department of Pathology
University of Utah School of Medicine
Director of Electron Microscopy and Immunostains
Intermountain Central Laboratory
Salt Lake City, Utah

Monica P. Revelo, MD, PhD
Professor
Department of Pathology
University of Utah School of Medicine
Medical Director of Renal and Cardiovascular Pathology
ARUP Laboratories
Salt Lake City, Utah

Additional Contributors

George P. Batsides, MD
Jagdish Butany, MBBS, MS, FRCPC
A. Brad Farris, III, MD
Billie Fyfe, MD
Pooja Gupta, MBBS, DNB
Brian J. Hall, MD
Elizabeth H. Hammond, MD
Amar Ibrahim, MB, ChB, MSc
Brandon T. Larsen, MD, PhD
Joseph J. Maleszewski, MD
Vidhya Nair, MBBS, MD, FRCPC
Victor E. Reuter, MD
Roy H. Rhodes, MD, PhD
Philippe Romeo, MD
Nikhil Sangle, MD, FRCPath
Satish K. Tickoo, MD

Elsevier
1600 John F. Kennedy Blvd.
Ste 1800
Philadelphia, PA 19103-2899

DIAGNOSTIC PATHOLOGY: CARDIOVASCULAR, THIRD EDITION

ISBN: 978-0-323-93620-0

Notices

Practitioners and researchers must always rely on their own experience and knowledge in evaluating and using any information, methods, compounds or experiments described herein. Because of rapid advances in the medical sciences, in particular, independent verification of diagnoses and drug dosages should be made. To the fullest extent of the law, no responsibility is assumed by Elsevier, authors, editors or contributors for any injury and/or damage to persons or property as a matter of products liability, negligence or otherwise, or from any use or operation of any methods, products, instructions, or ideas contained in the material herein.

Previous edition copyrighted 2018.

Library of Congress Control Number: 2022950799

Printed in Canada by Friesens, Altona, Manitoba, Canada

Last digit is the print number: 9 8 7 6 5 4 3 2 1

Dedications

For my parents, Hal and Jeneal.

DVM

To my family, mentors, and friends,
for their guidance, inspiration, support, and love.

MPR

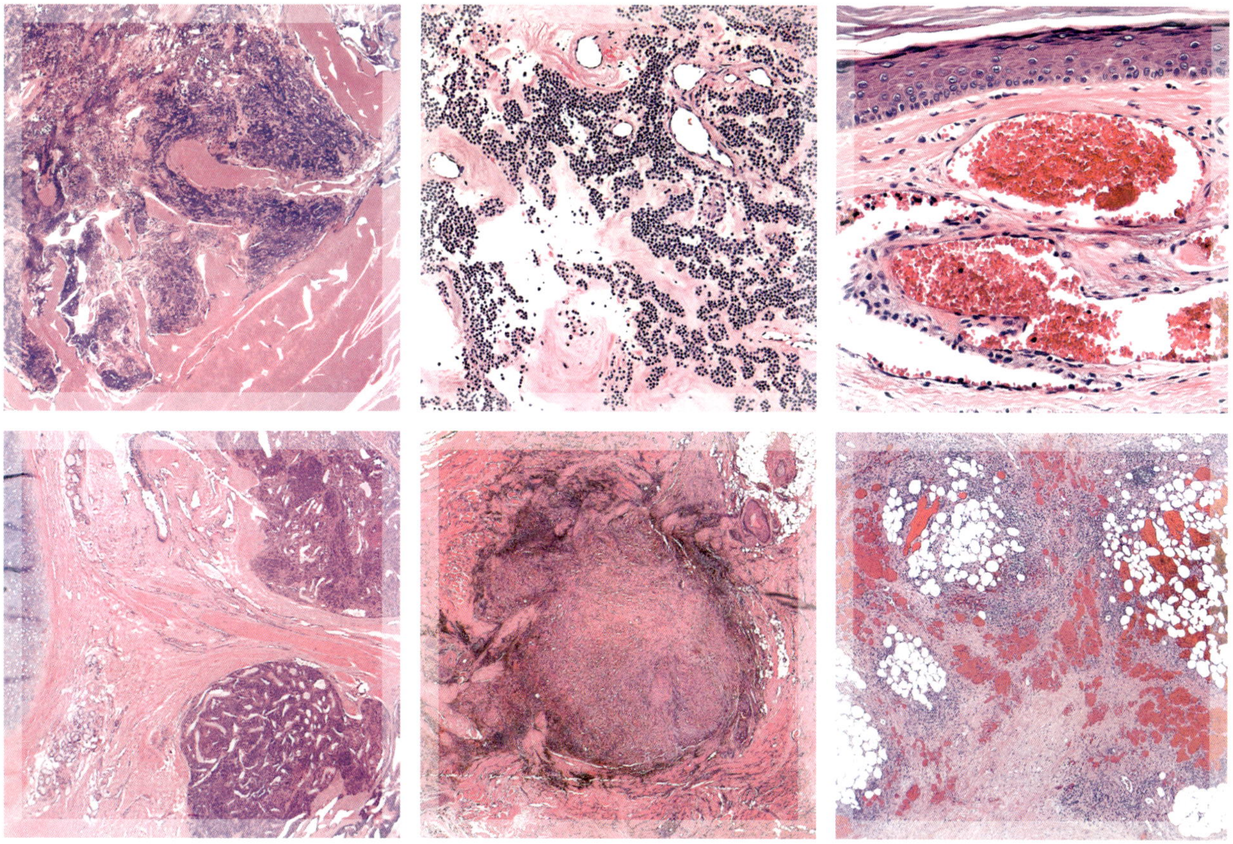

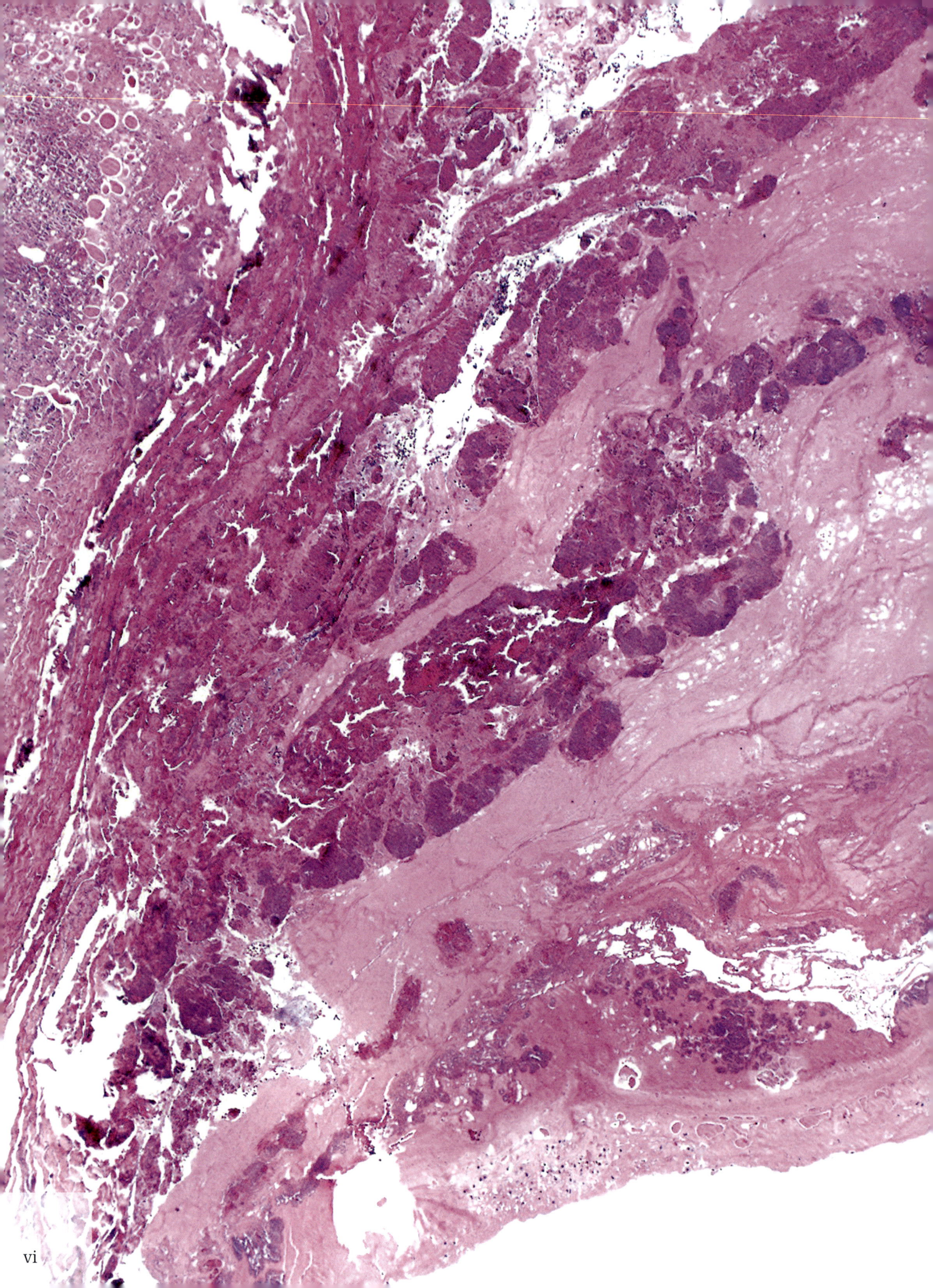

Preface

Cardiovascular pathology encompasses a diverse spectrum of disease processes, including congenital/heritable and acquired, inflammatory and degenerative, infectious and immune, endogenous and exogenous, systemic and localized, and even neoplastic conditions. Some diseases, such as atherosclerosis, ischemic, and valvular disease pose a substantial burden on our society (indeed, the leading cause of death in developed nations), whereas others are extremely rare and elusive. Despite the prevalence of cardiovascular disease in the population, cardiovascular tissue specimens received in pathology departments comprise a relatively minor proportion at most centers. Still, expertise in this area and diagnostic competence are critical because of the clinical impact attending many of these diagnoses.

This third-edition volume in the *Diagnostic Pathology* series covers the breadth of cardiovascular pathology, again with a focus on practical aspects of diagnosis. The sections are organized according to the manner in which they are most often encountered in practice (biopsy, explant and surgical specimens, and autopsy) as well as by anatomic site. Each section is succinct but thorough and provides a richly illustrated topical review. Most chapters address specific entities, although some are devoted to a recommended approach to specific diagnostic challenges in cardiovascular pathology (such as cardiomyopathy evaluation and examination of the conduction system). Many of the "bedrock" concepts in cardiovascular pathology have remained unchanged over past decades and even centuries, but many areas of the field are also rapidly evolving and are the focus of intensive and active research. Every effort was made to ensure that the content in each section is up-to-date. Notably, this edition includes chapters on COVID-19-related cardiovascular pathology and new devices that have come into common use since the previous edition.

Dylan V. Miller, MD
Professor (Clinical)
Department of Pathology
University of Utah School of Medicine
Director of Electron Microscopy and Immunostains
Intermountain Central Laboratory
Salt Lake City, Utah

Monica P. Revelo, MD, PhD
Professor
Department of Pathology
University of Utah School of Medicine
Medical Director of Renal and Cardiovascular Pathology
ARUP Laboratories
Salt Lake City, Utah

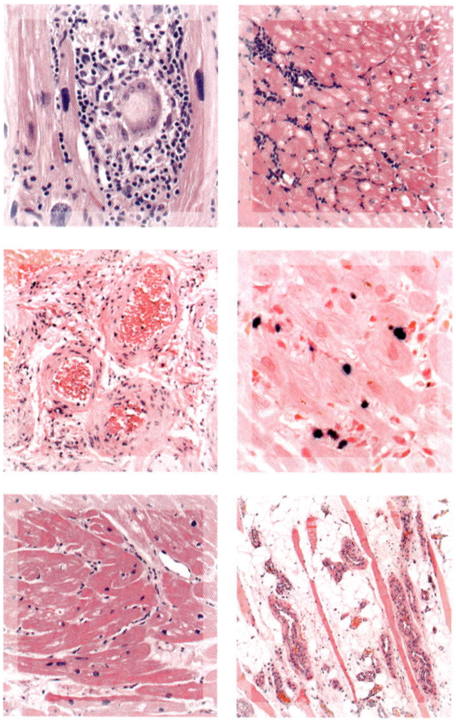

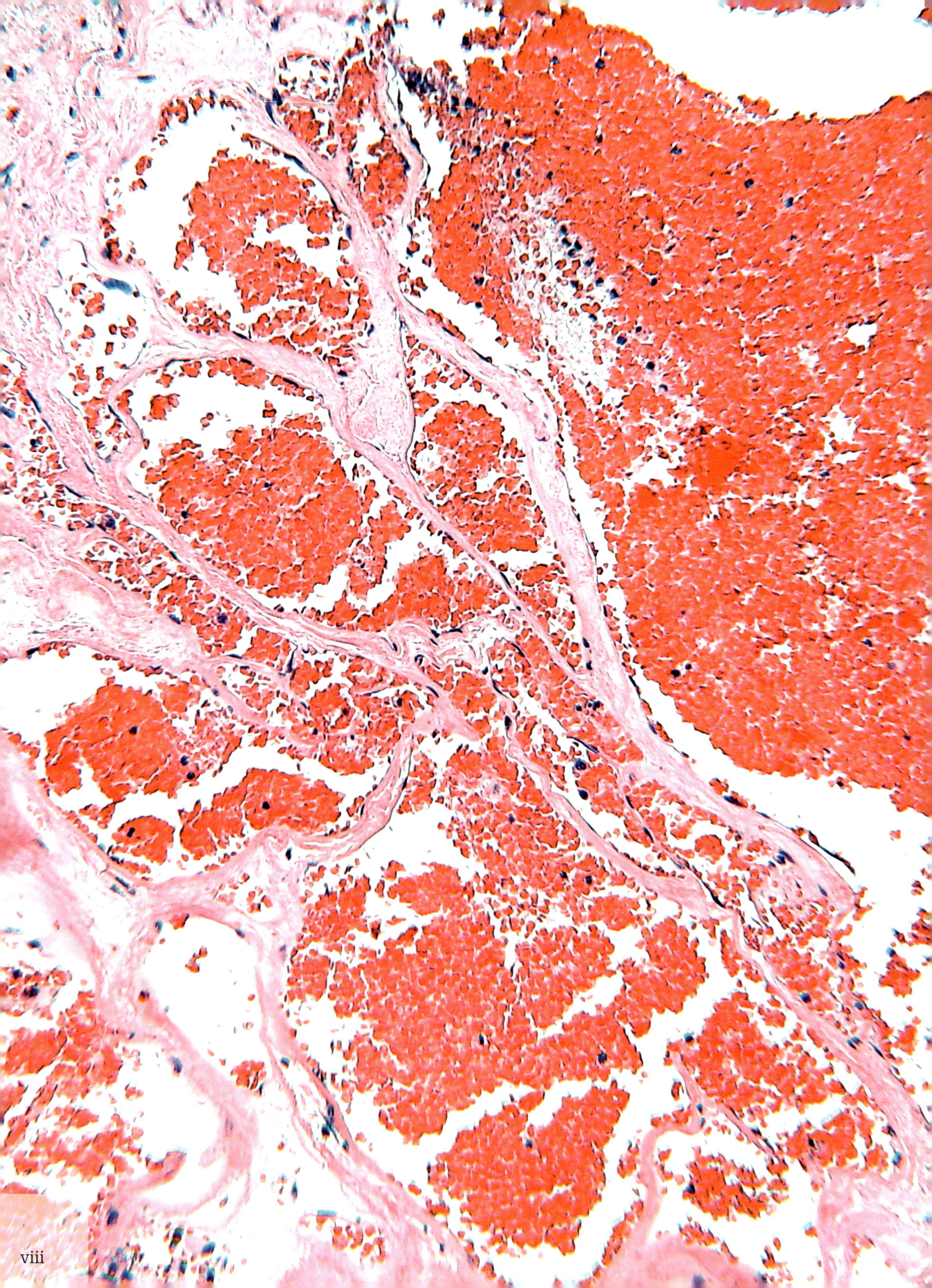

Acknowledgments

LEAD EDITOR
Nina Themann, BA

TEXT EDITORS
Arthur G. Gelsinger, MA
Rebecca L. Bluth, BA
Terry W. Ferrell, MS
Megg Morin, BA
Kathryn Watkins, BA
Shannon Kelly, MA

ILLUSTRATIONS
Lane R. Bennion, MS
Richard Coombs, MS
Laura C. Wissler, MA

IMAGE EDITORS
Jeffrey J. Marmorstone, BS
Lisa A. M. Steadman, BS

ART DIRECTION AND DESIGN
Cindy Lin, BFA

PRODUCTION EDITORS
Emily C. Fassett, BA
John Pecorelli, BS

ELSEVIER

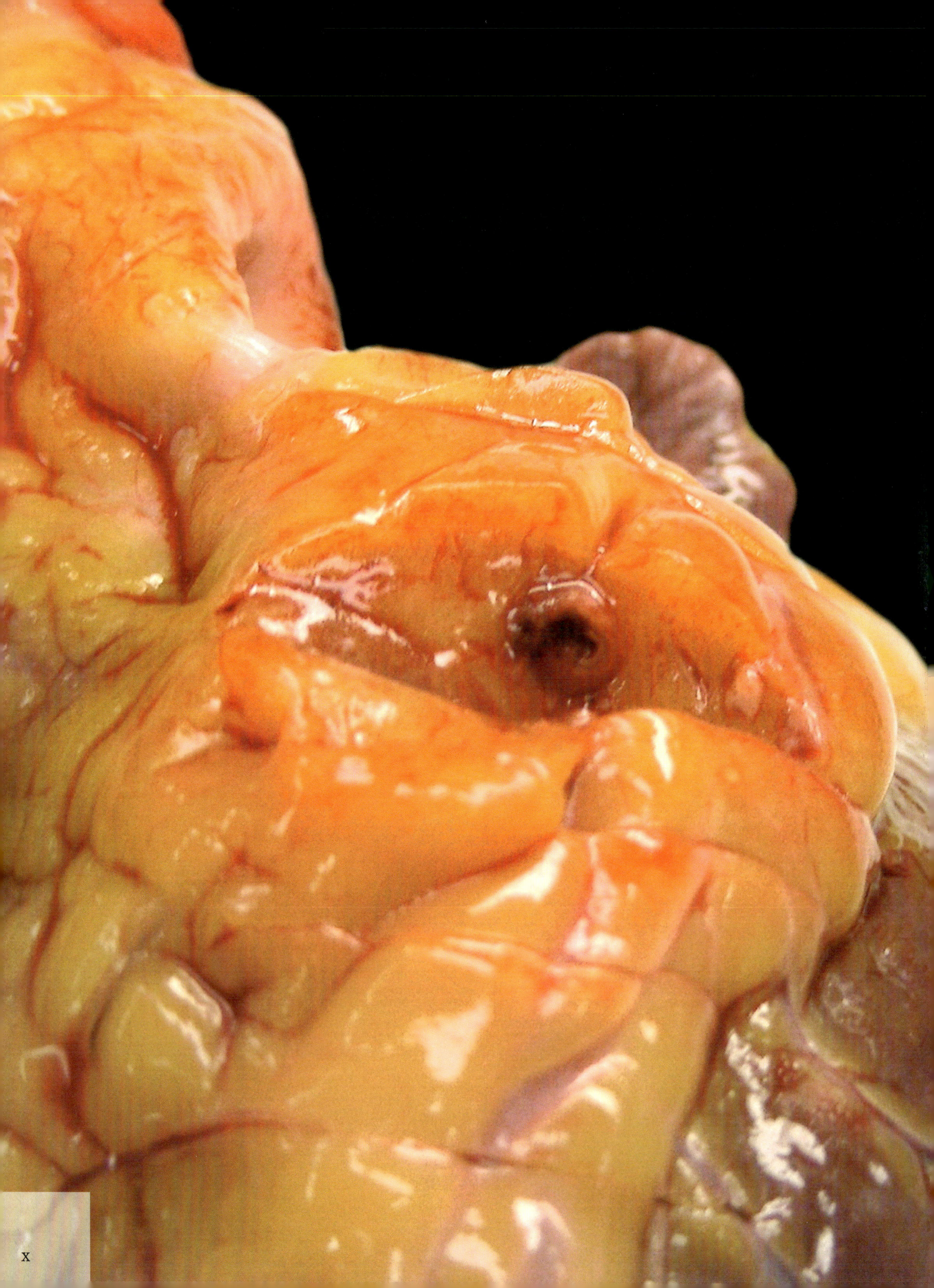

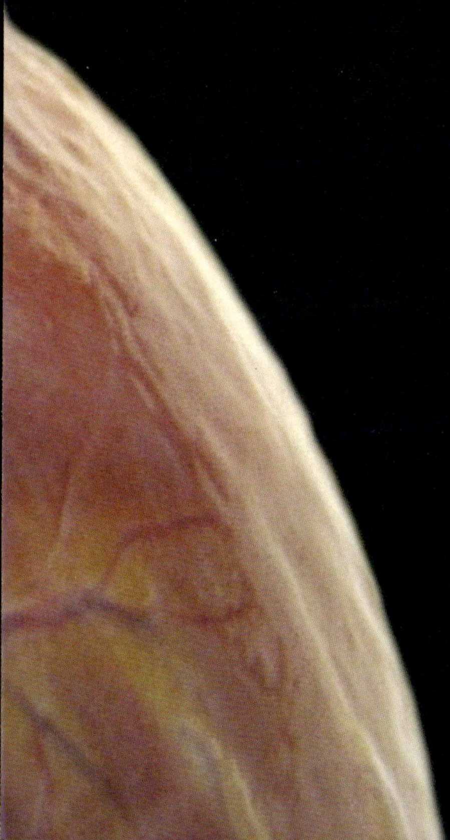

TABLE OF CONTENTS

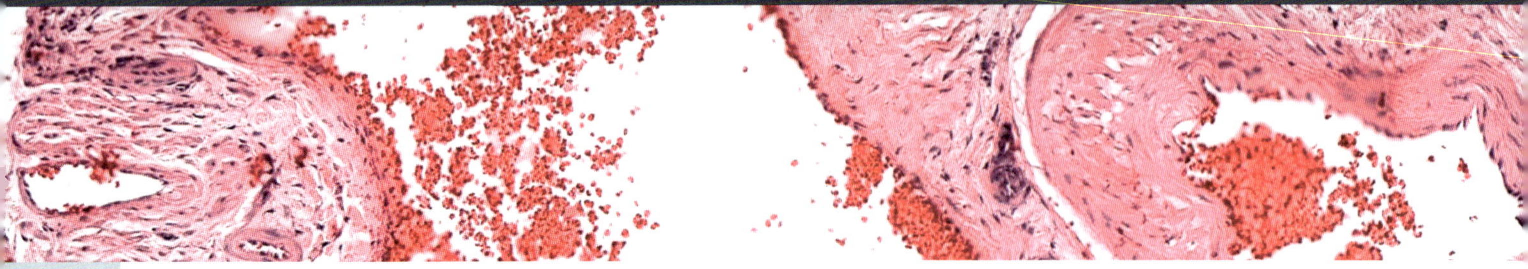

TABLE OF CONTENTS

TABLE OF CONTENTS

TABLE OF CONTENTS

VASCULAR

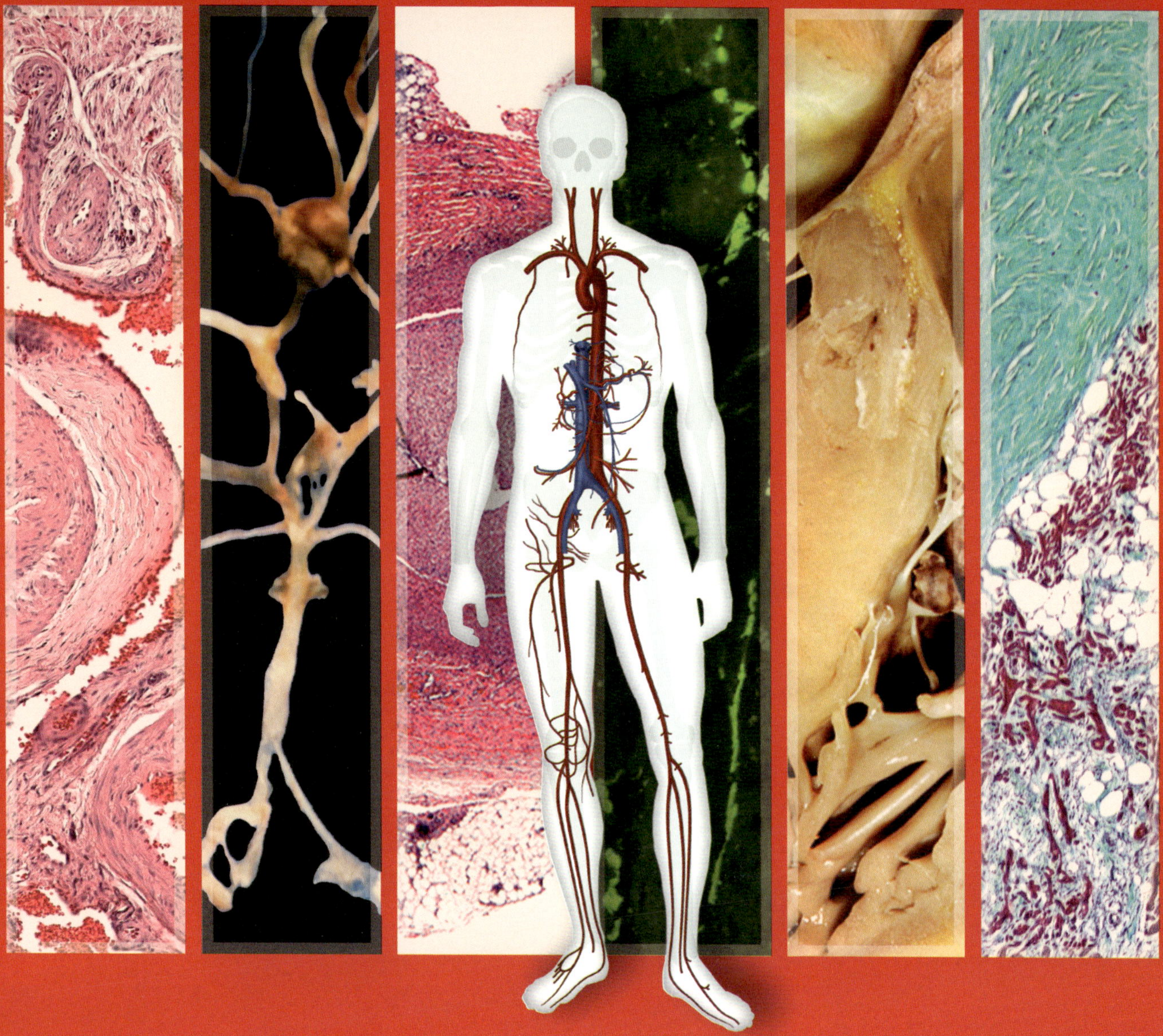

Diagnostic Pathology

Cardiovascular

Miller | Revelo

ELSEVIER

THIRD EDITION

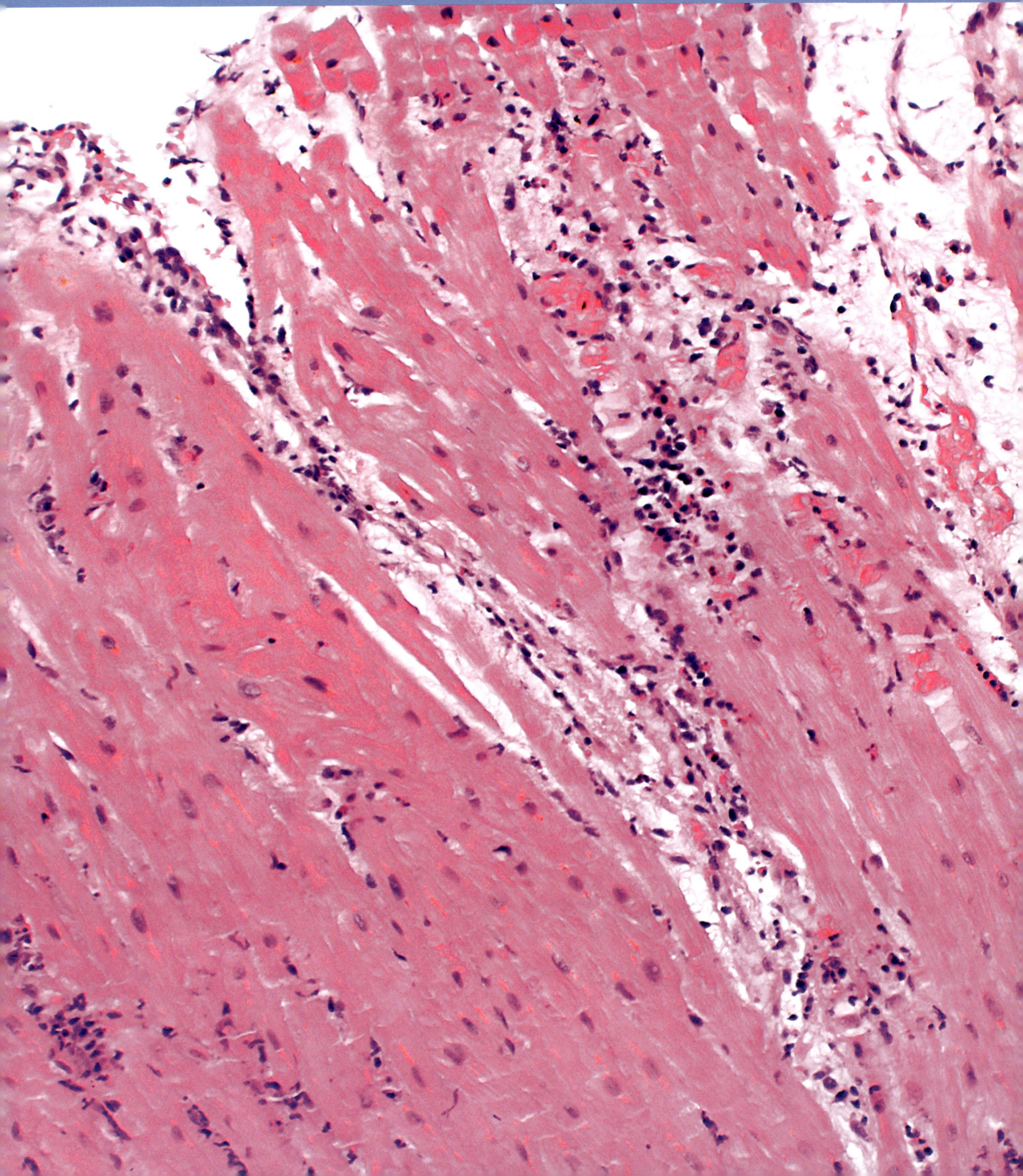

SECTION 1

Heart, Endomyocardial Biopsy

Congenital/Genetic

Acquired

Inflammatory

Transplant Rejection

Endocardial Fibroelastosis Syndrome

KEY FACTS

TERMINOLOGY
- Porcelain-like thickening of ventricular endocardium by layers of collagen and elastic fibers

ETIOLOGY/PATHOGENESIS
- Endocardial fibroelastosis (EFE) should be regarded as endocardial response to variety of stimuli rather than specific disease entity

CLINICAL ISSUES
- 80% of cases occur in 1st year of life
- 33% mortality and 50% heart failure at 10 years
- Unexplained congestive heart failure in infants
- Left ventricle hypertrophy/dilatation
- Depressed systolic function
- Exclusion of other structural abnormalities or injury

MACROSCOPIC
- Enlarged globular heart
- Left ventricle most frequently involved with endocardial thickening and porcelain appearance
- Flattened trabeculae and papillary muscles involved by fibrotic process

MICROSCOPIC
- Thickened endocardium with collagen and elastic fiber deposition
- Duplication of elastic fibers
- Generally unremarkable myocardium
- Trichrome and elastic stains highlight endocardial changes

TOP DIFFERENTIAL DIAGNOSES
- Eosinophilic endomyocardial disease (fibrotic stage)
- Congenital malformations
- Injury
    - Electric shock
    - Global ischemia/infarction (healed)

Gross Findings

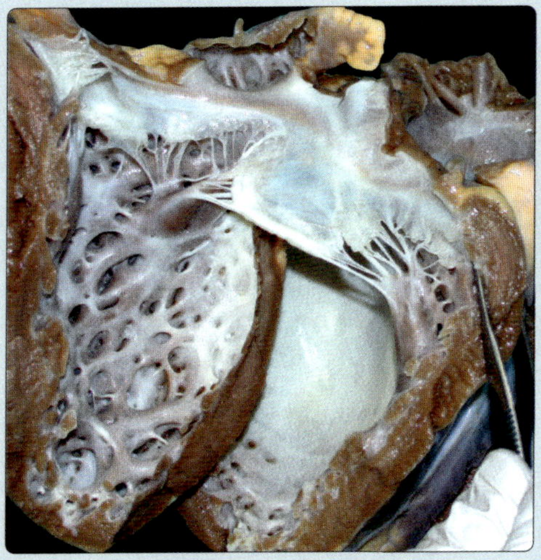

Gross Findings

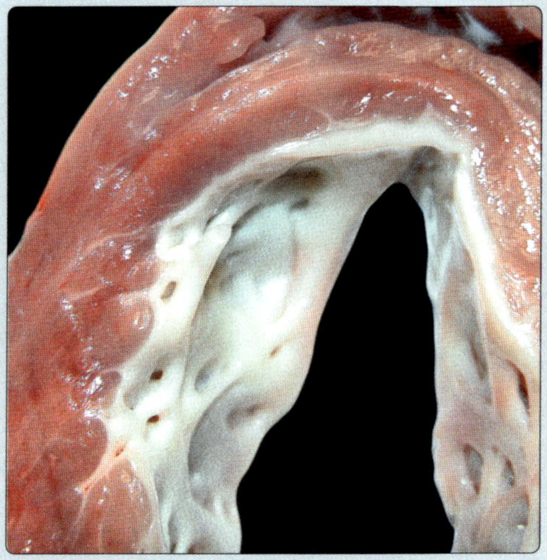

(Left) *Gross specimen shows the left ventricle with white opaque, thickened endocardium and flat trabeculae. The mitral valve is normal.* **(Right)** *Closer view of the left ventricular endocardium shows marked, rubbery endocardial thickening. The myocardium is unremarkable.*

Trichrome Stain

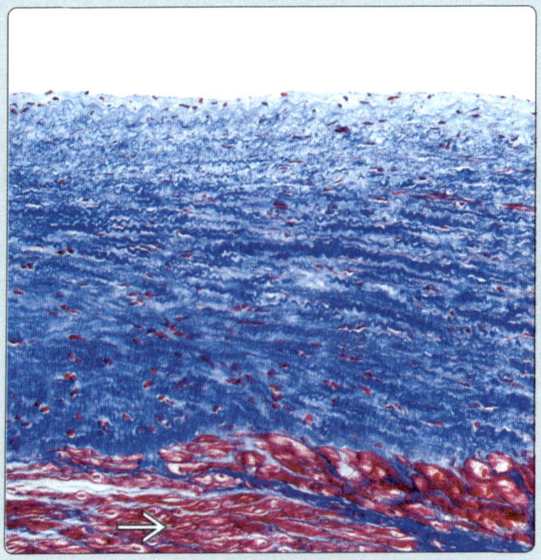

Elastic Stain

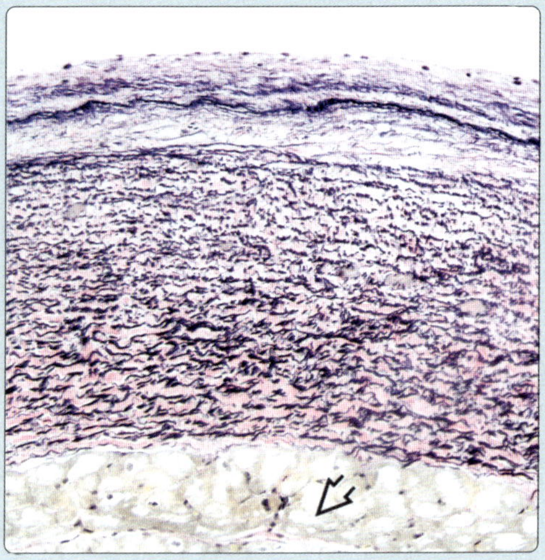

(Left) *Endocardium with a marked fibrous, thickened appearance is shown. The underlying myocardium ➡ is unremarkable.* **(Right)** *Endocardium with well-oriented, thickened elastic fibers resembling the thick elastic lamina of the aorta is shown. The underlying myocardium ⇨ is unremarkable.*

TERMINOLOGY

Abbreviations

- Endocardial fibroelastosis (EFE)

Definitions

- Porcelain-like thickening of ventricular endocardium by layers of collagen and elastic fibers

ETIOLOGY/PATHOGENESIS

General Considerations

- EFE is endocardial response to variety of stimuli rather than specific disease entity
  - Putative causes and associations include
    - Congenital malformations (common in hypoplastic left heart syndrome)
    - Myocarditis
    - Lysosomal storage diseases
    - Immunologic diseases
    - X-linked recessive form
    - Mitochondrial cardiomyopathy
    - Pre- and postnatal left ventricular outflow tract obstruction
    - Autosomal dominant dilated cardiomyopathy
    - Mumps viral infection
- Primary form is not related to cardiac anomalies
- Animal models point to aberrant endothelial to mesenchymal transition as mechanism leading to EFE associated with flow disturbances

CLINICAL ISSUES

Epidemiology

- Incidence
  - 80% of cases occur in 1st year of life

Presentation

- Unexplained congestive heart failure in infants < 2 years of age
- Left ventricle hypertrophy and dilatation
- Tachypnea and tachycardia
- Depressed systolic function

Prognosis

- 33% mortality and 50% heart failure at 10 years

IMAGING

Ultrasonographic Findings

- Systolic and diastolic dysfunction
- Endocardial thickening
- Ultrasound signal from endocardium unusually strong

MR Findings

- Endocardial rim: Hypointense signal in perfusion sequence, hyperintense signal in myocardial delay enhancement

MACROSCOPIC

General Features

- Enlarged globular heart
- Left ventricle most frequently involved with endocardial thickening and porcelain appearance
- Flattened trabeculae and papillary muscles involved by fibrotic process

MICROSCOPIC

Histologic Features

- Thickened endocardium with collagen deposition and thickening and duplication of elastic fibers
- Generally unremarkable myocardium

ANCILLARY TESTS

Histochemistry

- Elastic stain
  - Staining pattern: Markedly thickened endocardium with layered wavy elastic fibers

DIFFERENTIAL DIAGNOSIS

Eosinophilic Endomyocardial Disease (Fibrotic Stage)

- Thickened endocardium with prominent eosinophils showing degranulation
- Myocardial involvement with necrosis (early), fibrosis (later), and eosinophils
- Calcification and mural thrombosis (prominent eosinophils in thrombus)
- Atrioventricular valves involved
- Associated with hypereosinophilic syndrome

Congenital Malformations

- Mitral valve defects
- Anomalous left main coronary artery arising from pulmonary trunk
- Other anomalies with turbulent flow

Injury

- Electric shock
- Global ischemia/infarction (healed)

DIAGNOSTIC CHECKLIST

Pathologic Interpretation Pearls

- Ventricular endocardial thickening with opaque porcelain appearance
- Deposit of collagen and elastic fibers in endocardium

SELECTED REFERENCES

1. Islam S et al: The mechanobiology of endothelial-to-mesenchymal transition in cardiovascular disease. Front Physiol. 12:734215, 2021
2. Oh NA et al: Abnormal flow conditions promote endocardial fibroelastosis via endothelial-to-mesenchymal transition, which is responsive to losartan treatment. JACC Basic Transl Sci. 6(12):984-99, 2021
3. Weixler V et al: Flow disturbances and the development of endocardial fibroelastosis. J Thorac Cardiovasc Surg. 159(2):637-46, 2020
4. Alperi A et al: Young male with long-term impaired ejection fraction - endocardial fibroelastosis: the importance of cardiac magnetic resonance. Arch Cardiol Mex. 89(1):167-8, 2019
5. Chan JL et al: Surgical management of adult endocardial fibroelastosis. J Thorac Cardiovasc Surg. 154(5):e81-4, 2017
6. Seki A et al: Primary endocardial fibroelastosis: an underappreciated cause of cardiomyopathy in children. Cardiovasc Pathol. 22(5):345-50, 2013
7. Maredia N et al: Assessment of endocardial fibroelastosis by cardiac MRI. Can J Cardiol. 24(5):e33, 2008

Arrhythmogenic Cardiomyopathy

KEY FACTS

TERMINOLOGY

- Rare, inheritable disorder of myocardium characterized by replacement of right &/or left ventricle myocardium by fibrofatty tissue

ETIOLOGY/PATHOGENESIS

- Multiple mutations affect > 12 different genes encoding desmosomal proteins, including plakoglobin, plakophilin 2, and desmoplakin and nondesmosomal proteins
- Inheritance is mainly autosomal dominant with incomplete penetrance
- Combination of genetic and environmental factors affect pathogenesis of disease
- Less commonly, inheritance is autosomal recessive (Naxos disease, Carvajal syndrome)

CLINICAL ISSUES

- Palpitation, especially in young person
- Family history of sudden death
- T-wave inversion in anterior precordial leads (V1-V6)
- Epsilon waves; best visualized in leads V1-V3
- Pharmacologic treatment is most commonly used treatment for arrhythmogenic right ventricular dysplasia
- Heart transplantation is final option for biventricular involvement and uncontrollable hemodynamic compromise

MICROSCOPIC

- Areas of loss of myocardial fibers (> 60%)
- Replaced mainly by fibrous tissue
- Associated with adipocytes and several inflammatory cells
- No granulomas or giant cells (pathognomonic for sarcoidosis) are observed

ANCILLARY TESTS

- Plakoglobin signal is significantly reduced at intercalated discs in affected areas of right ventricle
- Plakoglobin signal is also reduced in regions that appear normal, such as left ventricle, IVS, and subendocardium

Arrythmogenic Cardiomyopathy (Short-Axis)

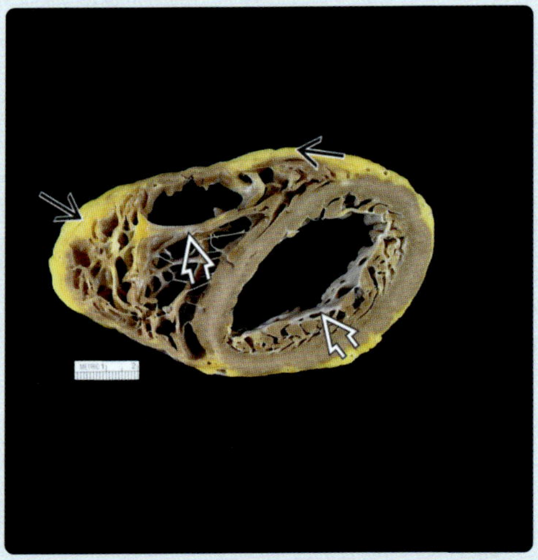

Light Microscopy Features of Arrhythmogenic Cardiomyopathy

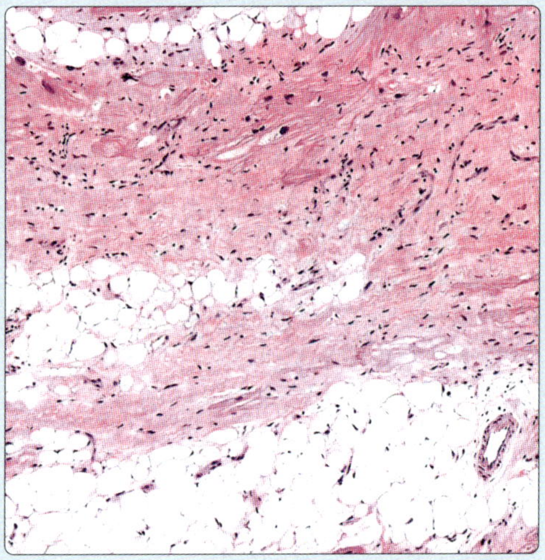

(Left) *Examination of the heart reveals areas of full-thickness fat infiltration affecting the wall of the right ventricle (RV) with focal areas of endocardial fibrosis.* **(Right)** *Section through the wall of the RV shows fibrosis, infiltration by mature adipocytes, and a decreased number of cardiac muscle fibers, indicating the histologic features of arrhythmogenic cardiomyopathy (ACM).*

Movat Stain of Right Ventricle in Case of Arrhythmogenic Cardiomyopathy

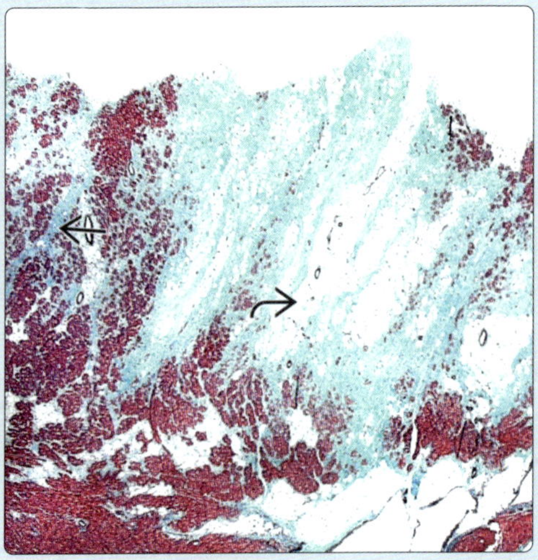

Movat Stain of Left Ventricle in Case of Arrhythmogenic Cardiomyopathy

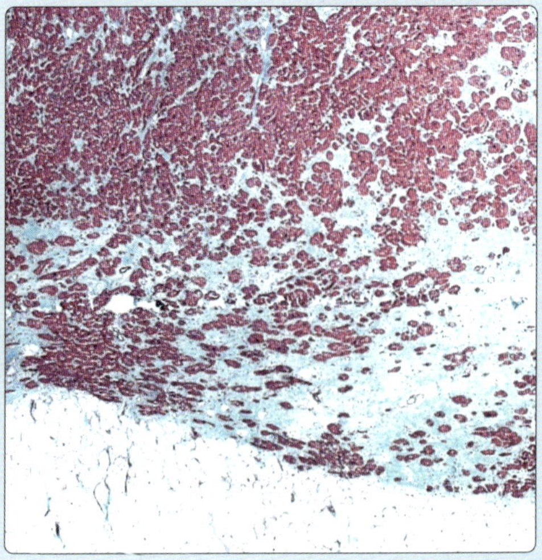

(Left) *Section from the RV shows transmural replacement of myocytes by mature fat cells and fibrous tissue. There is loss of myocytes through large parts of the wall of the RV. In areas with better preserved myocardium, fibrosis is also seen.* **(Right)** *Section shows focal infiltration by adipose cells and fibrous tissue through the epicardium of the left ventricle (LV). These findings are less severe compared to those found through the wall of the RV seen in the left side of the image.*

TERMINOLOGY

Abbreviations

- Arrhythmogenic cardiomyopathy (ACM)

Synonyms

- Arrhythmogenic right ventricular cardiomyopathy (ARVC)

Definitions

- Rare, inheritable disorder of myocardium characterized by replacement of right ventricle (RV) myocardium by fibrofatty tissue, but left ventricle (LV) or biventricular involvement is possible, leading to ventricular arrhythmias

ETIOLOGY/PATHOGENESIS

Etiology

- Genetic factors
  - Multiple mutations affect 5 major genes encoding desmosomal proteins, including
    - *JUP* (junction plakoglobin): Rare mutation, < 5% of cases
    - *PKP2* (plakophilin 2): Most common mutation with predominant RV involvement
    - *DSP* (desmoplakin): Phenotypic expression with either isolated RV, isolated LV, or biventricular ACM
    - *DSG2* (desmoglein 2): Most commonly biventricular involvement
    - *DSC2* (desmocollin 2): Also associated with biventricular involvement
  - Extradesmosomal mutations
    - *TMEM43* (transmembrane protein 43): High penetrance, risk of sudden cardiac death and heart failure
    - *TGFB3* (transforming growth factor β 3): Few cases reported
    - *TTN* (titin)
    - *LMNA* (lamin A/C)
    - *DES* (desmin)
    - *CTNNA3* (catenin α 3): Reported in Italian families
    - *CDH2* (cadherin 2): Reported in South African families
    - *PLN* (phospholamban)
    - *FLNC* (filamin C)
    - *SCN5A* (sodium voltage-gated channel α subunit 5)
  - ACM is hereditary disease in ≥ 50% of cases, and > 30% of patients report positive family history
  - Inheritance: Mainly autosomal dominant with incomplete penetrance and variable expression
  - Less commonly, inheritance is autosomal recessive
    - Naxos disease: Plakoglobin mutation, characterized by palmar and plantar keratoses and thick, woolly hair
    - Carvajal syndrome: Desmoplakin mutation, predominant LV involvement
- Environmental factors
  - Combination of genetic and environmental factors, especially exercise, appears to play role in pathogenesis of disease

Pathogenesis

- 3 main hypotheses explain pathogenesis of disease
  - Hypothesis 1: Occurs due to mutations in genes encoding desmosomal proteins, causing disruption of intercalated discs and connections between myocardial cells
  - Hypothesis 2: Occurs due to genetic defects in immune system that increase myocardial susceptibility to viral infections causing inflammation (myocarditis)
    - Both mechanisms can lead to myocardial cell death, apoptosis, and fibrofatty tissue replacement
  - Hypothesis 3: Occurs due to transdifferentiation of cardiac progenitor cells in myocardium into fibrofatty tissue
    - Dysregulation of canonical wingless-Int (WNT), Hippo, and TGF-β signaling pathways have been involved in fibroadipogenesis
- Tissue transformation is most common in triangle of dysplasia, located between infundibulum, RV apex, and inferior or diaphragmatic aspect of RV
- Transmural loss of myocardium occurs in parts of right ventricular free wall
- LV and interventricular septum (IVS) are usually spared, although they may be involved in more extensive cases (up to 50% of cases show some LV free wall involvement)
- Predominant LV or biventricular involvement also occurs
- Specialized conduction system is usually spared

CLINICAL ISSUES

Epidemiology

- Incidence
  - Ranges from 1/1,000-1/5,000 with wide geographic variability
    - Members of certain families from Greece and Italy have higher incidence
  - Accounts for 3-4% of sports-related deaths; exercise is considered common precipitant of arrhythmia
  - Studies of sudden cardiac death in athletes demonstrate that ACM was cause in 10-15% of cases
  - Can occur at any age, but usually manifests in young or middle-aged men (33 ± 14 years)
  - M:F = 3:1

Presentation

- Right-sided ACM
  - High index of suspicion for ACM should be raised in presence of palpitation, especially in young person, family history of sudden death, death at early age
  - Most common symptoms: Palpitation, fatigue, syncope
  - Cardiac arrest following physical exertion (participation in sports) can be initial manifestation of disease
  - Nonspecific complaints, such as abdominal pain and mental confusion, may occur
  - 50% of ACM patients have no clinical signs on physical examination
  - Important diagnostic clues
    - Widely split S2
    - Added heart sound (S3 or S4 heart sounds)
    - Murmur (rarely noted)
    - Asymmetry of chest wall (if RV is greatly dilated)
  - 50-90% of patients will have characteristic findings on resting ECG, including
    - T-wave inversion in anterior precordial leads (V1-V6)

- Epsilon waves; best visualized in leads V1-V3
  - Small deflections just beyond QRS complex
  - Any wave in V1-V3 that exceeds QRS duration in lead V6 by > 25 milliseconds
- Left-sided ACM
  - Ventricular arrhythmia and relative preservation of RV function
  - Sudden cardiac death
  - Unexplained syncope
  - Characteristic findings on ECG, including
    - Lateral or inferolateral T-wave inversion (leads V5, V6, L1, and aVL)
    - Low-voltage QRS complex on peripheral leads
    - Right bundle branch block/polymorphic ventricular arrhythmias

Treatment

- ACM is incurable; major treatment objective is to prevent arrhythmias and sudden death
- Available therapies include
  - Patient education
    - Considered initial step in management
    - Avoidance of excessive physical exertion that may trigger tachycardic event
    - Gradually increased physical activities under close medical supervision following effective control of arrhythmias
  - Pharmacologic treatment
    - Most commonly used treatment for ACM
    - Intravenous amiodarone has been effective in terminating acute ventricular arrhythmia in ACM patients
      - However, no single drug has been shown to be completely effective in controlling arrhythmias
  - Radiofrequency ablation: Epicardial/endocardial
    - Has been used in drug-refractory ACM, persistent ventricular tachycardia (VT), repeated tachycardia following placement of internal defibrillator, and localized foci of arrhythmia
    - Successful in 30-65% of patients
    - Relapses can occur due to disease progression that creates new reentrant circuit
  - Automatic implantable cardioverter defibrillator (AICD)
    - Provides antitachycardia pacing when needed and generates defibrillation shocks when arrhythmias occur
    - Should be strongly considered in patients with young age of onset, drug-refractory arrhythmias, cardiac arrest, or LV involvement
    - Most significant relative contraindication to AICD placement is incessant VT
  - Surgical treatment
    - Right ventriculotomy is performed by disconnecting RV from rest of heart
    - Heart transplantation is final option for biventricular involvement and uncontrollable hemodynamic compromise

Prognosis

- Increased risk of arrhythmias and worse prognosis in patients with myocardial tissue that has
  - Inflammatory cell infiltrates
  - Foci of necrotic or degenerative myocytes surrounded by inflammatory cells
- Increased risk of sudden death present in patients with
  - History of cardiac arrest
  - Hemodynamically unstable VT
  - Recurrent episodes of syncope
  - LV involvement
  - Young age
  - Multiple mutations and increased penetrance
- QRS dispersion ≥ 40 milliseconds is associated with increased risk of syncope and sustained VT
- QRS dispersion ≥ 40 milliseconds is not associated with increased risk of sudden death
  - However, shows trend toward correlation with sudden death when associated with LV involvement

IMAGING

Ultrasonographic Findings

- Patients with mutations of plakoglobin and plakophilin 2 genes have following findings
  - Regional RV wall motion abnormalities were found in 80-100% of cases
  - LV wall motion abnormalities were found in only 23%
  - Dilatation of RV outflow tract (> 33 mm) or inflow tract (> 40 mm) found in 58%
  - Trabeculation abnormalities observed in 54%
  - Moderator band hyperreflexive in 34%
  - RV aneurysms (akinetic or dyskinetic regions with diastolic bulging) found in 60%
  - Dimensions of RV are increased in most cases affected by ACM

MR Findings

- Myocardial infiltration by fat and fibrous tissue
- Wall thinning and RV dilatation
- Structural abnormalities of ventricular wall
- Late gadolinium enhancement in subepicardial and midmyocardial distribution (inferior or inferior lateral wall in LV dominant)

MACROSCOPIC

General Features

- Single or multiple aneurysm localized in triangle of dysplasia
- LV involvement characterized by subepicardial and midmural layers fibrous/fatty replacement of free wall
- In end-stage disease there is marked biventricular chamber dilatation with multiple free-wall aneurysms

MICROSCOPIC

Histologic Features

- Characterized by
  - Areas of myocardial fiber loss (> 60%)
    - Replaced mainly by fibrous tissue extending from epicardium to endocardium
    - Associated with adipocytes and several inflammatory cells
  - Myocardial muscle cells with abnormal dyssymmetric and dysmorphic nuclei

- Lack of granulomas or giant cells (pathognomonic for sarcoidosis)

ANCILLARY TESTS

Immunohistochemistry

- Plakoglobin signal
  - Significantly reduced at intercalated discs
    - Reduced not only in affected areas of RV but also in regions that appear normal, such as LV, IVS, and subendocardium
  - Strongly positive in patients suffering from other diseases, such as hypertrophic cardiomyopathy, dilated cardiomyopathy

Electron Microscopy

- Mislocalization and decrease in number of desmosomes
- Intercalated disc remodeling
- Increased intercellular gap widening

DIFFERENTIAL DIAGNOSIS

Sarcoidosis

- Tests for sarcoidosis (e.g., chest radiograph, serum angiotensin-converting enzyme, alkaline phosphatase, calcium, phosphorus, erythrocyte sedimentation rate, C-reactive protein) are usually negative in ACM
- Identification of nonnecrotizing granulomas in heart biopsy will favor sarcoidosis

DIAGNOSTIC CHECKLIST

Pathologic Interpretation Pearls

- Pathologic features range from grossly normal heart at one end, in which only careful histopathologic investigation can reveal features of ACM in 1 or both ventricles, to heart with massive biventricular disease
- Fatty infiltration of RV is not sufficient morphologic hallmark for ACM, and replacement-type fibrosis, myocyte atrophy, and degenerative changes should always be identified
- Endomyocardial biopsy has low sensitivity for diagnosis because samples are taken from RV septum, area not usually involved
- Samples from RV free wall can be diagnostic but high risk of perforation exists so are not usually recommended

SELECTED REFERENCES

1. Ciarambino T et al: Cardiomyopathies: an overview. Int J Mol Sci. 22(14), 2021
2. Cipriani A et al: Differential diagnosis of arrhythmogenic cardiomyopathy: phenocopies versus disease variants. Minerva Med. 112(2):269-80, 2021
3. Mattesi G et al: Arrhythmogenic left ventricular cardiomyopathy: genotype-phenotype correlations and new diagnostic Criteria. J Clin Med. 10(10), 2021
4. McKenna WJ et al: Epidemiology of the inherited cardiomyopathies. Nat Rev Cardiol. 18(1):22-36, 2021
5. Simonit F et al: Pitfalls in arrhythmogenic left ventricular cardiomyopathy (ALVC). A review of the literature with considerations on a single case of sudden death in a juvenile athlete. J Forensic Leg Med. 82:102208, 2021
6. Zorzi A et al: Role of exercise as a modulating factor in arrhythmogenic cardiomyopathy. Curr Cardiol Rep. 23(6):57, 2021
7. Brun F et al: FLNC truncations cause arrhythmogenic right ventricular cardiomyopathy. J Med Genet. 57(4):254-7, 2020
8. Cipriani A et al: Arrhythmogenic right ventricular cardiomyopathy: characterization of left ventricular phenotype and differential diagnosis with dilated cardiomyopathy. J Am Heart Assoc. 9(5):e014628, 2020
9. Eijgenraam TR et al: Current understanding of fibrosis in genetic cardiomyopathies. Trends Cardiovasc Med. 30(6):353-61, 2020
10. Feliu E et al: Importance of cardiac magnetic resonance findings in the diagnosis of left dominant arrythmogenic cardiomyopathy. Rev Esp Cardiol (Engl Ed). 73(11):885-92, 2020
11. Gao S et al: Established and emerging mechanisms in the pathogenesis of arrhythmogenic cardiomyopathy: a multifaceted disease. Int J Mol Sci. 21(17), 2020
12. Hamilton-Craig C et al: The Cardiac Society of Australia and New Zealand position statement on the diagnosis and management of arrhythmogenic right ventricular cardiomyopathy (2019 update). Heart Lung Circ. 29(1):4-8, 2020
13. Leopoulou M et al: Naxos disease - a narrative review. Expert Rev Cardiovasc Ther. 18(11):801-8, 2020
14. Segura-Rodríguez D et al: Myocardial fibrosis in arrhythmogenic cardiomyopathy: a genotype-phenotype correlation study. Eur Heart J Cardiovasc Imaging. 21(4):378-86, 2020
15. Smith ED et al: Desmoplakin cardiomyopathy, a fibrotic and inflammatory form of cardiomyopathy distinct from typical dilated or arrhythmogenic right ventricular cardiomyopathy. Circulation. 141(23):1872-84, 2020
16. Austin KM et al: Molecular mechanisms of arrhythmogenic cardiomyopathy. Nat Rev Cardiol. 16(9):519-37, 2019
17. Bennett RG et al: Arrhythmogenic cardiomyopathy in 2018-2019: ARVC/ALVC or both? Heart Lung Circ. 28(1):164-77, 2019
18. Blusztein DI et al: Arrhythmogenic right ventricular cardiomyopathy: a review of living and deceased probands. Heart Lung Circ. 28(7):1034-41, 2019
19. Goff ZD et al: Sudden death related cardiomyopathies - arrhythmogenic right ventricular cardiomyopathy, arrhythmogenic cardiomyopathy, and exercise-induced cardiomyopathy. Prog Cardiovasc Dis. 62(3):217-26, 2019
20. Miles C et al: Sudden death and left ventricular involvement in arrhythmogenic cardiomyopathy. Circulation. 139(15):1786-97, 2019
21. Protonotarios A et al: Arrhythmogenic cardiomyopathies (ACs): diagnosis, risk stratification and management. Heart. 105(14):1117-28, 2019
22. Towbin JA et al: 2019 HRS expert consensus statement on evaluation, risk stratification, and management of arrhythmogenic cardiomyopathy: executive summary. Heart Rhythm. 16(11):e373-407, 2019
23. Gandjbakhch E et al: Clinical diagnosis, imaging, and genetics of arrhythmogenic right ventricular cardiomyopathy/dysplasia: JACC state-of-the-art review. J Am Coll Cardiol. 72(7):784-804, 2018
24. Oomen AWGJ et al: Diagnosis of arrhythmogenic right ventricular cardiomyopathy: progress and pitfalls. Heart Lung Circ. 27(11):1310-7, 2018
25. Wang M et al: Endomyocardial biopsy in differential diagnosis between arrhythmogenic right ventricular cardiomyopathy and dilated cardiomyopathy: an in vitro simulated study. Cardiovasc Pathol. 34:15-21, 2018
26. Corrado D et al: Arrhythmogenic cardiomyopathy. Circ Res. 121(7):784-802, 2017
27. Corrado D et al: Arrhythmogenic right ventricular cardiomyopathy. N Engl J Med. 376(1):61-72, 2017
28. Femia G et al: Systematic review: impact of the new task force criteria in the diagnosis of arrhythmogenic right ventricular cardiomyopathy. Int J Cardiol. 241:311-7, 2017
29. Hoorntje ET et al: Arrhythmogenic cardiomyopathy: pathology, genetics, and concepts in pathogenesis. Cardiovasc Res. 113(12):1521-31, 2017
30. Mazurek S et al: Genetic and epigenetic regulation of arrhythmogenic cardiomyopathy. Biochim Biophys Acta Mol Basis Dis. 1863(8):2064-9, 2017
31. Saffitz JE: Molecular mechanisms in the pathogenesis of arrhythmogenic cardiomyopathy. Cardiovasc Pathol. 28:51-8, 2017
32. Corrado D et al: Treatment of arrhythmogenic right ventricular cardiomyopathy/dysplasia: an international task force consensus statement. Circulation. 132(5):441-53, 2015
33. Groeneweg JA et al: Clinical presentation, long-term follow-up, and outcomes of 1001 arrhythmogenic right ventricular dysplasia/cardiomyopathy patients and family members. Circ Cardiovasc Genet. 8(3):437-46, 2015
34. Lazzarini E et al: The ARVD/C genetic variants database: 2014 update. Hum Mutat. 36(4):403-10, 2015
35. Philips B et al: 2015 update on the diagnosis and management of arrhythmogenic right ventricular cardiomyopathy. Curr Opin Cardiol. 31(1):46-56, 2015
36. Que D et al: Traditional vs. genetic pathogenesis of arrhythmogenic right ventricular cardiomyopathy. Europace. 17(12):1770-6, 2015
37. Avramides D et al: Arrhythmogenic right ventricular cardiomyopathy/dysplasia. Hellenic J Cardiol. 52(5):452-61, 2011
38. Sen-Chowdhry S et al: Arrhythmogenic cardiomyopathy: etiology, diagnosis, and treatment. Annu Rev Med. 61:233-53, 2010

Overview of Genes Implicated in Arrhythmogenic Cardiomyopathy

Gene	Chromosomal Locus	Encoded Protein	Percentage of Index Cases	Mode of Inheritance	Predominantly Affected Ventricle	Characteristics
PKP2	12p11.21	Plakophilin 2	20-46%	AD/AR also reported	RV, biventricular	Most prevalent
DSP	6p24.3	Desmoplakin	3-15%	AR	LV, biventricular	Cardiocutaneous syndrome (Carvajal)
DSG2	18q12.1	Desmoglein 2	3-20%	AD/AR also reported	RV, biventricular	Frequent LV involvement
DSC2	18q12.1	Desmocollin 2	1-8%	AD/AR also reported	RV, biventricular	Cardiocutaneous form
JUP	17q21.2	Junction plakoglobin	0-1% (except in Naxos, Greece)	AR	RV, biventricular	Cardiocutaneous syndrome (Naxos disease)
Area composite						
CTNNA3	10q21.3	αT-catenin	0-2%	AD	RV, biventricular	Low penetrance
CDH2	18q12.1	Cadherin 2	0-2%	AD	RV, biventricular	
Other or overlapping syndromes						
PLN	6q22.31	Phospholamban	0-1% (except in Dutch population)	AD	LV, biventricular	Dutch founder mutation
TMEM43	3p25.1	Transmembrane protein 43	0-2% (except in Canadian population)	AD	RV, biventricular	Canadian (Newfoundland) founder mutation
SCN5A	3p22.2	Nav 1.5	2%	AD	LV, biventricular	Overlap with Brugada syndrome
LMNA	1q22	Lamin A/C	0-4%	AD	LV, biventricular	Overlap with DCM
DES	2q35	Desmin	0-2%	AD	LV	Overlap with DCM
FLNC	7q32.1	Filamin C	3%	AD	LV dominant, biventricular	7/219 Southern European ACM cases
TTN	2q31.2	Titin	0-10%	AD	RV, LV, biventricular	Overlap with DCM
TGFB3	14q24.3	Transforming growth factor beta 3	2 families	AD	RV	

ACM = arrhythmogenic cardiomyopathy; DCM = dilated cardiomyopathy; RV = right ventricle; LV = left ventricle; AD = autosomal dominant; AR= autosomal recessive.

Left Ventricle View of Arrhythmogenic Cardiomyopathy

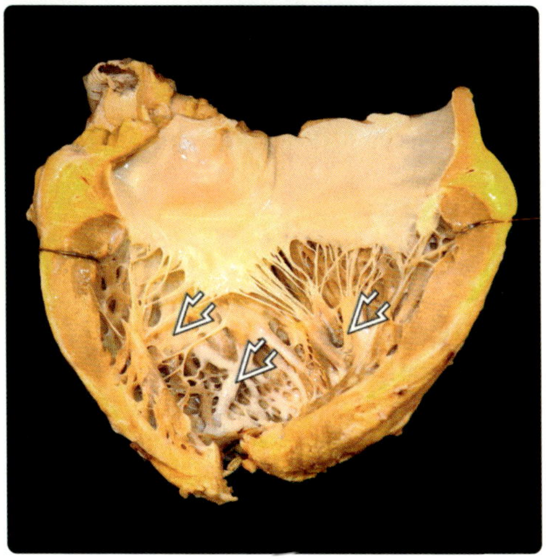

Transverse View of Ventricles in Arrhythmogenic Cardiomyopathy

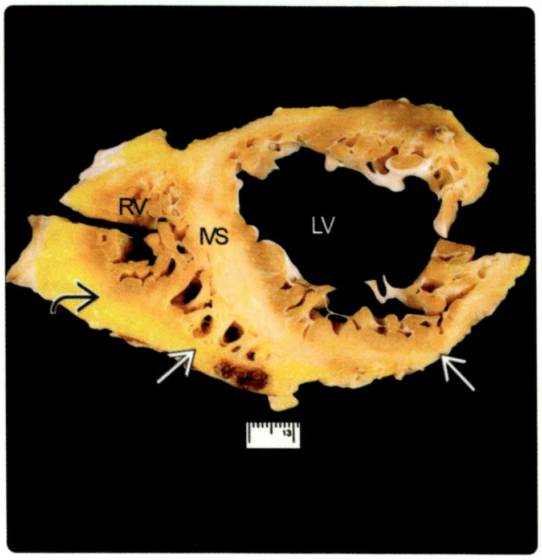

(Left) *The LV reveals multifocal areas of infiltration by fat and fibrous tissue, dilatation of the LV chamber, and areas of endocardial fibrosis affecting a larger area when compared to the RV.* **(Right)** *Transverse section of the heart shows biventricular dilatation, fibrosis of the LV wall and interventricular septum (IVS), and transmural extensive epicardial fibrosis. The RV wall is extensively infiltrated by fat.*

Movat Stain of Right Ventricle With Arrhythmogenic Cardiomyopathy

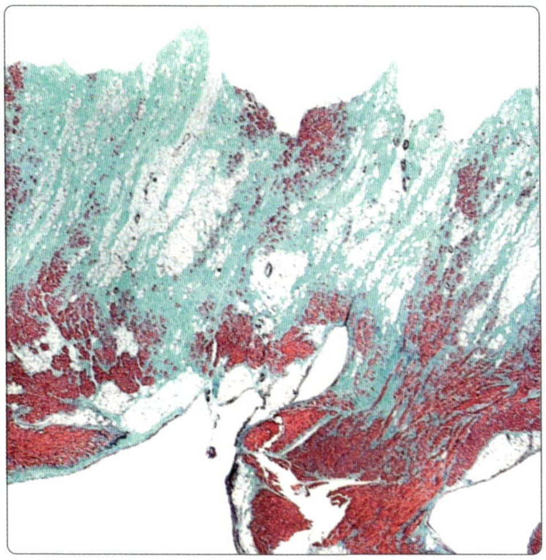

Movat Stain of Ventricular Trabeculae Carnea

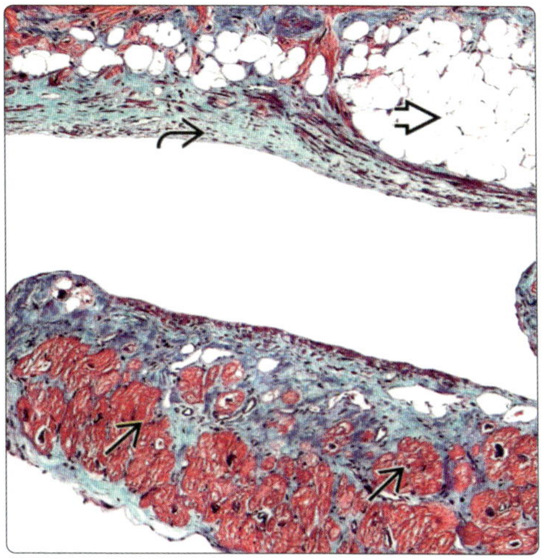

(Left) *Section from the RV shows transmural replacement of myocytes by mature fat cells and fibrous tissue. There is loss of myocytes through large parts of the wall of the RV.* **(Right)** *Section of the RV trabeculae carnea, found in the trabeculae carneae, shows mild endocardial fibrosis, endocardial fat infiltration, and loss of myocytes. Both the compacted wall and trabecular myocardium can show these changes.*

Movat Stain of Left Ventricle in Arrhythmogenic Cardiomyopathy

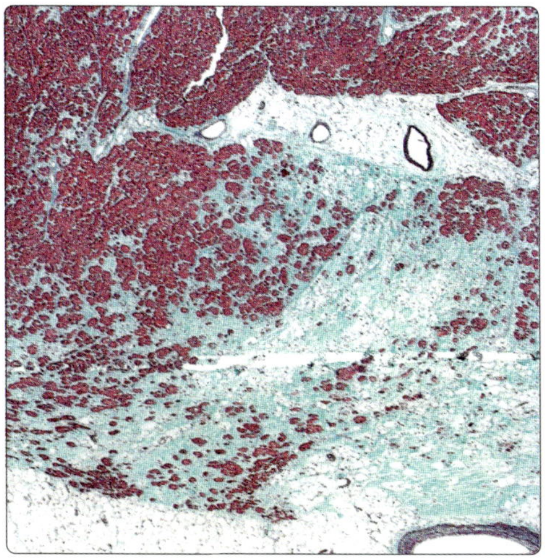

Movat Stain of Left Ventricle in Arrhythmogenic Cardiomyopathy

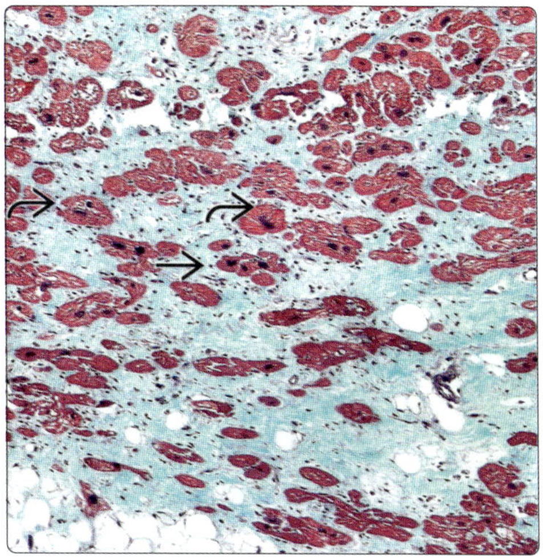

(Left) *Section shows infiltration by adipose cells and fibrous tissue through the epicardium of the LV. These findings are less severe compared to those found through the wall of the RV.* **(Right)** *This LV section shows loss of myocytes and extensive fibrofatty infiltration. Residual myocytes show features of hypertrophy admixed with some atrophic myocytes.*

Fatty Acid Metabolic Disorders

KEY FACTS

TERMINOLOGY

- Inherited disorders due to defects in mitochondrial fatty acid β-oxidation pathways; there are ≥ 20 diseases with distinct enzyme or transporter deficiencies

ETIOLOGY/PATHOGENESIS

- Medium-chain acyl-coenzyme A dehydrogenase: A985G
- Long-chain 3-hydroxyacyl-coenzyme A dehydrogenase: G1528C
- Carnitine transporter defect: *SLC22A5*
- Carnitine palmitoyl transferase 1A (*CPT1A*) and 2 (*CPT2*), mitochondrial trifunctional protein (MTP), very long-chain acyl-coenzyme A dehydrogenase deficiency: Heterogeneous mutations

CLINICAL ISSUES

- Cardiac: Sudden infant death, cardiomyopathies, arrhythmias
- Metabolic: Hypoketotic hypoglycemia
- Other: Rhabdomyolysis, hepatic failure
- High lethality in severe neonatal forms
- Good prognosis with early diagnosis and preventive treatment

MACROSCOPIC

- Enlarged heart
- Biventricular hypertrophy
- Mild endocardial fibrosis

MICROSCOPIC

- Vacuoles in myocardial fibers
- Positive stain for neutral lipids

ANCILLARY TESTS

- Electron microscopy
    - Accumulation of fat vacuoles
    - Myocytes occupied by bizarre-shaped mitochondria with crystalline inclusions

Gross Findings in Case of Fatty Acid Metabolic Disorder

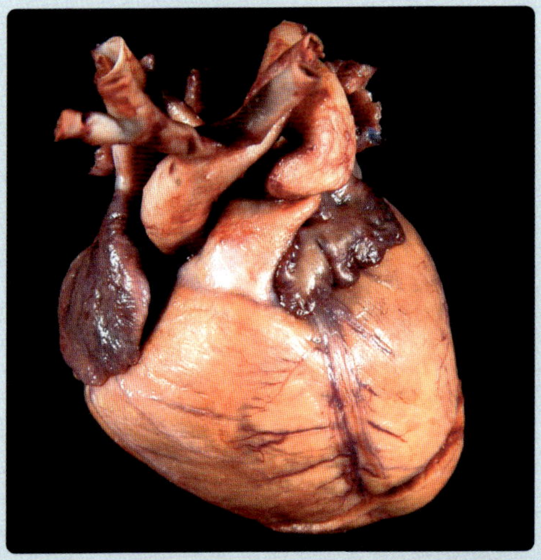

Gross Findings in Case of Fatty Acid Metabolic Disorder

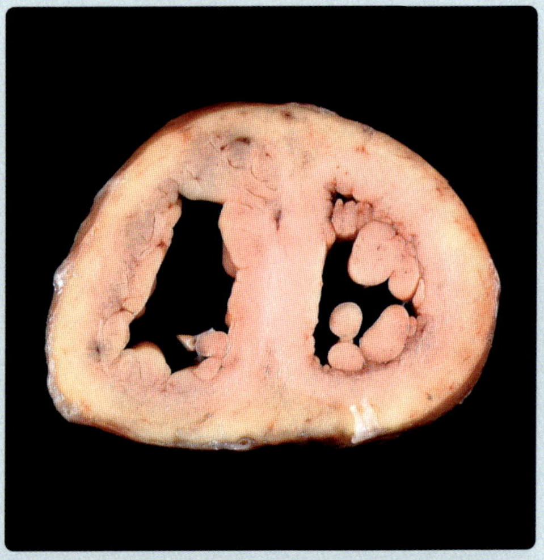

(Left) *Anterior view of the heart from a 2-day-old male patient with a fatty acid metabolic disorder shows enlargement and a globular shape.* **(Right)** *Transversal section of the heart from 2-day-old male patient with a fatty acid metabolic disorder shows biventricular hypertrophy.*

Electron Microscopy in Fatty Acid Metabolic Disorder

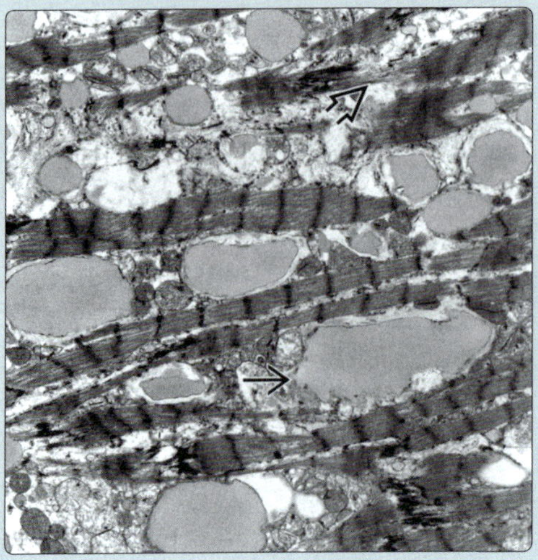

Electron Microscopy in Fatty Acid Metabolic Disorder

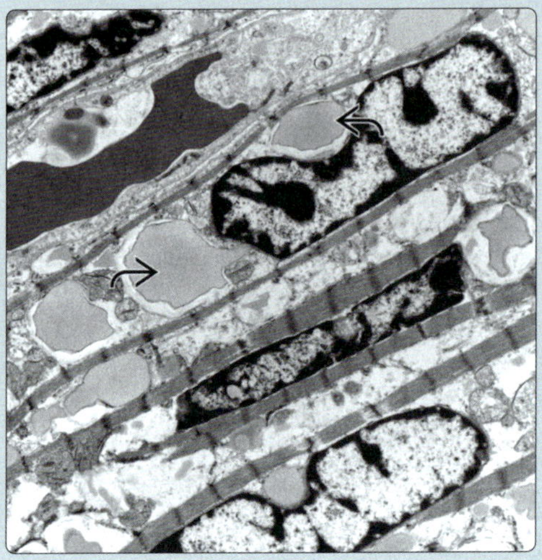

(Left) *Higher power view of myocardium shows fat vacuoles within myocyte cytoplasm* → *and focal loss of myofibrils* ⇨. **(Right)** *Electron micrograph of myocytes shows significant nuclear enlargement and prominent perinuclear fat vacuoles* ↷.

TERMINOLOGY

Definitions

- Heterogeneous inherited autosomal recessive disorders due to defects in mitochondrial fatty acid β-oxidation pathways; there are ≥ 20 diseases with distinct enzyme or transporter deficiencies

ETIOLOGY/PATHOGENESIS

Most Common Genetic Abnormalities

- Medium-chain acyl-coenzyme A dehydrogenase (MCAD): A985G
- Long-chain 3-hydroxyacyl-coenzyme A dehydrogenase (LCHAD): G1528C
- Carnitine transporter deficiency (CTD): *SLC22A5*
- Carnitine palmitoyl transferase 1A (*CPT1A*) and 2 (*CPT2*), mitochondrial trifunctional protein (MTP), very long-chain acyl-coenzyme A dehydrogenase (VLCAD) deficiency: Heterogeneous mutations

Metabolic Abnormalities

- Not fully established
- Inadequate energy supply due to fatty acid oxidation blockage combined with hypoketotic hypoglycemia are central to pathophysiology of tissue injury
- Toxic effects of fatty acids and their carnitine derivatives accumulation
  - Causing inhibition of respiratory chain complexes with increased formation of oxygen radicals and imbalance in calcium homeostasis
- Mitochondrial dysfunction
- High ammonia levels

CLINICAL ISSUES

Epidemiology

- MCAD: 1:10,000 to 1:27,000 newborns
- LCHAD: 1:250,000 newborns
- VLCAD: 1:30,000 to 1:100,000 newborns
- CTD: 1:142,000 newborns
- MTP: 1:750,000 newborns

Presentation

- Wide clinical spectrum of disease partly explained by genotype/phenotype correlation
  - Cardiac
    - Sudden infant death (20-30% in MCAD)
    - Cardiomyopathy
    - Arrhythmias/conduction anomalies
    - Heart failure
  - Metabolic
    - Episodic hypoketotic hypoglycemia
    - Metabolic acidosis
  - Other
    - Skeletal muscle: Rhabdomyolysis, weakness
    - Neurologic: Lethargy, seizures, coma, peripheral neuropathy, pigmentary retinopathy
    - Hepatic failure
    - Maternal hemolysis, elevated liver enzymes, and low platelets (HELLP syndrome)

Laboratory Tests

- Newborn screening card for initial detection
- Acylcarnitine profile in plasma
- Urinary organic acid profile and acylglycine analysis
- Enzymatic studies in cultured fibroblasts or lymphocytes
- DNA analysis

Treatment

- Preventive: Avoid fasting and catabolic states (all types)
- Long-chain triglyceride-restricted diet (VLCAD)
- Medium-chain triglyceride supplementation (LCHAD, VLCAD, MTP)
- Carnitine supplementation (CTD)
- Triheptanoin supplementation (LCHAD, VLCAD, MTP, *CPT2*)

Prognosis

- High lethality in severe neonatal forms &/or cardiomyopathy
- Good if early diagnosis and preventive treatment

MACROSCOPIC

General Features

- Enlarged heart with biventricular hypertrophy
- Mild endocardial fibrosis

MICROSCOPIC

Histologic Features

- Microvesicular fat accumulation in myocardial fibers and skeletal muscle
- Positive stain for neutral lipids

ANCILLARY TESTS

Histochemistry

- Oil Red O
  - Staining pattern: Cytoplasmic vacuoles

Electron Microscopy

- Accumulation of fat vacuoles
- Bizarre-shaped mitochondria in myocyte cytoplasm
- Mitochondria cristae may be disrupted by crystalline inclusions

SELECTED REFERENCES

1. Ribas GS et al: Evidence that oxidative disbalance and mitochondrial dysfunction are involved in the pathophysiology of fatty acid oxidation disorders. Cell Mol Neurobiol. 42(3):521-32, 2022
2. Vockley J et al: Response to triheptanoin therapy in critically ill patients with LC-FAOD: report of patients treated through an expanded access program. Mol Genet Metab. 136(2):152-62, 2022
3. Baker JJ et al: Diagnosis and clinical management of long-chain fatty-acid oxidation disorders: a review. touchREV Endocrinol. 17(2):108-11, 2021
4. Yoo HW: Inborn errors of mitochondrial fatty acid oxidation: overview from a clinical perspective. J Lipid Atheroscler. 10(1):1-7, 2021
5. Brailova M et al: Inherited metabolic diseases and cardiac pathology in adults: diagnosis and prevalence in a cardiometabo Study. J Clin Med. 9(3):694, 2020
6. Elizondo G et al: Effects of fasting, feeding and exercise on plasma acylcarnitines among subjects with CPT2D, VLCADD and LCHADD/TFPD. Mol Genet Metab. 131(1-2):90-7, 2020
7. Vockley J: Long-chain fatty acid oxidation disorders and current management strategies. Am J Manag Care. 26(7 Suppl):S147-S154, 2020
8. Wanders RJA et al: Mitochondrial fatty acid oxidation disorders: laboratory diagnosis, pathogenesis, and the complicated route to treatment. J Lipid Atheroscler. 9(3):313-33, 2020

Mitochondrial Myopathies

KEY FACTS

TERMINOLOGY

- Heterogeneous group of maternally inherited diseases resulting from dysfunction in mitochondrial DNA-encoded gene products

ETIOLOGY/PATHOGENESIS

- Kearns-Sayre syndrome: Heteroplasmic single deletion of mtDNA with reduction in cytochrome C oxidase
- Myoclonic epilepsy with red ragged fibers: tRNA gene for lysine, A8344G
- Mitochondrial myopathy, encephalopathy, lactic acidosis, and stroke-like episodes syndrome: A3243G, tRNA-Leu gene
- Leber hereditary optic neuropathy: Homoplasmic point mutation in ND4 protein-coding subunit, position G11778A

CLINICAL ISSUES

- Incidence: 1:22,500 (for cardiomyopathy-associated mitochondrial myopathy)
- 20-40% prevalence of cardiomyopathy in pediatric patients with mitochondrial diseases
- Onset ranges from neonatal period to adult life
- M:F = 1.5:1.0

MICROSCOPIC

- Myocyte vacuolization
- Myocyte necrosis
- Interstitial fibrosis

ANCILLARY TESTS

- Trichrome stain demonstrates ragged red fibrils
- Electron microscopy
  - Crystalloid or osmophilic globular inclusion bodies
  - Mitochondria with concentric cristae configuration
  - Increased numbers and size of mitochondria aggregated under sarcolemma
  - Myofibril loss

Myocardial Changes in Mitochondrial Myopathy

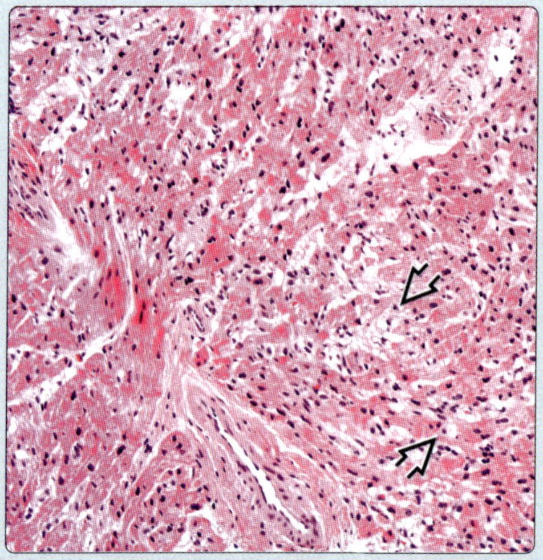

Myocardial Changes in Mitochondrial Myopathy

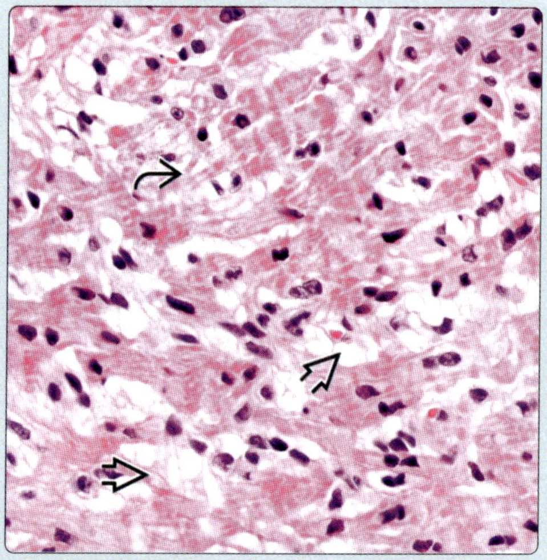

(Left) *Low-power H&E stain shows the myocardium with focal vacuolar change in the myocyte cytoplasm.* **(Right)** *Higher power H&E stain shows myocytes with fine vacuoles within the cytoplasm. There is focal loss of cross striations.*

Trichrome Stain in Mitochondrial Myopathy

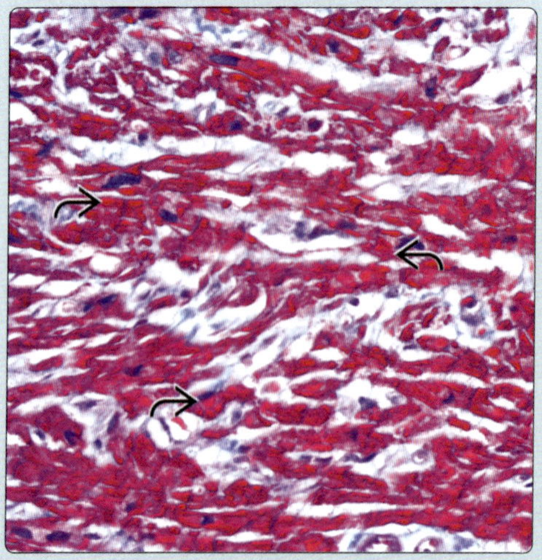

Mitochondria With Cristae Abnormalities

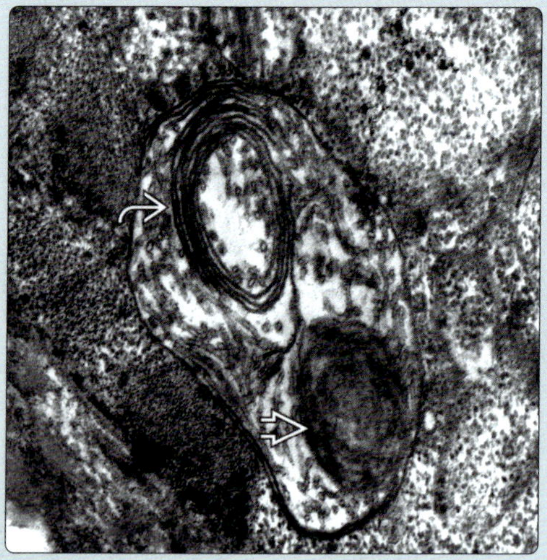

(Left) *Trichrome stain shows ragged red fibers with red-purple perinuclear deposits. This change is also seen in the skeletal muscle and is a characteristic feature of mitochondrial myopathies.* **(Right)** *Electron micrograph from a patient with cardiomyopathy shows an enlarged mitochondria with abnormal cristae concentrically arranged. There is also an osmophilic body.*

TERMINOLOGY

Definitions

- Heterogeneous group of maternally inherited diseases resulting from dysfunction in mitochondrial DNA-encoded gene products, leading to defective oxidative phosphorylation

ETIOLOGY/PATHOGENESIS

Genetic

- Kearns-Sayre syndrome (KSS): Heteroplasmic, large-scale single deletion of mtDNA with reduction in cytochrome C oxidase
- Myoclonic epilepsy with red ragged fibers (MERRF): tRNA gene for lysine, A8344G
- Mitochondrial myopathy, encephalopathy, lactic acidosis, and stroke-like episodes syndrome (MELAS): A3243G, tRNA-Leu gene
- Leber hereditary optic neuropathy (LHON): Homoplasmic point mutation in ND4 protein-coding subunit, position G11778A
- Chronic progressive external ophthalmoplegia (CPEO): mtDNA deletions, rearrangements, point mutations (genes *MT-TI*, *MT-TL1*)
- Leigh syndrome: MT-ATPase 6 T8993G (most prevalent mutation)

CLINICAL ISSUES

Epidemiology

- Incidence
  - 1:22,500 (for cardiomyopathy-associated mitochondrial myopathy)
    - 20-40% prevalence of cardiomyopathy in pediatric patients with mitochondrial diseases
- Age
  - Onset ranges from neonatal period to adult life
- Sex
  - M:F = 1.5:1.0

Presentation

- KSS: Progressive external ophthalmoplegia, pigmentary retinopathy, dilated cardiomyopathy, and conduction abnormalities (PR-interval prolongation with progression to atrioventricular block)
  - Less frequent features are dementia, deafness, limb weakness, and renal and endocrine dysfunction
- MERRF: Myoclonus, seizures, ataxia, dementia, muscle weakness, hypertrophic cardiomyopathy (20-30%); other features include symmetric trunk lipomatosis
- MELAS: Encephalopathy, subacute stroke-like events, hypertrophic/dilated cardiomyopathy, arrhythmia, sudden death; other features include recurrent vomiting, limb weakness, and short stature
- LHON: Severe, subacute, painless loss of central vision; prevalence in young males; short PR interval; supraventricular tachycardia
- CPEO: Ophthalmoplegia, bilateral ptosis, proximal and oropharyngeal muscle weakness, PR-interval prolongation preceding 2nd- or 3rd-degree atrioventricular block
  - Less frequent features are depression, deafness, diabetes mellitus, and short stature
- Leigh syndrome: Severe subacute psychomotor delay and necrotizing symmetric lesions in brainstem, thalamus, cerebellum, spinal cord, and optic nerve, associated with hypertrophic or dilated cardiomyopathy

Laboratory Tests

- Mutational analysis of mitochondrial DNA for identification of point mutations
- Whole-genome/exome sequencing

Treatment

- Adjuvant therapy
  - Use of antioxidants and supplements is controversial with modest therapeutic benefits
  - Avoid medications that interfere with respiratory chain and precipitate acute metabolic crisis (metformin, statins, valproic acid, antibiotics [aminoglycosides, tetracyclines, macrolides], high-dose acetaminophen)
- Pacemaker
- Defibrillator
- Supportive heart failure medication
- Left ventricular assist device
- Heart transplantation when predominant cardiac involvement present

Prognosis

- Progressive deterioration and premature death, especially in neonatal presentation
- Cardiomyopathy is associated with poor prognosis

IMAGING

Ultrasonographic Findings

- Ventricular dysfunction (MELAS, KSS)
- Asymmetric/symmetric septal hypertrophy and left ventricular diffuse hypokinesis (MERRF, MELAS)

Electrocardiography

- ST depression
- Short PR interval
- T wave inversion
- Ventricular premature beats
- Left anterior fascicular/right bundle branch block (complete/incomplete)

MACROSCOPIC

General Features

- Increased heart weight
- Dilated or hypertrophic heart
- Asymmetric septal hypertrophy
- Endocardial fibroelastosis

MICROSCOPIC

Histologic Features

- Heart
  - Myocyte fusiforme enlargement with vacuolization/clearing
  - Cross striations replaced by fine granules
  - Myocyte necrosis
  - Interstitial fibrosis
  - Endocardial fibrosis

Clinical Features of Main Mitochondrial Disorders Associated With Cardiomyopathies

Syndrome	General Features	Cardiac Manifestations	Common Mutations
Kearns-Sayre syndrome	Progressive ophthalmoplegia, pigmentary retinopathy, deafness, limb weakness, renal/endocrine dysfunction; onset < 21 years of age	PR interval prolongation progressing to complete atrioventricular block; His-ventricular interval prolongation; Wolff-Parkinson-White syndrome; dilated cardiomyopathy	mtDNA heteroplasmic deletions, rearrangements or, rarely, duplications; common deletion 1.3-8.8 kb
Myoclonic epilepsy with red ragged fibers	Myoclonus, seizures, ataxia, dementia, muscle weakness, symmetric trunk lipomatosis; onset in childhood or early adulthood	Wolff-Parkinson-White syndrome; hypertrophic cardiomyopathy (20-30% of cases)	tRNA gene for lysine, A8344G; less frequently T8356C
Mitochondrial myopathy, encephalopathy, lactic acidosis, and stroke-like episodes syndrome	Encephalopathy, subacute stroke-like events, recurrent vomiting, limb weakness, and short stature; onset < 40 years of age	Wolff-Parkinson-White syndrome in both children and adults; sudden death; concentric, nonobstructive hypertrophic cardiomyopathy; dilated cardiomyopathy	A3243G, tRNA-Leu gene 3271, 3291; *MT-ND1* T3308C; *MT-ND5* gene mutations; T9957C; large-scale deletions
Leber hereditary optic neuropathy	Severe, subacute, painless loss of central vision; onset in 3th-4th decades of life	Short PR interval; supraventricular tachycardia	Homoplasmic point mutation in *ND4* protein-coding subunit, position G11778A
Chronic progressive external ophthalmoplegia	Ophthalmoplegia, ptosis, proximal muscle weakness; onset in childhood or early adulthood	PR interval prolongation preceding 2nd- or 3rd-degree atrioventricular block	mtDNA deletions, rearrangements, point mutations (*MT-TI*, *MT-TL1*)
Leigh syndrome	Severe subacute psychomotor delay and necrotizing symmetric lesions in brainstem, thalamus, cerebellum, spinal cord, and optic nerve; onset in infancy and childhood; less common in early adulthood	Hypertrophic or dilated cardiomyopathy	MT-ATPase 6 T8993G; mutations described in all 14 genes coding for core subunits of: Complex I (*MT-ND1* to 6; *NDUFS1*, 2, 4, 7, 8; *NDUFV1*); complex II (*SDHA*, SDH); complex III (*SURF1*); others (*SUCLA2*)

- Skeletal muscle
  - Ragged red fibers: Subsarcolemmal accumulation of mitochondria
    - > 2% of sample is diagnostic cutoff
  - Cytochrome oxidase-negative fibers
  - Internal nuclei
  - Atrophic/hypertrophic fibers
  - Large quantities of lipid droplets
  - Inflammation

ANCILLARY TESTS

Histochemistry

- Trichrome
  - Reactivity: Ragged red fibrils
  - Staining pattern: Red-purple perinuclear deposits
- Succinate dehydrogenase
  - Reactivity: Positive
  - Staining pattern: Subsarcolemmal

Electron Microscopy

- Increased numbers and size of mitochondria aggregated under sarcolemma
- Mitochondria with concentric cristae configuration
- Crystalloid or osmophilic globular inclusion bodies
- Myofibril loss
- Giant organelles
- Lipid accumulation

DIAGNOSTIC CHECKLIST

Pathologic Interpretation Pearls

- On trichrome stain, ragged red fibrils (in MERRF)
- Electron microscopy shows increased numbers and size of mitochondria aggregated under sarcolemma with abnormal concentric cristae configuration

SELECTED REFERENCES

1. Ebihara T et al: Neonatal-onset mitochondrial disease: clinical features, molecular diagnosis and prognosis. Arch Dis Child Fetal Neonatal Ed. 107(3):329-34, 2022
2. Lioncino M et al: Cardiovascular involvement in mtDNA disease: diagnosis, management, and therapeutic options. Heart Fail Clin. 18(1):51-60, 2022
3. Shimura M et al: Development of Leigh syndrome with a high probability of cardiac manifestations in infantile-onset patients with m.14453G > A. Mitochondrion. 63:1-8, 2022
4. Baban A et al: Myocardial and arrhythmic spectrum of neuromuscular disorders in children. Biomolecules. 11(11):1578, 2021
5. Bakare AB et al: Leigh syndrome: a tale of two genomes. Front Physiol. 12:693734, 2021
6. Imai-Okazaki A et al: Long-term prognosis and genetic background of cardiomyopathy in 223 pediatric mitochondrial disease patients. Int J Cardiol. 341:48-55, 2021
7. Montano V et al: Clinical features of mtDNA-related syndromes in adulthood. Arch Biochem Biophys. 697:108689, 2021
8. Orsucci D et al: Mitochondrial syndromes revisited. J Clin Med. 10(6), 2021
9. Takeda A et al: Advanced pathological study for definite diagnosis of mitochondrial cardiomyopathy. J Clin Pathol. 74(6):365-71, 2020

Ragged Red Fiber

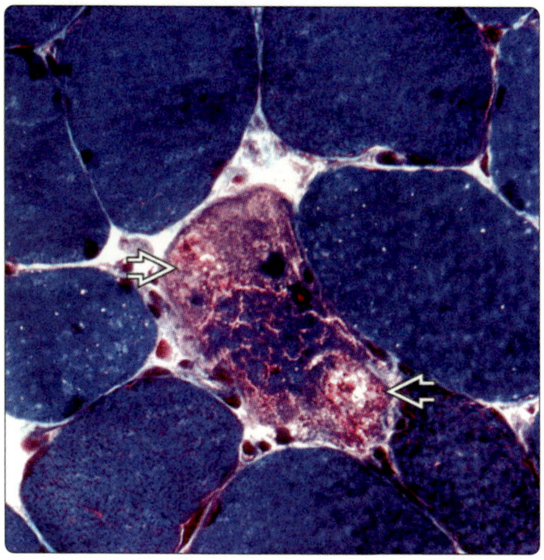

Myocardium: Toluidine Blue Stain

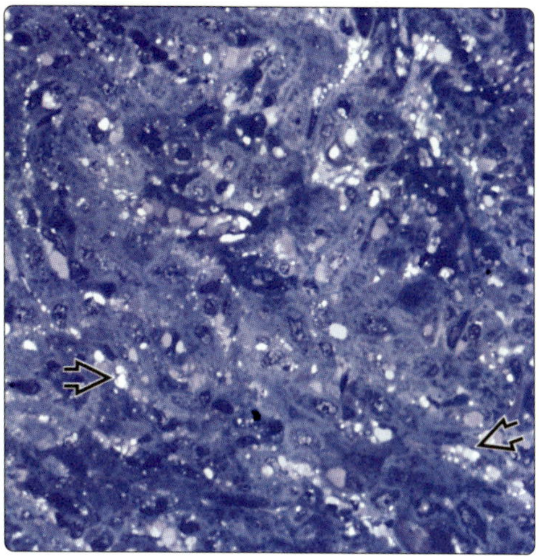

(Left) *Skeletal muscle shows a ragged red fiber ➡ resulting from subsarcolemmal loss of normal contractile elements and accumulation of abnormal mitochondria. (Courtesy C. Palmer, MD.)* **(Right)** *Thick section of plastic embedded myocardium for electron microscopy examination shows myocytes with fine vacuoles within the cytoplasm ⇨.*

Mitochondrial Abnormalities

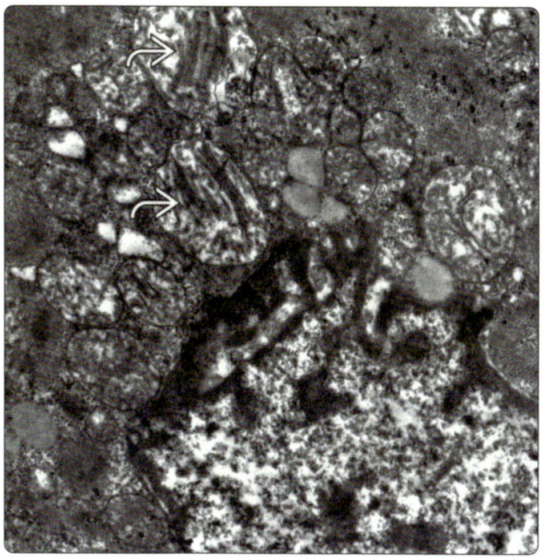

Mitochondrial Abnormalities

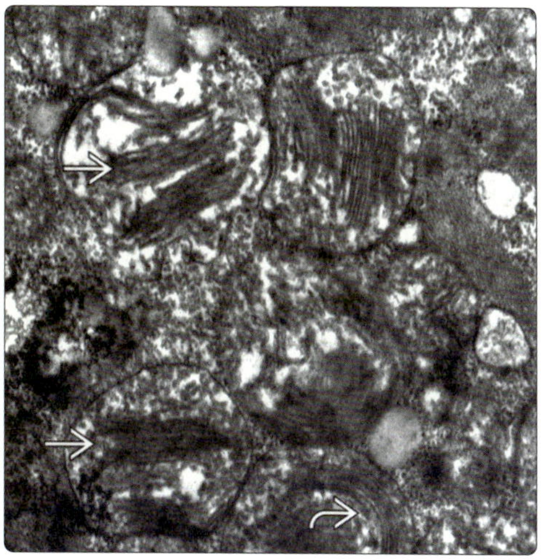

(Left) *Higher power electron micrograph of a myocyte demonstrates mitochondria of different sizes and shapes. The enlarged mitochondria contain abnormal parallel lamellae ↪.* **(Right)** *Low-power electron micrograph of a myocyte demonstrates mitochondria of different sizes and shapes. The enlarged mitochondria contain abnormal parallel ➡ or concentric lamellae ↪.*

Mitochondrial Abnormalities

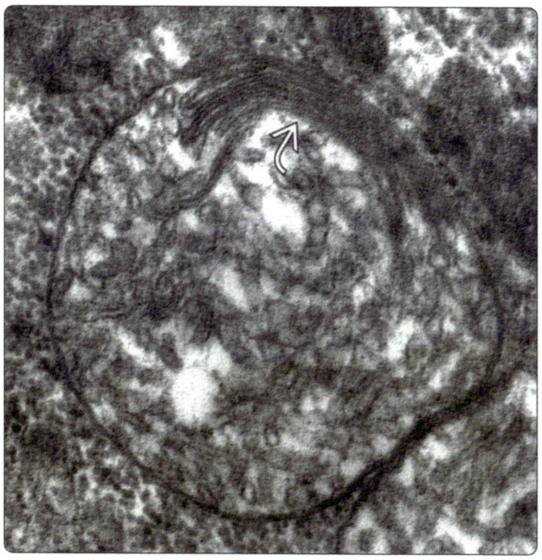

Mitochondrial Abnormalities

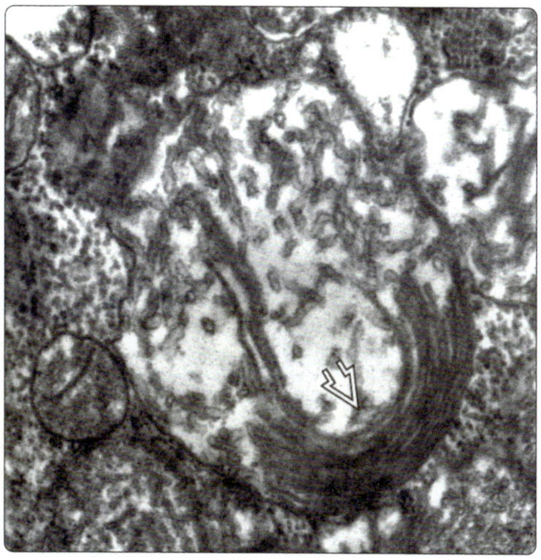

(Left) *On high-power view, an isolated mitochondria shows a round shape and contains a whorl of abnormal cristae ↪. The electron microscopy abnormalities are similar in the different mitochondrial diseases.* **(Right)** *On high-power view, the mitochondria show variable sizes and shapes. The larger mitochondria contains a whorl of abnormal cristae ➡.*

Muscular Dystrophies

KEY FACTS

TERMINOLOGY

- Muscular dystrophy (MD): Heterogeneous group of inherited disorders characterized by progressive skeletal muscle wasting and weakness with frequent cardiac involvement

ETIOLOGY/PATHOGENESIS

- Duchenne (DMD) and Becker (BMD): X-linked
- Myotonic dystrophy (DM): Autosomal dominant
- Emery-Dreifuss MD (EDMD): X-linked recessive and autosomal dominant
- Limb-girdle MD (LGMD): Autosomal recessive
- Facioscapulohumeral MD: Autosomal dominant
- Fukuyama MD: Autosomal recessive

CLINICAL ISSUES

- Cardiomyopathy: Dilated/hypertrophic
- Sudden death
- Atrial (fibrillation, flutter, standstill) and ventricular arrhythmias
- Conduction system abnormalities (atrioventricular or branches blocks)

MACROSCOPIC

- Enlarged or atrophic heart with dilated chambers
- Thickening of posterobasal left ventricle (DMD/BMD)

MICROSCOPIC

- Interstitial fibrosis with predilection of posterior basal segment of left ventricle (DMD)
- Fat infiltration of conduction system
- Myocyte necrosis and degeneration

ANCILLARY TESTS

- DMD/BMD: Dystrophin reduced/absent in sarcolemma
- EDMD1: Emerin absent
- LGMD2C-F: Sarcoglycans α, β, δ, and γ variably reduced/absent

Proteins Involved in Muscular Dystrophies That Affect Heart

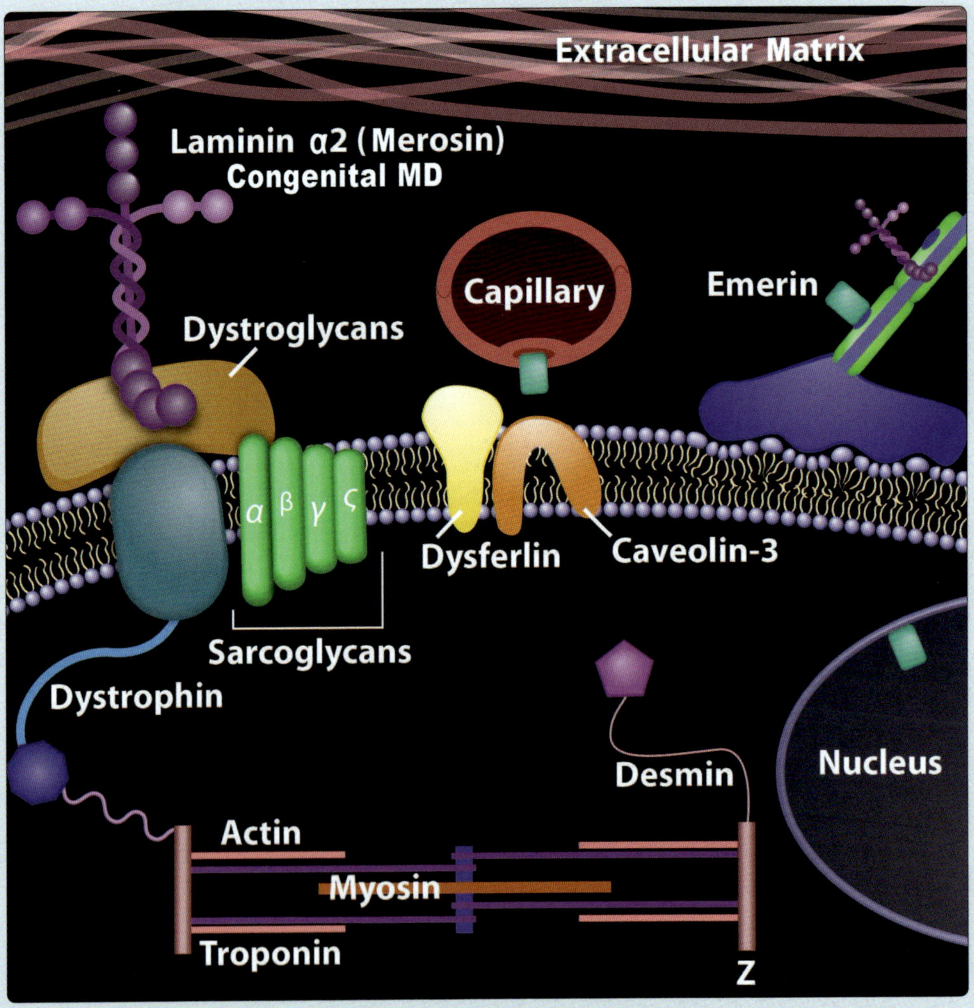

Graphic shows proteins linked to muscular dystrophies (MDs) affecting the heart. X-linked inherited dystrophin abnormalities are seen in Duchenne and Becker MDs. Sarcoglycan subunit mutations are found in limb-girdle-type MD with variable cardiac involvement. Emerin mutations lead to lack of nuclear emerin protein, which is responsible for X-linked Emery-Dreifuss MD. Mutations in laminins A and C are involved in autosomal dominant and recessive Emery-Dreifuss MD. Primary deficiency of laminin α2 is associated with congenital MD.

TERMINOLOGY

Abbreviations

- Muscular dystrophy (MD)

Definitions

- Heterogeneous group of inherited disorders characterized by dystrophic changes in skeletal muscle with progressive wasting and weakness of variable distribution with frequent cardiac involvement

ETIOLOGY/PATHOGENESIS

Most Common Genetic Associations

- Dystrophinopathies
  - Duchenne MD (DMD): X-linked
  - Becker MD (BMD): X-linked
  - X-linked dilated cardiomyopathy
- Myotonic dystrophy (DM): Autosomal dominant
- Emery-Dreifuss MD (EDMD)
  - EDMD1, EDMD6: X-linked recessive
  - EDMD2, EDMD4, EDMD5, EDMD7: Autosomal dominant
  - EDMD3: Autosomal recessive
- Limb-girdle MD (LGMD): Autosomal recessive
  - LGMD2C: Mutation in γ-sarcoglycan gene
  - LGMD2D: Mutation in α-sarcoglycan gene
  - LGMD2E: Mutation in β-sarcoglycan gene
  - LGMD2F: Mutation in δ-sarcoglycan gene
- Congenital MD: Autosomal recessive
- Facioscapulohumeral MD (FSHD): Autosomal dominant
- Fukuyama MD: Autosomal recessive

Basic Mechanisms of Myocyte Injury

- Reduced or absent membrane-associated proteins (dystrophin, sarcoglycans, emerin) lead to cell membrane fragility
- ↑ susceptibility to contraction-induced damage
- Influx of extracellular calcium and unbalanced production of nitric oxide and activation of proteases
- Induction of myocyte necrosis, inflammation, and replacement fibrosis

CLINICAL ISSUES

Epidemiology

- Incidence
  - DMD: 19.8:100,000 live male births
  - BMD: 3:100,000 live male births
  - DM: 1:8,000 general population
  - EDMD: 0.39:100,000
  - LGMD: 1:178,000 general population
  - FSHD: 1:20,000 general population

Presentation

- Cardiac clinical manifestations severity is variable
  - Cardiomyopathy: Dilated/hypertrophic
  - Sudden death
  - Atrial (fibrillation, flutter, standstill) and ventricular arrhythmias
  - Conduction system abnormalities: Atrioventricular or branches block
- Skeletal muscle
  - Progressive weakness of variable muscle groups
  - Pseudohypertrophy of calves
  - Myotonia
  - Elbow, Achilles tendon, and neck contractures
- Other organs
  - Cataracts, developmental delay, skull deformities, gonadal atrophy

Laboratory Tests

- Creatine kinase: DMD, elevated 10x, BMD, elevated 5x
- Cardiac troponin I (cTnI): Elevated but of uncertain significance
- Genetic testing

Treatment

- Surgical approaches
  - Left ventricular assist device
  - Cardiac transplantation
- Drugs
  - Corticosteroids, ACE inhibitors, β-blockers, mineralocorticoid receptor antagonist
- Other
  - Pacemaker, defibrillator, stem cell transplant, gene therapy

Prognosis

- Clear genotype-phenotype correlation with long-term prognosis has not been established
- Progressive cardiac involvement is leading cause of death

IMAGING

MR Findings

- Left ventricle free wall shows late gadolinium enhancement, initially subepicardial and later transmural
- More sensitive to detect early cardiac involvement

MACROSCOPIC

General Features

- Enlarged or atrophic heart
- Dilated chambers
- Thickening of posterior lateral left ventricle wall (most common in DMD/BMD)
- Normal valvular leaflets and coronary arteries
- Patchy myocardial scarring

MICROSCOPIC

Histologic Features

- Interstitial fibrosis with predilection of posterior lateral left ventricle wall with involvement of posterolateral papillary muscle (DMD/BMD)
- Fat infiltration of conduction system (sinus node, atrioventricular node, and His-Purkinje system)
- Myocyte necrosis and degeneration
- Focal myocyte hypertrophy

ANCILLARY TESTS

Immunohistochemistry

- DMD/BMD: Dystrophin reduced/absent in sarcolemma
- EDMD1: Emerin absent

Clinical and Pathologic Findings in Most Common Muscular Dystrophies

Type	Cardiac Symptoms	Genetics	Pathology Findings	EKG	Echo	Prognosis
Duchenne MD	Conduction defects; dilated/hypertrophied cardiomyopathy	Dystrophin; Xp21.2	Dilated chambers; myocyte necrosis; interstitial fibrosis; fat infiltration	Tall R waves or R:S ratio > V1 or V2; Q waves in lateral leads; complete right/left bundle branch block; arrhythmias	Systolic dysfunction; dilated cardiomyopathy; wall motion abnormalities	Progressive heart disease/failure; cardiac death: 10-20%; mean age at death: 19 y
Becker MD	Congestive heart failure; arrhythmias	Dystrophin; Xp21.2	Similar to Duchenne MD; right ventricle more involved	Similar to Duchenne MD	Similar to Duchenne MD	Progressive heart disease/failure; cardiac death: 50%; mean age at death: 45 y
X-linked dilated cardiomyopathy	Congestive heart failure in teenage male patients	Dystrophin; Xp21.2	Similar to Duchenne MD	Similar to Duchenne MD	Dilated cardiomyopathy	Rapidly progressive heart disease/failure; cardiac death: 100%; mean age at death: 22 y
Emery-Dreifuss MD: X-linked; autosomal dominant	Conduction defects; dilated cardiomyopathy; AV blocks	*EMD*, Xq28, *LMNA*; 1q21.2 *SYNE1-2, FHL1, TMEM43*	Dilated chambers; fatty/fibrous infiltration	AV block; atrial arrhythmias (flutter/fibrillation); low P-wave amplitude	Atrial and ventricular dilation; left ventricular dysfunction	High risk of sudden death (mean age at death: 50 y); good after pacemaker placement or ICD
Myotonic dystrophy	Conduction defects; ventricular dysfunction	*DMPK*; CTG amplified; 19 (type 1); CCTG amplified; 3q21 (type 2)	Heart hypertrophy; myocyte degeneration; fatty/fibrous infiltration of conduction system; diffuse interstitial fibrosis	AV block; atrial/ventricular arrhythmias; His-Purkinje conduction delay	Left ventricular dilation, dysfunction	Larger CTG expansions may have greater involvement of conduction tissue, sudden death; cardiac death 20-30%, mean age at death: 54 y
Limb-girdle MD	Varies with type of mutation	α, β, γ, δ sarcoglycans genes	Dilated chambers	Atrial arrhythmias; low P-wave amplitude; AV blocks; Q waves lateral leads	Dilated cardiomyopathy; left ventricular dysfunction	Slowly progressive heart failure; high risk of sudden death; mean age at death: 45 y
Facioscapulo-humeral MD	Arrhythmias; conduction defects	Deletion of integral number of repeats (D4Z4) with DNA shortening	Minor abnormalities	Minor abnormalities	Minor abnormalities	Cardiac death unusual
Fukuyama MD	Conduction defects; dilated cardiomyopathy; bundle branch blocks	Mutations: *FKTN, FKRP* (c.826C>A), *LARGE* genes	Extensive interstitial fibrosis	Atrial arrhythmias; right bundle branch block	Left ventricular dysfunction and dilatation; reduced fractional shortening	Cardiac death common

AV = atrioventricular; ICD = implantable cardioverter defibrillator; MD = muscular dystrophy.

- LGMD2C-F: Sarcoglycans α, β, δ, and γ variably reduced/absent

Electron Microscopy

- Foci of severe clumping of intercalated discs
- Marked pericellular fibrosis
- Increased numbers of mitochondria with abnormal cristae
- Abnormal Z bands
- Sarcoplasmic reticulum dilation

DIFFERENTIAL DIAGNOSIS

Idiopathic Dilated Cardiomyopathy

- In muscular dystrophies, skeletal muscle involvement is prominent clinical feature
- Immunohistochemical stains for emerin, dystrophin, and sarcoglycans differentiated EDMD1, DMD/BMD, and LGMD2C-F from idiopathic dilated cardiomyopathy

SELECTED REFERENCES

1. Groh WJ et al: 2022 HRS expert consensus statement on evaluation and management of arrhythmic risk in neuromuscular disorders. Heart Rhythm. 19(10):e61-120, 2022

Chamber Dilatation and Focal Endocardial Thickening in Duchenne Muscular Dystrophies

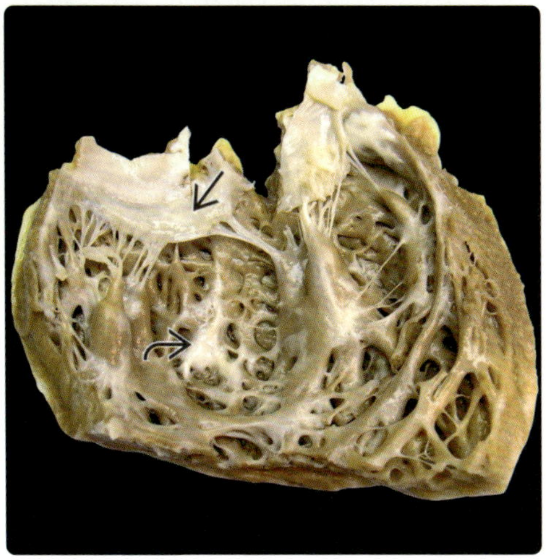

Short-Axis View

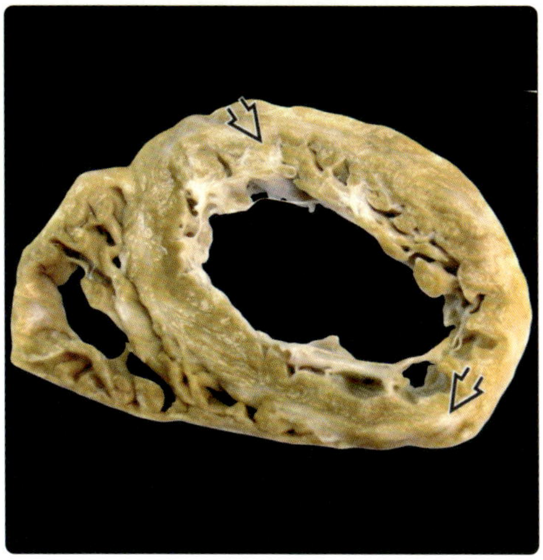

(Left) *Heart explant from a patient with Duchenne MD (DMD) shows left ventricle dilatation and focal endocardial thickening* ↪*. The mitral valve shows thin leaflets* →*.* **(Right)** *Transverse section of ventricles from the heart explant of a patient with DMD shows left chamber dilatation and white areas of discoloration* ⇨ *in the myocardium, consistent with fibrosis.*

Interstitial Fibrosis

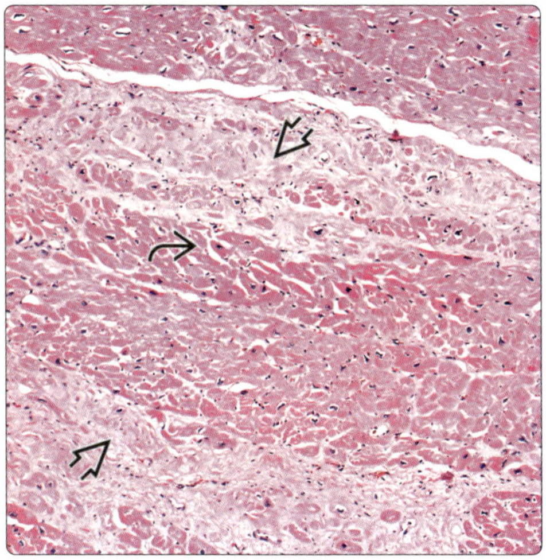

Myocyte Hypertrophy

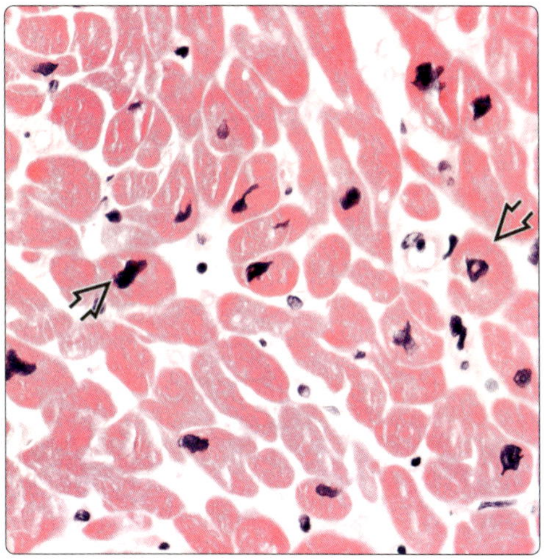

(Left) *Low-power H&E stain of myocardium from a patient with DMD shows extensive areas of interstitial fibrosis* ⇨ *and focal myocyte hypertrophy* ↪*. Inflammation is not present.* **(Right)** *High-magnification H&E stain of a myocardial section of a patient with DMD demonstrates scattered enlarged hypertrophic myocytes* ⇨*.*

Dystrophin Immunostain (Control)

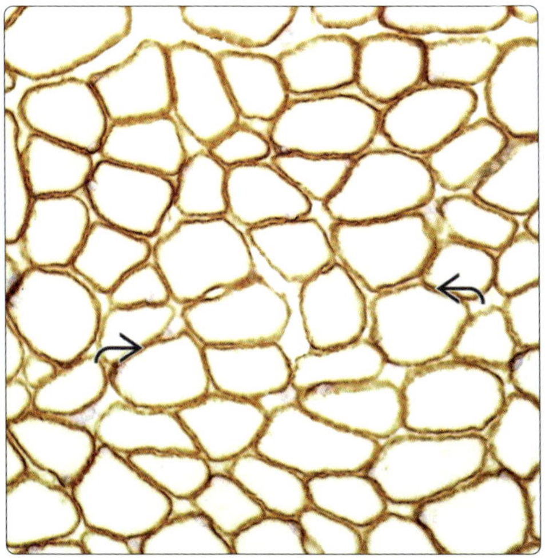

Dystrophin Immunostain (Patient)

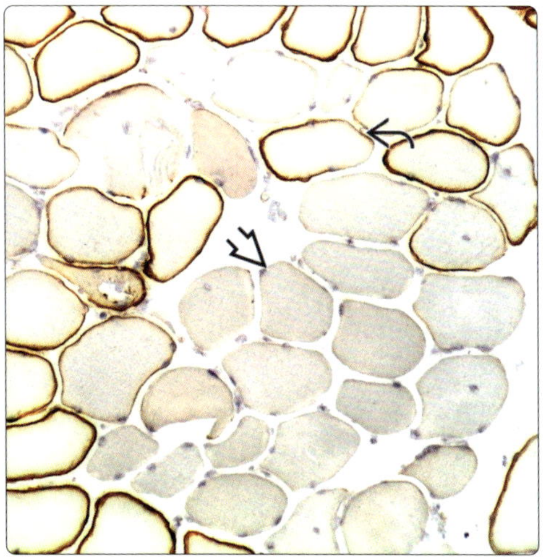

(Left) *Control immunohistochemical stain for dystrophin in the skeletal muscle shows diffuse positive sarcolemmal stain surrounding myofibers* ↪*.* **(Right)** *Dystrophin immunohistochemical stain in the skeletal muscle of a patient with DMD shows areas with complete loss of sarcolemmal staining* ⇨ *and other areas with weak incomplete sarcolemmal staining* ↪*.*

Glycogen Storage Diseases

KEY FACTS

TERMINOLOGY

- Inherited lysosomal enzyme deficiencies that cause glycogen accumulation resulting in cellular dysfunction with progressive damage of liver, heart, and skeletal muscle; mode of inheritance autosomal recessive or dominant

CLINICAL ISSUES

- Infantile
  - Cardiac
    - Hypertrophic cardiomyopathy
    - Congestive heart failure
    - Death
  - Other organs
    - Fetal hydrops, ketotic hypoglycemia, hepatomegaly with elevated liver enzymes, hypotonia, muscle weakness, respiratory distress
- Late onset (childhood, juvenile, adult)
  - Cardiac
    - Hypertrophic/dilated cardiomyopathy
    - Sudden death
  - Other organs
    - Skeletal myopathy and respiratory failure

MACROSCOPIC

- Massive cardiomegaly and marked ventricular walls thickening
- Endocardial fibroelastosis (20%)

MICROSCOPIC

- Marked vacuolar change of myocyte cytoplasm with lacework appearance and paucity of myofibrils
- Variable degree of interstitial fibrosis

ANCILLARY TESTS

- Myocardial glycogen deposits washed out after diastase treatment
- EM shows cytoplasmic accumulation of glycogen in myocytes with granular or fibrillary appearance

MR Findings: Glycogen Storage Disease

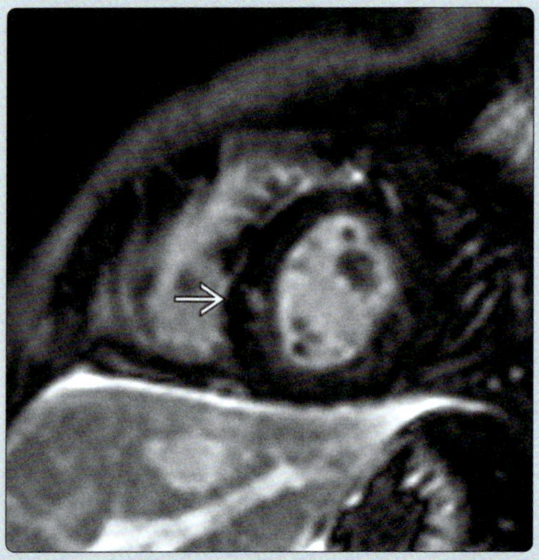

Histology: Glycogen Storage Disease

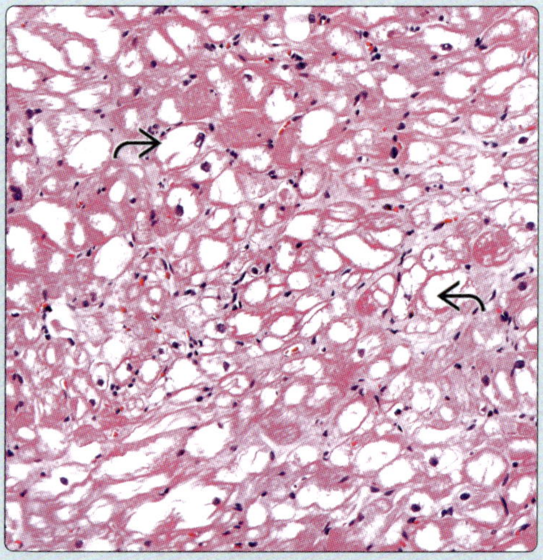

(Left) *Short-axis delayed-enhancement MR in a 3-year-old boy with glycogen storage disease shows midwall septal delayed enhancement ➡, a feature consistent with restrictive cardiomyopathy. (Courtesy G. Reddy, MD.)* **(Right)** *H&E-stained section at low magnification shows myocardium with marked cytoplasmic vacuolization of myocytes with an empty appearance and paucity of myofibrils ↪.*

Histology: Glycogen Storage Disease

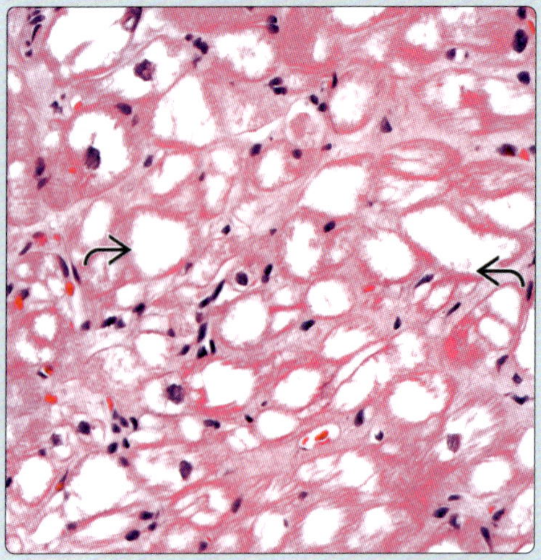

PAS-Diastase Stain: Glycogen Storage Disease

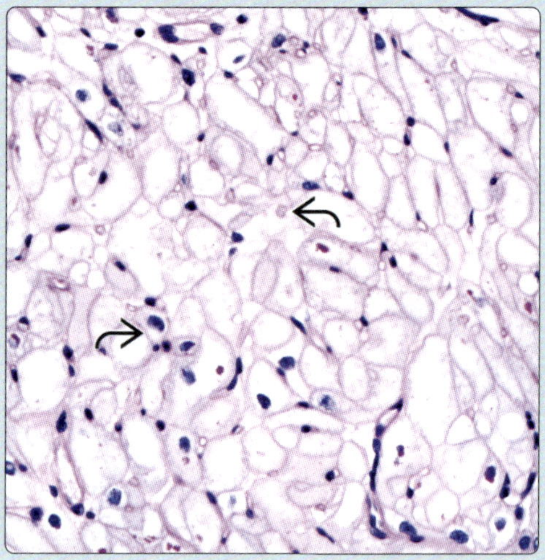

(Left) *H&E-stained section at higher magnification shows myocytes with a lacework appearance, empty-appearing cytoplasm, and loss of myofibrils ↪.* **(Right)** *Myocardial section stained with PAS-diastase shows myocytes with clear/empty cytoplasm due to loss of glycogen after diastase treatment ↪, demonstrating that the material within the cytoplasm is glycogen.*

TERMINOLOGY

Definitions

- Inherited lysosomal enzyme deficiencies that cause glycogen accumulation resulting in cellular dysfunction with progressive damage of liver, heart, and skeletal muscle; mode of inheritance autosomal recessive or dominant

ETIOLOGY/PATHOGENESIS

Inherited Enzyme Deficiency

- Glycogen storage disease II (Pompe disease): Acid α-1,4-glucosidase (GAA) > 600 pathogenic variants
- Glycogen storage disease III (Cori disease): Glycogen debranching enzyme (GDE); amylo-1,6-glucosidase and 4-α-glucanotransferase activity
- Glycogen storage disease IV (Andersen disease): α-1,4-glucan 6-glycosyl transferase
- AMP-activated protein kinase deficiency: γ-2 regulatory subunit of enzyme controlling uptake of glucose (PRKAG2)

CLINICAL ISSUES

Epidemiology

- Incidence
  - Glycogen storage disease II
    - Infantile: 1:140,000
    - Late onset: 1:57,000
  - Glycogen storage disease III: 1:100,000
  - Glycogen storage disease IV: 1:600,000-1:800,000
  - AMP-activated protein kinase deficiency: Unknown

Presentation

- Infantile
  - Cardiac: Congestive heart failure, hypertrophic cardiomyopathy, death
  - Other organs: Fetal hydrops, ketotic hypoglycemia, hepatomegaly with elevated liver enzymes, hypotonia and muscle weakness, respiratory distress
- Late onset (childhood, juvenile, adult)
  - Cardiac: Hypertrophic/dilated cardiomyopathy, arrhythmias, sudden death
  - Other organs: Skeletal myopathy, respiratory failure

Laboratory Tests

- Analysis of α-1,4-glucosidase activity in cultured fibroblasts and amylo-1,6-glucosidase activity in liver and muscle
- Molecular genetic testing for characteristic mutations
- Newborn screening available for Pompe disease

Treatment

- Enzyme replacement therapy for Pompe disease is available with recombinant human GAA
  - Better outcome if initiated very early within 1st days of life
- Heart failure medication
- Ketogenic diet

Prognosis

- Variable depending upon age of onset
- Infantile forms can lead to death within 1st year of life

IMAGING

Ultrasonographic Findings

- Marked thickening of ventricular walls
- Features of restrictive cardiomyopathy
- Reduced diastolic function

MR Findings

- Marked thickening of ventricular walls
- Abnormal delayed contrast enhancement
- Normal pericardium excludes constrictive pericarditis

EKG

- Abnormalities include short PR interval, marked left axis deviation, marked increased QRS voltage, inverted T waves

MACROSCOPIC

General Features

- Massive cardiomegaly (infantile)
- Marked thickening of ventricular walls
- Endocardial fibroelastosis (20%)

MICROSCOPIC

Histologic Features

- Marked vacuolar change of myocyte cytoplasm with lacework appearance and paucity of myofibrils
- Cytoplasm vacuolization in vascular smooth muscle cells and in conduction system
- Variable degree of interstitial fibrosis

ANCILLARY TESTS

Histochemistry

- PAS-diastase
  - Reactivity: Myocardial deposits washed out after diastase treatment
  - Staining pattern: Myocyte cytoplasm appears clear

Electron Microscopy

- Free cytoplasmic accumulation of glycogen in myocytes with granular or fibrillary appearance
- Glycogen accumulation within lysosomes in other organs

DIFFERENTIAL DIAGNOSIS

Fabry Disease

- Positive Sudan black stain of vacuoles on frozen sections
- Electron microscopy shows myelinoid figures

Mitochondrial Myopathy

- Negative PAS-diastase staining
- Electron microscopy shows abnormal mitochondria with crystallized and curvilinear cristae and osmophilic inclusions

SELECTED REFERENCES

1. Monda E et al: Hypertrophic cardiomyopathy in children: pathophysiology, diagnosis, and treatment of non-sarcomeric causes. Front Pediatr. 9:632293, 2021
2. van Kooten HA et al: Cardiovascular disease in non-classic Pompe disease: a systematic review. Neuromuscul Disord. 31(2):79-90, 2021
3. Berling É et al: Narrative review of glycogen storage disorder type III with a focus on neuromuscular, cardiac and therapeutic aspects. J Inherit Metab Dis. 44(3):521-33, 2021

Fabry Disease, Heart

KEY FACTS

TERMINOLOGY

- X-linked storage disease caused by deficiency in activity of lysosomal enzyme, resulting in progressive cellular accumulation of globotriaosylceramide (Gb3) in lysosomes in different tissues; heart may be only organ involved

ETIOLOGY/PATHOGENESIS

- X-linked recessive mutation in *GLA* gene on long arm of X chromosome (Xq22.1)
- > 245 different mutations

CLINICAL ISSUES

- Mutation prevalence: 1:40,000 males
- Hemizygous males develop severe multisystemic disease
- Heterozygous females can transmit disease but may be asymptomatic or may develop less severe symptoms later
- Cardiac: Angina, arrhythmias/conduction abnormalities, sudden death
- Cutaneous: Angiokeratomas, hypohidrosis/hyperhidrosis
- Kidney: Proteinuria, hypertension, renal failure
- Neurologic: Acroparesthesias, transient ischemic attack, stroke
- Ophthalmologic: Cornea verticillata, posterior subcapsular cataract

MACROSCOPIC

- Cardiomegaly with concentric or asymmetric left ventricular hypertrophy

MICROSCOPIC

- Marked myocyte perinuclear vacuolization and displacement of contractile elements to periphery
- Myocyte hypertrophy
- Variable degree of interstitial fibrosis

ANCILLARY TESTS

- Electron microscopy shows intralysosomal aggregates of myelin figures

Myocyte Vacuolar Changes

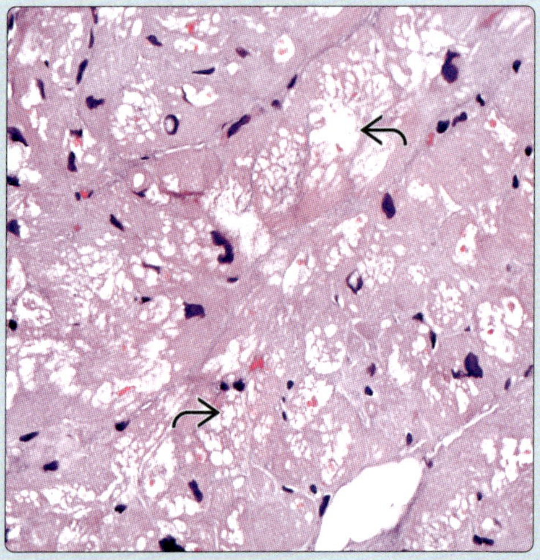

Myofibrillar Loss Highlighted on Trichrome Stain

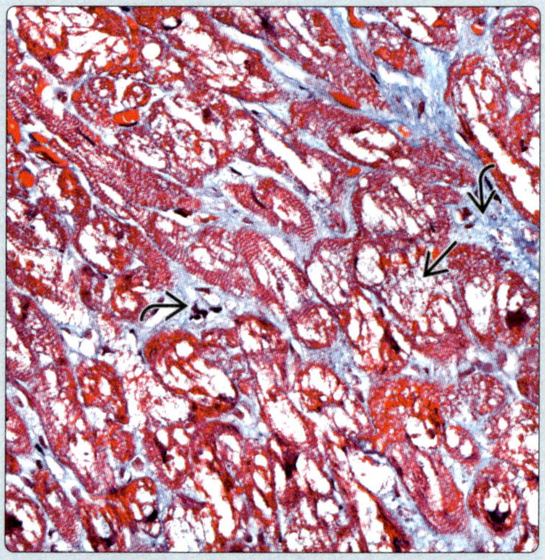

(Left) *H&E-stained section of the myocardium from a patient with Fabry disease shows enlarged, hypertrophic myocytes with extensive vacuolar change in the cytoplasm. Inflammation is not present.* **(Right)** *Trichrome stain of the myocardium from a patient with Fabry disease highlights perimyocyte fibrosis and the loss of myofibrils.*

Electron Microscopy Thick Section

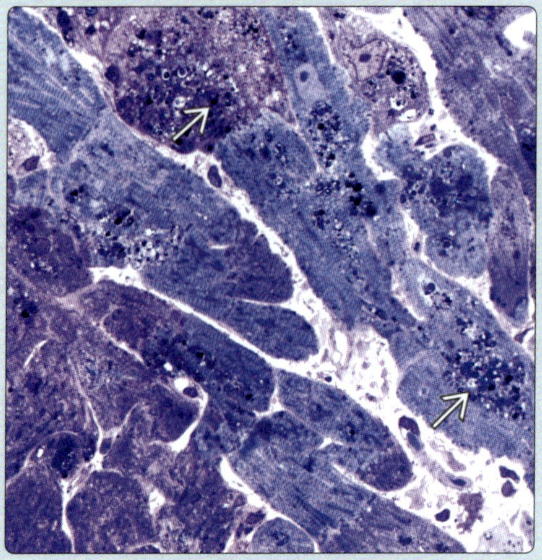

Ultrastructural Findings

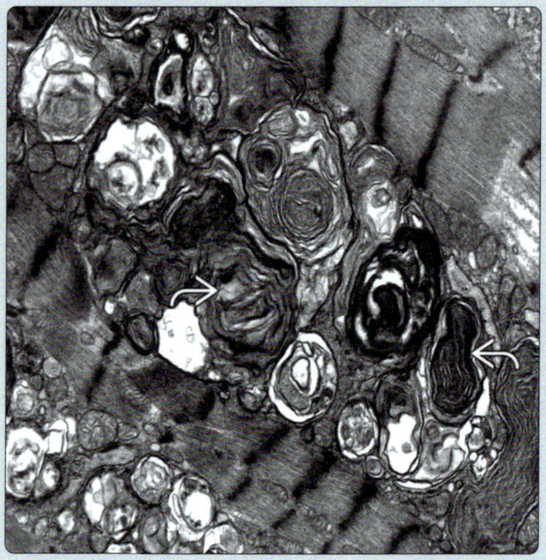

(Left) *Toluidine blue-stained section of the myocardium from a patient with Fabry disease shows accumulation of osmophilic material within the myocyte cytoplasm.* **(Right)** *Electron micrograph of the myocardium from a patient with Fabry disease shows myelin figures with characteristic lamellated, concentric appearance.*

TERMINOLOGY

Synonyms

- Anderson-Fabry disease (AFB)
- Angiokeratoma corporis diffusum

Definitions

- X-linked storage disease caused by deficiency in activity of lysosomal enzyme α-galactosidase A (*GLA*), resulting in progressive cellular accumulation of globotriaosylceramide (Gb3) and its deacylated form globotriaosylsphingosine (lyso-Gb3) in lysosomes in various cell types

ETIOLOGY/PATHOGENESIS

Genetics

- X-linked recessive mutation in *GLA* on long arm of X chromosome (Xq22.1)
- > 1,000 different variants (majority missense)

Mechanisms of Cardiac Injury

- Accumulation of GB3 in myocytes, conduction system cells, valvular fibroblasts, endothelial and vascular smooth muscle cells
- Activation of signaling pathways leading to myocyte hypertrophy, apoptosis, necrosis, and fibrosis
- Inflammation and oxidative stress
- Autophagy and mitochondrial dysfunction
- Microvascular dysfunction
- Accumulation of lyso-GB3
    - Inhibits *GLA* activity
    - Promotes smooth muscle cell proliferation

CLINICAL ISSUES

Epidemiology

- Incidence
    - Most common lysosomal storage disease
    - Mutation prevalence: 1:40,000 males
    - Neonatal screening data suggest that actual prevalence is close to 1:3,100 newborns in Italy; 1:5,495 and 1:8,454 in Washington and Illinois, respectively
    - Prevalence in late-diagnosed hypertrophic cardiomyopathy is 0.8-1.2%
- Age
    - Cardiac symptoms manifest at ~ 40 years of age in women and ~ 33 years of age in men
- Sex
    - Hemizygous males develop severe multisystemic disease
    - Heterozygous females can transmit disease; may be asymptomatic or develop less severe symptoms later

Presentation

- Classic: Onset in childhood/adolescence
    - Cardiac
        - Angina, arrhythmias, conduction abnormalities, sudden death, heart failure
    - Other organs
        - Cutaneous: Angiokeratomas, hypohidrosis/hyperhidrosis
        - Kidney: Proteinuria, hypertension, renal failure
        - Neurologic: Acroparesthesias, transient ischemic attack, stroke, neurosensorial deafness
        - Ophthalmologic: Cornea verticillata, posterior subcapsular cataract
- Variant: Onset in adulthood
    - Affects patients with less severe mutations (p.N215S, p.F113L, and IVS4+919G>A) and residual α-galactosidase A activity
    - Isolated cardiac or renal involvement can occur
        - Cardiac damage occurs at least 15 years later than in classic form
        - Severity of cardiac involvement is similar to or greater than in classic phenotype

Laboratory Tests

- Measurement of α-galactosidase A in leukocytes/urine or dried blood spot
- Measurement of lyso-Gb3 levels in plasma is useful for diagnosis and monitoring response to enzyme replacement or chaperone therapy
- High-sensitivity troponin and N-terminal pro-B-type natriuretic peptide are elevated and associated with adverse prognosis
- Genomic sequencing analysis for pathogenic mutations

Treatment

- Early initiation of enzyme replacement therapy (ERT) is desirable
- Oral molecular chaperone therapy for patients with specific "amenable" pathogenic mutations
- Substrate reduction therapy currently in preclinical phase
- Septal myomectomy if left ventricle (LV) outflow obstruction nonresponsive to ERT
- Conventional treatment for heart failure: ACE inhibitors, β-blockers, ARBs, anticoagulants, pacemaker, defibrillator, transplantation

Prognosis

- Early intervention with ERT slows progression of disease
- Cardiomyopathy is common cause of morbidity/mortality
    - Fibrosis progresses over time and correlates to arrhythmia and sudden death
- Death at mean age of 50 years in men, 70 years in women
    - Due to cardiovascular complications (40%), kidney failure, &/or cerebrovascular disease (10%)
- Does not recur after cardiac transplantation (due to intrinsic enzyme in donor heart)

IMAGING

Ultrasonographic Findings

- LV with diffuse concentric or asymmetric septal hypertrophy
- Reduced LV longitudinal strain
- Large left atrium
- Papillary muscle hypertrophy and right ventricular wall thickening
- Valvular thickening ± regurgitation (mitral/aortic)
- Initially preserved systolic function and diastolic dysfunction
- In end-stage disease, wall motion abnormalities are present

MR Findings

- Regional or global myocardial hypertrophy

- Low T1 signal in early stage of disease
- Late gadolinium enhancement in basal inferolateral LV segments is characteristic
- Useful for follow-up ERT efficacy

EKG

- Shortened PR interval
- Increased voltage
- High-degree atrioventricular block
- Arrhythmia
  - Sinus bradycardia
  - Atrial fibrillation
  - Nonsustained ventricular tachycardia
  - Ventricular tachycardia or ventricular fibrillation are common when hypertrophic cardiomyopathy &/or myocardial fibrosis have developed

MACROSCOPIC

General Features

- Cardiomegaly with concentric or asymmetric LV hypertrophy
- Prominent papillary muscles
- Mitral and aortic valve abnormalities
  - Thickening
- Aortic root or ascending dilatation

MICROSCOPIC

Histologic Features

- Marked myocyte perinuclear vacuolization and displacement of contractile elements to periphery
- Myocyte hypertrophy
- Variable degree of interstitial fibrosis involving specially basal posterolateral segment
- Variable degree of interstitial inflammation
- Vascular smooth muscle cells with cytoplasmic vacuolar change
- Vascular intima and media thickening and luminal narrowing

ANCILLARY TESTS

Histochemistry

- Sudan Black B (frozen tissue) (+)

Electron Microscopy

- Intralysosomal aggregates of concentric or parallel lamellae with alternating dense and light bands (myelin figures or zebra bodies) are characteristic

DIFFERENTIAL DIAGNOSIS

Glycogen Storage Diseases

- PAS-diastase stain shows washed-out myocytes
- Glycogen accumulation in electron microscopy examination
- Absent myelin figures/zebra bodies

Hydroxychloroquine Toxicity

- History of long-term hydroxychloroquine use
- Presence of myelin figures and curvilinear bodies in electron microscopy

Hypertrophic Cardiomyopathy

- Myocyte hypertrophy without significant vacuolization of cytoplasm
- Myofibrillary disarray
- Abnormal coronary branches
- Absence of myelin figures/zebra bodies

SELECTED REFERENCES

1. Germain DP et al: Challenging the traditional approach for interpreting genetic variants: lessons from Fabry disease. Clin Genet. 101(4):390-402, 2022
2. Rubino M et al: Diagnosis and management of cardiovascular involvement in Fabry disease. Heart Fail Clin. 18(1):39-49, 2022
3. Azevedo O et al: Fabry disease and the heart: a comprehensive review. Int J Mol Sci. 22(9), 2021
4. Chimenti C et al: Hypertrophy of unaffected cardiomyocytes correlates with severity of cardiomyopathy in female patients with Fabry disease. Orphanet J Rare Dis. 16(1):169, 2021
5. Passaro G et al: Arterial involvement in Fabry disease: state of the art and future diagnostic purposes. Eur Rev Med Pharmacol Sci. 25(2):845-55, 2021
6. Pieroni M et al: Cardiac involvement in Fabry disease: JACC review topic of the week. J Am Coll Cardiol. 77(7):922-36, 2021
7. Yim J et al: Fabry Cardiomyopathy: current practice and future directions. Cells. 10(6), 2021
8. Augusto JB et al: Myocardial edema, myocyte injury, and disease severity in Fabry disease. Circ Cardiovasc Imaging. 13(3):e010171, 2020
9. Del Pinto R et al: The role of immunity in Fabry disease and hypertension: a review of a novel common pathway. High Blood Press Cardiovasc Prev. 27(6):539-46, 2020
10. Linhart A et al: An expert consensus document on the management of cardiovascular manifestations of Fabry disease. Eur J Heart Fail. 22(7):1076-96, 2020
11. Miller JJ et al: Progress in the understanding and treatment of Fabry disease. Biochim Biophys Acta Gen Subj. 1864(1):129437, 2020
12. Sestito S et al: The heart in Anderson-Fabry disease. J Biol Regul Homeost Agents. Special Issue: Focus on Pediatric Cardiology. 34(4 Suppl. 2):63-9, 2020
13. Hagège A et al: Fabry disease in cardiology practice: literature review and expert point of view. Arch Cardiovasc Dis. 112(4):278-87, 2019
14. Knott KD et al: Quantitative myocardial perfusion in Fabry disease. Circ Cardiovasc Imaging. 12(7):e008872, 2019
15. Nordin S et al: Proposed stages of myocardial phenotype development in Fabry disease. JACC Cardiovasc Imaging. 12(8 Pt 2):1673-83, 2019
16. Perry R et al: Echocardiography in infiltrative cardiomyopathy. Heart Lung Circ. 28(9):1365-75, 2019
17. Perry R et al: The role of cardiac imaging in the diagnosis and management of Anderson-Fabry disease. JACC Cardiovasc Imaging. 12(7 Pt 1):1230-42, 2019
18. Wanner C et al: Therapeutic goals in Fabry disease: recommendations of a European expert panel, based on current clinical evidence with enzyme replacement therapy. Mol Genet Metab. 126(3):210-11, 2019
19. Yogasundaram H et al: Elevated inflammatory plasma biomarkers in patients with Fabry disease: a critical link to heart failure with preserved ejection fraction. J Am Heart Assoc. 7(21):e009098, 2018
20. Arends M et al: Characterization of classical and nonclassical Fabry disease: a multicenter study. J Am Soc Nephrol. 28(5):1631-41, 2017
21. Yogasundaram H et al: Clinical features, diagnosis, and management of patients with Anderson-Fabry cardiomyopathy. Can J Cardiol. 33(7):883-97, 2017

Myocardial Findings

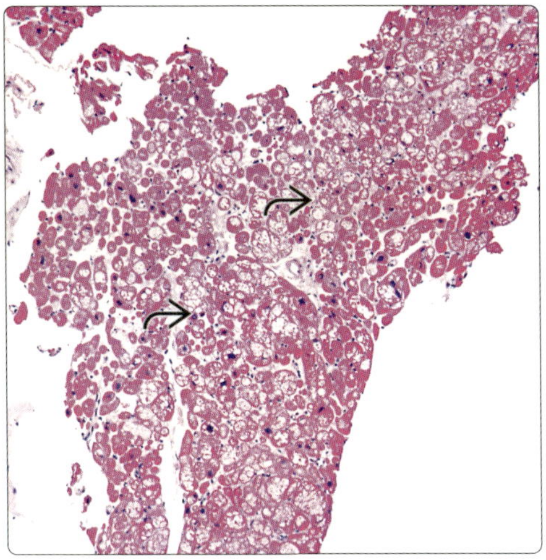

Myocyte Vacuolar Changes

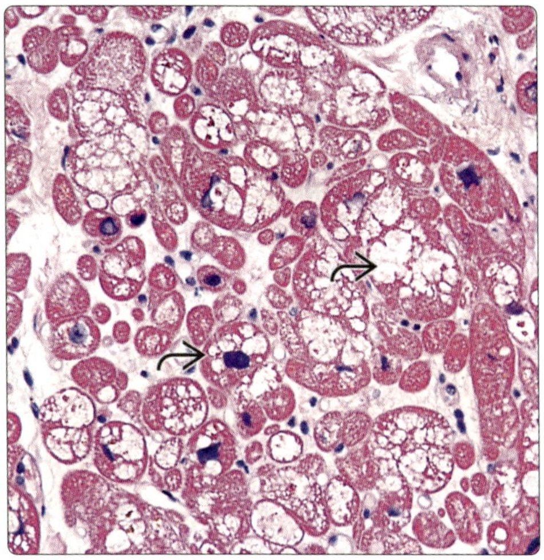

(Left) *Low-power view of H&E-stained section of the myocardium from a patient with Fabry disease shows diffusely enlarged and hypertrophic myocytes with extensive vacuolar change in the cytoplasm* →*. Inflammation is not present.* **(Right)** *High-power view of H&E-stained section of the myocardium from a patient with Fabry disease shows enlarged and hypertrophic myocytes with extensive vacuolar change in the cytoplasm* →*.*

Electron Microscopy Thick Section

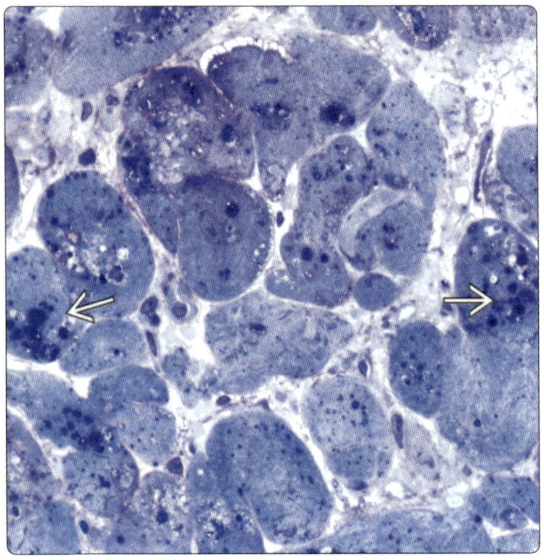

Electron Microscopy Findings in Myocardium

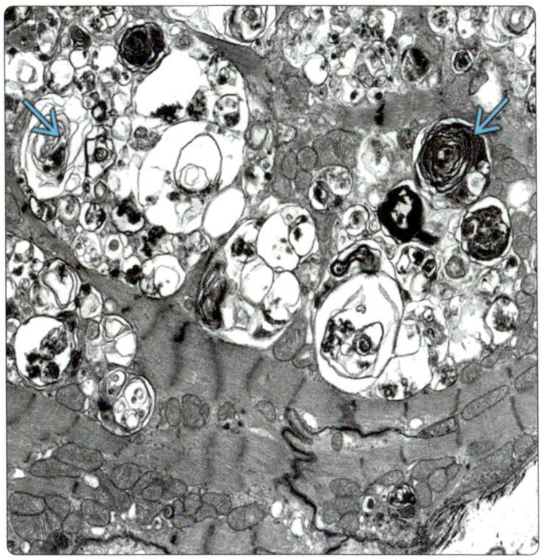

(Left) *Toluidine blue-stained section of the myocardium from a patient with Fabry disease shows accumulation of osmophilic material within the myocyte cytoplasm* →*.* **(Right)** *Electron micrograph of the myocardium from a patient with Fabry disease shows numerous myelin figures within the myocyte cytoplasm* → *and disruption of myofibrils.*

Glomerular Findings in Thick Section

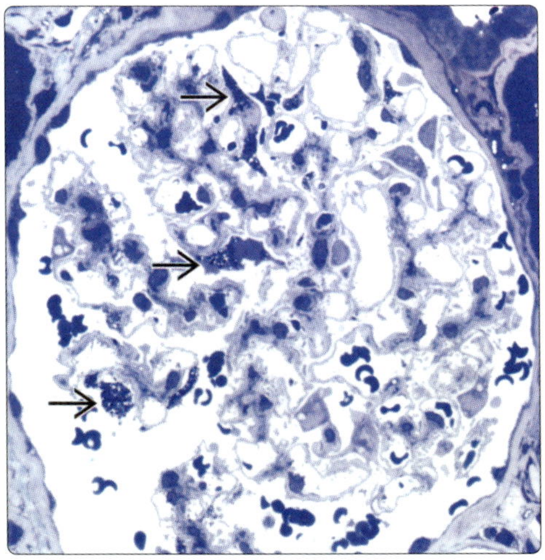

Podocyte Myelin Figures

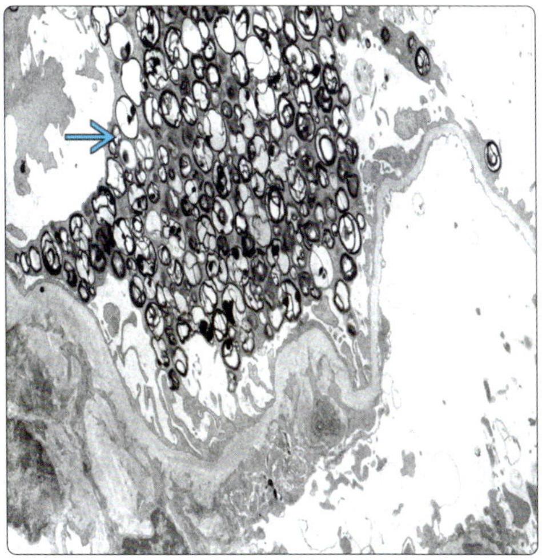

(Left) *Toluidine blue-stained thick section demonstrates podocytes* → *with vacuolar change in the cytoplasm and accumulation of osmophilic material. This material can be seen in endothelial, mesangial, and tubular cell cytoplasm.* **(Right)** *Electron micrograph of glomerulus from a patient with Fabry disease shows numerous myelin figures within the podocyte cytoplasm* → *and foot process effacement. The glomerular basement membranes do not demonstrate other abnormalities.*

LAMP2 Mutation (Danon Disease)

KEY FACTS

TERMINOLOGY

- X-linked dominant lysosomal disorder caused by primary deficiency of LAMP2 that leads to glycogen accumulation, which results in cardiac hypertrophy and electrophysiological abnormalities

ETIOLOGY/PATHOGENESIS

- X-linked dominant disorder
- Mutations affect *LAMP2* gene, which encodes LAMP2 protein
- Mutations include frame shifts, splicing sites, deletions, and insertions

CLINICAL ISSUES

- Most commonly affects teenage males
- Prevalence of 1-4% in some studies
- Geographic distribution of *LAMP2* mutations is broad
  - Disease has been reported in USA, Italy, Australia, Sweden, UK, Japan, and China
- Disease is characterized by cardiac or extracardiac features, including
  - Severe concentric left ventricular (LV) hypertrophy
    - Abnormal EKG findings, especially Wolff-Parkinson-White syndrome with very high voltage of LV
  - Intellectual disability or learning difficulties reported in 70% of patients
  - Skeletal myopathy or muscle weakness
    - Markedly elevated serum hepatic enzymes and CK
- Early morbidity and limited life expectancy
- No specific treatment except heart transplantation

MACROSCOPIC

- Cardiomegaly
- Severe concentric LV hypertrophy

MICROSCOPIC

- Intracytoplasmic vacuoles containing autophagic material and glycogen in cardiac and skeletal muscle cells

Gross Appearance

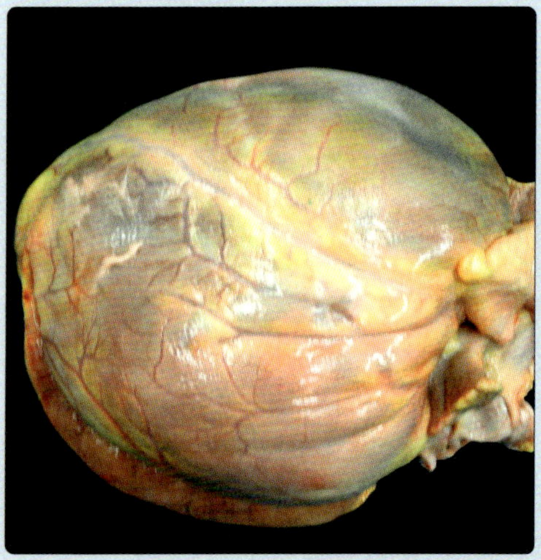

***LAMP2* Cardiomyopathy**

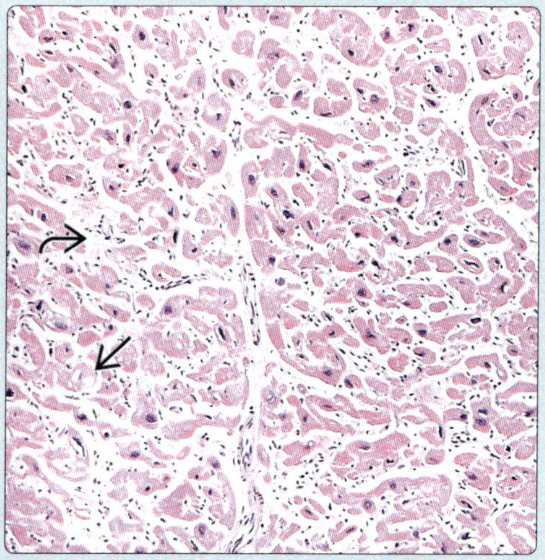

(Left) *Heart explanted from a patient affected with genetically confirmed Danon disease (LAMP2 mutation) shows cardiomegaly (weight = 910 g) and marked left ventricular hypertrophy.* **(Right)** *Myocardium in LAMP2 cardiomyopathy shows myocardial fiber hypertrophy and scant interstitial fibrosis ↪. Occasional intracytoplasmic vacuoles are seen ➡.*

***LAMP2* Cardiomyopathy**

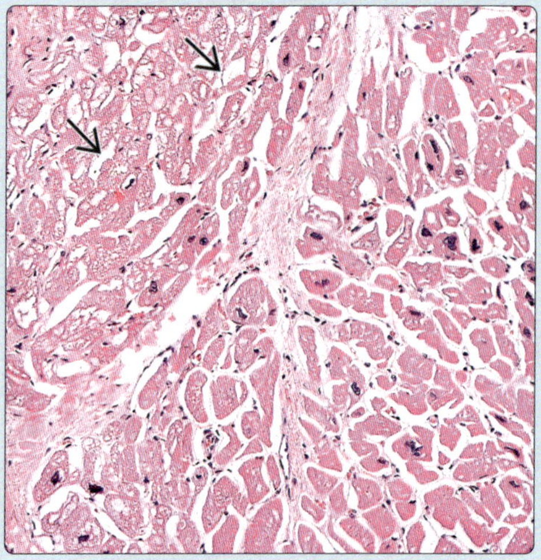

Electron Microscopic Features

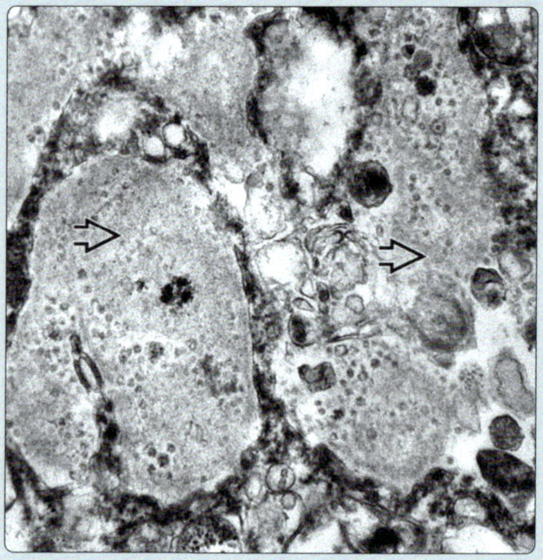

(Left) *LAMP2 cardiomyopathy shows hypertrophic myocardial fibers containing multiple cytoplasmic vacuoles (clear spaces) ➡ and focal interstitial fibrosis.* **(Right)** *Electron micrograph in LAMP2 mutation shows myocardial fibers with loss of myofibrils ⇨. Abundant ribosomes are evident.*

LAMP2 Mutation (Danon Disease)

TERMINOLOGY

Abbreviations

- Lysosome-associated membrane protein 2 (LAMP2)

Synonyms

- Danon disease

Definitions

- X-linked dominant lysosomal disorder caused by primary deficiency of LAMP2 that leads to glycogen accumulation, which results in cardiac hypertrophy and electrophysiological abnormalities

ETIOLOGY/PATHOGENESIS

Genetic

- X-linked dominant disorder
- Mutations (> 160 have been described) affect *LAMP2* gene, which encodes LAMP2 protein (3 isoforms LAMP2A, LAMP2B, LAMP2C), which leads to disruption of autophagy
- Mutations include frame shifts, splicing sites, deletions, and insertions; major isoform affected LAMP2B

CLINICAL ISSUES

Epidemiology

- Incidence
  - Geographic distribution of *LAMP2* mutations is broad
  - Disease has been reported in USA, Italy, Australia, Sweden, UK, Japan, and China
  - Prevalence is variable from 1-4% to 6-8%

Presentation

- Most commonly affects teenage males
  - Females typically present clinically 15 years later than males and are less severely affected
  - Affected females can present with dilated or hypertrophic cardiomyopathy during early 40s
- Disease is characterized by cardiac or extracardiac features, including
  - Severe concentric left ventricular (LV) hypertrophy
  - Abnormal EKG findings, especially Wolff-Parkinson-White syndrome with very high voltage of LV, atrial fibrillation
  - Skeletal myopathy or muscle weakness
  - Intellectual disability or learning difficulties (reported in 70% of patients)
    - Intellectual disability or skeletal myopathy can be present in female carriers but less commonly than in affected males
  - Markedly elevated serum hepatic enzymes and CK
  - Eye abnormalities: Retinitis pigmentosa

Treatment

- No specific treatment for Danon disease except heart transplantation, which significantly enhances survival
- Implantable cardioverter defibrillators fail to terminate lethal ventricular tachyarrhythmias in most patients

Prognosis

- Very poor with early morbidity and limited life expectancy (survival > 25 years is uncommon)
- Death occurs due to heart failure; can occur suddenly

IMAGING

Ultrasonographic Findings

- Echocardiography can detect different structural and functional abnormalities affecting heart, including
  - Size of each heart chamber
  - Severe muscle hypertrophy of both ventricles
  - Degree of obstruction of LV outflow tract
  - Heart valve insufficiency (tricuspid and mitral)
  - Decreased LV ejection fraction with global hypokinesis

MR Findings

- Cardiac MR similar to echocardiographic findings

MACROSCOPIC

General Features

- Cardiomegaly
- Severe concentric LV hypertrophy

MICROSCOPIC

Histologic Features

- Intracytoplasmic vacuoles in cardiac and skeletal muscle cells and fibrosis

ANCILLARY TESTS

Genetic Testing

- 3 frameshift mutations of *LAMP2* gene are important
  - c.808_809 insG in exon 6
  - c.320_321 insCATC in exon 3
  - c.257_258 delCC in exon 3
- All frameshift mutations lead to premature stop codon on cDNA analysis

Electron Microscopy

- Intracytoplasmic vacuoles containing autophagic material and glycogen in cardiac and skeletal muscle cells

DIFFERENTIAL DIAGNOSIS

Fabry Disease

- X-linked recessive disorder
- α-galactosidase A deficiency
- Frozen sections demonstrate that deposits are positive for PAS and Sudan staining
- Skin, cornea, and kidney involvement common

SELECTED REFERENCES

1. Wang XY et al: Clinical and molecular characterization of seven patients with Danon disease. Exp Ther Med. 21(4):395, 2021
2. Cenacchi G et al: Review: Danon disease: review of natural history and recent advances. Neuropathol Appl Neurobiol. 46(4):303-22, 2020
3. Di Nora C et al: Heart transplantation in Danon disease: long term single centre experience and review of the literature. Eur J Med Genet. 63(2):103645, 2020
4. Brambatti M et al: Danon disease: gender differences in presentation and outcomes. Int J Cardiol. 286:92-8, 2019
5. Demirdas S et al: Delayed diagnosis of Danon disease in patients presenting with isolated cardiomyopathy. Circ Genom Precis Med. 12(3):e002395, 2019
6. López-Sainz Á et al: Clinical findings and prognosis of Danon disease. An analysis of the Spanish multicenter Danon Registry. Rev Esp Cardiol (Engl Ed). 72(6):479-86, 2019

Amyloid Deposition, Heart

KEY FACTS

TERMINOLOGY

- Acquired or inherited extracellular deposition disorder in which infiltrating misfolded protein is found
  - Immunoglobulin amyloidosis (AL amyloid, AH amyloid)
  - Nonimmunoglobulin amyloidosis: AA, ATTR (wildtype/mutant), others

CLINICAL ISSUES

- Heart failure with normal angiogram, often with abnormal myocardial relaxation on echo and low voltage on EKG
- Prognosis is generally poor and varies according to amyloid type
- Combined heart and bone marrow transplants have shown improved outcomes compared with heart transplant alone for AL amyloidosis

MACROSCOPIC

- Organs show waxy color and may be brittle on sectioning
- Gross changes only seen in late stages of infiltration

MICROSCOPIC

- H&E shows pale pink, circumferential perimyocyte staining; vascular wall staining may also be seen

ANCILLARY TESTS

- Congo red shows pink stain with apple green birefringence on polarized light
- Immunofluorescence or immunohistochemistry can identify some amyloid protein subtypes
- Amyloid consists of short, straight fibrils 7.5-10.0 nm in diameter visible on electron microscopy
- Mass spectrometry provides highest sensitivity and specificity for identification of amyloid protein subtypes

TOP DIFFERENTIAL DIAGNOSES

- Idiopathic cardiomyopathy with fibrosis
- Light chain deposition disease
- Hypertrophic cardiomyopathy

(Left) *Cross section of left ventricle wall shows yellow-white areas in the myocardium and in subendocardial distribution in this case of apolipoprotein amyloidosis.* **(Right)** *Amorphous, pale eosinophilic material is seen in the interstitium ➩, forming nodules. The myocytes are trapped in the amyloid deposits ➩.*

Left Ventricle Wall Involved by Amyloidosis

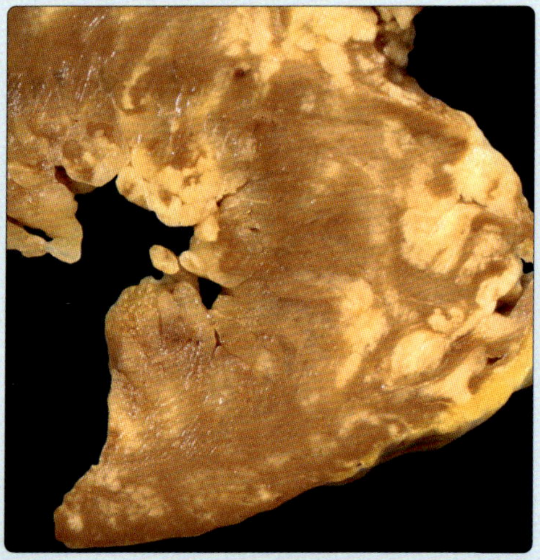

Myocardium Involved by Amyloid

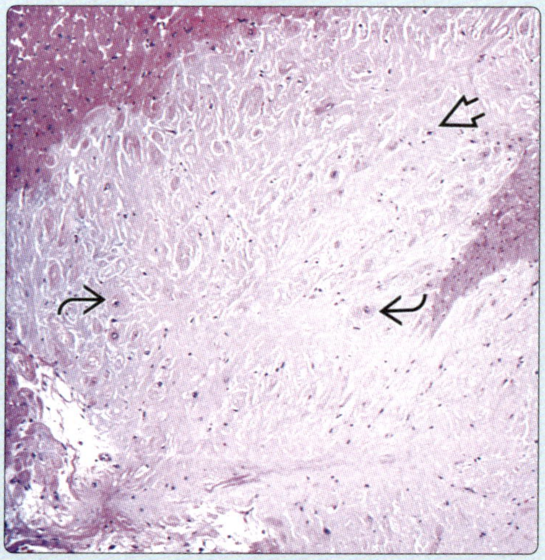

(Left) *Myocardial biopsy stained with Congo red shows perimyocytic deposits of pink-red material ➩ that would be apple green birefringent under polarized light. This feature is diagnostic of amyloid.* **(Right)** *Transmission electron micrograph shows randomly oriented, straight, nonbranching fibrils adjacent to the sarcolemmal membrane ➩ with diameters ranging up to 10 nm, characteristic of amyloid.*

Perimyocyte Congo Red Staining Pattern

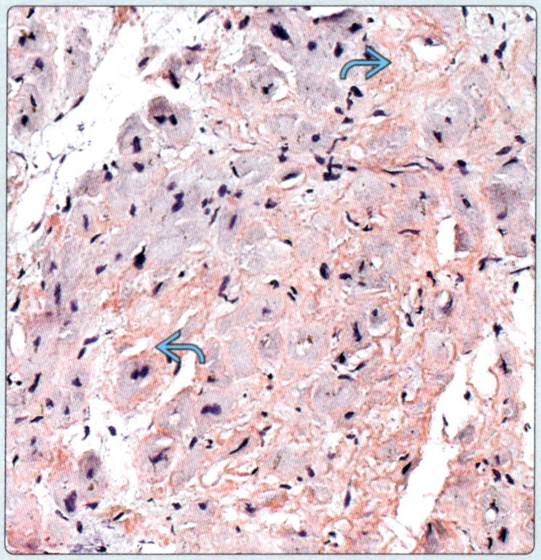

Morphology of Amyloid Fibers on Electron Microscopy

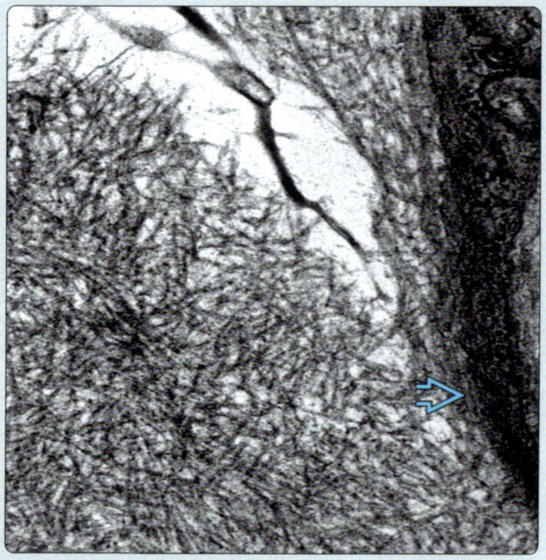

TERMINOLOGY

Abbreviations

- Immunoglobulin light chain amyloidosis (AL)
- Immunoglobulin heavy chain amyloidosis (AH amyloid)
- Transthyretin amyloidosis (ATTR)

Synonyms

- Immunoglobulin amyloidosis is also called primary amyloidosis
- Nonimmunoglobulin amyloidosis is also called secondary amyloidosis

Definitions

- Extracellular deposition disorder characterized by infiltration of multiple organs by insoluble deposits of fibrillar protein that arise from genetic mutations or excess production and form β-pleated sheet aligned in antiparallel array
- Amyloid: Name of class of infiltrating proteins that have undergone fibrillary modification in response to chemical, electrical, or mechanical stimuli

ETIOLOGY/PATHOGENESIS

Immunoglobulin-Related Amyloidosis

- AL amyloid
  - Infiltrating proteins are monoclonal light chains with substitutions in light chain variable regions produced by neoplastic plasma cells
  - Clonal B cells in bone marrow have clonal dominance of light chain isotype
  - More commonly λ than κ (6:1)
  - 85% of new cases are AL amyloid
- AH amyloid
  - Infiltrating protein is usually γ-heavy chain

Nonimmunoglobulin Amyloidosis

- Amyloid seen in old age is related to transthyretin wildtype (ATTRwt) accumulation in various organs
  - 2nd most common cause of clinically significant cardiac amyloidosis (~ 25% of cases)
  - More common in older men (> 70 years) than women (25-50:1)
  - Autopsy studies found that 25% of individuals ≥ 80 years of age can be affected
  - Association with aortic stenosis (~ 16%)
- Abnormal liver processing of serum A-associated protein (SAA)
  - ~ 5% of cases
  - Chronic infections, collagen vascular disease, or malignancy may be triggers for excessive protein production
  - Significant cardiac involvement appears to be rare
- Dialysis-associated amyloidosis in which precursor protein is β2-microglobulin
  - In autopsy studies, heart involvement occurs in ~ 80% of cases
- Atrial natriuretic factor-type amyloidosis (AANF)
  - Isolated atrial amyloid deposition
  - Common in older patients
  - Frequently associated with atrial fibrillation

Familial (Hereditary) Amyloidosis

- Accumulation of mutated transthyretin (ATTRm)
  - Autosomal dominant trait with variable penetrance (> 130 variations, including polymorphisms and mutations)
  - Val30Met most common mutation in USA
  - V122I variant confers higher risk of developing cardiac amyloidosis
    - 3-4% of African Americans have this mutation
- Apolipoprotein (AApo AI, AApo AII, and AApo AIV)
  - May occur with wildtype protein in atherosclerotic plaques, particularly in patients with aortic stenosis
  - May occur as hereditary form associated with germline mutation
  - Some mutations predispose patients to cardiac amyloidosis
- Gelsolin
- Lysozyme
- β2-microglobulin

CLINICAL ISSUES

Epidemiology

- Incidence
  - AL amyloidosis: 6-10 cases per 1 million
    - Almost 80% of patients with AL amyloidosis have some degree of cardiac involvement
  - ATTRm
    - 3.5-4.0% of African Americans have V122I mutation
    - T60A 2nd most common mutation
  - ATTRwt: 1-2% in African Americans and 0.4% in non-Hispanic
- Sex
  - AL amyloidosis: > 60% males
  - ATTRwt and ATTRm: Predominantly males
  - AANF: F > M

Presentation

- Heart failure with normal angiogram
  - Occurs in 25% of cases
  - Often associated with abnormal myocardial relaxation
- Abnormal EKG finding
  - EKG shows low voltage in limb leads or poor R-wave progression in precordial leads
  - Pseudoinfarct pattern characterized by QS waves in any 2 consecutive leads
- Arrhythmia
  - Commonly atrial fibrillation or conduction abnormalities, such as 1st-/2nd-degree or advanced heart block
- Syncope
  - Secondary to arrhythmia
- Sudden cardiac death
  - Related to electromechanical dissociation
- Orthostatic hypotension secondary to autonomic neuropathy
- Extracardiac findings
  - Skin/soft tissue
    - Purpura
    - Back pain
    - Macroglossia
    - Peripheral edema

- Neurologic
  - Carpal tunnel (usually bilateral)
    - Often precedes clinical presentation of heart failure
  - Autonomic or peripheral polyneuropathy (orthostatic hypotension, numbness, stabbing/burning pain, weakness)
  - Spinal stenosis
- Renal
  - Nephrotic syndrome/proteinuria
  - Renal failure
- Gastrointestinal
  - Diarrhea
  - Constipation
  - Nausea
  - Early satiety
  - Hepatomegaly

Laboratory Tests

- Serum free light chain levels and ratio and serum/urine electrophoresis with immunofixation are diagnostic and monitoring tools for AL amyloidosis
- N terminal pro B-type-natriuretic peptide (NT-pro-BNP) marker of cardiac involvement
- Troponin marker of cardiac involvement
- Genetic testing to determine mutations for ATTRm diagnosis

Treatment

- Symptomatic treatment of heart failure
  - Avoid dioxin, calcium channel blockers, and β-blockers, which worsen symptoms
- AL amyloidosis
  - Plasma cell disorder should be sought and treated with high-dose chemotherapy and autologous stem cell transplant
  - Cardiac transplantation is alternative with variable success
    - Amyloid recurrence can occur as early as 5 months after transplantation
    - Combined heart and autologous stem cell transplant has shown improved outcomes compared with heart transplant alone for AL amyloidosis with reported 5-year survival rate of ~ 65%
  - Antibodies to serum amyloid protein (SAP) can trigger clearance of amyloid deposits
  - Experimental antibodies targeting specific epitopes of misfolded LC are in clinical trials
  - Doxycycline can disrupt amyloid fibrils
- ATTR amyloidosis
  - Isolated liver or combined heart and liver transplant for ATTRm
  - Diflunisal and tafamidis have shown efficacy in stabilizing TTR and improving neuropathy in familial ATTR
  - TTR gene silencers (patisiran, inotersen) block TTR synthesis
  - Doxycycline can disrupt amyloid fibrils
- Other forms of amyloid cannot be treated

Prognosis

- Prognosis is generally poor and varies according to amyloid type and extent of tissue involvement
- Median survival is 13 months without treatment for AL amyloidosis, 2.5 years for ATTRm and 3.6 years for ATTRwt

IMAGING

Ultrasonographic Findings

- Abnormal global or regional myocardial relaxation early in disease process with restrictive pattern and increasing filling pressures later
- Concentric thickening of ventricular walls (LV wall > 12 mm) with abnormal granular echotexture (starry-sky appearance)
- Biatrial enlargement
- Small left ventricular cavity size and preserved ejection fraction
- Reduced longitudinal strain with relative apical sparing on strain imaging using speckle tracking echocardiography

MR Findings

- Diffuse heterogeneous enhancement of thickened subendocardial myocardium on delayed enhanced images
- Zebra pattern: Biventricular subendocardial enhancement lending striped appearance to ventricular septum
- T1 mapping and measurement of extracellular volume fraction is useful in detecting amyloid deposits
- High sensitivity and specificity for diagnosis (> 86%)

Tc-99m Pyrophosphate Scintigraphy

- Noninvasive imaging study specific for ATTR
- Heart:contralateral ratio > 2 is consistent with diagnosis of ATTR amyloidosis
- Other imaging Tc-diphosphonates tracers are available outside USA

MACROSCOPIC

General Features

- Organs show waxy color and may be brittle on sectioning
- Gross changes only seen in late stages of infiltration
- Amyloid deposits can be seen within myocardium, vessels, endocardium, valves, epicardium, and parietal pericardium
- Ventricular walls are typically thickened
  - Concentric
  - Septal thickening, especially posterobasal ventricular septum
- Atrial involvement may be mild or marked
- Endomyocardial biopsy often has no distinguishing characteristics

MICROSCOPIC

Histologic Features

- Pale, homogeneous, pink circumferential staining of myocytes widens interstitial regions; filamentous appearance common in AANF
- Arterioles may show deposits in some cases, especially in AL amyloidosis
- May also form nodules in interstitium
- Endocardial deposits may be prominent
- Fibrosis, myocyte hypertrophy &/or atrophy may be seen
- Pattern of amyloid distribution is not specific of amyloid protein type

Predominant Pattern/Injury Type

- Infiltrative

Predominant Cell/Compartment Type

- Interstitium

ANCILLARY TESTS

Histochemistry

- Congo red
  - Reactivity: Positive
  - Staining pattern: Perimyocytic or vascular walls
  - Congo red shows pink stain with apple green birefringence on polarized light, which is diagnostic
    - May be negative or hard to appreciate in early cases
- Methyl violet
  - Reactivity: Positive
  - Staining pattern: Perimyocytic
- Sulfated Alcian blue
  - Reactivity: Positive
  - Staining pattern: Perimyocytic
- Thioflavin T
  - Reactivity: Positive
  - Staining pattern: Perimyocytic
  - Staining is only visualized using UV light
- Trichrome
  - Pale or blue-gray

Immunohistochemistry

- Either κ- or λ-light chain perimyocytic, interstitial, or arteriole staining
  - Most commonly λ-light chain specific

Immunofluorescence

- Either κ- or λ-light chain perimyocytic, interstitial, or arteriole staining
  - Most commonly λ-light chain specific

Electron Microscopy

- Amyloid consists of short, nonbranching, straight fibrils 7.5-10.0 nm in diameter
- Fibrils are associated with electron-dense, dot-like structures (P component)
- Fibrils found associated with sarcolemma and less frequently with vascular basal lamina
- Transmission electron microscopy (TEM) is most sensitive and specific method of diagnosis, positive in cases where Congo red is negative or inconclusive

Laser Microdissection/Mass Spectrometry

- Provides highest sensitivity and specificity for accurate identification of amyloid protein types
- Considered gold standard for amyloid typing

DIFFERENTIAL DIAGNOSIS

Idiopathic Cardiomyopathy With Fibrosis

- Negative Congo red staining
- Fibrosis stains densely blue with Masson trichrome
- Fibrous tissue on TEM contains collagen fibers

Light Chain Deposition Disease

- Negative Congo red stain
- Ultrastructural appearance is of flocculent, dark, granular material in vascular walls or perimyocytic location

Hypertrophic Cardiomyopathy

- Asymmetric septal hypertrophy
- Myocyte disarray
- Negative Congo red stain

DIAGNOSTIC CHECKLIST

Clinically Relevant Pathologic Features

- Type of amyloid must be defined because it affects patient treatment

Pathologic Interpretation Pearls

- Laser microdissection and mass spectrometry of biopsy material has become gold standard for amyloid-type identification
- TEM is most sensitive method of detection in early cases

SELECTED REFERENCES

1. Addison D et al: Recent advances and current dilemmas in the diagnosis and management of transthyretin cardiac amyloidosis. J Am Heart Assoc. 10(9):e019840, 2021
2. Garcia-Pavia P et al: Diagnosis and treatment of cardiac amyloidosis: a position statement of the ESC Working Group on Myocardial and Pericardial Diseases. Eur Heart J. 42(16):1554-68, 2021
3. Korosoglou G et al: Diagnostic work-up of cardiac amyloidosis using cardiovascular imaging: current standards and practical algorithms. Vasc Health Risk Manag. 17:661-73, 2021
4. Nitsche C et al: Prevalence and outcomes of concomitant aortic stenosis and cardiac amyloidosis. J Am Coll Cardiol. 77(2):128-39, 2021
5. Smith A et al: Cardiac amyloidosis in non-transplant cardiac surgery. J Card Surg. 36(8):2901-10, 2021
6. Zhang KW et al: A multi-modal diagnostic model improves detection of cardiac amyloidosis among patients with diagnostic confirmation by cardiac biopsy. Am Heart J. 232:137-45, 2021
7. Fayyaz AU et al: Amyloidosis in surgically resected atrial appendages: a study of 345 consecutive cases with clinical implications. Mod Pathol. 33(5):764-74, 2020
8. McVeigh T et al: Understanding and recognizing cardiac amyloidosis. JAAPA. 33(10):16-20, 2020
9. Penalver J et al: Transthyretin cardiac amyloidosis and aortic stenosis: connection and therapeutic implications. Curr Cardiol Rev. 16(3):221-30, 2020
10. Damy T et al: Transthyretin cardiac amyloidosis in continental Western Europe: an insight through the transthyretin amyloidosis outcomes survey (THAOS). Eur Heart J. 43(5):391-400, 2019
11. Hanna M et al: Progress in diagnosing and managing cardiac amyloidosis. Cleve Clin J Med. 86(1):29-37, 2019
12. Lee SP et al: Contemporary imaging diagnosis of cardiac amyloidosis. J Cardiovasc Imaging. 27(1):1-10, 2019
13. Morris AD et al: The pathology and changing epidemiology of dialysis-related cardiac beta-2 microglobulin amyloidosis. Cardiovasc Pathol. 42:30-35, 2019
14. Sidana S et al: Clinical features, laboratory characteristics and outcomes of patients with renal versus cardiac light chain amyloidosis. Br J Haematol. 185(4):701-7, 2019
15. Ternacle J et al: Aortic stenosis and cardiac amyloidosis: JACC review topic of the week. J Am Coll Cardiol. 74(21):2638-51, 2019
16. Yamamoto H et al: Transthyretin cardiac amyloidosis: an update on diagnosis and treatment. ESC Heart Fail. 6(6):1128-39, 2019
17. Aimo A et al: Therapies for cardiac light chain amyloidosis: an update. Int J Cardiol. 271:152-60, 2018
18. Bhogal S et al: Cardiac amyloidosis: an updated review with emphasis on diagnosis and future directions. Curr Probl Cardiol. 43(1):10-34, 2018
19. Halatchev IG et al: Wild-type transthyretin cardiac amyloidosis (ATTRwt-CA), previously known as senile cardiac amyloidosis: clinical presentation, diagnosis, management and emerging therapies. J Thorac Dis. 10(3):2034-45, 2018
20. Kyriakou P et al: Diagnosis of cardiac amyloidosis: a systematic review on the role of imaging and biomarkers. BMC Cardiovasc Disord. 18(1):221, 2018
21. Maleszewski JJ et al: Neoplasia and the heart: pathological review of effects with clinical and radiological correlation. J Am Coll Cardiol. 72(2):202-27, 2018

Immunohistochemistry

Antibody	Reactivity	Staining Pattern	Comment
Immunologic Amyloid (Primary Amyloid)			
κ light chain	Positive	Interstitial	One or other light chain is positive in perimyocytic/artery distribution
λ light chain	Positive	Interstitial	Most commonly positive
IgG	Positive	Interstitial	Most common heavy chain is γ
Nonimmunologic Amyloid (Secondary Amyloid)			
SAA	Positive	Interstitial	Associated with chronic infection, inflammatory process, or malignancy
Prealbumin	Positive	Interstitial	Found in wildtype ATTR cardiac amyloid
β-2-microglobulin	Positive	Interstitial	Associated with dialysis
Familial Amyloid			
Prealbumin	Positive	Interstitial	Autosomal dominant inheritance, mutant ATTR
Lysozyme	Positive	Interstitial	Amyloid protein occurring in familial form

Immunofluorescence

Antibody	Reactivity	Staining Pattern	Comment
κ	Positive, linear	Interstitium/artery wall	20% of cases
λ	Positive, linear	Interstitium/artery wall	If light chain is positive (80% λ-light chain), may require dilution to illustrate monoclonality

Diagnostic Findings in Different Tests for Amyloidosis

Diagnostic Test	Characteristic Findings	Sensitivity/Specificity
Strain imaging using speckle tracking echocardiography	Significant decrease in longitudinal strain in mid and basal region with relative apical preservation	90-95%/80-85%
Tc-99m pyrophosphate	Heart:contralateral ratio > 1.5, consistent with ATTR amyloidosis	97%/100%
CMR	Global transmural or diffuse subendocardial late gadolinium enhancement	80%/95%
Endomyocardial biopsy (considered gold standard)	Amorphous deposits of Congo red-positive material; 8- to 10-nm fibrils on EM	Close to 100%
Laser capture microdissection and mass spectrometry on tissue biopsy	Can identify different amyloid types	Close to 100%

22. Nativi-Nicolau J et al: Amyloidosis cardiomyopathy: update in the diagnosis and treatment of the most common types. Curr Opin Cardiol. 33(5):571-9, 2018
23. Larsen BT et al: Correlation of histomorphological pattern of cardiac amyloid deposition with amyloid type: a histological and proteomic analysis of 108 cases. Histopathology. 68(5):648-56, 2016
24. Bejar D et al: Infiltrative cardiomyopathies. Clin Med Insights Cardiol. 9(Suppl 2):29-38, 2015
25. Maleszewski JJ: Cardiac amyloidosis: pathology, nomenclature, and typing. Cardiovasc Pathol. 24(6):343-50, 2015
26. Maurer MS: Noninvasive identification of ATTRwt cardiac amyloid: the re-emergence of nuclear cardiology. Am J Med. 128(12):1275-80, 2015
27. Rosenbaum AN et al: Current indications, strategies, and outcomes with cardiac transplantation for cardiac amyloidosis and sarcoidosis. Curr Opin Organ Transplant. 20(5):584-92, 2015
28. Austin BA et al: Comparison of functional status, electrocardiographic, and echocardiographic parameters to mortality in endomyocardial-biopsy proven cardiac amyloidosis. Am J Cardiol. 103(10):1429-33, 2009
29. Eriksson M et al: Hereditary apolipoprotein AI-associated amyloidosis in surgical pathology specimens: identification of three novel mutations in the APOA1 gene. J Mol Diagn. 11(3):257-62, 2009
30. Eriksson M et al: Prevalence of germline mutations in the TTR gene in a consecutive series of surgical pathology specimens with ATTR amyloid. Am J Surg Pathol. 33(1):58-65, 2009

Amyloid Deposition, Heart

Cardiac Amyloidosis

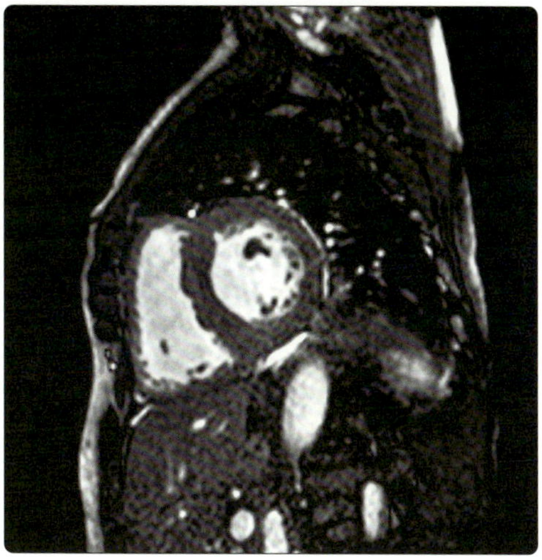

Cardiac Amyloidosis

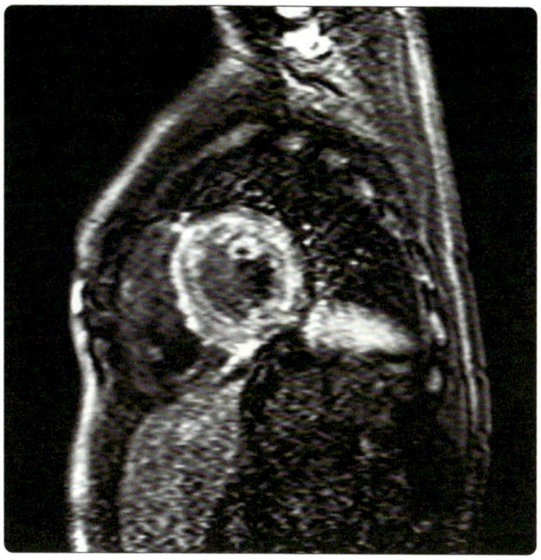

(Left) *Short-axis SSFP MR shows concentric left ventricular myocardial thickening in a patient with biopsy-proven cardiac amyloidosis. (Courtesy A. Fuisz, MD.)* **(Right)** *Short-axis DE MR shows delayed enhancement that is most prominent in the subendocardial region, a characteristic feature of amyloidosis involving the heart. (Courtesy A. Fuisz, MD.)*

Fibril Formation

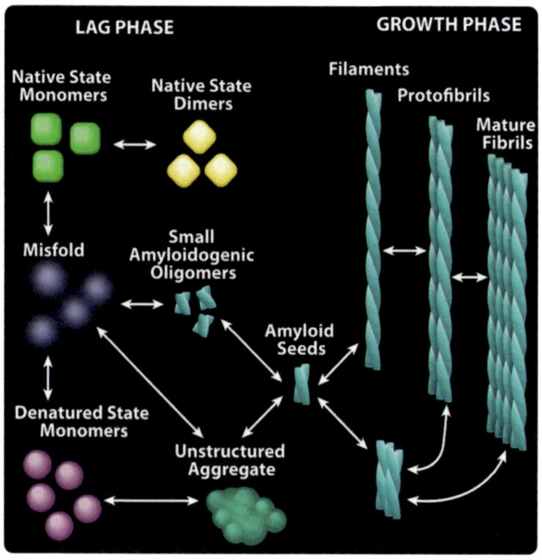

Amyloid Appearance

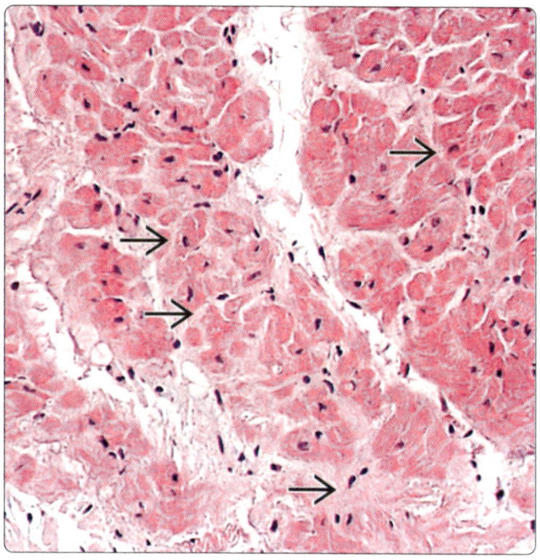

(Left) *Stages of amyloid fibrillogenesis involve refolding and highly ordered self-assembly into protofilaments of the various misfolded precursors or unstable proteins. The larger, mature fibrils resemble steel cables with 3-6 filaments wrapped around one another.* **(Right)** *Myocardium shows characteristic light pink perimyocytic amorphous material, suggestive of amyloid. The myocytes show slight hypertrophy.*

Myocardium Involved by Amyloid

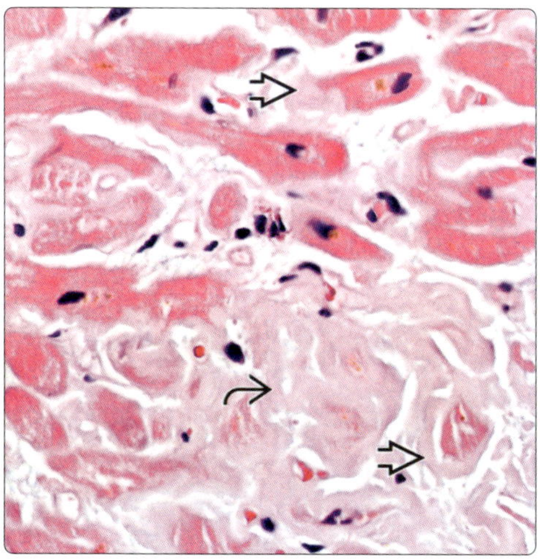

Trichrome Stain

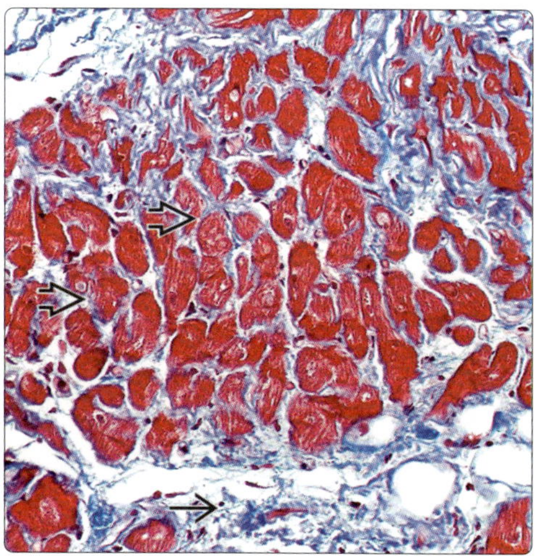

(Left) *H&E-stained section of myocardium shows characteristic light pink perimyocytic and interstitial amorphous material, suggestive of amyloid. The myocytes are separated by this material and show irregular shapes.* **(Right)** *Section of myocardium shows pale blue material around myocytes, somewhat lighter in color than the surrounding fibrosis. This lighter blue material corresponds to the amyloid deposits.*

Congo Red-Positive Material in Arteries and Interstitium

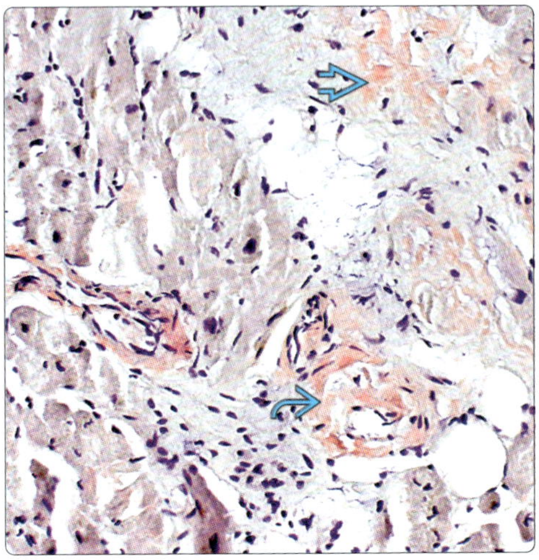

Polarized Light Apple Green Birefringence of Amyloid Material

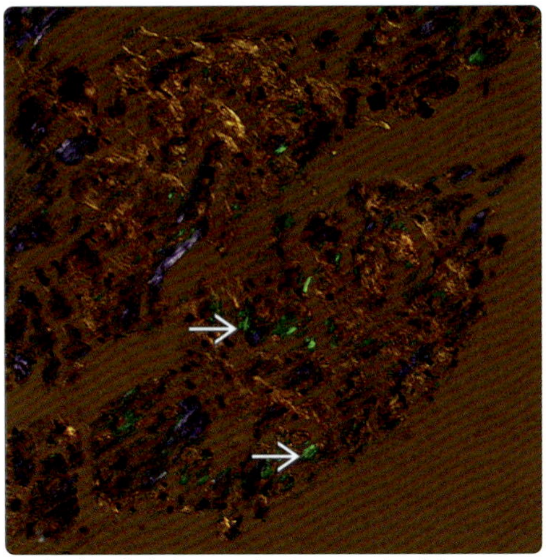

(Left) *Congo red-stained section of myocardium shows both perimyocytic and vascular deposits of pink amorphous material. The deposit in the interstitium is focal and patchy, and the irregular distribution may cause misdiagnosis if the sample is small.* **(Right)** *Positive Congo red stain shows distinct deposits in this endomyocardial biopsy photographed with polarized light in a case of light chain amyloidosis.*

Congo Red-Positive Material in Myocardial Interstitium

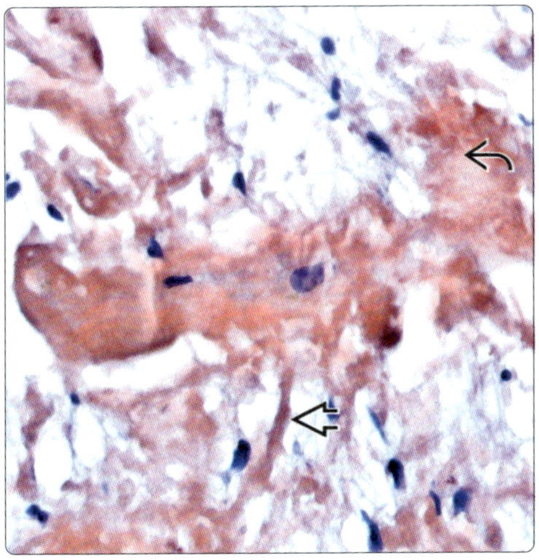

Polarized Light Apple Green Birefringence of Amyloid Material in Myocardial Interstitium

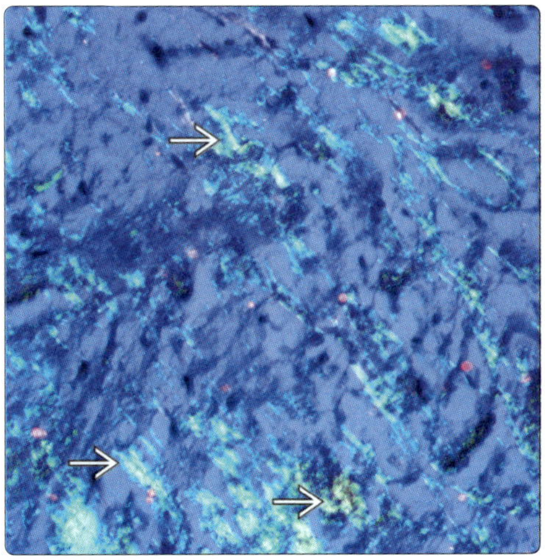

(Left) *Section of myocardium shows perimyocytic and interstitial deposits of pink amorphous material. The deposit in the interstitium is extensive and forms large aggregates. This is usually seen in advanced stages of the disease.* **(Right)** *Congo red stain shows larger deposits with apple green birefringence in this endomyocardial biopsy photographed under polarized light in a case of advanced light chain amyloidosis.*

Congo Red-Positive Material in Artery Wall

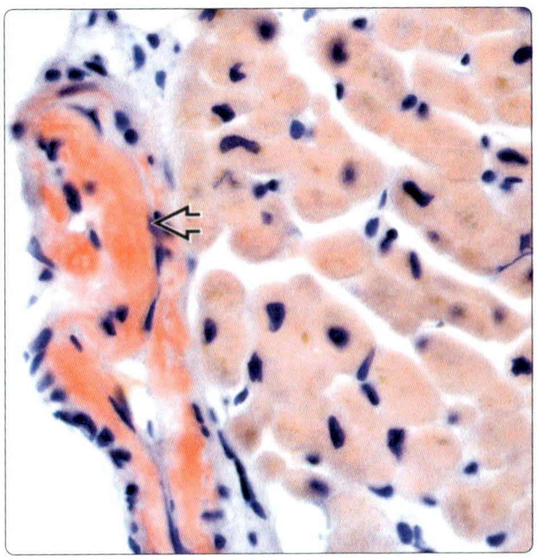

Polarized Light Apple Green Birefringence of Amyloid Material in Vessel Wall

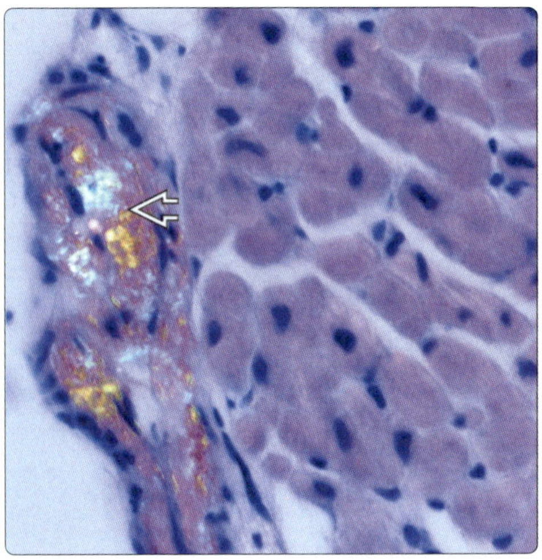

(Left) *Section of myocardial biopsy shows pink staining in the wall of a small intramyocardial artery branch. In some cases of amyloidosis, there is exclusive involvement of the arteries. The myocytes are unremarkable.* **(Right)** *Congo red stain of myocardial biopsy under polarized light shows a deposit of amyloid with characteristic apple green birefringence in the wall of an intramyocardial artery branch. In some cases, amyloid deposition exclusively involves arteries.*

Immunofluorescence Stain for λ-Light Chain

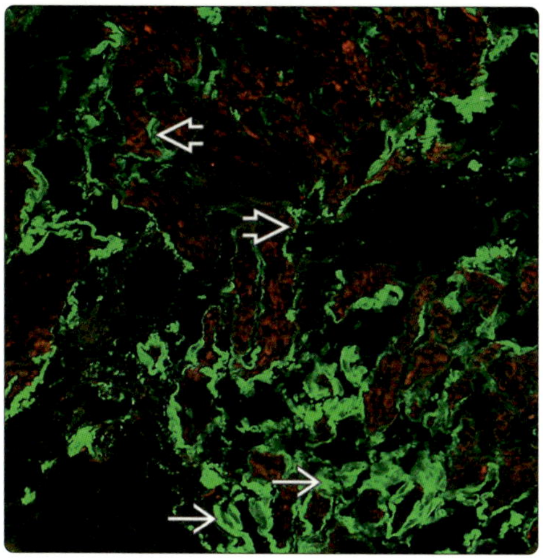

Immunofluorescence Stain for κ-Light Chain

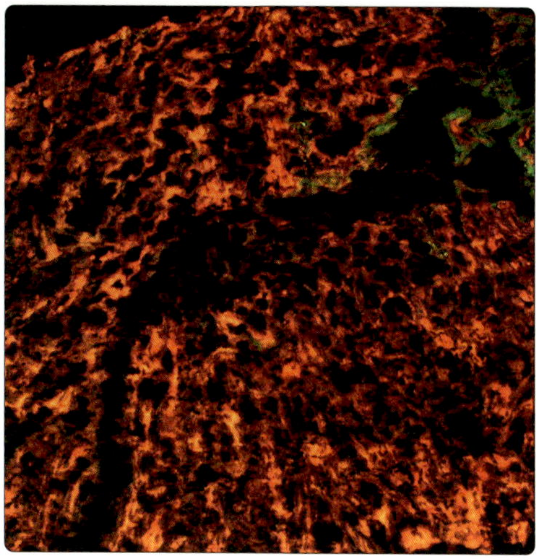

(Left) *Positive immunofluorescence shows strong λ-light chain staining surrounding myocytes ➡ and forming aggregates within the interstitium ➡. λ-light chain is the most common type of immunoglobulin amyloidosis involving the heart.* **(Right)** *Immunofluorescence stain for κ-light chain in a case of amyloidosis shows no perimyocytic or interstitial staining; however, λ-light chain was positive, indicating that there was monoclonal light chain restriction.*

Positive Immunohistochemical Stain for κ-Light Chain

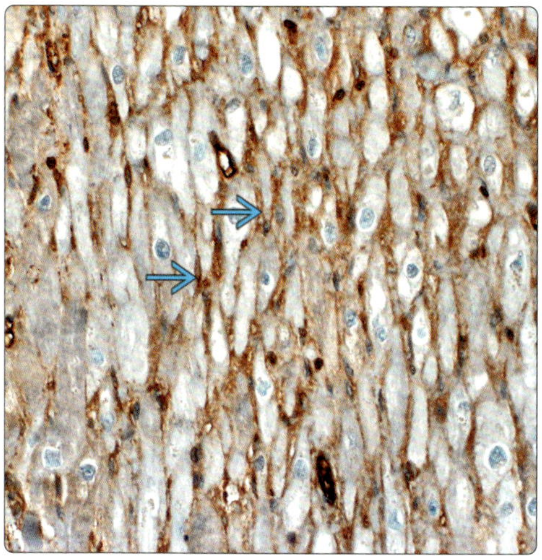

Negative Immunohistochemical Stain for λ-Light Chain

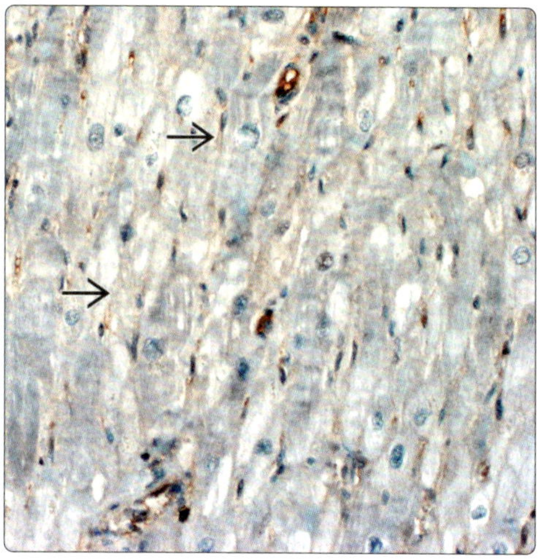

(Left) *Immunohistochemical stain of myocardial tissue shows strong positive perimyocytic staining ➡. In cases in which frozen tissue is not available, immunohistochemistry is contributory for identifying the type of amyloid.* **(Right)** *Immunohistochemical stain of myocardial tissue for λ-light chain shows neither perimyocytic nor interstitial staining with this marker ➡.*

Transmission Electron Microscopy of Myocardium Involved by Amyloid

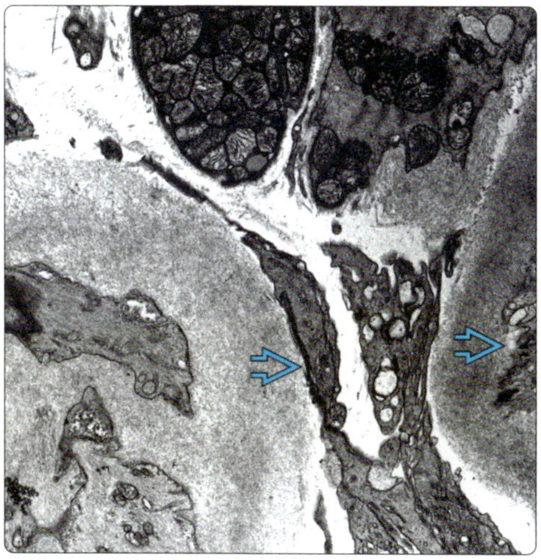

Transmission Electron Microscopy Features of Amyloid Fibers

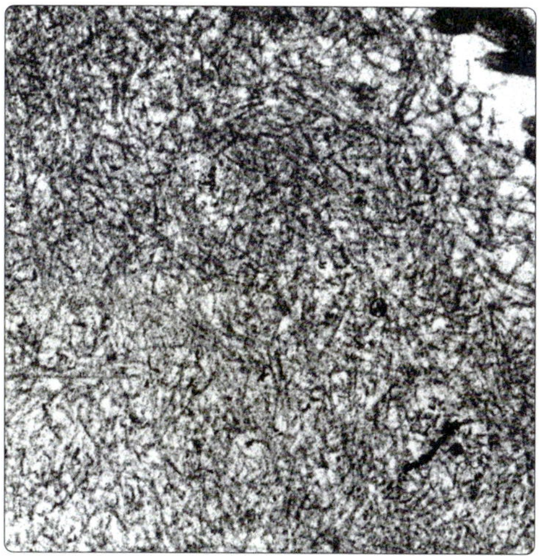

(Left) *Low-power view of myocardial section shows the cotton candy appearance of fibrillary material distributed around sarcolemma of myocytes ➡. High-magnification evaluation is required to characterize the size of the fibrils.* **(Right)** *High magnification of perimyocyte deposits shows straight, randomly oriented fibrils adjacent to sarcolemmal membrane with diameters ranging up to 10 nm, which are characteristic of amyloid.*

Hemochromatosis, Heart

KEY FACTS

TERMINOLOGY

- Systemic autosomal recessive disorder of iron metabolism with iron overload in different organs leading to hepatic cirrhosis, diabetes mellitus, arthritis, hypogonadism, &/or cardiomyopathy

CLINICAL ISSUES

- Cardiac involvement most often manifests as heart failure, mainly systolic, and often with arrhythmias
- Potentially lethal, but iron-depleting treatments forestall complications
- ~ 0.5% of White population homozygous and 10% heterozygous for C282Y, but penetrance highly variable
- Evolves slowly and progressively with symptoms often appearing ~ 5th decade if untreated
- Women become symptomatic later because of menses, delivery, and lactation

MACROSCOPIC

- Dilated heart with thickened ventricular walls
- Rust-brown myocardial discoloration may be present

MICROSCOPIC

- Hemosiderin deposits in myocytes (ventricles > atria)
- Golden brown, granular material limited to myocyte sarcoplasm
- Perinuclear concentration more frequent, especially in early phase
- Intensity of deposition usually higher at subepicardial level, followed by endomyocardial and finally mid wall levels

ANCILLARY TESTS

- Prussian blue demonstrates hemosiderin pigment as bright blue granulation

Hemosiderin Deposits

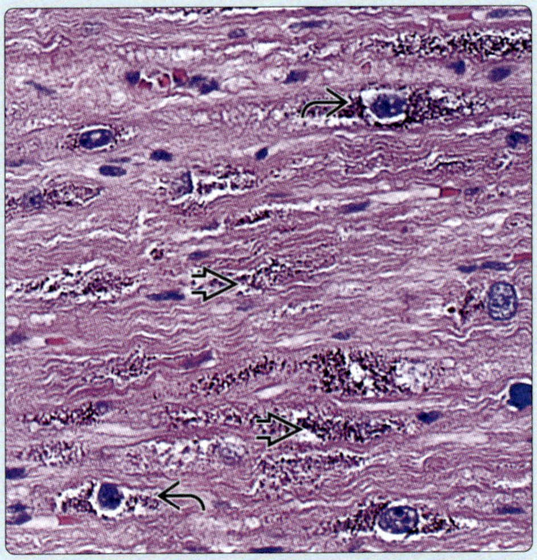

Intracytoplasmic Iron Deposits on Prussian Blue Stain

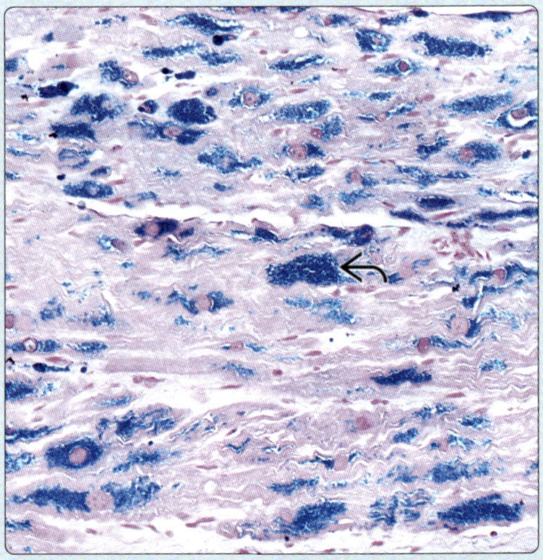

(Left) *Cardiac hemochromatosis is characterized on endomyocardial biopsy as golden brown granular intracellular pigment ⇨, often concentrated around the nucleus ↩.* **(Right)** *Prussian blue-stained section of myocardial biopsy shows iron deposits as blue granules ↩. Stainable iron pigment is not found in normal cardiac myocytes.*

Hemosiderin Deposits

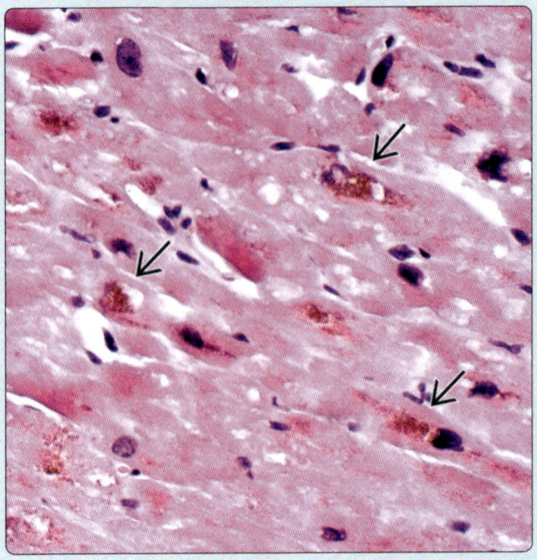

Lipofuscin Pigment on Prussian Blue Stain

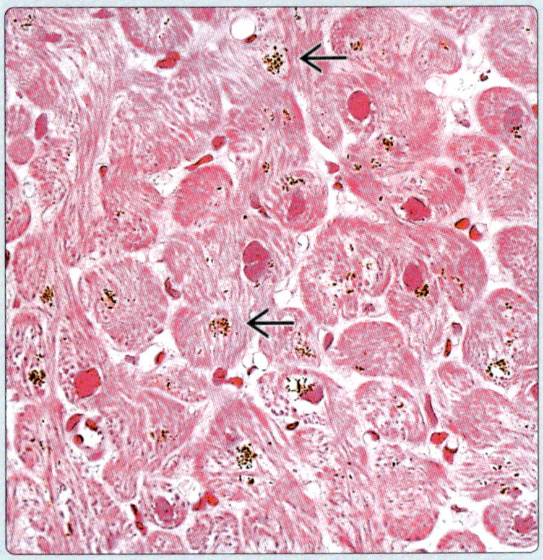

(Left) *H&E shows intracytoplasmic hemosiderin deposits ➡ in a patient with hemochromatosis (proven clinically, since other iron overload syndromes are histologically indistinguishable).* **(Right)** *Lipofuscin pigment ➡ is also golden brown and granular with perinuclear localization but does not stain blue by Prussian blue (as shown in this case).*

TERMINOLOGY

Definitions

- Systemic autosomal recessive disorder of iron metabolism with iron overload in different organs leading to hepatic cirrhosis, diabetes mellitus, arthritis, hypogonadism, &/or cardiomyopathy

ETIOLOGY/PATHOGENESIS

Iron Overload Syndrome

- Primary
  - Hereditary hemochromatosis
    - Autosomal recessive disease with highly variable penetrance
    - *HFE* gene mutation (C282Y) on chromosome 6p21.3 is most frequent (95%), though other mutations have also been described
- Secondary
  - Histologically indistinguishable from primary hemochromatosis; requires clinical correlation
  - Transfusional: Sickle cell disease, chronic hemolytic anemia, and aplastic anemia
  - Ineffective erythropoiesis: Thalassemia, sideroblastic anemia, and myelodysplastic syndrome
  - Chronic liver diseases
  - Excessive oral or parenteral iron intake (e.g., chronic hemodialysis)

Pathophysiology

- Nonbounded iron is deposited in heart, liver, pancreas, central nervous system, pituitary, &/or joints
- Cellular damage mediated through oxidation and generation of free radicals

CLINICAL ISSUES

Epidemiology

- Incidence
  - ~ 0.5% of White population homozygous and 10% heterozygous for C282Y, but penetrance highly variable
  - 3.7/1,000 adults affected; M > F

Presentation

- Evolves slowly and progressively with symptoms often appearing ~ 5th decade if untreated
- Women become symptomatic later because of menses, delivery, and lactation
- Symptoms secondary to organ dysfunction include liver failure/cirrhosis, diabetes, skin pigmentation, arthropathy, and hypogonadism
- Cardiac involvement most often manifests as heart failure, mainly systolic, and often with arrhythmias
  - Dilated phenotype most common
  - Restrictive cardiomyopathy may also occur

Laboratory Tests

- Transferrin saturation (> 45%) and ferritin concentration (> 300 µg/L for men and > 200 µg/L for women) used as screening tests
- Biopsy
  - Liver biopsy, reserved for quantitative iron studies and prognosis (staging fibrosis)
  - Endomyocardial biopsy may be useful if other noninvasive techniques are nondiagnostic or to confirm cause of cardiac failure
    - Laboratory values and liver iron cannot predict myocardial iron content
- Genetic testing

Treatment

- Dietary management, phlebotomy, chelating agents, calcium channel blockers
- Combined heart-liver transplantation may be only option for refractory severe heart failure

Prognosis

- Cardiac involvement and associated dysfunction represent important cause of death
- Early recognition and intervention with iron-depleting treatments significantly improve outcomes

IMAGING

MR Findings

- Some modalities (T2*, R2*) may be used for clinical assessment of liver/cardiac iron content

MACROSCOPIC

General Features

- Dilated heart with thickened ventricular walls
- Rust-brown myocardial discoloration may be present

MICROSCOPIC

Histologic Features

- Normal heart has no visible iron deposition
- Hemosiderin deposits in myocytes (ventricles > atria)
  - Golden brown, granular sarcoplasmic material
  - Perinuclear pattern frequent, especially in early phase
- Deposition in conduction system possible but infrequent (sinus node)
- Intensity of deposition usually higher at subepicardial level, followed by endomyocardial and finally mid wall levels

ANCILLARY TESTS

Histochemistry

- Prussian blue demonstrates hemosiderin pigment as bright blue granulation

DIFFERENTIAL DIAGNOSIS

Aging Changes

- Lipofuscin is brown to yellow granular pigment considered as cellular residue without effect on myocyte that accumulates near cell nucleus (iron stain negative)

SELECTED REFERENCES

1. Girelli D et al: Hemochromatosis classification: update and recommendations by the BIOIRON Society. Blood. 139(20):3018-29, 2022
2. Anderson GJ et al: Revisiting hemochromatosis: genetic vs. phenotypic manifestations. Ann Transl Med. 9(8):731, 2021
3. Danilowicz-Szymanowicz L et al: Pathogenesis, diagnosis, and clinical implications of hereditary hemochromatosis-The cardiological point of view. Diagnostics (Basel). 11(7), 2021

Anthracycline Cardiotoxicity

KEY FACTS

TERMINOLOGY

- Cardiac dysfunction due to anthracycline toxicity

CLINICAL ISSUES

- Acute/subacute: Within 2 weeks, EKG changes, arrhythmias, ventricular dysfunction; reversible, often resolving within 1 week
- Early chronic: Within 1 year, asymptomatic or CHF; progressive, irreversible, may be fatal
- Late chronic: > 1 year, otherwise as early chronic
- Risk factors
  - Strongest predictor is cumulative dose
  - Extremes of age
  - Radiation therapy to mediastinum
  - Concurrent cardiotoxic chemotherapy
  - Preexisting cardiac disease, kidney failure
  - Genetic susceptibility
- Prognosis
  - Generally poor, related to severity at initial diagnosis

MACROSCOPIC

- Enlarged, flabby heart with ventricular dilatation
- Endocardial sclerosis, mural thrombi may be present

MICROSCOPIC

- Focal/diffuse myofibrillar loss, vacuolization
- Interstitial fibrosis, minimal inflammation
- Evaluation of toluidine blue-stained thick sections by light microscopy (≥ 10 blocks, even if this limits paraffin sample) is essential for grading toxicity

ANCILLARY TESTS

- EM detects both early and advanced stages
- Severity grading is based on findings on Toluidine blue-stained thick sections
- EM findings
  - Sarcotubular dilatation
  - Vacuolization
  - Myofibrillar loss

Anthracycline Cardiotoxicity

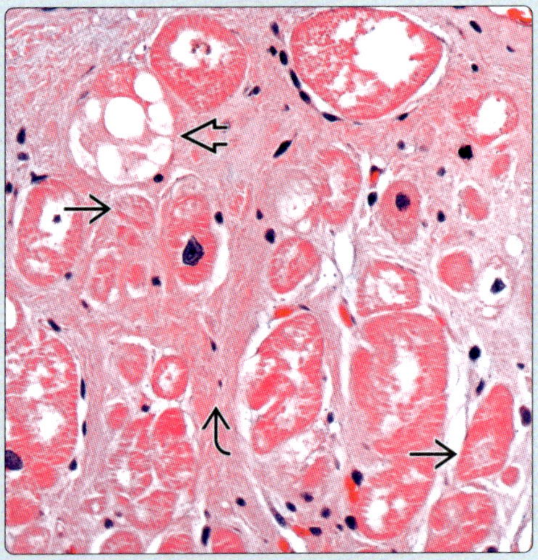

Toluidine Blue: Myocardium With Anthracycline Cardiotoxicity

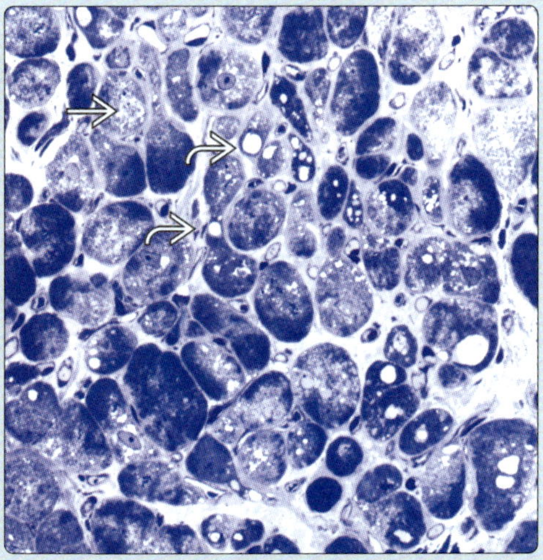

(Left) *At high magnification, vacuolization may occasionally be striking. Also present is myofibrillar loss and cardiomyocyte dropout. Note the bands of interstitial fibrosis between the cardiomyocytes without significant inflammation.* **(Right)** *Plastic-embedded thick section shows loss of myofilaments and membrane-bound sarcoplasmic vacuoles. Severity grading is based on the prevalence of these changes.*

EM Findings in Anthracycline Cardiotoxicity

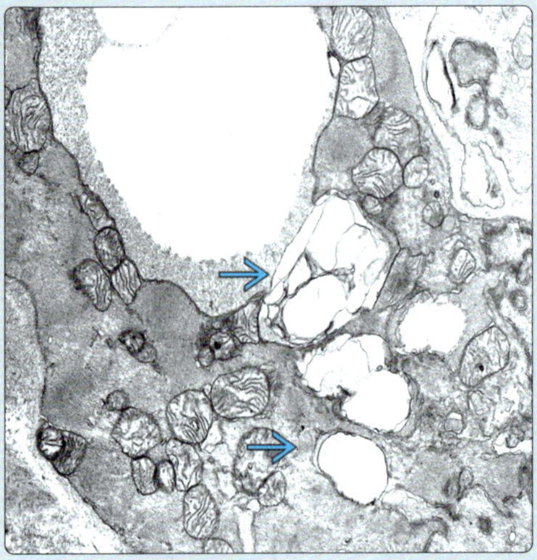

EM Findings in Anthracycline Cardiotoxicity

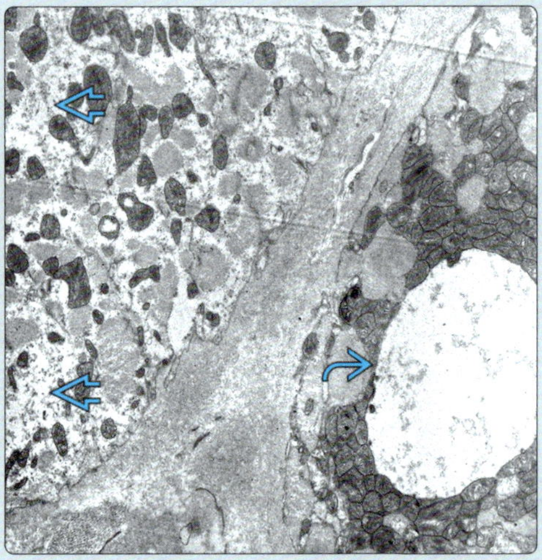

(Left) *Membrane-bound sarcoplasmic vacuoles are the hallmark of anthracycline cardiotoxicity. The number and size of vacuoles increases with the severity of the process, and grading severity is based on the prevalence of these changes.* **(Right)** *Ultrastructural examination of myocardium in a patient with late-onset anthracycline toxicity shows sarcoplasmic membrane-bound vacuoles and myofibrillar loss.*

TERMINOLOGY

Definitions

- Cardiac dysfunction induced by anthracyclines (e.g., doxorubicin, daunorubicin)

ETIOLOGY/PATHOGENESIS

Mechanisms of Cardiotoxicity

- Mitochondrial DNA damage mediated through topoisomerase-2 beta with generation of free radicals, lipid peroxidation, and membrane/protein damage
- Induction of apoptosis, interference with myofilament synthesis, autophagy deregulation, and impairment of hypertrophic response

CLINICAL ISSUES

Presentation

- Acute/subacute
    - From initiation to 2 weeks after last dose
    - Cardiac abnormalities include
        - EKG changes, arrhythmias, conduction defects
        - Transient ventricular dysfunction
    - Reversible, often resolving within 1 week
- Early chronic
    - Up to 1 year after last dose, usually ~ 3 months
    - Usually manifests as dilated cardiomyopathy
    - Asymptomatic or progresses to heart failure
- Late chronic
    - > 1 year after last dose; may be many years
    - Dilated cardiomyopathy (typically irreversible)
    - Ranges from asymptomatic to severe heart failure

Prognosis

- Generally poor, related to severity at initial diagnosis
- 1-5% mortality after developing heart failure

Risk Factors

- Cumulative dose is strongest predictor
    - Incidence < 1% at < 400 mg/m², 26% at 550 mg/m²
- Extremes of age
- Female sex
- Radiation therapy to mediastinum
- Concurrent cardiotoxic chemotherapy
- Preexisting cardiac disease, kidney failure
- Genetic susceptibility

Prevention

- Cumulative dose limited to < 450 mg/m²
- Adjunctive therapy with cardioprotective agents
- Administration by prolonged infusion instead of bolus

IMAGING

General Features

- Surveillance criteria by echocardiography, radionuclide ventriculography, or cardiac MR
    - In adults, 10% decline in left ventricular ejection fraction (LVEF) below normal, absolute LVEF ≤ 45%, 20% total decline in LVEF
    - In children, 10% decline in LVEF, absolute LVEF < 55%, drop in fractional shortening (FS) ≥ 10%, absolute FS < 29%

MACROSCOPIC

General Features

- Enlarged, flabby heart with ventricular dilatation
- Endocardial sclerosis, mural thrombi may be present

MICROSCOPIC

Histologic Features

- Focal or diffuse cardiomyocyte degeneration
    - Myofibrillar loss (best seen in plastic-embedded toluidine blue-stained thick sections)
    - Cytoplasmic vacuolization
- Interstitial fibrosis
- Minimal or no inflammation

ANCILLARY TESTS

Electron Microscopy

- Focal or diffuse cardiomyocyte degeneration
    - Sarcotubular dilatation
        - In later stages, large membrane-bound clear spaces, diffuse vacuolization
    - Myofibrillar loss
        - Partial or total, with only Z bands remaining
        - Must be distinguished from contraction bands; in true myofibrillar loss, Z band remnants present

DIFFERENTIAL DIAGNOSIS

Nonspecific Myofibrillar Loss or Vacuolization

- Seen in variety of processes with cardiac injury
- Clinicopathologic correlation is essential

GRADING

Light Microscopy of Toluidine Blue-Stained Thick Sections

- At least 10 plastic-embedded blocks should be prepared from biopsy tissue (even if this compromises sample available for paraffin embedding)
- In grid sections from 5-6 blocks
    - Grade 0.5: < 4 cardiomyocytes with vacuoles, no myofibrillar loss or necrosis
    - Grade 1.0: 4-10 with vacuoles, < 3 with myofibrillar loss, no necrosis
    - Grade 1.5: ≥ 10 with vacuoles, 3-5 with myofibrillar loss, < 2 with necrosis
    - Grade 2.0: ≥ 10 with vacuoles, 6-8 with myofibrillar loss, 2-5 with necrosis

SELECTED REFERENCES

1. Adhikari A et al: Anticancer drug-induced cardiotoxicity: insights and pharmacogenetics. Pharmaceuticals (Basel). 14(10), 2021
2. Bernaba BN et al: Pathology of late-onset anthracycline cardiomyopathy. Cardiovasc Pathol. 19(5):308-11, 2010
3. Mackay B et al: Assessment of anthracycline cardiomyopathy by endomyocardial biopsy. Ultrastruct Pathol. 18(1-2):203-11, 1994

Catecholamine Cardiomyopathy

KEY FACTS

TERMINOLOGY

- Cardiomyopathy due to excessive catecholamine release, commonly associated with pheochromocytoma

ETIOLOGY/PATHOGENESIS

- Progressive reduction of coronary flow due to vasospasm
- Increased oxygen demand, intracellular calcium, apoptosis
- Direct myocyte injury

CLINICAL ISSUES

- Incidence is unknown but reported in ~ 10% of pheochromocytoma series
- Cardiac clinical manifestations include chest pain, tachyarrhythmias, palpitations, myocarditis, dilated/hypertrophic cardiomyopathy, cardiogenic shock, and acute myocardial infarction
- Recovery of cardiomyopathy occurs with adequate clinical support and surgical removal of pheochromocytoma or catecholamine-producing neoplasm
- Sudden death can occur if untreated

MICROSCOPIC

- Acute changes
  - Focal contraction band necrosis
  - Mild mononuclear &/or neutrophilic interstitial infiltration
  - Platelet aggregates in microcirculation
- Chronic changes
  - Increased interstitial fibrosis
  - Medial thickening of small and medium-sized coronary arteries

ANCILLARY TESTS

- Electron microscopy examination shows
  - Hypercontracted sarcomeres
  - Swollen mitochondria and endoplasmic reticulum

Early Changes in Catecholamine Cardiomyopathy

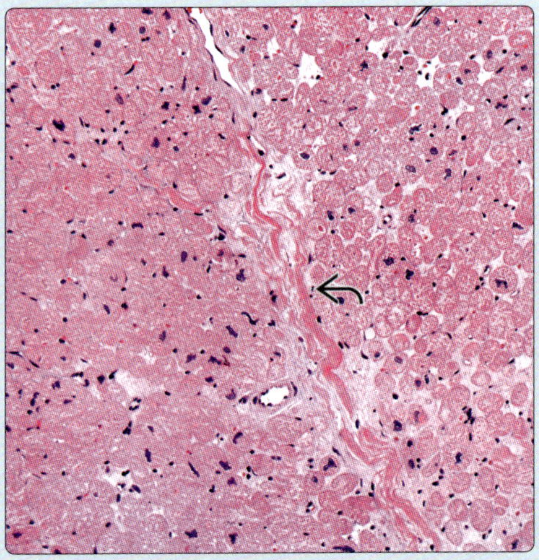

Histologic Features of Catecholamine Cardiomyopathy

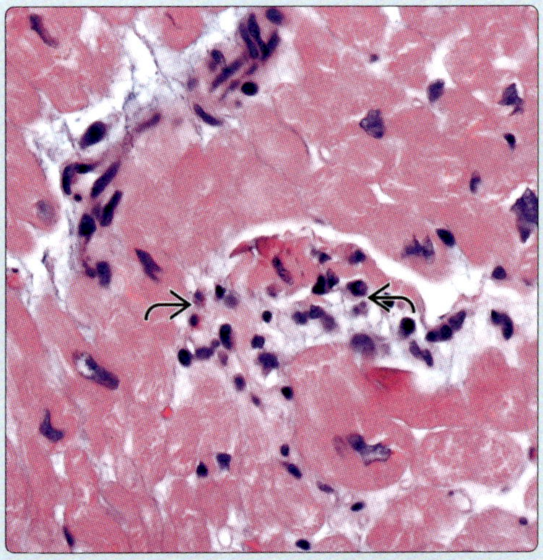

(Left) *H&E-stained section of myocardium shows ischemic-like injury of myocytes with a wavy, pink appearance.* **(Right)** *H&E-stained section shows myocardium with a focus of myocytes with necrosis surrounded by scant inflammatory infiltrate containing neutrophils.*

Subendocardial Changes in Catecholamine Cardiomyopathy

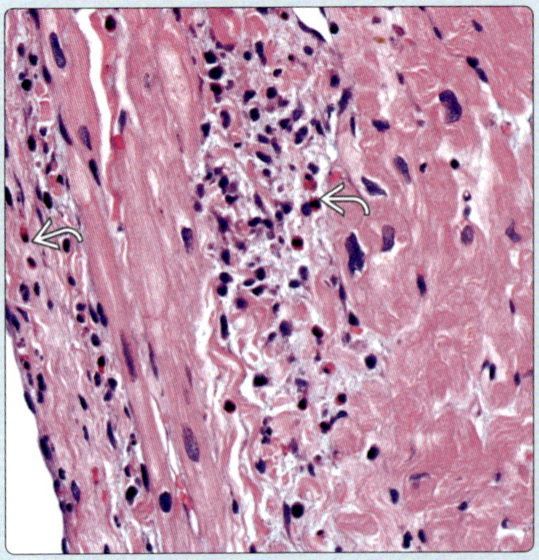

Subendocardial Changes in Catecholamine Cardiomyopathy

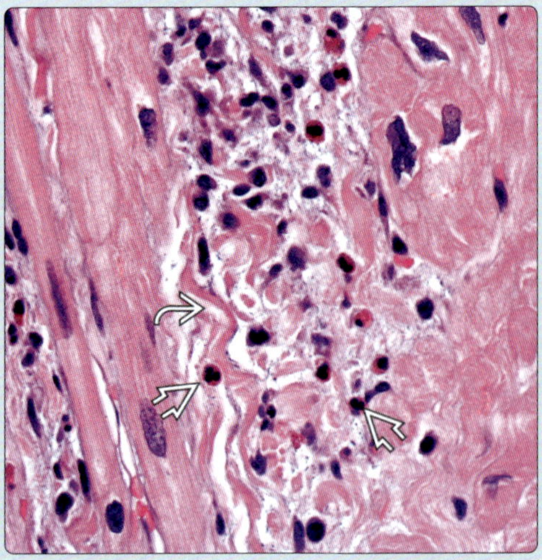

(Left) *H&E-stained section shows subendocardial and deeper myocytes with ischemic injury associated with mixed inflammatory infiltrate with frequent neutrophils.* **(Right)** *H&E-stained section shows a higher magnification of myocardium with wavy, eosinophilic myocytes and surrounding neutrophils.*

TERMINOLOGY

Definitions

- Cardiomyopathy due to excessive catecholamine release, commonly associated with pheochromocytoma

ETIOLOGY/PATHOGENESIS

Catecholamine Cardiotoxicity

- Direct myocyte injury: Calcium overload, free radical production, increased sarcolemmal permeability, mitochondrial dysfunction, apoptosis
- Secondary myocardial damage due to progressive reduction of coronary flow due to vasospasm and increased oxygen demand

CLINICAL ISSUES

Epidemiology

- Incidence
  - Unknown but reported in ~ 10% of pheochromocytoma series

Presentation

- General
  - Headaches
  - Diaphoresis
  - Shortness of breath
  - Anxiety
  - Pulmonary edema
  - Hypertension (paroxysmal or sustained)
- Cardiac
  - Chest pain
  - Palpitations
  - Tachyarrhythmias: Sinus tachycardia, supraventricular/ventricular tachycardia
  - Myocarditis
  - Dilated/hypertrophic cardiomyopathy
  - Cardiogenic shock
  - Acute myocardial infarction

Laboratory Tests

- Plasma metanephrines (free)
- Quantitative 24-hour urinary metanephrines
- Plasma fractionated catecholamine levels to confirm results from metanephrine studies

Treatment

- Surgical approaches
  - Removal of pheochromocytoma or catecholamine-producing neoplasm
- Drugs
  - Stabilization and optimization of patient with α-/β-adrenergic blockade

Prognosis

- Recovery from cardiomyopathy occurs with adequate clinical support and surgical removal of pheochromocytoma or catecholamine-producing neoplasm
- Sudden death can occur if untreated

IMAGING

Ultrasonographic Findings

- Normal or decreased systolic function

MR Findings

- Diffuse patchy myocardial enhancement on T1
- Increased left ventricle wall thickness
- Myocardial edema

Electrocardiogram

- Marked prolongation of QT interval
- Deep and wide symmetrically inverted T waves
- Ventricular arrhythmias

MICROSCOPIC

Histologic Features

- Acute changes
  - Multifocal contraction band necrosis
  - Mild mononuclear &/or neutrophilic interstitial infiltration
  - Platelet aggregates in microcirculation
- Chronic changes
  - Fibrosis in interstitium and conduction system
  - Medial thickening of small and medium-sized coronary arteries

ANCILLARY TESTS

Electron Microscopy

- Hypercontracted sarcomeres
- Swollen mitochondria and endoplasmic reticulum

DIFFERENTIAL DIAGNOSIS

Transient Apical Ballooning Syndrome (Takotsubo Cardiomyopathy)

- No history of pheochromocytoma
- Hyperkinesis of basal segments
- Apical hypokinesis
- Complete recovery after several days

Cocaine Cardiomyopathy

- History of cocaine abuse
- Association with
  - Ischemic/hemorrhagic strokes
  - Aortic dissection
  - Infective endocarditis

SELECTED REFERENCES

1. Du Y et al: Catecholamine-induced cardiotoxicity: a critical element in the pathophysiology of stroke-induced heart injury. Life Sci. 287:120106, 2021
2. Kundu N et al: Paraganglioma presenting as acute catecholamine cardiomyopathy. ANZ J Surg. 91(10):2209-11, 2021
3. Santos JRU et al: Catecholamine-induced cardiomyopathy in pheochromocytoma: how to manage a rare complication in a rare disease? Horm Metab Res. 51(7):458-69, 2019
4. Chow LTC et al: Coronary artery myointimal dysplasia in patients with pheochromocytoma-possible causal relationship: pathophysiology and clinical implication with reference to Takotsubo cardiomyopathy and spontaneous coronary dissection. Cardiovasc Pathol. 37:45-53, 2018
5. Miura M et al: The histological features of a myocardial biopsy specimen in a patient in the acute phase of reversible catecholamine-induced cardiomyopathy due to pheochromocytoma. Intern Med. 56(6):665-71, 2017

KEY FACTS

TERMINOLOGY

- Deleterious effects on heart from either acute or chronic intake of cocaine that include myocardial infarction (MI), ischemia, arrhythmia, dilated cardiomyopathy, myocarditis, and others

CLINICAL ISSUES

- Acute MI
  - True incidence of cocaine-induced infarction is unknown
  - Most reports involve acute intoxication in chronic user
- Sudden death and cardiac arrhythmias
  - May or may not be associated with myocardial ischemia or infarction
- Heart failure
- Drug-induced Brugada syndrome

MICROSCOPIC

- Acute cocaine toxicity
  - Contraction band necrosis
  - Hypercontracted myocytes or myofilaments
- Chronic cocaine use
  - May show myocarditis with monocyte-predominant infiltrate in cases temporally related to cocaine use
  - Variable interstitial fibrosis
  - Myocardial contraction bands are commonly seen and appear to correlate with level of cocaine in urine and blood
  - Intima smooth muscle hyperplasia of coronary arteries
- Arrhythmias
  - Foci of necrotic myocytes surrounded by normal-appearing myocytes or "microfocal myocardial damage"
  - Hypercontracted myofilaments

TOP DIFFERENTIAL DIAGNOSES

- Other causes of myocarditis
- Noncocaine-related heart failure

Histologic Features of Cocaine Cardiotoxicity

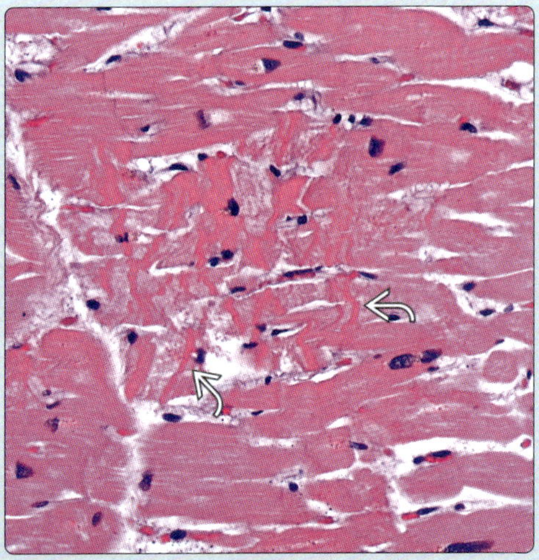

Chronic Cocaine Cardiotoxicity

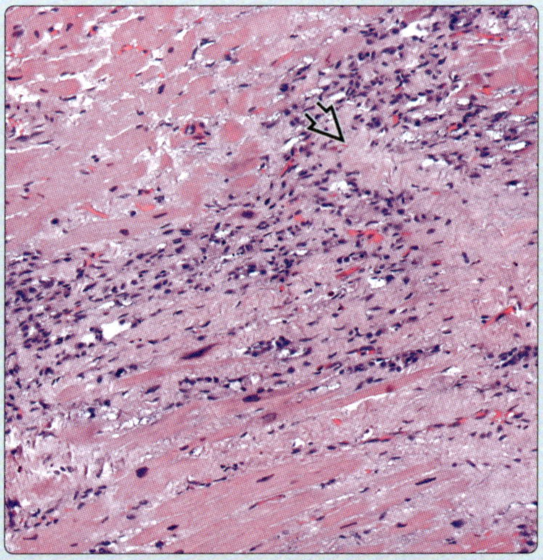

(Left) *Contraction band necrosis, although not specific for cocaine cardiotoxicity, is often seen in both acute and chronic cases. This case was not subtle and demonstrated numerous similar foci in other areas. (Courtesy E. Christensen, MD.)* **(Right)** *H&E section of chronic cocaine cardiotoxicity shows interstitial focal replacement fibrosis and surrounding chronic inflammation. These changes resemble those of sustained catecholamine exposure, as seen in pheochromocytoma. (Courtesy E. Christensen, MD.)*

Chronic Cocaine Cardiotoxicity

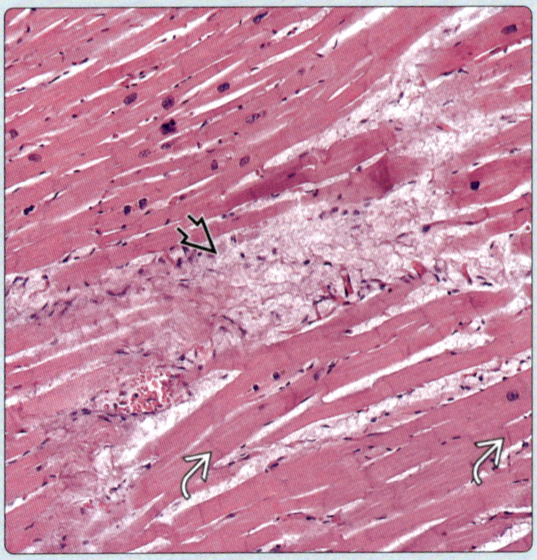

Coronary Artery Changes in Chronic Cocaine Toxicity

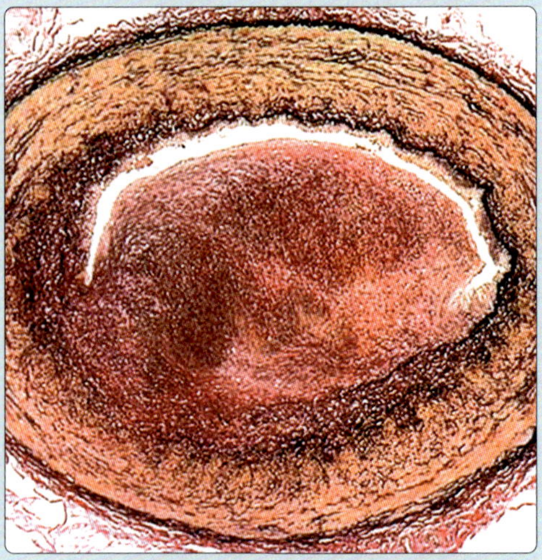

(Left) *H&E section of the myocardium in a case of chronic cocaine cardiotoxicity shows focal interstitial fibrosis, adjacent myocyte hypertrophy, and focal contraction band necrosis. (Courtesy E. Christensen, MD.)* **(Right)** *EVG stain of a coronary artery shows cocaine-related intimal smooth muscle proliferation resembling what is seen in chronic vasculopathy. This has been reported in only a few cases. (Courtesy W. D. Edwards, MD.)*

TERMINOLOGY

Abbreviations

- Cocaine cardiotoxicity (CC)

Definitions

- Deleterious cardiac effects from acute or chronic cocaine use, including myocardial infarction (MI), ischemia, arrhythmia, dilated cardiomyopathy, myocarditis, others

ETIOLOGY/PATHOGENESIS

Environmental Exposure

- Acute cocaine administration
  - Increased heart rate &/or blood pressure, coronary vasoconstriction, reduced cardiac myocyte contractility
- Chronic cocaine administration
  - Thought to increase risk for coronary vasospasm (may persist for several days after drug use)

CLINICAL ISSUES

Epidemiology

- Incidence
  - True incidence of cocaine-induced infarction is unknown
- Age
  - For cocaine-induced infarction, patients tend to be young (~ 30s)

Presentation

- Acute MI is best-documented cardiovascular complication
  - Only few reports are from 1st-time users
  - Most reports involve acute intoxication in chronic user
- Sudden death and cardiac arrhythmias due to acute or chronic cocaine use
  - ± myocardial ischemia or infarction
- Heart failure
  - Changes of heart in autopsies of cocaine users can show similar findings as heart failure patients
    - Myocyte damage, left ventricular hypertrophy, and dilated cardiomyopathy
- Ischemic chest pain without MI also reported
- Drug-induced Brugada syndrome due to acute cocaine overdose has been reported

Treatment

- Options, risks, complications
  - No one therapy universally agreed upon
  - In patients with cardiomyopathy, coronary artery disease, and structural heart changes, standard therapy is typically appropriate (with exception of β-blockers)
- Drugs
  - Mixed adrenergic blockers (carvedilol) for chronic use

Prognosis

- Long-term effects may be partly reversible in some cases

MACROSCOPIC

General Features

- In cocaine-induced infarction
  - 1/3 of cases show normal coronary arteries
  - 1/3 of cases show thrombus with underlying atherosclerotic narrowing of coronary arteries
  - Coronary narrowing of left and right coronary arteries is commonly seen
    - In one study, narrowing affected left anterior descending artery in 9 of 9 patients
- In cocaine-associated heart failure
  - Dilated cardiomyopathy and left ventricular hypertrophy
- May also see myocarditis, aortic dissection, or spontaneous coronary artery dissection

MICROSCOPIC

Histologic Features

- Acute cocaine toxicity
  - Contraction band necrosis
  - Hypercontracted myocytes
  - Rhexis of myofibrils
- Chronic cocaine use
  - May show myocarditis with monocyte-predominant infiltrate in cases temporally related to cocaine use
  - Myocardial contraction bands are commonly seen and appear to correlate with level of cocaine in urine and blood
    - May have focal-associated neutrophilic infiltrate
  - Usually small scattered foci of myocyte necrosis
  - Variable interstitial fibrosis
  - Rare case reports of cocaine-associated intimal smooth muscle hyperplasia in coronary arteries
- Arrhythmias
  - Foci of necrotic myocytes surrounded by normal-appearing myocytes or "microfocal myocardial damage"
    - Eventually, damaged cells are replaced by fibrosis
  - Hypercontracted myofilaments

DIFFERENTIAL DIAGNOSIS

Other Causes of Myocarditis

- Clinical history of chronic cocaine use in absence of other commonly implicated causes of myocarditis is necessary
  - Viral infections, nonviral infectious organisms (Lyme or Chagas diseases, etc.), or other drugs

Noncocaine-Related Heart Failure

- Also shows contraction band necrosis, myocyte necrosis, myocardial disarray, and interstitial fibrosis
- Clinical history of chronic cocaine abuse necessary to differentiate

SELECTED REFERENCES

1. Rallidis LS et al: Causes, angiographic characteristics, and management of premature myocardial infarction: JACC state-of-the-art review. J Am Coll Cardiol. 79(24):2431-49, 2022
2. Arenas DJ et al: Cocaine, cardiomyopathy, and heart failure: a systematic review and meta-analysis. Sci Rep. 10(1):19795, 2020
3. Carrier M et al: Association of recreational drug consumption, cardiac toxicity and heart transplantation Can J Surg. 62(5):356-7, 2019
4. Kim ST et al: Acute and chronic effects of cocaine on cardiovascular health. Int J Mol Sci. 20(3): 584, 2019
5. Bachi K et al: Vascular disease in cocaine addiction. Atherosclerosis. 262:154-62, 2017
6. Havakuk O et al: The cardiovascular effects of cocaine. J Am Coll Cardiol. 70(1):101-13, 2017

Immune Checkpoint Inhibitor Toxicity

KEY FACTS

TERMINOLOGY

- Cancer immunotherapy leading to immune-related adverse events (irAEs) involving several organs, including heart

ETIOLOGY/PATHOGENESIS

- Increased T-cell activity against antigens present in myocytes
- Increased levels of autoantibodies and cytokines
- Increased complement-mediated inflammation

CLINICAL ISSUES

- Incidence of immune checkpoint inhibitor (ICI)-associated myocarditis estimated range: 0.27-1.1%
- Most cases of cardiac toxicity occur ~ 30 days after treatment initiation but can occur any time post treatment
- Mortality associated with ICI myocarditis: 27-46%
- Presentation
  - Asymptomatic
  - Fulminant myocarditis
  - Conduction abnormalities (atrioventricular block)
  - Arrhythmia (atrial fibrillation, ventricular tachycardia)
  - Vasculitis: Giant cell arteritis, isolated aortitis, CNS vasculitis, cryoglobulinemic vasculitis
  - Pericarditis (0.3%)

MICROSCOPIC

- Myocardium: Interstitial inflammatory infiltrate composed of lymphocytes associated with myocyte necrosis/injury
- Pericardium: Inflammatory infiltrate composed of CD4(+) and CD8(+) lymphocytes and macrophages; pericardial thickening with fibrinous hemorrhagic exudate
- Arteries: Perivascular lymphocytic inflammation and wall necrosis; giant cells may be present in giant cell arteritis

ANCILLARY TESTS

- CD4 and CD8 (majority) (+) stain seen in infiltrating lymphocytes
- CD68 for macrophage identification

Histologic Changes in ICI Myocarditis

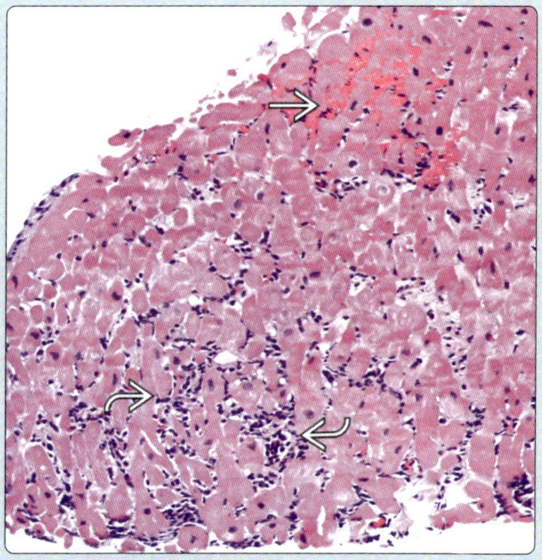

Histologic Changes in ICI Myocarditis

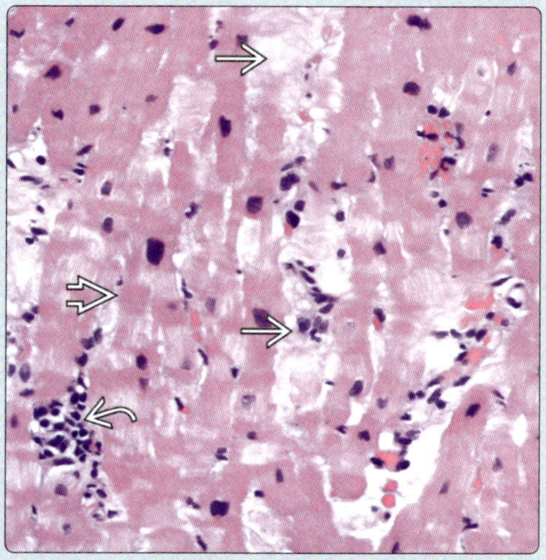

(Left) *H&E of a patient with malignant melanoma receiving treatment with PD-1 inhibitor shows interstitial mononuclear inflammatory infiltrates surrounding myocytes* →*. Focal interstitial hemorrhage is also present* →. **(Right)** *H&E of the myocardium from a patient with malignant melanoma treated with PD-1 inhibitor shows interstitial mononuclear inflammatory infiltrates surrounding myocytes* →*, focal interstitial edema* →*, and a few myocytes exhibiting contraction bands* →.

Histologic Changes in ICI Myocarditis

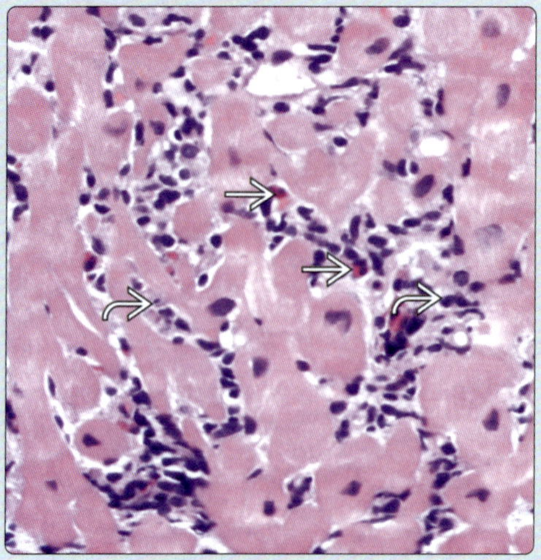

Histologic Changes in ICI Myocarditis

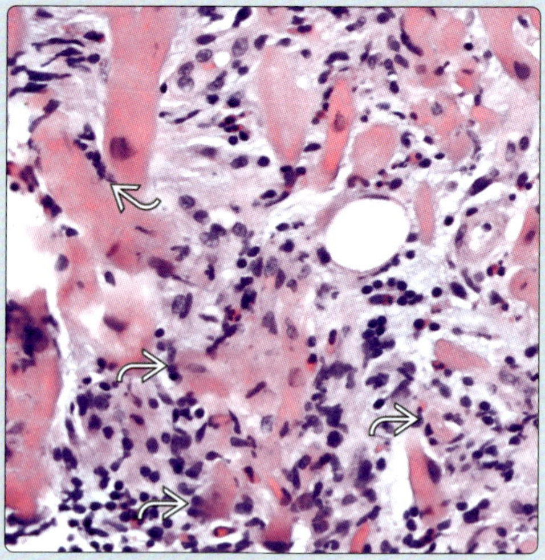

(Left) *H&E of the myocardium from a patient with malignant melanoma treated with PD-1 inhibitor shows interstitial mononuclear inflammatory infiltrates encroaching the myocytes* → *and causing injury. Isolated eosinophils are also seen* →. **(Right)** *On higher magnification, H&E of the myocardium from a patient with malignant melanoma treated with PD-1 inhibitor shows interstitial mononuclear inflammatory infiltrates encroaching the myocytes* → *and causing injury.*

TERMINOLOGY

Abbreviations

- Immune checkpoint inhibitor (ICI)

Definitions

- Cancer immunotherapy leading to immune-related adverse events (irAEs) involving several organs, including heart
  - ICIs are monoclonal antibodies directed to
    - Cytotoxic T-lymphocyte antigen 4 (CTLA-4, ipilimumab)
    - Programmed cell death 1 (PD-1, nivolumab, pembrolizumab, cemiplimab)
    - Programmed cell death ligand 1 (PD-L1, atezolizumab, avelumab, durvalumab)

ETIOLOGY/PATHOGENESIS

Immune-Mediated Side Effect

- Increased T-cell activity against antigens present in myocytes
- Increased levels of autoantibodies and cytokines
- Increased complement-mediated inflammation

Risk Factors for Developing Immune Checkpoint Inhibitor Immune-Related Adverse Event

- Female sex
- Higher BMI
- Sleep apnea
- History of radiation to chest
- Use of combination therapy
- Underlying autoimmune disease

CLINICAL ISSUES

Epidemiology

- Cardiac toxicity is extremely rare irAE, but true incidence is unknown
  - Incidence of ICI-associated myocarditis estimated range: 0.27-1.1%
  - Myocarditis is reported in 0.54% for monotherapy and 1.22% for combination therapy
  - Most cases of cardiac toxicity occur within 3 months of starting therapy but can occur any time post treatment

Presentation

- Asymptomatic
- Fulminant myocarditis
  - Association with myositis (23-25%) and myasthenia gravis (10%)
- Conduction abnormalities (atrioventricular block)
- Arrhythmia (atrial fibrillation, ventricular tachycardia)
- Noninflammatory left ventricle dysfunction
  - Takotsubo-like syndrome
  - Left ventricle dysfunction/heart failure (0.53-2.5%)
    - Usually presenting as late adverse event
- Pericarditis (0.3%)
  - Pericardial effusion
  - Cardiac tamponade
  - Perimyocarditis
- Acute coronary syndrome
  - Accelerated atherosclerosis
  - Coronary vasculitis
- Vasculitis
  - Giant cell arteritis
  - Isolated aortitis
  - CNS vasculitis
  - Cryoglobulinemic vasculitis

Laboratory Tests

- Elevated troponin I, T
  - Higher levels (≥ 1.5 ng/dL) of troponin T associated with worse prognosis
- Brain natriuretic peptide (BNP) can be elevated

Treatment

- Hold ICIs permanently
- Immunosuppression with high-dose steroids
- Supportive treatment of cardiac complications
- In cases of steroid-refractory myocarditis, Thymoglobulin, mycophenolate mofetil, and tacrolimus can be used
- Rechallenging with ICI may be considered in cases of mild cardiotoxicity after normalization of abnormal tests

Prognosis

- Mortality associated with ICI myocarditis: 27-46%
- Clinical risk factors linked to worse prognosis
  - High serum troponin levels
  - Reduced left ventricle ejection fraction
  - Conduction disorders
  - Combination therapy

IMAGING

Ultrasonographic Findings

- Myocarditis
  - Left ventricle dysfunction with regional wall motion abnormalities
  - Reduced or preserved ejection fraction
  - Low global longitudinal strain by speckle tracking
  - Intracardiac thrombi
- Pericarditis
  - Pericardial thickening &/or effusion

MR Findings

- Myocarditis
  - Myocardial edema
  - Late gadolinium enhancement (diffuse, subendocardial, transmural, subepicardial)
  - T2 hyperintensity
  - Local or global wall motion abnormalities with decrease in left ventricle ejection fraction in some cases
- Pericarditis
  - Pericardial thickening with enhancement and pericardial effusion

CT Angiogram

- Shows diffuse wall thickening and luminal narrowing of affected vessel with vasculitis

Electrocardiogram

- New PR interval prolongation
- Atrioventricular block
- Supraventricular and ventricular arrhythmias
- ST-depression

- Diffuse T-wave inversion
- ST-segment elevation
- New Q waves

MICROSCOPIC

Histologic Features

- Myocardium
  - Interstitial inflammatory infiltrate composed predominantly of T lymphocytes
    - CD8(+) lymphocytes comprise majority of inflammatory infiltrate
    - Rare eosinophils may be present
    - Conduction system can be involved
  - Myocyte injury/necrosis
- Pericardium
  - Inflammatory infiltrate composed of CD4(+) and CD8(+) lymphocytes and macrophages
  - Pericardial thickening
  - Fibrinous hemorrhagic exudate
- Arteries
  - Perivascular lymphocytic inflammation
  - Wall necrosis
  - Giant cells may be present in giant cell arteritis

ANCILLARY TESTS

Immunohistochemistry

- CD4 and CD8 (majority) (+) stain seen in infiltrating lymphocytes
- Reduction of FOXP3(+) regulatory T cells
- CD68 for macrophage identification
- PD-L1 expression in myocytes and CD8(+) lymphocytes

DIFFERENTIAL DIAGNOSIS

Lymphocytic Myocarditis

- No history of ICI use
- Viral agent could be identified by PCR studies

Hypersensitivity Myocarditis

- History of recent medication use but no ICIs
- Skin rash
- Peripheral eosinophilia
- Predominantly eosinophilic myocardial inflammation

Acute Cellular Rejection

- Heart transplant recipients are at higher risk of developing malignancies
- ICIs are being used in this group of patients
- Differentiation between cellular rejection and ICI myocarditis is extremely difficult

DIAGNOSTIC CHECKLIST

Clinically Relevant Pathologic Features

- Diagnosis is challenging due to low event rate and lack of well-established criteria

Pathologic Interpretation Pearls

- Endomyocardial biopsy is confirmatory of diagnosis but is infrequently performed, and sensitivity is low

SELECTED REFERENCES

1. Arcari L et al: Cardiac magnetic resonance imaging in immune check-point inhibitor myocarditis: a systematic review. J Imaging. 8(4):99, 2022
2. Baranseh J et al: Pro-BNP in the differential diagnosis of dyspnea in patients treated with immune-checkpoint inhibitors: case report. J Oncol Pharm Pract. ePub, 2022
3. Brumberger ZL et al: Cardiotoxicity risk factors with immune checkpoint inhibitors. Cardiooncology. 8(1):3, 2022
4. Gilon D et al: The diagnosis and management of immune checkpoint inhibitor cardiovascular toxicity: myocarditis and beyond. Vaccines (Basel). 10(2):304, 2022
5. Gosangi B et al: Imaging features of toxicities associated with immune checkpoint inhibitors. Eur J Radiol Open. 9:100434, 2022
6. Li C et al: Immune checkpoint inhibitors-associated cardiotoxicity. Cancers (Basel). 14(5):1145, 2022
7. Park BC et al: Hypersensitivity reactions and immune-related adverse events to immune checkpoint inhibitors: approaches, mechanisms, and models. Immunol Allergy Clin North Am. 42(2):285-305, 2022
8. Rubio-Infante N et al: A systematic review of the mechanisms involved in immune checkpoint inhibitors cardiotoxicity and challenges to improve clinical safety. Front Cell Dev Biol. 10:851032, 2022
9. D'Souza M et al: The risk of cardiac events in patients receiving immune checkpoint inhibitors: a nationwide Danish study. Eur Heart J. 42(16):1621-31, 2021
10. Jacobs F et al: Pericarditis during chemoimmunotherapy for non-small cell lung cancer: an adverse event to prevent and recognise. Eur J Cancer. 149:114-6, 2021
11. Stoycheva D et al: External cues to drive B cell function towards immunotherapy. Acta Biomater. 133:222-30, 2021
12. Totzeck M et al: Are we underestimating the potential for cardiotoxicity related to immune checkpoint inhibitors? Eur Heart J. 42(16):1632-5, 2021
13. Dolladille C et al: Late cardiac adverse events in patients with cancer treated with immune checkpoint inhibitors. J Immunother Cancer. 8(1):e000261, 2020
14. Durrechou Q et al: Management of immune checkpoint inhibitor toxicities. Cancer Manag Res. 12:9139-58, 2020
15. Liu S et al: Immune checkpoint inhibitor-associated myocarditis with persistent troponin elevation despite abatacept and prolonged immunosuppression. JACC CardioOncol. 2(5):800-4, 2020
16. Salido Iniesta M et al: A different type of acute myocarditis: a case report of acute autoimmune myocarditis mediated by anti-PD-1 T lymphocyte receptor (pembrolizumab). Eur Heart J Case Rep. 4(5):1-6, 2020
17. Sławiński G et al: Immune checkpoint inhibitors and cardiac toxicity in patients treated for non-small lung cancer: a review. Int J Mol Sci. 21(19):7195, 2020
18. Thomas R et al: A review of the imaging manifestations of immune check point inhibitor toxicities. Clin Imaging. 64:70-9, 2020
19. Ibraheim H et al: Pathology of immune-mediated tissue lesions following treatment with immune checkpoint inhibitors. Rheumatology (Oxford). 58(Suppl 7):vii17-28, 2019
20. Ederhy S et al: Takotsubo-like syndrome in cancer patients treated with immune checkpoint inhibitors. JACC Cardiovasc Imaging. 11(8):1187-90, 2018
21. Inayat F et al: New drugs and new toxicities: pembrolizumab-induced myocarditis. BMJ Case Rep, 2018
22. Mahmood SS et al: Myocarditis in patients treated with immune checkpoint inhibitors. J Am Coll Cardiol. 71(16):1755-64, 2018
23. Varricchi G et al: Cardiotoxicity of immune checkpoint inhibitors. ESMO Open. 2(4):e000247, 2017
24. Johnson DB et al: Fulminant myocarditis with combination immune checkpoint blockade. N Engl J Med. 375(18):1749-55, 2016

Histologic Changes in ICI Myocarditis

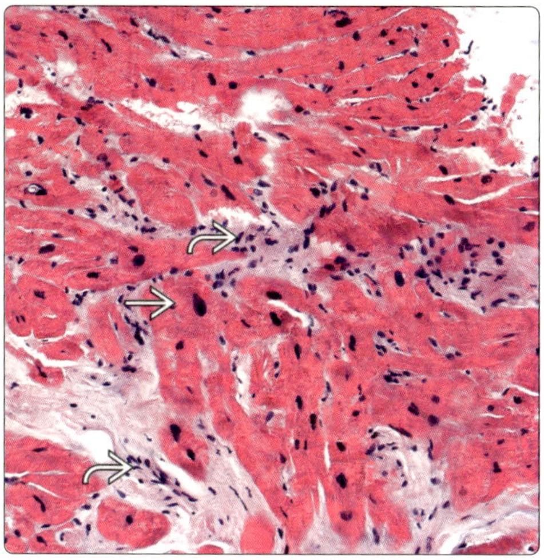

Histologic Changes in ICI Myocarditis

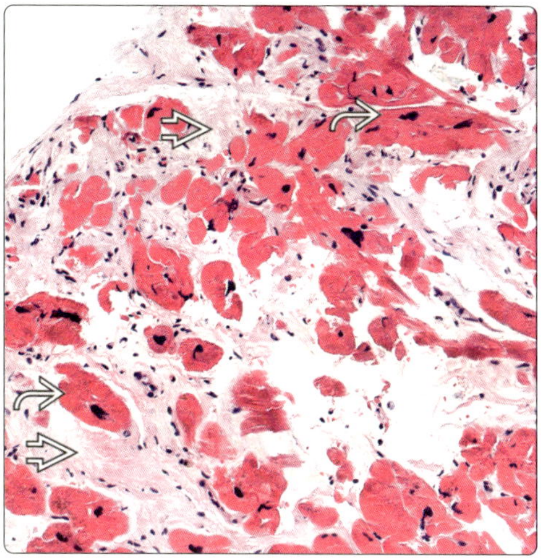

(Left) *H&E of the myocardium from a patient with malignant melanoma treated with PD-1 inhibitor shows interstitial fibrosis admixed with scant interstitial mononuclear inflammatory infiltrate ➡ and focal myocyte hypertrophy ➡. In this case, the findings of immune checkpoint inhibitor (ICI) toxicity are in subacute stage.* **(Right)** *H&E of the myocardium from a patient with malignant melanoma treated with PD-1 inhibitor shows interstitial fibrosis ➡ and myocyte hypertrophy ➡. In this case, the findings of ICI toxicity is in a chronic stage.*

Lymphocytic Myocarditis

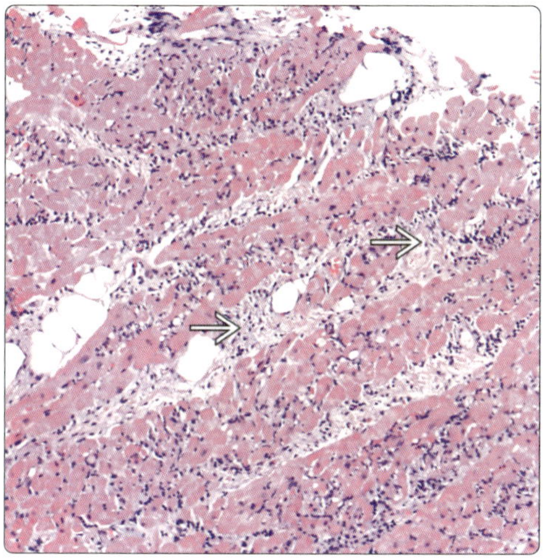

Lymphocytic Myocarditis

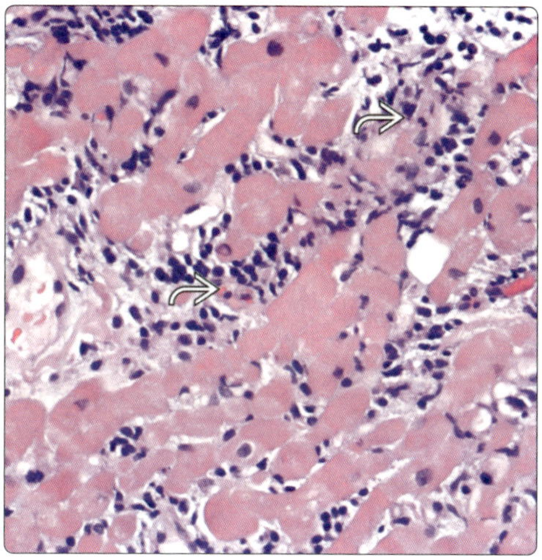

(Left) *H&E of the myocardium from a patient with suspected viral myocarditis shows interstitial edema and mononuclear inflammatory infiltrates surrounding myocytes ➡.* **(Right)** *Higher magnification of the same image shows the myocardium with interstitial mononuclear inflammatory infiltrates associated with myocyte necrosis ➡, characteristic of lymphocytic myocarditis. Without appropriate clinical history, lymphocytic myocarditis cannot be differentiated from ICI myocarditis on morphology.*

Hypersensitivity Myocarditis

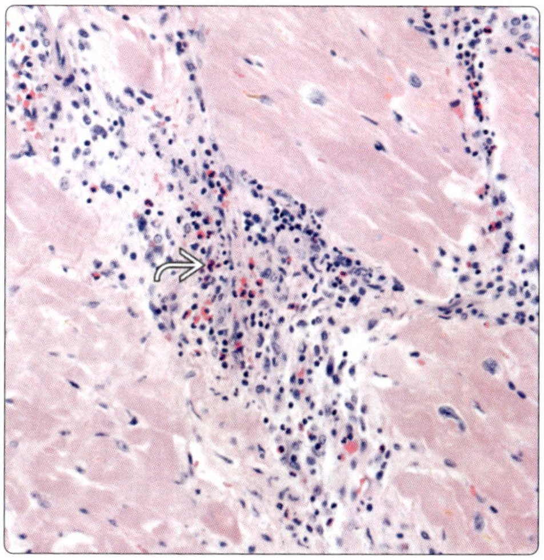

Hypersensitivity Myocarditis

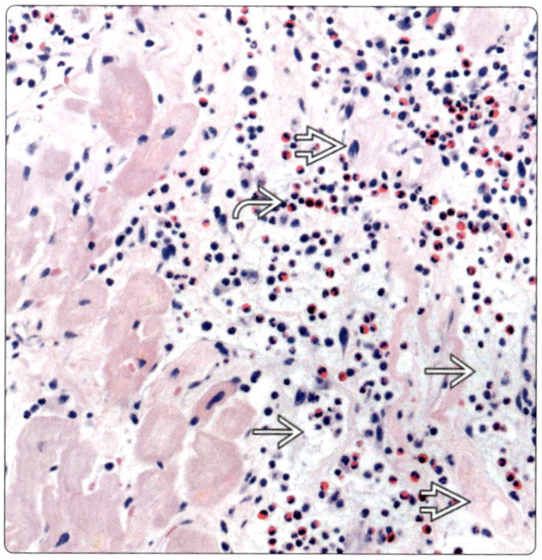

(Left) *H&E of the myocardium from a patient with hypersensitivity myocarditis secondary to antiinflammatory medication shows interstitial edema and numerous eosinophils ➡ admixed with mononuclear cells.* **(Right)** *Higher magnification of the same image shows interstitial edema ➡ and numerous eosinophils ➡ admixed with mononuclear cells and associated with myocyte injury ➡, characteristic of hypersensitivity myocarditis. In ICI myocarditis, eosinophils are very rare.*

Lymphocytic Myocarditis

KEY FACTS

TERMINOLOGY

- Inflammatory process involving myocardium with degeneration &/or necrosis of myocytes secondary to viral infection or postviral autoimmune response

ETIOLOGY/PATHOGENESIS

- Viruses have been implicated
  - RNA virus: Coxsackie A and B, influenza A and B, hepatitis C
  - DNA virus: Adenovirus, herpesvirus [varicella-zoster, cytomegalovirus (CMV), Epstein-Barr], parvovirus B19

CLINICAL ISSUES

- True incidence is unknown
- 10% of acute-onset heart failure
- Slight male predominance
- Fulminant myocarditis; patients can recover
- Progress to dilated cardiomyopathy
- Sudden death from circulatory failure in acute phase

MACROSCOPIC

- Dilatation of left ventricle
- Myocardium with flabby consistency
- Mural thrombi in any chamber
- Cut myocardial surface with marked variegate mottled appearance and pale foci alternating with minute hemorrhagic lesions

MICROSCOPIC

- Dallas criteria: 1st diagnostic biopsy ± fibrosis
  - No myocarditis: No inflammation or myocardial abnormalities
  - Borderline myocarditis: Sparse inflammatory infiltrate, but damage of myocytes not demonstrated
  - Myocarditis: Significant inflammation with myocyte damage (necrosis, myocyte vacuolization)

ANCILLARY TESTS

- Immunohistochemistry for CD3 and CD68

Pathogenesis of Viral Myocarditis

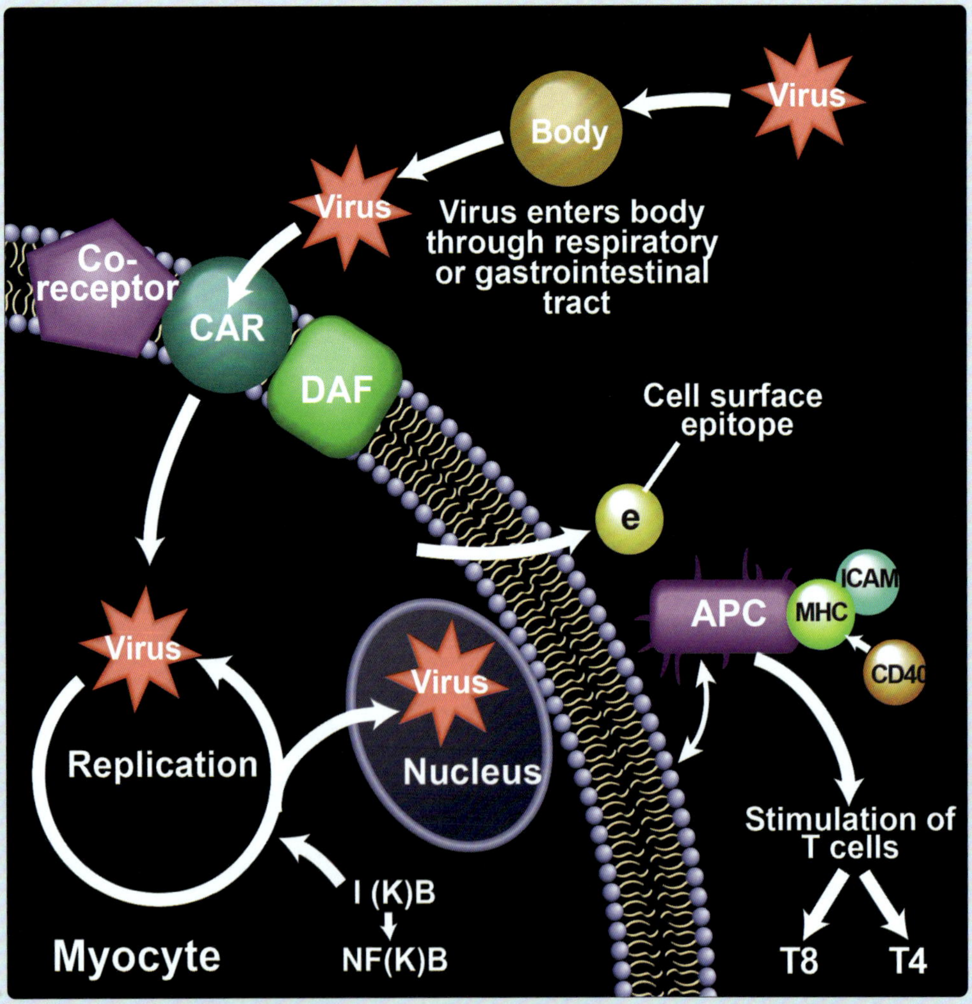

Graphic depicts pathogenesis of viral myocarditis. The virus enters myocytes through Coxsackie adenoviral receptor (CAR), coreceptor, and decay accelerating factor (DAF). Within the myocyte, the virus replicates and is transmitted to the nucleus, where it redirects cell activity. Antigen-presenting cells (APC) expressing MHC, CD40, and ICAM couple with infected myocytes and stimulate cytotoxic cells capable of ingesting myocytes or antibody-producing cells, which affect cell function or enhance cell damage by cytotoxic cells.

TERMINOLOGY

Definitions

- Inflammatory process involving myocardium with degeneration &/or necrosis of myocytes secondary to viral infection or postviral autoimmune response

ETIOLOGY/PATHOGENESIS

Infectious Agents

- RNA virus
    - Coxsackie A and B
    - Influenza A and B
    - Hepatitis C
    - SARS-CoV-2
- DNA virus
    - Adenovirus
    - Herpesvirus [varicella-zoster, cytomegalovirus (CMV), Epstein-Barr]
    - Parvovirus B19

CLINICAL ISSUES

Epidemiology

- Incidence
    - True incidence is unknown
    - Estimated that 10% of acute-onset heart failure is due to acute myocarditis
    - Myocarditis is cause of sudden cardiovascular death in ~ 2% of infants, 5% of childhood, and 10-20% young adults
- Age
    - Young individuals are more susceptible to viral infections
- Sex
    - Slight male predominance

Presentation

- New onset of congestive heart failure
- Atrial/ventricular arrhythmias
- Sudden death
- Embolic events
- Fatigue
- Chest pain
- Palpitations
- Sinus tachycardia
- Gallops, murmurs
- Pericardial friction rub
- Fever

Laboratory Tests

- White blood cell count usually elevated
- Elevated cardiac-specific troponin in 1/3 of cases
- Elevated creatine kinase isoform MB in 10% of cases
- Nonspecific markers of inflammation
    - C-reactive protein (CRP) elevated
    - Erythrocyte sedimentation rate (ESR) elevated
- Autoantibodies to sarcolemma, α-myosin, mitochondria, endothelial antigens
- Rising IgM/IgG titers to specific virus
- Molecular identification of viral DNA/RNA in blood &/or heart biopsy

Treatment

- Limit physical activity
- Standard supportive heart failure therapy
- Standard antiarrhythmic therapy
- Intravenous immunoglobulin in children
- Immunosuppressive therapy not beneficial
- Antiviral therapy only limited studies; use is controversial
- Interferon-β therapy has shown improvement in some patients

Prognosis

- Mild cases of myocarditis may be asymptomatic, and patients can recover without sequelae
- Fulminant myocarditis more likely to have sequelae, but complete recovery is possible after support
- Progress to dilated cardiomyopathy in ~ 1/4 of cases
- Sudden death from circulatory failure in acute phase in some cases

IMAGING

Ultrasonographic Findings

- Segmental/global wall motion abnormalities
- Normal diastolic volumes
- Increased left ventricle wall thickness
- Right/left ventricular dysfunction

MR Findings

- Global relative gadolinium enhancement in myocardium compared to skeletal muscle
- Increased T2 signal in areas of myocardial inflammation
- Delayed enhancement in subepicardial region

EKG

- Elevation/depression of ST segment
- T-wave changes
- Pathologic Q waves
- Atrial/ventricular arrhythmias: Premature beats, tachycardia, fibrillation, conduction delays

MACROSCOPIC

General Features

- Dilatation of left ventricle
- Cut myocardial surface with markedly variegated mottled appearance and pale foci alternating with minute hemorrhagic lesions
- Myocardium with flabby consistency
- Mural thrombi in any chamber
- Pericarditis may be present

MICROSCOPIC

Histologic Features

- Dallas criteria
    - 1st diagnostic biopsy ± fibrosis
        - No myocarditis: No inflammation or myocardial abnormalities
        - Borderline myocarditis: Sparse inflammatory infiltrate, but damage of myocytes is not demonstrated
        - Myocarditis: Significant inflammation with myocyte damage (necrosis, myocyte vacuolization)

Clinical and Morphologic Findings in Lymphocytic Myocarditis

Parameter	Fulminant	Subacute	Chronic Active	Chronic Persistent
Onset	Distinct	Indistinct	Indistinct	Indistinct
Left ventricle dysfunction	Severe	Moderate	Moderate	None
Initial biopsy findings	Multiple foci of active myocarditis	Active, borderline	Active, borderline	Active, borderline
Clinical outcome	Ranges from recovery to death	Incomplete recovery, progress to dilated cardiomyopathy	Restrictive cardiomyopathy	Normal left ventricle function
Histopathologic outcome	Complete resolution	Complete resolution	Chronic inflammation, fibrosis	Ongoing inflammation
Response to immunosuppressive therapy	No benefit	Variable	Initial response, late relapses	No benefit

- 2nd/follow-up biopsy ± fibrosis
  - Ongoing (persistent) myocarditis: Morphology similar to that in prior biopsy
  - Resolving (healing) myocarditis: Fewer abnormalities than in prior biopsy
  - Resolved (healed) myocarditis: Fibrosis, no inflammation

Cytologic Features

- Most inflammatory cells are T lymphocytes; few are B lymphocytes and macrophages, and mast cells are rare

ANCILLARY TESTS

Immunohistochemistry

- CD3 staining for T lymphocytes
- CD68 staining for macrophages
- IHC criteria for diagnosis of myocarditis
  - ≥ 14 leukocytes/mm², including up to 4 CD68(+)/mm² and ≥ 7 CD3(+) T cells

PCR

- Viral genomic material detected in nucleic acid extract from myocardial tissue
- Quantitative PCR (qPCR) to measure viral load may help differentiate between active and latent viral infection

DIFFERENTIAL DIAGNOSIS

Giant Cell Myocarditis

- Mixed myocardial inflammatory infiltrate with presence of giant cells
- Extensive areas of myocardial necrosis
- History of thymoma or autoimmune disorders

Hypersensitivity Myocarditis

- History of recent medication use
- Skin rash, peripheral eosinophilia
- Eosinophilic myocardial infiltrates

Sarcoidosis

- Noncaseating granulomas in myocardium, endocardium, or pericardium
- Hypercalcemia
- Lung or other organ involvement

Cytomegalovirus Myocarditis

- Viral inclusions identified in endothelial cells
- CMV DNA detection in myocardial tissue

Bacterial Myocarditis

- Interstitial infiltrate composed predominantly of neutrophils
- Microabscesses may be identified

DIAGNOSTIC CHECKLIST

Pathologic Interpretation Pearls

- Diagnosis of myocarditis requires lymphocytic interstitial inflammation associated with myocyte necrosis or injury
- Endomyocardial biopsy has low sensitivity for diagnosis of myocarditis but is highly specific

SELECTED REFERENCES

1. Domínguez F et al: Endomyocardial biopsy-confirmed myocarditis and inflammatory cardiomyopathy: clinical profile and prognosis. Rev Esp Cardiol (Engl Ed). ePub, 2022
2. Kondo T et al: Differences in prognosis and cardiac function according to required percutaneous mechanical circulatory support and histological findings in patients with fulminant myocarditis: insights from the CHANGE PUMP 2 study. J Am Heart Assoc. 11(4):e023719, 2022
3. Seidel F et al: Clinical characteristics and outcome of biopsy-proven myocarditis in children - results of the German prospective multicentre registry "MYKKE". Int J Cardiol. 357:95-104, 2022
4. Zheng SY et al: Role of toll-like receptors and th responses in viral myocarditis. Front Immunol. 13:843891, 2022
5. Amioka N et al: Pathological and clinical effects of interleukin-6 on human myocarditis. J Cardiol. 78(2):157-65, 2021
6. Kawada JI et al: Immune cell infiltration landscapes in pediatric acute myocarditis analyzed by CIBERSORT. J Cardiol. 77(2):174-8, 2021
7. Khawaja A et al: The innate immune response in myocarditis. Int J Biochem Cell Biol. 134:105973, 2021
8. Murphy L et al: The role of endomyocardial biopsy in suspected myocarditis in the contemporary era: a 10-year National Transplant Centre experience. Cardiovasc Pathol. 54:107366, 2021
9. Sinagra G et al: Viral presence-guided immunomodulation in lymphocytic myocarditis: an update. Eur J Heart Fail. 23(2):211-6, 2021
10. Buja LM et al: Clinicopathological manifestations of myocarditis in a heart failure population. Cardiovasc Pathol. 45:107190, 2020
11. Li L et al: Demographic, clinical and pathological features of sudden deaths due to myocarditis: results from a state-wide population-based autopsy study. Forensic Sci Int. 272:81-6, 2017
12. Aretz HT et al: Myocarditis. A histopathologic definition and classification. Am J Cardiovasc Pathol. 1(1):3-14, 1987

MR Findings in Myocarditis

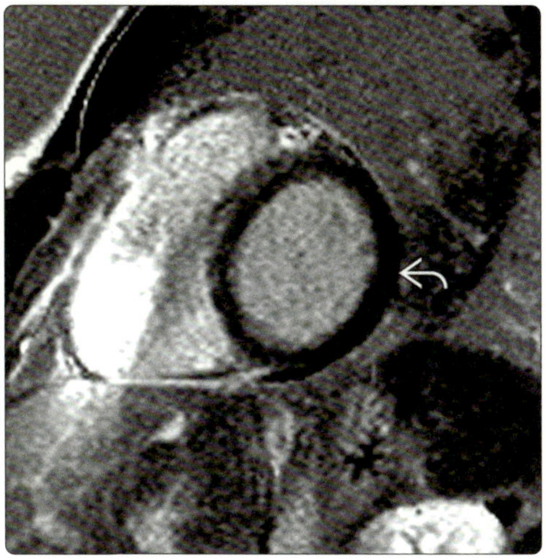

Negative Biopsy in Case of Clinical Myocarditis

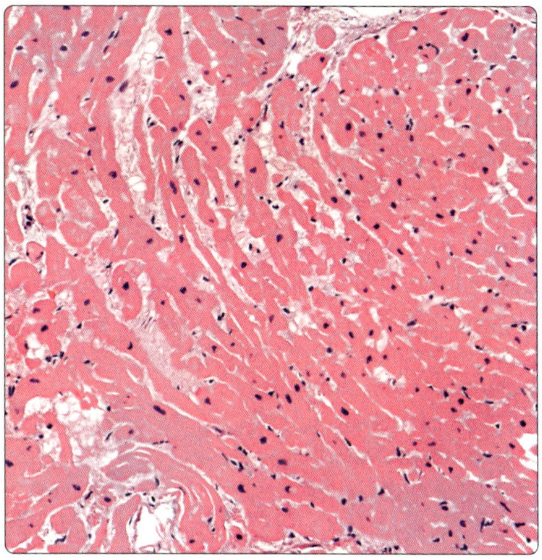

(Left) *Short-axis heart MR in a patient with a clinical diagnosis of myocarditis shows delayed contrast enhancement, which is a characteristic finding in MR. (Courtesy C. McGann, MD.)* **(Right)** *H&E of a patient with a clinical diagnosis of myocarditis does not demonstrate interstitial inflammatory infiltrate, and the myocytes appear unremarkable. In this case, the biopsy is negative for myocarditis.*

Borderline Myocarditis

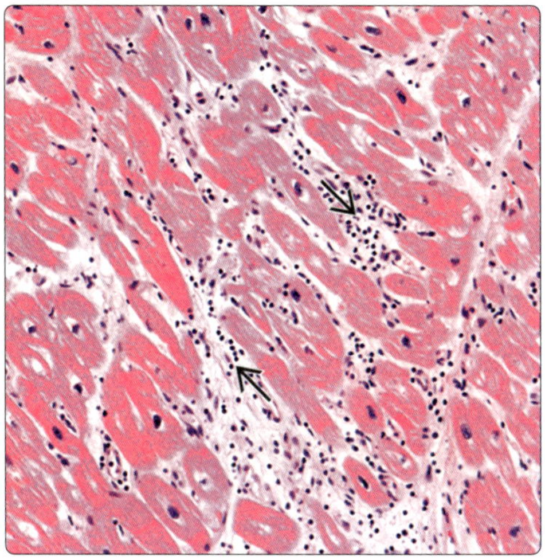

Histologic Changes of Myocarditis

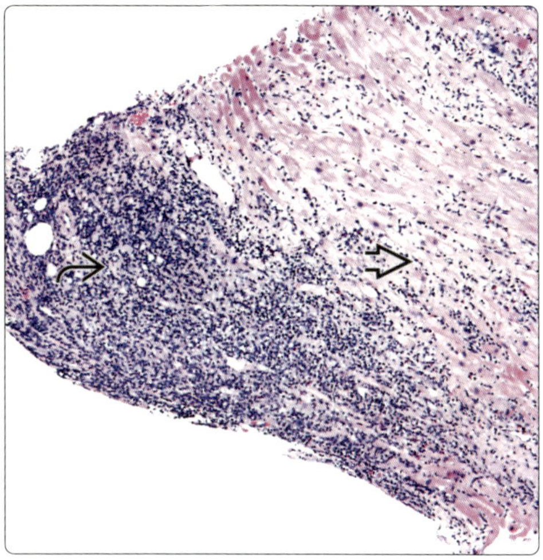

(Left) *H&E of a patient with a clinical diagnosis of myocarditis shows sparse mononuclear inflammatory infiltrate in the interstitium; however, the myocytes appear unremarkable. The diagnosis of borderline myocarditis can be made.* **(Right)** *H&E shows marked predominantly mononuclear inflammatory infiltrate involved extensively in this biopsy sample. There is myocyte injury with vacuolization of the cytoplasm. The findings are diagnostic of lymphocytic myocarditis.*

Histologic Changes of Myocarditis

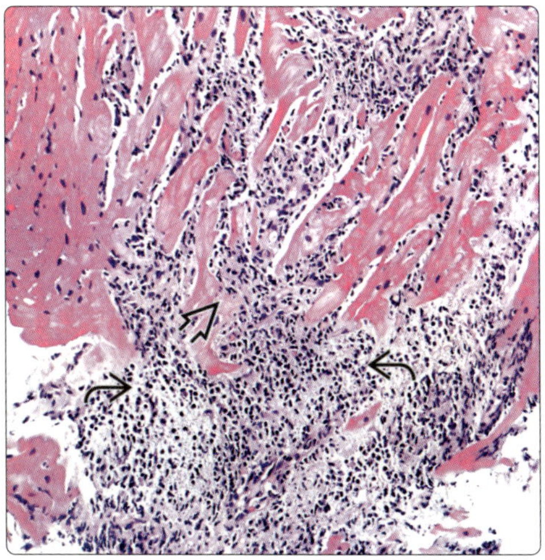

Histologic Changes of Myocarditis

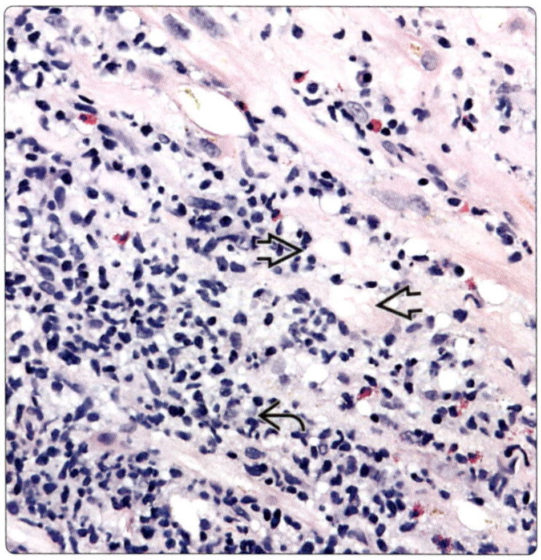

(Left) *H&E of a patient with the diagnosis of myocarditis shows marked mononuclear inflammatory infiltrate in the interstitium and myocyte damage, diagnostic of lymphocytic myocarditis.* **(Right)** *H&E shows marked predominantly mononuclear inflammatory infiltrate with rare eosinophils, and there is myocyte injury with vacuolization of the cytoplasm. In this case, the biopsy is diagnostic of lymphocytic myocarditis.*

Giant Cell Myocarditis

KEY FACTS

TERMINOLOGY

- Uncommon aggressive inflammatory process targeting myocardium with prominent giant cells

ETIOLOGY/PATHOGENESIS

- Unknown but associated with autoimmune disorders

CLINICAL ISSUES

- Most commonly involves young to middle-aged adults
- Rarely seen in small children and infants
- Slight male predominance
- Clinical presentation: Rapidly progressive or fulminant heart failure (75%), ventricular arrhythmias (14%), heart block (5%), other symptoms mimicking acute ischemia (6%)
- Treatment: Immunosuppression, transplantation
- Prognosis is poor; may recur in native and transplanted heart

MACROSCOPIC

- In explanted or autopsy hearts, gross findings are nonspecific
  - Cardiomegaly with dilated and flabby appearance
  - Irregular myocardial scarring or mottling

MICROSCOPIC

- Chronic inflammation with prominent giant cells and occasional eosinophils
- Obvious cardiomyocyte degeneration and necrosis
- In later stages, extensive fibrosis, sparse inflammation, and rare to no giant cells

DIAGNOSTIC CHECKLIST

- Giant cells
- Mixed inflammation around individual cardiomyocytes
- Obvious cardiomyocyte necrosis
- Epicardium uninvolved
- Eosinophils not abundant

Histologic Features of Giant Cell Myocarditis

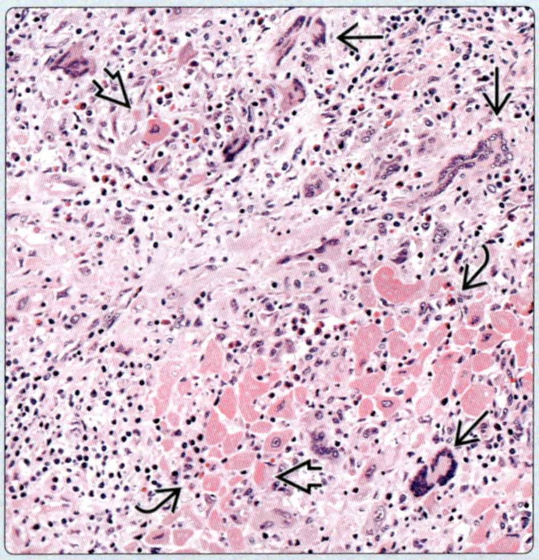

Histologic Features of Giant Cell Myocarditis

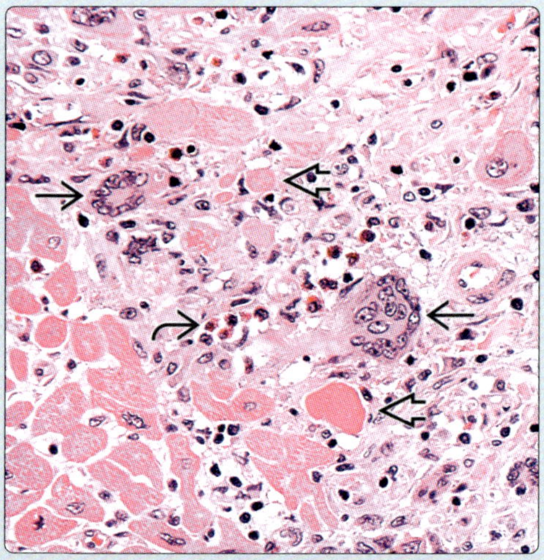

(Left) *On medium power, a dense mixed chronic inflammatory infiltrate surrounds individual cardiomyocytes ⇨ with prominent multinucleated giant cells → and obvious cardiomyocyte necrosis ↪.* **(Right)** *On high power, giant cells → are striking, and cardiomyocyte necrosis ↪ is readily apparent. Eosinophils may also be focally increased ⇨.*

Histologic Features of Giant Cell Myocarditis

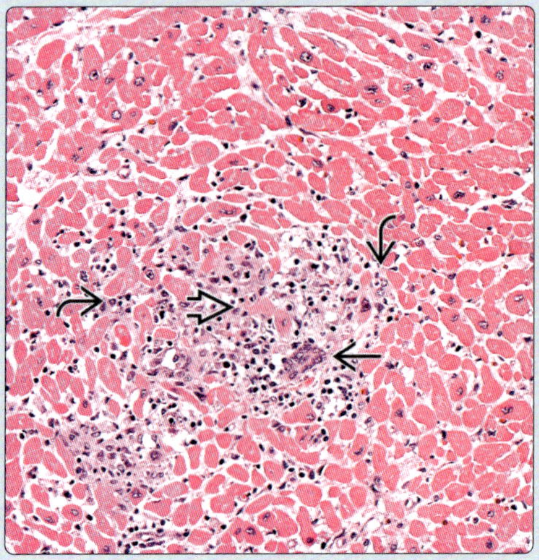

Trichrome Stain of Giant Cell Myocarditis

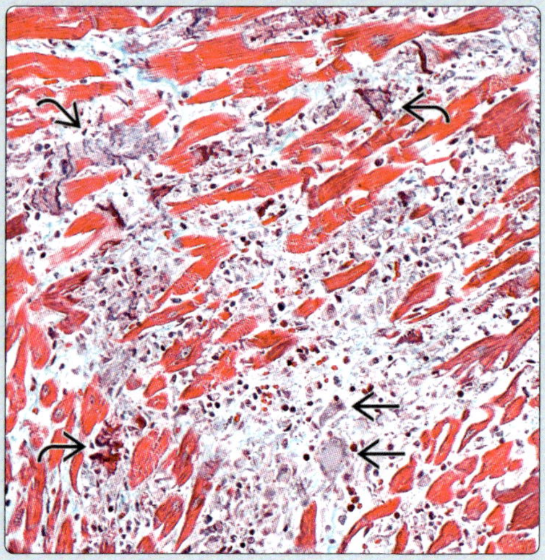

(Left) *In some cases, lesions are small, but giant cells →, cardiomyocyte necrosis ↪, and perimyocytic inflammation ⇨ are still present. The areas of inflammation do not show a well-circumscribed border.* **(Right)** *Trichrome stain shows focal cardiomyocyte degeneration with contraction band necrosis ↪ with associated inflammation and giant cells →. In later stages, fibrosis predominates with cardiomyocyte loss and scattered mononuclear inflammatory cells. Giants cells are rare or absent.*

TERMINOLOGY

Abbreviations

- Giant cell myocarditis (GCM)

Synonyms

- Fiedler myocarditis

Definitions

- Uncommon aggressive inflammatory process targeted at cardiomyocytes with prominent giant cells

ETIOLOGY/PATHOGENESIS

Unknown

- Associations with autoimmune disease or neoplasia
  - Myasthenia gravis/thymoma
  - Inflammatory bowel disease/celiac disease
  - Connective tissue disorders: Systemic lupus erythematosus, Sjögren syndrome, polymyositis
  - Autoimmune hepatitis

CLINICAL ISSUES

Epidemiology

- Incidence
  - 0.007-0.051% in autopsy studies
  - 0.13 cases/100,000 persons/year
- Age
  - Most commonly involves young to middle-aged adults
  - Rarely seen in small children and infants
- Sex
  - No predominance

Presentation

- Rapidly progressive or fulminant heart failure (75%)
- Ventricular arrhythmias (14-29%)
- Heart block (5-8%)
- Other symptoms mimicking acute ischemia (6-19%)

Treatment

- High-dose immunosuppression: Cyclosporine, corticosteroids, thymoglobulin, mycophenolate mofetil, alemtuzumab
- Left ventricular assist devices
- Heart transplantation
- Heart failure management and antiarrhythmic medication

Prognosis

- Without immunosuppression: Very poor; average transplant-free survival of 3 months
- With immunosuppression: Still poor; average transplant-free survival of 13 months
- May recur in native and transplanted heart (20-25%)

IMAGING

Ultrasonographic Findings

- Diffuse left ventricular or biventricular dysfunction
- Normal ventricular size and wall thickness in acute presentation

MACROSCOPIC

General Features

- In explanted or autopsy hearts, gross findings are nonspecific
  - Cardiomegaly with dilated and flabby appearance
  - Irregular myocardial scarring or mottling

MICROSCOPIC

Histologic Features

- Diffuse/multifocal myocardial infiltration by abundant lymphocytes, prominent multinucleated giant cells, occasional neutrophils, eosinophils, plasma cells
  - T lymphocytes more numerous than B lymphocytes, predominantly CD8 positive
  - Giant cells macrophage derived, CD68 positive
- Infiltrate surrounds individual cardiomyocytes
- Obvious cardiomyocyte degeneration and necrosis
- Later stages: Extensive fibrosis, collagen deposition, sparse inflammation, less cardiomyocyte necrosis, rare to no giant cells
- Epicardium typically uninvolved

DIFFERENTIAL DIAGNOSIS

Cardiac Sarcoidosis

- Syncope and heart block are more common presenting symptoms
- Epithelioid granulomas with giant cells
- Little to no cardiomyocyte necrosis
- May involve epicardium
- Fibrosis is typically more extensive
- Eosinophils are generally not seen
- Zone of inflammation is more discrete with well-circumscribed border

Eosinophilic (Hypersensitivity) Myocarditis

- Usually drug induced
- Interstitial infiltrate is rich in eosinophils
- Cardiomyocyte necrosis is less prominent
- Giant cells are usually rare to absent but may be prominent in fulminant cases

Bacterial Myocarditis

- Neutrophilic infiltrates are more prominent, often with microabscess formation
- Granulomas with caseating necrosis may occur, particularly with mycobacteria
- Stains for acid-fast bacilli are useful to rule out mycobacterial infections

SELECTED REFERENCES

1. Bang V et al: Management of patients with giant cell myocarditis: JACC review topic of the week. J Am Coll Cardiol. 77(8):1122-34, 2021
2. Liu S et al: Clinical identification and characteristic analysis of giant cell myocarditis in 12 cases. Front Cardiovasc Med. 8:649094, 2021
3. Nordenswan HK et al: Manifestations and outcome of cardiac sarcoidosis and idiopathic giant cell myocarditis by 25-year nationwide cohorts. J Am Heart Assoc. 10(6):e019415, 2021
4. Vaidya GN et al: Heart transplantation for giant cell myocarditis: a case series. Transplant Proc. 53(1):348-52, 2021
5. Xu J et al: Giant cell myocarditis: a brief review. Arch Pathol Lab Med. 140(12):1429-34, 2016

Eosinophilic (Löffler) Myocarditis

KEY FACTS

TERMINOLOGY

- Rare disease characterized by eosinophilic infiltration of endocardium and myocardium, often with mural thrombus and peripheral blood eosinophilia leading to development of restrictive cardiomyopathy

ETIOLOGY/PATHOGENESIS

- Drugs/hypersensitivity reaction
- Infection: Parasitic, viral, fungal
- Hypereosinophilic syndrome
- Hematologic malignancies
- Idiopathic

CLINICAL ISSUES

- Adults; peak incidence in 5th decade
- Male predominance (80-95%)
- In hypereosinophilic syndrome, cardiac involvement is major cause of mortality and morbidity
- Progression to restrictive cardiomyopathy

MICROSCOPIC

- Stage 1: Acute (necrotic)
  - Mixed inflammatory cell infiltrate with frequent eosinophils in interstitial or perivascular distribution
  - Eosinophil degranulation and breakdown products (Charcot-Leyden crystals)
- Stage 2: Subacute (thrombotic)
  - Mural thrombosis containing eosinophils, usually apical and extending toward base of heart
  - Thrombosis, fibrinoid change, and inflammation involving small intramural coronary vessels
- Stage 3: Chronic (fibrotic)
  - Endocardial thickening and fibrous plaques
  - Valvular endocardial thickening
  - Interstitial fibrosis

TOP DIFFERENTIAL DIAGNOSES

- Eosinophilic granulomatosis with polyangiitis
- Other myocarditis

(Left) *Myocardial biopsy of a patient with eosinophilic myocarditis shows prominent eosinophils ↷ in the endocardium as well as inflammatory cells in the myocardial interstitium →.* **(Right)** *Myocardial biopsy of a patient with eosinophilic myocarditis shows prominent eosinophils → in the interstitial inflammatory infiltrate surrounding myocytes.*

Endocardial Changes in Eosinophilic Myocarditis

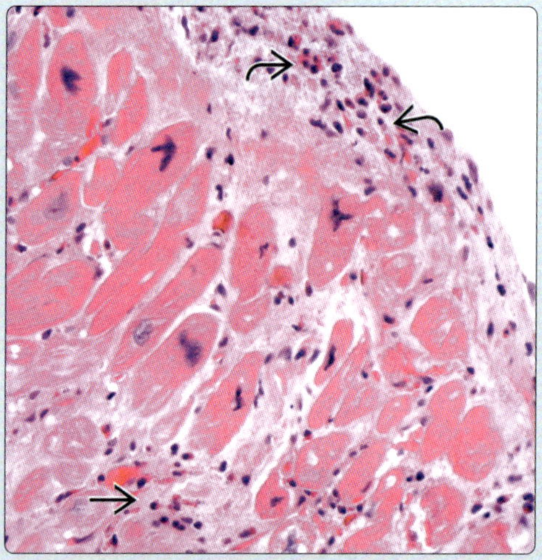

Myocardial Changes in Eosinophilic Myocarditis

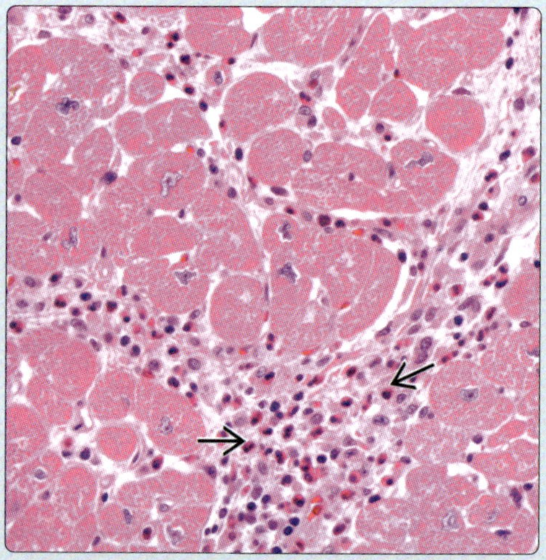

(Left) *Myocardial biopsy of a patient with eosinophilic myocarditis shows prominent eosinophils → at higher magnification in the interstitial inflammatory infiltrate and focal myocyte injury ⇗.* **(Right)** *Myocardial biopsy of a patient with eosinophilic myocarditis shows interstitial inflammation and edema with eosinophils ➡ dominating the infiltrate, some of which show degranulation.*

Myocardial Changes in Eosinophilic Myocarditis

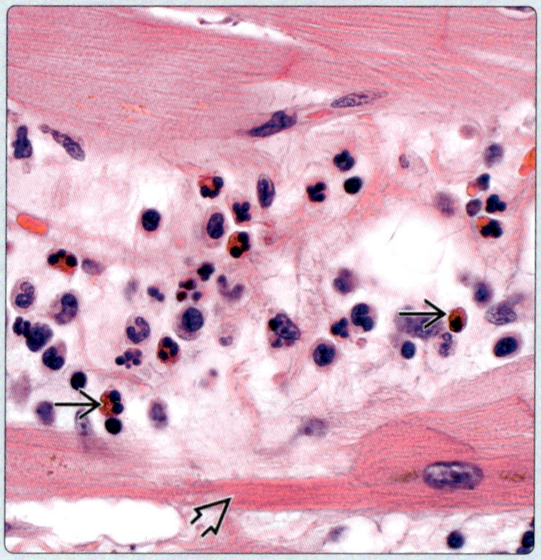

Myocardial Changes in Eosinophilic Myocarditis

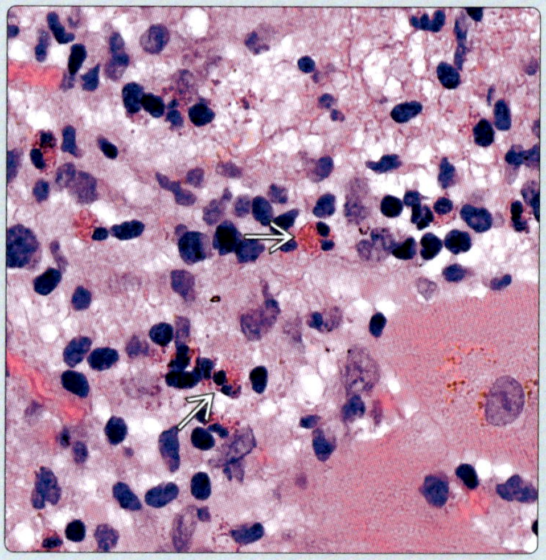

TERMINOLOGY

Definitions

- Rare disease characterized by eosinophilic infiltration of endocardium and myocardium, often with mural thrombus and peripheral blood eosinophilia leading to development of restrictive cardiomyopathy

ETIOLOGY/PATHOGENESIS

Environmental Exposure

- Hypersensitivity reaction: (34.1%) Antibiotics, diuretics, anticonvulsants, antiinflammatories, inotropic agents, vaccines

Infectious Agents

- Parasitic infection (tropical form), HIV infection, fungal infection

Hypereosinophilic Syndrome (8.4%)

- Absolute eosinophil count > 1.5 x 10^9/L, ≥ 6 months
- Systemic tissue involvement by eosinophils
- Other causes excluded

Neoplastic Disorders

- Eosinophilic leukemia, lymphomas

Systemic Immunologic Disorders

- Systemic, lupus, ANCA-related small vessel vasculitis

Idiopathic (> 30%)

- All other causes excluded

CLINICAL ISSUES

Epidemiology

- Incidence
  - 0.5% in unselected autopsy series
  - 0.1% in suspected myocarditis
  - Up to 20% in explanted hearts from heart transplant recipients (reflecting frequent use of inotropic agents)
- Age
  - Adults; peak incidence in 4th decade
- Sex
  - No predominance

Presentation

- Heart symptoms: Chest pain, cardiogenic shock (right- or left-sided heart failure), arrhythmias, sudden death, atrioventricular valve dysfunction
- Other organ symptoms: Skin rash, fever, peripheral blood eosinophilia, systemic embolization of mural thrombus (e.g., stroke, renal failure, limb ischemia)

Laboratory Tests

- Hypereosinophilia (75% cases)

Prognosis

- Progression to restrictive cardiomyopathy
- In hypereosinophilic syndrome, cardiac involvement is major cause of mortality and morbidity
- No recurrence reported after heart transplantation

IMAGING

Ultrasonographic Findings

- Localized thickening of posterobasal left ventricle
- Limited motion of posterior mitral valve leaflet
- Atrioventricular valve regurgitation
- Obliteration of apex by mural thrombus

MR Findings

- Increased T2 signal intensity in ventricular apices
- Diffuse delayed subendocardial hyperenhancement
- Intraventricular apical thrombus

Electrocardiogram

- Nonspecific ST segment and T-wave abnormalities
- Atrial fibrillation
- Right bundle branch block

MICROSCOPIC

Histologic Features

- Stage 1: Acute (necrotic)
  - Mixed inflammatory cell infiltrate with frequent eosinophils in interstitial or perivascular distribution
  - Myocyte necrosis (focal/extensive)
  - Eosinophilic granulomas
  - Eosinophil degranulation and breakdown products (Charcot-Leyden crystals)
- Stage 2: Subacute (thrombotic)
  - Mural thrombosis containing eosinophils, usually apical and extending toward base of heart
  - Thrombosis, fibrinoid change, and inflammation involving small intramural coronary vessels
- Stage 3: Chronic (fibrotic)
  - Endocardial thickening and fibrous plaques
  - Valvular endocardial thickening
  - Interstitial fibrosis

DIFFERENTIAL DIAGNOSIS

Eosinophilic Granulomatosis With Polyangiitis

- History of asthma or allergic rhinitis
- Necrotizing small vessel vasculitis with kidney involvement
- Positive MPO-ANCA in 30-40% of cases

Other Forms of Myocarditis

- Giant cell myocarditis very frequently shows increased eosinophils, but giant cells and extensive myocyte necrosis are prominent
- Lymphocytic and other forms of myocarditis may have eosinophils, particularly early in evolution, but clinical presentation is different

SELECTED REFERENCES

1. Jain V et al: Eosinophilic myocarditis: when allergies attack the heart! Cardiol Rev. 30(2):70-4, 2022
2. Murphy L et al: The role of endomyocardial biopsy in suspected myocarditis in the contemporary era: a 10-year National Transplant Centre experience. Cardiovasc Pathol. 54:107366, 2021
3. Leone O et al: The spectrum of myocarditis: from pathology to the clinics. Virchows Arch. 475(3):279-301, 2019
4. Brambatti M et al: Eosinophilic myocarditis: characteristics, treatment, and outcomes. J Am Coll Cardiol. 70(19):2363-75, 2017

(Left) *Four-chamber view of an explanted heart shows biventricular and predominantly right atrium dilatation and an organized thrombus coating the endocardium of the right ventricle.* **(Right)** *Mural thrombus from a patient with eosinophilic myocarditis shows progressive organization and prominent entrapped eosinophils.*

Explanted Heart of Patient With Eosinophilic Myocarditis

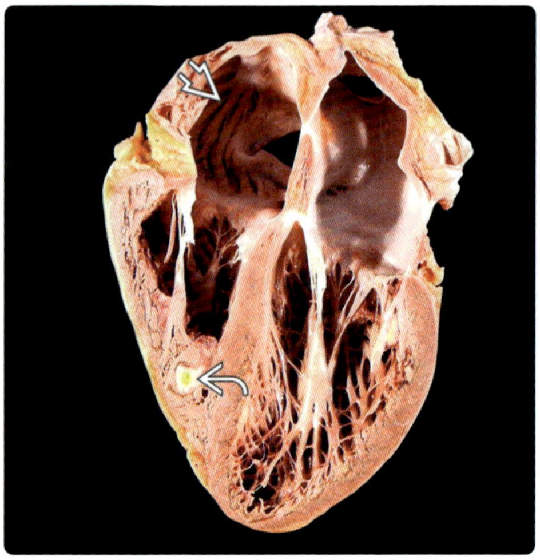

Mural Thrombus, Histology

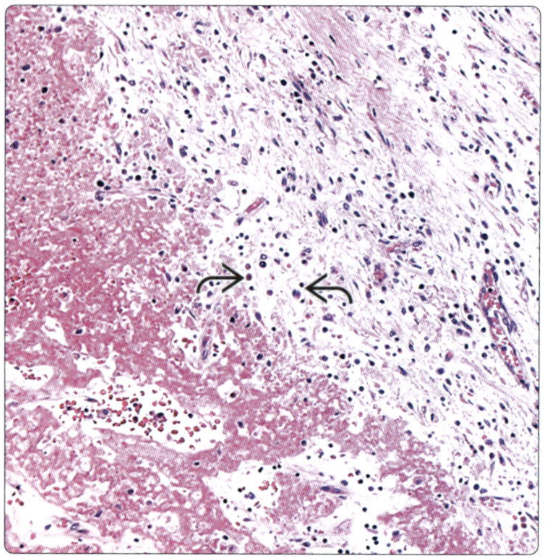

(Left) *In some cases of eosinophilic myocarditis, eosinophils may be particularly sparse, and significant myocyte damage may not be present.* **(Right)** *High-power view of early-stage eosinophilic myocarditis shows eosinophil-rich interstitial infiltrate with prominent eosinophil degranulation and focal myocyte injury.*

Eosinophilic Myocarditis, Acute Stage

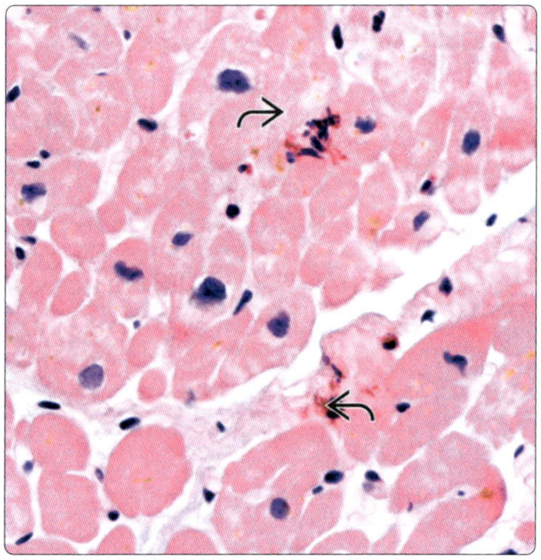

Eosinophilic Myocarditis, Acute Stage

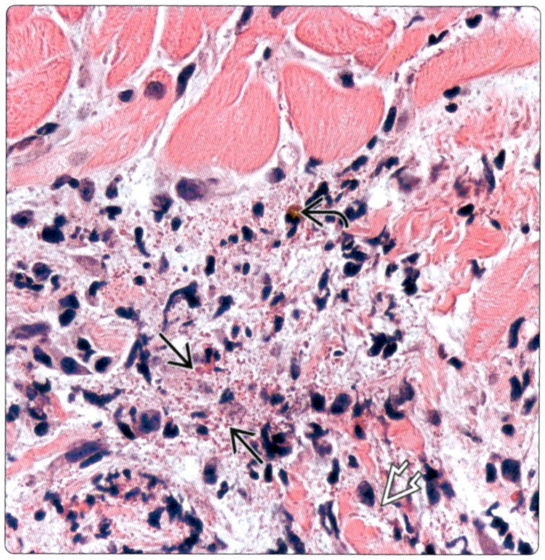

(Left) *H&E-stained section of a myocardial biopsy of a patient with early-stage eosinophilic myocarditis shows Charcot-Leyden crystals with associated foreign-body reaction in a sea of eosinophils.* **(Right)** *H&E-stained section of a patient with acute (necrotic) phase of eosinophilic myocarditis shows numerous eosinophils infiltrating the endocardium and extensive intramyocardial hemorrhage.*

Eosinophilic Myocarditis, Acute Stage

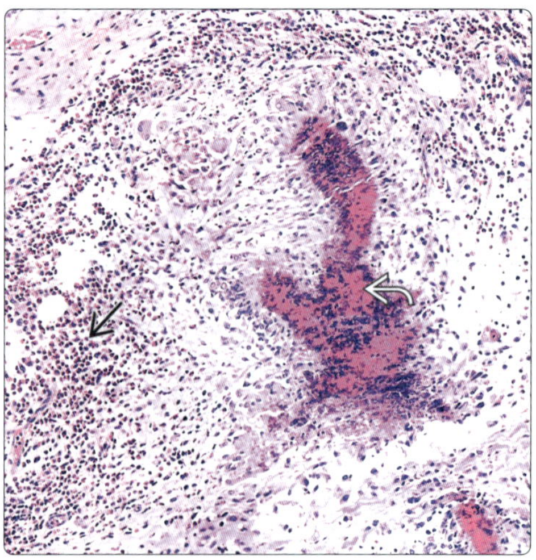

Eosinophilic Myocarditis, Acute Stage

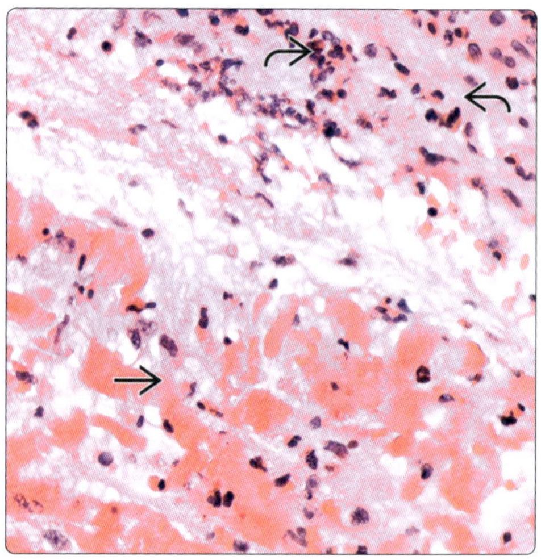

Inconclusive Biopsy for Diagnosis of Eosinophilic Myocarditis

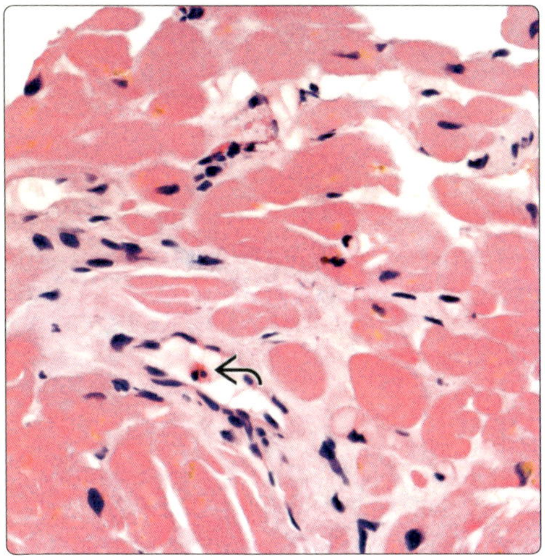

Eosinophilic Myocarditis With Endocardial Involvement

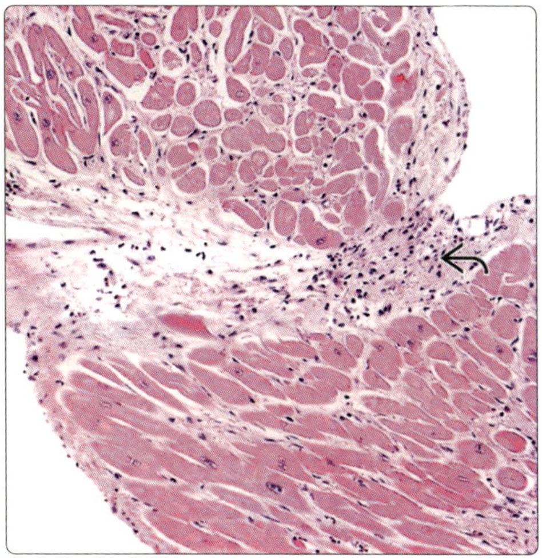

(Left) *Eosinophilic myocarditis may be patchy with sparing of areas, such as this relatively preserved myocardium. The single intravascular eosinophil is not sufficient to diagnose myocarditis.* **(Right)** *H&E-stained section of the myocardium from a patient with eosinophilic myocarditis shows relatively sparse eosinophils, mostly localized in the endocardium.*

Eosinophilic Myocarditis, Subacute Stage

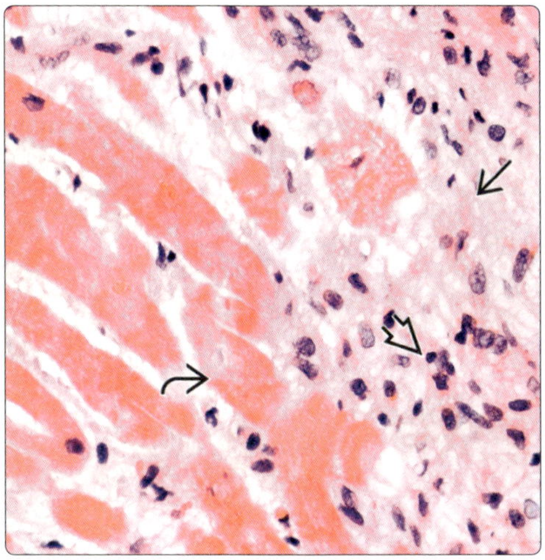

Eosinophilic Myocarditis, Subacute Stage

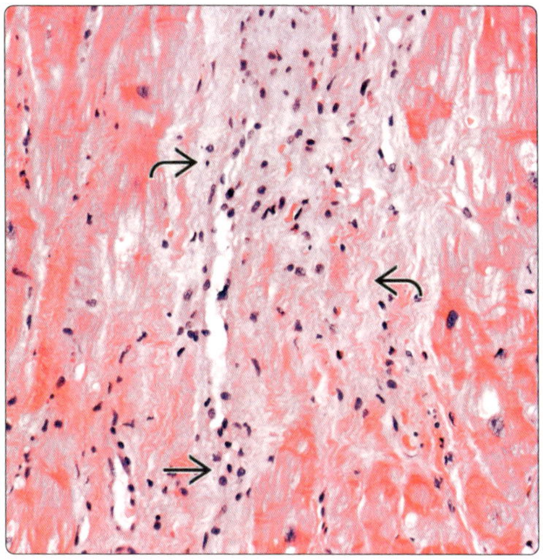

(Left) *In the subacute phase of eosinophilic myocarditis, eosinophils may be sparse among the organizing interstitial inflammation. Myocyte damage and early interstitial fibrosis are also seen in this field.* **(Right)** *Subacute (thrombotic) phase of eosinophilic myocarditis shows interstitial fibrosis with focal inflammatory infiltrate with rare eosinophils.*

Eosinophilic Myocarditis, Chronic Stage

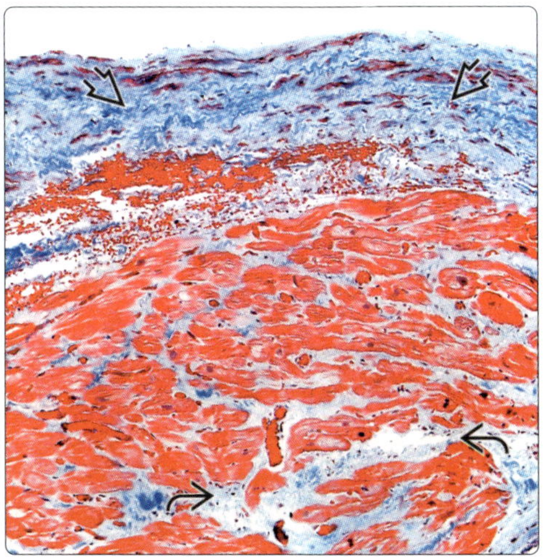

Immunofluorescence Findings in Eosinophilic Myocarditis

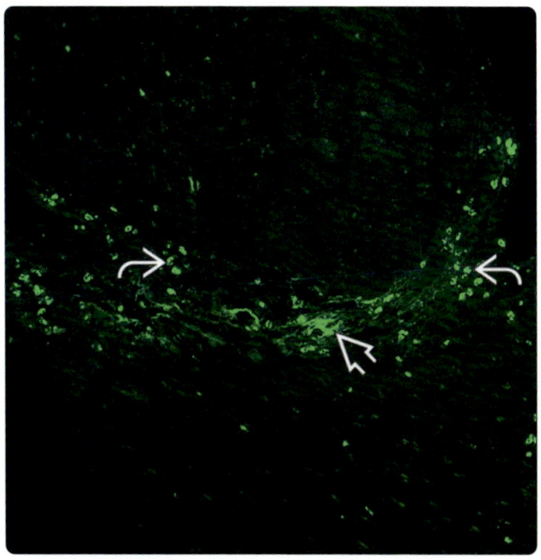

(Left) *Chronic (fibrotic) phase of eosinophilic endomyocardial disease shows dense fibrosis of the endocardium and patchy myocardial fibrosis. Inflammatory infiltrate is not identified.* **(Right)** *Immunofluorescence staining for eosinophil major basic protein shows bright staining of eosinophils but also more diffuse staining of released protein from degranulation.*

Sarcoidosis, Heart

KEY FACTS

TERMINOLOGY

- Chronic disorder of unknown etiology characterized by nonnecrotizing granulomatous inflammation involving multiple organs and systems, including heart

CLINICAL ISSUES

- Conduction disturbances [atrioventricular (AV) delay, bundle branch block]
- Arrhythmias (atrial, ventricular)
- Congestive heart failure
- Sudden death
- Hypercalcemia
- Increased serum angiotensin-converting enzyme
- 10.9 per 100,000 White Americans
- 35.5 per 100,000 Black Americans
- 20-30% heart involvement in autopsy series
- Young/middle-aged adults (30-50 years)
- Females slightly more affected than males

MACROSCOPIC

- Diffuse yellow, white-gray, irregular myocardial coloration
- Diffuse or focal areas of fibrosis
- Focal expanding yellow areas in basal interventricular septum
- Regional left ventricle aneurysm

MICROSCOPIC

- Nonnecrotizing epithelioid granulomas with giant cells with intracytoplasmic inclusions
- Diffuse or focal interstitial fibrosis
- Small coronary arteries may be involved
- Multinucleated giant cell inclusions
  - Schaumann bodies: Oval, concentrically laminated, calcified, intracytoplasmic inclusion
  - Asteroid bodies: Stellate-shaped with cytoplasmic clearing

(Left) *Left ventricle short-axis DE MR shows patchy, subepicardial delayed enhancement* ➔ *in a patient with cardiac sarcoidosis. (Courtesy R. Cury, MD and A. Sarwar, MD.)* **(Right)** *Transverse section of the left ventricle of the heart involved by sarcoidosis shows white areas of discoloration of myocardium involving free and posterolateral wall* ➔*.*

Findings in Sarcoidosis

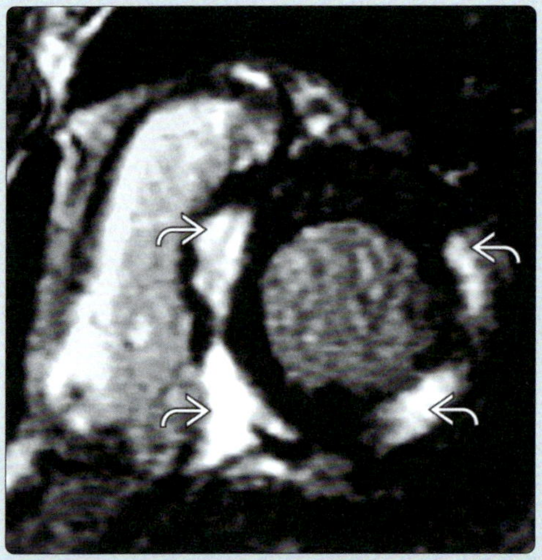

Left Ventricle Involved by Sarcoidosis

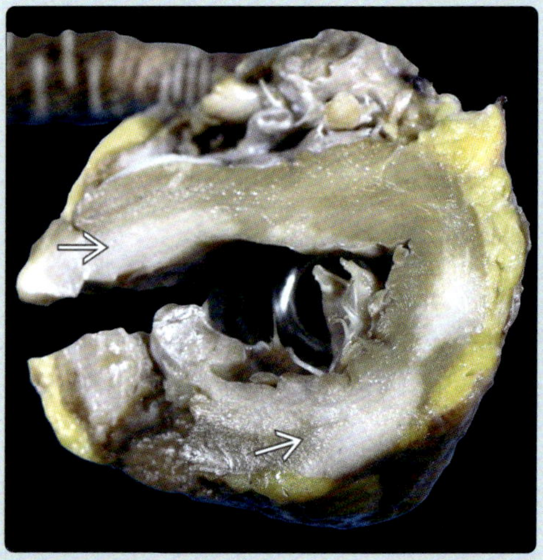

(Left) *Low-power view of myocardial biopsy shows nonnecrotizing granulomas with numerous multinucleated giant cells* ➔ *admixed with mononuclear inflammatory infiltrate* ➔*.* **(Right)** *Small but well-formed granuloma shows a central multinucleated giant cell* ➔ *in the interstitial space between otherwise intact myocytes. There is a sharp line of demarcation between the myocardium and granuloma, and no myocyte injury is seen.*

Nonnecrotizing Granulomatous Inflammation

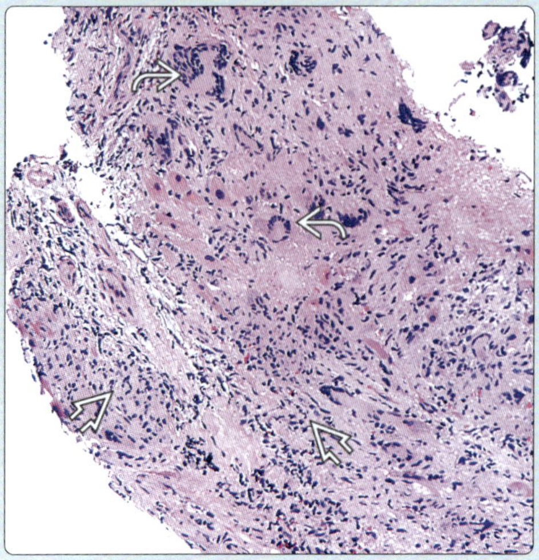

Cardiac Sarcoid: Higher Magnification

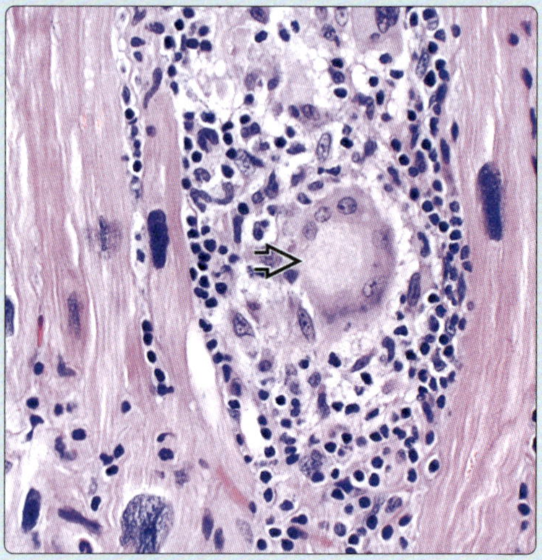

TERMINOLOGY

Definitions

- Chronic disorder of unknown etiology characterized by nonnecrotizing granulomatous inflammation involving multiple organs and systems, including heart

CLINICAL ISSUES

Epidemiology

- Incidence
  - Incidence/prevalence of sarcoidosis varies widely by sex, age, ethnicity, and geographic location
    - 10.9 per 100,000 White Americans
    - 35.5 per 100,000 Black Americans
  - Cardiac involvement occurs in 5-10% of systemic sarcoidosis and may be primary and only presenting feature
    - Autopsy studies and advanced imaging indicate prevalence of 20-25% heart involvement
- Age
  - Young/middle-aged adults (30-50 years)
- Sex
  - Females slightly more affected than males
- Ethnicity
  - Black Americans more commonly involved in USA
  - High incidence of sarcoidosis has been reported in Scandinavia, Japan, and Ireland

Presentation

- Conduction disturbances [atrioventricular (AV) delay, bundle branch block]
- Arrhythmias (atrial, ventricular)
- Sudden death (15%)
- Congestive heart failure (2x higher than general population)
- Asymptomatic in 20-25% of patients

Laboratory Tests

- Elevated serum/urine calcium level
- Increased serum angiotensin-converting enzyme
- Increased levels of IL-2, IL-10, IL-6, and interferon-γ

Treatment

- Surgical approaches
  - Heart transplant, pacemaker, implantable cardioverter defibrillator
- Drugs
  - Corticosteroids are mainstay of treatment; methotrexate and TNF-α inhibitors are also recommended
  - Standard heart failure medication and antiarrhythmics

Prognosis

- Poor when heart failure has developed
- 13-25% of deaths from sarcoidosis due to heart involvement
- 10-year survival in 60-90% of cases

IMAGING

Ultrasonographic Findings

- Left ventricle (LV) dilatation and dysfunction
- LV wall focal/diffuse motion abnormalities
- Wall thinning/thickening and echogenicity increase (basal interventricular septum)

MR Findings

- Structural (wall thinning, chamber dilatation, aneurysm) and ventricular function abnormalities
- Late gadolinium enhancement in multifocal, nonischemic pattern involving basal to midseptum of LV that could extend to right ventricle (RV)
- Increased signal intensity in T2 in ventricular septum

FDG PET

- Mismatch pattern of perfusion defects and myocardial inflammation are characteristic

EKG

- T-wave abnormalities, intraventricular/atrioventricular blocks; Q waves present

MACROSCOPIC

General Features

- Diffuse/focal yellow, white-gray, irregular, tumor-like myocardial infiltrates
- Diffuse or focal areas of fibrosis most prominent in LV free wall and basal septum
- Ventricular dilatation and regional LV aneurysm
- Pericardial thickening

MICROSCOPIC

Histologic Features

- Noncaseating epithelioid granulomas and multinucleated giant cells in transmural or focal distribution
- Transmural or focal interstitial fibrosis in scarring stage
- Rare/absent eosinophils
- Multinucleated giant cell inclusions
  - Schaumann bodies: Oval, concentrically laminated, calcified, intracytoplasmic inclusion
  - Asteroid bodies: Stellate-shaped with cytoplasmic clearing

DIFFERENTIAL DIAGNOSIS

Giant Cell Myocarditis

- Absence of well-formed granulomas
- Numerous eosinophils and necrosis present
- Significant fibrosis not seen acutely

Fungal/Mycobacterial Infections

- Granulomas with central necrosis
- Positive special stains for GMS or AFB

DIAGNOSTIC CHECKLIST

Pathologic Interpretation Pearls

- Heart biopsy is highly specific but has low sensitivity (20-30%) due to patchy distribution of granulomatous inflammation

SELECTED REFERENCES

1. Kouranos V et al: Cardiac sarcoidosis: state-of-the-art review. Heart. 107(19):1591-9, 2021

Acute Rheumatic Carditis

KEY FACTS

TERMINOLOGY

- Acute, immunologically mediated, multisystemic inflammatory disease occurring few weeks after episode of untreated pharyngeal infection with group A β-hemolytic streptococci, causing pancarditis

CLINICAL ISSUES

- 100 per 100,000 in resource-poor countries
- Heart failure, murmurs
- Pericardial rub/effusion
- Jones criteria
  - Major: Carditis (clinical/subclinical, 50%), mono-/polyarthritis (50-70%), chorea (20%), erythema marginatum (5%), and subcutaneous nodules (3%)
  - Minor: Fever, arthralgias, previous rheumatic fever/rheumatic heart disease, prolonged PR interval in EKG, elevated sedimentation rate, and C-reactive protein (CRP)
  - 2 major or 1 major and 2 minor criteria and evidence of prior streptococcal infection are needed for diagnosis

MACROSCOPIC

- Pericardium: Serofibrinous exudate ("bread and butter" pericarditis)
- Endocardium: Valve swelling and small, flat vegetations along closure line of mitral and aortic valve cusps

MICROSCOPIC

- Myocardium with Aschoff nodules and nonspecific lymphocytic infiltrate
- Valvular vegetations containing predominantly platelets and lymphocytic and histiocytic leaflet infiltrates
- Pericardium with nonspecific inflammatory infiltrate

DIAGNOSTIC CHECKLIST

- Finding Aschoff nodules and Anitschkow cells should prompt review of clinical history for other major Jones criteria

Aschoff Nodule

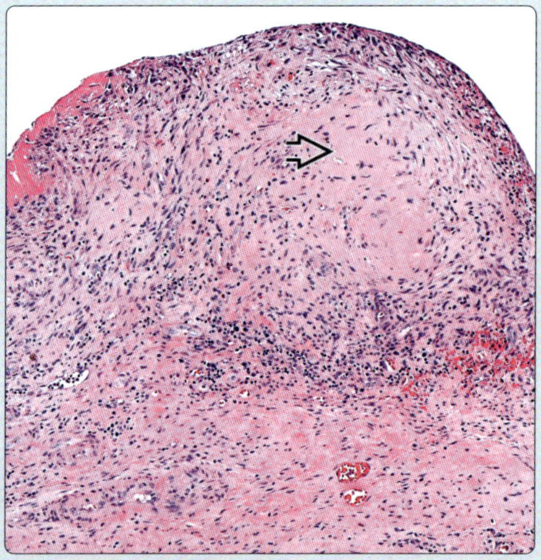

Morphologic Components of Aschoff Nodule

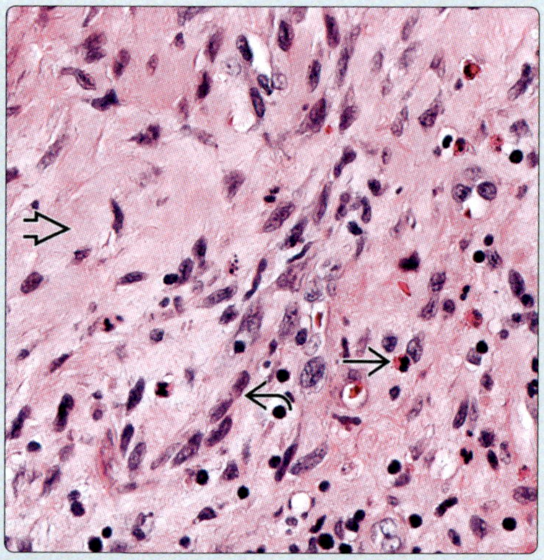

(Left) *H&E-stained section of the myocardium shows an Aschoff nodule with characteristic central eosinophilic connective tissue change → surrounded by mixed inflammatory infiltrate with numerous lymphocytes and histiocytes.* **(Right)** *H&E-stained section of the myocardium at higher power shows an Aschoff nodule with characteristic eosinophilic connective tissue change → surrounded by histiocytes →, lymphocytes, and eosinophils →.*

Anitschkow Cells

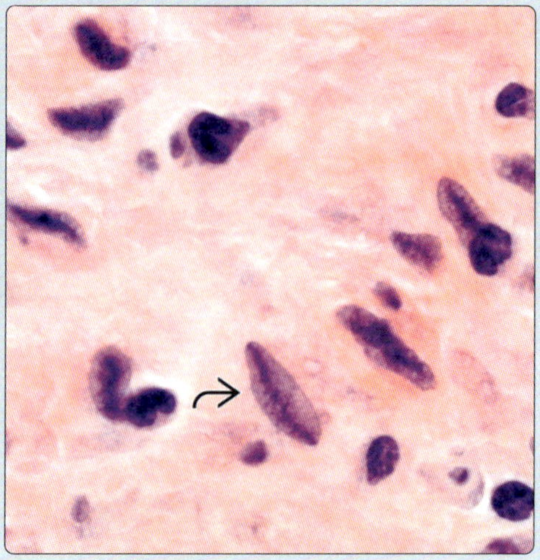

Aschoff Nodule and Anitschkow Cells

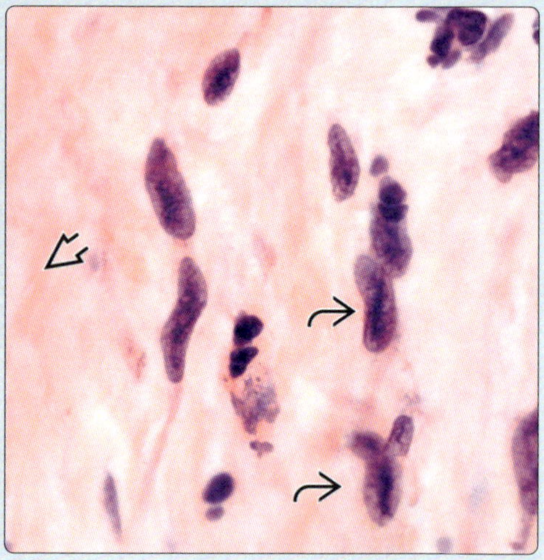

(Left) *H&E-stained section of the myocardium at higher power shows the central portion of an Aschoff nodule with an eosinophilic center surrounded by histiocytes with a central chromatic bar → (Anitschkow cells).* **(Right)** *H&E-stained section of the myocardium at higher power shows an Aschoff nodule with central eosinophilic connective tissue change → surrounded by histiocytes with a central bar of nuclear chromatin (Anitschkow cells) →, characteristic of acute rheumatic fever (ARF).*

TERMINOLOGY

Abbreviations

- Acute rheumatic fever (ARF)

Definitions

- Acute, immunologically mediated, multisystemic inflammatory disease occurring few weeks after episode of untreated pharyngeal infection with group A β-hemolytic streptococci, causing pancarditis

ETIOLOGY/PATHOGENESIS

Infectious Agents

- Heart injury is due to humoral and cellular immune-mediated reaction to streptococcal antigens
- Strains of M types 1, 3, 5, 6, and 18 are more rheumatogenic
- Susceptibility to rheumatic fever has been linked to different HLA class II subtypes in different populations (DR7, DQA1, DQB1)
- Cross reactivity between streptococcal antigens and human heart tissue (myosin and tropomyosin in heart muscle; laminin and vimentin in heart valves) mediates tissue injury
- Immune complexes and complement activation may contribute to valve inflammation

CLINICAL ISSUES

Epidemiology

- Incidence
  - 100 per 100,000 in resource-poor countries
  - < 2 per 100,000 in resource-rich countries
- Age
  - 5-15 years
- Sex
  - No predilection
- In resource-poor countries, ARF is major cause of death from cardiac disease in young people
- Recurrence is most common in first 5 years after initial episode; can occur in up to 75% of patients not receiving secondary prophylaxis
- Progression to rheumatic heart disease occurs in ~ 60% of untreated cases

Presentation

- Heart: Heart failure, arrhythmias and conduction abnormalities, chest pain, pericardial rub/effusion, new-onset murmurs
- Skin: Erythema marginatum, subcutaneous nodules
- Joint: Arthralgias &/or polyarthritis
- Systemic: Fever

Laboratory Tests

- Elevated erythrocyte sedimentation rate (ESR) > 60 mm/hr
- Elevated C-reactive protein (CRP) > 3 mg/dL
- Elevated antistreptolysin-O (ASO) titer
- Throat swab for rapid antigen detection test &/or culture positive for *Streptococcus*

Treatment

- Drugs
  - Antibiotics (penicillin 10-day course) for acute pharyngitis and prevention of development of ARF
  - Antiinflammatories (salicylates, corticosteroids)
  - Secondary prophylaxis with antibiotics (benzathine penicillin G) to prevent recurrence

Prognosis

- Good with treatment

Diagnostic Criteria (Jones Criteria, Modified 2015)

- Major criteria include carditis (clinical/subclinical-diagnosed by echocardiography, 50%), mono-/polyarthritis (50-70%), chorea (20%), erythema marginatum (5%), and subcutaneous nodules (3%)
- Minor criteria include fever, arthralgias, prolonged PR interval in EKG, and elevated ESR and CRP
- 2 major or 1 major and 2 minor criteria and evidence of prior streptococcal infection (positive culture of throat swab &/or rising ASO titre) are needed for diagnosis

MACROSCOPIC

General Features

- Pericardium: Serofibrinous exudate ("bread and butter" pericarditis)
- Endocardium: Valve swelling and small, flat vegetations along closure line of mitral and aortic valve cusps

MICROSCOPIC

Histologic Features

- Pericardium
  - Nonspecific inflammatory infiltrate
- Myocardium
  - Aschoff nodule
    - Central focus of smudged, slightly eosinophilic-appearing connective tissue (fibrinoid necrosis)
    - Multinucleated giant cells (Aschoff giant cells) and histiocytes with long central bar of nuclear chromatin (Anitschkow/"caterpillar" cells)
    - Most commonly present in interventricular septum, left ventricle wall, and left atrial appendage
  - Nonspecific lymphocytic infiltrate
- Valvular endocardium
  - Vegetations containing predominantly platelets on rough zone of valve leaflets
  - Lymphocytic and histiocytic leaflet infiltrates
  - Rarely Aschoff nodules
  - Neovascularization of leaflets

SELECTED REFERENCES

1. Dooley LM et al: Rheumatic heart disease: a review of the current status of global research activity. Autoimmun Rev. 20(2):102740, 2021
2. Lahiri S et al: Acute rheumatic fever. Pediatr Rev. 42(5):221-32, 2021
3. Ralph AP et al: The 2020 Australian guideline for prevention, diagnosis and management of acute rheumatic fever and rheumatic heart disease. Med J Aust. 214(5):220-7, 2021
4. Arvind B et al: Rheumatic fever and rheumatic heart disease in children. Indian J Pediatr. 87(4):305-11, 2020
5. Sable C: Update on prevention and management of rheumatic heart disease. Pediatr Clin North Am. 67(5):843-53, 2020
6. Gewitz MH et al: Revision of the Jones Criteria for the diagnosis of acute rheumatic fever in the era of Doppler echocardiography: a scientific statement from the American Heart Association. Circulation. 131(20):1806-18, 2015
7. Webb RH et al: Acute rheumatic fever. BMJ. 351:h3443, 2015

(Left) *H&E-stained section of the mitral valve shows an Aschoff nodule with characteristic central eosinophilic connective tissue change* ⇨ *surrounded by mixed inflammatory infiltrate with numerous lymphocytes and histiocytes.* **(Right)** *H&E-stained section of the mitral valve at higher power shows an Aschoff nodule with central eosinophilic connective tissue change* ⇨ *surrounded by mixed inflammatory infiltrate with numerous lymphocytes and histiocytes. It is unusual to find these nodules in the valves.*

Mitral Valvulitis

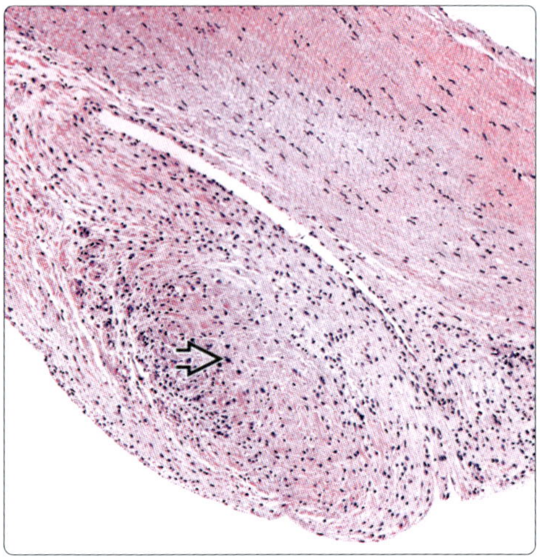

Aschoff Nodule Involving Mitral Valve

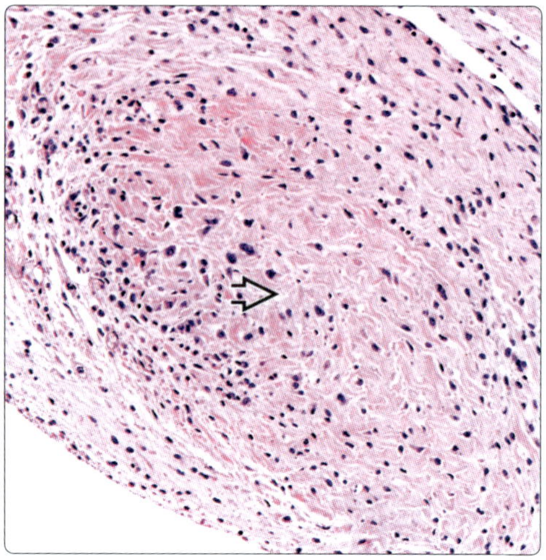

(Left) *H&E-stained section of the mitral valve at higher power shows the inflammatory infiltrate of an Aschoff nodule composed of numerous lymphocytes and histiocytes, some of which are multinucleated giant cells (Aschoff giant cells)* ⇨*.* **(Right)** *H&E-stained section of the mitral valve at higher power shows nonspecific inflammatory infiltrate composed of lymphocytes, neutrophils, and histiocytes. There is also vascular proliferation and congestion.*

Aschoff Giant Cells

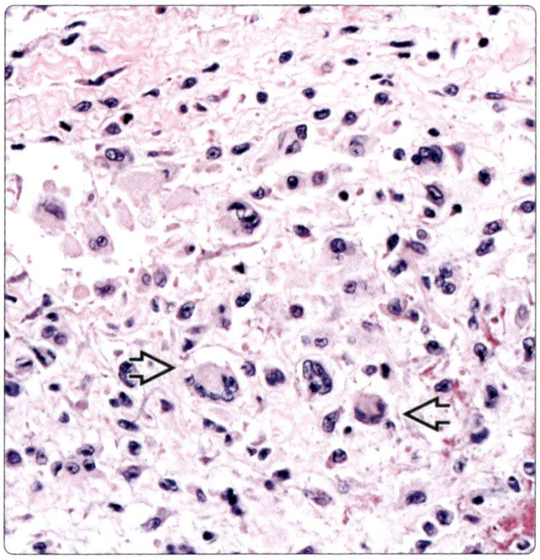

Histologic Changes of Heart Valve

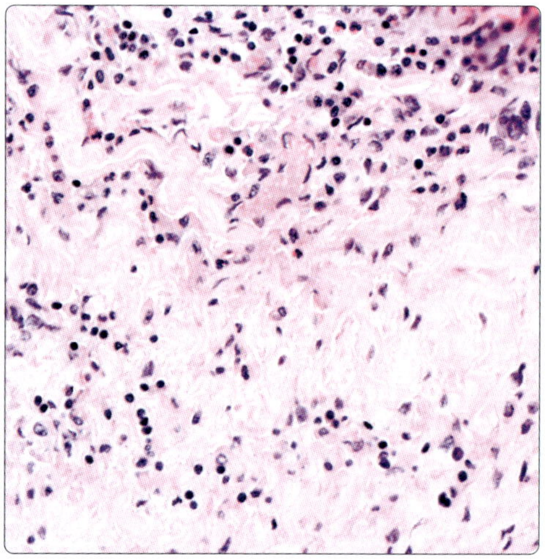

(Left) *H&E-stained section of the myocardium shows an Aschoff nodule with central eosinophilic connective tissue change* ⇨ *surrounded by mixed inflammatory infiltrate with numerous lymphocytes and histiocytes. There is also interstitial edema.* **(Right)** *H&E-stained section of the myocardium shows the mixed inflammatory infiltrate of an Aschoff nodule with numerous lymphocytes and histiocytes, some of them forming multinucleated giant cells (Aschoff giant cells)* ⇨ *admixed with Anitschkow cells* →*.*

Myocardium Involvement

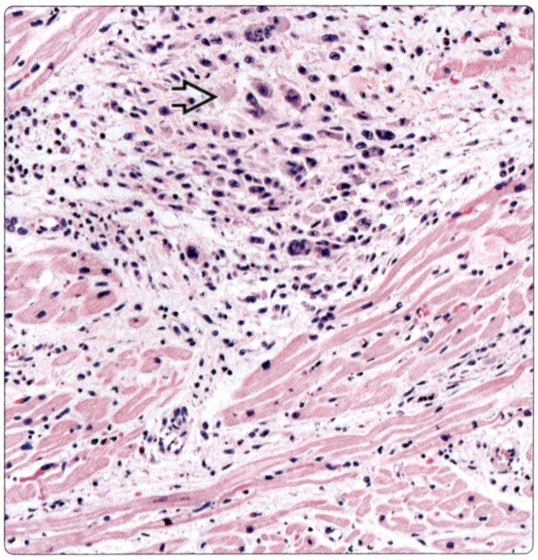

Aschoff Giant Cells and Inflammatory Components of Aschoff Nodule

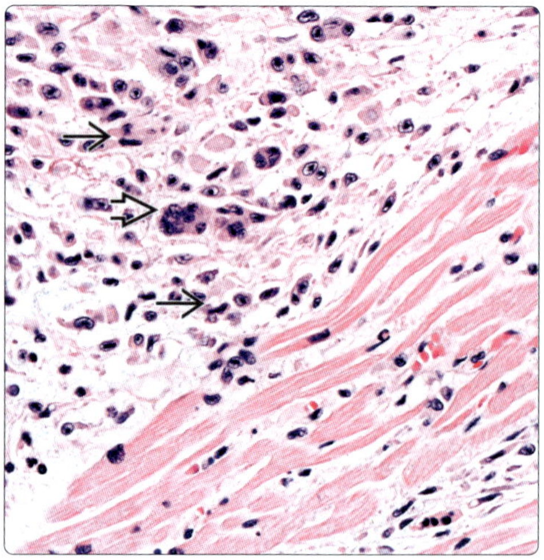

Myocardial Changes

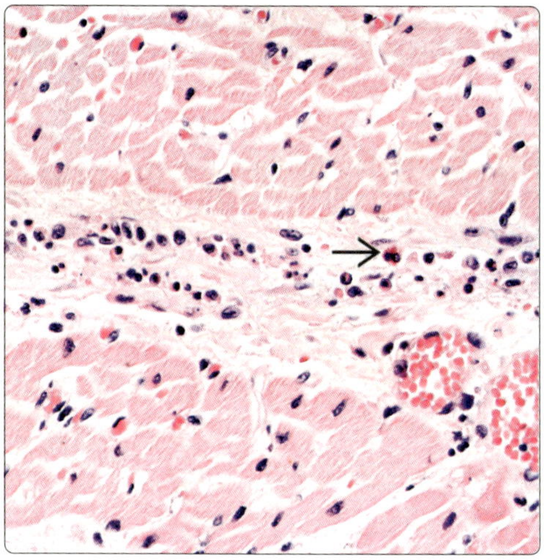

Histologic Features of Aschoff Nodule

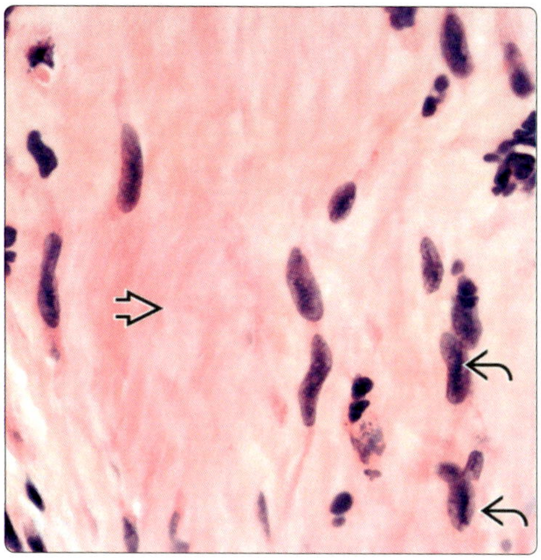

(Left) *H&E-stained section of the myocardium shows interstitial edema, vascular congestion, and a mixed inflammatory infiltrate with numerous lymphocytes and histiocytes as well as occasional eosinophils →. Occasionally, well-defined Aschoff nodules are not seen.* **(Right)** *H&E-stained section of the myocardium shows an Aschoff nodule with central eosinophilic connective tissue change ⇨ surrounded by histiocytes with a central bar of nuclear chromatin (Anitschkow cells) ↶, characteristic of ARF.*

Histologic Components of Aschoff Nodule

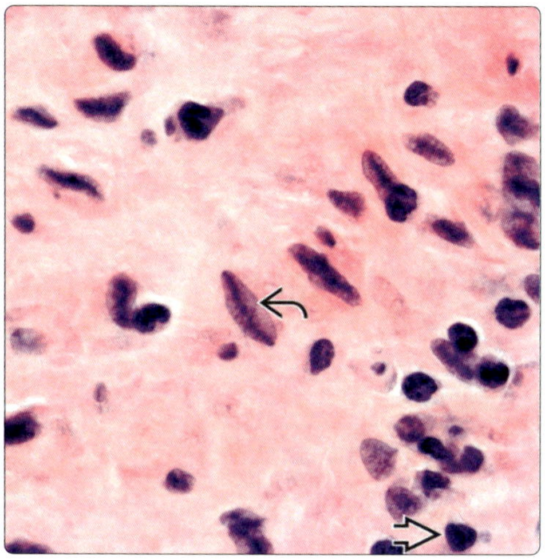

Cross Section of Anitschkow Cells

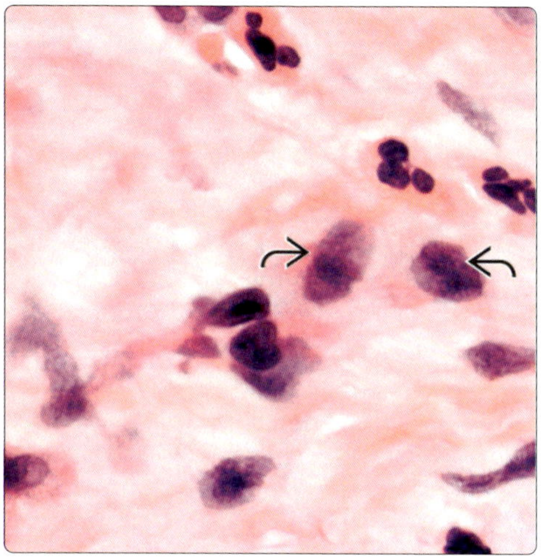

(Left) *H&E-stained section of the myocardium at higher power shows the inflammatory component of an Aschoff nodule composed of lymphocytes ⇨ and histiocytes with a central bar of nuclear chromatin (Anitschkow cells) ↶, characteristic of ARF.* **(Right)** *H&E-stained section of the myocardium shows the inflammatory component of an Aschoff nodule with Anitschkow cells ↶ in cross section with an owl-eyes appearance.*

Pericardial Involvement

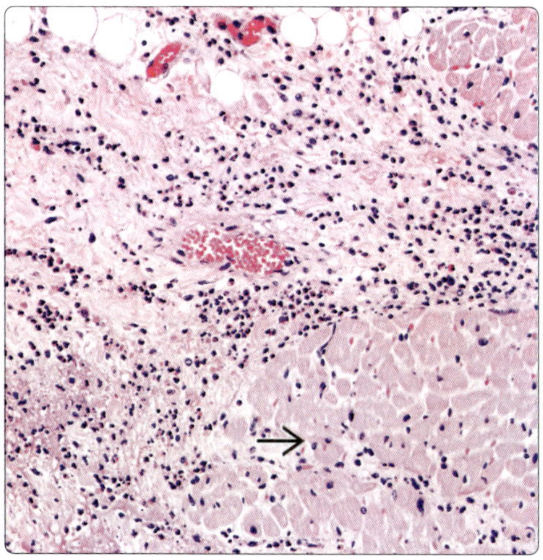

Pericardial Involvement

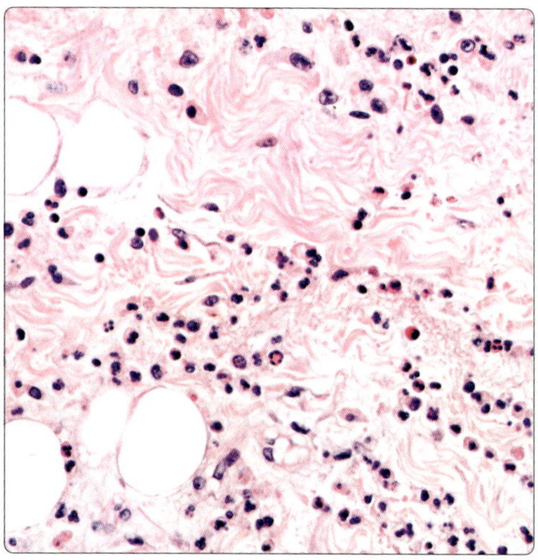

(Left) *H&E-stained section of the pericardium shows nonspecific inflammatory infiltrate composed of lymphocytes, neutrophils, and histiocytes. There is also vascular proliferation and congestion. The adjacent myocardium appears uninvolved →.* **(Right)** *H&E-stained section of the pericardium at higher power shows nonspecific inflammatory infiltrate composed of lymphocytes, neutrophils, and histiocytes. In ARF, all of the heart layers are involved by this process.*

Eosinophilic Granulomatosis With Polyangiitis

KEY FACTS

TERMINOLOGY

- Multisystemic disorder characterized by necrotizing small/medium-sized vessel vasculitis with extravascular granulomas, eosinophilic infiltrates in multiple organs, peripheral eosinophilia, asthma

ETIOLOGY/PATHOGENESIS

- Possible mechanisms include
  - Antineutrophil cytoplasmic antibodies (ANCA)
  - Th1-/Th2-mediated immune response
  - Direct damage caused by eosinophils
  - IL mediated

CLINICAL ISSUES

- 0.5-6.8 cases/1 million/year
- Heart involvement occurs in 15-60% of cases and more often is ANCA negative
- Presentation
  - Arrhythmias
  - Acute pericarditis
  - Eosinophilia: > 10% of differential white blood cell count
  - Restrictive cardiomyopathy (late)
  - Positive MPO-ANCA in 30-40% of cases
  - Cardiac involvement is associated with 50% mortality
  - Kidney manifestations include acute renal failure with rapidly progressive glomerulonephritis

MICROSCOPIC

- Perivascular eosinophilic infiltrates in myocardium and endocardium
- Granulomas
- Eosinophilic infiltrates
- Coronary artery vasculitis

TOP DIFFERENTIAL DIAGNOSES

- Granulomatosis with polyangiitis
- Parasitic infection
- Hypereosinophilic syndrome

Myocardial Changes

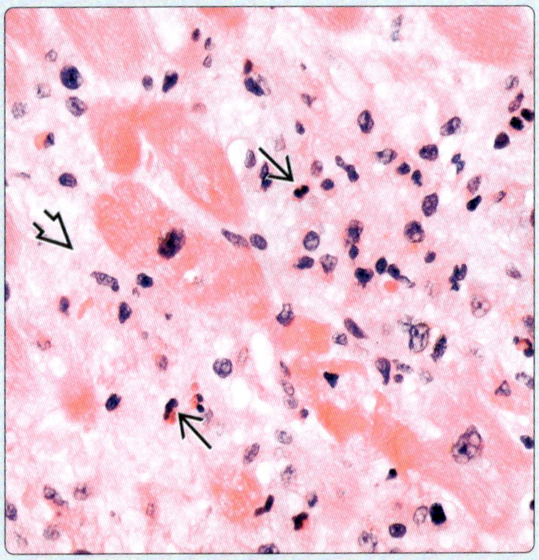

Myocardial Changes

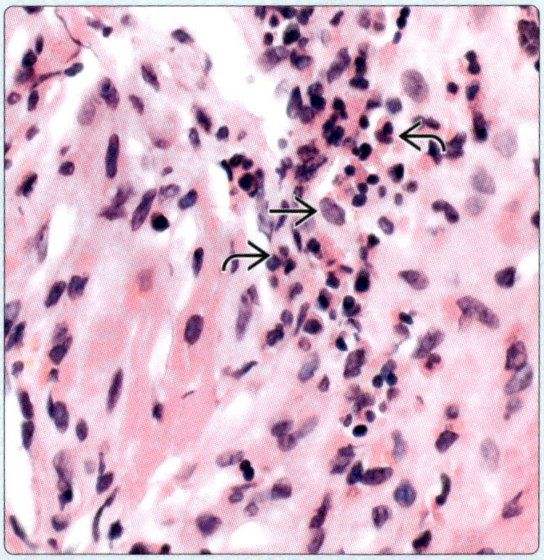

(Left) *H&E-stained section of the myocardium shows interstitial edema ⇨ and interstitial inflammatory infiltrate with frequent eosinophils →.* **(Right)** *H&E-stained section of the myocardium shows interstitial inflammatory infiltrate with prominent eosinophils ↪ and associated myocyte injury →.*

Endocardial and Myocardial Changes

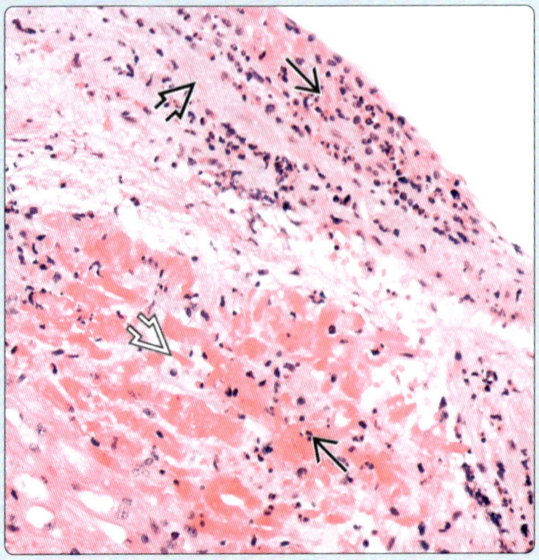

Vascular Changes

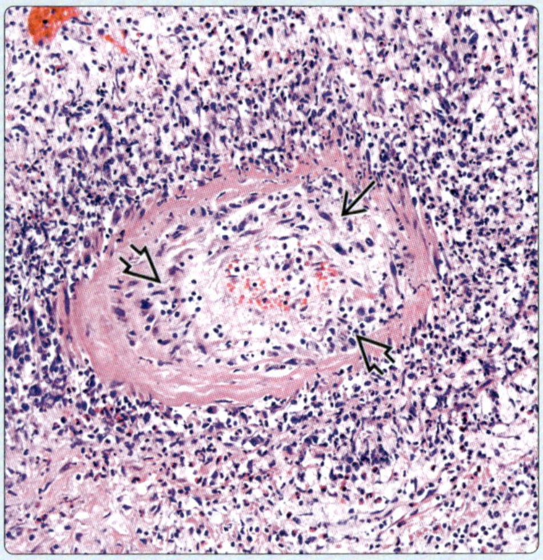

(Left) *Endocardium and myocardium show extensive inflammatory infiltrate with numerous eosinophils →. Endocardial thickening ⇨ and myocyte necrosis ➡ are also present.* **(Right)** *Small vessel cross section from the kidney shows fibrinoid change in the wall, endothelial swelling ⇨ with luminal occlusion, and transmural mixed inflammatory infiltrate with frequent eosinophils → as well as marked mixed perivascular inflammation.*

TERMINOLOGY

Abbreviations

- Eosinophilic granulomatosis with polyangiitis (EGPA)

Definitions

- Multisystemic disorder characterized by necrotizing small/medium-sized vessel vasculitis with extravascular granulomas, eosinophilic infiltrates in multiple organs, peripheral eosinophilia, asthma

ETIOLOGY/PATHOGENESIS

Unknown

- Genetic and environmental factors are contributory to development of EGPA
  - HLA-DQ has been identified as risk allele and is associated with ANCA-positive EGPA
  - Variants at *GATA3*, *TSLP*, *LPP*, and *BACH2* contribute to eosinophilic inflammation
  - Variants at *IRF1/IL5* and *GPA33* are associated with ANCA-negative EGPA
- Possible mechanisms include
  - Antineutrophil cytoplasmic antibodies (ANCA)
  - Th1-/Th2-mediated immune response
  - Direct damage caused by eosinophils
  - IL-5 mediated

CLINICAL ISSUES

Epidemiology

- Incidence
  - 0.5-6.8 cases/1 million/year
  - Heart involvement occurs in 15-30% of cases and, more often, is ANCA negative
- Age
  - Peak incidence: 35-50 years
- Sex
  - No predilection

Presentation

- Prodromic phase: Asthma, rhinosinusitis
- Eosinophilic phase: Peripheral eosinophilia and eosinophilic infiltration of organs
  - Heart: Arrhythmias, sudden death; acute pericarditis/effusion &/or tamponade; myocarditis/myocardial infarction, valvular disease, intraventricular thrombosis, restrictive cardiomyopathy (late)
  - Lung: Respiratory failure, noncavitating nodules, alveolar hemorrhagic syndrome
  - Gastrointestinal: Hemorrhage, abdominal pain, vomiting
- Vasculitic phase
  - Renal disease: Rapidly progressive glomerulonephritis
  - Peripheral neuropathy; sensorial/motor/central nervous system manifestations
  - Skin lesions: Purpura

Laboratory Tests

- Elevated C-reactive protein and IgE levels
- Eosinophilia: > 10% of differential white blood cell count
- Positive ANCA in 30-40% of cases, typically anti-MPO

Treatment

- Drugs
  - Steroids, cyclophosphamide, IL-5 blockers, methotrexate, rituximab

Prognosis

- Cardiac involvement associated with 50% mortality
- Higher eosinophilic count is associated with increased disease activity and cardiac involvement

IMAGING

Radiographic Findings

- Chest x-ray
  - Multifocal lung interstitial infiltrates
  - Noncavitating pulmonary nodules

MR Findings

- Heart shows late gadolinium enhancement
- Apical, midleft ventricle segment and subendocardial enhancement

MICROSCOPIC

Histologic Features

- Heart
  - Perivascular eosinophilic infiltrates in myocardium, endocardium, and pericardium
  - Granulomas
  - Myocyte necrosis and myocytolysis
  - Mural thrombi
  - Acute fibrinous pericarditis
  - Coronary artery vasculitis
- Kidney
  - Necrotizing crescentic glomerulonephritis
  - Interstitial nephritis with numerous eosinophils
- Lungs, other organs
  - Eosinophilic infiltrates
  - Granulomas

DIFFERENTIAL DIAGNOSIS

Hypereosinophilic Syndrome

- Negative history of asthma or vasculitis
- Association with myeloproliferative disorders
- Endocardial fibrosis (late)
- Ventricular apical necrosis and mural thrombosis

SELECTED REFERENCES

1. Sartorelli S et al: Revisiting characteristics, treatment and outcome of cardiomyopathy in eosinophilic granulomatosis with polyangiitis (Churg-Strauss). Rheumatology (Oxford). 61(3):1175-84, 2022
2. Garcia-Vives E et al: Heart disease in eosinophilic granulomatosis with polyangiitis (EGPA) patients: a screening approach proposal. Rheumatology (Oxford). 60(10):4538-47, 2021
3. Lagan J et al: Myocardial involvement in eosinophilic granulomatosis with polyangiitis evaluated with cardiopulmonary magnetic resonance. Int J Cardiovasc Imaging. 37(4):1371-81, 2021
4. Uzzo M et al: Novel targets for drug use in eosinophilic granulomatosis with polyangiitis. Front Med (Lausanne). 8:754434, 2021
5. Zampieri M et al: Cardiac involvement in eosinophilic granulomatosis with polyangiitis (formerly Churg-Strauss syndrome): prospective evaluation at a tertiary referral centre. Eur J Intern Med. 85:68-79, 2021
6. Moiseev S et al: International consensus on ANCA testing in eosinophilic granulomatosis with polyangiitis. Am J Respir Crit Care Med. ePub, 2020

KEY FACTS

TERMINOLOGY

- Inflammation of myocardium due to infection

CLINICAL ISSUES

- Epstein-Barr virus (EBV) accounts for ~ 1% of all cases of viral myocarditis
- Cytomegalovirus (CMV) myocarditis is more common in immunosuppressed (especially HIV and transplant) patients but can occur in immunocompetent patients as well
- CMV myocarditis can also affect pericardium (myopericarditis) and lead to dilated cardiomyopathy
- Nonspecific chest pain with EKG abnormalities and elevated cardiac enzymes
- In immunosuppressed patients, CMV myocarditis carries 60% risk of mortality

IMAGING

- Cardiac MR can detect myocyte injury, indicative of myocarditis

MICROSCOPIC

- Somewhat nonspecific histologic findings
- Mononuclear cell infiltrate of varying intensity
- Myocyte necrosis
- Disarray of myocardial cells
- CMV myocarditis may show cytoplasmic and nuclear basophilic inclusions resembling owl eyes and perinuclear halo and cytomegaly

ANCILLARY TESTS

- Both EBV and CMV myocarditis are typically diagnosed using serology and excluding other possible infections or etiologies
- FISH can detect EBV virus in myocytes
- Positive IgM for either virus indicates acute infection

TOP DIFFERENTIAL DIAGNOSES

- Myocarditis due to other causes

(Left) *Epstein-Barr virus (EBV) myocarditis may show nonspecific histologic findings with a predominantly lymphocytic infiltrate and disarray of myocardial cells. (Courtesy P. Morrow, MD.)* **(Right)** *EBER in situ hybridization (ISH) demonstrates positive brown staining of lymphocytes ➔, confirming infection with EBV. (Courtesy P. Morrow, MD.)*

Histologic Findings in EBV Myocarditis

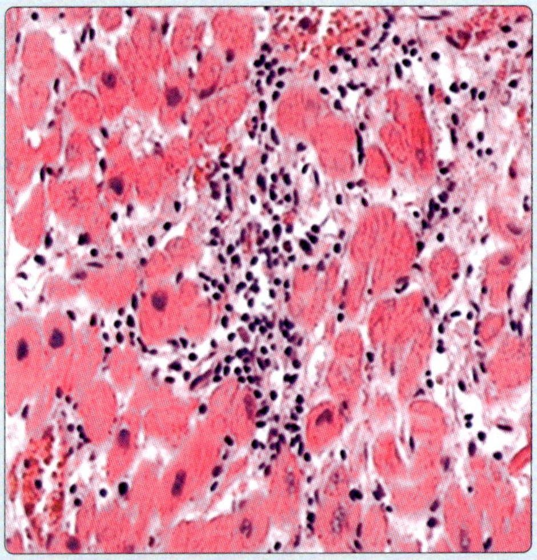

In Situ Hybridization for EBER

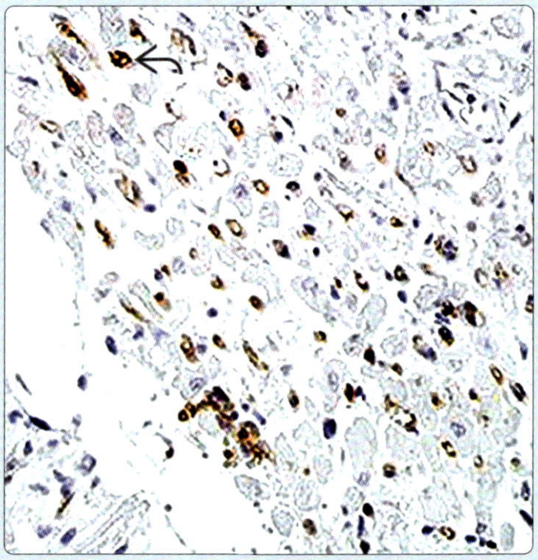

(Left) *Viral myocarditis demonstrates a sparse mononuclear infiltrate with some myocyte necrosis ➔. Without proper clinical context and appropriate serologic studies, this would be indistinguishable from other causes of myocarditis.* **(Right)** *In cytomegalovirus myocarditis, characteristic nuclear basophilic inclusions can be seen ➔. (Courtesy M. Graham, MD.)*

Histologic Findings in Viral Myocarditis

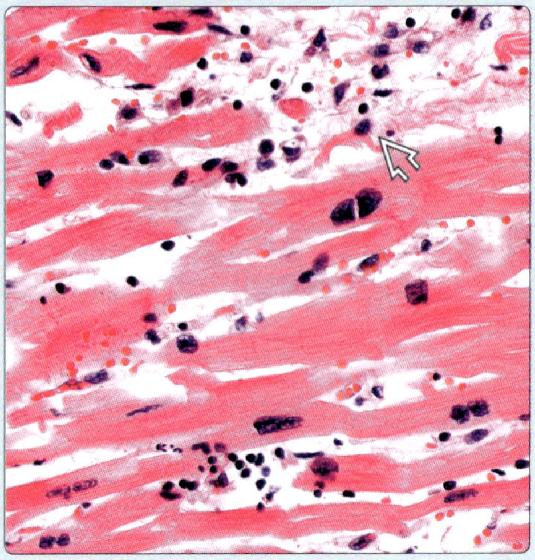

Histologic Findings in Cytomegalovirus Myocarditis

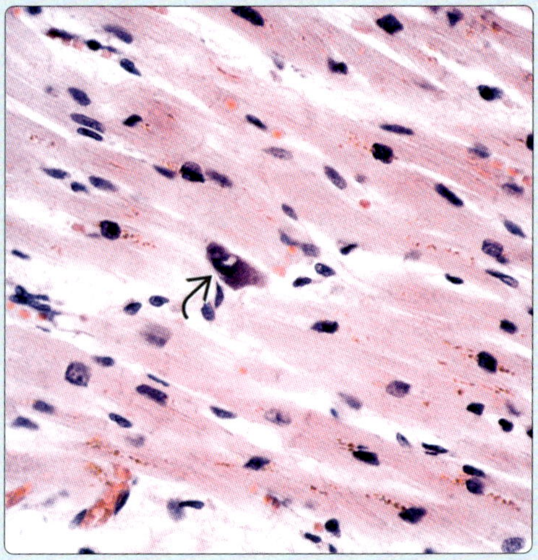

TERMINOLOGY

Definitions

- Many viruses have etiologic role in myocarditis; this document focuses on 2 specific viruses as prototypical of the remainder
  - Inflammation of myocardium due to infection with Epstein-Barr virus (EBV) or Cytomegalovirus (CMV)

ETIOLOGY/PATHOGENESIS

Infectious Agents

- EBV is member of herpesvirus family; causes recurring and persistent infection infrequently resulting in myocarditis
- CMV is also member of herpesvirus family with estimated seroprevalence of 40-70% in adult population
  - More frequently in immunosuppressed (e.g., HIV and transplant) patients

CLINICAL ISSUES

Epidemiology

- Incidence
  - EBV accounts for ~ 1% of all cases of viral myocarditis
  - CMV accounts for 1-7% of all cases of viral myocarditis, depending on study

Presentation

- Similar for both EBV and CMV myocarditis
  - Chest pain with EKG abnormalities and elevated cardiac enzymes
  - Congestive heart failure
  - Palpitations
  - Rarely, sudden death
  - Fever
  - Anecdotal reports of dilated cardiomyopathy in children with EBV myocarditis
  - CMV myocarditis can also affect pericardium (myopericarditis) and lead to dilated cardiomyopathy

Prognosis

- In immunosuppressed patients, CMV myocarditis carries 60% risk of mortality

IMAGING

MR Findings

- Cardiac MR can detect myocyte injury, capillary leakage, and edema, indicative of myocarditis

MICROSCOPIC

Histologic Features

- EBV and CMV myocarditis
  - Somewhat nonspecific histologic findings
  - Mononuclear cell infiltrate of varying intensity
  - Myocyte necrosis

Cytologic Features

- CMV myocarditis may show cytoplasmic and nuclear basophilic inclusions resembling owl eyes
  - May also show perinuclear halo and cytomegaly

ANCILLARY TESTS

In Situ Hybridization

- In situ hybridization (ISH) can detect EBV (EBER transcripts)

PCR

- For viral identification as well as quantification of viral loads

Serologic Testing

- EBV and CMV myocarditis are typically diagnosed using serology and excluding other possible infections or etiologies
  - Positive IgM for either indicates acute infection
  - Increase in IgG titer in convalescent sera also supportive

Culture

- Can be used for both, but less specific due to high seroprevalence of both viruses in immunocompetent patients (presence does not prove causality)

DIFFERENTIAL DIAGNOSIS

Myocarditis Due to Other Causes

- Viruses are most common cause of myocarditis
  - Coxsackie B virus, influenza virus, Adenovirus, echovirus, HIV, and Parvovirus B19 are other important causes of myocarditis and must be ruled out with ancillary tests and serology
    - Adenovirus may show smudged nuclei with brick-like nuclear inclusions
  - COVID-19 virus is somewhat controversial; definitive cases are relatively rare
- General histologic findings (inflammatory infiltrate, myocyte necrosis/disarray) would be similar

COVID-19 Myocarditis

- Clinically suspected far more often than it is found histologically; data still emerging

DIAGNOSTIC CHECKLIST

Pathologic Interpretation Pearls

- Clinicopathologic correlation with particular attention to serologic studies and other ancillary tests necessary for diagnosis of responsible virus
  - Relying on histology or cytology features alone is not recommended

SELECTED REFERENCES

1. Ammirati E et al: State-of-the-art of endomyocardial biopsy on acute myocarditis and chronic inflammatory cardiomyopathy. Curr Cardiol Rep. 24(5):597-609, 2022
2. Khidr SS et al: Clinical course, viral etiology, and the diagnostic workup for patients with suspected myocarditis: a single-center prospective study. BMC Cardiovasc Disord. 22(1):396, 2022
3. Zheng SY et al: Role of toll-like receptors and Th responses in viral myocarditis. Front Immunol. 13:843891, 2022
4. Shauer A et al: Acute viral myocarditis: current concepts in diagnosis and treatment. Isr Med Assoc J. 15(3):180-5, 2013
5. Vanstechelman F et al: Cytomegalovirus myocarditis in an immunocompetent patient. Acta Cardiol. 67(2):257-60, 2012
6. Mutlu H et al: A rare case of Epstein-Barr virus-induced dilated cardiomyopathy. Heart Lung. 40(1):81-7, 2011
7. Burke M: Viral myocarditis. Histopathology. 17(3):193-200, 1990

Toxoplasmosis, Heart

KEY FACTS

TERMINOLOGY

- Protozoan parasitic infection caused by *Toxoplasma gondii*, which can produce myocarditis as isolated process or as part of disseminated infection

ETIOLOGY/PATHOGENESIS

- Primary infection or reactivation of *T. gondii*
- Risk factors include
  - Immunodeficiency: Primary or acquired
  - Age: Young infants and older adults

CLINICAL ISSUES

- Heart clinical manifestations include
  - Myocarditis: Chest pain, atrial fibrillation, ventricular arrhythmias, heart block, heart failure, sudden death
  - Pericarditis: Pericardial effusion, cardiac tamponade
- May be life threatening in transplanted patients when acquired from donor organ and in immunocompromised hosts

MICROSCOPIC

- Interstitial mononuclear inflammation
- Tachyzoites (smaller, motile, asexually reproducing form) within intracellular vacuoles
- *Toxoplasma* cysts (< 30 μm) containing bradyzoites (larger, crescent-shaped, slowly replicating form)
- Spherical in shape except in muscle cells, where cysts show elongated appearance

ANCILLARY TESTS

- Immunohistochemistry stain demonstrates *Toxoplasma* antigen in inclusions
- PCR enhances diagnostic sensitivity on endomyocardial biopsy

TOP DIFFERENTIAL DIAGNOSES

- *Histoplasma* myocarditis
- Chagas disease

(Left) *H&E section of myocardial biopsy from a patient with Toxoplasma myocarditis shows focal lymphocytic interstitial inflammatory infiltrates →.* **(Right)** *High-power view of myocardial biopsy shows Toxoplasma cysts within myocyte sarcoplasm → containing bradyzoites. Inflammatory reaction is not noted. The inflammatory reaction occurs when the myocyte ruptures and the microorganism is released to the interstitium.*

***Toxoplasma* Myocarditis, Low-Power View**

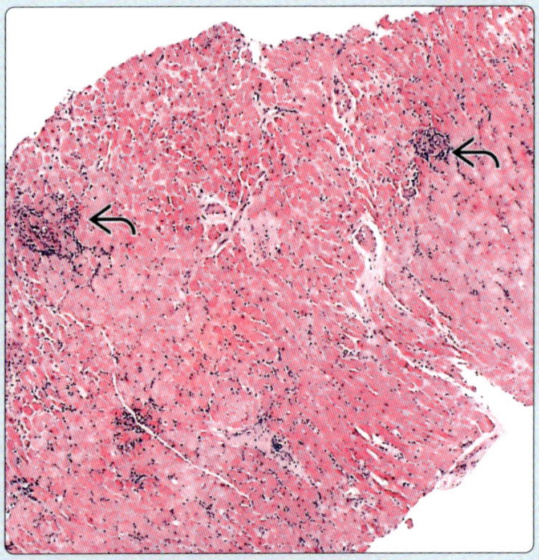

***Toxoplasma* Myocarditis, Intramyocardial Cysts**

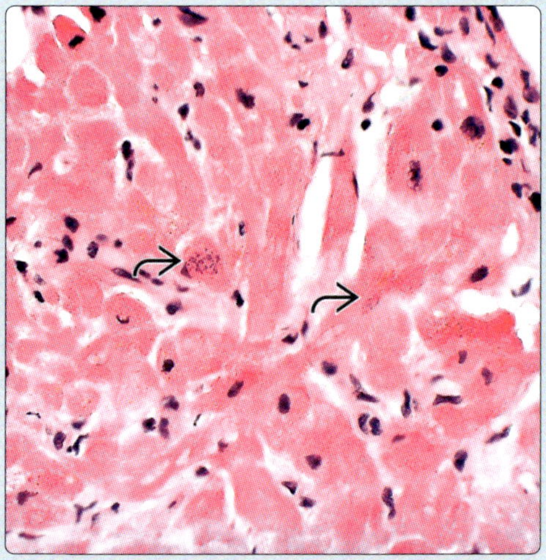

(Left) *High-power view of Toxoplasma myocarditis shows focal lymphocytic inflammatory infiltrate, macrophages, and myocyte injury →. A Toxoplasma cyst is present within the myocyte sarcoplasm →.* **(Right)** *High-power view of Toxoplasma myocarditis shows focal mononuclear inflammatory infiltrate and a Toxoplasma cyst within the myocyte sarcoplasm →.*

Histologic Changes in *Toxoplasma* Myocarditis

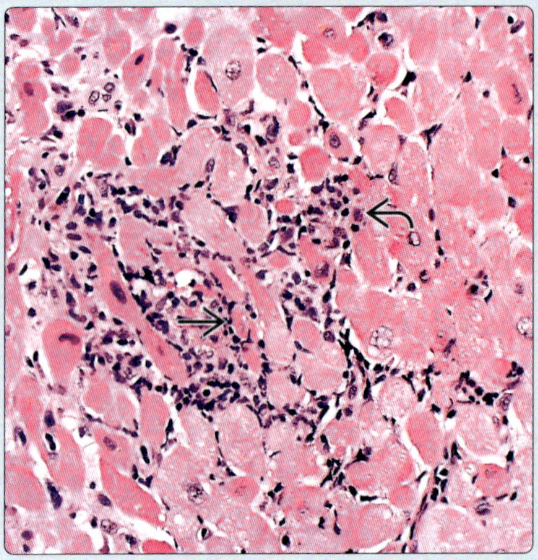

***Toxoplasma* Myocarditis, High-Power View**

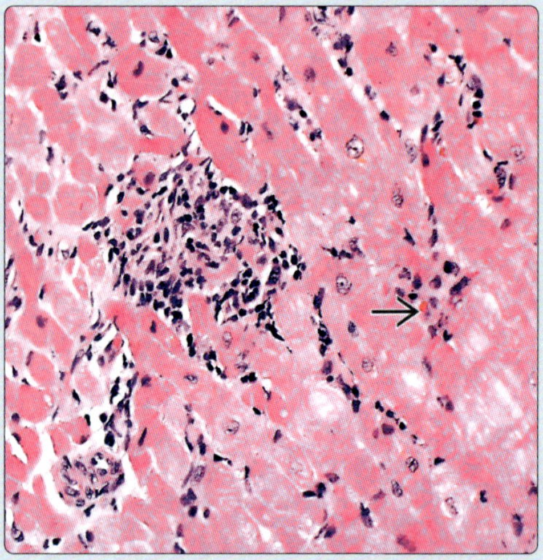

TERMINOLOGY

Definitions

- Protozoan parasitic infection caused by *Toxoplasma gondii*, which can produce myocarditis as isolated process or as part of disseminated infection

ETIOLOGY/PATHOGENESIS

Infectious Agents

- Primary infection with *T. gondii*
  - May be asymptomatic in immunocompetent hosts
  - Life threatening in immunodeficient hosts
- Reactivation of latent *T. gondii* infection
  - Most frequent type of infection in immunodeficient host

Life Cycle

- Mammals and birds are intermediate hosts
- Cats are complete or final hosts
- Animals and humans acquire infection by eating meat of contaminated animals or by ingesting oocysts deposited in soil, sand, or litter pans of cats
  - After ingestion, oocysts develop into tachyzoites that divide rapidly in intestine and disperse through lymphatics to other organs
  - After effective immune response tachyzoites convert into bradyzoites, which reside in tissue cysts
- In immunocompetent hosts, acute or chronic infection may be asymptomatic

Risk Factors

- Immunodeficiency: Primary or acquired
- Age: Young infants and older adults
- In heart transplantation: Recipient with seronegative status
- Patients with heart disease more susceptible to chronic infection

CLINICAL ISSUES

Epidemiology

- Seroprevalence in USA is ~ 10-20% and ~ 60% in underdeveloped countries
- 1/3 of human population is infected

Presentation

- Heart
  - Myocarditis: Chest pain, atrial fibrillation, ventricular arrhythmias, heart block, heart failure, sudden death
  - Pericarditis: Pericardial effusion, cardiac tamponade
- Other organs
  - Acute febrile disease
  - Lymphadenopathy
  - Acute and chronic encephalitis in immunosuppressed host
  - Uveitis
  - Polymyositis
  - Pneumonitis
  - Neonatal disease with jaundice and encephalitis

Laboratory Tests

- IgG and IgM titers for *T. gondii* by indirect fluorescent antibody test are sensitive and specific for diagnosis
  - False-positive results may occur
  - Low titers in case of immunocompromised host with acute infection have been seen
- PCR testing for *T. gondii* DNA in peripheral blood

Treatment

- Drugs
  - Corticosteroids in cases of severe myocarditis
  - Anti-*Toxoplasma* medication (sulfadiazine, pyrimethamine, atovaquone)
- Prevention
  - Protection of pregnant women, young children, and immunocompromised hosts from exposure to possible contaminated soil and cats
  - Prophylaxis in transplanted patients with trimethoprim-sulfamethoxazole

Prognosis

- May be life threatening in transplanted patients when acquired from donor organ
- Sudden death has been reported in immunocompromised hosts

MICROSCOPIC

Histologic Features

- Focal interstitial mononuclear inflammation
- Tachyzoites (smaller, motile, asexually reproducing form) within intracellular vacuoles
- *Toxoplasma* cysts (< 30 μm) containing bradyzoites (larger, crescent-shaped, slowly replicating form)
  - Spherical cysts become elongated in muscle cells

ANCILLARY TESTS

Histochemistry

- Periodic acid-Schiff
  - Reactivity: Positive
  - Staining pattern: Highlights wall of bradyzoites

Immunohistochemistry

- Demonstrates *Toxoplasma* antigen in inclusions

PCR

- Enhances diagnostic sensitivity on endomyocardial biopsy

DIFFERENTIAL DIAGNOSIS

Histoplasma Myocarditis

- PAS(+) cell wall of *Histoplasma*
- Other fungal stains will also identify microorganism

Chagas Disease

- Presence of kinetoplast in *Trypanosoma cruzi*
- PAS(+) material in *Toxoplasma* but not in *T. cruzi*

SELECTED REFERENCES

1. Zhou Z et al: Toxoplasmosis and the heart. Curr Probl Cardiol. 46(3):100741, 2021
2. Lévêque MF et al: Molecular diagnosis of toxoplasmosis at the onset of symptomatic primary infection: a straightforward alternative to serological examinations. Int J Infect Dis. 79:131-3, 2019
3. Petty LA et al: Cardiac toxoplasmosis after heart transplantation diagnosed by endomyocardial biopsy. Transpl Infect Dis. 17(5):719-22, 2015
4. Sahasrabudhe NS et al: Pathology of Toxoplasma myocarditis in acquired immunodeficiency syndrome. Indian J Pathol Microbiol. 46(4):649-51, 2003

Chagas Disease, Heart

KEY FACTS

TERMINOLOGY

- Zoonotic, tropical, protozoan parasitic disease transmitted by reduviid bugs to humans that, in its chronic phase, can lead to death due to cardiac involvement

ETIOLOGY/PATHOGENESIS

- Caused by infection with flagellate protozoan parasite *Trypanosoma cruzi*

CLINICAL ISSUES

- Acute phase
- Undifferentiated (or undetermined) phase
- Chronic phase

MACROSCOPIC

- Apical aneurysm with thrombus formation is common, distinctive finding of chronic Chagas
- Epicardial plaques (milk spots)

MICROSCOPIC

- In acute phase, parasite pseudocysts within myocardial fibers are numerous
  - Severe myocarditis with numerous neutrophils, lymphocytes, histiocytes, and plasma cells
  - Amastigotes are round to oval, 1.5-5.0 µm in size, and contain bar-shaped kinetoplasts
- Extensive fibrosis and myocytolysis in late chronic phase with few organisms

ANCILLARY TESTS

- Diagnosis is typically made in acute phase by visualizing trypomastigotes on fresh blood smears, thick drop preparations, or buffy coat smears
- Positive serology can be helpful in diagnosing patients in chronic phase
- Tissue-based PCR confirm Chagas infection in 60% of cases

(Left) *The infected host part of the Trypanosoma cruzi life cycle begins when reduviid bugs bite and release trypomastigotes that then migrate to muscle, encyst, and transform to amastigotes. Amastigotes then transform back into trypomastigotes, are released back into the bloodstream, and are reingested by another bug to continue the cycle.* **(Right)** *Periorbital swelling (Romaña sign) → is a classic clinical sign of Chagas disease in patients from endemic areas. (Courtesy A. Rassi, Jr., MD.)*

***Trypanosoma cruzi* Life Cycle**

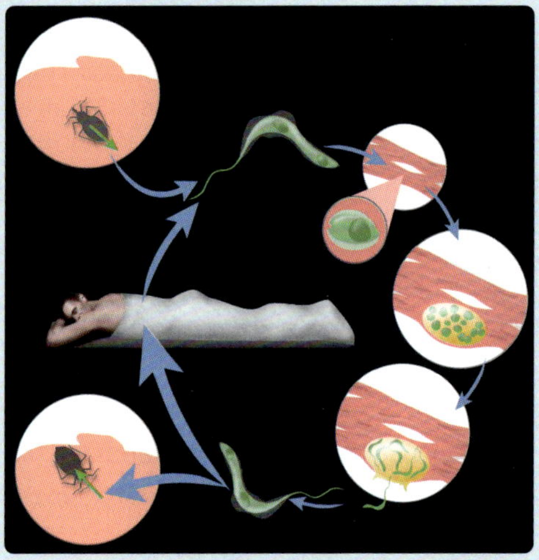

Romaña Sign in Patient With Chagas Disease

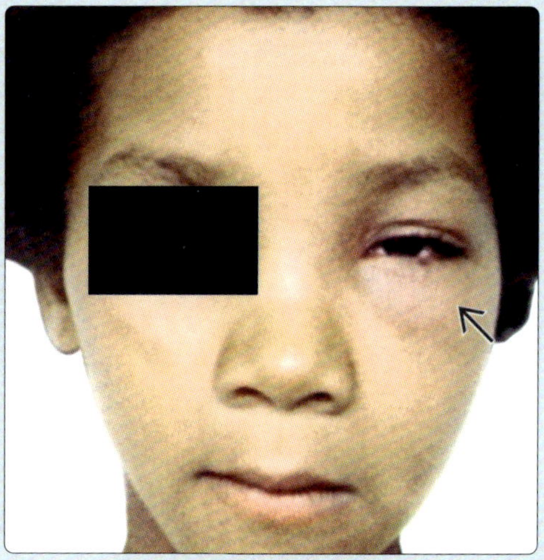

(Left) *Gross photograph of late-stage chronic Chagas disease shows the classic apical thinning → with thrombus formation → located in the left ventricle. (Courtesy M. C. Furian Ferreira, MD.)* **(Right)** *H&E of a case of acute-phase Chagas disease demonstrates numerous parasites → forming pseudocysts or pseudoleishmanic cysts that are often perinuclear in location. (Courtesy B. Pritt, MD.)*

Left Ventricular Changes in Chronic Chagas Disease

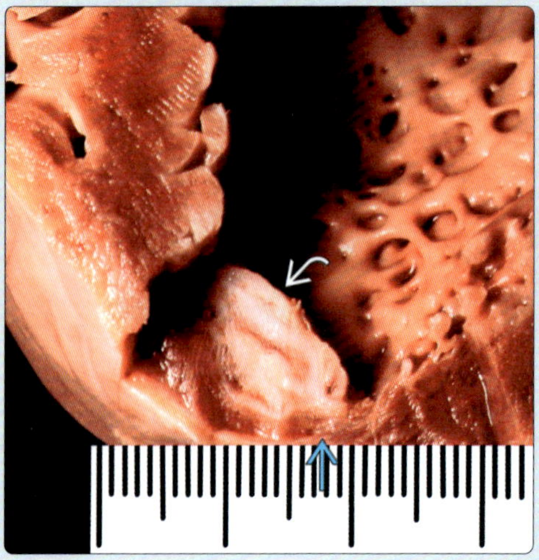

Acute Myocardial Findings in Chagas Disease

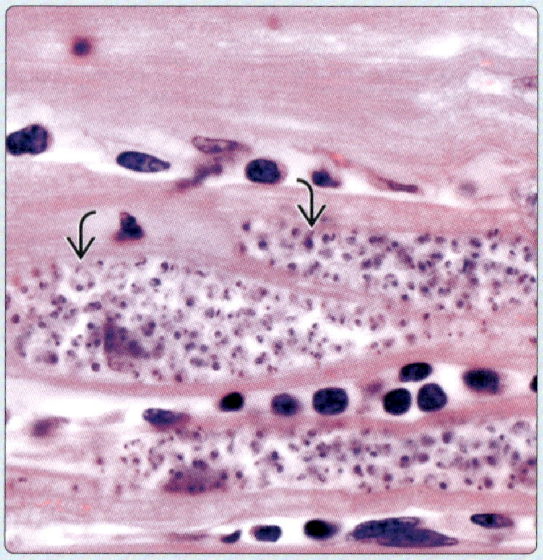

TERMINOLOGY

Definitions

- Zoonotic, tropical, protozoan parasitic disease transmitted by reduviid bugs to humans; in its chronic phase, can lead to death due to cardiac involvement

ETIOLOGY/PATHOGENESIS

Environmental Exposure

- Reduviid bug, or "kissing bug," is more often found in tropical or subtropical, typically rural, locations where thatched roofs or poor-quality houses with cracks or crevices are prevalent

Infectious Agents

- Caused by infection with flagellate protozoan parasite *Trypanosoma cruzi*
- Mode of transmission
  - Transmitted to humans by "assassin bug" of family Reduviidae, subfamily Triatominae, genus *Triatoma* ("Mexican bed bugs")
- Blood transfusions, organ transplantation, vertical transmission from mother to infant, oral contamination, and laboratory exposure are also ways in which *T. cruzi* infection can be acquired

Pathogenesis of Chronic Heart Disease

- Very complex process that is still being studied
- Most likely explanation is combination of low-grade chronic systemic infection with associated autoimmune reaction

CLINICAL ISSUES

Epidemiology

- Incidence
  - ~ 300,000 people currently infected in USA
  - Estimated 5.7 million people infected in Latin America
  - Cardiomyopathy associated with chronic disease; estimated to account for 21,000 deaths each year in endemic areas
- Ethnicity
  - Endemic in southern USA, Mexico, Central America, and South America

Presentation

- After infection, all patients enter acute phase and then undifferentiated, or undetermined, stage
  - Only 20-30% of patients enter final chronic, determined phase
- Acute phase
  - Affects minority of patients
  - Usually lasts 1-3 months with incubation period of 1-2 weeks
  - Myocarditis
    - Affects nearly all patients with acute Chagas disease but not always symptomatic
      - Up to 10% die in acute phase, especially children
    - Tachycardia (more than can be accounted by fever alone), muffled heart sounds, arterial hypotension, low pulse pressure, and cardiac murmurs are possible clinical manifestations
  - Localized cutaneous inflammation at portal site &/or subcutaneous edema
    - Chagoma: Sign of portal entry through skin
    - Romaña sign: Sign of portal entry through eye, giving rise to periorbital swelling
  - Prolonged fever, lymphadenopathy, hepatosplenomegaly, and, rarely, meningoencephalitis
  - Resolves spontaneously, even without treatment in most patients
- Undifferentiated or undetermined phase
  - 60-70% of infected patients will never show clinical signs of disease
    - These patients remain infected but are asymptomatic throughout life
- Chronic phase
  - 30-40% of patients develop chronic, determined phase after infection
  - Cardiac involvement is most frequent and serious consequence of chronic disease
  - Signs and symptoms
    - Palpitations, atypical chest pain, presyncope, syncope, dyspnea upon exertion, edema, and thromboembolic events
  - Digestive tract and nervous system involvement
    - Destruction of nerves and dilatation of GI tract can lead to megaesophagus or megacolon and cause digestive problems &/or severe weight loss
- Congenital disease
  - Signs can include prematurity, hepatosplenomegaly, meningitis, &/or encephalitis

Laboratory Tests

- Leukocytosis and lymphocytosis are common findings

Treatment

- Options, risks, complications
  - Treatment is recommended in acute and congenital infection, reactivated infection, early chronic Chagas disease, and infected adults without advanced cardiomyopathy
  - Treatment is contraindicated in patients with megaesophagus and swallowing impairment
  - Symptomatic treatment of heart disease parallels medical treatment for heart failure of other causes
- Surgical approaches
  - Transplantation for end-stage chronic Chagas cardiomyopathy is increasingly being used
    - Survival probability is increased vs. end-stage patients who do not receive heart transplant
  - Risk of Chagas disease reactivation in transplanted hearts (risk correlates with increasing amount of immunosuppressive therapy)
    - However, can be easily treated with benznidazole or allopurinol
    - Morbidity is high with disease reactivation, but mortality is low
  - Chagas transplant patients have equal incidence of rejection as non-Chagas heart transplant recipients
- Drugs
  - Only 2 drugs approved for treatment: Benznidazole and nifurtimox
    - Numerous side effects associated with both drugs

Prognosis

- Acute Chagas disease
  - Most patients return to full or near-normal cardiac status, but
    - ~ 30% develop chronic fibrosing myocarditis
  - Death can occur rarely (~ 5-10% of symptomatic patients) as result of
    - Congestive heart failure, secondary to severe acute myocarditis
    - Meningoencephalitis
- Chronic Chagas disease
  - Normal life expectancy for patients in early stages of cardiomyopathy
  - Life expectancy for late-stage symptomatic or advanced cardiomyopathy with cardiomegaly or systolic dysfunction ≤ 30% at 5 years
    - Causes of death include heart failure (25-30%) and sudden death (55-65%)
  - Survival probability for transplant recipients at 1 year is 71% and at 10 years is 46%

MACROSCOPIC

General Features

- Epicardial plaques (milk spots)
- Chronic phase
  - Early stage
    - Circumscribed apical thinning without thrombosis is characteristic
    - Striking hypertrophy of left ventricular wall proximal to apical thinning
    - Slightly dilated ventricles with conical shape
  - Late stage
    - Severe dilatation and hypertrophy of all cavities
    - Thinning of left ventricular wall is characteristic
    - Extensive apical thinning, usually with mural thrombosis

MICROSCOPIC

Histologic Features

- Acute phase
  - Severe myocarditis with interstitial cellular infiltrate composed of numerous neutrophils, lymphocytes, histiocytes, and plasma cells
  - Parasite pseudocysts within myocardial fibers are numerous and characteristic (termed pseudoleishmanic cysts)
  - Degeneration/necrosis of myocytes to varying degrees &/or early interstitial fibrosis can be seen
- Latent phase
  - Pathologic lesions not well studied
- Chronic phase
  - Early stage
    - Usually shows interstitial mononuclear infiltrate
    - Fibrosis and myocytolysis, particularly of inner ventricular wall
  - Late stage
    - Extensive fibrosis and myocytolysis
    - Variable mixed chronic inflammatory infiltrate with lymphocytes, plasma cells, eosinophils, and histiocytes
    - Parasites are more difficult to find, even with specific immunohistochemical or special stains
  - Occasionally, noncaseating granulomas ± giant cells can be found

Cytologic Features

- Amastigotes are round to oval and 1.5-5.0 μm in size
  - Intracytoplasmic, bar-shaped kinetoplast within organisms is diagnostic
- Trypomastigotes (found in peripheral blood) are flagellated with undulating membrane
  - Measure 20 μm long and 3 μm wide

ANCILLARY TESTS

PCR

- Tissue-based PCR confirms Chagas infection in 60% of cases

Serologic Testing

- Anti-*T. cruzi* IgG and IgM antibody testing is available by ELISA, indirect hemagglutination assay (IHA), and indirect immunofluorescence assay (IFA)
  - IgM may be useful in acute infection (first 60-90 days)
  - IgG is useful in confirming chronic disease
    - ≥ 2 positive tests using ELISA, IHA, or IFA confirm diagnosis of chronic disease

DIFFERENTIAL DIAGNOSIS

Histoplasmosis

- Round (*T. cruzi* is more oval) and without kinetoplast
- PAS or GMS stain may be helpful
  - *Histoplasma capsulatum* will contain pseudocapsule (*T. cruzi* will not)
- Clinical history may help, as histoplasmosis is typically found in areas bordering Ohio or lower Mississippi river valleys

Toxoplasmosis

- Small, basophilic to amphophilic crescent-shaped tachyzoites 2-6 μm in size within myocytes
- Elongated larger cysts (up to 100 μm) containing crescent-shaped bradyzoites may be present
- Immunohistochemical stain specific to *T. gondii* is available
- Clinical history (immunosuppression vs. travel) helpful

SELECTED REFERENCES

1. Nonaka CKV et al: Circulating miRNAs as potential biomarkers associated with cardiac remodeling and fibrosis in Chagas disease cardiomyopathy. Int J Mol Sci. 20(16):4064, 2019
2. Vieira JL et al: Chagas cardiomyopathy in Latin America review. Curr Cardiol Rep. 21(2):8, 2019
3. Benziger CP et al: Chagas cardiomyopathy: clinical presentation and management in the Americas. Cardiol Clin. 35(1):31-47, 2017
4. Hsu RC et al: Chagas cardiomyopathy in New Orleans and the southeastern United States. Ochsner J. 16(3):304-8, 2016
5. Kransdorf EP et al: Pathology of chronic Chagas cardiomyopathy in the United States: a detailed review of 13 cardiectomy cases. Am J Clin Pathol. 146(2):191-8, 2016
6. Lewis MD et al: Putting infection dynamics at the heart of Chagas disease. Trends Parasitol. 32(11):899-911, 2016
7. Bonney KM et al: Autoimmune pathogenesis of Chagas heart disease: looking back, looking ahead. Am J Pathol. 185(6):1537-47, 2015
8. Gurgel CB et al: [Apical lesions in Chagas' heart disease patients: an autopsy study.] Rev Soc Bras Med Trop. 43(6):709-12, 2010
9. Rassi A Jr et al: Chagas disease. Lancet. 375(9723):1388-402, 2010

Acute Chagas Myocarditis

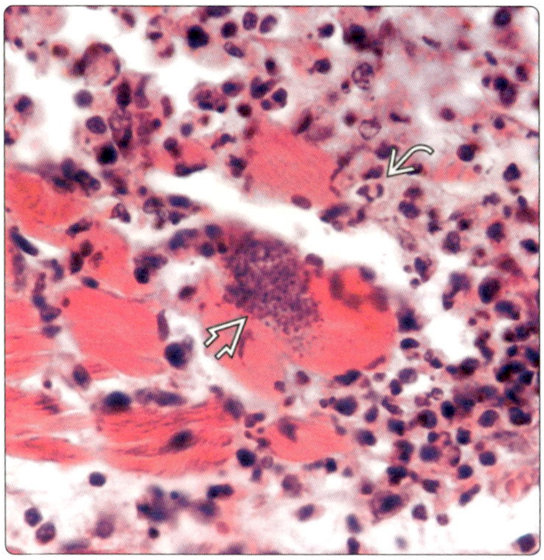

Chagas Reactivation Post Heart Transplant

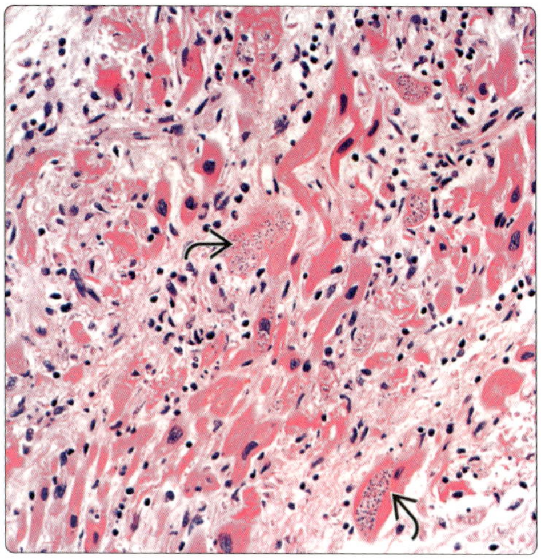

(Left) *Severe myocarditis of acute Chagas disease shows a mixed infiltrate with frequent neutrophils ➡ surrounding degenerating myocytes containing parasites ➡. (Courtesy M. C. Furian Ferreira, MD.)* **(Right)** *Reactivation of Chagas disease 3 months post transplant shows myofiber degeneration, inflammation, and numerous organisms ➡. Although mortality is low and reactivation is treatable, this disease can be quite morbid. (Courtesy D. Luthringer, MD.)*

Chagas Reactivation Post Heart Transplant

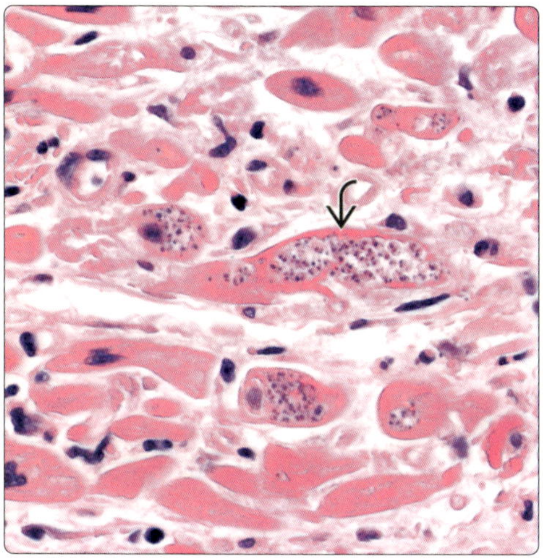

Chronic Chagas Disease Changes in Left Ventricle

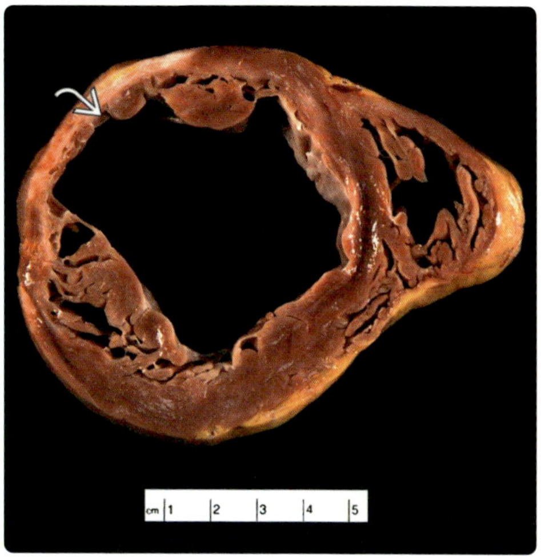

(Left) *Higher power H&E of reactivation Chagas disease after heart transplant demonstrates numerous intracellular organisms ➡. Although mortality is low and reactivation is treatable, this disease can be quite morbid. (Courtesy D. Luthringer, MD.)* **(Right)** *Cross section of heart from a patient with chronic Chagas disease demonstrates aneurysmal dilatation of the left ventricle ➡ that extended all the way to the apex of the heart. (Courtesy D. Luthringer, MD.)*

Histologic Changes in Chronic Chagas Disease

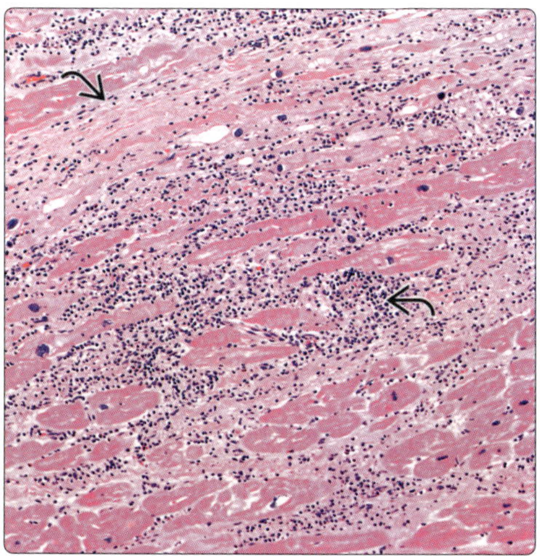

Histologic Changes in Chronic Chagas Disease

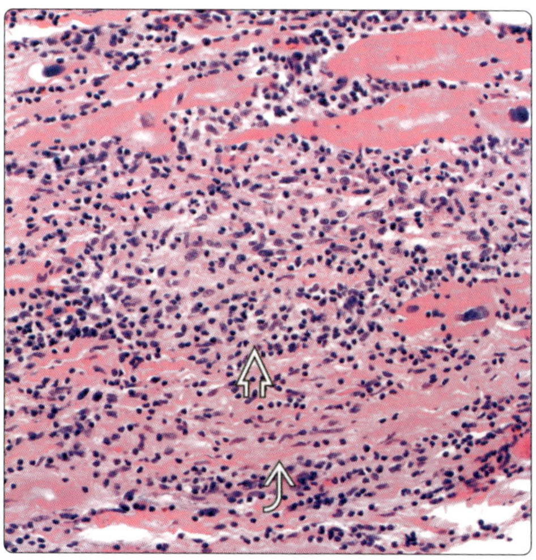

(Left) *Low-power H&E of a myocardial biopsy of chronic Chagas disease demonstrates moderate interstitial fibrosis and mixed chronic inflammatory infiltrate ➡. (Courtesy D. Luthringer, MD.)* **(Right)** *Occasionally, poorly formed noncaseating granulomas ➡ can be seen in biopsies of patients with chronic Chagas disease along with significant myocytolysis and some fibrosis ➡. Organisms are often not found, even with sensitive staining methods. (Courtesy D. Luthringer, MD.)*

Lyme Disease and Rickettsial Myocarditis

KEY FACTS

TERMINOLOGY

- Myocarditis as result of infection with *Borrelia burgdorferi*, *Rickettsia rickettsii*, or *Coxiella burnetii*

ETIOLOGY/PATHOGENESIS

- *B. burgdorferi sensu lato* sp. is spirochete transmitted by *Ixodes* tick and responsible for manifestations of Lyme disease (LD)
- Most common rickettsial bacteria in North America is *R. rickettsii*, which causes Rocky Mountain spotted fever (RMSF)
- *C. burnetii* is rickettsial organism responsible for Q fever

CLINICAL ISSUES

- LD occurs in USA, Canada, South America, and temperate areas of Europe and Asia
- Lyme carditis is rare manifestation (1-10% of cases in USA, 0.5-4.0% in Europe)
- In LD, most common cardiac manifestations are conduction and rhythm disturbances
- Myocarditis and cardiomyopathy are other possible presentations

MICROSCOPIC

- Lyme carditis
    - Transmural lymphocyte (neutrophils and histiocytes seen in hyperacute disease) inflammatory infiltrate is most common finding
- Q fever myocarditis
    - Mononuclear and lymphocytic myocardial infiltrates
    - Degeneration and necrosis of myofibrils
- RMSF myocarditis
    - More often causes endothelialitis ± thrombosis

DIAGNOSTIC CHECKLIST

- Histologic findings are nonspecific and not sufficient to rule out other causes of myocarditis

(Left) *Low-power H&E of an endomyocardial biopsy demonstrates myocarditis with inflammatory infiltrates composed mostly of lymphocytes. Although nonspecific, this could be consistent with Lyme or Q fever myocarditis.* **(Right)** *H&E of a case of Lyme disease (LD) myocarditis demonstrates a more intense lymphohistiocytic infiltrate causing myocardial fiber degeneration/necrosis and disarray.*

Histology of Lyme Myocarditis

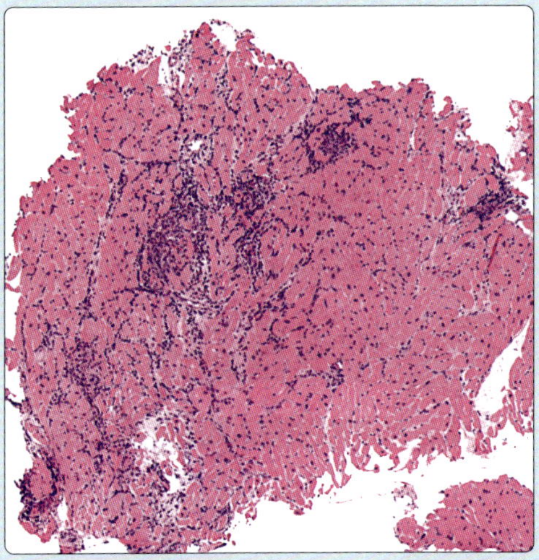

Myocyte Changes in Lyme Myocarditis

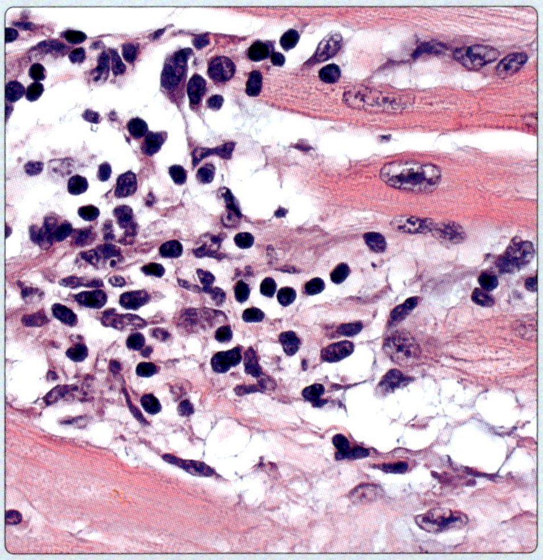

(Left) *H&E of myocarditis in a patient with LD demonstrates lymphocyte-predominant interstitial infiltrate ➙ admixed with histiocytes and focal myocardial fiber degeneration ⇨.* **(Right)** *High-power H&E of a Lyme carditis case demonstrates focal myocyte necrosis ⇨ and surrounding lymphohistiocytic chronic inflammatory infiltrate ➙.*

Lyme Myocarditis

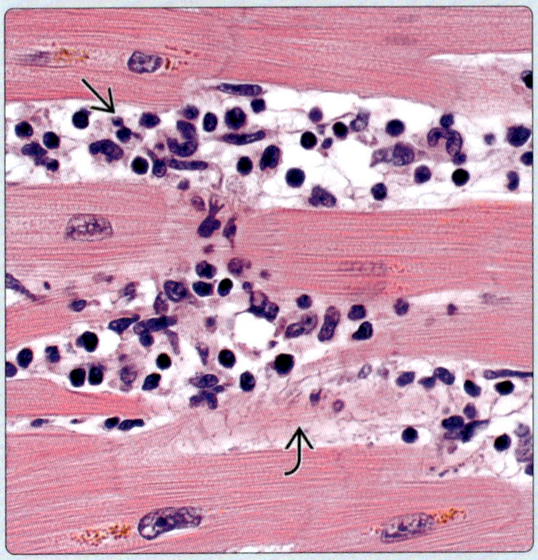

Myocyte Changes in Lyme Myocarditis

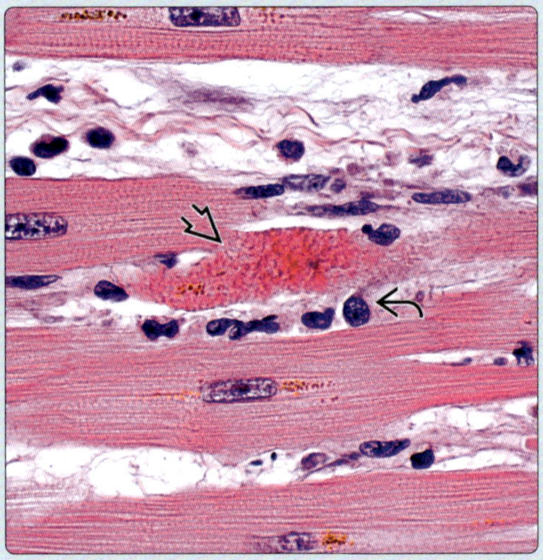

TERMINOLOGY

Abbreviations

- Lyme disease (LD)

Synonyms

- Lyme carditis

Definitions

- Myocarditis as result of infection with *Borrelia burgdorferi*, *Rickettsia rickettsii*, or *Coxiella burnetii*

ETIOLOGY/PATHOGENESIS

Infectious Agents

- *B. burgdorferi sensu lato* sp. is spirochete transmitted by *Ixodes* tick and responsible for manifestations of LD
- Most common rickettsial bacteria in North America is *R. rickettsii*, which causes Rocky Mountain spotted fever (RMSF)
    - Transmitted by ticks, and bacteria invade and proliferate in endothelial cells of small vessels
    - Endothelial damage and dysfunction leads to activation of acute-phase response, coagulation abnormalities, cytokine activation, and resultant immune dysregulation
    - Host response not as well understood, but cell-mediated response thought to be important
- *C. burnetii* is rickettsial organism responsible for Q fever

CLINICAL ISSUES

Epidemiology

- Incidence
    - Lyme carditis is rare manifestation (1-10% of cases in USA, 0.5-4.0% in Europe)
    - LD occurs in USA, Canada, South America, and temperate areas of Europe and Asia
        - In USA, most cases of LD are concentrated in states in Northeast, Wisconsin, or Minnesota
        - However, nearly all states (except HI, AR, MS, WY, and OK) have had confirmed cases in past 10 years
    - Heart involvement in both RMSF and Q fever is quite rare
        - In 2 different large case series, < 1% of Q fever patients experienced myocarditis
    - Chronic Q fever accounts for < 5% of acutely infected patients
- Sex
    - Lyme carditis
        - M:F = 3:1

Presentation

- In 1st stage of LD (localized, acute), erythema chronicum migrans (ECM) is classic clinical manifestation
    - ECM (seen in ~ 80% of patients) occurs as erythematous target-like patch typically > 5 cm in diameter 7-14 days after tick bite and increases in size over days to weeks
    - Lymphadenitis, headache, myalgias, fever, and malaise may also be present during this stage
- 2nd-stage LD (disseminated) results from hematogenous spread, occurs weeks to months after 1st stage, and may show cardiac arrhythmias, secondary annular plaques (usually smaller), migratory arthritis, and meningitis
- 3rd stage of LD (late, chronic) occurs 2-3 years after 1st stage and is characterized by
    - Acrodermatitis chronica atrophicans (typically seen in Europe), which presents as reddish blue discoloration of skin without scaling
    - Neuropathy, arthritis, meningoencephalitis, and other nonspecific signs can occur
- In LD, most common cardiac manifestations are conduction and rhythm disturbances
    - Atrioventricular (AV) block is most common conduction abnormality
        - Can rapidly progress from 1st to 3rd degree
        - Escape rhythms with severe AV block, brief asystoles, and fluctuating bundle branch blocks can also occur
    - Myocarditis and cardiomyopathy are other possible presentations
    - Pericarditis with pericardial effusion has been reported
    - Anecdotal reports of dilated cardiomyopathy, but this has been disputed by several studies
- For RMSF, incubation period varies from 2 days to 2 weeks
    - Early symptoms are nonspecific with fever, malaise, chills, headaches, anorexia, and myalgias
    - Classic clinical triad is sudden onset of fever, rash, and headache
    - Rash develops in most patients 3-5 days after exposure and consists of macular, blanching, nonpruritic rash
        - Later, it becomes papular, and petechiae may be present
        - Rarely, it may progress to ischemia and skin necrosis
        - Centripetal spread from wrists inward actually occurs in minority of patients
        - Palm and sole involvement, although characteristic, may not be present until late stage or absent altogether
- Cardiac involvement in RMSF is rare
    - Cardiac dysfunction related to myocarditis can occur
    - Signs of pericarditis or arterial occlusion can also occur
    - In severe RMSF, cardiac failure can ensue
        - Myocardial infarctions and heart block can also occur
- Clinically, Q fever symptoms are nonspecific in both acute and chronic forms
    - Acute
        - Often no symptoms
        - Mild symptoms can include flu-like symptoms, malaise, severe headaches, myalgias, and others
        - Most patients recover, but rarer serious complications include pneumonia, myocarditis, granulomatous hepatitis, or meningoencephalitis
    - Chronic
        - Most often presents as endocarditis or aneurysmal or vascular graft infection
        - Chronic hepatitis or arthritis are also possible presentations
        - Myocarditis is rare complication (~ 20 cases reported in literature)
            - However, it can be fatal
        - Most common symptoms
            - Dyspnea
            - Chest pain
            - Palpitations

Laboratory Tests

- RMSF
  - Most patients have thrombocytopenia, and liver enzyme tests are often elevated
  - Hyponatremia is also quite common, occurring in ~ 1/2 of patients

Treatment

- Options, risks, complications
  - With suspicious clinical features and appropriate epidemiology, RMSF treatment should be started before serology or ancillary tests are positive
    - However, without suspicious clinical symptoms, prophylactic therapy is not recommended after tick bite since even in endemic areas, ≤ 1% of ticks are infected with *R. rickettsii*
- Drugs
  - Doxycycline is drug of choice for all patients with LD, RMSF, and acute Q fever; however, there are 2-3 clinical contraindications
    - Major exception is patients with history of serious hypersensitivity reactions to tetracyclines
    - Relative contraindication is pregnant women
    - For children with suspected LD under 8 years of age, doxycycline is contraindicated
  - Chloramphenicol is only alternative therapy for RMSF
  - Oral amoxicillin or cefuroxime can also be used for LD
  - In patients with Lyme carditis and severe conduction abnormalities, IV ceftriaxone or high-dose penicillin G recommended
  - Cotrimoxazole is 2nd-line therapy for acute Q fever in pregnant women and young children
  - Chronic Q fever often requires multiple drugs (difficult to treat)
    - Doxycycline with quinolones or doxycycline with hydroxychloroquine are 2 main therapy options
- Pacemaker
  - Temporary transvenous pacing may be necessary in selected cases

Prognosis

- Lyme carditis
  - > 90% of patients completely recover
  - Mortality related to Lyme myocarditis is exceedingly rare
- RMSF
  - Poorly understood geographic variation of RMSF virulence
    - Mortality rates in preantibiotic era varied significantly even between neighboring states
  - Untreated mortality rate of RMSF is ~ 20%; treated mortality rate is ~ 5%
    - Fatality rate appears to be higher in children ≤ 4 years and adults ≥ 40 years
- Q fever myocarditis
  - With proper antibiotics, most recover
    - In one series, 2 of 7 patients died from acute congestive heart failure despite adequate treatment

IMAGING

Ultrasonographic Findings

- Findings are variable and nonspecific
  - Minimal left or right ventricle dilatation
  - Left ventricle may show normal function or diffuse hypokinesis
  - Depressed left ventricular systolic function

MR Findings

- Areas of increased signal intensity
- Focal late gadolinium enhancement

MICROSCOPIC

Histologic Features

- Lyme carditis
  - Transmural lymphocyte-predominant infiltrate (with mixed neutrophils and histiocytes in hyperacute disease) is most common finding
    - Has characteristic band-like appearance in endocardium
    - May lead to myocyte necrosis
  - Endocardial and interstitial fibrosis may be seen
  - Small and large vessel damage may be seen as endothelial swelling in smaller vessels and increased collagen deposition around larger vessels
  - Myocardial fiber degeneration and fibrinous pericarditis have also been reported
- RMSF myocarditis
  - More often causes endothelialitis (or endotheliitis) ± thrombosis
  - Typically does not cause true myocarditis
- Q fever myocarditis
  - Mononuclear and lymphocytic myocardial infiltrates
  - Degeneration and necrosis of myofibrils

ANCILLARY TESTS

Histochemistry

- Warthin-Starry or Steiner silver stain may identify spirochete within cardiac tissue

Immunohistochemistry

- Staining with anti-*C. burnetii* serum can be useful in cases of Q fever myocarditis

PCR

- LD: Very specific and can detect multiple species of *Borrelia*
  - More sensitive than culture

Serologic Testing

- LD: Recommendation in USA is screening with ELISA and, if positive or equivocal, confirmation with Western blot for diagnosis
- Q fever: Phase I and II IgG and IgM titers directed against *C. burnetii* by indirect fluorescent antibody
  - Acute: Phase I and II IgM increased, phase I IgG increased
  - Chronic: Phase I IgG increased
    - Phase I IgG titer ≥ 1:800 is diagnostic of chronic endocarditis

Culture

- Most specific for diagnosis of LD but very low sensitivity, so not clinically useful

DIFFERENTIAL DIAGNOSIS

Lymphocytic Myocarditis

- Immunohistochemistry in case of Q fever may be helpful
- PCR for coxsackievirus in case of lymphocytic myocarditis

Cytomegalovirus Myocarditis

- Characteristic viral inclusions in endothelial cells
- Immunohistochemistry for cytomegalovirus (CMV) is positive in infected cells
- CMV DNA is detected in myocardial tissue

Giant Cell Myocarditis

- Mixed inflammatory infiltrate with giant cells
- Extensive myocardial necrosis
- History of thymoma or autoimmune disease

DIAGNOSTIC CHECKLIST

Clinically Relevant Pathologic Features

- Clinical history, proper signs/symptoms, and supportive serologic/ancillary testing are necessary to distinguish LD and RMSF from other causes of myocarditis

Pathologic Interpretation Pearls

- Histologic findings are nonspecific and not sufficient to rule out other causes of myocarditis

SELECTED REFERENCES

1. Marx GE et al: Fatal lyme carditis in New England: two case reports. Ann Intern Med. 172(3):222-4, 2020
2. Fishe JN et al: Lyme myocarditis presenting as chest pain in an adolescent girl. Pediatr Emerg Care. 32(7):459-61, 2016
3. Kostić T et al: Manifestations of Lyme carditis. Int J Cardiol. 1(232):24-32, 2016
4. Muehlenbachs A et al: Cardiac tropism of Borrelia burgdorferi: an autopsy study of sudden cardiac death associated with Lyme carditis. Am J Pathol. 186(5):1195-205, 2016
5. Jansweijer JA et al: Tricky ticks: the importance of Lyme carditis recognition. Neth Heart J. 23(11):531-2, 2015
6. Karatolios K et al: Suspected inflammatory cardiomyopathy. Prevalence of Borrelia burgdorferi in endomyocardial biopsies with positive serological evidence. Herz. 40 Suppl 1:91-5, 2015
7. Robinson ML et al: Lyme carditis. Infect Dis Clin North Am. 29(2):255-68, 2015
8. Shah P et al: Third-degree heart block as initial presentation of Lyme disease. Acta Cardiol. 70(6):744-5, 2015
9. Dubrey SW et al: Lyme disease in the United Kingdom. Postgrad Med J. 90(1059):33-42, 2014
10. Forrester JD et al: Third-degree heart block associated with lyme carditis: review of published cases. Clin Infect Dis. 59(7):996-1000, 2014
11. Krause PJ et al: Cardiology patient pages. Lyme disease and the heart. Circulation. 127(7):e451-4, 2013
12. Koene R et al: Acute heart failure from lyme carditis. Circ Heart Fail. 5(2):e24-6, 2012
13. Olarte L et al: Bartonella vinsonii endocarditis in an adolescent with congenital heart disease. Pediatr Infect Dis J. 31(5):531-4, 2012
14. Dubrey SW et al: Lyme disease and the heart in the UK. Br J Hosp Med (Lond). 72(11):621-2, 624-5, 2011
15. Mener DJ et al: Tick tock. Am J Med. 124(4):306-8, 2011
16. Schmit VL et al: Analysis of Borrelia burgdorferi surface proteins as determinants in establishing host cell interactions. Front Microbiol. 2:141, 2011
17. Lalosevic D et al: Borrelia-like organism in heart capillaries of patient with Lyme-disease seen by electron microscopy. Int J Cardiol. 145(3):e96-8, 2010
18. Cihakova D et al: Pathogenesis of myocarditis and dilated cardiomyopathy. Adv Immunol. 99:95-114, 2008
19. Lelovas P et al: Cardiac implications of Lyme disease, diagnosis and therapeutic approach. Int J Cardiol. 129(1):15-21, 2008
20. Mansueto P et al: Immunology of human rickettsial diseases. J Biol Regul Homeost Agents. 22(2):131-9, 2008
21. Vogiatzis I et al: Q fever myocarditis. Hippokratia. 12(1):46-9, 2008
22. Bartůnek P et al: Lyme borreliosis infection as a cause of dilated cardiomyopathy. Prague Med Rep. 107(2):213-26, 2006
23. Doyle A et al: Myocardial involvement in rocky mountain spotted fever: a case report and review. Am J Med Sci. 332(4):208-10, 2006
24. Karakousis PC et al: Chronic Q fever in the United States. J Clin Microbiol. 44(6):2283-7, 2006
25. Bernabeu-Wittel M et al: [Rickettsioses.] Enferm Infecc Microbiol Clin. 23(3):163-72, 2005
26. Haddad FA et al: Lyme disease and the heart. Front Biosci. 8:s769-82, 2003
27. Lepidi H et al: Cardiac valves in patients with Q fever endocarditis: microbiological, molecular, and histologic studies. J Infect Dis. 187(7):1097-106, 2003
28. Lo R et al: Complete heart block due to lyme carditis. J Invasive Cardiol. 15(6):367-9, 2003
29. Fournier PE et al: Myocarditis, a rare but severe manifestation of Q fever: report of 8 cases and review of the literature. Clin Infect Dis. 32(10):1440-7, 2001
30. Paparone PW: Cardiovascular manifestations of Lyme disease. J Am Osteopath Assoc. 97(3):156-61, 1997
31. Nagi KS et al: Cardiac manifestations of Lyme disease: a review. Can J Cardiol. 12(5):503-6, 1996
32. Pebody RG et al: Epidemiological features of Coxiella burnetii infection in England and Wales: 1984 to 1994. Commun Dis Rep CDR Rev. 6(9):R128-32, 1996
33. Stein A et al: Q fever endocarditis. Eur Heart J. 16 Suppl B:19-23, 1995
34. Brouqui P et al: Immunohistologic demonstration of Coxiella burnetii in the valves of patients with Q fever endocarditis. Am J Med. 97(5):451-8, 1994
35. Rallis TM et al: Rocky Mountain spotted fever following cardiac transplantation. West J Med. 158(6):625-8, 1993
36. Cox J et al: Cardiovascular manifestations of Lyme disease. Am Heart J. 122(5):1449-55, 1991
37. McAlister HF et al: Lyme carditis: an important cause of reversible heart block. Ann Intern Med. 110(5):339-45, 1989
38. Walker DH et al: The pathology of fatal Mediterranean spotted fever. Am J Clin Pathol. 87(5):669-72, 1987
39. Olson LJ et al: Cardiac involvement in Lyme disease: manifestations and management. Mayo Clin Proc. 61(9):745-9, 1986
40. Salvi A et al: Acute rickettsial myocarditis and advanced atrioventricular block: diagnosis and treatment aided by endomyocardial biopsy. Int J Cardiol. 7(4):405-9, 1985
41. Feltes TF et al: M-mode echocardiographic abnormalities in Rocky Mountain spotted fever. South Med J. 77(9):1130-2, 1984
42. Marin-Garcia J et al: Myocardial disease in Rocky Mountain spotted fever: clinical, functional, and pathologic findings. Pediatr Cardiol. 5(2):149-54, 1984
43. Marin-Garcia J: Left ventricular dysfunction in Rocky Mountain spotted fever. Clin Cardiol. 6(10):501-6, 1983
44. Marin-Garcia J et al: Cardiac manifestations of Rocky Mountain spotted fever. Pediatrics. 67(3):358-61, 1981
45. Walker DH et al: Pathogenesis of myocarditis in Rocky Mountain spotted fever. Arch Pathol Lab Med. 104(4):171-4, 1980
46. Bradford WD et al: Myocardial involvement in Rocky Mountain spotted fever. Arch Pathol Lab Med. 102(7):357-9, 1978

KEY FACTS

TERMINOLOGY

- Cardiac diseases associated with SARS-CoV-2 infection include
  - Acute ischemia (acute elevation of troponin, acute myocardial infarction, "mild unspecific cardiac injury")
  - Myocarditis, pericarditis
  - Acute exacerbation of heart failure
  - Microvascular injury with thrombosis
  - Coronary artery dissection

CLINICAL ISSUES

- 20% of hospitalized patients with COVID-19 have evidence of myocardial injury (defined as elevated troponin I levels)
- Patients > 64 years of age at higher risk of severe COVID-19
- Male patients at higher risk of severe COVID-19 and cardiovascular complications
- Clinical manifestations
  - Chest pain: 5-21%
  - Palpitations: 10%
  - Arrhythmia (atrial fibrillation, bradyarrhythmia, ventricular tachycardia/fibrillation, high-degree atrioventricular block): 23%
  - Venous thromboembolic events: 20-26%
  - Cardiogenic shock
  - Sudden cardiac death

MACROSCOPIC

- Cardiomegaly is common finding
- Dilated right and left ventricular chambers, right > left

MICROSCOPIC

- Microthrombi (10.8%)
- Endothelial cells swelling and neutrophilic endothelialitis
- Acute ischemic changes: Contraction band necrosis, hypereosinophilic myocytes, areas of granulation tissue
- Single myocyte necrosis (13.7%)
- Nonmyocarditis inflammation (12.6%)
- Pericardial inflammatory infiltrate (6.9%)

Acute Myocardial Infarction in COVID-19

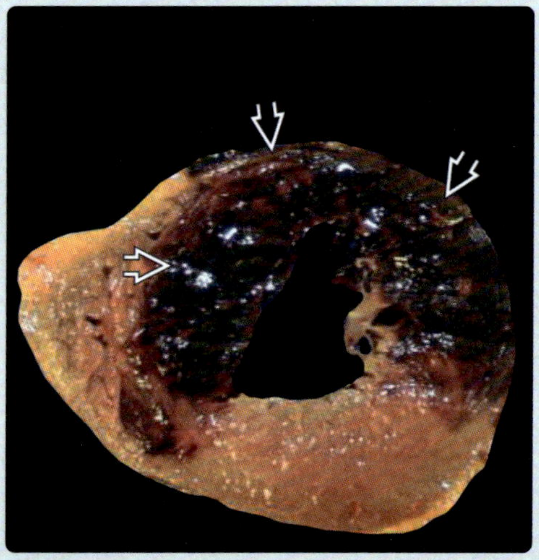

Biventricular Dilatation in COVID-19

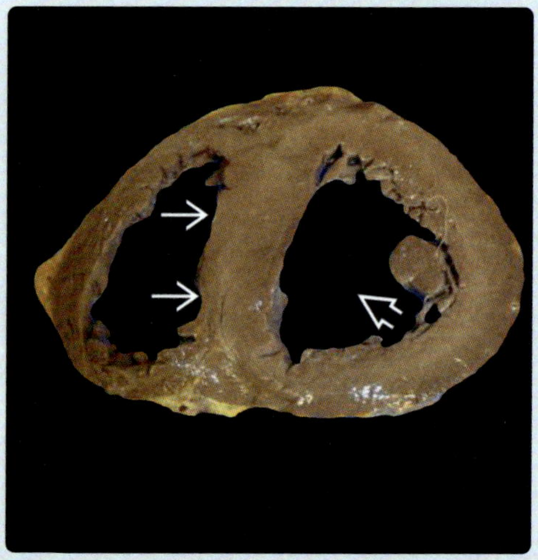

(Left) *Autopsy of a heart from a COVID-19-positive patient shows a hemorrhagic anterior wall (transmural) myocardial infarction. (Courtesy C.J. Sang, MD.)* **(Right)** *Autopsy of a heart from a COVID-19-positive patient shows dilatation of the left ventricle. Features of elevated right-sided pressures are also apparent with a straightened septum and enlarged right ventricle with thickened walls. (Courtesy C.J. Sang, MD.)*

Myocardial Fibrin Immunostain in COVID-19

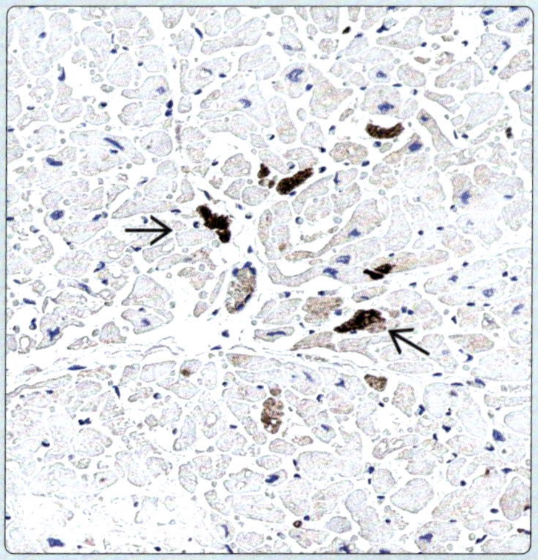

Myocardial CD68 Immunostain in COVID-19

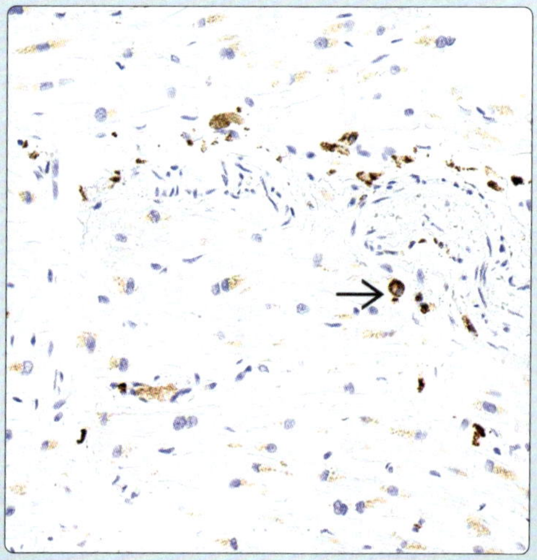

(Left) *Microvascular thrombi are one (rare) finding occurring in heart tissue from COVID-19-positive patients at autopsy. Immunostaining for fibrin highlights thrombi within the microvasculature. (Courtesy M.E.H. Hammond, MD and M. Belenky, MD.)* **(Right)** *CD68 staining has been used to highlight an overall increase in macrophage lineage cells as part of the immune response observed in hearts from COVID-19-positive patients. (Courtesy M.E.H. Hammond, MD and M. Belenky, MD.)*

TERMINOLOGY

Abbreviations

- Severe acute respiratory syndrome coronavirus 2 (SARS-CoV-2)
- Coronavirus disease 2019 (COVID-19)

Definitions

- Cardiac diseases associated with SARS-CoV-2 infection include
  - Acute ischemia (acute elevation of troponin, acute myocardial infarction, "mild unspecific cardiac injury")
  - Myocarditis, pericarditis
  - Acute exacerbation of heart failure
  - Microvascular injury with thrombosis
  - Coronary artery dissection

ETIOLOGY/PATHOGENESIS

Infectious Agents

- SARS-CoV-2 belongs to Beta-CoV-2b lineage of Sarbecovirus subgenus
  - Enveloped virus with nonsegmented, single-stranded positive-sense RNA, measuring 60-160 nm in diameter with spikes ranging 9-12 nm
  - Infection of cardiovascular system occurs by ACE2 receptor expressed in myocytes and pericytes, and less so in fibroblasts, endothelial cells, and leukocytes
- Myocardial and vascular damage can occur due to
  - Direct viral infection of myocytes (less common)
  - Indirect mechanisms, including
    - Cytokine storm/immune injury (high concentration of circulating proinflammatory cytokines and ferritin)
    - Endothelial dysfunction and microthrombosis
      - Due to direct viral infection of endothelial cells, leading to cell death and exposure of basement membranes
      - ACE2 receptor downregulation may promote prothrombotic state, decreasing levels of circulating angiotensin
      - Indirectly activated by inflammatory immune response
      - Increased clotting factors and blood viscosity
      - Venous stasis due to prolonged immobilization
    - Supply/demand mismatch
      - Coronary plaque rupture/erosion
      - Spontaneous coronary artery dissection
      - Vasculitis

CLINICAL ISSUES

Epidemiology

- Incidence
  - 1/3 of patients admitted to ICU presented with cardiovascular manifestations
  - 1/3 of all COVID-19-related deaths had underlying cardiovascular diseases
  - 13-41% of hospitalized patients with COVID-19 have evidence of myocardial injury (defined as elevated troponin I levels)
- Age
  - Patients > 64 years of age at higher risk of severe COVID-19
- Sex
  - Male patients at higher risk of severe COVID-19 and cardiovascular complications
- Ethnicity
  - Black patients more affected
- Risk factors
  - Hypertension
  - Diabetes mellitus
  - Obesity
  - Cardiovascular diseases
  - Chronic kidney diseases
  - Hypercholesterolemia
  - Chronic respiratory diseases
  - Cancer
  - Old age

Presentation

- Clinical presentation is heterogeneous, ranging from asymptomatic to severe symptoms
  - Chest pain: 5-21%
  - Palpitations: 10%
  - Arrhythmia (atrial fibrillation, bradyarrhythmia, ventricular tachycardia/fibrillation, high-degree atrioventricular block): 23%
  - Venous thromboembolic events: 20-26%
  - Acute coronary syndrome
  - Acute-onset heart failure
  - Stress cardiomyopathy
  - Cardiogenic shock
  - Sudden cardiac death

Laboratory Tests

- Biomarkers of myocyte injury (troponin I, N-terminal pro B-type natriuretic peptide) frequently elevated
  - Higher troponin levels seen in severely ill patients and those who died
- Markers of coagulopathy: D-dimer, thrombin, von Willebrand factor, fibrinogen are frequently elevated
- Biomarkers of acute inflammation: IL-6, IL-1B, interferon-γ, C-reactive protein

Natural History

- Incubation: Up to 14 days
- Zoonosis, uncertain source (suspected bats and pangolins)
- Human-to-human transmission
- Overall case mortality: 2.3%

Treatment

- Drugs
  - IL-6, IL-1 receptor antagonists
  - Antiviral therapy: Remdesivir
  - Anticoagulation
  - Antiinflammatory: Corticosteroids
  - Convalescent serum

Prognosis

- Cardiovascular diseases are common in COVID-19-infected patients and they increase risk of severe disease and mortality

Post-COVID Syndrome

- Post acute COVID syndrome: Persistent symptoms after 3 weeks of acute infection
- Chronic COVID syndrome: Persistent symptoms after 12 weeks of acute infection
  - Findings in imaging studies include: Pericardial effusion, perimyocarditis, myocardial edema, interstitial fibrosis

IMAGING

MR Findings

- Detects myocardial edema
- Diffuse late gadolinium enhancement is characteristic in myocarditis
- Useful test for long-term follow-up post-COVID-19 infection

CT Findings

- More specific to determine CAD, intracardiac thrombus, coronary dissection, intracardiac device dysfunction
- Identification of extracardiac causes of chest pain (aortic dissection, pulmonary embolism)

Echocardiography: TTE/TEE

- Can demonstrate ventricular dysfunction, wall motion abnormality, ejection fraction
  - Right ventricular dysfunction most common abnormality
- Identification of cardiac tamponade, intracardiac thrombi, pericardial effusion, valvular abnormalities, chamber dilatation, wall thickness

MACROSCOPIC

General Features

- Cardiomegaly is common finding
- Dilated right and left ventricular chambers, right > left

MICROSCOPIC

Histologic Features

- Microthrombi (10.8%)
- Endothelial cells swelling and neutrophilic endothelialitis
- Acute ischemic changes: Contraction band necrosis, hypereosinophilic myocytes, areas of granulation tissue
- Single myocyte necrosis (13.7%)
- Lymphocytic interstitial inflammation fulfilling criteria of myocarditis is rarely seen in autopsy studies (1.4-7.2%)
- Nonmyocarditis inflammation (12.6%)
- Pericardial inflammatory infiltrate (6.9%), fibrosis
- Interstitial fibrosis

Noncoronavirus-Related Findings

- Variable degree of coronary artery atherosclerosis
- Interstitial fibrosis and myocyte hypertrophy secondary to CAD
- Amyloidosis reported in ~ 13.6% of autopsy studies

ANCILLARY TESTS

Immunohistochemistry

- CD3 and CD68 are helpful to characterize inflammatory infiltrate
  - CD68 > CD3 cells reported in autopsy studies

In Situ Hybridization

- In several autopsy reports, presence of virus in interstitial cells within cardiac tissue but not in myocytes was confirmed

Electron Microscopy

- Demonstration of viral particles in heart tissue is controversial, but some studies have described them within myocytes, endothelial cells, fibroblasts, and macrophages
  - Particles with spherical morphology, measuring 60-160 nm in diameter with spikes 9-12 nm long, giving appearance of solar corona

Molecular Testing

- Identification of viral RNA in myocardial tissue has been reported in several autopsy cases

DIAGNOSTIC CHECKLIST

Pathologic Interpretation Pearls

- Myocyte single cell necrosis is common finding
- Myocarditis is not frequent in SARS-CoV-2 infection
- Demonstration of SARS-CoV-2 in heart tissue with different methodologies is rare

SELECTED REFERENCES

1. Almamlouk R et al: COVID-19-associated cardiac pathology at post-mortem evaluation: a collaborative systematic review. Clin Microbiol Infect. 28(8):1066-75, 2022
2. Martínez-Salazar B et al: COVID-19 and the vasculature: current aspects and long-term consequences. Front Cell Dev Biol. 10:824851, 2022
3. Raman B et al: Long COVID: post-acute sequelae of COVID-19 with a cardiovascular focus. Eur Heart J. 43(11):1157-72, 2022
4. Vander Heide RS: Diffuse mononuclear inflammatory response to COVID-19: friendly fire or smoldering enemy? Cardiovasc Pathol. 58:107416, 2022
5. Xie Y et al: Long-term cardiovascular outcomes of COVID-19. Nat Med. 28(3):583-90, 2022
6. Beckerman JK et al: Coronavirus disease 2019 (COVID-19)-associated constrictive pericarditis. BMJ Case Rep. 14(5):e242018, 2021
7. Fremont-Smith M et al: Models for COViD-19 early cardiac pathology following SARS-CoV-2 infection. Int J Infect Dis. 113:331-5, 2021
8. Halushka MK et al: Myocarditis is rare in COVID-19 autopsies: cardiovascular findings across 277 postmortem examinations. Cardiovasc Pathol. 50:107300, 2021
9. Hooper JE et al: A postmortem portrait of the Coronavirus disease 2019 (COVID-19) pandemic: a large multi-institutional autopsy survey study. Arch Pathol Lab Med. 145(5):529-35, 2021
10. Kawakami R et al: Pathological evidence for SARS-CoV-2 as a cause of myocarditis: JACC review topic of the week. J Am Coll Cardiol. 77(3):314-25, 2021
11. Luo J et al: Cardiovascular disease in patients with COVID-19: evidence from cardiovascular pathology to treatment. Acta Biochim Biophys Sin (Shanghai). 53(3):273-82, 2021
12. Sang CJ 3rd et al: Cardiac pathology in COVID-19: a single center autopsy experience. Cardiovasc Pathol. 54:107370, 2021
13. Sawalha K et al: Systematic review of COVID-19 related myocarditis: insights on management and outcome. Cardiovasc Revasc Med. 23:107-13, 2021
14. Tajbakhsh A et al: COVID-19 and cardiac injury: clinical manifestations, biomarkers, mechanisms, diagnosis, treatment, and follow up. Expert Rev Anti Infect Ther. 19(3):345-57, 2021
15. Basso C et al: Pathological features of COVID-19-associated myocardial injury: a multicentre cardiovascular pathology study. Eur Heart J. 41(39):3827-35, 2020
16. Fox SE et al: Cardiac endotheliitis and multisystem inflammatory syndrome after COVID-19. Ann Intern Med. 173(12):1025-7, 2020
17. Fox SE et al: Unexpected features of cardiac pathology in COVID-19 infection. Circulation. 142(11):1123-5, 2020

Focal Myocarditis in COVID-19-Positive Patient

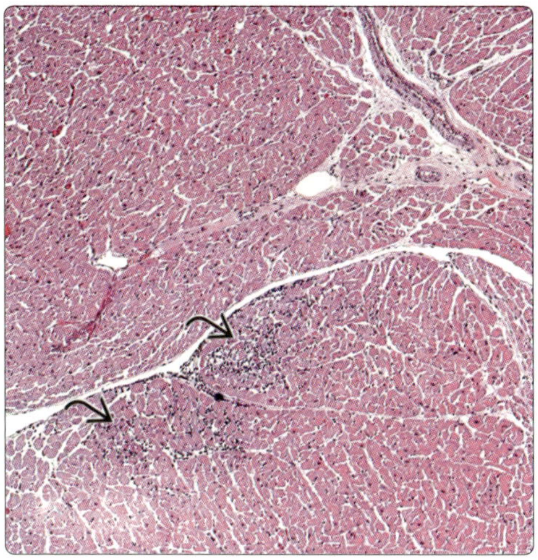

Subtle Early Ischemic Myocardial Changes in COVID-19

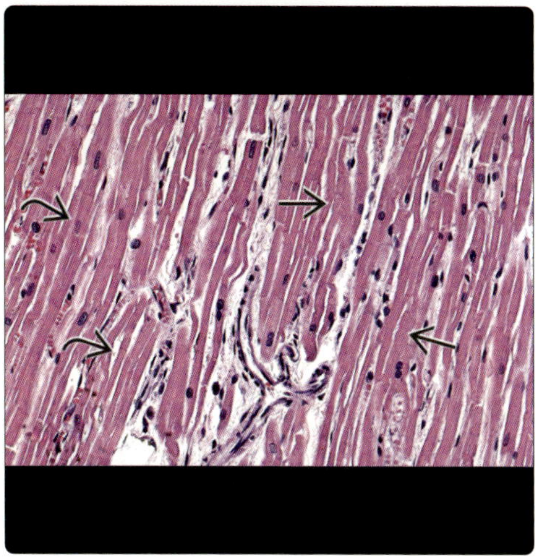

(Left) *While rare, myocarditis has been observed in hearts from COVID-19-positive patients. This example shows focal inflammatory infiltrate ↪ with myocyte injury. (Courtesy M.E.H. Hammond, MD and M. Belenky, MD.)* **(Right)** *Subtle changes, such as nuclear "drop out" ↪ and homogenization of the sarcoplasm →, have also been observed in hearts from COVID-19-positive patients. (Courtesy M.E.H. Hammond, MD and M. Belenky, MD.)*

Myocardial Vascular Smooth Muscle Changes in COVID-19

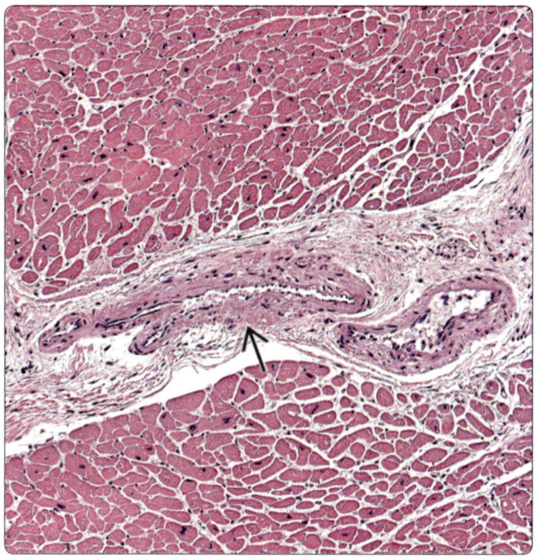

Myocardial Microthrombi in COVID-19

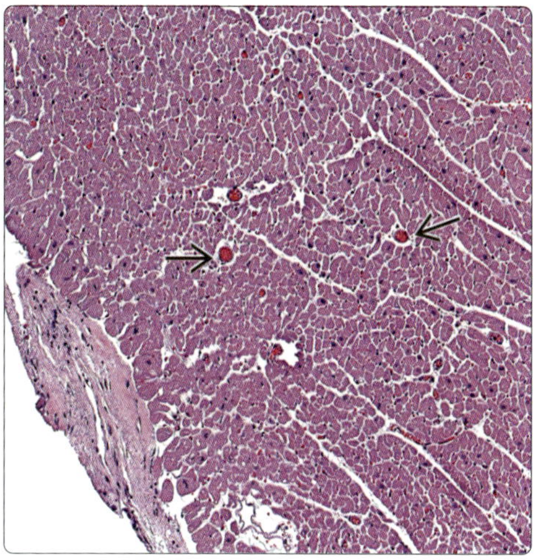

(Left) *Another change observed in autopsied hearts from COVID-19-positive patients is disruption → of the vascular smooth muscle wall of the small arteries. (Courtesy M.E.H. Hammond, MD and M. Belenky, MD.)* **(Right)** *Small, recent microthrombi → are seen in the myocardium of this patient who died from a critical illness related to COVID-19 infection. (Courtesy M.E.H. Hammond, MD and M. Belenky, MD.)*

Myocardial Inflammation in COVID-19

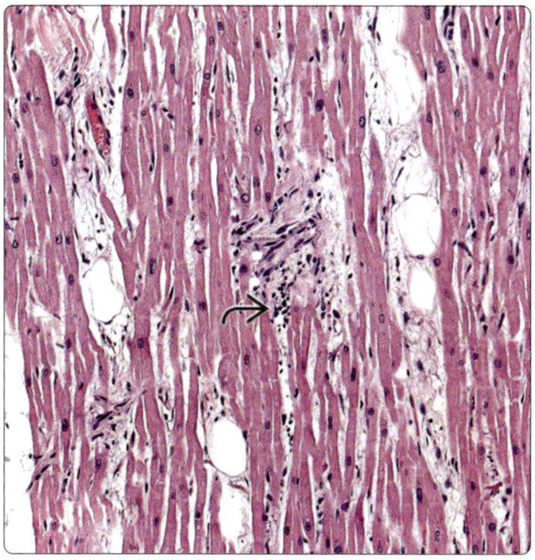

Increased Myocardial Macrophages in COVID-19

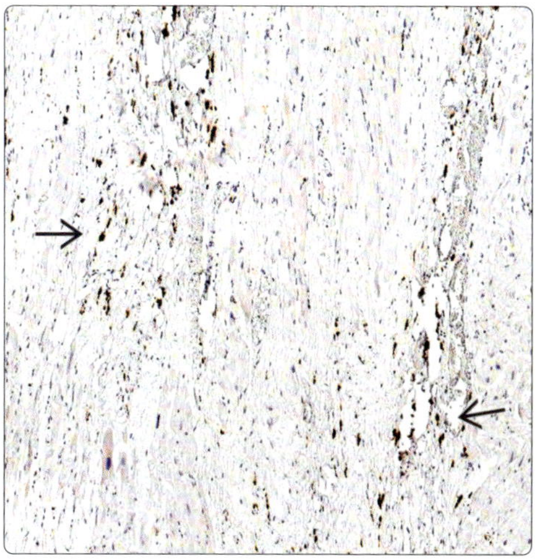

(Left) *True myocarditis is exceptionally rare in COVID-19-positive patients, but subtle (and less specific) inflammatory infiltrates ↪ are reported with increased frequency in autopsied hearts from COVID-19-positive patients. (Courtesy M.E.H. Hammond, MD and M. Belenky, MD.)* **(Right)** *An increase in macrophage lineage [CD68(+)] inflammatory cells → has been observed in autopsy hearts from COVID-19-positive patients. (Courtesy M.E.H. Hammond, MD and M. Belenky, MD.)*

Lupus Erythematosus, Heart

KEY FACTS

TERMINOLOGY

- Chronic inflammatory autoimmune disease affecting skin, joints, kidneys, lungs, heart, nervous system, serous membranes, &/or other organs of body

CLINICAL ISSUES

- Course characterized by periods of remission and chronic or acute relapses
- Cardiovascular complications are among most important causes of mortality
- Atherosclerotic coronary disease is common
- Pericardial abnormalities associated with markers of ongoing inflammation
- Verrucous endocarditis
- Myocarditis
- Phospholipid antibody syndrome
- Prognosis is improving with early diagnosis and treatment

MACROSCOPIC

- Pericardial involvement is frequent, and fibrinous exudate may be seen
- In chronic phase, pericardium becomes thickened, opaque, and coated with shaggy fibrous tissue
- Nonbacterial verrucous endocarditis (Libman-Sacks endocarditis) involving mitral/aortic valves

MICROSCOPIC

- Pericardium: Acute, subacute, or chronic inflammation
- Myocardium: Nonspecific lymphocytic inflammation with hematoxylin bodies and fibrinoid degeneration of collagen fibrils
- Valves: Active lesions (Libman-Sacks endocarditis) consist of deposits of fibrin-like material, which may contain hematoxylin bodies, focal necrosis, and mononuclear inflammation
- Coronary arteries
  - Atherosclerotic plaques, vasculitis, thrombosis

Microscopic Features of Systemic Lupus Erythematosus Involving Myocardium

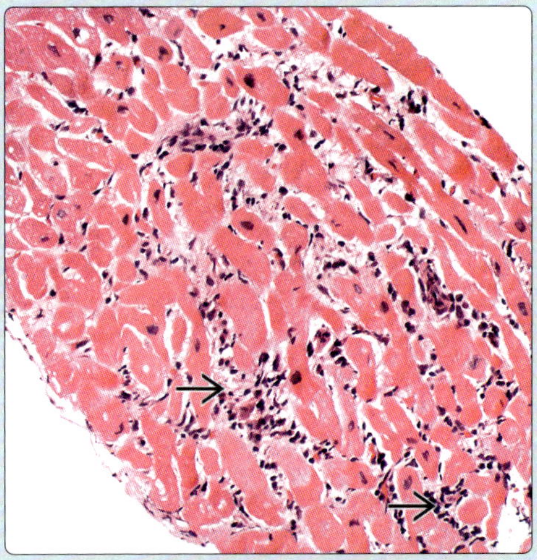

Electron Microscopy Features of Systemic Lupus Erythematosus

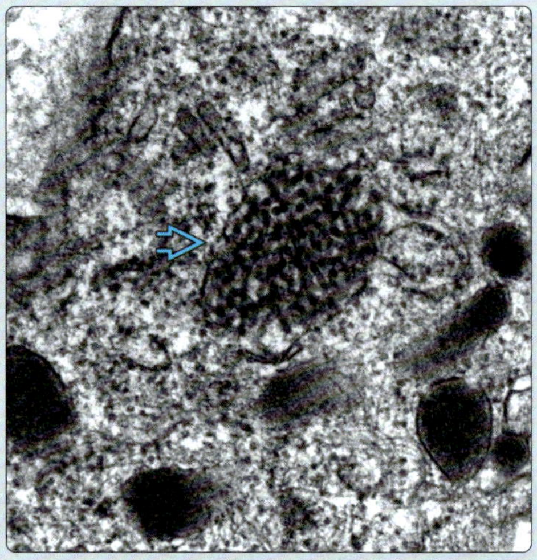

(Left) *H&E-stained section of myocardial biopsy from a patient with a diagnosis of systemic lupus erythematosus (SLE) shows focal interstitial mononuclear inflammation ➔ and edema with nonspecific pattern resembling myocarditis of other etiologies.* **(Right)** *Transmission electron microscopy (TEM) of coronary artery shows a reticular aggregate ➔ in the endothelial cell cytoplasm, a feature characteristic of high levels of α-interferon seen in patients with SLE.*

Microscopic Features of Systemic Lupus Erythematosus Involving Myocardium

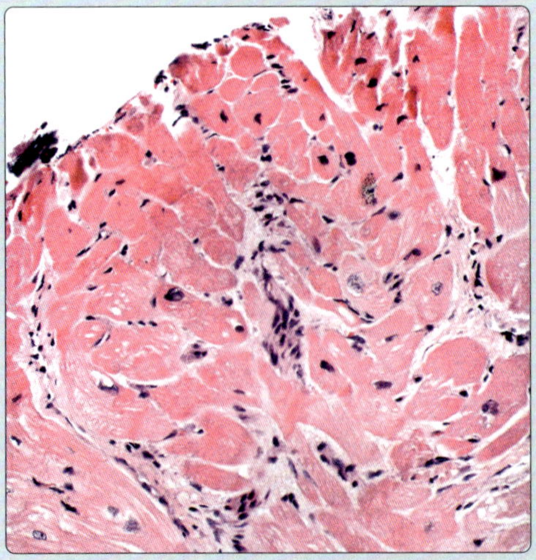

Microscopic Features of Systemic Lupus Erythematosus Involving Myocardium

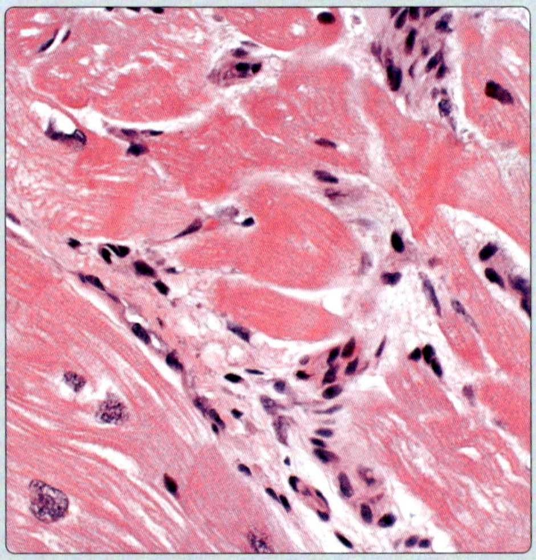

(Left) *H&E-stained section of myocardial biopsy from a patient with a diagnosis of SLE presenting with acute chest pain shows focal myocyte eosinophilic change, consistent with ischemia secondary to vascular injury in coronary artery branches.* **(Right)** *High magnification of an H&E-stained section of myocardial biopsy from a patient with a diagnosis of SLE shows perimyocyte capillaries with endothelial swelling and reduction of the lumina. There is also scant interstitial edema.*

TERMINOLOGY

Abbreviations

- Systemic lupus erythematosus (SLE)

Definitions

- Chronic inflammatory autoimmune disease affecting skin, joints, kidneys, lungs, heart, nervous system, serous membranes, &/or other organs
    - Immunologic abnormalities, especially production of antinuclear antibodies (ANAs)

ETIOLOGY/PATHOGENESIS

Autoimmune

- Autoantibodies to nuclear antigens in 95% of SLE patients
    - Double-stranded (ds) DNA
    - Antibodies to histones: Anti-Smith (Sm)
    - Antibodies to nonhistone proteins bound to RNA: SS-A(Ro), SS-B(La)
- Autoantibodies against elements of blood: Red cells, platelets, lymphocytes
- Antiphospholipid antibodies

Genetic Factors

- 20% of unaffected 1st-degree relatives reveal autoantibodies
- Higher risk of concordance (> 20%) in monozygotic twins in comparison to dizygotic twins (1-3%)
- HLA-DQ locus linked to production of anti-dsDNA, anti-Sm, and antiphospholipid antibodies
- Inherited C1q, C2, or C4 deficiencies leading to impaired removal of circulating immune complexes by mononuclear phagocyte system

Environmental Factors

- Ultraviolet light
- Drugs: Hydralazine, procainamide, D-penicillamine
- Sex hormones

Pathogenesis

- Genetically susceptible individuals
- Possible environmental triggers
- Activation of helper T cells and B cells
- Production of pathogenic autoantibodies, immune complexes, and T lymphocytes being deposited in otherwise healthy tissue
- Failure of multiple regulatory networks to interrupt process

CLINICAL ISSUES

Epidemiology

- Incidence
    - Overall SLE incidence: ~ 7/100,000/year
    - Symptomatic myocarditis: ~ 9% of SLE patients
- Age
    - 20-30 years
- Sex
    - Women affected 10x more frequently than men
- Ethnicity
    - 3x higher for African American women than for European American women

Presentation

- Course characterized by periods of remission and chronic or acute relapses
- 1 or several clinical manifestations may be initial presentation
    - Fever
    - Fatigue
    - Weight loss
    - Photosensitivity rash
    - Arthralgia or arthritis
    - Raynaud phenomenon
    - Serositis: Pleuritis, pericarditis, peritonitis
    - Alopecia
    - Phlebitis
    - Recurrent miscarriage
    - Anemia
- Kidney manifestations: Nephritic/nephrotic syndrome, acute/chronic renal failure
- Neurologic symptoms: Seizures, psychosis
- Heart
    - Atherosclerotic coronary disease
        - Myocardial infarction (50x increased risk in comparison with patients without SLE)
        - Angina
        - Sudden death
    - Pericardial abnormalities associated with markers of ongoing inflammation
        - Acute/chronic pericarditis most common cardiac manifestation of SLE
        - Effusion
        - Cardiac tamponade and constrictive pericarditis are rare manifestations
    - Verrucous endocarditis most commonly involves mitral valve
        - Most cases are asymptomatic
        - Occasionally, murmurs or embolic events can occur
        - 1-2% will require surgery
    - Myocarditis may be initial clinical manifestation of SLE or subclinical in majority of cases
        - Arrhythmias, conduction disturbances (QT prolongation, ST-segment elevation), heart block
        - Dilated cardiomyopathy
        - Heart failure (40%)
        - Cardiogenic shock could be initial manifestation of SLE
    - Antiphospholipid antibody syndrome
        - Myocardial perfusion defects associated with presence of lupus anticoagulant and with elevated levels of anticardiolipin and anti-β2GPI antibodies of IgG class
        - Valve abnormalities: Vegetations, thickening, valve dysfunction
        - Thrombotic and atherosclerotic coronary artery occlusion
        - Intracardiac thrombosis; right side most commonly involved
        - Ventricular hypertrophy and dysfunction
        - Pulmonary systolic pressure elevation secondary to chronic recurrence of embolic/thrombotic events involving lung

Laboratory Tests

- Elevated antinuclear, antiphospholipid, anti-Sm, and anti-dsDNA antibodies
- Cytopenias on complete blood count (CBC)
- Hematuria and proteinuria
- Elevated cardiac troponin I level in myocarditis

Treatment

- Drugs
  - Immunosuppressive medication: Steroids, mycophenolate mofetil, cyclophosphamide, azathioprine
  - Hydrochloroquine
  - Standard heart failure medication

Prognosis

- Improving with early diagnosis and treatment
- Cardiovascular complications are among most important causes of mortality

IMAGING

MR Findings

- Myocarditis: T1 abnormalities and increased T2-weighted edema images, early or late gadolinium enhancement, focal lesion with nonischemic regional distribution
- Pericarditis: Increased pericardial signal intensity on late gadolinium enhancement and T2 STIR

Echocardiogram

- Pericardial effusion
- Valvular abnormalities
  - Verrucous vegetations (mitral and aortic), leaflet thickening, or motion abnormalities
- Decreased ejection fraction
- Increased chamber size
- Global, regional, or segmental wall motion abnormalities
- Prolonged isovolumetric relaxation time

MACROSCOPIC

General Features

- Pericardial involvement is most common heart-related finding
  - In acute phase, fibrinous, serous exudate may be seen
  - In chronic phase, pericardium becomes thickened, opaque, and coated with shaggy fibrous tissue
  - Partial or total obliteration of serosal cavity can occur
- Valvular abnormalities
  - Nonbacterial verrucous endocarditis (Libman-Sacks endocarditis)
    - Single/multiple 1- to 3-mm warty deposits on either side or both sides of leaflets of any heart valve (mitral and aortic more commonly involved)

MICROSCOPIC

Histologic Features

- Heart
  - Pericardium
    - Nonspecific acute, subacute, or chronic inflammation
    - Variable degree of fibrosis
  - Myocardium
    - Nonspecific lymphocytic perivascular inflammation with hematoxylin bodies and interstitial edema
    - Fibrinoid degeneration of collagen fibrils and myocyte necrosis
    - Intramural coronary artery branch thickening and luminal narrowing
    - In chronic stage, interstitial fibrosis not associated with coronary changes may be seen
  - Valvular endocardium
    - Deposits of fibrin-like material, which may contain hematoxylin bodies, focal necrosis, and mononuclear inflammation
    - Healed lesions characterized by vascularized leaflets, fibrosis, and calcifications
  - Coronary arteries
    - Atherosclerotic plaques, vasculitis, thrombosis, immune complex deposits

ANCILLARY TESTS

Immunofluorescence

- Fine granular immune complex-type deposits (immunoglobulins and complement) seen in walls and perivascular tissues of myocardial blood vessels and perimyocytes

DIFFERENTIAL DIAGNOSIS

Bacterial Endocarditis

- Negative autoantibodies
- Large vegetations localized on valve cusps and extending into chordae
- Vegetations contain neutrophils; microorganisms may be identified
- Positive blood cultures

Viral Myocarditis

- Preceding viral illness
- Negative autoantibodies
- No evidence of systemic involvement
- Inflammatory process limited to myocardium
- Absence of immune complex-type deposits

Acute Rheumatic Carditis

- Negative autoantibodies
- Smaller vegetations confined to leaflet lines of closure
- Aschoff nodules
- Chronic valvular disease

SELECTED REFERENCES

1. Battisha A et al: Cardiogenic shock in autoimmune rheumatologic diseases: an insight on etiologies, management, and treatment outcomes. Heart Fail Rev. 27(1):93-101, 2022
2. Tayem MG et al: A review of cardiac manifestations in patients with systemic lupus erythematosus and antiphospholipid syndrome with focus on endocarditis. Cureus. 14(1):e21698, 2022
3. Zagelbaum Ward NK et al: Cardiac manifestations of systemic lupus erythematous: an overview of the incidence, risk factors, diagnostic criteria, pathophysiology and treatment options. Cardiol Rev. 30(1):38-43, 2022
4. Guglin M et al: The spectrum of lupus myocarditis: from asymptomatic forms to cardiogenic shock. Heart Fail Rev. 26(3):553-60, 2021
5. Butt S et al: Cardiac conduction defects in systemic lupus erythematosus. Cureus. 12(10):e10882, 2020
6. Gartshteyn Y et al: Endomyocardial biopsies in the diagnosis of myocardial involvement in systemic lupus erythematosus. Lupus. 29(2):199-204, 2020

Microscopic Features of Systemic Lupus Erythematosus Involving Myocardium

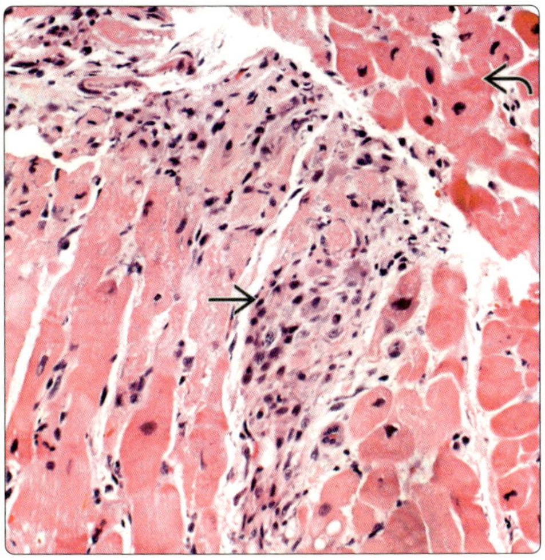

Microscopic Features of Systemic Lupus Erythematosus Involving Myocardium

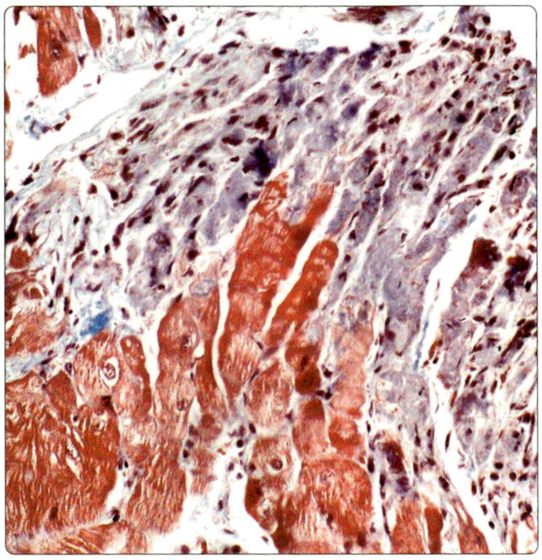

(Left) *H&E-stained section of a myocardial biopsy from a patient with a diagnosis of SLE shows focal myocyte eosinophilic change* ⮫*, consistent with ischemia. In the adjacent area, there is mild lymphocytic inflammatory infiltrate and early fibrous organization* ➔*.* **(Right)** *Trichrome-stained section of a myocardial biopsy in the same patient shows connective tissue proliferation and scant lymphocytic inflammatory infiltrate in an area of myocyte necrosis secondary to ischemia.*

Microscopic Features of Systemic Lupus Erythematosus Involving Myocardium

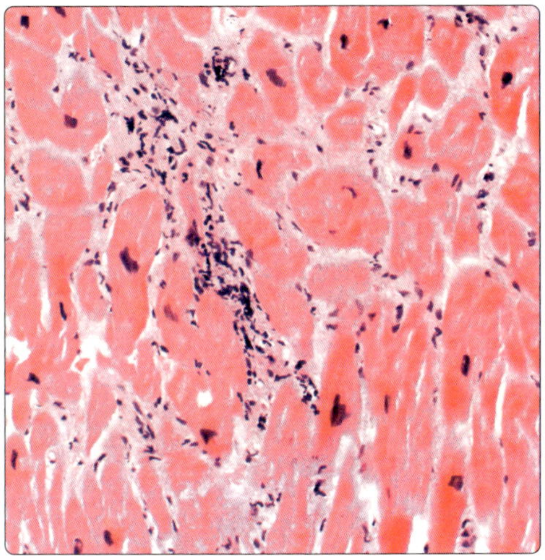

Microscopic Features of Systemic Lupus Erythematosus Involving Myocardium

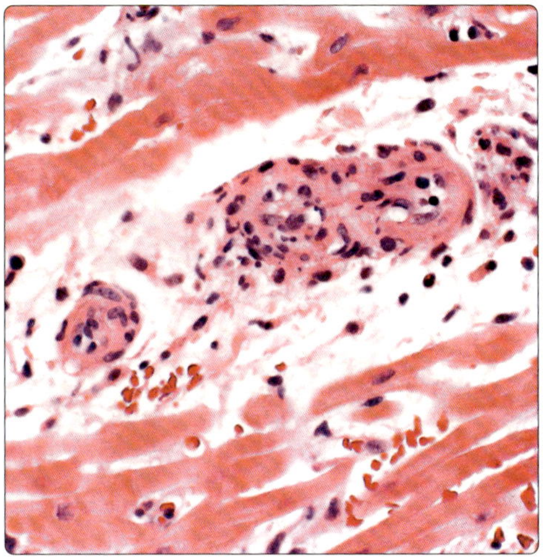

(Left) *H&E-stained section of myocardial biopsy from a patient with a diagnosis of SLE presenting with fever and heart failure shows focal interstitial inflammatory infiltrate composed of mononuclear cells, which is nonspecific but resembles myocarditis.* **(Right)** *H&E-stained section of myocardial biopsy from a patient with a diagnosis of SLE shows interstitial edema and small intramyocardial artery branches with endothelial swelling, reduction of the lumen, and scant perivascular inflammation.*

Microscopic Features of Systemic Lupus Erythematosus Involving Myocardium

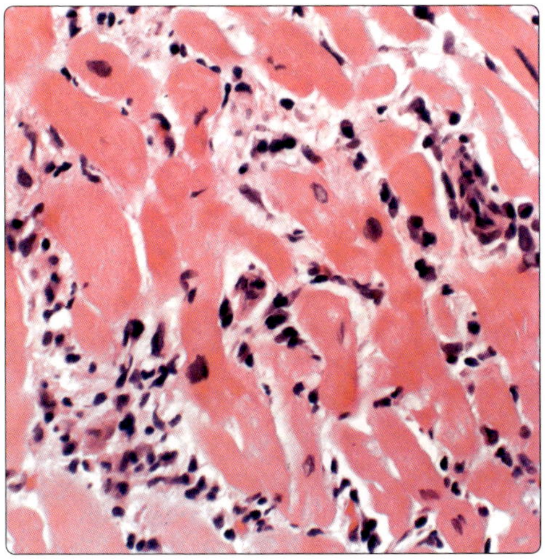

Microscopic Features of Systemic Lupus Erythematosus Involving Myocardium

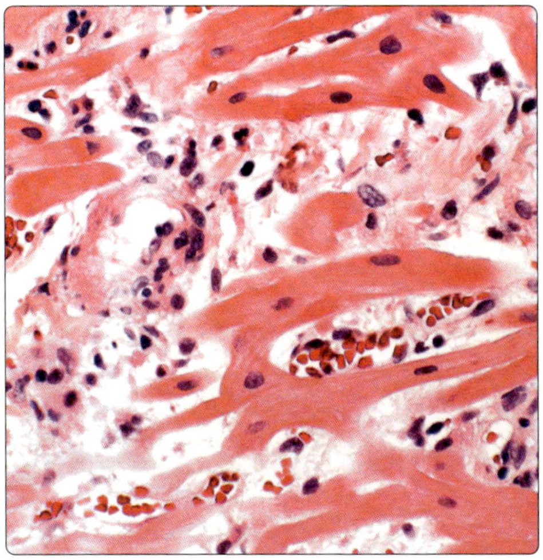

(Left) *H&E-stained section of myocardial biopsy from a patient with a diagnosis of SLE shows focal interstitial and perivascular inflammatory infiltrate composed of mononuclear cells, which, although nonspecific in this clinical setting, is likely secondary to lupus involvement of the heart.* **(Right)** *H&E-stained section of myocardial biopsy from a patient with a diagnosis of SLE shows edema and sparse interstitial inflammatory infiltrate composed of mononuclear cells, resembling acute myocarditis.*

(Left) *Trichrome-stained section of myocardium from a patient with a diagnosis of SLE who died from renal failure shows patchy mononuclear interstitial inflammation → with myocyte injury.* **(Right)** *Higher magnification of a trichrome-stained section of myocardium from a patient with a diagnosis of SLE who died from renal failure shows patchy mononuclear interstitial inflammation → with myocyte injury. There is pale blue staining in areas of edema. Myocarditis is identified more frequently at autopsy.*

Microscopic Features of Systemic Lupus Erythematosus Involving Myocardium

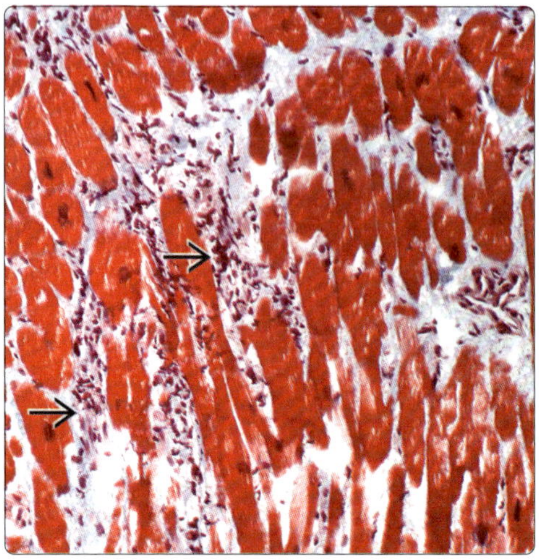

Microscopic Features of Systemic Lupus Erythematosus Involving Myocardium

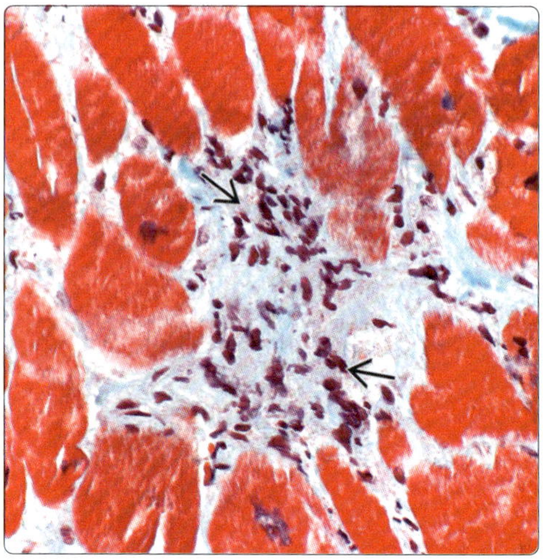

(Left) *Trichrome-stained section of myocardium from a patient with a diagnosis of SLE shows focal interstitial fibrosis → and myofibrillar loss ⇨, which may be seen in cases with longstanding SLE.* **(Right)** *Trichrome-stained section of myocardium from a patient with a diagnosis of SLE who died from renal failure shows marked interstitial fibrosis →, which may be seen in cases with longstanding SLE and is usually not associated with coronary artery stenosis.*

Microscopic Features of Systemic Lupus Erythematosus Involving Myocardium

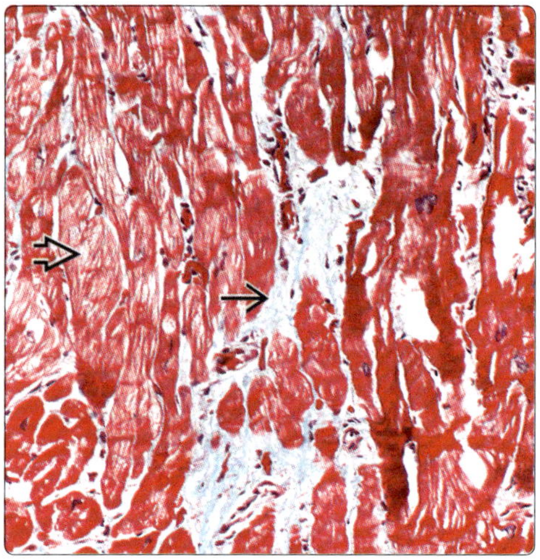

Microscopic Features of Systemic Lupus Erythematosus Involving Myocardium

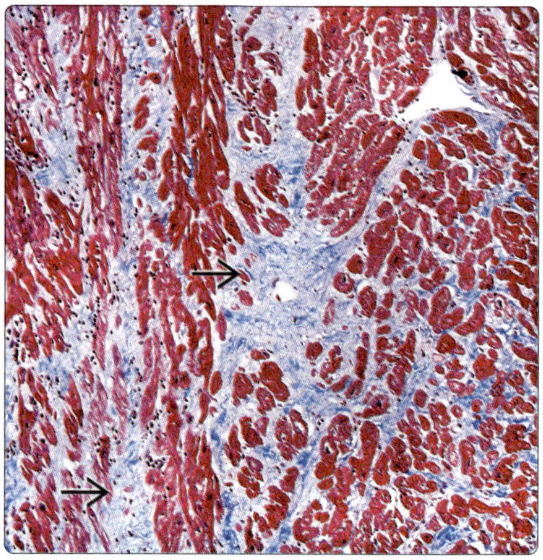

(Left) *C1q immunofluorescence stain of myocardial biopsy from a patient with a diagnosis of SLE shows granular staining in perimyocytic distribution. Deposits of this immunoreactant and IgG are commonly found in patients with SLE.* **(Right)** *IgG immunofluorescence stain of myocardial biopsy from a patient with a diagnosis of SLE shows granular perimyocytic deposits.*

C1q Immunofluorescence

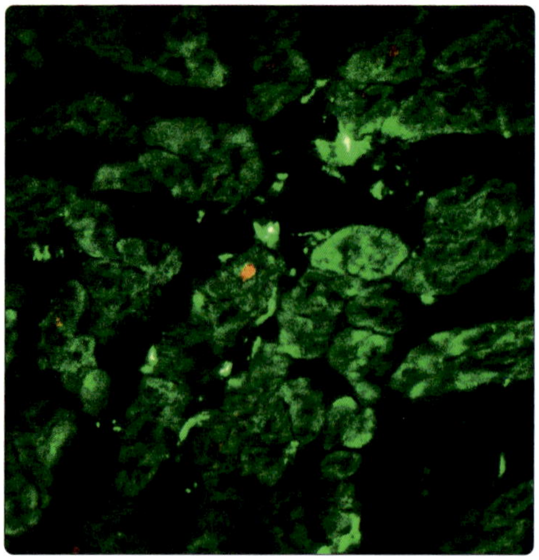

IgG Immunofluorescence

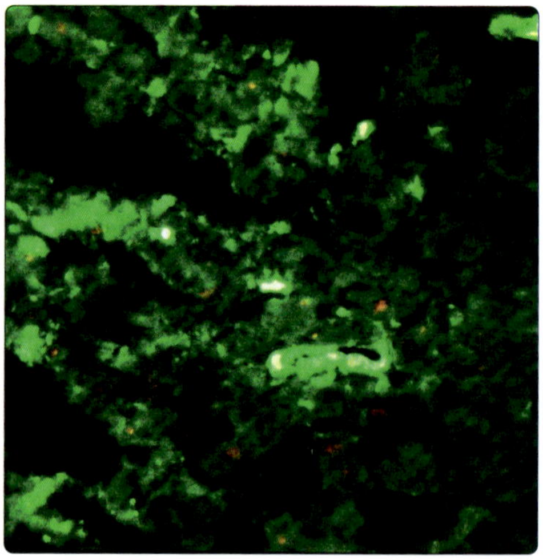

IgG Immunofluorescence

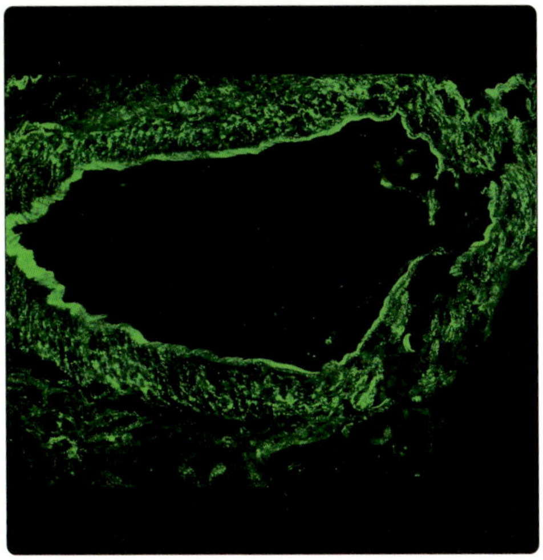

C1q Immunofluorescence

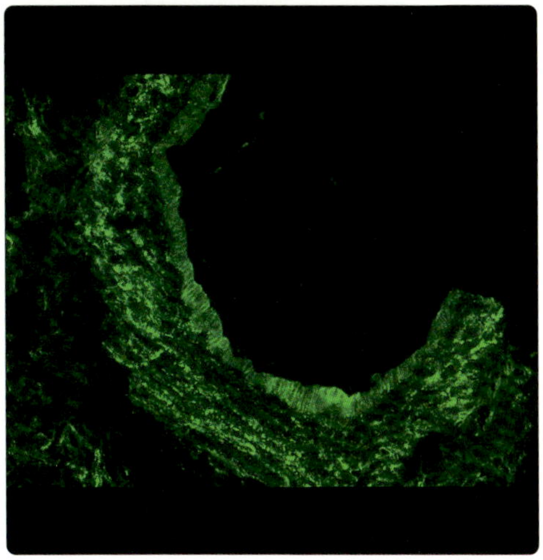

(Left) *IgG immunofluorescence stain of coronary artery from a patient with a diagnosis of SLE shows granular staining in the wall. Similar findings may be seen in other vessels.* **(Right)** *C1q immunofluorescence stain of coronary artery from a patient with a diagnosis of SLE shows granular staining in the wall. Associations between this immunoreactant and IgG are commonly found in patients with SLE.*

Ultrastructure of Small Artery With Deposits

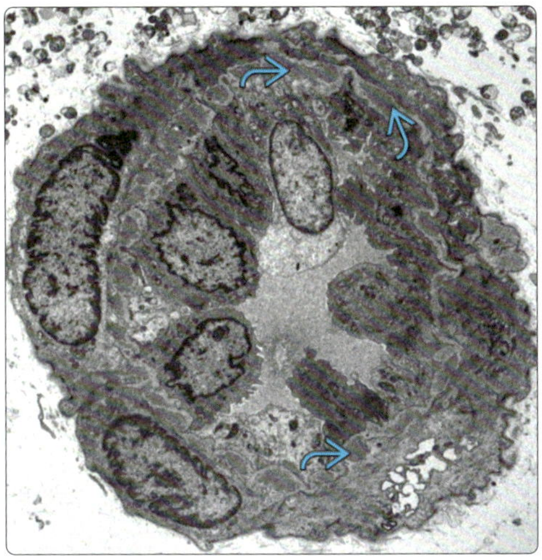

Electron-Dense Deposits in Coronary Artery

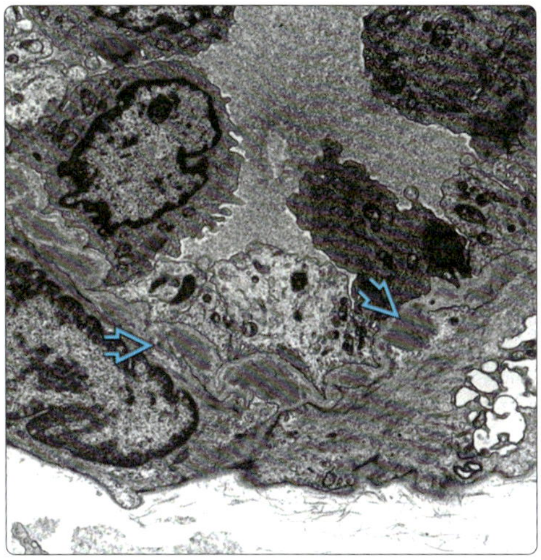

(Left) *Electron micrograph of an intramyocardial penetrating artery branch shows numerous circumferential deposits near the internal elastic lamina. These correspond to the granules seen on immunofluorescence staining.* **(Right)** *TEM of coronary artery from a patient with SLE shows electron-dense deposits in subendothelial distribution. The deposits are granular and do not display substructure.*

Electron-Dense Deposits in Coronary Artery

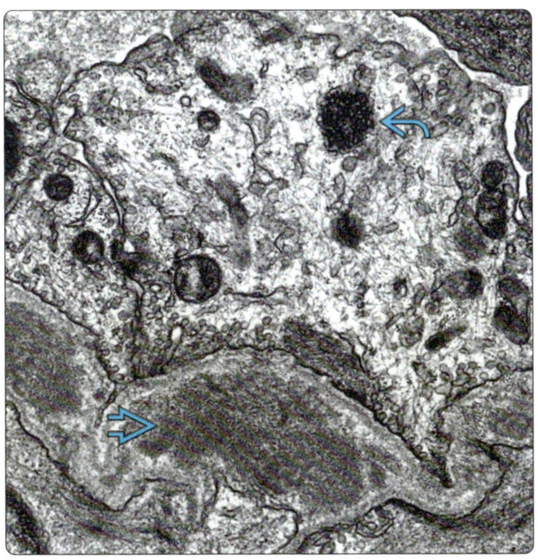

Hematoxylin Body

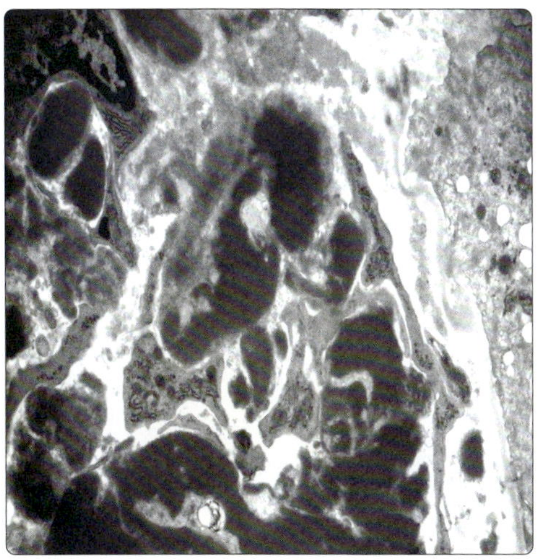

(Left) *TEM of coronary artery at high magnification shows electron-dense deposits in subendothelial distribution. In the endothelial cell cytoplasm, a reticular aggregate is seen . Together, these findings are very characteristic of SLE, though clinical diagnosis may not be established.* **(Right)** *Electron-dense nuclear fragments comprise the bulk of these hematoxylin bodies seen by electron microscopy. These are composed of nuclear histone proteins, nucleic acids, and bound antinuclear antibodies.*

Acute Cellular Transplant Rejection, Heart

KEY FACTS

TERMINOLOGY

- Acute cellular rejection (ACR): Host response producing destruction of transplanted hearts, mediated by T lymphocytes and characterized by their presence in apposition to myocytes

CLINICAL ISSUES

- Most acute rejection episodes occur within first 6 months post transplant
- 20-30% of recipients may experience episode of ACR within 1st year post transplant
- ACR is uncommon after 1 year post transplant
- Cellular and antibody-mediated rejection (mixed rejection) can occur simultaneously in 25% of cases
- Asymptomatic presentation is most common
- Symptoms occur only with moderate or severe ACR and include symptoms associated with heart failure
- Relationship of ACR to chronic allograft vasculopathy is tenuous

MACROSCOPIC

- At least 4 samples should be received and sectioned at 3 levels; 1 sample should be frozen for immunofluorescence if needed

MICROSCOPIC

- Histologic features are graded using International Society of Heart Lung Transplantation grading schema, updated 2004

ANCILLARY TESTS

- Antibody-mediated rejection can be ruled in or out by either doing immunofluorescence for complement components or immunohistochemistry for C4d and CD68

TOP DIFFERENTIAL DIAGNOSES

- Quilty effect
- Ischemic injury and repair
- Biopsy site inflammation
- Lymphoproliferative disorder

Morphologic Features of Mild Acute Cellular Rejection

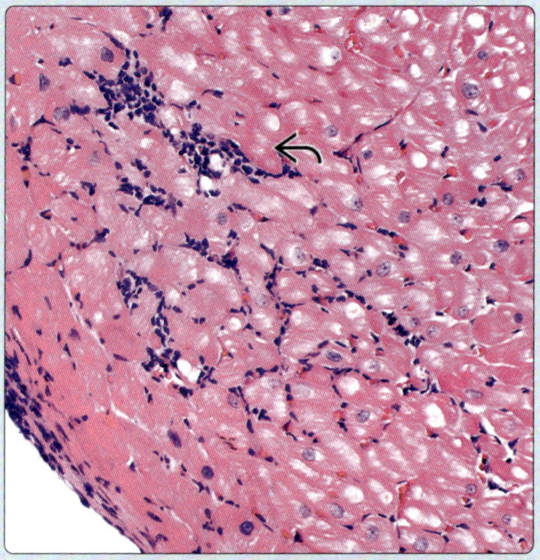

Morphologic Features of Severe Acute Cellular Rejection

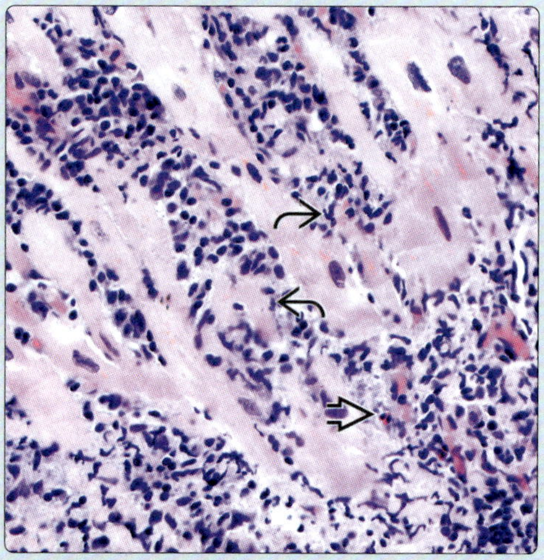

(Left) *Myocardium shows lymphoid inflammatory infiltrate in the interstitium associated with at least 1 focus of myocyte distortion ↪ and injury diagnostic of mild transplant rejection [International Society for Heart and Lung Transplantation (ISHLT) 1R].* **(Right)** *H&E-stained section of myocardium shows marked lymphoid inflammatory infiltrate with rare eosinophils ⇨ in the interstitium associated with multifocal myocyte distortion ↪ and injury diagnostic of severe rejection (ISHLT 3R).*

Morphologic Features of Moderate Acute Cellular Rejection

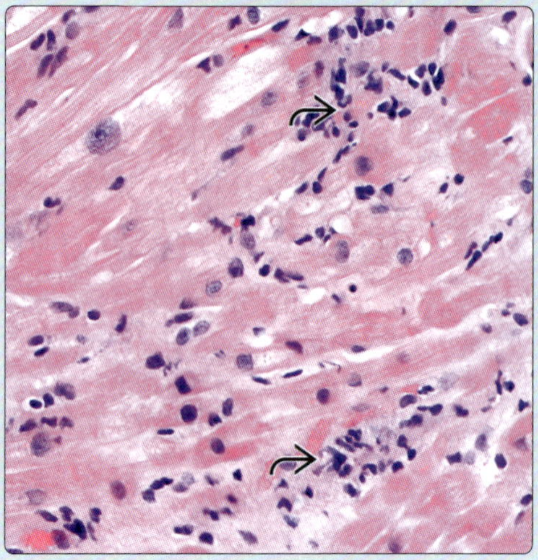

Morphologic Features of Moderate Acute Cellular Rejection

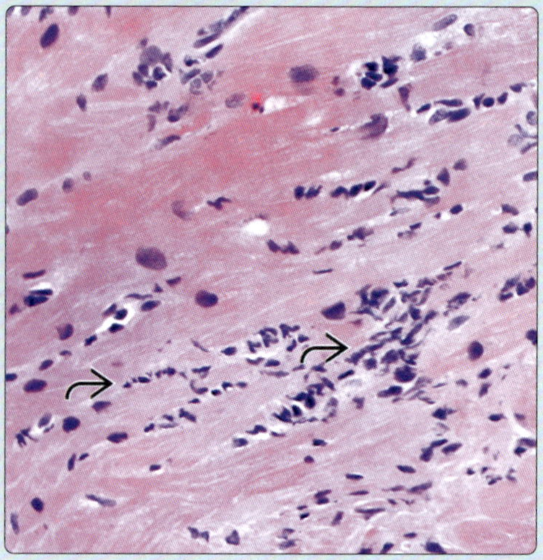

(Left) *H&E-stained section of myocardium shows lymphoid inflammatory infiltrate in the interstitium associated with myocyte distortion ↪ and injury diagnostic of moderate rejection (ISHLT 2R). There are also vacuolar changes in myocyte cytoplasm.* **(Right)** *H&E-stained section of myocardium at higher magnification shows lymphoid inflammatory infiltrate in the interstitium associated with multifocal myocyte distortion ↪ and injury diagnostic of moderate rejection (ISHLT 2R).*

TERMINOLOGY

Abbreviations

- Acute cellular rejection (ACR)

Definitions

- Host response producing destruction of transplanted hearts, mediated by T lymphocytes and macrophages, and characterized by their apposition to myocytes with associated myocyte damage

ETIOLOGY/PATHOGENESIS

Pathogenesis

- Hosts recognize allografted organ as foreign because it often contains foreign complex human leukocyte antigens (HLAs) that lead to T-cell stimulation and cytokine release
  - Recipient T-cells are directly stimulated by simultaneous exposure to both foreign HLA antigens (class I and class II) and foreign allograft peptides
    - Foreign peptides are extremely biologically diverse as are HLA antigens, and these factors amplify numbers of stimulated T cells
    - Class I antigens (HLA-A, -B, and -C) are constitutively expressed on most cells in heart, especially vascular endothelium
    - Class II antigens (HLA-DP, -DQ, and -DR) are constitutively expressed on vascular endothelium, macrophages, monocytes, and B lymphocytes
    - Presentation of antigen occurs to T cells directly or indirectly via antigen-presenting cells and endothelial cells
  - T-cell antigen stimulation leads to production of multiple methods of graft destruction
    - Activated T cells produce cytokines that upregulate class II antigens on vascular endothelium to promote inflammatory and procoagulant responses
    - Activated T cells activate CD8(+) T cells and macrophages, which can then participate in cytotoxic killing of graft myocytes
    - Activated T cells activate B cells, which can produce donor-specific antibody that can bind to vascular endothelium, fix complement, and mediate injury
  - Other antigens are also involved due to cellular necrosis and endothelial sloughing that happens during initial posttransplant period
    - Activated endothelial cells express more class II antigens, which may be presented in context of foreign endothelial peptides
    - Vimentin is antigen that may also provoke response
  - Innate allorecognition is potentially involved in initiation and maintenance of alloimmune response

CLINICAL ISSUES

Epidemiology

- Incidence
  - 20-30% of recipients may experience episode of ACR within 1st year post transplant
  - Current maintenance immunosuppression has resulted in waning incidence and severity of ACR
  - Cellular and antibody-mediated rejection (AMR) can occur simultaneously in ~ 25% of patients

Presentation

- Asymptomatic presentation is most common
- Symptoms occur only with moderate or severe ACR and include symptoms associated with heart failure

Natural History

- Most ACR is mild and self-limited because of effective maintenance immunosuppression
- Most acute rejection episodes occur within first 6 months post transplant
- ACR is uncommon after 1 year post transplant
- Relationship of ACR to chronic allograft vasculopathy is tenuous
  - Little increased risk of coronary artery vasculopathy in patients with more frequent ACR
  - No change in incidence of coronary artery vasculopathy despite more effective maintenance immunosuppression

Treatment

- Drugs
  - Currently used immunosuppressive drugs are highly effective in controlling ACR

Prognosis

- Most asymptomatic ACR (85%) resolves without treatment
- Combination of corticosteroids and antithymocyte globulin reverses 90% of symptomatic ACR episodes
- Graft loss is rare, occurring in ~ 6% overall, although it is as high as 12% in 1st year post transplant

Surveillance

- Biopsies are done weekly for 2 months, monthly for 4 months, and then yearly unless rejection is suspected
- Evidence exists that biopsy surveillance after 5 years is not necessary; controversial data suggest that monitoring may be unnecessary after 1 year
- Gene expression profiling of RNA derived from peripheral blood mononuclear cells (AlloMap) is routinely used for surveillance in some settings
  - Low AlloMap scores define patients with low probability of moderate or severe ACR at time of testing (score < 30)
- Donor-derived cell-free DNA
  - Threshold of ≥ 0.25% has excellent sensitivity and specificity for diagnosis of rejection (performed after 28 days post transplant)

IMAGING

General Features

- Surveillance by imaging has been investigated but has not been found to have sufficient evidence to recommend routine use

MACROSCOPIC

General Features

- Adequate sample should contain at least 3 fragments of myocardium
- Samples should be aggregated into small mass and sectioned at 3 different levels to assure complete examination

- 1 frozen sample should be saved for immunofluorescence if AMR is suspected

MICROSCOPIC

Histologic Features

- Perivascular/interstitial mononuclear inflammation, predominantly composed of activated lymphocytes and macrophages
- Myocyte damage in association with mononuclear inflammation
  - Damage is not myocyte necrosis but rather encroachment of inflammatory cells into myocyte borders leading to architectural distortion
- In severe ACR, neutrophils &/or eosinophils may be present; such rejection is usually mixed with AMR
- Histologic features are graded using International Society of Heart Lung Transplantation 2004 grading schema

ANCILLARY TESTS

Immunohistochemistry

- CD3 and CD20 may be used to rule out posttransplant lymphoproliferative disorder and Quilty effect
- C4d can be used when frozen tissue is not available to rule out AMR
- CD68 to identify intravascular macrophages, which would support diagnosis of AMR

Immunofluorescence

- In cases where endothelial cells are swollen and interstitial edema is seen, immunofluorescence (C4d, C3d) should be done to rule out AMR

Molecular

- Molecular microscope diagnostic system (MMDx) measures gene expression using microarrays and applies machine learning algorithms to assign probability or diagnoses of cellular/antibody-mediated rejection in fresh myocardial biopsy samples
- Nano string technology has also been used for analysis of expression of 34-gene set for diagnosis of rejection in paraffin-embedded samples
- MicroRNA expression on tissue biopsies

DIFFERENTIAL DIAGNOSIS

Quilty Effect

- Endocardial infiltrates of mixed lymphocytes and macrophages associated with capillary proliferation and lymphoid follicle-like substructure
- Quilty infiltrates can invade subjacent myocardium and be mistaken for rejection
- In 46% of cases, acute rejection is also found
- CD21(+) cells (dendritic follicular cell marker) are frequently found
- Controversy exists about whether Quilty effect is associated with poor allograft outcome

Postperfusion Injury

- Mixed infiltrate is associated with myocyte disarray and coagulation necrosis secondary to perfusion-related damage to myocardium
- Only minority of cells are activated lymphocytes, and evidence of repair is obvious
- Lesions present in 1st weeks post transplant

Biopsy Site

- Areas of repair secondary to biopsy site injury can also cause confusion
- Only minority of infiltrating cells are lymphocytes, and myocyte distortion is found only near endocardial surface
- Fibrosis with entrapped myocytes and variable amount of mononuclear inflammation seen in later stages

Posttransplant Lymphoproliferative Disorder

- EBV virus-related proliferation of B lymphocytes can be confused with acute rejection
- Infiltrates express CD19 and CD20 and may be monoclonal for light chains on immunohistochemistry
- EBV in situ hybridization studies or PCR for EBV can be useful

DIAGNOSTIC CHECKLIST

Clinically Relevant Pathologic Features

- Edema and vasculitis strongly suggest that AMR is also present; immunohistochemistry or immunofluorescence should be done to look for C4d expression

Pathologic Interpretation Pearls

- Myocyte-distorting lymphoid infiltrates are necessary to diagnose treatment requiring rejection; this pattern is called moderate cellular rejection

SELECTED REFERENCES

1. Afzal A et al: Observed elevated donor-derived cell free DNA in orthotopic heart transplant recipients without clinical evidence of rejection. Clin Transplant. 36(3):e14549, 2022
2. Alam A et al: Evolving the surveillance and workup of heart transplant rejection: a real-world analysis of the Molecular Microscope Diagnostic System. Am J Transplant.22(10):2443-50, 2022
3. Awad MA et al: Current status and outcomes in heart transplantation: a narrative review. Rev Cardiovasc Med. 23(1):11, 2022
4. Qian X et al: Noninvasive biomarkers in heart transplant: 2020-2021 year in review. Curr Opin Organ Transplant. 27(1):7-14, 2022
5. Giarraputo A et al: A changing paradigm in heart transplantation: an integrative approach for invasive and non-invasive allograft rejection monitoring. Biomolecules. 11(2), 2021
6. Oh KT et al: Protocol endomyocardial biopsy beyond 6 months-It is time to move on. Am J Transplant. 21(2):825-9, 2021
7. Palmieri V et al: Novel biomarkers useful in surveillance of graft rejection after heart transplantation. Transpl Immunol. 67:101406, 2021
8. Duong Van Huyen JP et al: The XVth Banff Conference on Allograft Pathology the Banff Workshop Heart Report: Improving the diagnostic yield from endomyocardial biopsies and Quilty effect revisited. Am J Transplant. 20(12):3308-18, 2020
9. Kfoury AG et al: Mixed cellular and antibody-mediated rejection in heart transplantation: in-depth pathologic and clinical observations. J Heart Lung Transplant. 35(3):335-41, 2016
10. Crespo-Leiro MG et al: Performance of gene-expression profiling test score variability to predict future clinical events in heart transplant recipients. BMC Cardiovasc Disord. 15:120, 2015
11. Bernstein D et al: Gene expression profiling distinguishes a molecular signature for grade 1B mild acute cellular rejection in cardiac allograft recipients. J Heart Lung Transplant. 26(12):1270-80, 2007
12. Stewart S et al: Revision of the 1990 working formulation for the standardization of nomenclature in the diagnosis of heart rejection. J Heart Lung Transplant. 24(11):1710-20, 2005
13. Billingham ME: Endomyocardial biopsy diagnosis of acute rejection in cardiac allografts. Prog Cardiovasc Dis. 33(1):11-8, 1990
14. Kottke-Marchant K et al: Endomyocardial biopsy. Pathologic findings in cardiac transplant recipients. Pathol Annu. 25 Pt 1:211-44, 1990

Negative Biopsy for Acute Cellular Rejection

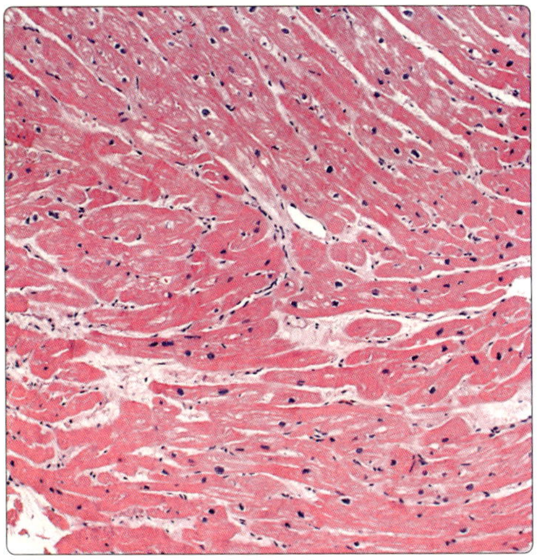

Negative Biopsy for Acute Cellular Rejection

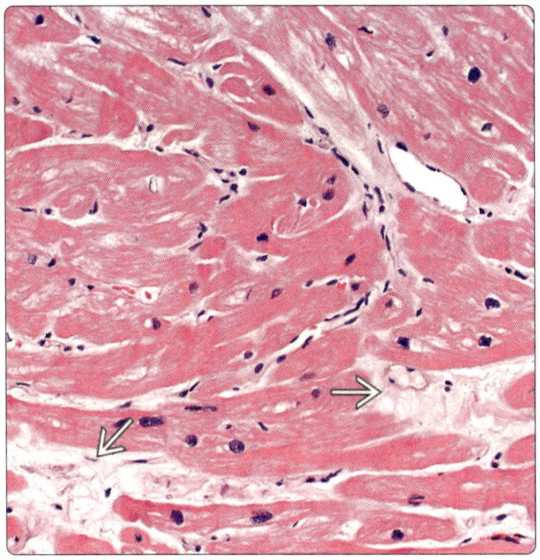

(Left) *H&E-stained section shows myocardium without inflammation, myocyte injury, or capillary endothelial activation. The biopsy is interpreted as negative for rejection (ISHLT 0R).* **(Right)** *H&E-stained section shows higher magnification of this entirely unremarkable myocardial biopsy fragment. Note that endothelial cells are flattened. Slight interstitial edema* ➡ *may be apparent focally; however, this is not associated with endothelial injury, so it is not significant (ISHLT 0R).*

Myocardium With Minimal Abnormalities

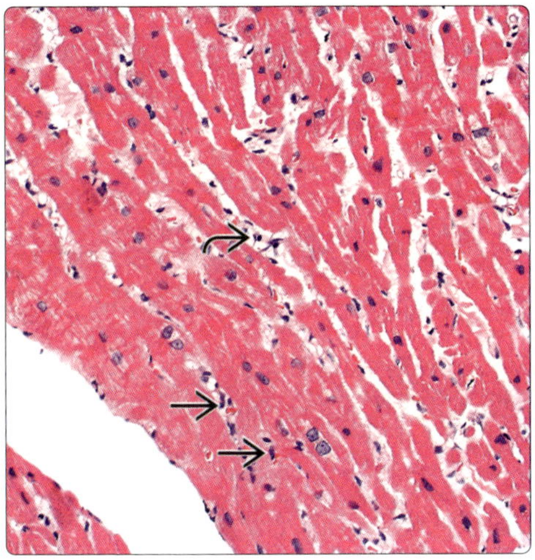

Morphologic Features of Mild Acute Cellular Rejection

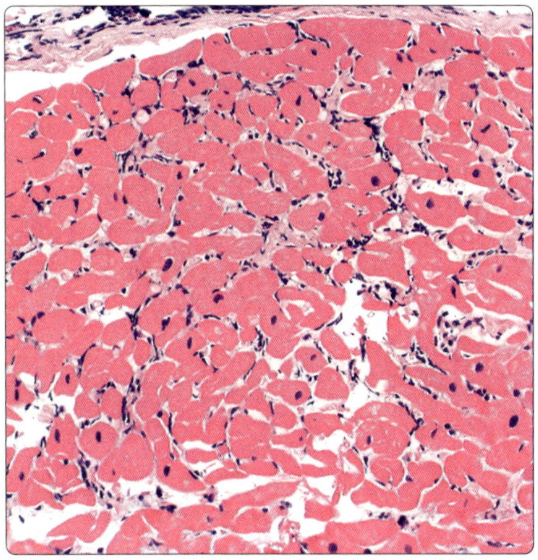

(Left) *H&E-stained section of myocardium shows slight endothelial prominence* ⇨ *with occasional inflammatory cells* ⇨ *within the interstitium. While this biopsy is not entirely normal, it is not diagnostic of cellular rejection because the amount of infiltrate is very slight (ISHLT 0R).* **(Right)** *H&E-stained section of myocardium shows interstitial accumulation of lymphocytes without myocyte distortion or injury. This pattern is typical of mild cellular rejection (ISHLT 1R).*

Morphologic Features of Mixed Rejection

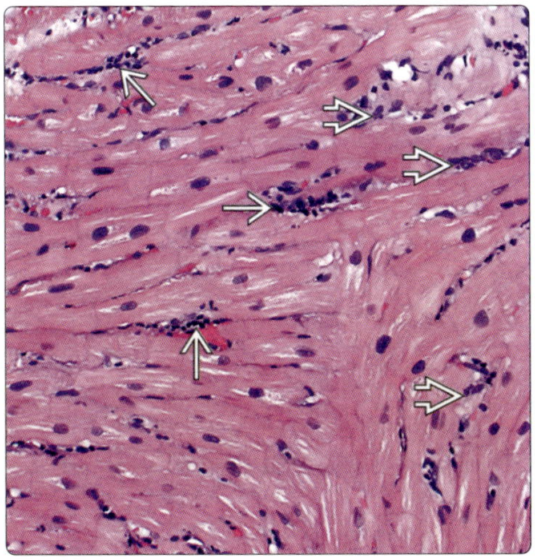

Morphologic Features of Mixed Rejection

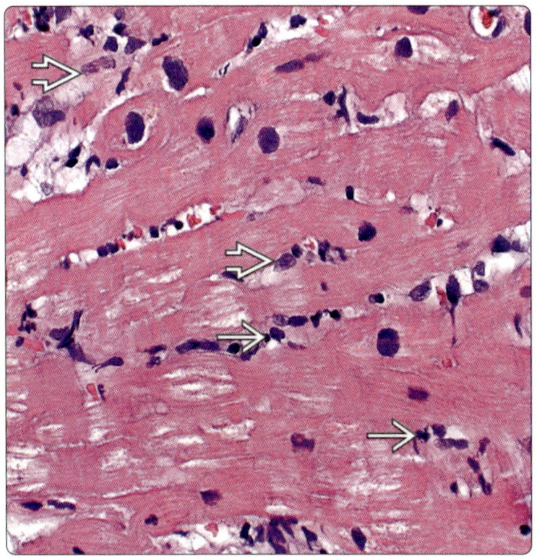

(Left) *H&E-stained section of myocardium shows obvious interstitial infiltrate* ➡ *and capillary endothelial changes* ➡. *The nature of this process is more difficult to define. The infiltrate contains lymphocytes and macrophages suggesting both cellular and antibody-mediated rejection. C3d and C4d were positive, confirming mixed rejection (ISHLT 1R, pAMR 2).* **(Right)** *H&E-stained section of myocardium at higher magnification shows detail of the inflammatory infiltrate* ➡ *and endothelial changes* ➡ *(ISHLT 1R, pAMR2).*

(Left) *H&E-stained section of myocardium shows interstitial lymphocytic inflammatory infiltrate with at least 2 foci of myocyte injury , consistent with moderate rejection (ISHLT 2R).* **(Right)** *H&E-stained section of myocardium at higher magnification shows moderate interstitial lymphocytic inflammatory infiltrate with at least 2 foci of myocyte injury , consistent with moderate rejection. In some areas, the infiltrate is more confluent, but still there are few myocytes in between (ISHLT 2R).*

Morphologic Features of Moderate Acute Cellular Rejection

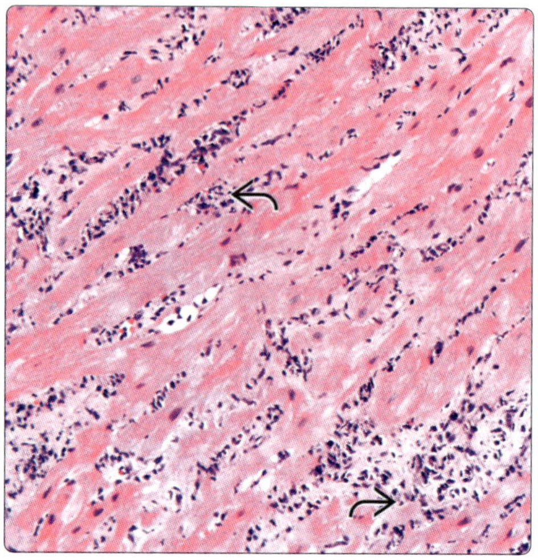

Morphologic Features of Severe Acute Cellular Rejection

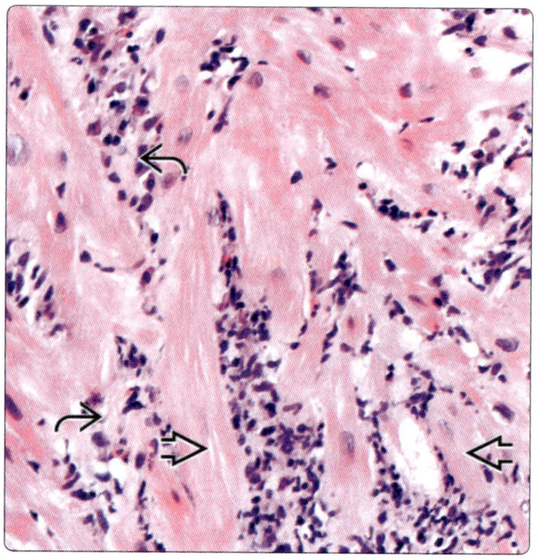

(Left) *H&E-stained section of myocardium shows marked confluent interstitial lymphocytic inflammatory infiltrate with several foci of myocyte injury, consistent with severe rejection (ISHLT 3R).* **(Right)** *H&E-stained section of myocardium at higher magnification shows confluent interstitial lymphocytic inflammatory infiltrate with several eosinophils and myocyte injury, which was present in several fragments, consistent with severe rejection (ISHLT 3R).*

Morphologic Features of Severe Acute Cellular Rejection

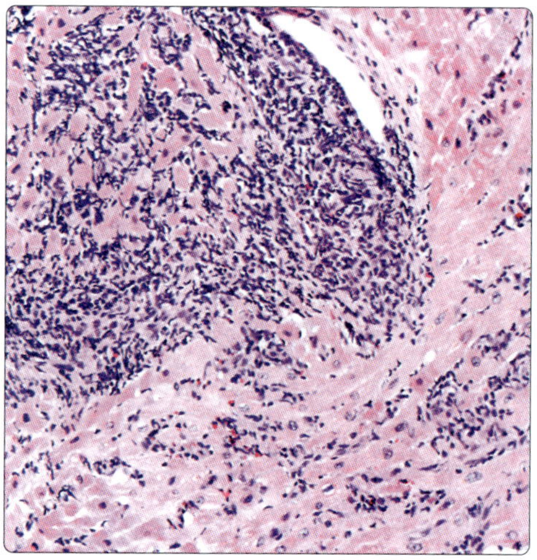

Morphologic Features of Severe Acute Cellular Rejection

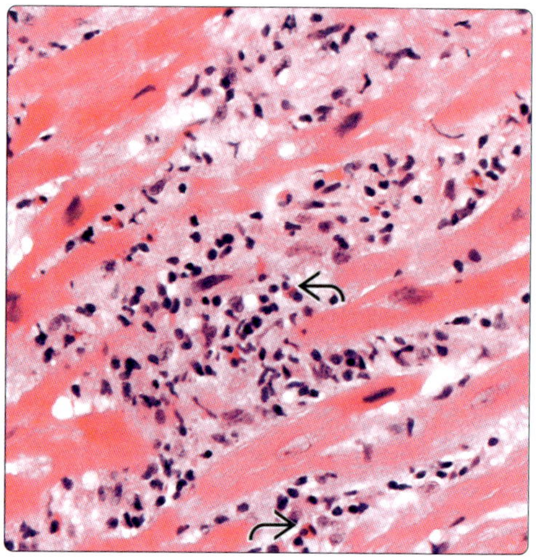

(Left) *H&E-stained section shows severe mixed cellular and antibody-mediated rejection with obvious vasculitis , mixed infiltrate , edema, and endothelial injury . C3d, C4d, and fibrin staining were positive (ISHLT 3R, pAMR 2).* **(Right)** *H&E-stained section shows severe rejection with obvious interstitial accumulation of flocculent material , which is fibrin and cellular debris. Infiltrate of inflammatory cells is mixed and extensive . Focal ischemic necrosis of myocytes is also seen (ISHLT 3R).*

Morphologic Features of Severe Acute Cellular and Antibody-Mediated Rejection

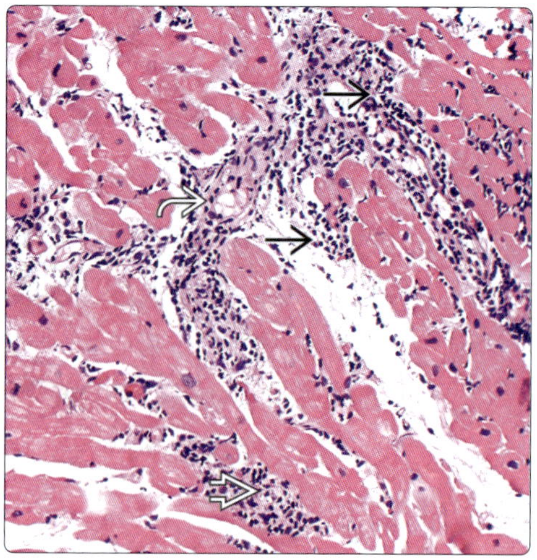

Morphologic Features of Severe Acute Cellular Rejection

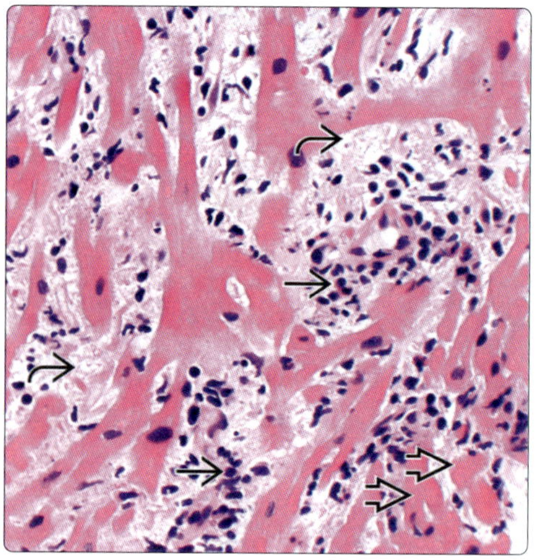

Quilty Effect

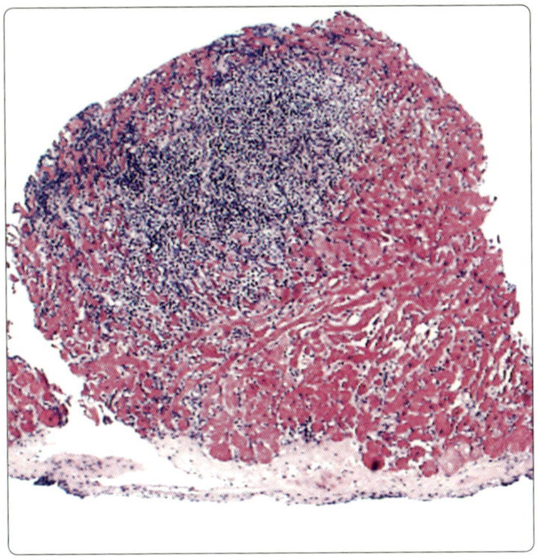

Quilty Effect

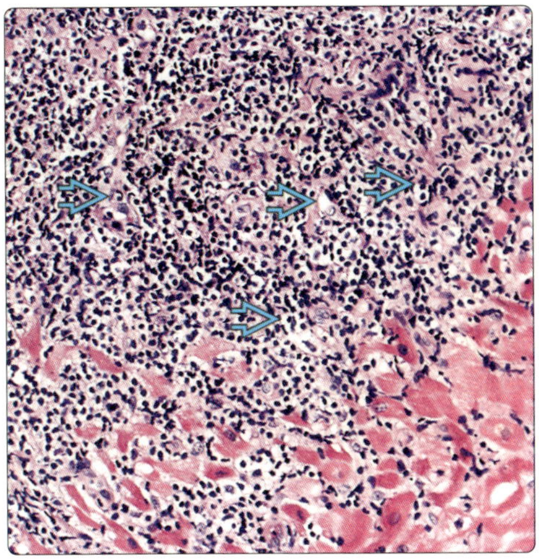

(Left) *This typical nodular Quilty effect shows the relationship to both endocardium and subjacent myocardium (ISHLT 0R).* **(Right)** *H&E-stained section of Quilty effect shows the characteristic features of the lesion composed of lymphocytes and plasma cells associated with proliferating capillaries ➩. The aggressive nature of the infiltrate is apparent. Sections through only the infiltrating part of the lesion are often misdiagnosed as acute cellular rejection (ISHLT 0R).*

Quilty Effect

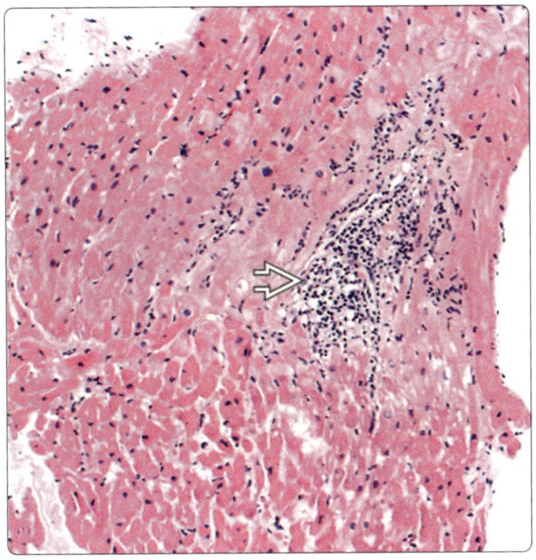

Myocardial Ischemic Changes

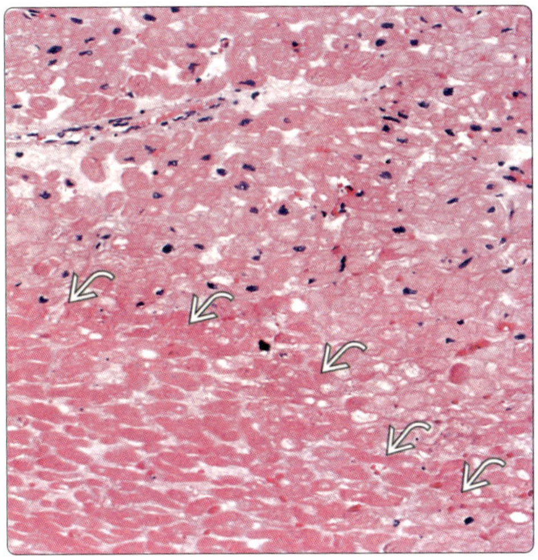

(Left) *H&E-stained section shows myocyte-distorting infiltrate ➩, suggestive of moderate cellular rejection. Further sections revealed that this infiltrate was in contiguity with typical Quilty effect. The biopsy was interpreted as negative for rejection (ISHLT 0R).* **(Right)** *H&E-stained section of myocardium 1 week after transplantation shows a large area of coagulation necrosis ➩. Such infarcted areas may be associated with inflammation in subsequent biopsies, leading to confusion with rejection (ISHLT 0R).*

C3d Immunofluorescence in Ischemic Myocytes

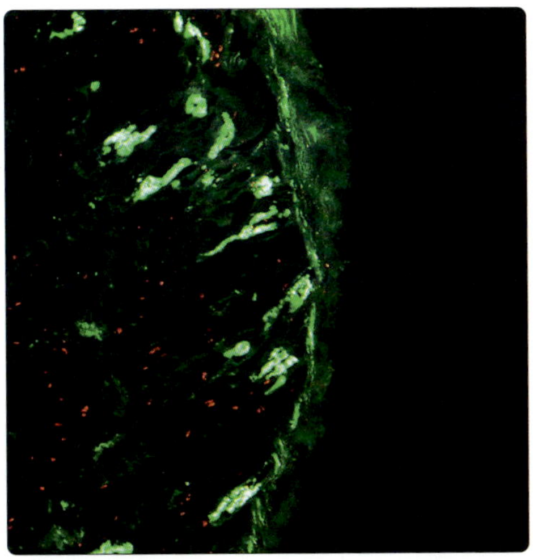

Myocardial Ischemic Changes

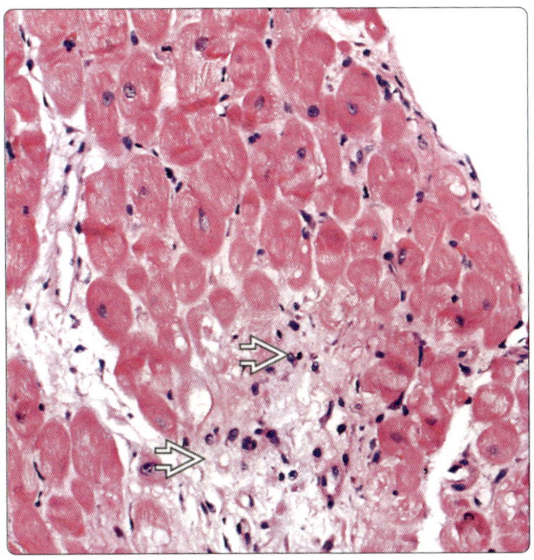

(Left) *C3d immunofluorescence shows binding to necrotic subendocardial myocytes of a 1-week posttransplant biopsy. Complement and immunoglobulin adherence to necrotic myocytes is a helpful clue that the changes seen are related to ischemic injury rather than rejection.* **(Right)** *H&E-stained section of myocardium with previous ischemic injury ➩ shows residual macrophages and necrotic myocyte dropout. Other areas of biopsy are unremarkable, supporting this interpretation (ISHLT 0R).*

Antibody-Mediated Transplant Rejection, Heart

KEY FACTS

TERMINOLOGY

- Damage to cardiac allograft related to antibody and complement activation in capillaries and arteries, which results in injury leading to either acute or chronic graft loss
- Synonyms: Humoral rejection/vascular rejection

ETIOLOGY/PATHOGENESIS

- Presensitization
- Multiple transfusions
- Prior transplantation, especially if donor-specific antibody from 1st transplant was positive
- Circulating donor-specific antibody binds antigens expressed on graft endothelium
- Bound antibody fixes complement and incites complement-mediated damage

CLINICAL ISSUES

- Patient may be asymptomatic
- Surveillance biopsies may detect antibody-mediated rejection (AMR) before patient develops significant symptoms
- Immunosuppressive strategies include steroids, mycophenolate mofetil, cyclophosphamide, rituximab, bortezomib, and plasmapheresis

MICROSCOPIC

- Obvious capillary endothelial swelling and injury ("activated intravascular mononuclear cells")
- Adherence of neutrophils or macrophages to capillary endothelium ("activated intravascular mononuclear cells")

ANCILLARY TESTS

- C4d must be diffusely (> 50% capillaries staining) present in capillaries of myocardium on initial biopsies for AMR; pattern may be patchy after capillary damage occurs
- Diffuse staining (> 50% capillaries staining) of capillaries of myocardium with C4d ± C3d establishes diagnosis according to most recent ISHLT classification

Histologic Findings in AMR

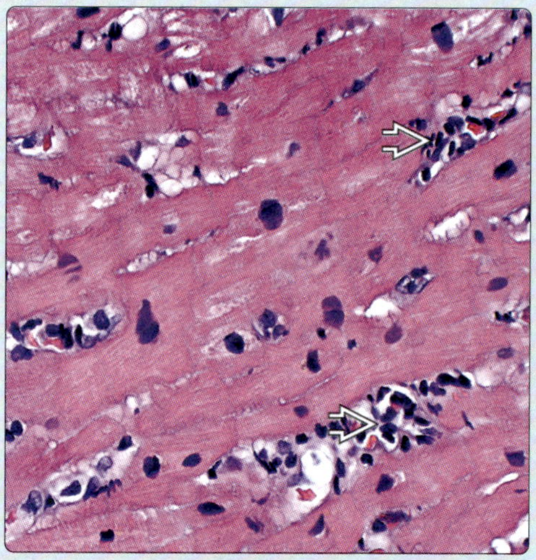

Immunofluorescence Findings in AMR

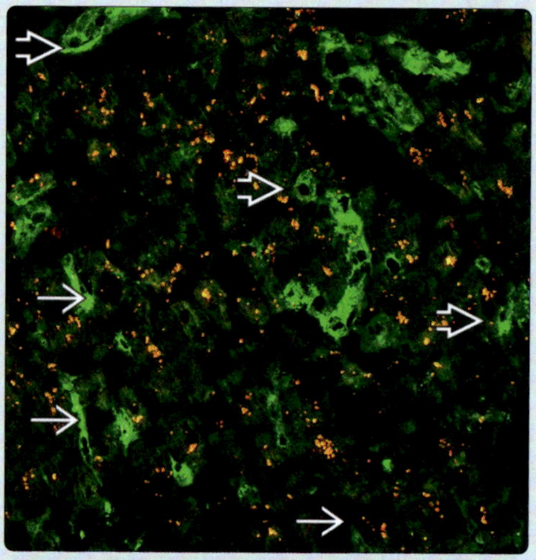

(Left) *Heart transplant biopsy shows accumulation of macrophages and rare neutrophils within capillaries, consistent with antibody-mediated rejection (AMR). HLA-DR, IgG, C3d, and C4d were also positive by immunofluorescence.* **(Right)** *C4d immunofluorescence stain is positive in capillaries (doughnut-like pattern in cross section and more linear profile in longitudinal section). Myocytes show only orange lipofuscin autofluorescence.*

Severe AMR

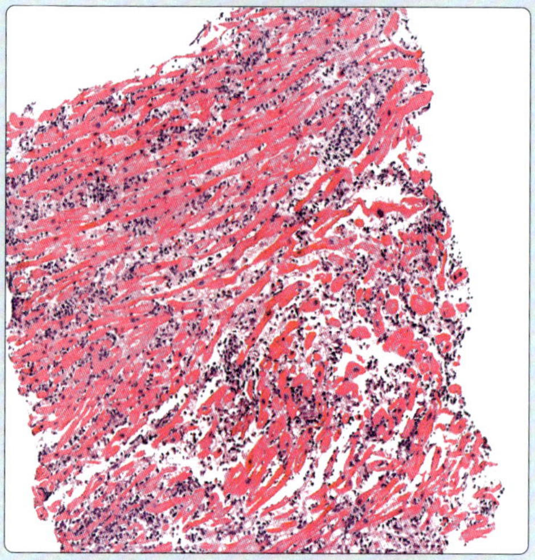

"Chronic" AMR: Ultrastructure

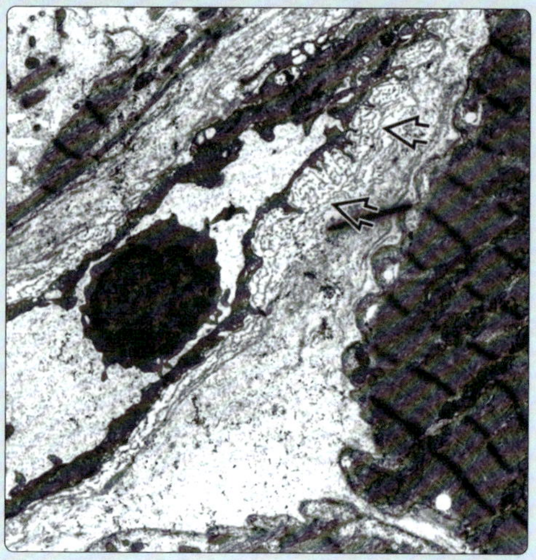

(Left) *Both intravascular inflammation and perivascular inflammatory cells are seen throughout this biopsy showing severe AMR (ISHLT pAMR3). Interstitial edema and karyorrhectic debris are also present.* **(Right)** *Electron photomicrograph shows biopsy from a patient with multiple repeated episodes of AMR who developed allograft vasculopathy. There is multilayering of the capillary basement membrane .*

TERMINOLOGY

Abbreviations

- Antibody-mediated rejection (AMR)

Synonyms

- Humoral rejection
- Vascular rejection

Definitions

- Damage to cardiac allograft related to antibody and complement activation in capillaries and arteries, which results in injury leading to either acute or chronic graft loss

ETIOLOGY/PATHOGENESIS

Risk Factors

- Intrinsic: Young age, female sex
- Presensitization
  - Multiparity
  - Multiple transfusions
  - Prior transplantation, especially if donor-specific antibody from 1st transplant was positive

Pathogenesis

- Endothelial cells are important participants in process because they can act as antigens, present antigens in context of HLA, and process antigens just like macrophages
- Capillary and other endothelia are potent sources of alloimmune antigens
  - HLA class I or II, endothelin-1 receptor, cardiac myosin, vimentin, angiotensin II type 1 receptor, and major histocompatibility class I chain A (MICA)
- Donor endothelial antigens are shed during transplantation, inducing de novo or anamnestic antibody formation
- Circulating donor-specific antibody binds antigens expressed on graft endothelium
  - Inducing production of proinflammatory cytokines and chemoattractants for neutrophils, macrophages, NK cells
  - Bound antibody fixes complement and incites complement-mediated damage
- In severe cases, damage leads to loss of endothelial antithrombotic compounds and exposed tissue factor
  - Vascular thrombosis, vascular permeability, positive fibrin staining, ischemic damage can result

CLINICAL ISSUES

Epidemiology

- AMR affects up to 15% of patients in 1st year post transplant

Presentation

- Hemodynamic compromise
  - Allograft failure
  - Echocardiogram with diastolic dysfunction
  - Abnormal angiogram (allograft vasculopathy)
- Patient may be asymptomatic
  - Surveillance biopsies may detect AMR before patient develops significant symptoms
- Timing
  - Most AMR is demonstrable by 3 months post transplant
  - Late cases (> 1 year post transplant) of AMR may occur

Treatment

- Immunosuppressive strategies include steroids, mycophenolate mofetil, cyclophosphamide, rituximab, bortezomib, complement inhibition, and plasmapheresis

Prognosis

- Depends of severity
  - When graft failure present
    - 1-year survival is 50%
  - Major risk factor for cardiac allograft vasculopathy (even asymptomatic cases)
- Allograft loss after cellular rejection is ~ 3% per year; allograft loss after symptomatic AMR is 15% per year

MACROSCOPIC

General Features

- Biopsies should be submitted fresh (saline) if immunofluorescence (IF) methods are used
- Biopsy must include at least 3-4 fragments to ensure that there is no sampling error (e.g., 3 pieces for paraffin and 1 piece for IF)
- Biopsies can be surveyed using immunohistochemistry (IHC) for CD68 and C4d if fresh tissue is not available

MICROSCOPIC

Histologic Features

- Obvious capillary endothelial swelling and injury ("activated intravascular mononuclear cells")
- Adherence of neutrophils or macrophages to capillary endothelium ("activated intravascular mononuclear cells")
- Occasional arteriolitis
- Interstitial edema
- Vascular thrombosis in severe cases

Predominant Cell/Compartment Type

- Capillaries

International Society for Heart and Lung Transplant 2013 Working Formulation

- Negative for pathologic AMR: pAMR 0
- Histopathologic AMR alone: pAMR 1 (H+)
  - Histologic findings present with negative IF/IHC
- Immunopathologic AMR alone: pAMR 1 (I+)
  - IF positive C4d (> 50% of capillaries) ± C3d with negative histology
  - IHC positive for CD68 (> 10% of capillaries) &/or C4d (> 50% of capillaries) with negative histology
- Pathologic AMR: pAMR 2
  - Both histological and immunopathologic findings present
- Severe pathologic AMR: pAMR 3
  - Includes cases showing interstitial hemorrhage, capillary fragmentation, mixed inflammatory infiltrate, endothelial pyknosis &/or karyorrhexis, marked edema, and immunopathologic findings

Immunohistochemistry

Antibody	Reactivity	Staining Pattern	Comment
C4d	Positive	Vascular	Capillary staining is only true positive and must be diffusely seen
CD68	Positive	Cytoplasmic	Macrophages are found adhering to capillary endothelium

Immunofluorescence

Antibody	Reactivity	Staining Pattern	Comment
C3d	Positive	Perimyocyte capillary	Intensity noted as trace to strong
C4d	Positive	Perimyocyte capillary	Intensity noted as trace to strong
Fibrin	Positive	Perimyocyte capillary	Intensity noted as trace to strong
HLA-DR	Positive	Perimyocyte capillary	Intensity noted as trace to strong

ANCILLARY TESTS

Immunohistochemistry

- Evaluation for C4d and CD68 can establish diagnosis; CD31 or CD34 definition of capillary location and damage is helpful
  - C4d must be diffusely (> 50% of capillaries staining) present in capillaries of myocardium on initial biopsies for AMR; pattern may be patchy after capillary damage occurs
  - CD68(+) macrophages must be within capillaries
  - C4d IHC is less sensitive than IF detection methods

Immunofluorescence

- Diffuse staining (> 50% of capillaries) of myocardium with C4d ± C3d establishes diagnosis according to most recent ISHLT classification
- HLA-DR staining can define capillary location and assist in definition of capillary damage when C3d or C4d is not diffuse as expected
- Fibrin accumulation has been shown to relate to increased severity of process, especially when it involves both capillaries and interstitium

Electron Microscopy

- Capillaries with swollen endothelium, increase in pinocytotic vesicles, and adherent macrophages are seen
- In chronic injury, reduplicated basal lamina in capillary wall is seen

Molecular Testing

- Molecular microscope diagnostic system (MMDx) measures gene expression using microarrays and applies ensemble machine-learning algorithms to assign probability or diagnoses of rejection on fresh myocardial samples

DIFFERENTIAL DIAGNOSIS

Acute Postperfusion Ischemic Injury

- Usually occurs in early weeks post transplant and rapidly resolves with time
- Process includes acute myocyte necrosis and inflammation
- Negative immunopathologic findings (IF/IHC)
- C3d can be found in necrotic myocardium, and fibrin aggregates can also be seen

Acute Mixed Cellular-Mediated and Antibody-Mediated Rejection

- Lymphoid infiltrates within interstitium and in apposition to myocytes
- Capillary endothelium is swollen, and endothelial cell injury may be present

DIAGNOSTIC CHECKLIST

Clinically Relevant Pathologic Features

- Activated intravascular mononuclear cells
  - Endothelial changes ± accumulation of monocyte-macrophages

Pathologic Interpretation Pearls

- IHC or IF must be done to demonstrate that complement components are deposited
  - C4d, C3d, CD68, HLA-DR, fibrin

SELECTED REFERENCES

1. Coutance G et al: Correlation between microvascular inflammation in endomyocardial biopsies and rejection transcripts, donor-specific antibodies, and graft dysfunction in antibody-mediated rejection. Transplantation. 106(7):1455-64, 2022
2. Halloran PF et al: Many heart transplant biopsies currently diagnosed as no rejection have mild molecular antibody-mediated rejection-related changes. J Heart Lung Transplant. 41(3):334-44, 2022
3. Moreno JD et al: Angiotensin II type 1 receptor antibody-mediated rejection following orthotopic heart transplant: a single-center experience. Transplantation. 106(2):373-80, 2022
4. Fujino T et al: Discordance between immunofluorescence and immunohistochemistry C4d staining and outcomes following heart transplantation. Clin Transplant. 35(4):e14242, 2021
5. Hurskainen M et al: Failing heart transplants and rejection-a cellular perspective. J Cardiovasc Dev Dis. 8(12), 2021
6. Patel JK et al: Complement inhibition for prevention of antibody-mediated rejection in immunologically high-risk heart allograft recipients. Am J Transplant. 21(7):2479-88, 2021
7. Cai Q et al: Upregulation of endothelial HLA class II is a marker of antibody-mediated rejection in heart allograft biopsies. Transplant Proc. 52(4):1192-7, 2020
8. Berry GJ et al: The 2013 International Society for Heart and Lung Transplantation Working Formulation for the standardization of nomenclature in the pathologic diagnosis of antibody-mediated rejection in heart transplantation. J Heart Lung Transplant. 32(12):1147-62, 2013
9. Hammond ME et al: Utility of histologic parameters in screening for antibody-mediated rejection of the cardiac allograft: a study of 3,170 biopsies. J Heart Lung Transplant. 24(12):2015-21, 2005
10. Hammond EH et al: Vascular (humoral) rejection in heart transplantation: pathologic observations and clinical implications. J Heart Transplant. 8(6):430-43, 1989

"Busy" Capillary Pattern in AMR

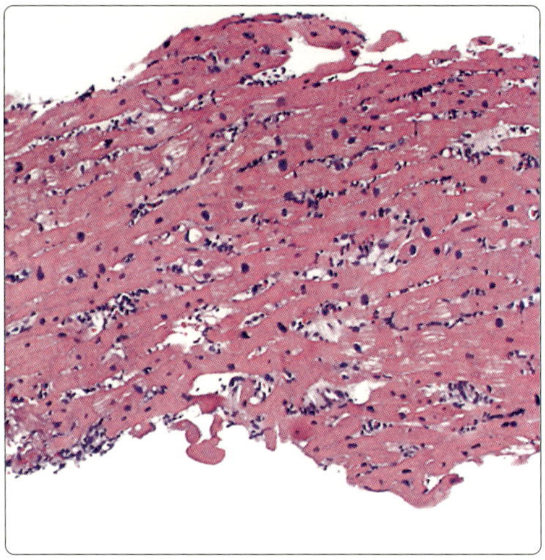

Intravascular Mononuclear Cells in AMR

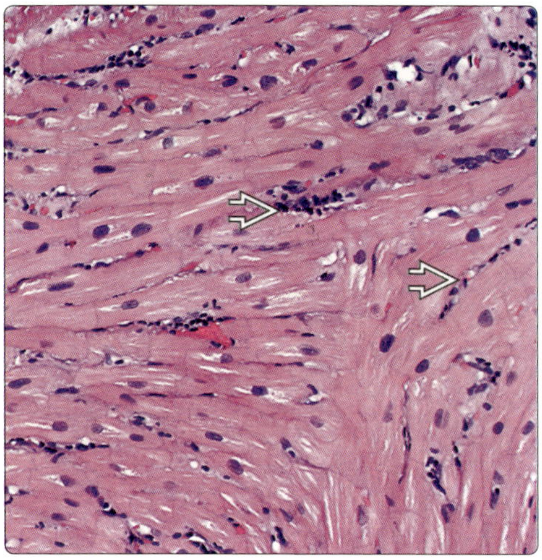

(Left) *Myocardial biopsy shows overall pattern of endothelial activation, scant interstitial edema, and adherence of macrophages within capillaries in a case of AMR. Note the absence of activated lymphocyte aggregates.* **(Right)** *Myocardial biopsy at higher magnification shows capillary changes* ➡ *of endothelial swelling and adherence of macrophages and neutrophils. There are no enlarged lymphocytes in the interstitium, and no evidence of myocyte injury is seen.*

Interstitial Edema in AMR

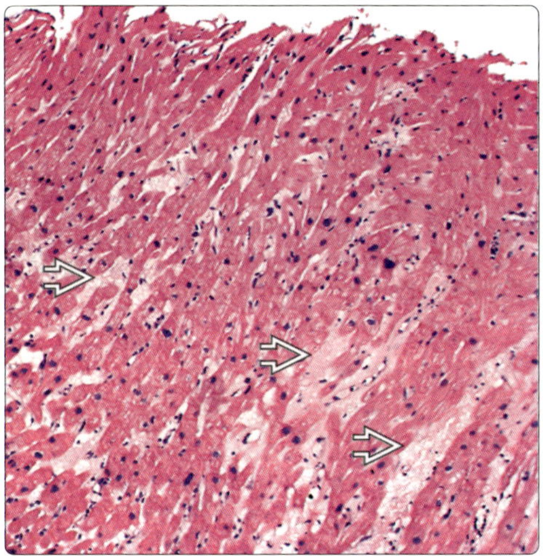

Edema and Capillary Injury in AMR

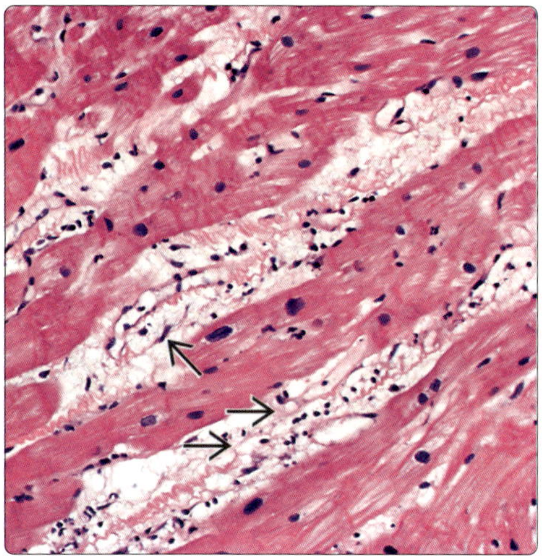

(Left) *H&E-stained section of a myocardial biopsy shows few capillary changes but obvious interstitial edema* ➡ *in this case of AMR associated with significant hemodynamic compromise.* **(Right)** *H&E-stained section of a myocardial biopsy at high magnification illustrates significant edema present in interstitial regions in this case of AMR. Fibrin, C4d, C3d, and IgG were positive by immunofluorescence in this case as well. Note that capillary endothelium is attenuated* ➡.

Mixed Rejection Pattern in AMR

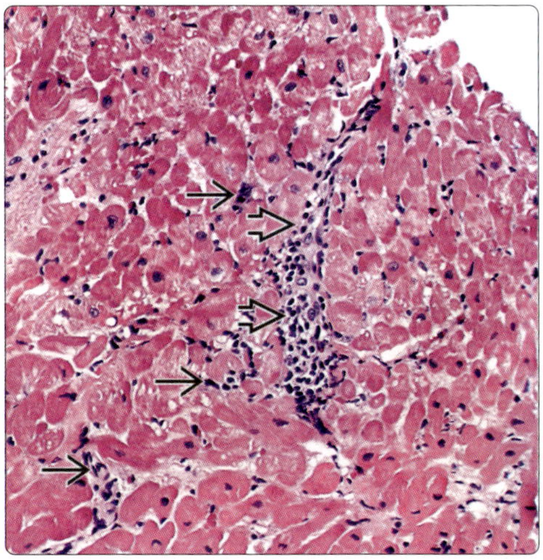

"Chronic" AMR: Trichrome Stain

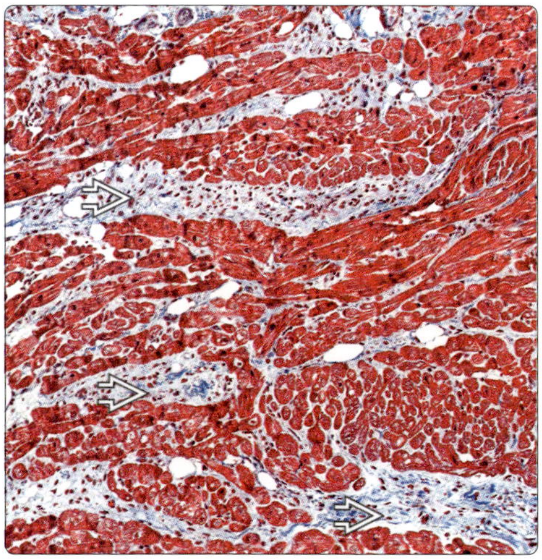

(Left) *H&E-stained section of a myocardial biopsy shows obvious vasculitis involving an arteriole* ➡ *in this case of AMR. The features overlap somewhat with cellular rejection. Capillaries show endothelial activation* ➡*; however, the myocytes appear uninvolved.* **(Right)** *Biopsy from a patient with recurrent episodes of AMR shows a paucity of patent vascular lumina. There are also bands of collagen fibrosis* ➡.

Immunofluorescence (C3d) in AMR

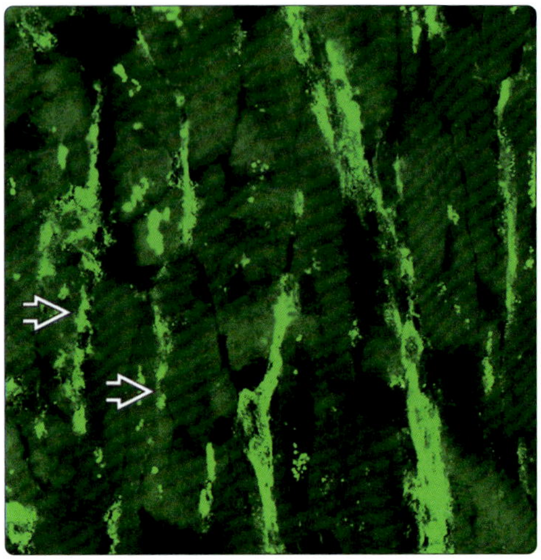

Immunofluorescence (C4d) in AMR

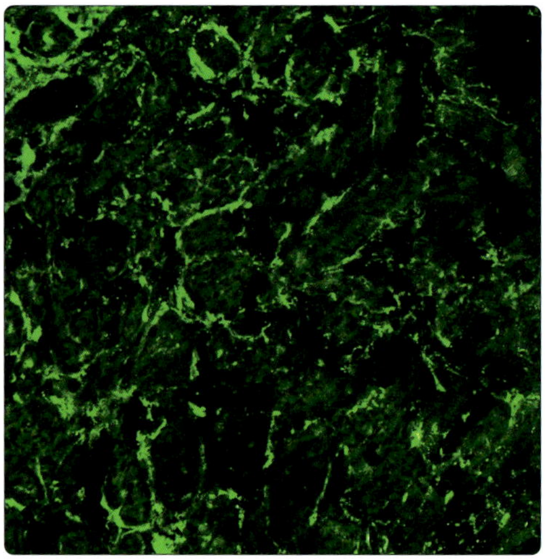

(Left) *C3d accumulation is seen in perimyocyte capillaries at high magnification. Focal interrupted staining ➡ is seen in some vessels. This sample is from the 2nd episode of AMR in this patient.* **(Right)** *C4d immunofluorescence stain is present in an interrupted linear pattern in capillaries in a heart biopsy from a patient with AMR. Fibrin accumulation was present as well as C3d-positive staining in the same capillaries.*

Fibrin Staining in Severe AMR

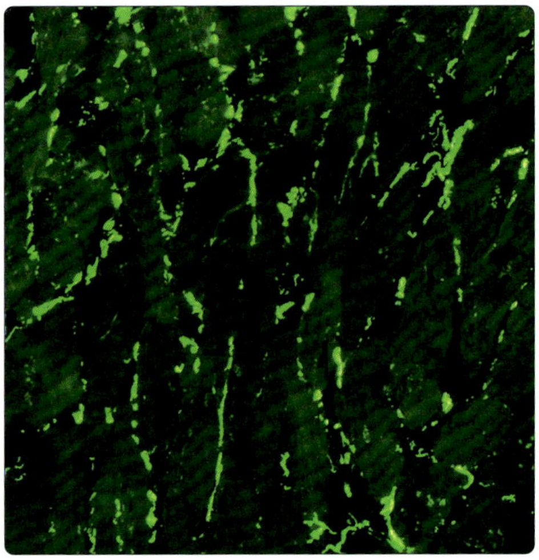

Fibrin Deposition in AMR

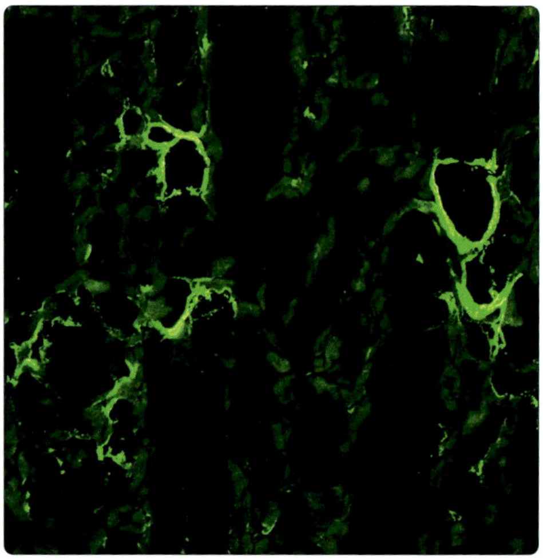

(Left) *Fibrin-stained section from a patient with repeated acute AMR shows diffusely distributed fibrin within capillaries.* **(Right)** *Section from a patient with longstanding AMR shows focal accumulation of fibrin in and around damaged capillaries. This contrasts to an earlier biopsy on the same patient, which showed diffuse intravascular fibrin accumulation. Capillary integrity at this time has been compromised, and most staining is around ectatic vessels.*

Immunohistochemistry (CD68) in AMR

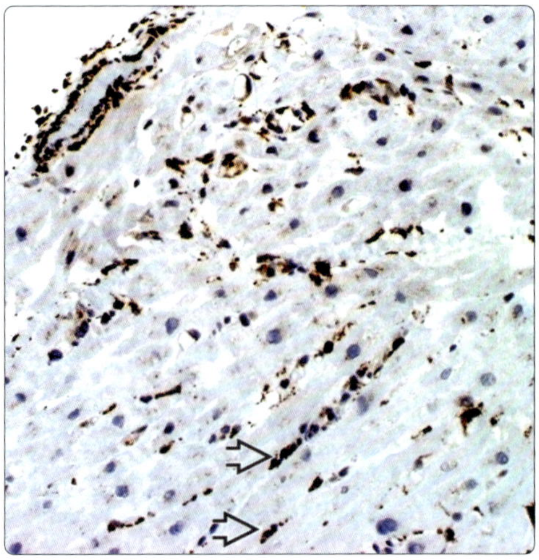

Immunohistochemistry (C4d) in AMR

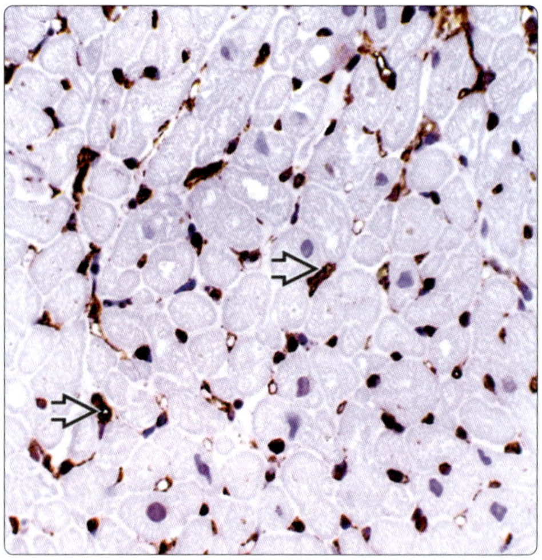

(Left) *CD68-stained section of a myocardial biopsy shows accumulation of macrophages (CD68 positive) ➡ within perimyocyte capillaries in this case of AMR.* **(Right)** *C4d-stained section of a myocardial biopsy in this case of AMR shows diffuse strong positive labeling of perimyocyte capillaries ➡. Sample was fixed for 12 hours in buffered formalin. Samples with fixation time < 6 hours often exhibit weak staining.*

Immunofluorescence (C4d) in "Chronic" AMR

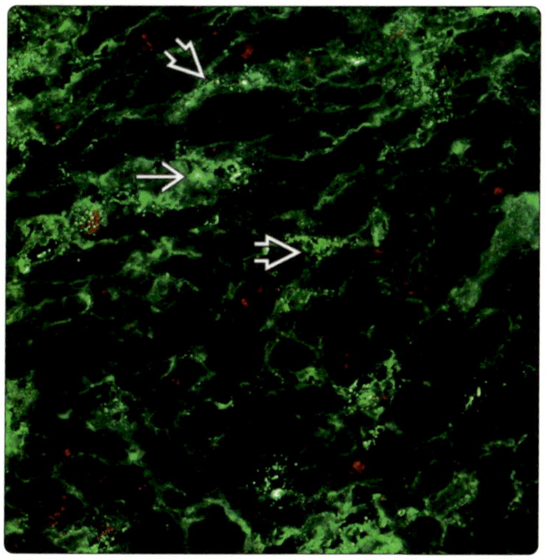

Immunofluorescence HLA-DR in "Chronic" AMR

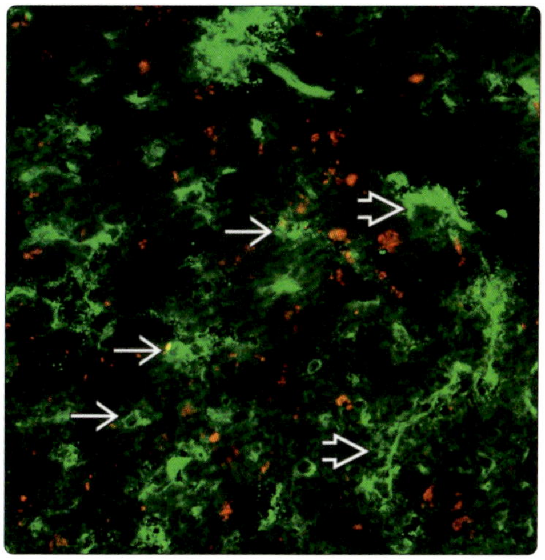

(Left) *C4d staining from a patient with repeated episodes of AMR shows interrupted vascular staining* ⇨ *and punctate deposits* ➡*, which related to the obvious vascular damage. Such a pattern is difficult to classify in the current system.* **(Right)** *Biopsy from a patient with repeated episodes of AMR stained with HLA-DR shows capillaries with an interrupted and feathered* ⇨ *appearance, suggesting capillary damage. In addition, adherent macrophages likely are also staining* ➡*.*

Immunofluorescence Findings in Ischemic Subendocardial Region

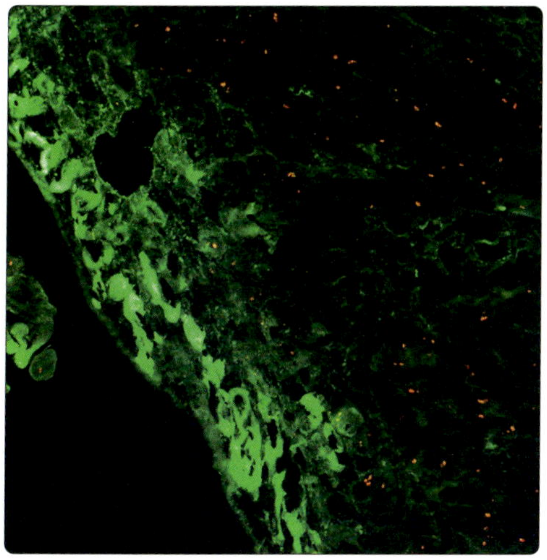

Immunofluorescence Findings in Perfusion Injury

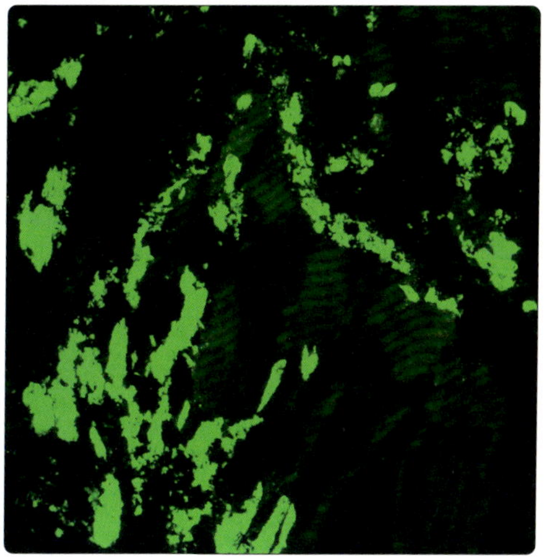

(Left) *Endocardial region shows necrotic myocytes with C3d staining found often in necrotic cells. This region is the predominant area at risk for ischemia early after transplant and also late when chronic allograft vasculopathy is suspected.* **(Right)** *C3d staining of myocytes documents the significant myocardial necrosis in this case of perfusion injury in a transplant. No vascular C3d is visualized, and these changes are not indicative of AMR.*

Histologic Findings in Reperfusion Injury

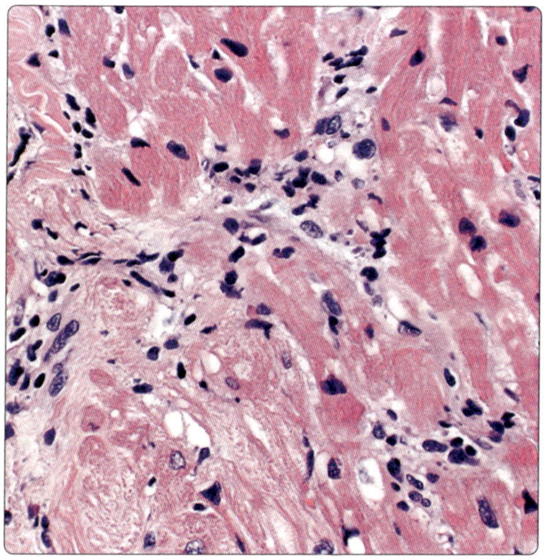

Fibrin Immunofluorescence

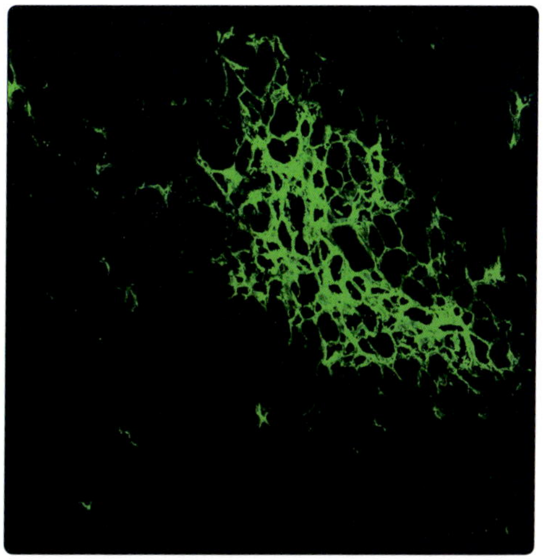

(Left) *H&E-stained section shows the type of inflammation seen in biopsies of transplanted hearts early after transplant where perfusion time was long. There is a mixed infiltrate and obvious vascular damage. Myocytes also look disordered. C3d showed myocardial necrosis without capillary accumulation.* **(Right)** *Biopsy shows perfusion injury with focal aggregate of fibrin in an area of disordered myocytes. No evidence of AMR was found in this biopsy.*

Quilty Lesions

KEY FACTS

TERMINOLOGY

- Raised aggregate of lymphocytes (T and B), macrophages, and small vessels located on endocardial surface of cardiac allografts; considered distinct from rejection
  - Named after patient in whom it was 1st identified

CLINICAL ISSUES

- Asymptomatic finding on posttransplant endomyocardial biopsy
- Found in ~ 15-20% of posttransplant biopsies
- Does not require augmented immunosuppression
- No known impact on cardiac allograft at present

MACROSCOPIC

- Small, white nodules on endocardial surface of explanted transplant heart

MICROSCOPIC

- Raised aggregate of lymphocytes along endocardial surface
  - Cellular infiltrate composed of lymphocytes (T and B), macrophages, occasional plasma cells
    - B cells often central with peripheral T lymphocytes
- CD21(+) follicular dendritic cell network may be present, particularly in larger Quilty lesions
- Many small vessels are present
- May infiltrate into underlying myocardium and be associated with myocyte damage
- Concomitant rejection may be noted in biopsies containing Quilty lesions

ANCILLARY TESTS

- CD21 helpful in distinguishing rejection from Quilty

TOP DIFFERENTIAL DIAGNOSES

- Acute rejection
- Posttransplant lymphoproliferative disorder
- Healing ischemic injury
- Endocardial thrombi/healing biopsy site

Left Ventricle Wall Involved by Quilty Lesions

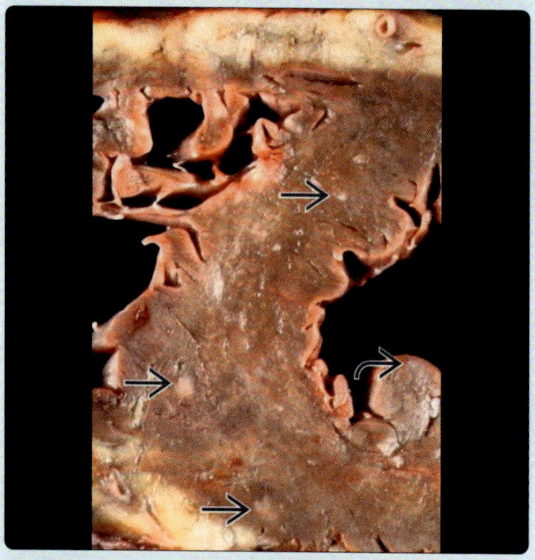

Endocardium and Myocardium Involved by Quilty Lesions

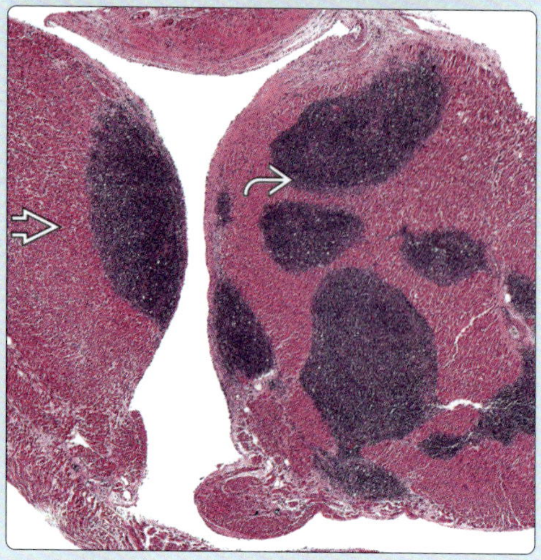

(Left) *Gross photograph of the left ventricle shows white-tan nodules in myocardium and endocardium, which on histology corresponded to aggregates of lymphocytes admixed with capillary proliferation, consistent with Quilty lesions.* **(Right)** *Low-power view shows the left ventricle involved by nodular aggregates of lymphocytes associated with capillary proliferation, consistent with Quilty lesions. Some of the aggregates were connected to endocardium, but many were completely localized in the myocardium.*

Quilty Lesion: Low-Power View

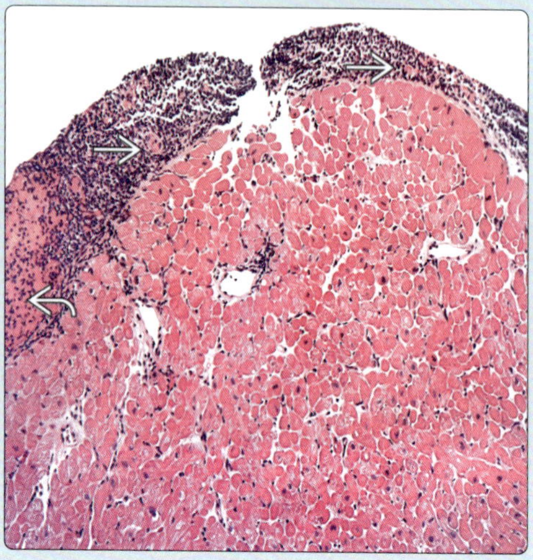

Quilty Lesion: High-Power View

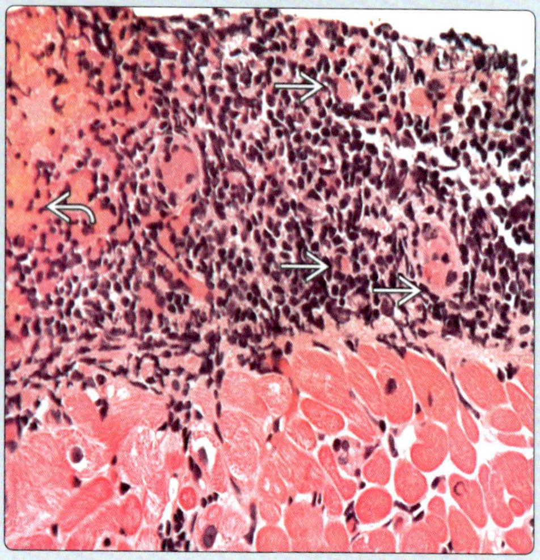

(Left) *Low-power view of a Quilty lesion shows a dense lymphoid infiltrate along the endocardium and many small vessels. Trauma to these vessels during biopsy may lead to areas of hemorrhage.* **(Right)** *High-power view of a Quilty lesion shows the density of the lymphoid infiltrate, the numerous small vessels, and a small area of biopsy-related hemorrhage.*

Quilty Lesions

TERMINOLOGY

Synonyms

- Endocardial lymphoid infiltrate, Quilty effect, Quilty A (old terminology for noninvasive Quilty), Quilty B (old terminology for invasive Quilty)

Definitions

- Raised aggregate of lymphocytes (T and B), macrophages, and small vessels located on endocardial surface of cardiac allografts; considered distinct from rejection
  - Named after patient in whom it was 1st identified
  - Morphologic features resemble tertiary lymphoid organ

ETIOLOGY/PATHOGENESIS

Unknown

- Not related to posttransplant lymphoproliferative disorder
- Not clearly associated with acute rejection
- Not related to viral infection

CLINICAL ISSUES

Presentation

- Asymptomatic finding on posttransplant endomyocardial biopsy
- Found in ~ 15-20% of posttransplant biopsies
- Tend to persist in subsequent biopsies

Treatment

- Does not require augmented immunosuppression

Prognosis

- Variable reports of increased incidence of rejection and cardiac allograft vasculopathy with Quilty but not reproducible findings
- Must be distinguished from rejection to avoid overimmunosuppression

MACROSCOPIC

General Features

- Small, white nodules on endocardial surface or in myocardium of explanted transplant heart

MICROSCOPIC

Histologic Features

- Raised aggregate of lymphocytes along endocardial surface
  - Cellular infiltrate composed of lymphocytes (T and B), macrophages, and occasional plasma cells
    - B cells are usually central with peripheral T cells
  - CD21(+) follicular dendritic cell network may be present, particularly in larger Quilty lesions
    - May help to distinguish Quilty lesion from rejection
  - Many small vessels are present
- May infiltrate into underlying myocardium and be associated with myocyte damage
  - This pattern had been termed Quilty B (or invasive Quilty) but was found not to have prognostic import
    - Now classified along with Quilty A (or noninvasive Quilty) as Quilty lesion (revised International Society for Heart and Lung Transplantation working formulation)
- Concomitant rejection may be noted in biopsies containing Quilty lesions

ANCILLARY TESTS

Immunohistochemistry

- CD3, CD20, and CD68 reveal mixture of cell types, but similar mixture may be seen in rejection
  - Centrally located B lymphocytes with peripheral T lymphocytes would be more suggestive of Quilty lesion
- CD21 may reveal follicular dendritic cells in Quilty lesions, helpful in distinguishing rejection from Quilty

DIFFERENTIAL DIAGNOSIS

Acute Rejection

- Diffuse infiltrate not contiguous with endocardium
  - Quilty has nodular infiltrate contiguous with endocardium
    - May need serial sections to denote continuity with endocardium in Quilty
- Activated lymphocytes and eosinophils in rejection, not Quilty
- Vascular stroma associated with Quilty

Posttransplant Lymphoproliferative Disorder

- Atypical lymphocytes, B cells [CD20(+)], usually EBER(+)

Healing Ischemic Injury

- Coagulative myocyte necrosis, lipofuscin macrophages, fibrin on endocardial surface, mixed infiltrate with polymorphonuclear leukocytes

DIAGNOSTIC CHECKLIST

Pathologic Interpretation Pearls

- Endocardial-based infiltrate often nodular
- Mixed T and B lymphocytes, macrophages, plasma cells
- Numerous small blood vessels associated with infiltrate
- May infiltrate into underlying myocardium and be associated with myocyte damage

SELECTED REFERENCES

1. Duong Van Huyen JP et al: The XVth Banff Conference on Allograft Pathology the Banff Workshop Heart Report: improving the diagnostic yield from endomyocardial biopsies and Quilty effect revisited. Am J Transplant. 20(12):3308-18, 2020
2. Cho H et al: Quilty lesions in the endomyocardial biopsies after heart transplantation. J Pathol Transl Med. 53(1):50-6, 2019
3. Szymanska S et al: Prevalence of the Quilty effect in endomyocardial biopsy of patients after heart transplantation - from cellular rejection to antibody-mediated rejection? Pol J Pathol. 67(3):216-20, 2016
4. Winters GL: Cardiac transplant biopsies. Surg Pathol Clin. 5(2):371-400, 2012
5. Mengel M et al: The molecular phenotype of heart transplant biopsies: relationship to histopathological and clinical variables. Am J Transplant. 10(9):2105-15, 2010
6. Sattar HA et al: The presence of a CD21+ follicular dendritic cell network distinguishes invasive Quilty lesions from cardiac acute cellular rejection. Am J Surg Pathol. 30(8):1008-13, 2006
7. Chu KE et al: The relationship of nodular endocardial infiltrates (Quilty lesions) to anti-HLA antibodies, coronary artery disease, and survival following heart transplantation. Cardiovasc Pathol. 14(4):219-24, 2005
8. Marboe CC et al: Nodular endocardial infiltrates (Quilty lesions) cause significant variability in diagnosis of ISHLT grade 2 and 3A rejection in cardiac allograft recipients. J Heart Lung Transplant. 24(7 Suppl):S219-26, 2005
9. Stewart S et al: Revision of the 1990 working formulation for the standardization of nomenclature in the diagnosis of heart rejection. J Heart Lung Transplant. 24(11):1710-20, 2005

Quilty Lesion: Trichrome Stain

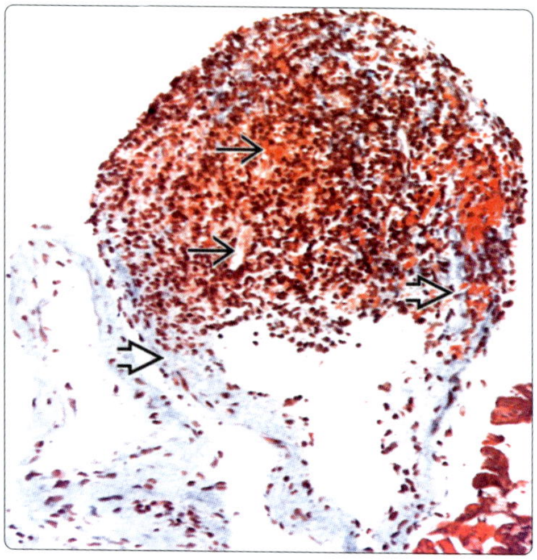

Quilty Lesion: CD68 Stain

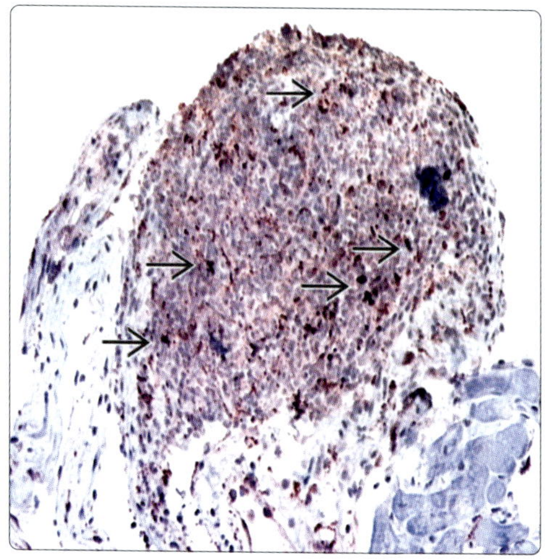

(Left) *Trichrome stain of a quite nodular Quilty lesion shows the endocardial connective tissue ⇨ and highlights the vascularity of the lesion →.* **(Right)** *CD68 stain of a Quilty lesion reveals positive staining of scattered macrophages →. A Quilty lesion contains B lymphocytes generally in the center of the lesion and T cells more peripherally (CD4 > CD8). Follicular dendritic cells [CD21(+)] have been demonstrated in Quilty lesions and may distinguish them from rejection.*

Quilty Lesion With Extension Into Myocardium

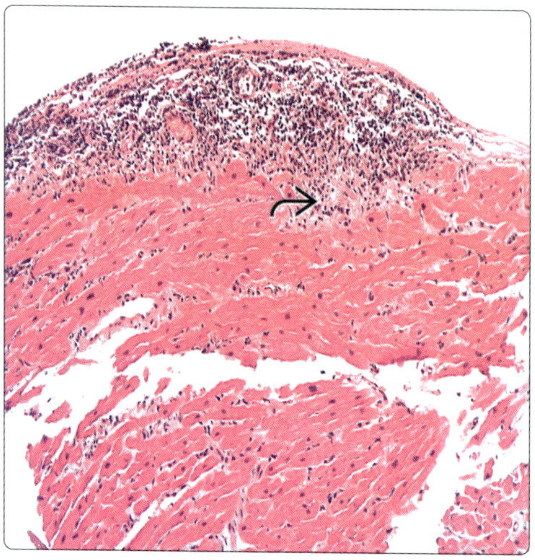

Quilty Lesion With Extension Into Myocardium

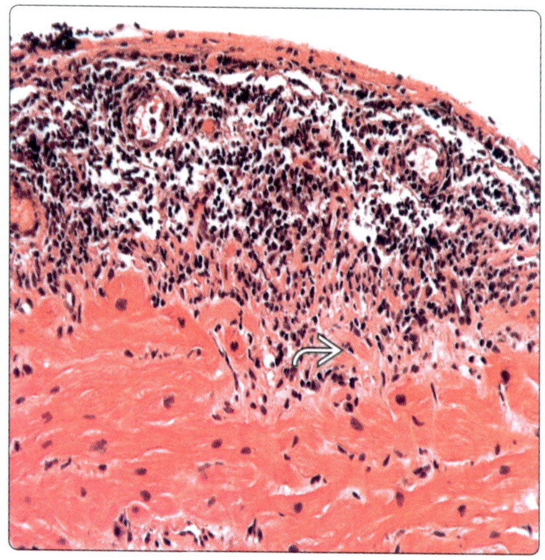

(Left) *Low-power view of an invasive Quilty lesion shows a small area where the infiltrate is beginning to extend into the underlying myocardium ↪.* **(Right)** *High-power view of an area of myocardial infiltration in a Quilty lesion shows myocyte injury ↪. It is important to recognize this area of injury as contiguous with the endocardial infiltrate and representative of an invasive Quilty lesions instead of cellular rejection.*

Quilty Lesion: Low-Power View

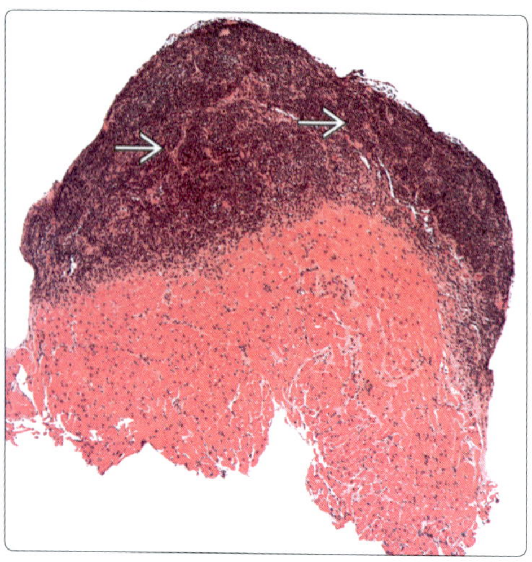

Epstein-Barr Virus-Encoded In Situ Hybridization

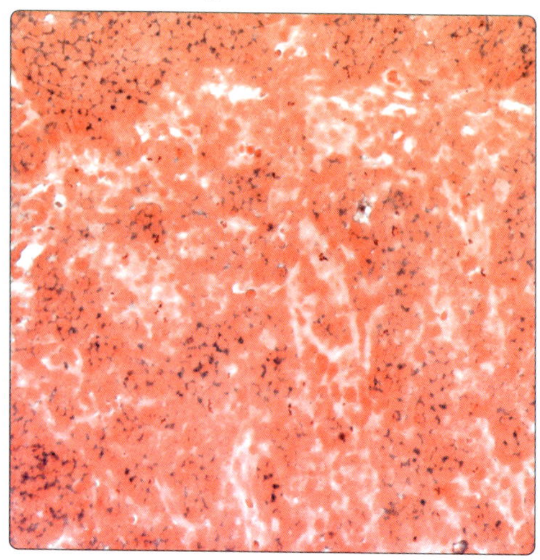

(Left) *H&E shows a large, dense Quilty lesion in a patient who was subjected to immunophenotyping. Note the vascularity present within the lymphoid infiltrate →.* **(Right)** *In situ hybridization for Epstein-Barr virus (EBV)-encoded small RNA was performed on this Quilty lesion to investigate for possible posttransplant lymphoproliferative disorder. It was negative. Studies have failed to show an association of Quilty lesion with EBV infection.*

Quilty Lesion: CD3 Stain

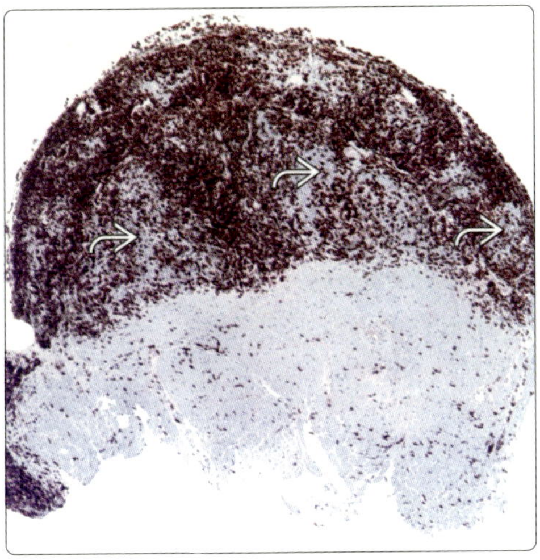

Quilty Lesion: CD20 Stain

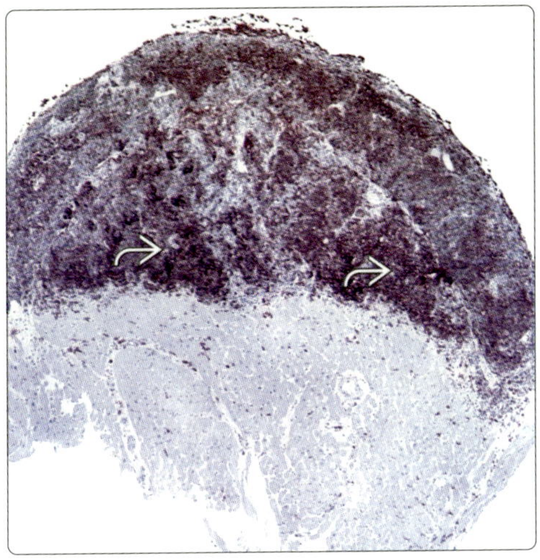

(Left) *CD3 stain of a large Quilty lesion reveals dense T-lymphocytic infiltrate with some central areas without staining* ↪*. Sparse CD3(+) infiltrate is also seen in the myocardium but is not contiguous with the endocardial infiltrate.* **(Right)** *CD20 stain of a Quilty lesion reveals B-lymphocyte staining more prominent in the central areas of the lesion* ↪*, which were not labeled with CD3 immunostain.*

Quilty Lesion: CD21 Stain

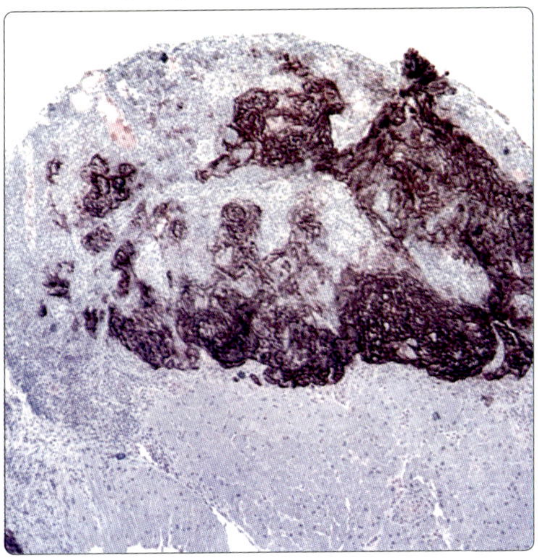

Ischemic Myocardial Injury

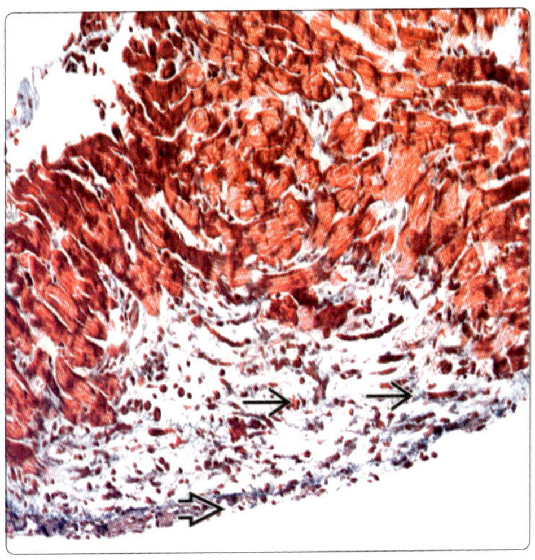

(Left) *CD21 stain for follicular dendritic cells reveals a well-formed dendritic cell network in this large Quilty lesion. This marker is helpful to distinguish Quilty lesion from rejection.* **(Right)** *Vessels from the granulation tissue in healing ischemic injury* → *could potentially mimic a Quilty lesion, but the lack of dense lymphocytic infiltrate, the directly subendocardial location* ⇨ *(endocardium), and the loss of myocytes should all point toward healing ischemic injury.*

Ischemic Myocardial Injury

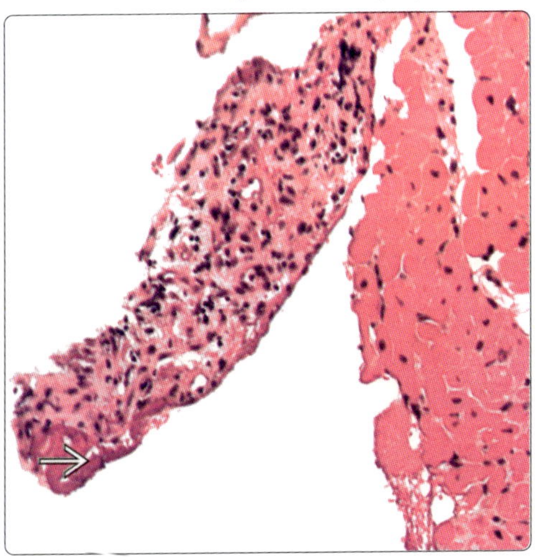

Organizing Thrombus

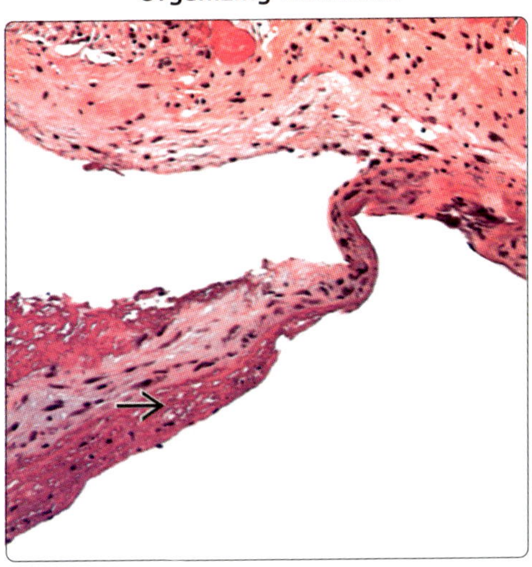

(Left) *As with healing ischemic injury, the inflammatory response to an organizing endocardial thrombus may also mimic Quilty lesions. Note the surface fibrin* ➡ *and lack of a dense lymphocytic infiltrate. Also, looking at all of the biopsy can help put changes in context. There was a large organizing thrombus in this biopsy.* **(Right)** *H&E shows a larger portion of an organizing endocardial thrombus* →*, which may be confused with a Quilty lesion when associated with inflammatory infiltrate.*

Previous Biopsy Sites, Heart Transplant

KEY FACTS

TERMINOLOGY

- Distinctive area of scarring along endocardium and subendocardium of right ventricle
  - Represents healing response to prior endomyocardial biopsy
  - Generally visualized in transplanted hearts subjected to multiple endomyocardial biopsy procedures

CLINICAL ISSUES

- Biopsy site is common finding in surveillance endomyocardial biopsies and can be seen in up to 69% of biopsies
- Biopsy sites generally form small scars along apex and septum of right ventricle
  - Usually of no clinical significance except for potentially affecting adequacy of posttransplant endomyocardial biopsy specimens
  - Represents healing injury that needs to be distinguished from rejection in posttransplant setting

MACROSCOPIC

- Usually located on septum and apex of right ventricle: Endocardial thrombi (recent biopsy site) or endocardial scars with slightly depressed center (healed biopsy site)

MICROSCOPIC

- Recent thrombus overlying areas of acute myocyte injury and interstitial hemorrhage
- Healed biopsy site has fibrosis with myocyte disarray at periphery and thick-walled vessels

TOP DIFFERENTIAL DIAGNOSES

- Healing perioperative ischemic myocyte injury
  - Look for more extensive coagulative myocyte necrosis in healing perioperative ischemic myocyte injury
- Acute rejection
  - Look for mixed inflammatory infiltrate and myocyte disarray to correctly distinguish healing biopsy site from rejection

Histologic Features of Healed Biopsy Site

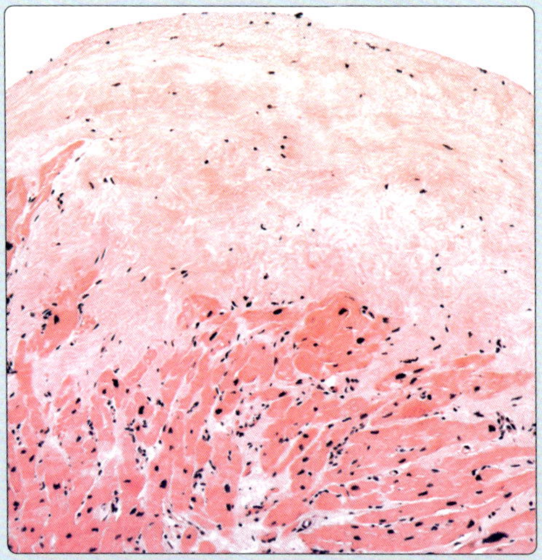

Trichrome Stain of Healed Biopsy Site

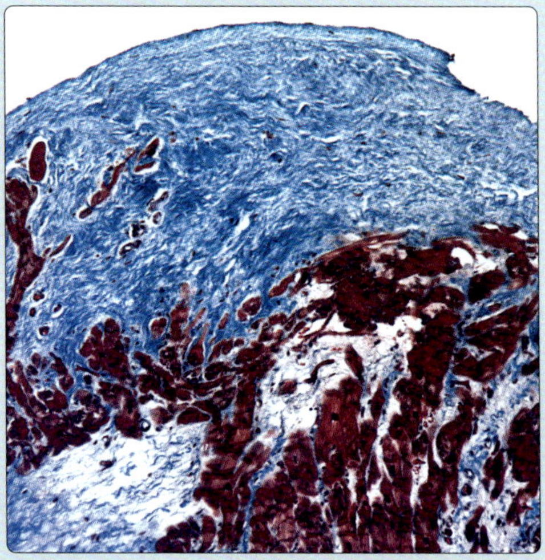

(Left) *H&E shows the classic appearance of a healed biopsy site with a small area of endocardial fibrosis with myocyte disarray at the base. Scant inflammatory infiltrate may be present, but it is not associated with myocyte injury, and this has to be differentiated from acute rejection.* **(Right)** *Trichrome stain highlights the endocardial fibrosis and myocyte disarray present at the base of the lesion in a healed biopsy site.*

Trichrome Stain of Healing Biopsy Site

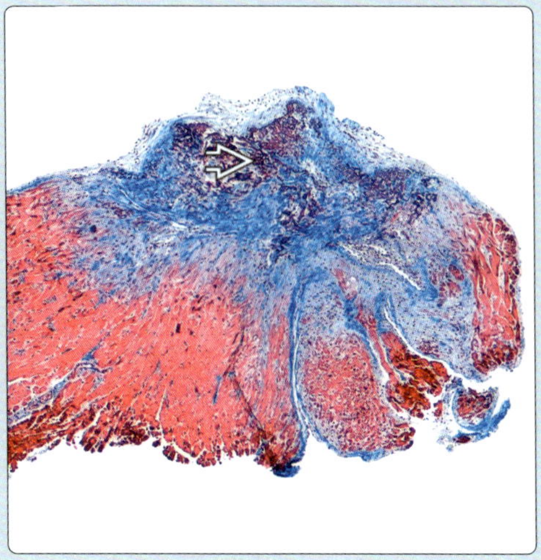

CD68 Immunostain of Healing Biopsy Site

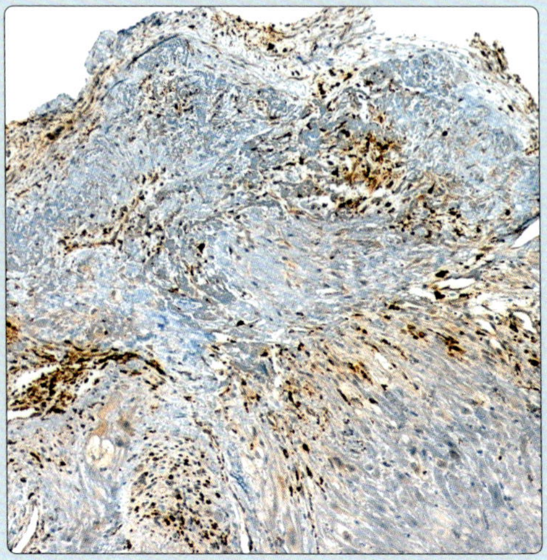

(Left) *Trichrome stain highlights the cup-shaped pattern of fibrosis present in a healing biopsy site. Note that fibrin is still present in its center* ➡. **(Right)** *CD68 immunostain highlights the large numbers of macrophages present within and around a healing biopsy site. This should not be mistaken for a rejection infiltrate. It represents the healing response to the biopsy procedure.*

TERMINOLOGY

Synonyms

- Healing biopsy site
- Prior/previous biopsy site

Definitions

- Distinctive area of scarring along endocardium and subendocardium of right ventricle
  - Represents healing response to prior endomyocardial biopsy
  - Generally visualized in transplanted hearts subjected to multiple endomyocardial biopsy procedures

ETIOLOGY/PATHOGENESIS

Iatrogenic

- Average transplant patient undergoes ≥ 14 biopsies in 1st posttransplant year

CLINICAL ISSUES

Epidemiology

- Incidence
  - Biopsy site is common finding in surveillance endomyocardial biopsies and can be seen in up to 69% of biopsies

Site

- Constant anatomy and fairly rigid bioptome predict that biopsy tissue will come from similar location within right ventricle each time heart is biopsied

Presentation

- Asymptomatic

Prognosis

- Biopsy sites generally form small scars along apex and septum of right ventricle
  - Usually of no clinical significance except for potentially affecting adequacy of posttransplant endomyocardial biopsy specimens
    - 3 fragments composed of at least 50% myocardium (not healing biopsy site tissue) is minimum for evaluation
  - Represents healing injury that needs to be distinguished from rejection in posttransplant setting

MACROSCOPIC

General Features

- Usually located on septum and apex of right ventricle
- Small endocardial thrombi (recent biopsy site)
- Small white endocardial scars that may demonstrate slightly depressed center (healed biopsy site)

MICROSCOPIC

Histologic Features

- Recent biopsy site
  - Recent thrombus overlying areas of acute myocyte injury and interstitial hemorrhage
    - Myocyte injury may include small areas of coagulative myocyte necrosis and contraction band injury
- Organizing biopsy site
  - Granulation tissue formation ± overlying organizing thrombus
  - Mixed inflammatory infiltrate, including lymphocytes, polymorphonuclear leukocytes, and occasional hemosiderin-laden macrophages
- Healed biopsy site
  - Fibrosis with myocyte disarray at periphery and thick-walled vessels
  - Mononuclear inflammation may be present

DIFFERENTIAL DIAGNOSIS

Healing Perioperative Ischemic Myocyte Injury

- Look for more extensive coagulative myocyte necrosis in healing perioperative ischemic myocyte injury
- May have overlying thrombus and mixed inflammatory infiltrate, but thrombus is more common in healing biopsy site
- Ischemic changes are particularly prominent in 1st biopsy post transplant but may be seen up to 4 weeks post transplant

Acute Rejection

- Look for mixed inflammatory infiltrate and myocyte disarray to correctly distinguish healing biopsy site from rejection
- Mononuclear inflammation is more common in rejection than in biopsy site
- Fibrin thrombi are unusual for acute rejection

DIAGNOSTIC CHECKLIST

Pathologic Interpretation Pearls

- Granulation tissue underlying surface fibrin with underlying mixed inflammation ± myocyte injury in recent biopsy site
- Fibrosis with myocyte disarray at periphery in healed biopsy site

SELECTED REFERENCES

1. Seferović PM et al: Heart Failure Association of the ESC, Heart Failure Society of America and Japanese Heart Failure Society position statement on endomyocardial biopsy. Eur J Heart Fail. 23(6):854-71, 2021
2. Strecker T et al: Endomyocardial biopsy for monitoring heart transplant patients: 11-years-experience at a german heart center. Int J Clin Exp Pathol. 6(1):55-65, 2013
3. Winters GL: Cardiac transplant biopsies. In Winters GL et al: Current Concepts in Cardiovascular Pathology. Surgical Pathology Clinics. 5:382-3, 2012
4. Nair V et al: Heart transplant biopsies: interpretation and significance. J Clin Pathol. 63(1):12-20, 2010
5. Tan CD et al: Update on cardiac transplantation pathology. Arch Pathol Lab Med. 131(8):1169-91, 2007
6. Cunningham KS et al: An approach to endomyocardial biopsy interpretation. J Clin Pathol. 59(2):121-9, 2006
7. Stewart S et al: Revision of the 1990 working formulation for the standardization of nomenclature in the diagnosis of heart rejection. J Heart Lung Transplant. 24(11):1710-20, 2005
8. Winters GL: The challenge of endomyocardial biopsy interpretation in assessing cardiac allograft rejection. Curr Opin Cardiol. 12(2):146-52, 1997
9. Rose AG et al: Endomyocardial biopsy site morphology. An experimental study in baboons. Arch Pathol Lab Med. 110(7):622-5, 1986
10. Sibley RK et al: Endomyocardial biopsy in the cardiac allograft recipient. A review of 570 biopsies. Ann Surg. 203(2):177-87, 1986

Posttransplant Lymphoproliferative Disorder, Heart

KEY FACTS

TERMINOLOGY

- Abnormal proliferation of lymphoid cells histologically ranging from benign polyclonal proliferation to lymphoma that develops in recipient of solid organ or bone marrow allograft

ETIOLOGY/PATHOGENESIS

- Epstein-Barr virus (EBV) is believed to play central role in development of posttransplant lymphoproliferative disorder (PTLD) (in one large study, > 80% of patients were positive)
- Immunosuppressive drugs, cytomegalovirus status, activation of cellular oncogenes, long-term antigenic stimulation by allograft, impaired T-cell regulation, and B-cell interleukins probably play role as well

CLINICAL ISSUES

- Incidence: 2-10%; higher incidence in pediatric patients
- Heart transplant-associated PTLD is very rare when compared with other organ transplants
- Risk factors that increase PTLD incidence include
  - Recipient &/or donor age < 18 years, increasing number of rejection episodes, EBV seronegative recipients, and increasing recipient patient survival
- Mean age at diagnosis in one large study: 40 years

MICROSCOPIC

- Early lesions show no architectural effacement and are characterized by small lymphocytes, plasma cells, and immunoblasts in hyperplastic follicles
- Polymorphic PTLD shows architectural effacement and full spectrum of lymphoid maturation
- Monomorphic PTLD shows architectural effacement and histologic characteristics of non-Hodgkin lymphoma
- Rarely, cases of Hodgkin lymphoma-type PTLD have been described

TOP DIFFERENTIAL DIAGNOSES

- Primary lymphoma

(Left) *Low-power H&E of polymorphic posttransplant lymphoproliferative disorder (PTLD) involving the heart demonstrates patchy lymphocytic inflammatory infiltrates ➔ involving the myocardium.* **(Right)** *High-power H&E of polymorphic PTLD involving the heart can sometimes mimic vasculitis with lymphocytes showing a full spectrum of maturation and some plasma cells ➔ surrounding vascular spaces.*

Polymorphic PTLD in Heart Allograft

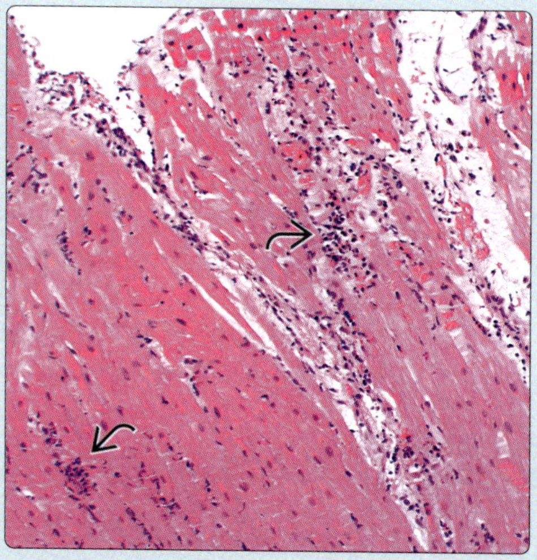

Polymorphic PTLD in Heart Allograft

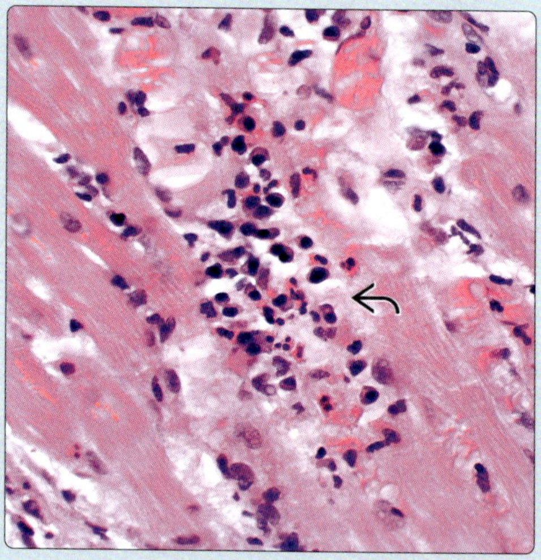

(Left) *H&E from a case of monomorphic PTLD shows a population of large transformed mononuclear cells resembling a large B-cell non-Hodgkin lymphoma. B-cell derived malignancies are the most common type of monomorphic PTLD.* **(Right)** *This case of PTLD involving the heart shows in situ hybridization positivity in lymphocytes ➔ for Epstein-Barr virus (EBV). EBV is thought to play a central role in the pathogenesis of PTLD.*

Monomorphic PTLD

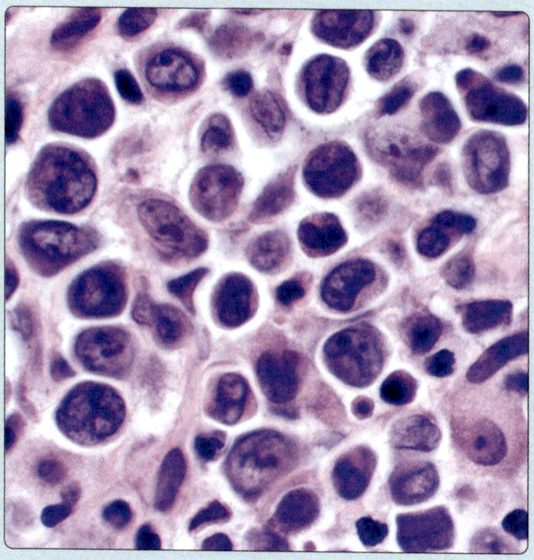

In Situ Hybridization for EBV

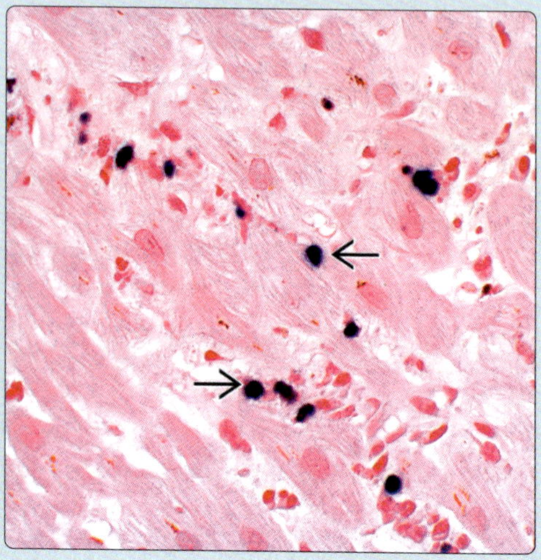

TERMINOLOGY

Abbreviations

- Posttransplant lymphoproliferative disorder (PTLD)

Definitions

- Abnormal proliferation of lymphoid cells histologically ranging from polyclonal proliferation to lymphoma that develops solid organ/bone marrow allograft recipients

ETIOLOGY/PATHOGENESIS

Infectious Agents

- Epstein-Barr virus (EBV) is believed to play central role in development of PTLD (in one large study, > 80% of patients were positive)
  - Immunosuppressive drugs, cytomegalovirus status, activation of cellular oncogenes, long-term antigenic stimulation by allograft, impaired T-cell regulation, and B-cell interleukins probably play role as well

CLINICAL ISSUES

Epidemiology

- Incidence
  - Varies from 2-10%; increased incidence in pediatric patients
  - Heart transplant-associated PTLD is very rare when compared with other organ transplants
  - Risk factors that increase PTLD incidence
    - Recipient &/or donor age < 18 years, increasing number of rejection episodes, EBV seronegative recipients of EBV seropositive donors, and increasing recipient patient survival
- Age
  - Mean age at diagnosis: 40 years
  - PTLD is more prevalent in pediatric patients
- Sex
  - Slightly more common in males

Presentation

- Generally nonspecific with features, such as low-grade fever, malaise, weight loss, and lethargy
- Occasionally, patients may present with organ-specific dysfunction or lymphadenopathy
- Often associated with multiorgan and disseminated PTLD (> 90% of cases in one large study)
- ~ 1/2 of patients present with early-onset PTLD (within first 12 months after transplant)
- Overall, EBV-negative and T-/NK-cell PTLD tends to present later (4-6 years following transplant)

Treatment

- Options, risks, complications
  - Prevention is best treatment with optimal immunosuppressive therapy being most important

Prognosis

- Overall mortality varies depending on study but is estimated at ~ 65%
- Heart transplant recipients with allograft PTLD have worse survival than PTLD associated with other organs

MACROSCOPIC

General Features

- Visible lesions only at advanced stage, particularly in monomorphic PTLD

MICROSCOPIC

Histologic Features

- Early lesions show no architectural effacement and are characterized by small lymphocytes, plasma cells, and immunoblasts in hyperplastic follicles
- Polymorphic PTLD shows architectural effacement and full spectrum of lymphoid maturation
- Monomorphic PTLD shows architectural effacement and histologic characteristics of non-Hodgkin lymphoma
- Rarely, cases of Hodgkin lymphoma-type PTLD have been described
- In one large study in cardiac PTLD, 60% of cases showed monomorphic PTLD, 30% showed polymorphic B-cell lymphoma, and 10% showed plasmacytic hyperplasia

ANCILLARY TESTS

Immunohistochemistry

- Most monomorphic PTLD are of nongerminal center type and exhibit CD19, CD20, CD79-α, PAX5, CD30, and restricted light chain
- Polymorphic PTLD shows heterogeneous B- &/or T-cell population ± light chain restriction
- Reed-Sternberg cells in Hodgkin-type PTLD are CD15(-), CD30(+), and CD20(+)

Flow Cytometry

- Can help distinguish immunophenotype

In Situ Hybridization

- Helpful in determining EBV status

PCR

- May be indicated for IgH/TCR rearrangement studies

DIFFERENTIAL DIAGNOSIS

Primary Lymphoma

- Differentiation of lymphoma from monomorphic PTLD is possible only when history of prior transplant is available
- EBV detection may be helpful

SELECTED REFERENCES

1. Asleh R et al: Post-transplant lymphoproliferative disorder following cardiac transplantation. Front Cardiovasc Med. 9:787975, 2022
2. Ramos-Gonzalez G et al: Presentation and outcomes of post-transplant lymphoproliferative disorder at a single institution pediatric transplant center. Pediatr Transplant. 26(5):e14268, 2022
3. Offor UT et al: Transplantation for congenital heart disease is associated with an increased risk of Epstein-Barr virus-related post-transplant lymphoproliferative disorder in children. J Heart Lung Transplant. 40(1):24-32, 2021
4. Toscano G et al: Post-transplant lymphoproliferative disorders: a rare case of primary pericardial involvement Epstein-Barr virus-correlated in heart transplantation. Transplant Proc. 47(7):2287-90, 2015
5. Khedmat H et al: Heart allograft involvement by posttransplant lymphoproliferative disorders: report from the PTLD. Int survey. Exp Clin Transplant. 9(4):258-64, 2011

Harvesting Injury/Acute Ischemia, Heart

KEY FACTS

TERMINOLOGY

- Ischemic myocardial injury diagnosed in first 6 weeks following transplantation
- May occur in donor, during organ transport (obligate ischemic injury) and after implantation

CLINICAL ISSUES

- Usually asymptomatic histologic finding on early routine posttransplantation biopsies
- Severe cases may be associated with early graft failure, graft loss, and death

MICROSCOPIC

- Coagulative myocyte necrosis, myocyte necrosis with contraction bands, individual cells, small clusters to confluent necrosis, focal or multifocal
- Necrotic myocytes may be noted on multiple biopsies during protracted healing phase
- Healing of ischemic injury in posttransplant setting may be protracted due to immunosuppressive therapy
  - Inflammation peaks in later biopsies than coagulative myocyte necrosis (weeks 2-3 vs. week 1 biopsies)
- Inflammation polymorphous with polymorphonuclear leukocytes, macrophages, lymphocytes, and occasional plasma cells
- Fat necrosis with inflammatory healing response

ANCILLARY TESTS

- Trichrome highlights ischemic myocytes that stain bluish to blue-gray
- C4d highlights ischemic myocyte injury and may stain rare microvessels in area of injury
  - Diffuse microvascular staining is indicative of antibody-mediated rejection

TOP DIFFERENTIAL DIAGNOSES

- Acute cellular rejection
- Antibody-mediated rejection

Histologic Changes in Graft Harvesting Injury

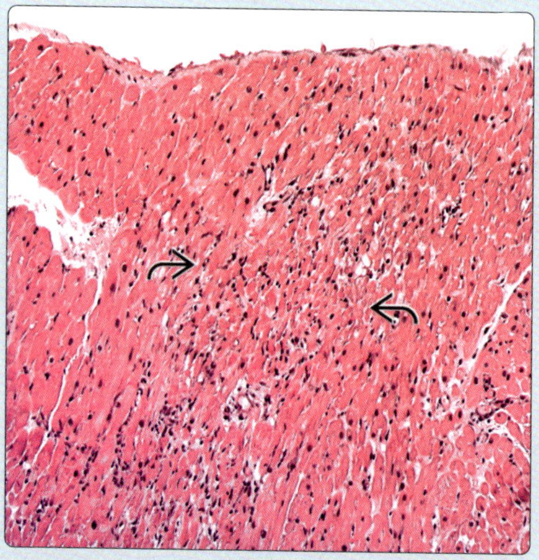

Trichrome Stain of Graft Harvesting Injury

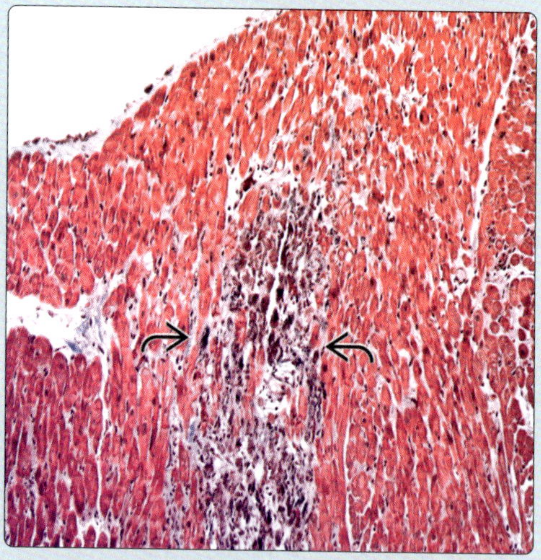

(Left) *Confluent area of coagulative myocyte necrosis ➩ in an initial posttransplant endomyocardial biopsy is consistent with harvesting injury of the graft.* **(Right)** *Trichrome stain is useful in highlighting ischemic myocyte injury ➩ in an initial posttransplant endomyocardial biopsy. Necrotic myocytes appear blue-gray in color.*

Histologic Changes in Persisting Graft Harvesting Injury

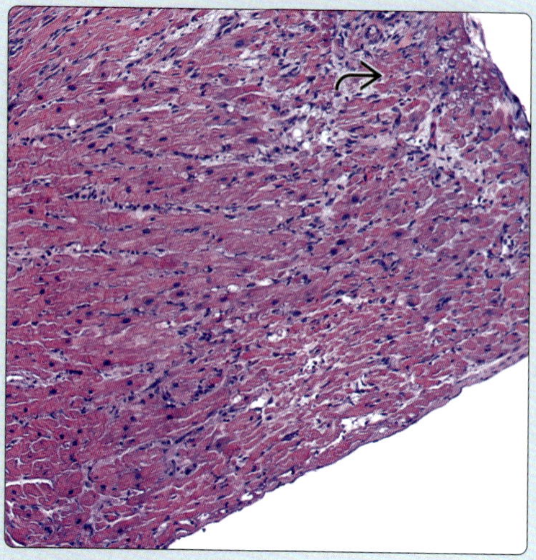

Trichrome Stain of Persisting Graft Harvesting Injury

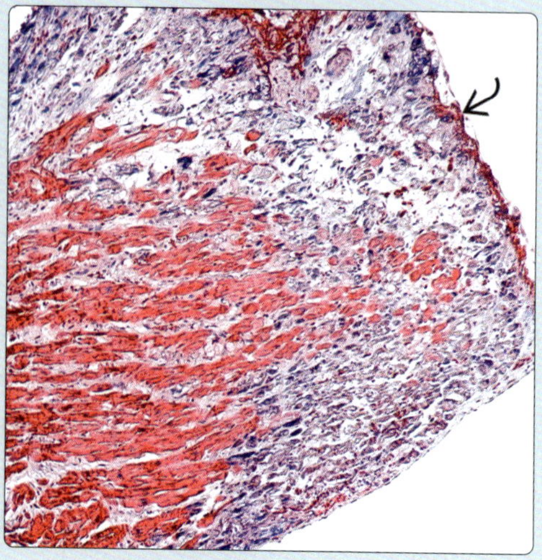

(Left) *H&E stain of a 2nd-week biopsy post transplant highlights the persistent presence of an ischemic myocyte injury, coagulative myocyte necrosis ➩, and polymorphous interstitial inflammation, consistent with harvesting injury of the graft.* **(Right)** *Trichrome stain of a 2nd-week biopsy post transplant highlights the persistent presence of an ischemic myocyte injury. This injury characteristically extends up to the endocardial surface ➩.*

TERMINOLOGY

Synonyms

- Peritransplant ischemia reperfusion injury, early posttransplant ischemic injury

Definitions

- Ischemic myocardial injury diagnosed in first 6 weeks following transplantation
  - May occur in donor, during organ transport (obligate ischemic injury) and after implantation
  - Process involves activation of complex metabolic, cytokine/chemokine, endothelial, and immune networks

ETIOLOGY/PATHOGENESIS

Ischemic Injury in Donor

- Donor trauma/shock and head injury
  - Ultrastructural analysis of myocardial tissue from brain-dead donors has shown evidence of myocyte injury of moderate to severe degree
    - Increased severity with increased use of inotropic support in donor

Ischemic Injury During Transport (Obligate Cold Ischemic Interval)

- Severity of early acute ischemia post transplant has been shown to directly correlate with cold ischemic interval
- Pattern of injury extending up to endocardial surface relates to ischemic injury in non-blood-filled heart

Reperfusion and Perioperative Injury

- Reperfusion may lead to free radical-induced myocardial injury
- Technical issues during surgery, hemorrhage, and use of inotropes in postoperative period may all potentiate early allograft ischemic injury

CLINICAL ISSUES

Presentation

- Usually asymptomatic histologic finding on early routine posttransplantation biopsies
- Severe cases may be associated with early graft failure, graft loss, and death

MACROSCOPIC

General Features

- Severe cases: Edema, hemorrhage, ischemic necrosis, subendocardial, often extending up to endocardial lining

MICROSCOPIC

Histologic Features

- Coagulative myocyte necrosis, myocyte necrosis with contraction bands
  - Injury frequently extends up to endocardial surface
  - Extent of injury is variable
    - Spotty individual or small clusters of myocyte necrosis to areas of confluent necrosis, focal or multifocal
  - Necrotic myocytes may be noted on multiple biopsies during protracted healing phase
  - Vacuolar alteration of ischemically injured but viable myocytes may also be seen
- Healing response to ischemic injury is polymorphous, including polymorphonuclear leukocytes, macrophages, lymphocytes, and occasional plasma cells
  - Myocyte coagulative necrosis is generally greater in amount than inflammation
  - Inflammation is interstitial, not encroaching on individual myocytes
  - Necrotic debris in background helps distinguish from rejection as necrotic background is generally not seen in rejection unless rejection is severe
  - Healing of ischemic injury in posttransplant setting may be protracted due to immunosuppressive therapy
- Additional features
  - Fat necrosis with inflammatory healing response
  - Endocardial inflammation and occasional fibrin deposition
  - Microvascular endothelial cell swelling limited to vicinity of myocyte injury
    - If microvascular changes are noted away from areas of localized ischemic myocyte injury, consider antibody-mediated rejection as there may be morphologic overlap
  - Acute cellular rejection may coexist with healing ischemic injury

ANCILLARY TESTS

Histochemistry

- Trichrome
  - Reactivity: Ischemic myocytes stain bluish to blue-gray

Immunohistochemistry

- C4d highlights ischemic myocyte injury
  - May stain rare microvessel in area of injury
  - If diffuse microvascular staining is noted, think antibody-mediated rejection

DIFFERENTIAL DIAGNOSIS

Acute Cellular Rejection

- Predominantly mononuclear infiltrate surrounding and encroaching on individual myocytes
- Necrotic background more common in early ischemic injury than in rejection (except in severe rejection)

Antibody-Mediated Rejection

- Microvascular changes of endothelial cell swelling and intracapillary mononuclear cells are diffuse and not limited to areas of myocyte necrosis
- Diffuse microvascular staining for C4d is indicative of antibody-mediated rejection

SELECTED REFERENCES

1. Ledwoch N et al: Identification of distinct secretory patterns and their regulatory networks of ischemia versus reperfusion phases in clinical heart transplantation. Cytokine. 149:155744, 2022
2. Frye CC et al: Sterile inflammation in thoracic transplantation. Cell Mol Life Sci. 78(2):581-601, 2021
3. Rohrbach S et al: Ischemia and reperfusion related myocardial inflammation: a network of cells and mediators targeting the cardiomyocyte. IUBMB Life. 67(2):110-9, 2015

(Left) *Fibrin along the endocardial surface and areas of interstitial hemorrhage, which are consistent with harvesting injury, are noted in an initial posttransplant endomyocardial biopsy.* **(Right)** *Trichrome stain of a 2nd-week biopsy post transplant highlights the persistent presence of an ischemic myocyte injury. This injury characteristically extends up to the endocardial surface.*

Initial Histologic Changes in Graft Harvesting Injury

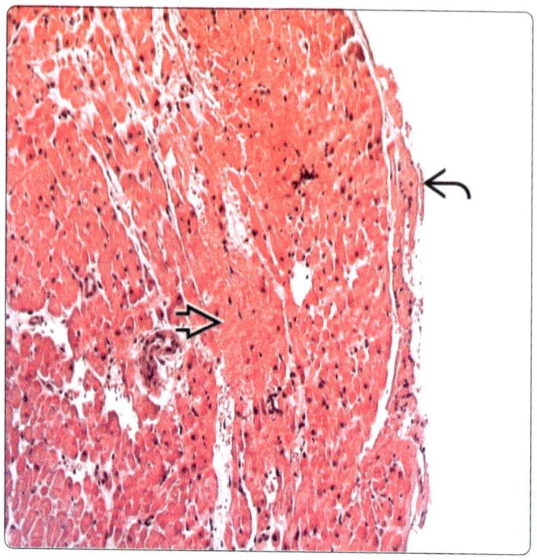

Trichrome Stain of Graft Harvesting Injury 2 Weeks Post Transplant

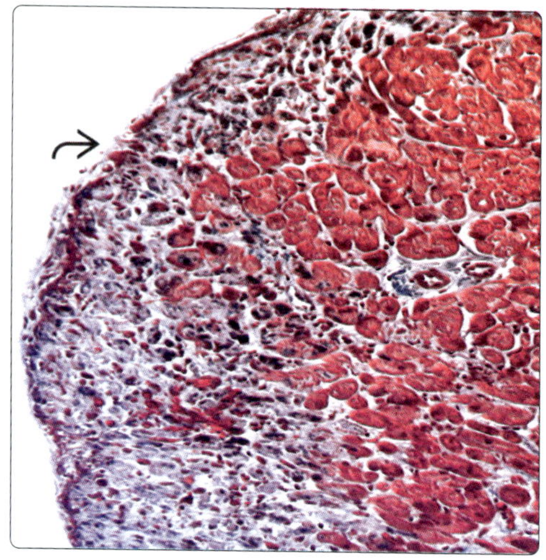

(Left) *C4d stain of early posttransplant biopsy is very helpful for highlighting areas of ischemic myocyte injury. C4d is known to stain ischemically injured myocytes in both the transplant and nontransplant setting.* **(Right)** *Healing response to ischemic injury is delayed in the posttransplant setting, likely due to immunosuppressive therapy. CD68 stain highlights the macrophages responding to the injured myocytes.*

C4d Stain of Graft Harvesting Injury

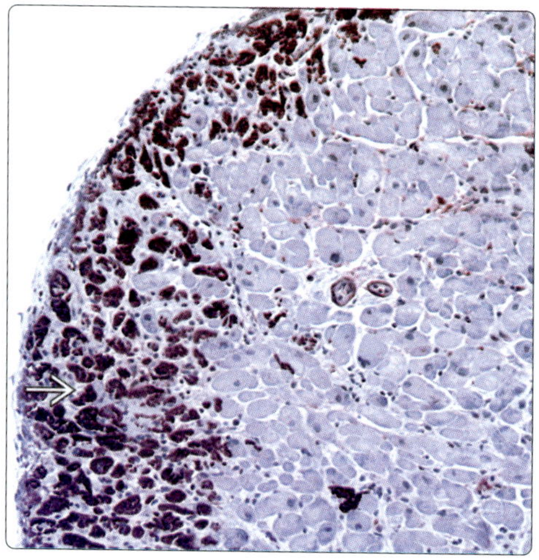

CD68 Stain of Graft Harvesting Injury

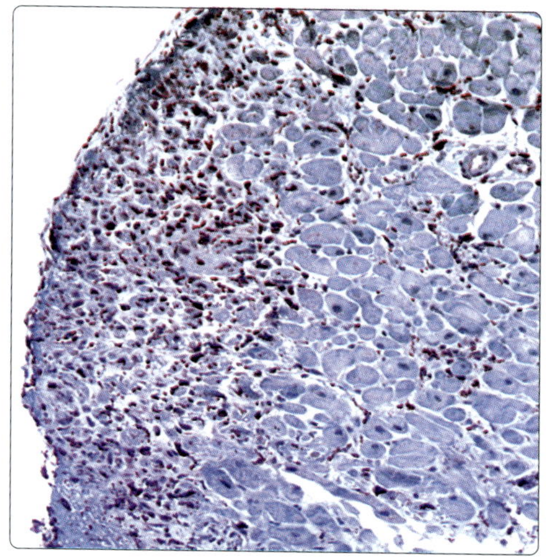

(Left) *C4d stain of subsequent endomyocardial biopsy from a patient with harvesting injury reveals the persistent presence of ischemically injured myocytes, even at the 4th posttransplant biopsy. This is due to delayed healing in the immunosuppressed transplant patient.* **(Right)** *Areas of fat necrosis are often seen in early posttransplant endomyocardial biopsies and are felt to be related to perioperative ischemic injury to the graft.*

C4d Stain of Late Graft Harvesting Injury

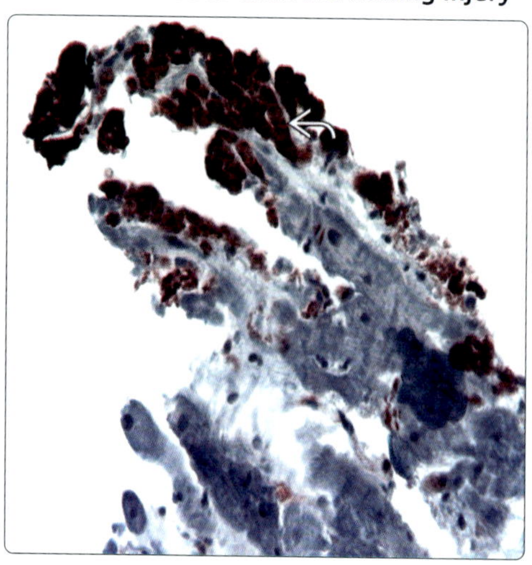

Fat Changes in Graft Harvesting Injury

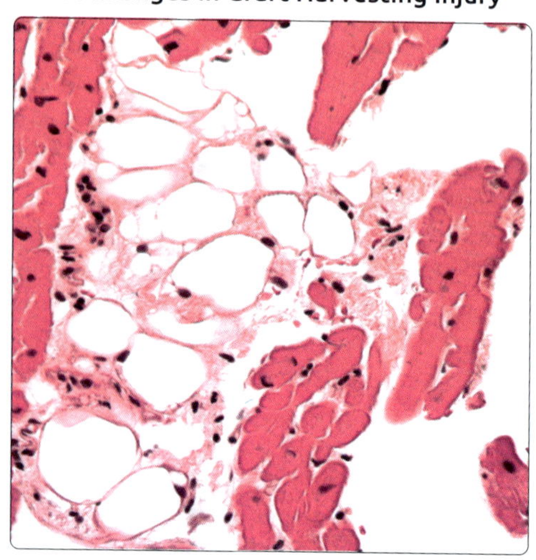

Fat Changes in Late Graft Harvesting Injury

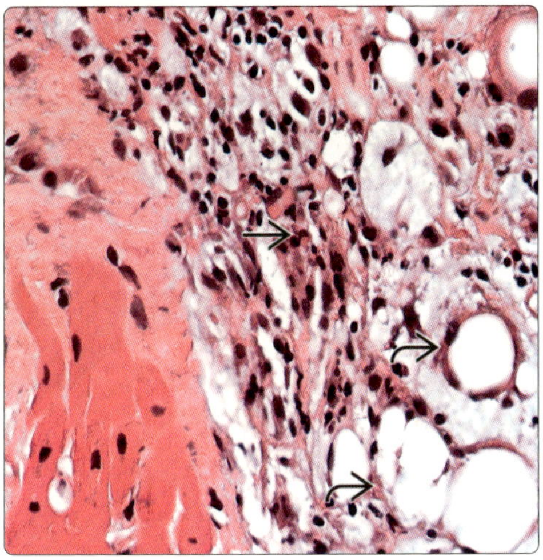

Histologic Changes in Healing Graft Harvesting Injury

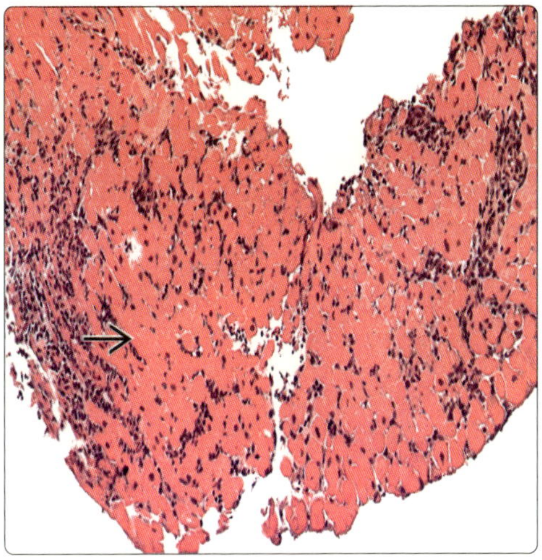

(Left) *Fat necrosis heals with mixed inflammation, including lymphocytes and occasional eosinophils ⇒. This infiltrate may mimic rejection, especially if the injured fat cells are not readily apparent (easily noted here ⇒).* **(Right)** *Healing response to ischemic myocyte injury may also mimic rejection in the early posttransplant setting. However, the presence of necrotic myocytes ⇒ and the mixed type of inflammatory infiltrate are clues of harvesting injury.*

Histologic Changes in Healing Graft Harvesting Injury

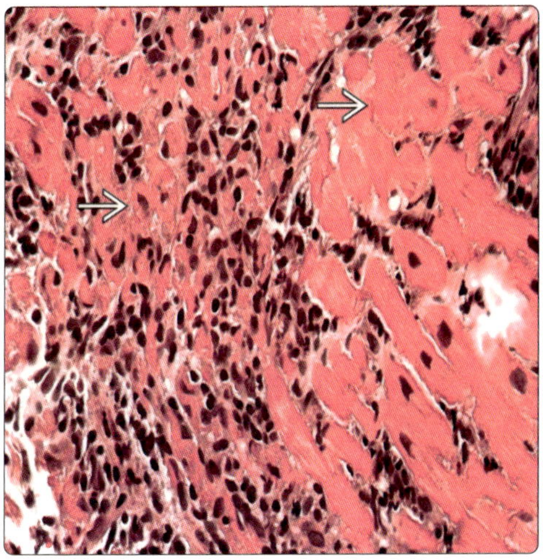

C4d Stain of Graft Harvesting Injury

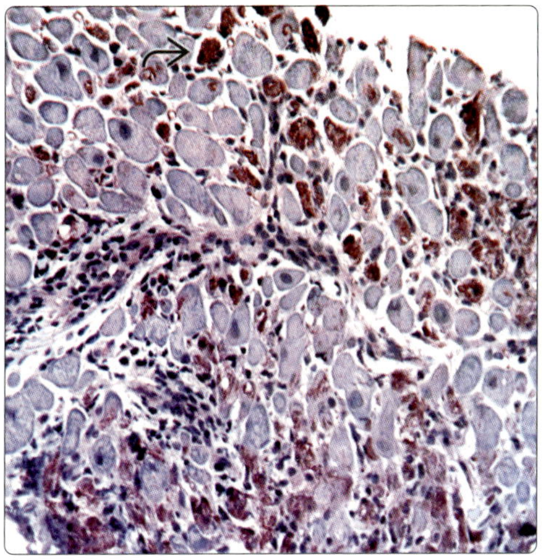

(Left) *Mixed inflammatory infiltrate with a necrotic background and myocyte necrosis > infiltrate is characteristic of healing ischemic injury. Coagulative myocyte necrosis can still be appreciated ⇒, even on H&E.* **(Right)** *C4d stain in this area of inflammation helps to highlight that the extensive ischemic myocyte necrosis is out of proportion to the infiltrate. There are also injured myocytes not surrounded by inflammatory cells ⇒.*

CD68 Stain of Graft Harvesting Injury

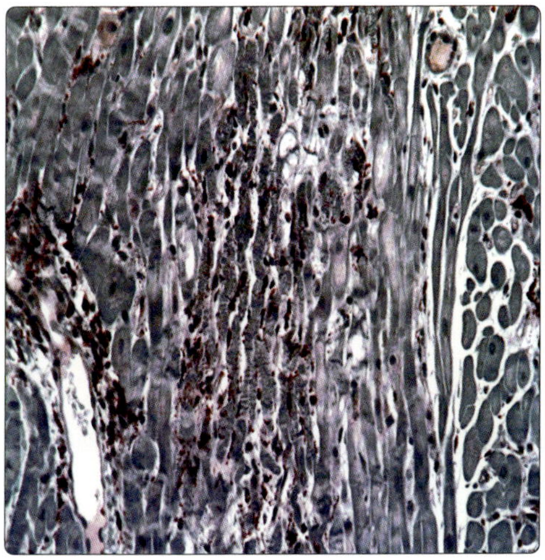

Histologic Changes in Late Allograft Ischemia

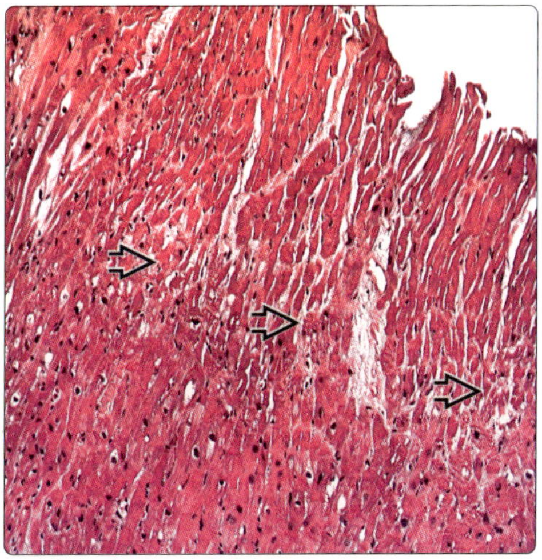

(Left) *CD68 stain can also help to distinguish the infiltrate of healing ischemic injury from a rejection infiltrate, as macrophages are more frequently identified in healing ischemic injury.* **(Right)** *Coagulative myocyte necrosis ⇒ may also be seen in older allografts (microinfarcts), usually related to chronic allograft vasculopathy, as was the case noted at subsequent autopsy of this patient 4 years post transplant.*

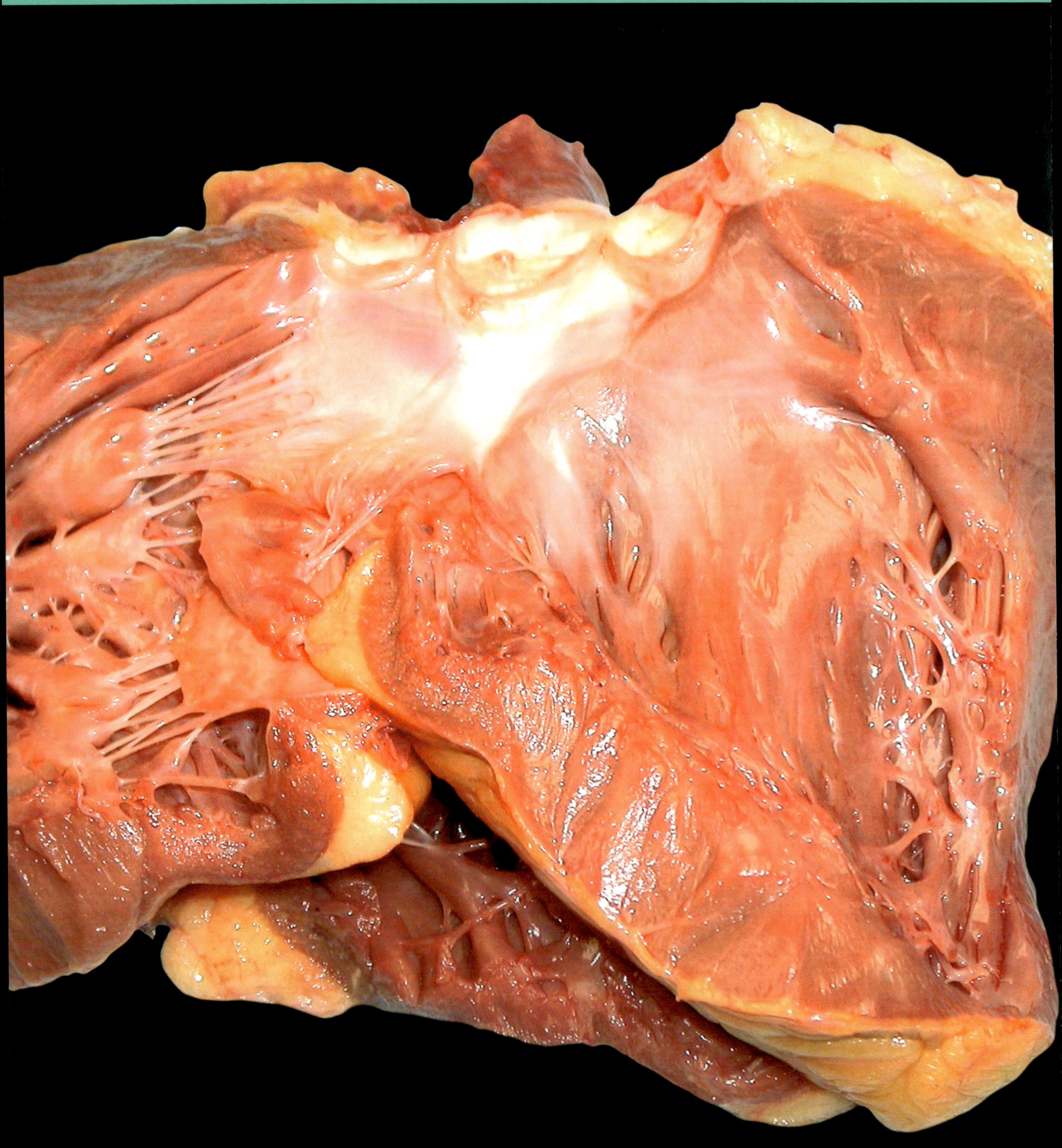

SECTION 2

Heart, Resection

Heart Explant

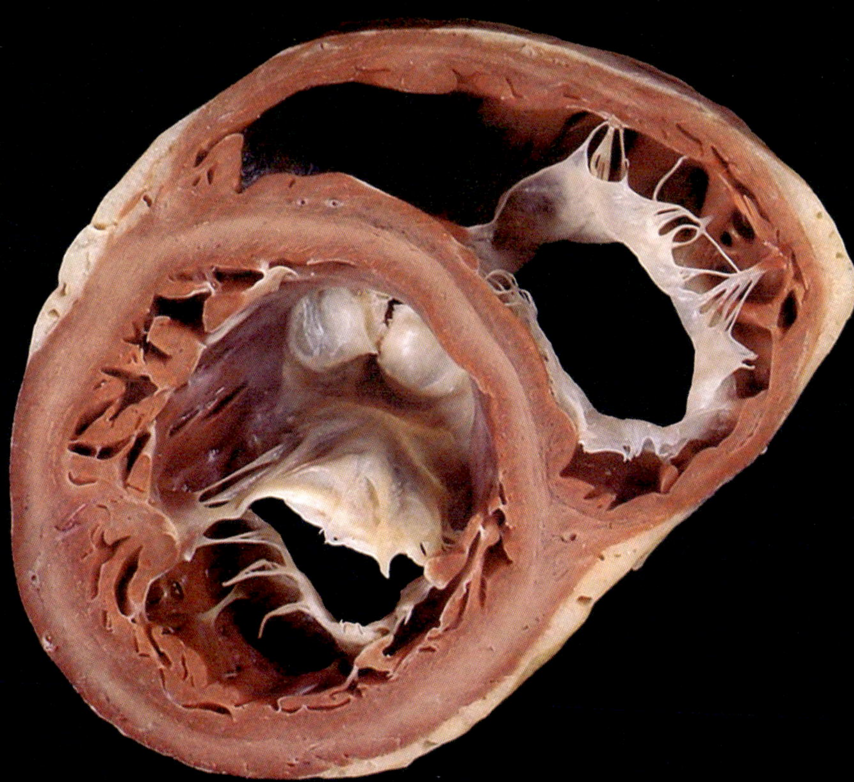

Hypertrophic Cardiomyopathy

KEY FACTS

TERMINOLOGY

- Asymmetric (septal) hypertrophy, hypertrophic (muscular) subaortic stenosis, obstructive cardiomyopathy
- Common inherited cardiovascular disease characterized by left &/or right ventricular hypertrophy, usually asymmetric, involving interventricular septum, causing impaired ventricle relaxation

ETIOLOGY/PATHOGENESIS

- Autosomal dominant mutations in genes encoding protein components of sarcomere and its constituent myofibrillar proteins
- 70% have mutations in 2 genes, β-myosin heavy chain (*MYH7*) and myosin-binding protein C (*MYBPC3*)

CLINICAL ISSUES

- ~ 0.6% (i.e., 1:200) in general population
- Palpitations, exertional dyspnea, atrial fibrillation, and sudden cardiac death

MACROSCOPIC

- Hypertrophy of left ventricle, asymmetric or symmetric
- Classic: Asymmetric septal hypertrophy (septum: Free wall thickness ratio > 1.3)
- Systolic anterior motion of mitral valve and subaortic endocardial fibrosis

MICROSCOPIC

- Diffuse myocyte hypertrophy
- Myocyte disarray and myocytes with bizarre, disorganized myofibrillar architecture
- Bizarre myocyte nuclei with nuclear enlargement, pleomorphism, and hyperchromatism
- Interstitial and replacement fibrosis

TOP DIFFERENTIAL DIAGNOSES

- Physiologic athlete's heart
- Hypertensive heart disease
- Storage disease

Gross Specimen With Changes of Hypertrophic Cardiomyopathy

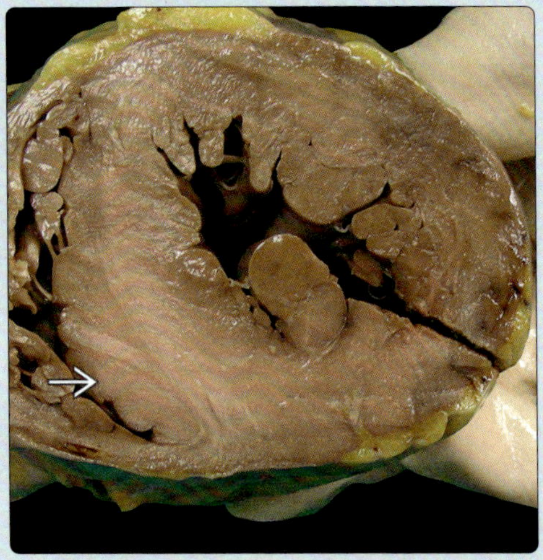

Gross Specimen of Case With Hypertrophic Cardiomyopathy

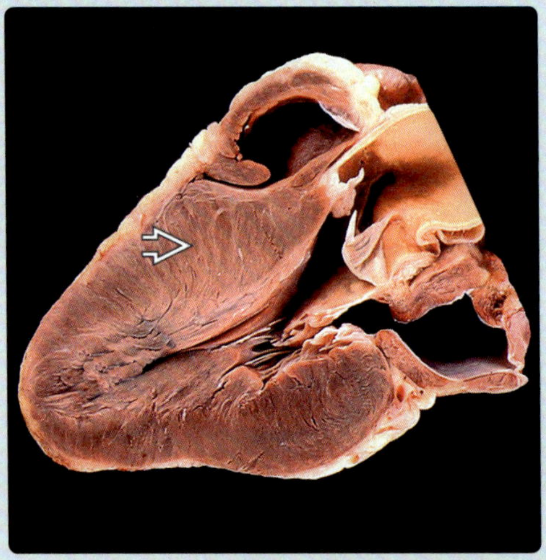

(Left) *Short-axis section of the heart shows marked thickening of the septum ➡, especially toward the posterior heart, characteristic of hypertrophic cardiomyopathy.* **(Right)** *Long-axis view of an autopsy heart specimen from a patient with hypertrophic cardiomyopathy shows asymmetric basal septal thickening ➡.*

Histologic Features of Hypertrophic Cardiomyopathy

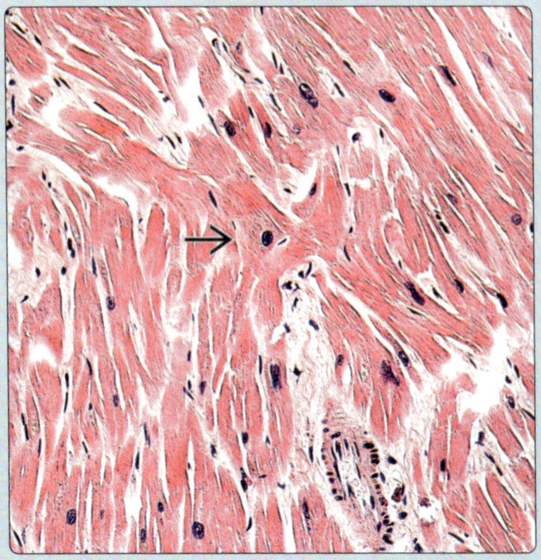

Trichrome Stain of Myocardium With Changes of Hypertrophic Cardiomyopathy

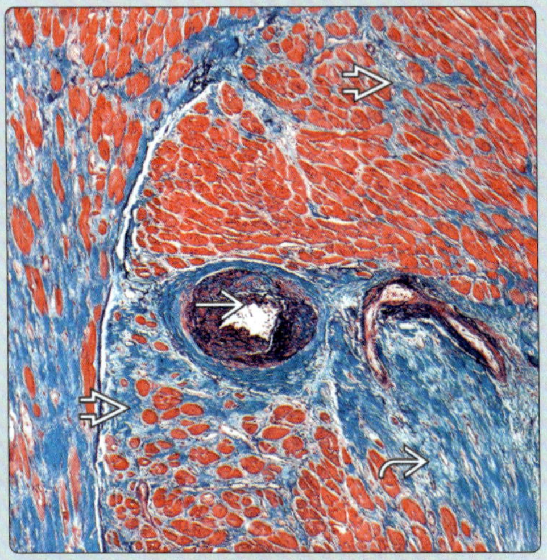

(Left) *H&E stain shows myocyte disarray with cartwheel or storiform pattern ➡. The typical appearance is that of branching myocytes with hypertrophy and nuclear enlargement.* **(Right)** *Masson trichrome stain shows features of hypertrophic cardiomyopathy, including fibrosis, myocyte hypertrophy, and intramural dysplastic vessels ➡. Fibrosis may be interstitial ➡ or replacement type ➡.*

TERMINOLOGY

Abbreviations

- Hypertrophic cardiomyopathy (HCM)
- Hypertrophic obstructive cardiomyopathy (HOCM)

Synonyms

- Asymmetric (septal) hypertrophy, hypertrophic (muscular) subaortic stenosis, obstructive cardiomyopathy

Definitions

- Common inherited cardiovascular disease characterized by left ventricular hypertrophy, usually asymmetric, involving interventricular septum, causing impaired ventricle relaxation
  - End-diastolic left ventricle (LV) wall thickness in adults ≥ 13 mm (≥ 15-mm cut point recommended by European Society of Cardiology) in absence of abnormal loading conditions or other secondary causes

ETIOLOGY/PATHOGENESIS

Genetics

- Autosomal dominant mutations in genes encoding sarcomeric and associated myofibrillar proteins
- There are at least 50 causative genes and over 1,400 mutations
- ~ 50% have mutations in either β-myosin heavy chain (*MYH7*) or myosin-binding protein C (*MYBPC3*)
- Troponin T (*TNNT2*), troponin I (*TNNI3*), and α-tropomyosin (*TPM1*) account for ≤ 10% of cases
- Other uncommon genes include: Cardiac α-actin (*ACTC1*), myosin light chain 2 (*MYL2*) and 3 (*MYL3*), cysteine and glycine-rich protein 3 (*CSRP3*)
- In 40% of cases, genetic mutations cannot be found

Nongenetic Factors

- Sustained dysregulated intracellular calcium handling
- Dysregulated autophagy response
- Altered glucose metabolism
- Altered cell to cell interaction

CLINICAL ISSUES

Epidemiology

- Incidence
  - ~ 1:200-500 in general population
- Age
  - Can present at any age (including coincidentally at autopsy in older adults)
- Sex
  - Male predominance: 3:2
  - Either underrecognized or clinical diagnosis is delayed in women
  - At presentation, women are older, more symptomatic, and frequently develop LV outflow obstruction with higher risk of progression to advanced heart failure
- Ethnicity
  - More frequently in Black patients

Presentation

- 1st manifestation may be sudden cardiac death (SCD) due to ventricular fibrillation
  - Risk factors for SCD include
    - Family history of SCD
    - Multiple gene mutations
    - Unexplained syncope
    - Maximal LV thickness > 30 mm
    - Abnormal blood pressure response to exercise
    - Repetitive nonsustained ventricular tachycardia
    - LV apical aneurysm
    - Myocardial fibrosis
- Syncopal attacks, palpitations, exertional dyspnea, chest pain
- Arrhythmias
  - Supraventricular (atrial fibrillation)
  - Ventricular (fibrillation/tachycardia)

Laboratory Tests

- Genetic testing to determine pathogenic mutation for patients with HCM
- Genetic screening of 1st-degree relatives is recommended

Treatment

- Surgical approaches
  - Implantable cardiac defibrillator (ICD) for primary or secondary prevention of SCD
  - Septal/apical myomectomy
  - Heart transplantation is option for symptomatic patients not responsive to optimal medical therapy
    - Survival after transplant is superior to that for ischemic cardiomyopathy and similar to other causes with low acute rejection episodes
- Drugs
  - β-blockers
  - Angiotensin-converting enzyme inhibitors
  - Angiotensin receptor blockers
  - Ca^{++} channel blockers
  - Selective inhibitor of cardiac myosin (mavacamten) in phase III clinical trials
- Endovascular alcohol septal ablation

Prognosis

- Most patients of HCM are asymptomatic and can have normal or near-normal life expectancy
- Mortality rates have ranged from < 1% to 3-6%
  - Younger patients, particularly children, have much higher mortality rate
- Most common causes of death include SCD, heart failure, and stroke

IMAGING

EKG

- Ventricular hypertrophy, ventricular tachycardia
- ST-/T-wave abnormalities or pathologic Q waves

Echocardiography

- Assess hypertrophy pattern, diastolic dysfunction
- Dynamic LV outflow obstruction [systolic anterior motion (SAM) of anterior mitral leaflet]
- Quantitative estimates of peak LV outflow gradient
- Assess aortic and mitral valve abnormalities (e.g., elongation, prolapse, calcification, flail)

Stress Test

- Assessment of functional capacity and response to therapy

Cardiac MR

- Magnitude of LV hypertrophy and anatomy of mitral valve
- Provides accurate measurements of maximal LV wall thickness
- Identify areas of LV (apex and anterolateral free wall) sometimes blind to echocardiography
- Characterize presence of apical aneurysm
- Late gadolinium enhancement is indicative of fibrosis, which is risk factor for SCD
- Definition of LV outflow tract anatomy in preoperative planning of invasive septal reduction
- Ruling out sarcoidosis, amyloidosis, etc.

Coronary Angiography

- Rule out concomitant coronary artery disease

MACROSCOPIC

General Features

- Hypertrophy of LV
  - Classic: Asymmetric septal hypertrophy (septum: Free wall thickness ratio > 1.3)
    - Thickening of basal anterior septum
  - Symmetric hypertrophic form accounts for 42% of cases
  - Dilated or burned-out phase accounts for 10% of cases
  - Rare variants
    - Midventricular
    - Apical
    - Concentric
- Subaortic endocardial fibrosis (mitral contact lesion)

MICROSCOPIC

Histologic Features

- Myocyte hypertrophy, size > 40 μm (normal: 15 μm)
  - Bizarre myocyte nuclei, nuclear enlargement, pleomorphism, and hyperchromatism
- Myocyte disarray (> 20% of myocardium in ≥ 2 tissue blocks)
- Myocytes with bizarre disorganized myofibrillar architecture
- Interstitial and replacement fibrosis
- Intramural coronary arteries show medial hypertrophy and luminal narrowing
- Endocardial thickening
- Reduced microvessel density

ANCILLARY TESTS

Immunohistochemistry

- BRG1 nuclear expression has been demonstrated in HCM

Genetic Testing

- DNA sequencing for identification of mutations
  - Sarcomere mutations do not predict sudden death, prognosis, or clinical course of individual patients
  - Useful for family screening and identification of phenocopies
  - Identifies clinically silent, genetically affected family members that have capability of disease transmission to offspring

DIFFERENTIAL DIAGNOSIS

Physiologic Athlete's Heart

- Symmetric LV hypertrophy without myocyte disarray
- Absence of familial distribution

Hypertensive Heart Disease

- Older age, history of hypertension
- Do not have familial distribution
- Absence of myocyte disarray

Fabry Disease

- Deficiency of lysosomal α-galactosidase A
  - Histologically, involved cells are vacuolated with cardiac myocytes having lace-like appearance
  - Deposits stain positive with toluidine blue, PAS, or Sudan Black B and are birefringent
  - Ultrastructurally, presence of numerous intralysosomal deposits of concentric lamellar bodies

Pompe Disease

- Deficiency of lysosomal acid α-1,4-glucosidase
  - Histologically, vacuolization of myocytes with storage of structurally normal glycogen
  - Ultrastructurally, increased glycogen both free and in cytoplasm membrane-bound lysosomes

LAMP2; Danon Disease

- X-linked lysosomal-associated membrane protein 2 (*LAMP2*)
  - Mild interstitial fibrosis and vacuolated cardiac myocytes containing glycogen
  - Ultrastructural examination reveals free and membrane-bound lysosomal glycogen
  - Similar features to Pompe disease

Sigmoid Septal Curvature

- Prominent subaortic bulge due to S curvature of septum in older adults
- Do not have familial distribution

SELECTED REFERENCES

1. Cui H et al: Survival following alcohol septal ablation or septal myectomy for patients with obstructive hypertrophic cardiomyopathy. J Am Coll Cardiol. 79(17):1647-55, 2022
2. Edelberg JM et al: The impact of mavacamten on the pathophysiology of hypertrophic cardiomyopathy: a narrative review. Am J Cardiovasc Drugs. 22(5):497-510, 2022
3. Hong Y et al: Risk factors of sudden cardiac death in hypertrophic cardiomyopathy. Curr Opin Cardiol. 37(1):15-21, 2022
4. Kwon S et al: Comparison of mortality and cause of death between adults with and without hypertrophic cardiomyopathy. Sci Rep. 12(1):6386, 2022
5. Maron BJ et al: Diagnosis and evaluation of hypertrophic cardiomyopathy: JACC state-of-the-art review. J Am Coll Cardiol. 79(4):372-89, 2022
6. Maron BJ et al: Management of hypertrophic cardiomyopathy: JACC state-of-the-art review. J Am Coll Cardiol. 79(4):390-414, 2022
7. Nagueh SF et al: Recommendations for multimodality cardiovascular imaging of patients with hypertrophic cardiomyopathy: an update from the American Society of Echocardiography, in collaboration with the American Society of Nuclear Cardiology, the Society for Cardiovascular Magnetic Resonance, and the Society of Cardiovascular Computed Tomography. J Am Soc Echocardiogr. 35(6):533-69, 2022
8. Nguyen MB et al: Pediatric hypertrophic cardiomyopathy: exploring the genotype-phenotype association. J Am Heart Assoc. 11(5):e024220, 2022

Most Prevalent Genes Associated With Hypertrophic Cardiomyopathy

Encoding Proteins/Gene	Protein	Frequency of Pathogenic Variants	Protein Function
Sarcomere thick filaments: *MYH7*	β-MYH	20%	Comprises 1/3 of sarcomere proteins, is main muscle motor molecule, and is essential for muscle contraction
Sarcomere thick filaments: *MYBPC3*	Myosin-binding protein C3	20%	MYBC3 protein is associated with thin and thick filaments and regulates actin/myosin interactions
Sarcomere thick filaments:*MYL2/MYL3*	Myosin light chain 2 and 3	< 1%	MYL2/MYL3 are part of myosin hexamer and interact with MYH7 hinge region
Sarcomere thick filaments:*TTN*	Titin	Low	Titin expands from M to Z lines
Sarcomere thin filaments:*TNNT2*	TNNT2	Low	Constitutes 5% of sarcomere proteins
Sarcomere thin filaments:*TNNI3, TNNC1, TPM1*	TNNI3, TNNC1, TPM1	< 5%	Components of thin filaments
Sarcomere thin filaments: *ACTC1*	ACTC1	Low	Major component of thin filaments
Z lines: *MYOZ2*	MYOZ2	Low	Involved in regulation of myofibrillogenesis and calcium-dependent signaling pathways
Z lines: *ACTN2*	ACTN2	Sporadic	Binds to actin thin filament protein and regulates sarcomere function
M line: *OSBCN*	Obscurin	Low	Obscurin interacts with TTN and MYBPC3
M line: *TRIM63*	TRIM63 (muscle ring finger 1)	Low	Protein is E3 ubiquitin ligase that tags thick filament protein for degradation by UPS
M line: *MYOM2*	MYOM2	Low	Protein crosslinks TTN and MYH7
Sarcomere-associated proteins: *FLNC*	FLNC	Sporadic	Protein crosslinks with actin and is presumed it regulates organization of cytoskeletal proteins
Sarcomere-associated proteins: *ALPK3*	α kinase3	Low	Protein implicated in myocyte differentiation
Sarcomere-associated proteins: *CAV3*	Caveolin 3	Low	CAV3 is involved in several myogenic mechanisms
Sarcomere-associated proteins: *CRYAB*	Crystallin αB	Low	Protein is member of small heat shock proteins with chaperon-like activity
Nonsarcomeric: *JPH2*	Juntophilin 2	Sporadic	Juntophilin major component of junctional/membrane complex involved in calcium homeostasis

9. Palyam V et al: Hypertrophic cardiomyopathy and atrial fibrillation: a review. Cureus. 14(1):e21101, 2022
10. Scherba JC et al: BRG1 is a biomarker of hypertrophic cardiomyopathy in human heart specimens. Sci Rep. 12(1):7996, 2022
11. Shintani Y et al: Clinical impact of the pathological quantification of myocardial fibrosis and infiltrating T lymphocytes using an endomyocardial biopsy in patients with hypertrophic cardiomyopathy. Int J Cardiol. 362:110-7, 2022
12. Ušaj M et al: Critical evaluation of current hypotheses for the pathogenesis of hypertrophic cardiomyopathy. Int J Mol Sci. 23(4):2195, 2022
13. Zhang MK et al: Microvascular rarefaction and myocardial fibrosis in hypertrophic obstructive cardiomyopathy: a histopathological comparison of pediatric and adult patients. Heart Surg Forum. 25(1):E042-7, 2022
14. Chou C et al: Pathogenic mechanisms of hypertrophic cardiomyopathy beyond sarcomere dysfunction. Int J Mol Sci. 22(16):8933, 2021
15. Cui H et al: Myocardial histopathology in patients with obstructive hypertrophic cardiomyopathy. J Am Coll Cardiol. 77(17):2159-70, 2021
16. De Gaspari M et al: Small vessel disease: another component of the hypertrophic cardiomyopathy phenotype not necessarily associated with fibrosis. J Clin Med. 10(4), 2021
17. Grassi S et al: Update on the diagnostic pitfalls of autopsy and post-mortem genetic testing in cardiomyopathies. Int J Mol Sci. 22(8):575, 2021
18. Ioakeimidis NS et al: Routine histopathology of septal myectomy for hypertrophic obstructive cardiomyopathy in a greek cohort. Histol Histopathol. 36(11):1145-53, 2021
19. Marian AJ: Molecular genetic basis of hypertrophic cardiomyopathy. Circ Res. 128(10):1533-53, 2021
20. Yotti R et al: Advances in the genetic basis and pathogenesis of sarcomere cardiomyopathies. Annu Rev Genomics Hum Genet. 20:129-53, 2019
21. Abecasis J et al: Surgical pathology of subaortic septal myectomy: histology skips over clinical diagnosis. Cardiovasc Pathol. 33:32-8, 2018
22. Hughes SE: The pathology of hypertrophic cardiomyopathy. Histopathology. 44(5):412-27, 2004

Area of Endocardial Fibrosis in Subaortic Region of Hypertrophic Cardiomyopathy

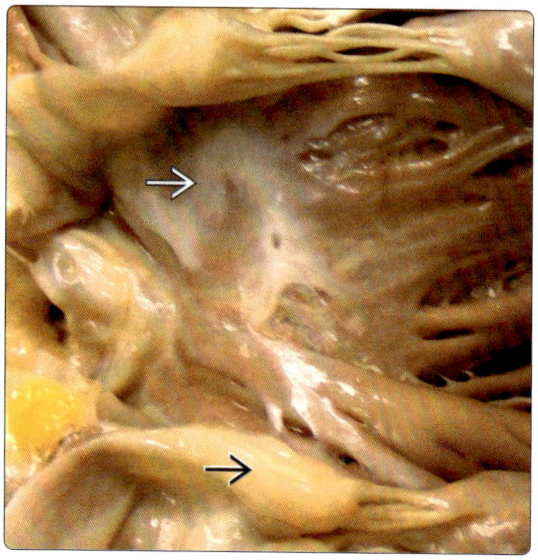

Histologic Features of Area of Endocardial Fibrosis in Subaortic Region

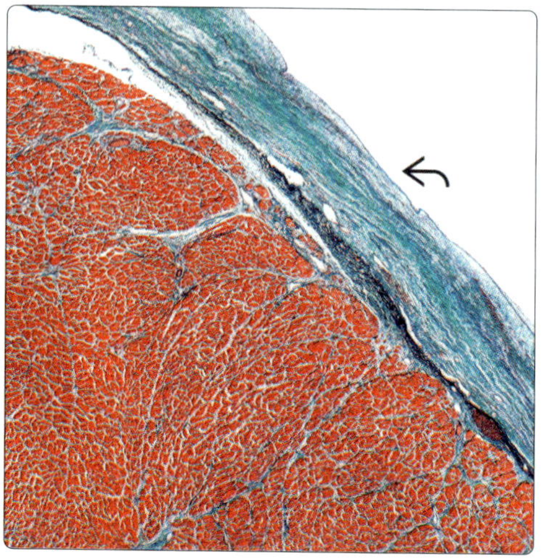

(Left) *Gross photograph shows a discrete area of endocardial fibrosis in the subaortic region of the left ventricular outflow tract* ➡*. This corresponds to a friction lesion adjacent to the anterior leaflet of the mitral valve* ⇨*.* **(Right)** *Masson trichrome staining demonstrates the prominent area of endocardial fibrosis* ⮐*. This histologic section corresponds to the subaortic area of fibrosis.*

Histologic Features of Myocytes in Hypertrophic Cardiomyopathy

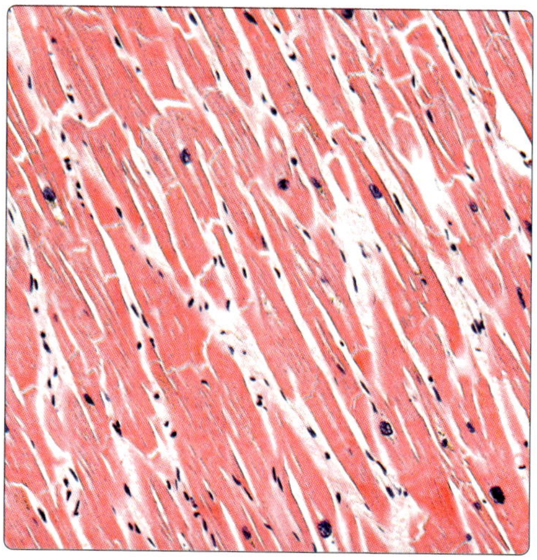

Histologic Features of Hypertrophic Cardiomyopathy

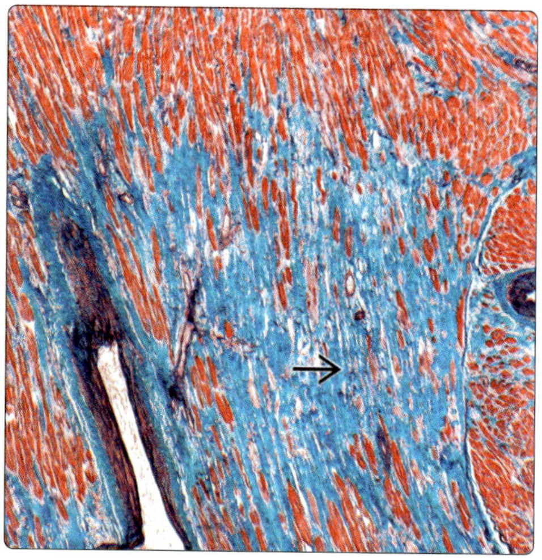

(Left) *H&E-stained section shows hypertrophy of cardiac myocytes. The hypertrophy is characterized by nuclear enlargement.* **(Right)** *Masson trichrome stain shows marked interstitial and replacement-type* ⇨ *fibrosis. These areas of scarring may be apparent grossly. They are most often seen along the ventricular septum.*

Vascular Changes in Hypertrophic Cardiomyopathy

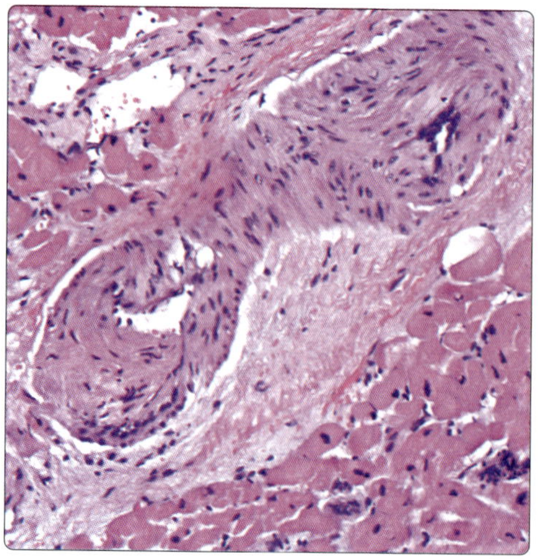

Vascular Changes in Hypertrophic Cardiomyopathy

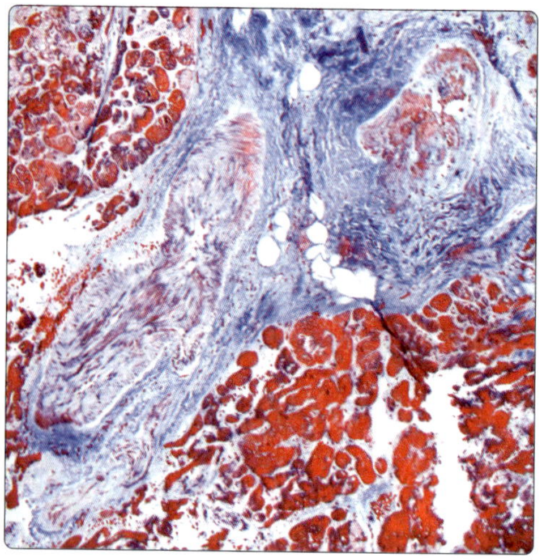

(Left) *Section of myocardium in a case of hypertrophic cardiomyopathy shows intramural vessels with dysplastic changes characterized by media thickening and reduction of luminal area. This frequently causes myocardial ischemia, which correlates with clinical manifestations.* **(Right)** *Trichrome-stained section of myocardium in a case of hypertrophic cardiomyopathy shows intramural coronary vessels with dysplastic changes and perivascular fibrosis.*

Gross Specimen From Case of Hypertrophic Cardiomyopathy

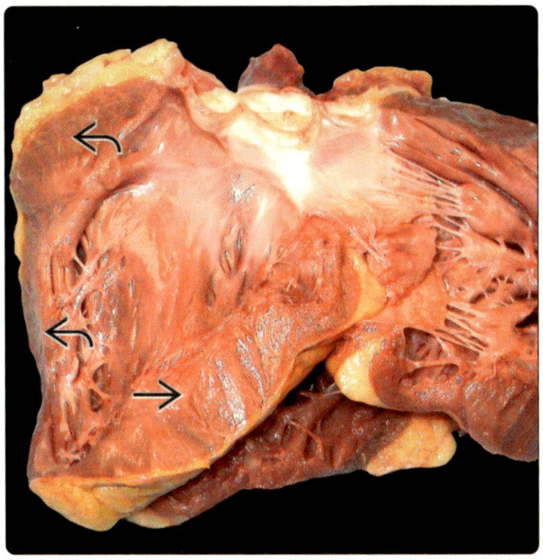

Gross Specimen From Myomectomy in Case of Hypertrophic Cardiomyopathy

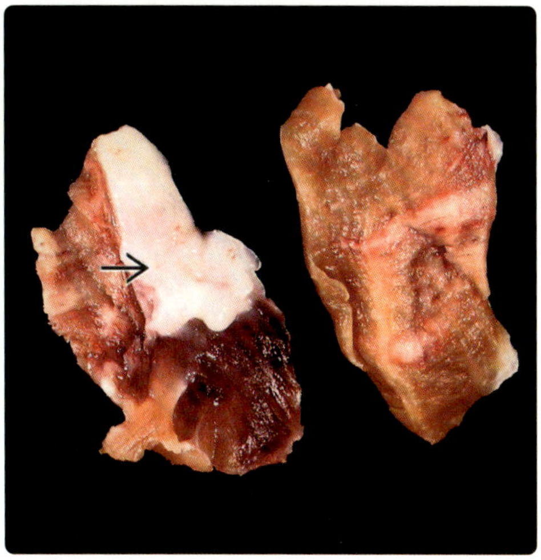

(Left) *An explanted heart specimen from an adult with hypertrophic cardiomyopathy shows thickening of the midseptum* → *relative to the left ventricle free wall* ↶ *(excluding the papillary muscle).* **(Right)** *Gross photograph shows septal myectomy specimens taken during transaortic surgery in a patient with hypertrophic cardiomyopathy. Marked endocardial thickening* → *can occasionally be seen in such specimens.*

Histologic Features of Hypertrophic Cardiomyopathy

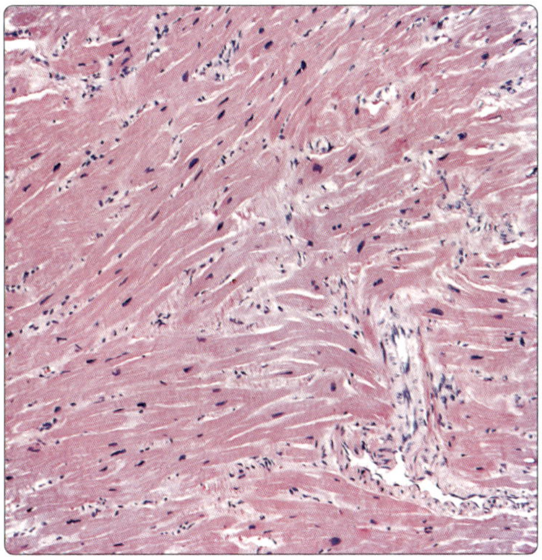

Histologic Features of Hypertrophic Cardiomyopathy

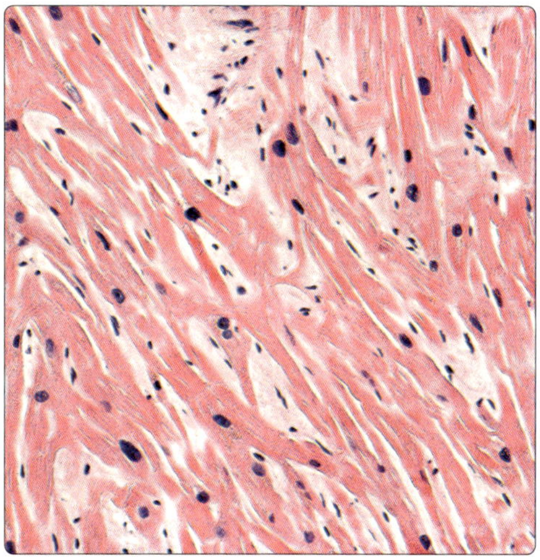

(Left) *H&E stain shows the usual type of myocyte architectural disarray with a seemingly random orientation of myocytes and myocyte bundles.* **(Right)** *Another pattern of myocyte disarray assumes a so-called herringbone pattern with alternating myocyte bundles intersecting at acute angles. This pattern can be more subtle, especially at lower magnification.*

Histologic Features of Hypertrophic Cardiomyopathy

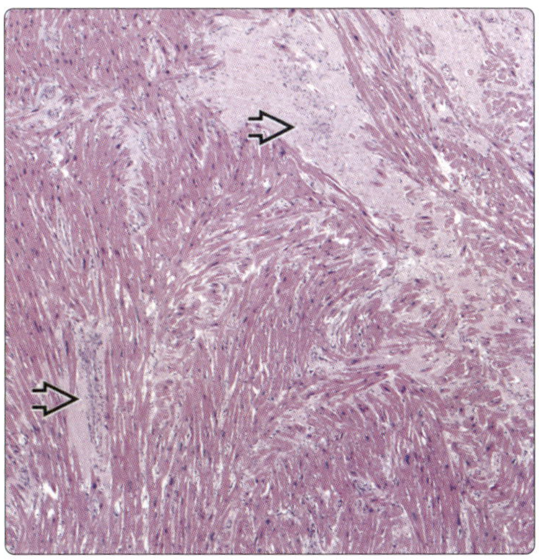

Histologic Features of Myocytes in Hypertrophic Cardiomyopathy

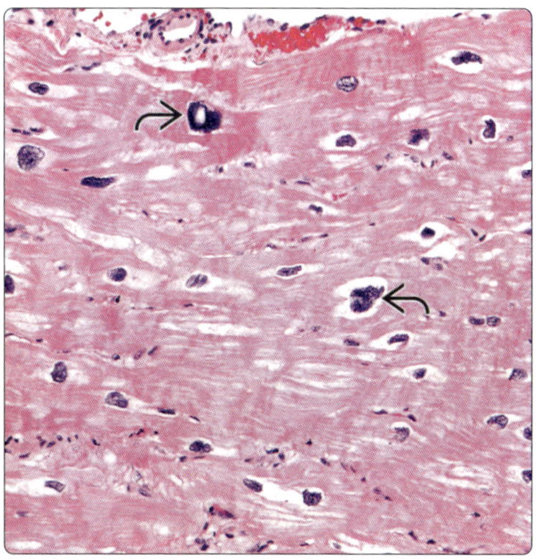

(Left) *Haphazard orientation of hypertrophic myocytes is present and characteristic of disarray. Patchy interstitial fibrosis is also seen focally surrounding coronary artery branches with thickened walls* ⇨. **(Right)** *H&E stain shows extreme individual myocyte hypertrophy with markedly hyperchromatic and bizarre myocyte nuclei* ↶.

Idiopathic Dilated Cardiomyopathy

KEY FACTS

TERMINOLOGY

- Progressive left ventricular dilatation and systolic (contractile) dysfunction in absence of other cardiac/coronary abnormalities, resulting in global systolic impairment

CLINICAL ISSUES

- All ages may be affected, but most common in middle-aged adults (4th/5th decades)
- M:F = 3:1
- Most common heart failure entity requiring heart transplantation

MACROSCOPIC

- Large and flabby appearance
- Markedly dilated chambers; ventricles > atria
- Ventricular wall thickness may be less than, equal to, or greater than normal
- Mural thrombi are common, particularly in ventricular apex
- Increase in weight up to 2-3x normal

MICROSCOPIC

- Severity of changes neither correlates with dysfunction nor with prognosis
- Myocyte changes
  - Hypertrophy (> 22 μ) and foci of myocyte attenuation
  - Vacuolization of myocyte cytoplasm/myofibrillar loss
- Interstitial, perivascular, replacement, and endocardial fibrosis of variable degree
- Nonspecific mononuclear inflammatory infiltrate
- Nonspecific thickening of pericapillary arterioles

TOP DIFFERENTIAL DIAGNOSES

- Ischemic cardiomyopathy
- Hereditary hemochromatosis
- Anthracycline toxicity

DCM: Long-Axis View

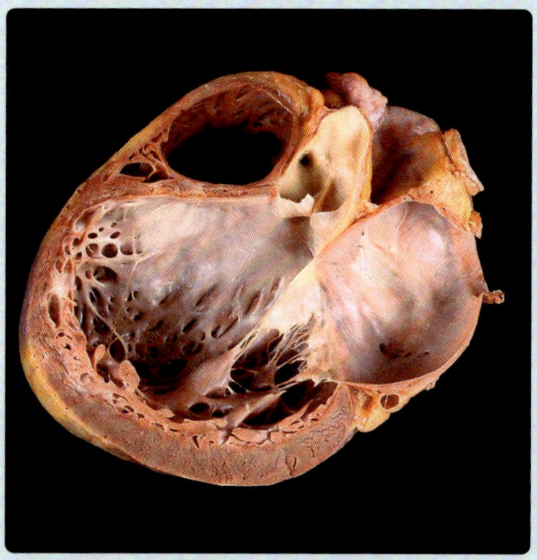

DCM: Short-Axis View

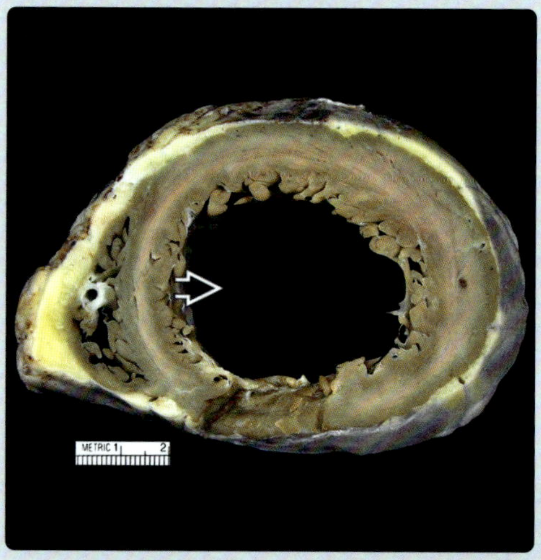

(Left) *Sagittally sectioned gross specimen shows marked dilatation of both atria and ventricles in a case of idiopathic dilated cardiomyopathy (DCM). Significant valvular disease is not evident.* **(Right)** *Gross heart autopsy specimen from a patient with idiopathic DCM shows marked dilatation of the left ventricle chamber ➡.*

Myocyte Hypertrophy and Interstitial Fibrosis: Trichrome Stain

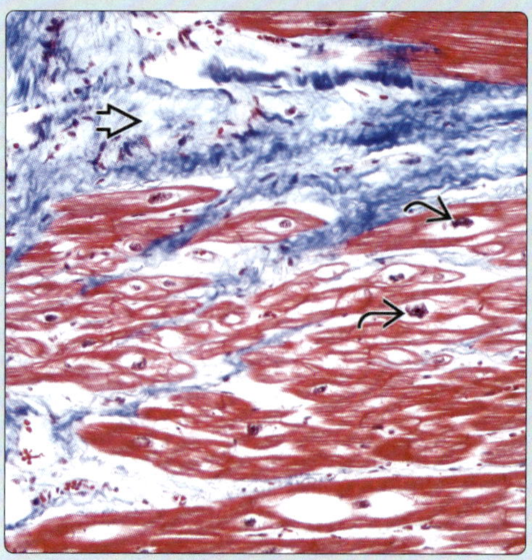

Idiopathic DCM: Postmortem Angiogram

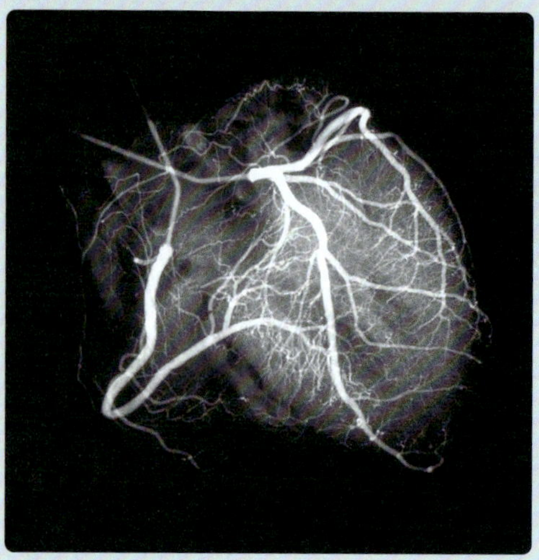

(Left) *While not specific, the main histologic abnormalities in idiopathic DCM are interstitial fibrosis ➡ and enlarged nuclei, indicating myocyte ↪ hypertrophy.* **(Right)** *Contrast injection into the coronary arteries demonstrates no stenotic lesions through the right and left circulation, ruling out ischemic cardiomyopathy.*

TERMINOLOGY

Abbreviations

- Dilated cardiomyopathy (DCM)

Synonyms

- Congestive cardiomyopathy

Definitions

- Progressive left ventricular dilatation and systolic (contractile) dysfunction in absence of other cardiac/coronary abnormalities, resulting in global systolic impairment
  - Right ventricular dilatation and dysfunction may also be present but are not necessary for diagnosis

ETIOLOGY/PATHOGENESIS

Environmental Exposure

- Alcohol-associated DCM
  - Ethanol or its metabolites (acetaldehyde) are toxic to myocardium
  - Secondary nutritional deficiencies induced by alcohol consumption
    - Thiamine deficiency (beriberi heart disease)
- Chemotherapeutic agents

Infectious Agents

- Viral agents (enterovirus, adenovirus, parvovirus B19, HHV-6)
  - Postviral myocardial infection initiates autoimmune reaction that leads to damage of myocardium
  - Antibody formation to sarcolemmal, mitochondrial heat-shock proteins, and surface receptors
- Parasitic infections (*Trypanosoma cruzi*)

Pregnancy-Associated Dilated Cardiomyopathy

- Multifactorial
  - Pregnancy-associated hypertension
  - Volume overload
  - Nutritional deficiency
  - Metabolic derangement
  - Immunologically mediated
  - ~ 29% carry deleterious cardiomyopathy gene variants

Familial

- 25-35% of DCM cases are familial
- Autosomal dominant in 90% of DCM cases
  - Abnormalities in genes coding for
    - α-actin
    - Desmin
    - Lamin A/C
    - Titin
    - Troponin T
- Autosomal recessive
  - Troponin I gene abnormalities
- X-linked and mitochondrial inheritance: 10%

Idiopathic

- When all secondary causes excluded
- Most cases of DCM fall in this category

CLINICAL ISSUES

Epidemiology

- Age
  - All ages may be affected, but most common in middle-aged adults (4th/5th decades)
- Sex
  - M:F = 3:1
- Ethnicity
  - Most common in Black males (3:1)
- Prevalence: 1:2,500
- Incidence: 5-8 cases/100,000 population/year
  - Most common heart failure entity requiring heart transplantation

Presentation

- Symptoms
  - Congestive heart failure, particularly left sided
  - Fatigue/weakness
  - Dyspnea, progressive
  - Systemic or pulmonary emboli
  - Chest pain, uncommon
- Signs
  - Right-sided heart failure: Peripheral edema, ascites, liver congestion
  - Presystolic gallops
  - Systolic murmurs due to mitral/tricuspid regurgitation
  - Arrhythmias and conduction abnormalities

Laboratory Tests

- Viral studies to rule out myocardial infection
- Endomyocardial biopsy
  - May be indicated to establish specific diagnosis of secondary causes of DCM
- Genetic testing
  - When familial cardiomyopathy is suspected
  - In young-onset (< 35 years) DCM or associated with high-risk features

Natural History

- Not well established
  - May present with minimal or no symptoms, and progression of disease is unclear, although long-term prognosis is not good
  - In symptomatic patients, course is usually progressive with 10-50% of patients with heart failure dying within 1 year in some series
  - More recently, estimated survival free from death or heart transplantation up to 85% at 10 years with appropriate therapies

Treatment

- Surgical approaches
  - Left ventricular assist devices are used when failure is refractory to clinical therapy &/or as bridge to heart transplant
  - Heart transplantation is indicated in end-stage heart failure
- Drugs
  - Standard therapy for heart failure
  - Antiarrhythmics
- Implantable devices

- Pacemaker
- Cardiac defibrillator

Prognosis

- Clinical predictors of higher risk for death include
  - Protodiastolic gallop
  - Ventricular arrhythmias
  - Advanced age
  - Failure to respond to inotropic stimulation
  - Greater ventricular enlargement and dysfunction correlate with poor prognosis, particularly if right ventricle is involved
  - Marked limitation of exercise capacity (reduced maximal systemic oxygen uptake below 10-12 mL/kg/min)

IMAGING

Radiographic Findings

- Chest x-rays
  - Moderate/marked cardiac enlargement
  - Pulmonary venous hypertension

Ultrasonographic Findings

- Global hypokinesis
- Left ventricular dilatation and dysfunction
- Abnormal diastolic mitral valve motion
- Ejection fraction < 50%
- Fractional shortening < 25-30%

MR Findings

- Useful to assess ventricular volumes, ejection fraction, and degree of cardiac fibrosis
- Late gadolinium enhancement in midwall distribution is finding frequently seen and has prognostic value being strong predictor for cardiovascular events, particularly arrhythmias

MACROSCOPIC

General Features

- Large and flabby appearance
- Markedly dilated chambers; ventricles > atria
- Left ventricle chamber measures > 4 cm in transverse section at level of papillary muscles
- Ventricular wall thickness may be less than, equal to, or greater than normal
- Mural thrombi are common, particularly in ventricular apex
- Mitral and tricuspid valves with changes of regurgitation
- Coronaries with no abnormalities or minor changes insufficient to explain myocardial abnormalities

Size

- Increase in weight up to 2-3x normal
- May exceed 1,000 g (cor bovinum)

MICROSCOPIC

Histologic Features

- Nonspecific changes without indication of specific etiology
- Severity of changes neither correlates with dysfunction nor with prognosis
  - Myocytes
    - Hypertrophy (> 22 μ) and foci of myocyte attenuation
    - Vacuolization of myocyte cytoplasm/myofibrillar loss
  - Interstitial, perivascular, replacement, and endocardial fibrosis of variable degree
    - Fibrosis increases from epicardium toward endocardium
    - More noticeable on left side of left ventricular septum
    - Irregular subendocardial scars
  - Nonspecific mild mononuclear inflammatory infiltrate
  - Nonspecific thickening of pericapillary arterioles

ANCILLARY TESTS

Electron Microscopy

- Increase in myocyte diameter
- Increase in nuclear size, Golgi complex, mitochondria, glycogen, and ribosomes
- Degenerative changes: Increase lipid droplets, lysosomes, lipofuscin, and T-tubule dilatation
- Myofibrillar loss

DIFFERENTIAL DIAGNOSIS

Ischemic Cardiomyopathy

- > 75% cross-sectional luminal narrowing of at least 1 coronary artery must be present, which explains myocardial changes and clinical presentation

Hereditary Hemochromatosis

- Usually restrictive physiology pattern
- Iron stain is positive

Anthracycline Toxicity

- History of treatment with anthracyclines
- Electron microscopy findings of extensive myocyte cytoplasm vacuolization

DIAGNOSTIC CHECKLIST

Pathologic Interpretation Pearls

- Diagnosis of idiopathic DCM should be restricted to cases of global cardiac dilatation in absence of significant coronary, valvular, cor pulmonale, and congenital heart disease
  - Clinical history of hypertensive disease should be ruled out

SELECTED REFERENCES

1. Cojan-Minzat BO et al: Non-ischemic dilated cardiomyopathy and cardiac fibrosis. Heart Fail Rev. 26(5):1081-101, 2021
2. Davis MB et al: Peripartum cardiomyopathy: JACC state-of-the-art review. J Am Coll Cardiol. 75(2):207-21, 2020
3. Hänselmann A et al: Dilated cardiomyopathies and non-compaction cardiomyopathy. Herz. 45(3):212-20, 2020
4. Imanaka-Yoshida K: Inflammation in myocardial disease: from myocarditis to dilated cardiomyopathy. Pathol Int. 70(1):1-11, 2020
5. Marrow BA et al: Emerging techniques for risk stratification in nonischemic dilated cardiomyopathy: JACC review topic of the week. J Am Coll Cardiol. 75(10):1196-207, 2020
6. Peters S et al: Familial dilated cardiomyopathy. Heart Lung Circ. 29(4):566-74, 2020
7. Saito T et al: Long-term prognostic value of ultrastructural features in dilated cardiomyopathy: comparison with cardiac magnetic resonance. ESC Heart Fail. 7(2):682-91, 2020
8. Donal E et al: Multimodality imaging in the diagnosis, risk stratification, and management of patients with dilated cardiomyopathies: an expert consensus document from the European Association of Cardiovascular Imaging. Eur Heart J Cardiovasc Imaging. 20(10):1075-93, 2019

Idiopathic DCM: Chamber Dilatation and Focal Fatty Replacement

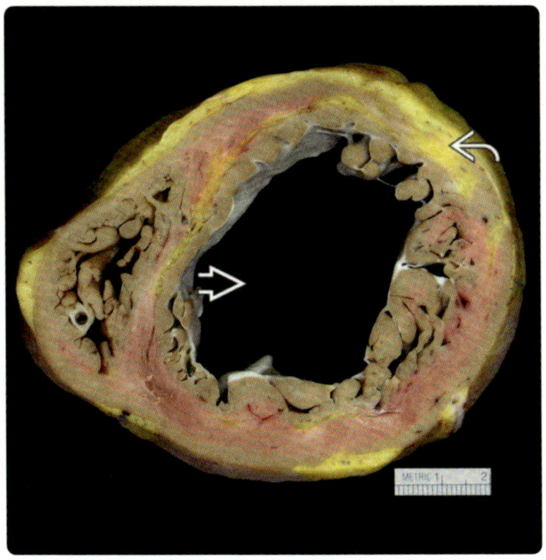

Ischemic Cardiomyopathy: Short-Axis View

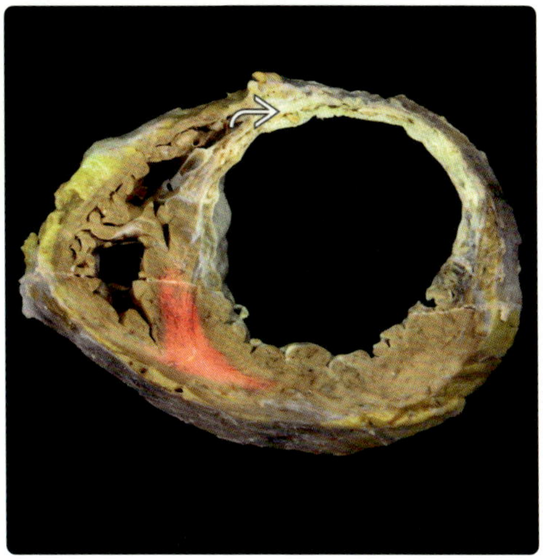

(Left) *Gross autopsy specimen shows DCM (chamber dilatation > 5 cm ⇨). The wall is of normal thickness with focal scar and fatty replacement ⇨ (but not arrhythmogenic cardiomyopathy). There is no obvious infarct.* **(Right)** *Marked left ventricular dilatation is also seen in advanced ischemic cardiomyopathy. However, in these cases, there is also evidence of prior infarct ⇨ causing the ventricle changes. Compensatory hypertrophy of noninfarcted myocardium may also occur.*

Idiopathic DCM: Short-Axis View

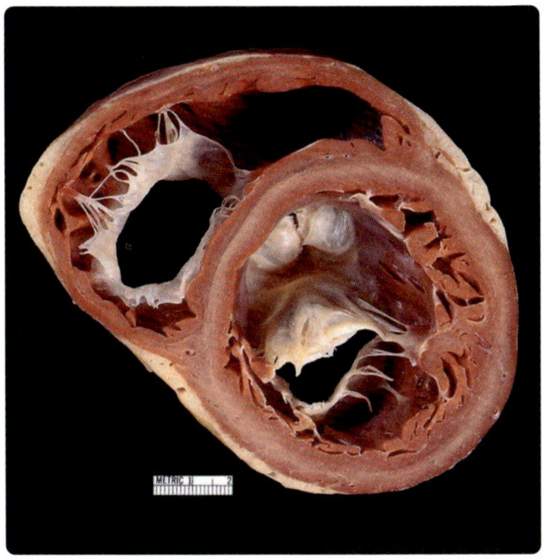

DCM: Myocyte Hypertrophy

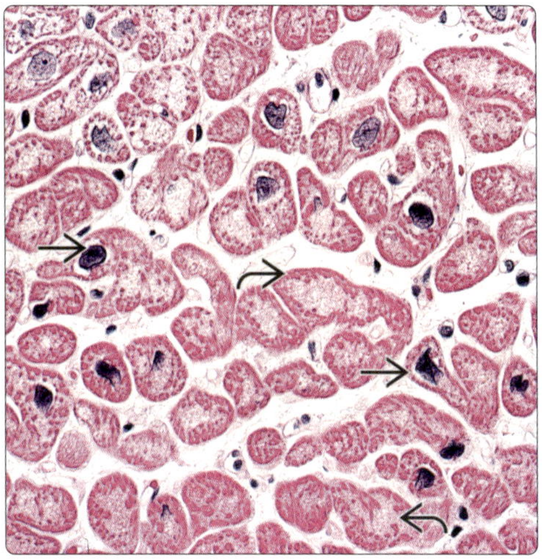

(Left) *Gross specimen shows biventricular chamber dilatation and thinning of ventricle walls, most evident in the right ventricle. Valvular abnormalities are not identified, except for secondary anulus dilatation. Regurgitation is a common complication in advanced cases of DCM.* **(Right)** *H&E of the myocardium shows myocyte hypertrophy with enlarged myocytes ⇨ with irregular nuclei →. Myocyte hypertrophy is frequently seen in DCM, although it is a nonspecific finding.*

DCM: Interstitial Fibrosis

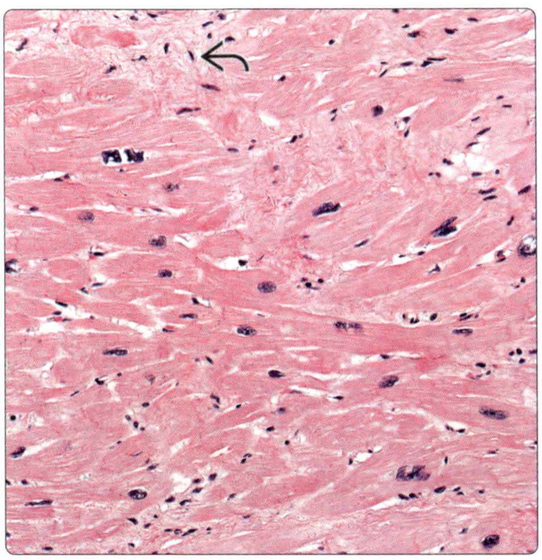

DCM: Replacement-Type Fibrosis

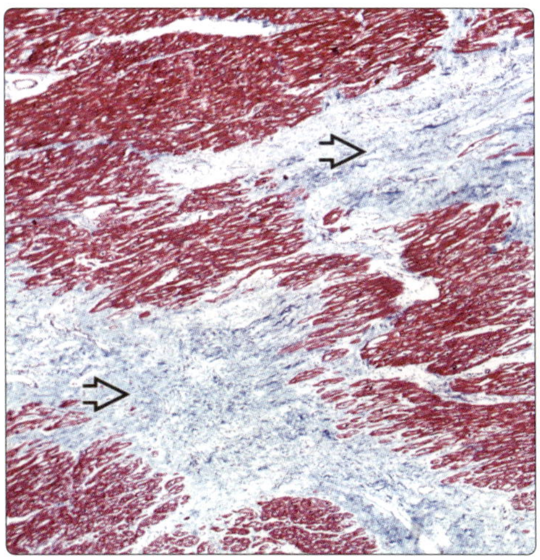

(Left) *H&E of the myocardium shows longitudinally oriented myocytes with enlarged irregular nuclei. Focal interstitial fibrosis ⇨ is also seen, although it is a nonspecific finding.* **(Right)** *Trichrome stain highlights extreme interstitial fibrosis ⇨ in a replacement-type pattern. The pattern raises the question of healed myocarditis in cases such as this.*

Ischemic Heart Disease

KEY FACTS

TERMINOLOGY

- Irreversible myocardial damage caused by prolonged ischemia, resulting from sustained imbalance of perfusion, supply, and demand

CLINICAL ISSUES

- Complications
  - Rupture of myocardium (tamponade, acquired ventricular septal defect, ruptured papillary muscle)
- Longer term
  - Ischemic dilated cardiomyopathy
  - Ventricular true aneurysms (often with mural thrombus)
- Median 30-day mortality: 16.6%
- Median 30-day readmission: 19.9%
- Treatment
  - Coronary artery bypass grafting
  - Percutaneous coronary intervention
  - Sublingual nitroglycerin
  - Thrombolytic agents (effective only in 1st hours after acute coronary thrombosis)

MACROSCOPIC

- 12-24 hours: Dark myocardial mottling
- 7-10 days: Grossly softened and depressed with more prominent hyperemic edges
- 3-8 weeks: Grayish white scar begins to form at edges and progresses to center

MICROSCOPIC

- 1-3 days: Coagulative necrosis with loss of nuclei, contraction bands, and heavy neutrophilic infiltration
- 3-7 days: Myocyte loss, karyorrhexis of neutrophils ("nuclear dust"), early phagocytosis by macrophages at infarct border
- 10-14 days: Well-established granulation tissue with new blood vessels and fibroblast infiltration
- 2-8 weeks: Increased collagen deposition with decreased cellularity

Transmural Acute Myocardial Infarction (5-7 Days)

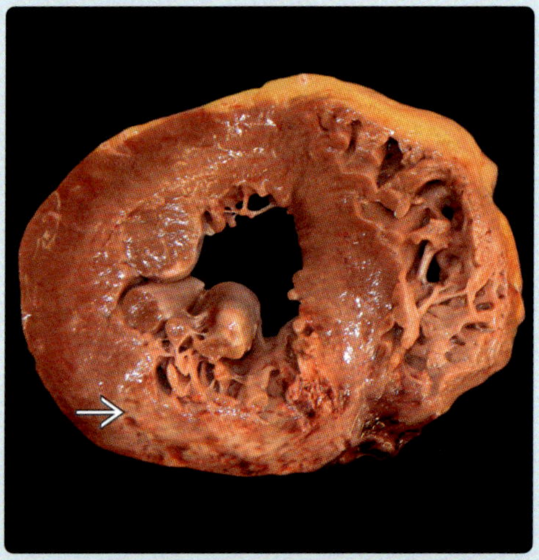

Acute Coronary Occlusion by Atherothrombosis

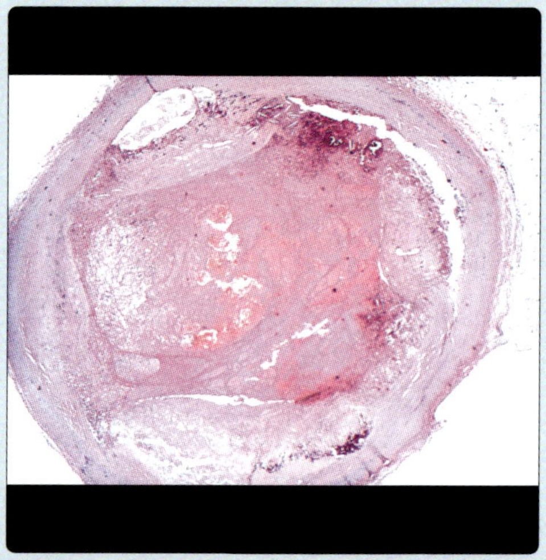

(Left) *Gross photograph shows acute transmural myocardial infarction ➔ involving the posterior/inferior wall of the left ventricle. There is a yellow necrotic area surrounded by a hyperemic border, typical of a 2- to 4-day-old infarct.* **(Right)** *H&E-stained section shows a coronary artery with recent thrombus occluding the lumen.*

Subendocardial Global Acute Myocardial Infarction

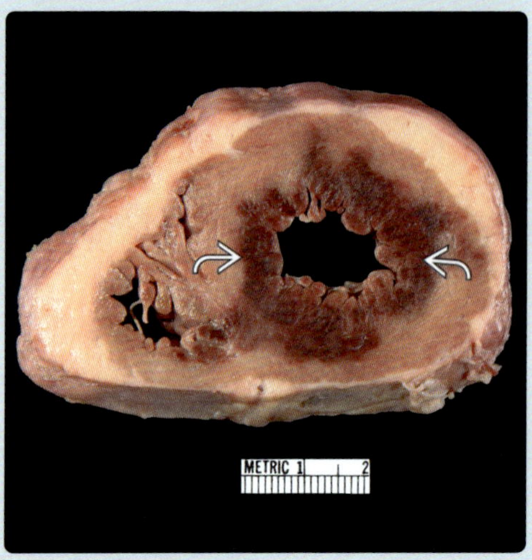

Contraction Bands in Acute Myocardial Infarction

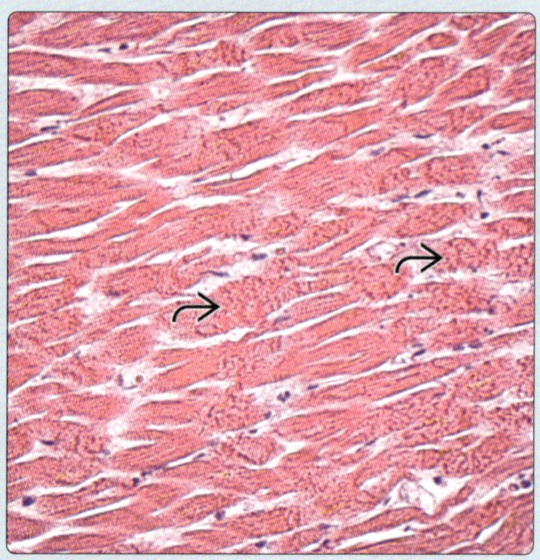

(Left) *There is circumferential mottling/hyperemia ➔ extending less than halfway into the myocardial wall. Since this pattern crosses all the coronary territories, it is most likely due to shock and global hypoperfusion.* **(Right)** *Sarcoplasmic contraction bands ➔ can be seen as one of the first changes in myocardial infarction. This is an irreversible change heralding myocyte cell death.*

TERMINOLOGY

Synonyms

- Myocardial ischemia, myocardial infarction

Definitions

- Myocardial infarction can be defined as irreversible myocardial muscle fiber damage caused by prolonged ischemia, resulting from sustained imbalance of perfusion, supply, and demand

ETIOLOGY/PATHOGENESIS

Coronary Artery Atherosclerosis

- Risk factors
  - Smoking
  - Hypertension
  - Elevated low-density lipoprotein cholesterol
  - Diabetes mellitus
  - Increasing age
  - Obesity
- Mechanism of coronary artery occlusion: Thrombosis of eroded or ulcerated atherosclerotic plaque
- Myocardial infarction with nonobstructive coronary arteries (MINOCA)

Nonatherosclerotic Coronary Disease

- Coronary artery vasculitis
- Coronary artery dissection
- Coronary artery spasm
- Coronary artery embolus (such as from endocarditis)

Other Causes of Mismatched Perfusion-Myocardial Demand

- Left ventricular hypertrophy (cardiomyopathy, hypertensive heart disease)
- Congenital heart disease
- Cardiac arrest (metabolic, neurogenic, arrhythmia)
- Impaired oxygen delivery (respiratory failure, severe anemia)

CLINICAL ISSUES

Epidemiology

- Incidence
  - Annual incidence of ischemic heart disease (acute coronary syndrome) has been estimated at 610,000
  - Recurrent myocardial infarction accounts for 325,000 episodes
- Age
  - Average: 64.5 years for men and 70.3 years for women
- Sex
  - M > F
  - Women thought to be "protected" in their reproductive years
- Ethnicity
  - Prevalence is highest in developed nations, presumably due to comparatively high-calorie diet, more sedentary lifestyle, and longer life expectancy
  - Significant variation in incidence across developed nations with rates (per 100,000), such as
    - 30 in Japan
    - 39.8 in France
    - 65.2 in Italy
    - 94.9 in Canada
    - 106.5 in United States
    - 216 in Slovakia

Presentation

- Cardiac arrest without recognized antecedent symptoms
- Typical symptoms
  - Chest pain (angina) on exertion or rest
  - Mandibular, upper arm, or epigastric discomfort; usually lasts > 20 minutes
  - Associated nausea, diaphoresis, syncope
- No symptoms
  - In older, female, diabetic, postoperative, and critically ill patients

Treatment

- Surgical approaches
  - Percutaneous coronary intervention (PCI) considered superior over fibrinolysis
    - Usually reserved for acute ST elevation myocardial infarction (salvageable myocardium)
    - Balloon angioplasty with coronary artery stenting with drug-eluting stents
  - Coronary artery bypass grafting
- Drugs
  - Sublingual nitroglycerin
  - Antiplatelet therapy (aspirin, clopidogrel)
  - Morphine for pain relief
  - Thrombolytic agents (effective only in 1st hours after acute coronary thrombosis)
    - 1st generation: Streptokinase, urokinase, acetylated plasminogen streptokinase activator complex
    - 2nd generation: tPA, tenecteplase

Prognosis

- Median 30-day mortality: 16.6%
- Median 30-day readmission: 19.9%
- Complications
  - Acute
    - Cardiogenic shock
    - Rupture of myocardium (tamponade, acquired ventricular septal defect, ruptured papillary muscle)
    - Ventricular pseudoaneurysm (contained rupture)
    - Arrhythmias
    - Pericarditis (Dressler syndrome)
  - Longer term
    - Congestive heart failure
    - Ischemic dilated cardiomyopathy
    - Ventricular true aneurysms (often with mural thrombus)
    - Mitral regurgitation (scar retraction of papillary muscle)
    - Recurrent ventricular arrhythmias
- Risk of 2nd myocardial infarction

IMAGING

Echocardiography

- Assesses myocardial thickness and motion

- Assesses myocardial perfusion and microvascular obstruction (coronary flow reserve)

Radionucleotide Imaging

- Commonly available to assess viability

Magnetic Resonance Imaging

- Accurate assessment of myocardial function and motion and perfusion (with contrast)

Coronary Angiography

- Assesses degree of obstruction/thrombosis and guides PCI

Intravascular Ultrasound/Intracoronary Optical Coherence Tomography

- New imaging technologies with higher sensitivity to identify atherosclerotic plaque abnormalities and burden

MACROSCOPIC

General Features

- In initial few minutes to hours (up to 8-12 hours), there is no grossly apparent abnormality
- Thereafter
  - 12-24 hours: Dark myocardial mottling
  - 1-3 days: Mottling with yellow-tan center
  - 3-7 days: Yellow-tan center with hyperemic edges
  - 7-10 days: Grossly softened and depressed with more prominent hyperemic edges
  - 10-14 days: Edges become more gray in color
  - 3-8 weeks: Grayish white scar begins to form at edges and progresses to center
  - 8-12 weeks: Grayish white scar with early remodeling (wall thinning and chamber dilatation)

Hemorrhagic Infarct

- After revascularization (durable or failed), restoration of blood flow to damaged tissue may result in hemorrhagic infarction
  - Dark red-brown in color due to hemorrhage into ischemic tissues

Vital Staining of Fresh Heart Tissue (Autopsy)

- Triphenyltetrazolium chloride (TTC) or nitro blue tetrazolium (NBT) dye test
  - Redox indicator catalyzed by dehydrogenase enzymes in viable myocardium (but not infarcted myocardium)
  - TTC will stain viable myocardium brick red (infarcted myocardium will remain unchanged)
  - NBT will stain viable myocardium dark blue-purple (infarcted myocardium will remain unchanged)

MICROSCOPIC

Histologic Features

- After 4 hours (variable), myocytes may appear wavy and elongated; interstitial edema
- Within 24 hours, interstitial edema, focal hemorrhage, myocyte contraction bands, and infiltration of neutrophils (margination)
  - Staining for C4d may be positive in acutely ischemic myocytes due to complement activation
- 1-3 days: Coagulative necrosis with loss of nuclei, contraction bands, and heavy neutrophilic infiltration
- 3-7 days: Myocyte loss, karyorrhexis of neutrophils ("nuclear dust"), early phagocytosis by macrophages at infarct border
- 7-10 days: Well-developed phagocytosis with distended macrophages, granulation tissue at infarct border
- 10-14 days: Well-established granulation tissue with new blood vessels and fibroblast infiltration
- 2-8 weeks: Increased collagen deposition with decreased cellularity
- > 2 months: Dense collagenous scar
- Reperfusion injury (after revascularization)
  - Prominent coagulative necrosis
  - Marked erythrocyte extravasation/hemorrhage
  - Small vessels may show small thrombi or atheroemboli

ANCILLARY TESTS

Immunohistochemistry

- C4d, C9: Positive staining in necrotic myocardium
- cTnT: Negative staining in necrotic myocardium

Electron Microscopy

- Sarcolemmal disruption
- Mitochondrial swelling, mitochondrial amorphous densities
- Relaxation of myofibrils
- Glycogen loss

DIFFERENTIAL DIAGNOSIS

Chest Pain

- Clinically, can be due to
  - Acute aortic dissection
  - Pericarditis
  - Gastrointestinal disorders (reflux, cholecystitis, gastritis)
  - Pneumonia
  - Pulmonary embolism
  - Pneumothorax

SELECTED REFERENCES

1. Kunkel KJ et al: 2021 update for the diagnosis and management of acute coronary syndromes for the perioperative clinician. J Cardiothorac Vasc Anesth. 36(8 Pt A):2767-79, 2022
2. Rallidis LS et al: Causes, angiographic characteristics, and management of premature myocardial infarction: JACC state-of-the-art review. J Am Coll Cardiol. 79(24):2431-49, 2022
3. Beijnink CWH et al: Cardiac MRI to visualize myocardial damage after ST-segment elevation myocardial infarction: a review of its histologic validation. Radiology. 301(1):4-18, 2021
4. Damluji AA et al: Mechanical complications of acute myocardial infarction: a scientific statement from the American Heart Association. Circulation. 144(2):e16-35, 2021
5. Kolte D et al: New insights into plaque erosion as a mechanism of acute coronary syndromes. JAMA. 325(11):1043-4, 2021
6. Mæhle BO et al: Acute and healed myocardial infarctions as cause of sudden death: age and sex differences. J Am Coll Cardiol. 77(6):826-7, 2021
7. Thygesen K et al: Fourth universal definition of myocardial infarction (2018). Circulation. 138(20):e618-51, 2018
8. Chang J et al: Pathology of myocardial infarction. Diagnostic Histopathology. 19(1):7-12, 2013
9. Jenkins CP et al: The utility of C4d, C9, and troponin T immunohistochemistry in acute myocardial infarction. Arch Pathol Lab Med. 134(2):256-63, 2010
10. Antman EM et al: ST-elevation myocardial infarction: pathology, pathophysiology, and clinical features. In Libby P et al: Braunwald's Heart Disease: A Textbook of Cardiovascular Medicine. Saunders Elsevier. 1207-32, 2008
11. Pasotti M et al: The pathology of myocardial infarction in the pre- and post-interventional era. Heart. 92(11):1552-6, 2006

Coronary Thrombosis

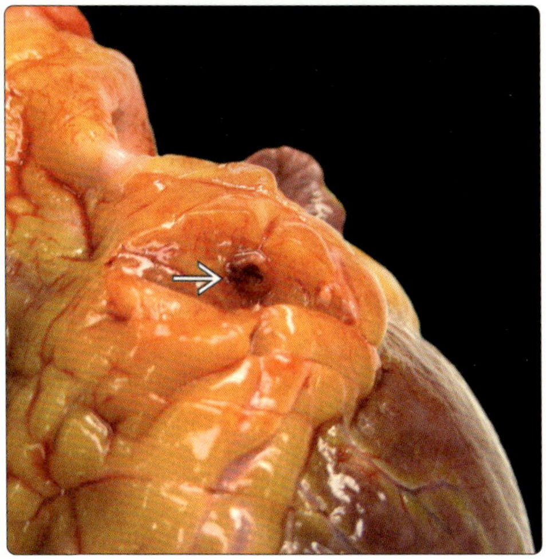

Mural Thrombus in Remodeled Infarction

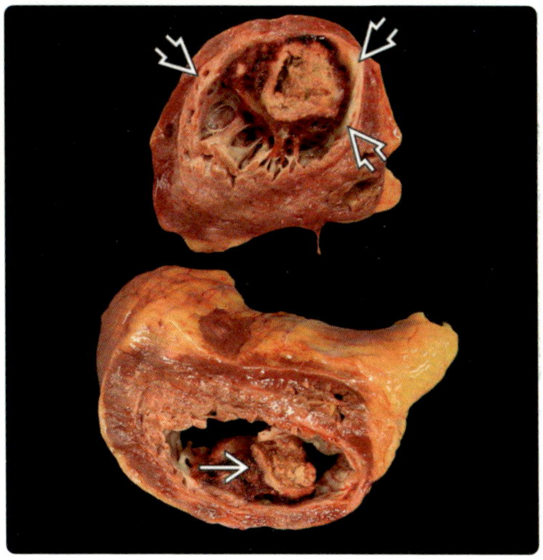

(Left) *Left anterior descending artery shows recent thrombus* ➡ *occluding the lumen. This artery supplies the anterolateral wall of the left ventricle.* **(Right)** *Gross photograph shows an aneurysm* ➡ *involving the apex of the left ventricle. The aneurysms are seen more frequently in healed transmural infarct than subendocardial infarct. A thrombus* ➡ *is seen in the cavity of the aneurysm. (Courtesy J. Fernandes, MD.)*

Early Histologic Changes in Acute Myocardial Infarction

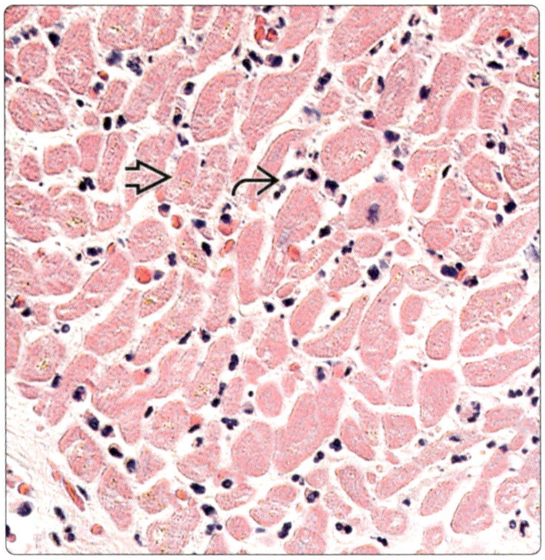

Early Histologic Changes in Acute Myocardial Infarction

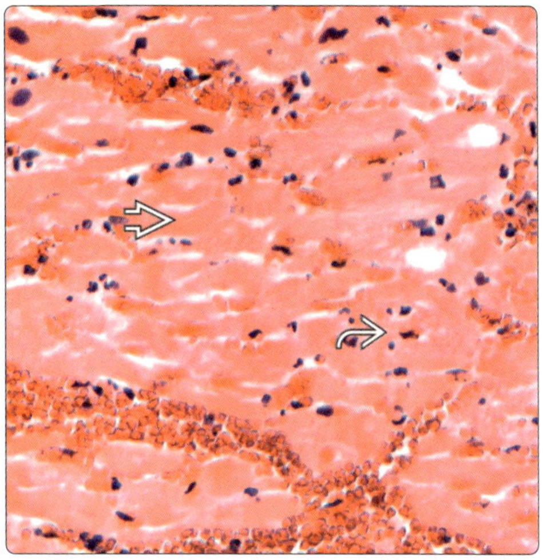

(Left) *Acute myocardial infarction that is 24-48 hours old shows hypereosinophilic myocytes* ➡ *and acute inflammatory infiltrate* ➡*.* **(Right)** *Acute reperfusion infarct shows hypereosinophilic myocytes* ➡*, hemorrhage, and neutrophilic apoptosis* ➡*. Reperfusion infarcts are usually hemorrhagic and can be extensive.*

Subacute Histologic Changes in Acute Myocardial Infarction

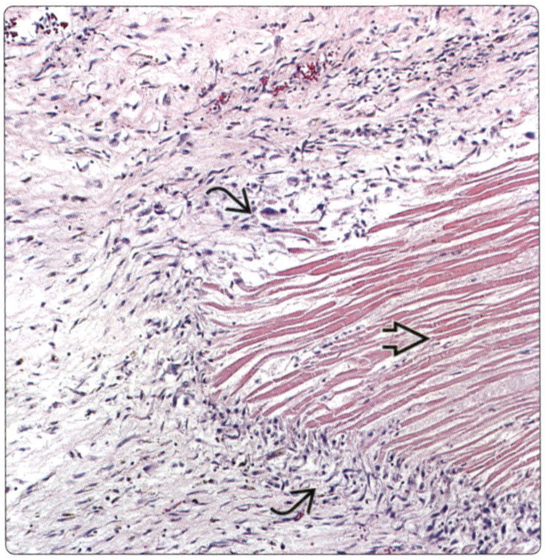

Late Histologic Changes in Myocardial Infarction

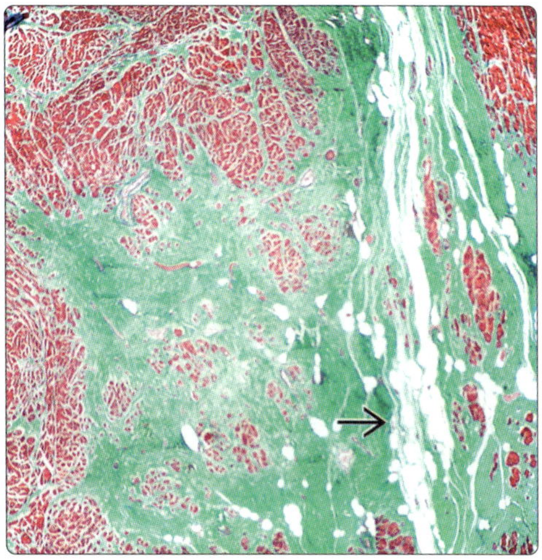

(Left) *Healing infarct that is 2 weeks old shows necrotic myocytes* ➡ *in the center surrounded by granulation tissue* ➡ *composed of fibroblasts, chronic inflammation, and neocapillaries.* **(Right)** *Masson trichrome stain shows a well-healed transmural infarct. There is dense fibrosis* ➡ *with focal fatty infiltration.*

TERMINOLOGY

Definitions

- Prosthetic intraluminal tubular metal scaffold device
- Designed to maintain lumen patency in setting of underlying intrinsic or extrinsic coronary artery narrowing
- Deployed by inflation of balloon-tipped endovascular catheter
  - Balloon inflation disrupts vessel wall plaque and expands lumen
  - Stent holds lumen open
- Self-expanding stents in development
- Different metal alloys used
  - Surgical grade stainless steel
  - Cobalt chromium
  - Platinum chromium
  - Nickel titanium (nitinol)
- "Bare metal" or coated with drug-eluting polymers to inhibit neointimal growth
  - Cypher (sirolimus)
  - Taxus (paclitaxel)
  - Xience V (everolimus)

CLINICAL IMPLICATIONS

Indications

- Primary therapy for coronary atherosclerosis
- Revascularization therapy in acute myocardial infarction
- Bailout procedure for abrupt or threatened artery closure due to arterial dissection or following angioplasty

Complications

- Reocclusion/restenosis of stented coronary artery segments (in-stent restenosis) occurs in 5-30% of cases
  - Early restenosis usually results from acute thrombosis
  - Late restenosis results from concentric neointimal growth or thrombosis
- Chronic total stent occlusion (at autopsy)
  - 6% for drug-eluting stents
  - 12% for bare metal stents

SPECIMEN HANDLING AND EVALUATION

Gross Specimen Evaluation

- Specimen radiographs should be used to delineate stents within cardiovascular specimens
- Radiographs are important to assess stent expansion and determine whether stent was abnormally compressed during deployment
- Total stented length and curvature should be documented since these correlate with risk of restenosis

Special Handling Required for Examination

- Evaluation for restenosis in specimens submitted for pathology is difficult because metallic stents cannot be cut by conventional methods (scissors, scalpels, or conventional microtome blades)
  - Disruption of normal histoarchitecture (especially stent-tissue interface) will occur if conventional methods are used
- Avoid attempts to cut through stents with scissors or scalpel
- Trim stented vessel by cutting proximal and distal to stent
- Fix stented segment in formalin prior to special handling

Methods of Stent Sectioning for Microscopy

- Plastic resin embedding and diamond or tungsten carbide blade microtomy
  - Stented vessel tissue fixed and embedded in rigid methacrylate resin (as used in transmission electron microscopy)
  - Cut using conventional microtome equipped with special blade hard enough to cut metal stents
- Diamond saw microtome
  - Stented vessel tissue fixed and embedded in plastic and cut with high-speed diamond saw with precision movement capable of cutting ~ 10-μm sections (as used in undecalcified bone mineral density samples)
- Sawing and grinding
  - Stented vessel tissue fixed and embedded in plastic then subject to 2-stage process of sawing into ~ 100-μm sections that are mounted with adhesive to glass slide

Arterial Ballooning and Stenting

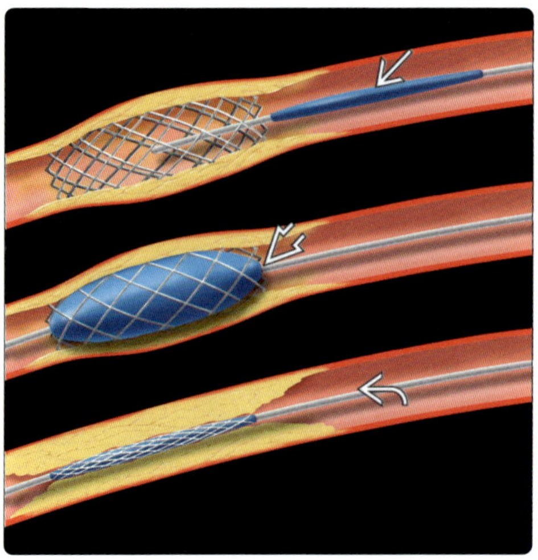

Chronically Occluded Stent

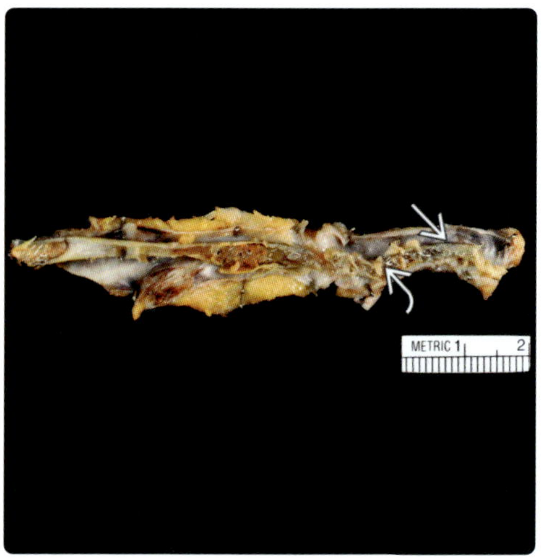

(Left) *Graphic shows a deployed stent within an atherosclerotic vessel ➡, balloon inflation with dilatation of the stenotic segment ➡, and retrieval of the catheter after stent placement ➡.* **(Right)** *Gross photograph of multiple stents in a coronary artery dissected from an explant heart shows exposed stent struts ➡ and struts enveloped in neointimal tissue ➡. This method of stent examination is not advised.*

- Slide is then placed in sanding/grinding device that progressively erodes thick section down to < 10-μm thickness
- Reverse electroplating
  - Prior to embedding, fixed stented vessel is placed in acid-salt solution, and electrodes are connected to stent metal
  - Current is applied in such a way that stent metal dissolves by electrolysis
  - Vessel can then be sectioned with scalpel and submitted for routine paraffin sectioning
- Acid dissolution
  - 3 N nitric acid and 12.8 N hydrofluoric acid
  - 28°C with mild shaking for 5 hours
  - Effective for all alloys except cobalt chromium
  - May affect antigen and nucleic acid stability for special studies
- Rotary tool micro-cutoff wheel
  - Rapid and inexpensive method
  - Freeze embedding in optimal cutting temperature (OCT) compound within wide plastic straw segment
  - Sectioning frozen block using rotary tool (e.g., Dremel) fitted with micro-cutoff wheel (1-mm thickness)
  - Thawing sections and removing stent shards under dissecting microscope
  - Submitting sections for routing paraffin embedding and histology

REPORTING CRITERIA

Required

- Stented artery segments should be examined in cross section using special methodologies
  - Evaluation of stented artery segments should include
    - Assessment of native vessel disease
    - Assessment of any neointimal growth within stent
    - Relationship of struts to vessel wall (well apposed, embedded/coated, or free in lumen)
- Artery sections immediately distal and proximal to stent should also be submitted and reviewed
- Estimated cross-sectional area stenosis as well as plaque composition (fibrous, calcific, smooth muscle, lipid, necrosis, etc.) should be reported
- Quantification of native vessel plaque and in-stent neointimal growth should be reported

PATHOLOGIC RESPONSES

Items to Consider

- Histologic findings after stenting are directly related to duration of stent implantation
- Features implicated in precipitation of stent thrombosis include
  - Malapposition of struts relative to vessel wall
  - Active inflammation around struts (especially eosinophils)
  - Fibrin surrounding struts
- Elastic lamina disruption, consequence of balloon inflation, is common and does not indicate vasculitis

Early Complications

- Rupture of thin-cap atheromas induced by balloon inflation can lead to atherothrombosis or atheroemboli
- Lipid core penetration by struts is associated with increased acute/chronic inflammation and neointimal growth
- Fibrin and platelet aggregation is seen commonly around struts during 1st week

Late Complications

- Smooth muscle-rich neointimal proliferation may significantly occlude lumen
- Late stent thrombosis is usually associated with malapposed struts or delayed incorporation
- Multinucleated giant cells around struts are more common after 30 days
  - Their contribution to neointimal growth is uncertain

SELECTED REFERENCES

1. Miller DV et al: A novel, rapid, and low cost method for preparing tissues with metallic stents for routine histology. Cardiovasc Pathol. 45:107177, 2020
2. Mori H et al: Pathology of chronic total occlusion in bare-metal versus drug-eluting stents: implications for revascularization. JACC Cardiovasc Interv. 10(4):367-78, 2017
3. Fishbein I et al: Paraffin processing of stented arteries using a postfixation dissolution of metallic and polymeric stents. Cardiovasc Pathol. 25(6):483-8, 2016
4. Stone JR et al: Recommendations for processing cardiovascular surgical pathology specimens: a consensus statement from the Standards and Definitions Committee of the Society for Cardiovascular Pathology and the Association for European Cardiovascular Pathology. Cardiovasc Pathol. 21(1):2-16, 2012
5. Nakazawa G et al: The pathology of neoatherosclerosis in human coronary implants bare-metal and drug-eluting stents. J Am Coll Cardiol. 57(11):1314-22, 2011
6. Bradshaw SH et al: A practical method to rapidly dissolve metallic stents. Cardiovasc Pathol. 18(3):127-33, 2009
7. Nakazawa G et al: A review of current devices and a look at new technology: drug-eluting stents. Expert Rev Med Devices. 6(1):33-42, 2009
8. Lüscher TF et al: Drug-eluting stent and coronary thrombosis: biological mechanisms and clinical implications. Circulation. 115(8):1051-8, 2007
9. Rippstein P et al: Comparison of processing and sectioning methodologies for arteries containing metallic stents. J Histochem Cytochem. 54(6):673-81, 2006
10. Farb A et al: Morphological predictors of restenosis after coronary stenting in humans. Circulation. 105(25):2974-80, 2002

(Left) *Plastic-embedded cross section of a stented coronary artery from an experimental model (without atherosclerosis) demonstrates proper apposition of stent struts to the vessel wall, causing some indentation and polygonal distortion of the circular lumen.* **(Right)** *Elastic-stained section of a stented coronary artery from an experimental model highlights a small dissection in the vessel resulting from balloon inflation during stent deployment. This is a recognized acute complication of the procedure.*

Plastic Resin-Embedded Stented Artery (H&E)

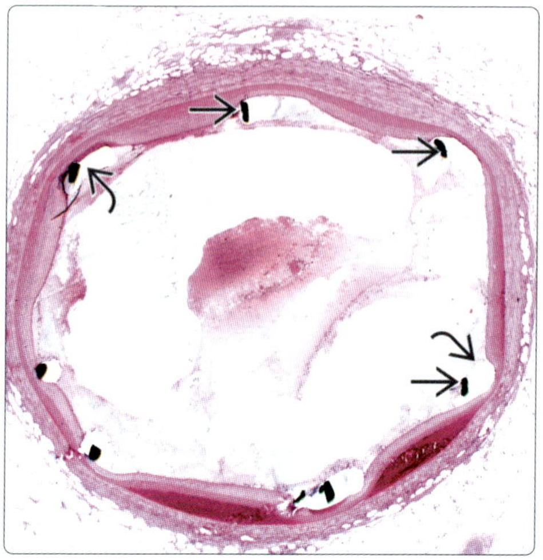

Plastic Resin-Embedded Stented Artery

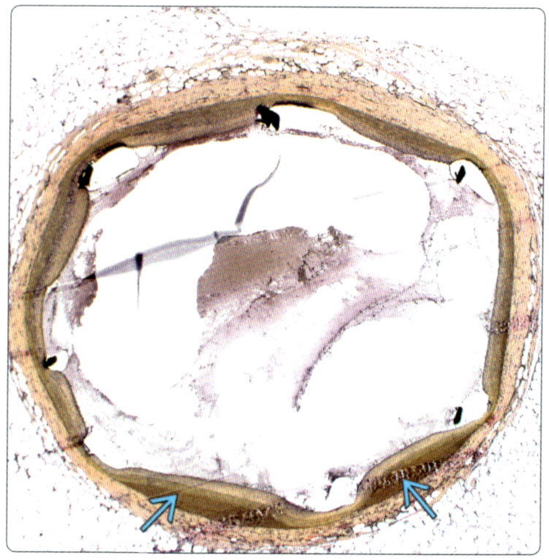

(Left) *Plastic-embedded cross section of a previously atherosclerotic (plaque) coronary artery is shown. There has been little to no neointimal formation, suggesting that the stent was placed very recently. The stent struts are well apposed to the wall.* **(Right)** *Elastic-stained plastic section of a stented coronary artery highlights the intimal localization of atherosclerosis and the absence of neointima formation.*

Stent Struts (Plastic Resin-Embedded Stented Artery)

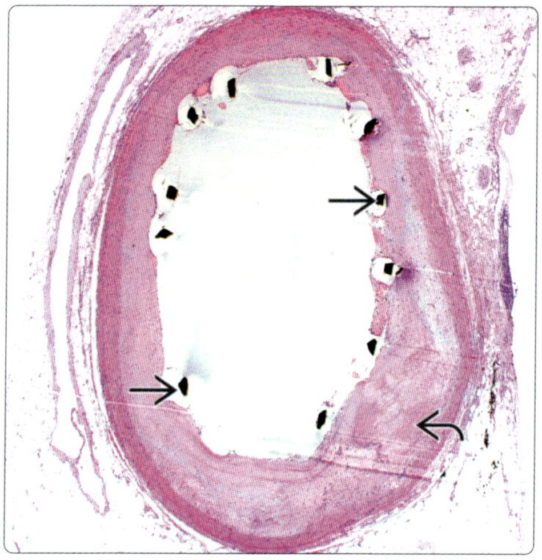

Stent Struts (Plastic Resin-Embedded Stented Artery)

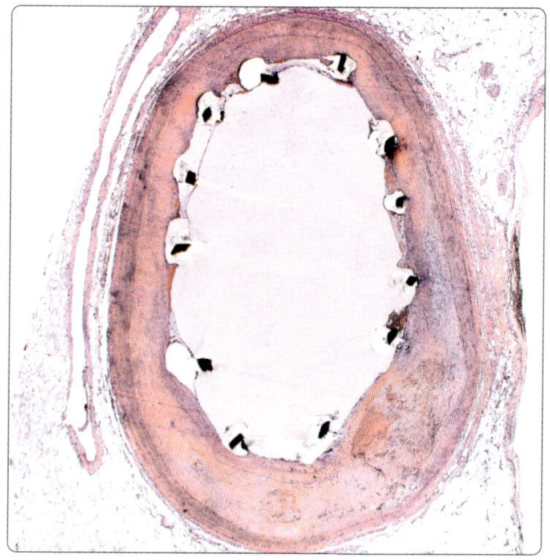

(Left) *Elastic-stained plastic section of a stented coronary artery shows a significant native plaque , which obstructs > 75% of the original lumen, and in-stent restenosis caused by concentric neointimal ingrowth , further restricting the lumen .* **(Right)** *Movat-stained plastic section shows a stent within a stent. There is a native plaque , a neointimal stenosis of the original (outer) stent , and a 2nd inner stent placed later, also showing significant stenosis.*

Native Vessel Plaque and In-Stent Stenosis

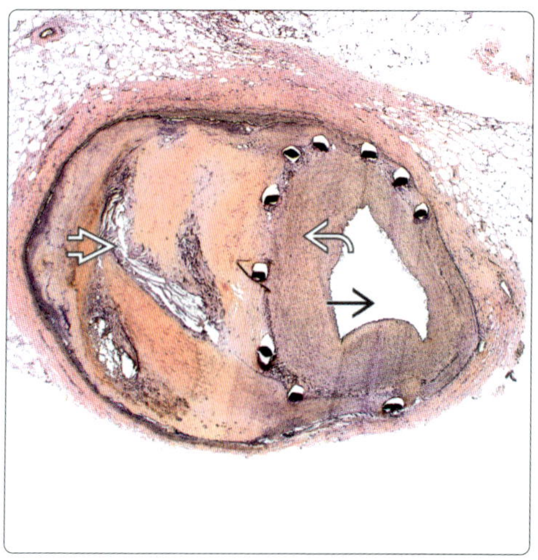

Stent Within Stent

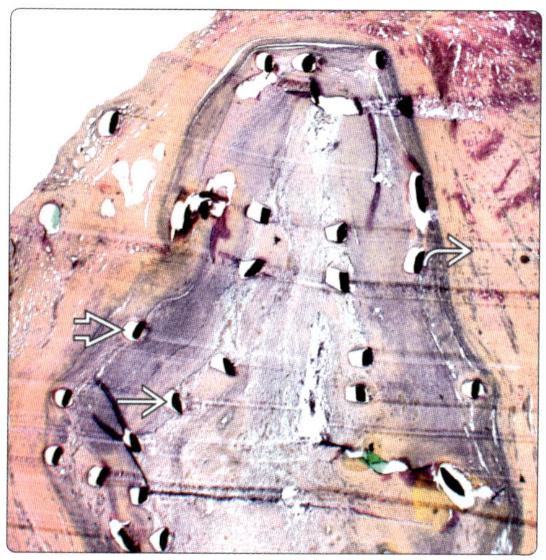

Stent Neointimal Fibrosis (High Magnification)

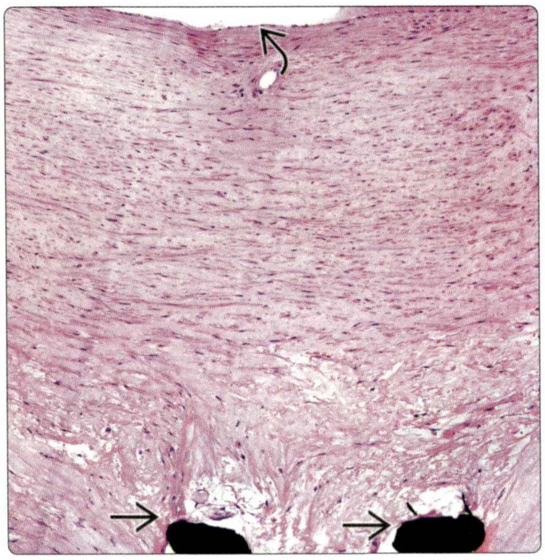

Inflammation and Revascularization Within Neointima

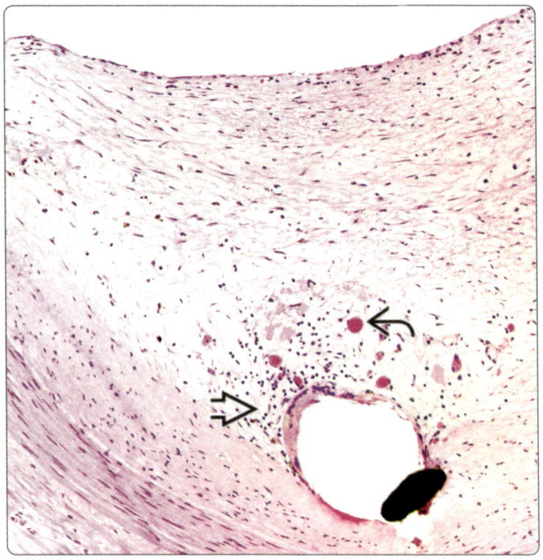

(Left) *Plastic-embedded coronary artery section shows 2 stent struts → marking the original stented lumen boundary and substantial smooth muscle-rich neointimal ingrowth extending to the residual lumen → at the top.* **(Right)** *Plastic section of a stented coronary artery shows neointimal growth with neovascularization → and inflammation → surrounding the strut.*

Foreign Body Reaction to Stent Strut

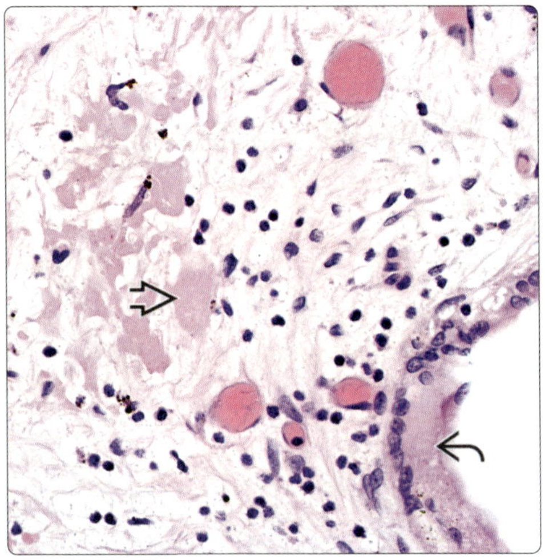

Fibrin Associated With Stent Strut

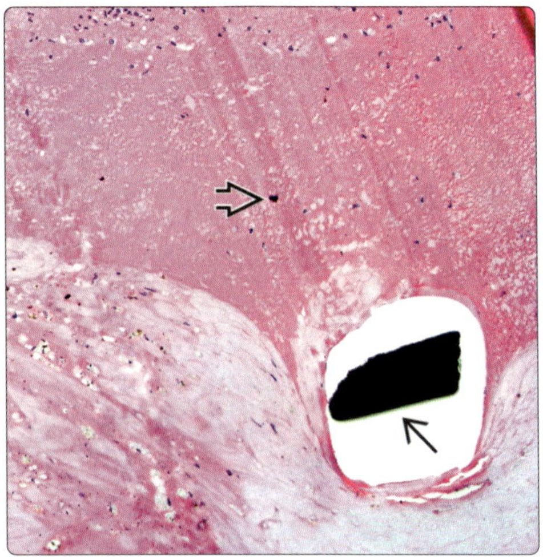

(Left) *Higher magnification of the peristrut neointimal tissue of a stented coronary artery highlights wisps of fibrin →, sparse mononuclear cells, and a giant cell foreign body reaction →.* **(Right)** *Plastic section of a stented coronary artery shows extreme amounts of fibrin and platelets surrounding the stent strut → and merging with a recent luminal thrombus →. Thrombosis is still a common stent complication.*

Stented Artery (After Electrolytic Stent Removal)

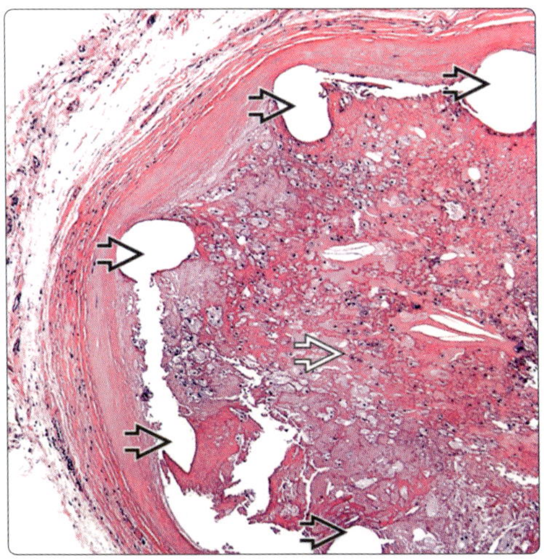

Apparatus for Stent Reverse Electroplating

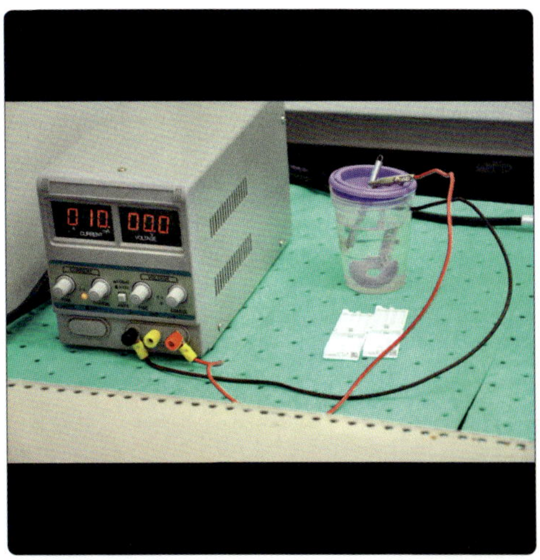

(Left) *Paraffin section of a stented coronary artery after reverse electroplating to remove the metallic struts shows empty "holes" →. Atherothrombosis →, which had resulted from rupture of a thin-cap soft core plaque during stent deployment, occludes the lumen.* **(Right)** *Photograph shows an apparatus for dissolving metallic stents from coronary artery specimens using reverse electroplating. A current is applied to the stent in an artery submerged in acid-salt solution after formalin fixation.*

Cardiac Allograft Vasculopathy

KEY FACTS

TERMINOLOGY

- Inflammatory fibroproliferative disorder characterized by concentric intima thickening involving epicardial and intramyocardial coronary arteries, leading to chronic ischemia with secondary myocyte changes and interstitial fibrosis

CLINICAL ISSUES

- Most common complication of heart transplantation in long-term survivors
- Asymptomatic (cardiac denervation, often absent chest pain)
- Acute coronary syndrome-like symptoms
- Systolic dysfunction acutely, diastolic dysfunction chronically
- Allograft failure (reduced cardiac output and pulmonary venous hypertension)
- Sudden death
- Retransplantation is only "cure"
- Leading cause of death (usually sudden) &/or retransplantation, but outcomes generally unpredictable

MACROSCOPIC

- Epicardial coronaries with cord-like orange-colored appearance
- Calcification is infrequent

MICROSCOPIC

- Myocardial changes: Myocyte cytoplasmic vacuolization
- Interstitial changes: Variable degrees of fibrosis
- Epicardial coronary arteries with
  - Marked concentric intima thickening
  - Intact elastic lamina or minimal breaks
  - Media layer of normal thickness or, in some cases, thinner
  - Perivascular inflammation
  - Advanced lesions may show features of more conventional atherosclerosis

(Left) *Selective left coronary artery angiogram in lateral camera angulation demonstrates a severe (~ 80%) narrowing of the midportion of the circumflex coronary artery. There is also severe pruning of the distal left anterior descending coronary artery and distal circumflex arteries. (Courtesy M. Everitt, MD.)* **(Right)** *Coronary CTA 3D volume rendering shows areas of luminal narrowing in the left anterior descending artery and diagonal branches in a patient 3 years post heart transplant.*

Angiographic Findings in Cardiac Allograft Vasculopathy

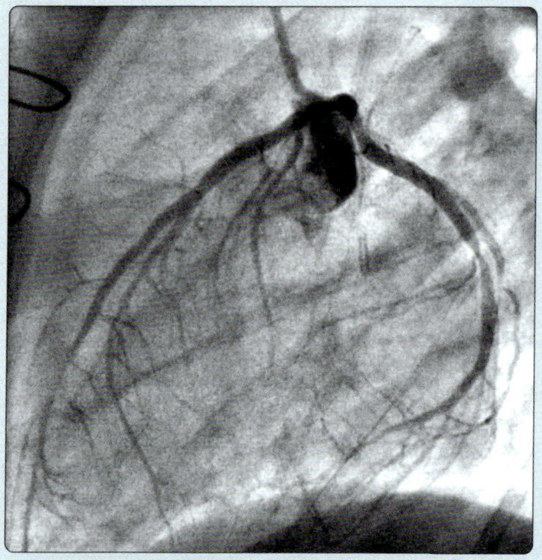

Coronary CTA 3D Findings in Cardiac Allograft Vasculopathy

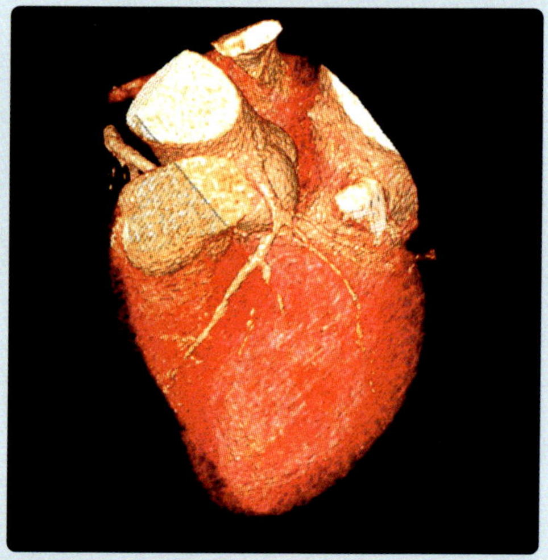

(Left) *Left ventricular section from a cardiac allograft removed at the time of retransplantation shows concentric narrowing of an epicardial coronary artery →, resulting in significant stenosis.* **(Right)** *Epicardial coronary artery branch shows a nearly complete luminal occlusion. The intima is expanded by a collagen-rich matrix and fibroblasts with chronic inflammatory cells around the endothelium →.*

Gross Findings in Cardiac Allograft Vasculopathy

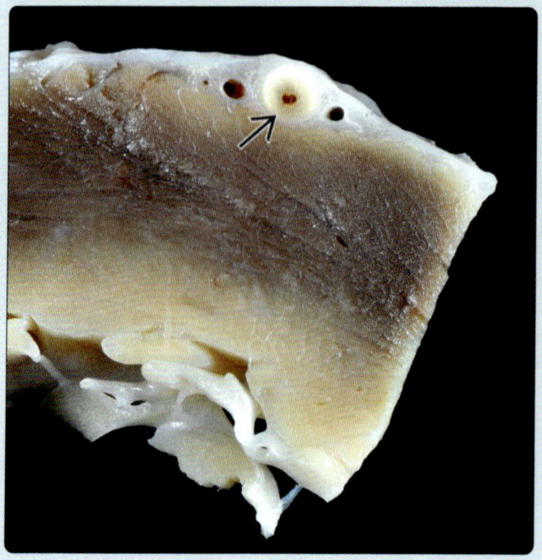

Epicardial Artery Changes in Cardiac Allograft Vasculopathy

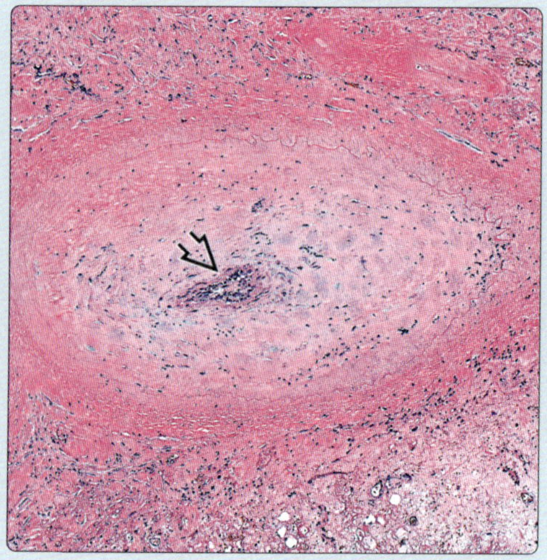

TERMINOLOGY

Abbreviations

- Cardiac allograft vasculopathy (CAV)

Definitions

- Inflammatory fibroproliferative disorder characterized by concentric intima thickening involving epicardial and intramyocardial coronary arteries, leading to chronic ischemia with secondary myocyte changes and interstitial fibrosis

ETIOLOGY/PATHOGENESIS

Risk Factors for Cardiac Allograft Vasculopathy Development

- Immunologic
  - Total number of human leukocyte antigen (HLA) mismatches (HLA-DR highest correlation)
  - Humoral immune response against graft antigens thought to incite inflammation, leading to progressive fibroproliferative response
  - Development of donor-specific antibodies (DSA) post transplant, in particular DSA to major histocompatibility complex (MHC) type II antigens (HLA-DQ)
  - Increased T-helper activity
  - "Chronic" rejection: Cumulative effects of multiple rejection episodes, especially of antibody-mediated rejection (AMR), leading to
    - Higher incidence and shorter time to CAV onset
  - Autoimmunity
    - Antibodies to myosin, vimentin, and MHC class I chain-related A (MICA) may also play role
- Nonimmunologic
  - Ischemia/reperfusion injury sustained during harvesting and organ preservation can result in
    - Endothelial injury, promoting platelet and phagocytic cell adherence
    - Secondary fibrin accumulation and local release of growth factors
    - Migration and proliferation of smooth muscle cells
  - Deficient fibrinolysis
  - Older donor/recipient age
  - Donor with explosive brain death
  - Usual atherosclerotic risk factors may also influence development and progression of CAV
  - Active CMV infection after transplantation
  - Hepatitis C (+) donor

CLINICAL ISSUES

Epidemiology

- Incidence
  - Most common complication of heart transplantation in long-term survivors
    - 8% at 1 year post transplant
    - 20% at 3 years post transplant
    - ~ 30% at 5 years post transplant
    - ~ 50% at 10 years post transplant
    - CAV and late graft failure account for majority of patient mortality (32.3%) at 5-10 years post transplant
    - Incidence varies by rejection history; patients with predominant AMR have 15% increased incidence over those with cellular rejection

Presentation

- Asymptomatic (cardiac denervation, often absent chest pain)
- Acute coronary syndrome-like symptoms
- Systolic dysfunction acutely, diastolic dysfunction chronically
- Allograft failure (reduced cardiac output and pulmonary venous hypertension)
- Arrhythmias
- Sudden death

Treatment

- Options, risks, complications
  - Management of CAV is focused on primary prevention, imaging surveillance, and early treatment
- Surgical approaches
  - Retransplantation is only "cure"
    - However, there is association with lower survival and increased CAV incidence
  - Percutaneous coronary intervention has no clear long-term benefit with poor long-term outcomes: 1/2 of patients developing cardiac events 2 years post intervention or restenosis
  - Mechanical circulatory support also considered in some cases
- Drugs
  - mTOR inhibitors may slow progression, stabilize, or partially reverse allograft vasculopathy
  - Anticoagulants may reduce endothelial injury and prevent progression via shallow thrombus formation
  - Statins, angiotensin-converting enzyme (ACE) inhibitors, and blood pressure control are beneficial

Prognosis

- Leading cause of death (usually sudden) &/or retransplantation, but outcomes generally unpredictable
  - If early post transplant (< 1-2 years), usually bad outcome
  - If late post transplant, course may be indolent
  - 4-year graft survival after CAV diagnosis is ~ 50%
  - Angiographic CAV predicts 5x greater relative risk of cardiac events

IMAGING

Coronary Angiogram

- Standard of care and identifies
  - Significant artery stenosis
  - Diffuse distal artery narrowing
  - Luminal irregularities
- Insensitive for detection of early disease

Intravascular US

- Most sensitive and specific in defining abnormalities in artery wall, including
  - Luminal area
  - Maximal intima thickness
  - Intimal cross-sectional area
  - Total and percentage of atheroma volume

ISHLT Angiographic Cardiac Allograft Vasculopathy Grading

Grade	Angiographic Lesion
ISHLT CAV0 (not significant)	No detectable angiographic lesion
ISHLT CAV1 (mild)	Left main < 50% stenosis, primary vessel† maximum lesion of < 70% stenosis, or any branch stenosis < 70% without allograft dysfunction
ISHLT CAV2 (moderate)	Left main ≥ 50% stenosis, single primary vessel ≥ 70% stenosis, or any isolated branch ≥ 70% stenosis without allograft dysfunction
ISHLT CAV3 (severe)	Left main ≥ 50% stenosis, 2 or more primary vessels ≥ 70% stenosis, isolated branch stenosis ≥ 70% in all 3 systems, or CAV1/CAV2 with allograft dysfunction or restrictive physiology

†"Primary vessel" denotes proximal and middle 1/3 of left anterior descending artery, circumflex, ramus, and dominant or codominant right coronary artery with posterior descending and posterolateral branches.
ISHLT = International Society for Heart and Lung Transplantation; CAV = cardiac allograft vasculopathy.

Dobutamine Stress Echocardiography

- Noninvasive test for CAV diagnosis; determines cardiac structure, systolic/diastolic function, wall motion abnormalities, myocardial perfusion; has poor sensitivity for early diagnosis of CAV

PET

- Alternative noninvasive CAV screening that can quantify myocardial blood flow
- Useful for early diagnosis and as marker of disease progression

MACROSCOPIC

General Features

- Epicardial coronaries with cord-like orange-colored appearance
- Calcification is infrequent

MICROSCOPIC

Histologic Features

- Epicardial coronary arteries
  - Marked diffuse, concentric, longitudinal intima thickening
    - Smooth muscle cell proliferation
    - Deposit of fibrous material
    - Lipid-laden macrophages may be common or rare
    - Variable number of inflammatory cells in subendothelial distribution
  - Intact elastic lamina or minimal breaks
  - Media layer of normal thickness or, in some cases, thinner
  - Adventitial and perivascular inflammation
  - Advanced lesions may show features of more conventional atherosclerosis, including
    - Disruption of internal elastic lamina
    - Intracellular and extracellular lipid accumulation
    - Necrosis, calcium deposition, and calcification
- Intramyocardial coronary artery branches
  - Myointimal proliferative changes ± foamy macrophages
  - Narrowing of lumina
  - Endothelialitis
  - Perivascular fibrosis
- Myocardial changes
  - Myocyte cytoplasmic vacuolization: Subendocardial and watershed zones of myocardium are predominantly affected
  - Myocyte hypertrophy
  - Focal myocyte necrosis
    - Acute: Eosinophilic granular appearance of myocytes
    - Healing: Granulation tissue
- Interstitial changes
  - Variable degrees of interstitial, perivascular, and replacement fibrosis

ANCILLARY TESTS

Histochemistry

- Elastic van Gieson
  - Staining pattern: Elastic lamina is highlighted in black

DIFFERENTIAL DIAGNOSIS

Coronary Atherosclerosis

- Eccentric intima proliferation and media attenuation
- Intracellular and extracellular lipid accumulation is prominent
- Disruption of internal elastic lamina is commonly seen
- Process affects focally epicardial arteries but not intramyocardial branches
- Calcification occurs frequently

DIAGNOSTIC CHECKLIST

Clinically Relevant Pathologic Features

- Patients with repeated AMR are more likely to have CAV, and index of suspicion should be higher in these patients

Pathologic Interpretation Pearls

- Intramyocardial coronary artery branches are usually absent in endomyocardial biopsy and cannot be evaluated
- Degree of small vessel vasculopathy does not correlate with degree of epicardial artery stenosis

SELECTED REFERENCES

1. Spartalis M et al: Cardiac allograft vasculopathy after heart transplantation: pathophysiology, detection approaches, prevention, and treatment management. Trends Cardiovasc Med. 32(6):333-8, 2022
2. Pober JS et al: Cardiac allograft vasculopathy: current review and future research directions. Cardiovasc Res. 117(13):2624-38, 2021

Gross Findings in Cardiac Allograft Vasculopathy

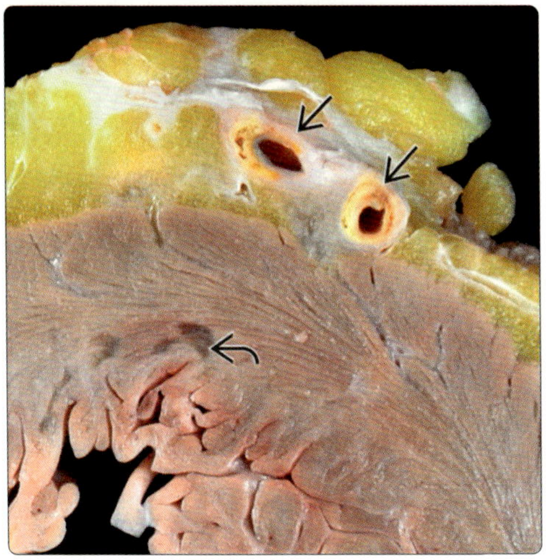

Gross Findings in Cardiac Allograft Vasculopathy

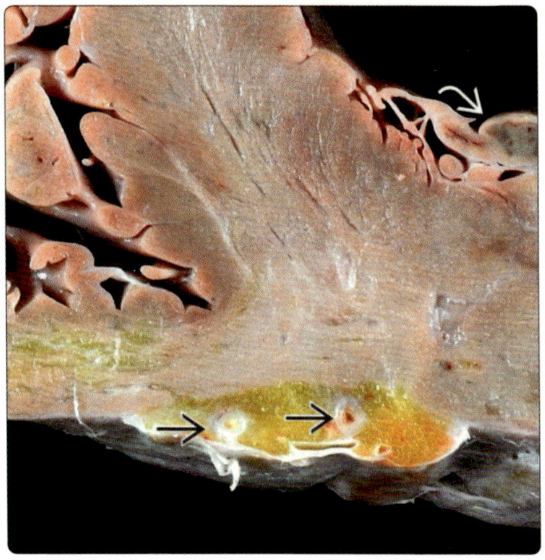

(Left) *Short-axis view of the left ventricle with cardiac allograft vasculopathy (CAV) at autopsy shows significant narrowing of epicardial coronary arteries* → *along with depressed scars* ↷ *representing old subendocardial ischemic damage in the myocardium supplied by these vessels.* **(Right)** *Gross specimen of heart allograft affected by CAV shows nearly complete occlusion of patent ductus arteriosus branches* →*. Old subendocardial infarction is seen in the inferior wall* ➡*.*

Epicardial Artery Changes in Cardiac Allograft Vasculopathy

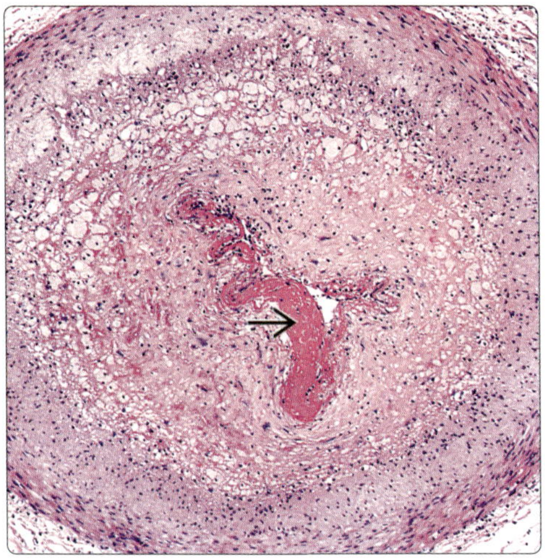

Epicardial Artery Changes in Cardiac Allograft Vasculopathy

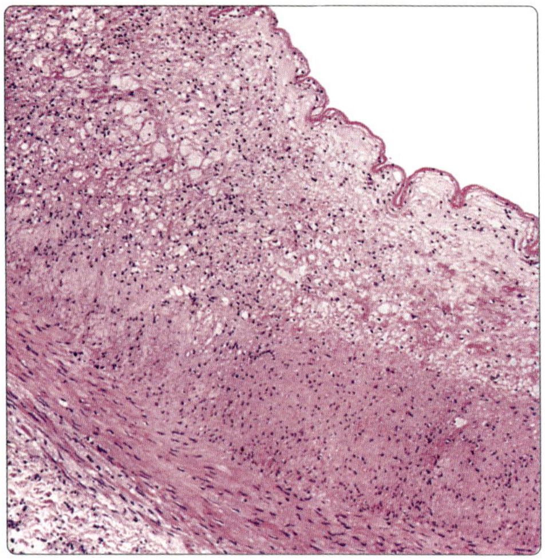

(Left) *Epicardial artery from a heart allograft affected by CAV shows marked accumulation of foamy cells in the intima with scant inflammatory cells. Deposit of fibrin is present in the lumen* →*.* **(Right)** *At higher magnification, coronary artery affected by CAV shows intima expanded by foamy macrophages admixed with scant inflammatory cells. The media layer is uninvolved.*

Epicardial Artery Changes in Cardiac Allograft Vasculopathy

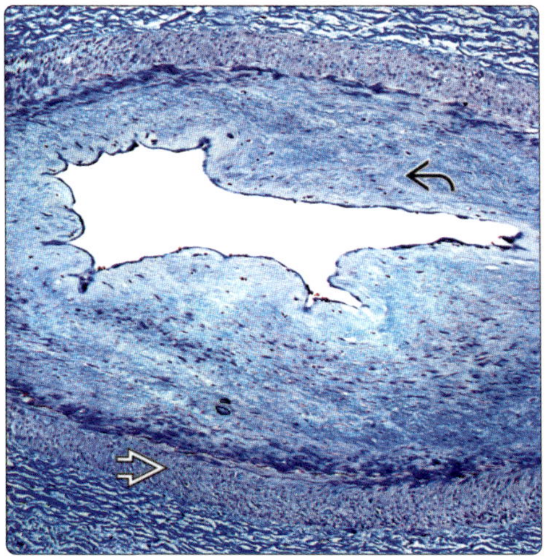

Epicardial Artery Changes in Cardiac Allograft Vasculopathy

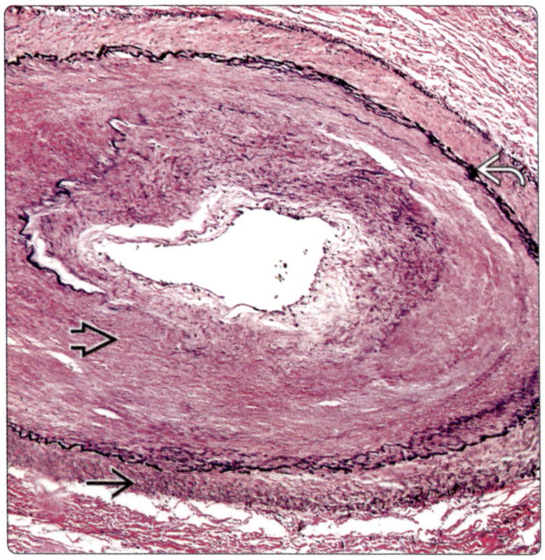

(Left) *Trichrome-stained section of epicardial coronary artery affected by CAV shows marked concentric intima thickening* ↷*. There is no inflammatory infiltrate within the wall, and the media appears intact* ➡*.* **(Right)** *Elastic-stained section of epicardial coronary artery with advanced CAV shows marked intima fibrosis* ⇒*. There is no significant inflammatory infiltrate within the wall, the media appear intact* →*, and the internal elastic lamina* ➡ *is well preserved.*

(**Left**) *The intimal expansion in this epicardial artery is more asymmetric and eccentric but also shows a prominent inflammatory component →.* (**Right**) *Epicardial artery shows CAV with a slit-like lumen and endothelial inflammation →. Collagen matrix, fibroblasts, and smooth muscle cells account for the intimal expansion. Because of the rapidity of CAV progression, it is thought the vessel has limited capacity for outward remodeling to preserve the luminal diameter.*

Epicardial Artery Changes in Cardiac Allograft Vasculopathy

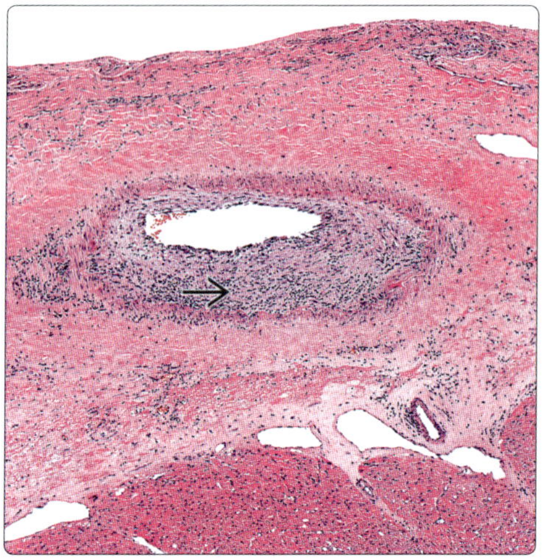

Epicardial Artery Changes in Cardiac Allograft Vasculopathy

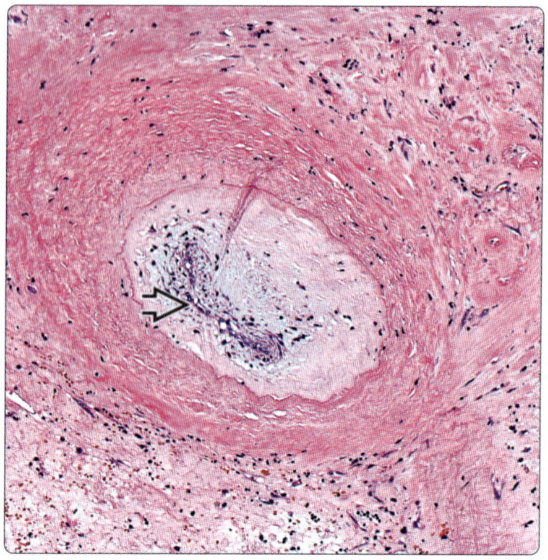

(**Left**) *Epicardial arteries involved by CAV show > 90% luminal occlusion. Intima is expanded by matrix, fibroblasts, smooth muscle cells, and scant inflammatory infiltrate. Dense perivascular fibrosis is also seen surrounding the vessels →.* (**Right**) *Inflammation is often prominent in association with CAV, such as this perivascular lymphocytic infiltrate →. Posttransplant lymphoproliferative disorder should be excluded when cytologic atypia &/or significant monomorphism is present.*

Epicardial Artery Changes in Cardiac Allograft Vasculopathy

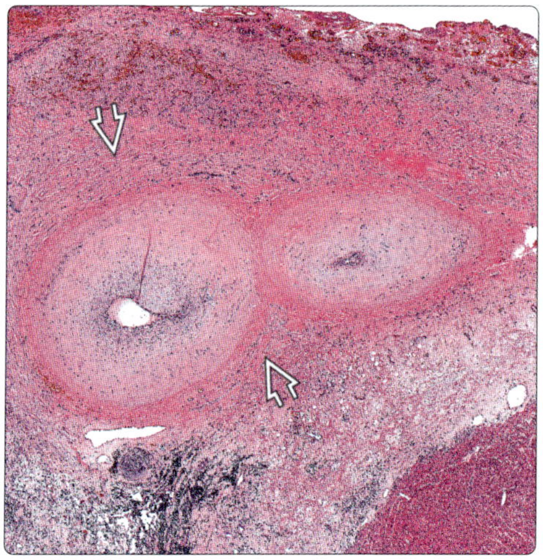

Epicardial Artery Changes in Cardiac Allograft Vasculopathy

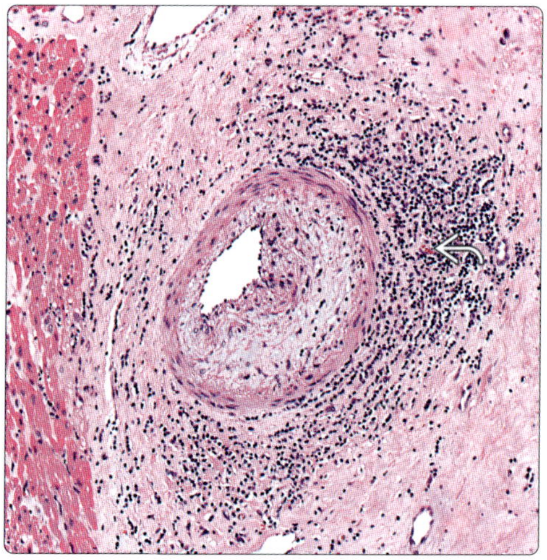

(**Left**) *Intramyocardial penetrating artery involved by CAV shows ~ 75% luminal occlusion. The morphologic features are similar to what is seen in epicardial arteries with intima expanded by collagen matrix, fibroblasts, and smooth muscle cells. Dense perivascular fibrosis admixed with inflammatory cells is also seen surrounding this vessel →.* (**Right**) *This intramyocardial vessel does not show significant narrowing but is involved by intimal → and focally transmural → "arteritis."*

Intramyocardial Artery Changes in Cardiac Allograft Vasculopathy

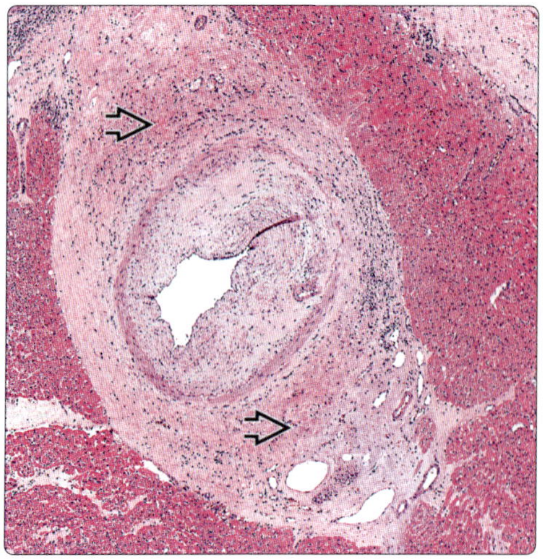

Intramyocardial Artery Changes in Cardiac Allograft Vasculopathy

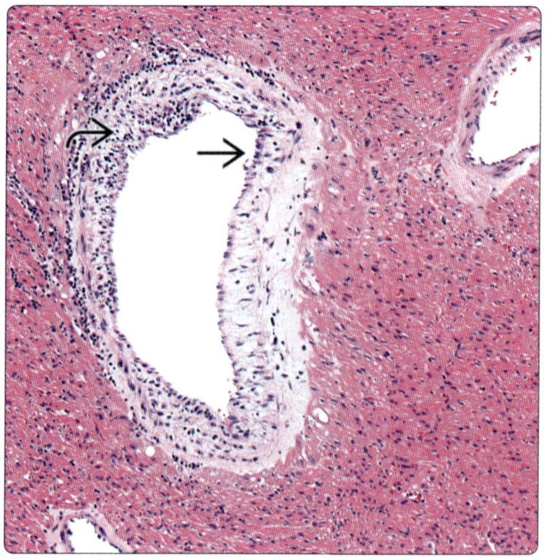

Myocardial Changes in Cardiac Allograft Vasculopathy

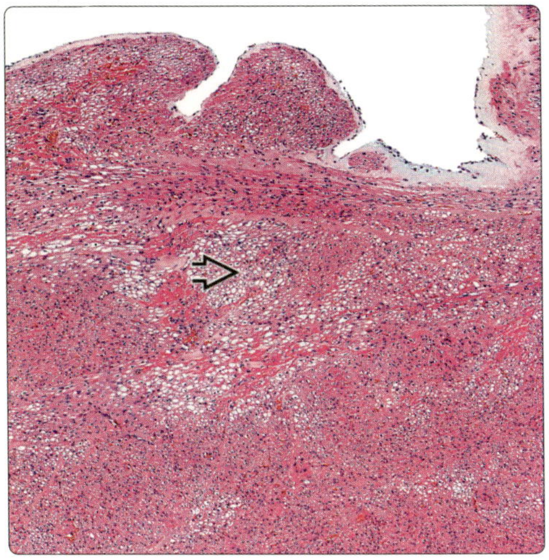

Myocardial Changes in Cardiac Allograft Vasculopathy

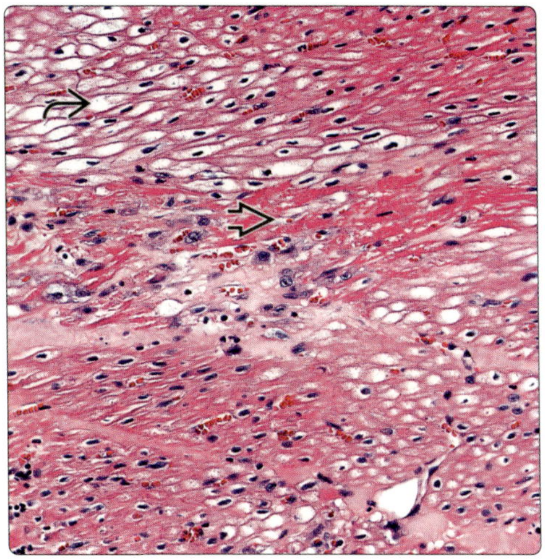

(Left) *Left ventricle from a heart removed during retransplantation for CAV shows prominent cytoplasmic vacuolization of subendocardial myocytes ⇨.* **(Right)** *At higher magnification, the myocardium from a heart removed during retransplantation for CAV shows prominent clearing of the myocytes sarcoplasm ⇨, representing loss of contractile elements. Islands of necrotic myocytes are also present ⇨.*

Intramyocardial Small Artery Changes in Cardiac Allograft Vasculopathy

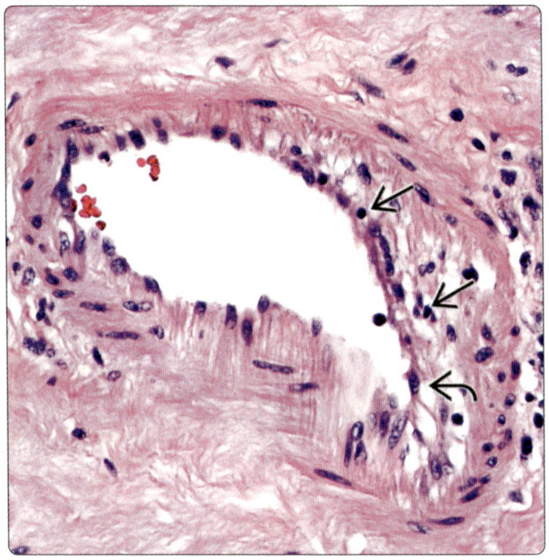

Intramyocardial Small Artery Changes in Cardiac Allograft Vasculopathy

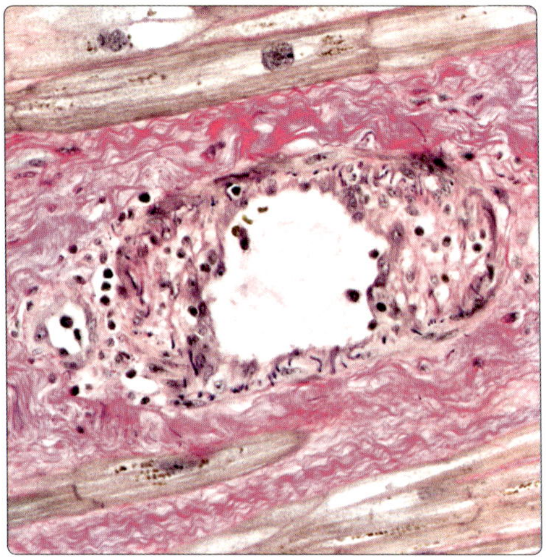

(Left) *Intramyocardial coronary branch from a transplant patient with chronic ischemia shows foamy macrophages in the intima ⇨, but there is no significant reduction of the lumina. Focal endothelialitis is seen ⇨.* **(Right)** *Elastic stain of an intramyocardial arteriole shows involvement by CAV. However, most of the time, they are not sampled in endomyocardial biopsy.*

Myocardial Changes in Cardiac Allograft Vasculopathy

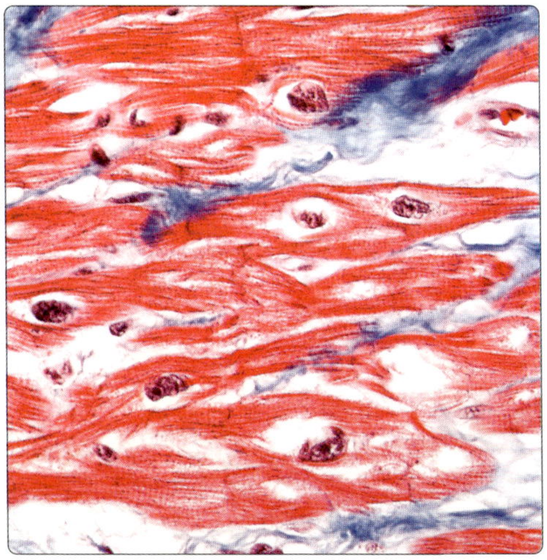

Interstitial Changes in Cardiac Allograft Vasculopathy

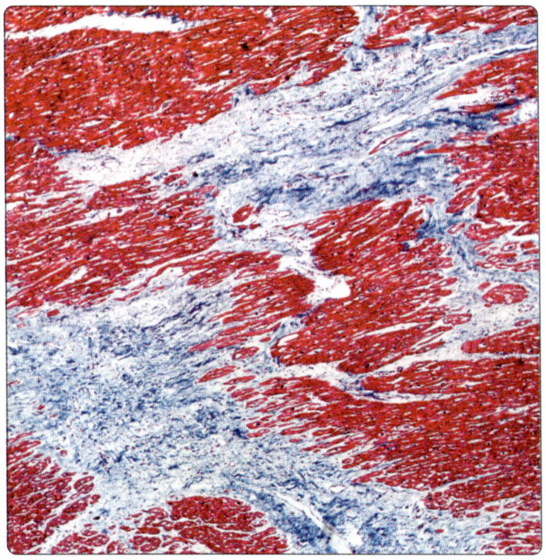

(Left) *Higher magnification of a trichrome-stained myocardium from an autopsied heart with coronaries involved by CAV shows sarcoplasmic (perinuclear) clearing and delicate wisps of interstitial fibrosis. The areas of clearing represent loss of contractile elements in the myocytes.* **(Right)** *Trichrome stain highlights interstitial fibrosis in the myocardium of a transplant patient with chronic myocardial ischemia secondary to CAV.*

KEY FACTS

TERMINOLOGY

- Damage to any cardiac structure (especially pericardium, coronary arteries, and valves) from radiation (iatrogenic or otherwise)

ETIOLOGY/PATHOGENESIS

- Volume of heart irradiated, total radiation dose (usually > 30 Gy), dose per fraction and techniques
- Less frequent due to radiation therapy advances

CLINICAL ISSUES

- Acute phase (weeks to months after exposure)
  - Pericarditis most common, usually fibrinous, with effusion
- Chronic phase (years to decades after exposure)
  - Coronary stenosis, cardiomyopathy, constrictive pericarditis, valve dysfunction

MACROSCOPIC

- Myocardium: Restrictive, dilated, or ischemic cardiomyopathy
- Endocardium: Endocardial fibrosis
- Pericardium: Thickening > 1 mm, fibrinous exudate, variable pericardial effusion
- Coronary arteries: Intimal fibrosis and periarterial fibrosis
- Valves: Fibrous thickening of leaflets &/or chordae

MICROSCOPIC

- Valves: Endocardial fibrosis of leaflets ± calcification
- Pericardium
  - Acute: Lymphocytic pericarditis affecting mostly parietal pericardium
  - Chronic: Fibrosis and calcification (constrictive)

Radiation-Induced Coronary Artery Narrowing

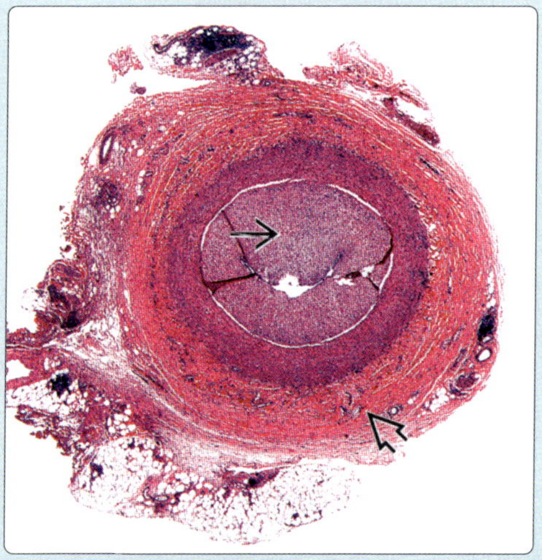

Radiation-Induced Aortic Valve Fibrosis

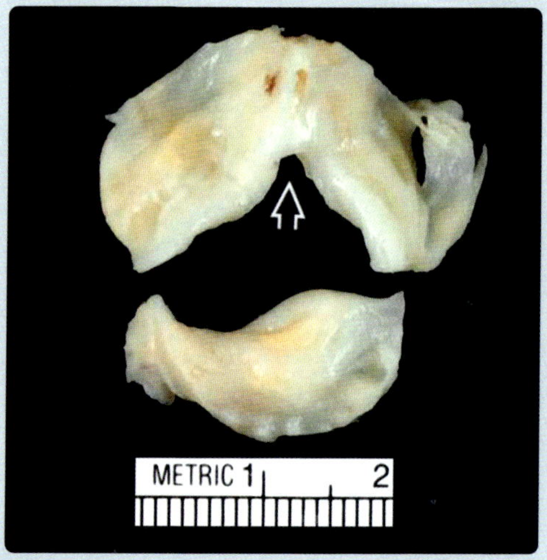

(Left) *Coronary artery shows chronic changes from radiation injury, including lumen stenosis primarily due to intimal fibrosis ➙ and adventitial fibrosis ➙.* **(Right)** *Aortic valve shows fibrotic thickening and acquired fusion of 2 cusps ➙, consistent with postinflammatory valve disease. The patient had prior mediastinal irradiation for lymphoma.*

Radiation-Induced Pericardial Calcification

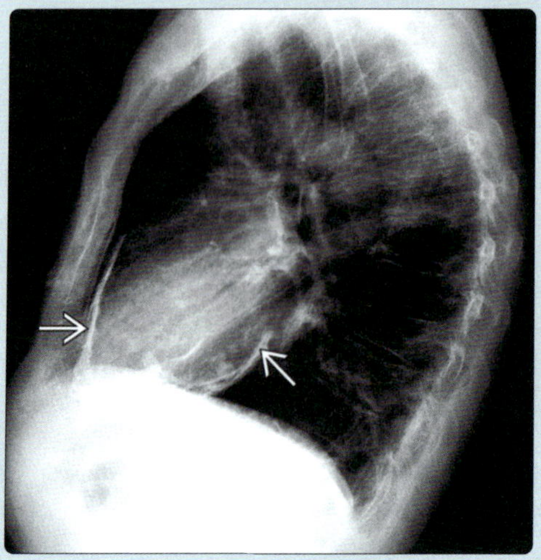

Radiation-Induced Constrictive Pericarditis

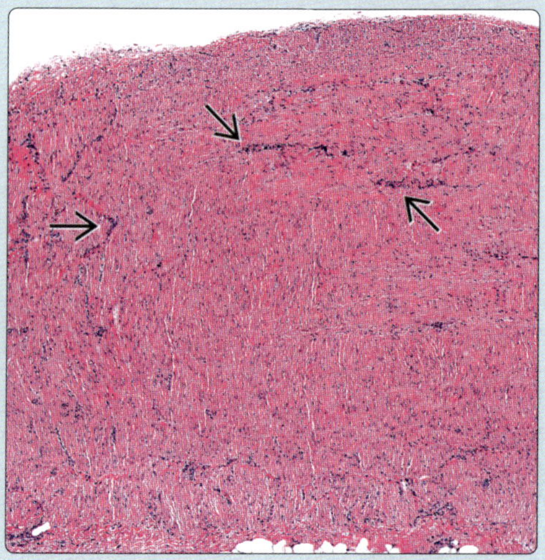

(Left) *Lateral chest radiograph shows pericardial calcification ➙ in a patient with a remote history of thoracic irradiation for malignancy.* **(Right)** *Pericardium from a patient with radiation-associated constrictive pericarditis shows a haphazard to focally storiform population of fibroblasts with dense collagen and prominent vasculature ➙.*

TERMINOLOGY

Definitions

- Damage to any cardiac structure (especially pericardium, coronary arteries, and valves) from radiation

ETIOLOGY/PATHOGENESIS

Complication of Cancer Treatment

- Irradiation of tumor in same field as heart, such as
  - Carcinoma of left breast
  - Mediastinal tumor, such as Hodgkin lymphoma
  - Malignancies affecting esophagus, thymus, or lung

Risk Factors

- Volume of heart irradiated, total radiation dose (usually > 30 Gy), dose per fraction and techniques
- Concomitant administration of cardiotoxic agent, such as anthracyclines
- Younger age at treatment

Pathogenesis

- Radiation-induced endothelial cell injury (vascular and valvular disease)
- Capillary destruction/obstruction with resultant ischemia and inflammation (myocardium and pericardium)

CLINICAL ISSUES

Presentation

- Acute phase (weeks to months after exposure)
  - Pericarditis, usually fibrinous, with effusion
  - Pancarditis also described
- Chronic phase (years to decades after exposure)
  - Coronary artery stenosis
    - Angina and infarction
  - Cardiomyopathy, systolic or diastolic heart failure
    - Focal wall motion anomaly, mild global hypokinesia, impaired relaxation
  - Valvular dysfunction
    - Regurgitation but also stenosis or mixed dysfunction
    - More common on left side, especially aortic valve
  - Arrhythmias: Bradycardia, heart block, sick sinus syndrome, ventricular fibrillation
  - Constrictive pericarditis (most common complication)
    - Interval between radiation and onset of symptoms ranges from months to 45 years; average: 7 years

Prognosis

- Contemporary radiation therapy minimizes irradiation to heart and substantially decreases cardiac radiation injury

MACROSCOPIC

Myocardium

- Restrictive, dilated, or ischemic cardiomyopathy

Endocardium

- Endocardial fibrosis

Pericardium

- Pericardial thickening of > 1 mm, fibrinous exudate, variable pericardial effusion

Coronary Artery

- Intimal fibrosis and periarterial fibrosis
  - Ostia, left main, proximal left anterior descending, and proximal right coronary most often involved

Valves

- Fibrous thickening of leaflets &/or chordae

Aorta

- Accelerated atherosclerosis with en plaque calcification and periarterial fibrosis

MICROSCOPIC

Histologic Features

- Acute vascular injury
  - Involves primarily small arteries, arterioles, capillaries, and venules with ectasia &/or endothelial damage (swelling and vacuolization)
  - Mural necrosis, thrombosis, and elastic laminar disruption
  - Perivascular tissue edema
- Chronic myocardial fibrosis
  - Interstitial and perivascular fibrosis, diffuse or patchy
    - Most prominent in left ventricle (lateral and anterior)
  - Microvessel loss, narrowing, and obstruction
  - Adventitial fibrosis around arterioles
- Coronary artery intimal lesions
  - May be identical to usual atherosclerosis or concentric fibroproliferative stenosis
  - Occasionally prominent fibrosis of media and adventitia with bizarre reactive fibroblasts
- Valves
  - Endocardial fibrosis of leaflets ± calcification
- Aorta
  - Intimal fibrocalcific atherosclerosis
  - Laminar medial necrosis with fibrosis and cellular loss
- Pericardium
  - Acute: Lymphocytic pericarditis (parietal pericardium)
  - Chronic: Fibrosis and calcification (constrictive)

DIFFERENTIAL DIAGNOSIS

Dilated Cardiomyopathy (Idiopathic or Secondary)

- Clinical history is essential, as morphologic changes might be identical

Constrictive Pericarditis (Nonradiation Induced)

- No clinical history of radiation
- Atypical fibroblasts are absent

SELECTED REFERENCES

1. Koutroumpakis E et al: Radiation-induced cardiovascular disease: mechanisms, prevention, and treatment. Curr Oncol Rep. 24(5):543-53, 2022
2. Yusuf SW et al: Radiation-induced heart disease: a clinical update. Cardiol Res Pract. 2011:317659, 2011
3. Veinot JP et al: Pathology of radiation-induced heart disease: a surgical and autopsy study of 27 cases. Hum Pathol. 27(8):766-73, 1996

MACROSCOPIC

Sinoatrial Node

- Specialized "pacemaker" myocyte collection in right atrium
- Subepicardial structure near superior vena cava, overlying terminal crest (vertical crest on interior wall of right atrium that separates sinus of vena cava from rest of right atrium)
- Found at union of smooth-walled "sinus venosus" portion and trabecular portion of right atrium
- Supplied by sinus node artery (usually branch from right coronary)

Atrioventricular Node

- Specialized conducting myocytes within tricuspid anulus near atrioventricular (AV) (membranous) septum
- Subendocardial structure found within "Koch triangle," anatomic area defined by these 3 vertices
  - Membranous septum
  - Roof of coronary sinus ostium
  - Tricuspid anulus at point directly below coronary sinus ostium
- Supplied by AV nodal artery (usually from posterior descending artery)

MICROSCOPIC

Sinoatrial Node

- Compact and polyhedral myocytes surrounded by dense collagenous tissue
- Sarcoplasm and cross striations less prominent
- Sinus nodal artery courses through sinus node
- Autonomic nerve fibers and ganglia seen in vicinity
- Increased ratio of dense collagen:myocytes with increasing age reported

Atrioventricular Node

- Compact "bulb" of smaller polyhedral myocytes merging with larger stellate to spindled myocytes with vacuolar sarcoplasm toward His bundle
- Mesothelial-like cells and cystic structures occasionally intermixed
- AV nodal artery courses through AV node
- Connective tissue surrounds node, "insulating" adjacent myocardium
- Autonomic nerves and lymphatics seen in vicinity
  - Rich supply of lymphatics may explain predilection for involvement in patients with sarcoidosis
  - Lymphatic drainage of endogenous toxins from distal infarcted myocardium causes "stunning" of AV node and transient heart block post myocardial infarction in some patients

His Bundle and Bundle Branches

- Constituent cells mostly smaller than myocardial myocytes and more vacuolated
- Right bundle branch is smaller and cord-like
- Left bundle branch is larger and splays out over leftward ventricular septum

Purkinje Cell

- Term applied to cells in left bundle branch and distal right bundle branch because they are larger than myocardial myocytes and have more vacuolar cytoplasm
- As with all conduction system cells, Purkinje cells are myocytes and contain myofibrils by electron microscopy
- Differ from normal cardiomyocytes by absence of T tubules and striking abundance of cell-cell junctions

Histochemical Stains

- Conduction system myocytes differ from contractile myocytes
  - Anaerobic oxidation predominates over aerobic
  - Unique cholinesterases expressed in conduction system myocytes
  - Abundant glycogen found in conduction system myocytes

Strategies for Processing and Examining Conduction System

- Given small size of these structures
  - It is difficult to grossly cut tissue blocks thinly enough to evaluate different segments in single histologic section

Atrioventricular Node

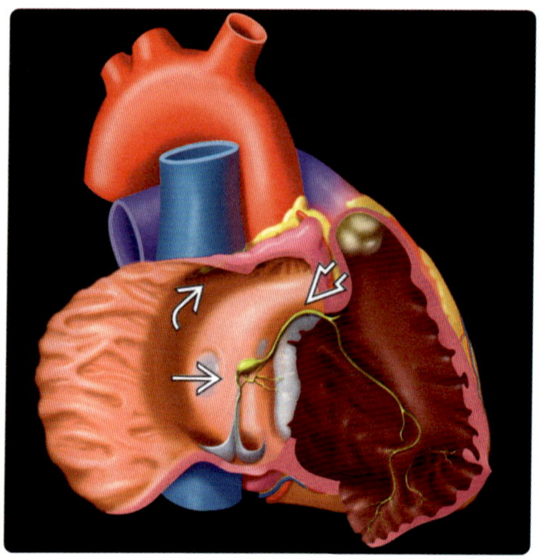

Triangle of Koch

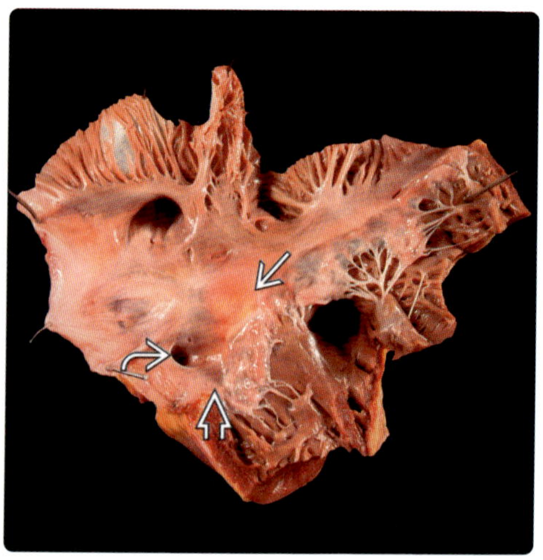

(Left) *This graphic shows the approximate locations of the sinoatrial node ➡ (subepicardial), atrioventricular (AV) node ➡ (subendocardial), and His bundle ➡.* **(Right)** *This view of the opened right heart shows the location of Koch triangle: A septum ➡, coronary sinus ostium ➡, and tricuspid anulus below the coronary sinus ostium ➡.*

 - Serial sectioning of paraffin blocks is necessary to identify structures and evaluate abnormalities
 - Some authors advocate exhaustive sectioning of paraffin blocks (1,200-1,600 total slides) to evaluate every conduction system cell

HISTOLOGIC PITFALLS

Atrioventricular Node and Bundle Branches

- Normally occurring smooth muscle bundles in endocardium should not be mistaken for Purkinje cells or conduction system tracts

INDICATIONS FOR EXAMINATION OF CONDUCTION SYSTEM

Sinoatrial Node

- Documented sinus node electrocardiographic abnormalities
  - Tachycardia-bradycardia syndrome
  - Sick sinus syndrome
  - Sinus arrest
  - **Not** atrial fibrillation or atrial flutter (in most cases, sinoatrial node is normal)
- Previous ablation procedure
- Sudden unexpected death without other cardiac cause(s) (pathologist's discretion)

Atrioventricular Node

- AV block
  - 1st degree
  - 2nd degree (Mobitz type 1 or Wenckebach type)
  - 2nd degree (Mobitz type 2)
  - 3rd degree
- Junctional arrhythmias
- Previous ablation procedure

His Bundle and Bundle Branches

- Variable, generally not indicated
- Very difficult to localize pathways of interest
- Previous ablation procedure

Preexcitation Electrocardiographic Changes

- Classic example is Wolff-Parkinson-White syndrome
- Anomalous connecting band of contractile myocardium between atria and ventricle
- Bypassing normal conduction delay coordinated in AV node
- Careful examination of entire coronary groove can be undertaken to identify "myocardial bridge"

Transient Antemortem Conduction Disturbances

- Usually not associated with identifiable structural abnormality

MAJOR DISEASES AFFECTING CARDIAC CONDUCTION SYSTEM

Congenital Atrioventricular Block

- Usually "benign" clinically
  - Eventual pacemaker therapy
- Lack of connection to atrial myocytes
- Fatty replacement of AV nodal structures
- Fibrosis and septation (bands of fibrosis dividing nodal myocyte groups)
- Increased fibrosis of basal ventricular septal "summit"

Sarcoidosis

- Predilection for subendocardium and conduction pathways
- May relate to density of lymphatics in these areas
- Identical to sarcoidosis elsewhere
  - Nonnecrotizing granulomas
  - Fibrosis and chronic inflammation
  - Infectious causes should be excluded

Myocarditis

- Conduction disturbance may occur in acute or chronic phase
- Sinus node dysfunction usually reflects direct involvement of sinoatrial node myocytes
- AV node dysfunction
  - Direct involvement by inflammation
  - Stunning through lymphatic drainage of toxic substrates
- Can occur in all myocarditis etiologies
  - Infections (viral, bacterial, fungal)
  - Toxins (drug, chemotherapy)
  - Hypersensitivity
  - Autoimmune
- Ventricular arrhythmias also common in myocarditis
  - Foci of electrical excitability in damaged ventricular myocardium

Cystic Tumor of Atrioventricular Node

- Biologically indolent
  - Slow growing
  - Never metastasizes
- May replace AV node entirely
- Wide age range at presentation
  - Diverse electrocardiogram manifestations
    - AV block (narrow QRS on electrocardiogram)
    - Ventricular arrhythmias (wide QRS on electrocardiogram)
  - Sudden death may be presenting sign
- Histopathology
  - Variably sized epithelial-lined cysts
  - Cyst lining ranging from squamoid (stratified) to simple cuboidal
  - Fibroblastic stroma and hemorrhage surrounding cysts
  - Often grossly inapparent

Lenègre Disease

- Idiopathic fibrosis of AV node
- Heritable component
- Several genes implicated
  - Cardiac morphogenesis
  - Cardiac structural proteins
  - Cardiac ion channels
- Histopathology
  - Fibrotic replacement, septation
  - Fatty infiltrate
  - Sparse inflammation in some cases

Others

- Amyloid

- Ischemic heart disease
  - AV nodal artery is typically primary branch of proximal right coronary artery
  - Right coronary artery territory infarction may be associated with direct AV node ischemic injury
  - Left bundle branches are most vulnerable in septal wall infarction
  - Chronic ischemia to nodal areas may result in increased fibrosis
- Metastasis
  - Any primary site possible
  - Disseminated lymphoma also reported
- Fabry disease

PATHOLOGY OF ENDOVASCULAR ABLATION PROCEDURES FOR ARRHYTHMIAS

Technical Aspects

- Increasingly common due to improved imaging guidance and catheter-based mapping and energy delivery
- Radiofrequency and high-frequency ultrasound energy
- Controlled "dose" delivery
- Catheter tip irrigation to limit scatter and improve precision

MR Mapping

- Used at some centers

3D Endovascular Electrophysiologic Mapping

- Used to identify target areas

Complications

- Possible injury to phrenic nerve, esophageal wall (in pulmonary vein isolation procedures)

Histopathologic Changes

- Acute
  - Cautery-like thermal injury
  - Infarct-like myocyte damage, edema, hemorrhage, distinct borders
  - Influx of neutrophils
- Chronic
  - Discrete punched-out areas of dense collagenous replacement fibrosis
  - Sharp interface with surrounding normal myocardium
  - Occasional mesenchymal heterotopia (chondroid, osseous)

SELECTED REFERENCES

1. Jansen H et al: Anatomy for ablation of atrioventricular nodal reentry tachycardia and accessory pathways. Herzschrittmacherther Elektrophysiol. 33(2):133-47, 2022
2. Tretter JT et al: Miniseries 1-part III: 'behind the scenes' in the triangle of Koch. Europace. 24(3):455-63, 2022
3. Karki R et al: Anatomy and pathology of the cardiac conduction system. Card Electrophysiol Clin. 13(4):569-84, 2021
4. Tan SY et al: Dissecting the cardiac conduction system: is it worthwhile? Pediatr Dev Pathol. 23(6):413-23, 2020
5. Cohle SD: Cystic tumour of the atrioventricular node: case report and literature review. Forensic Sci Res. 4(3):287-9, 2019
6. Frustaci A et al: Pathology and function of conduction tissue in Fabry disease cardiomyopathy. Circ Arrhythm Electrophysiol. 8(4):799-805, 2015
7. Ho SY: Anatomy of the atrioventricular junction, atrioventricular grooves, and accessory pathways. Card Electrophysiol Clin. 12(4):437-45, 2020
8. Jongbloed MR et al: Normal and abnormal development of the cardiac conduction system; implications for conduction and rhythm disorders in the child and adult. Differentiation. 84(1):131-48, 2012
9. Arbustini E et al: Autosomal dominant dilated cardiomyopathy with atrioventricular block: a lamin A/C defect-related disease. J Am Coll Cardiol. 39(6):981-90, 2002
10. Wang JN et al: Complete atrioventricular block following myocarditis in children. Pediatr Cardiol. 23(5):518-21, 2002
11. Gollob MH et al: Identification of a gene responsible for familial Wolff-Parkinson-White syndrome. N Engl J Med. 344(24):1823-31, 2001
12. Tan HL et al: A sodium-channel mutation causes isolated cardiac conduction disease. Nature. 409(6823):1043-7, 2001
13. McGuire MA et al: Atrioventricular junctional tissue. Discrepancy between histological and electrophysiological characteristics. Circulation. 94(3):571-7, 1996
14. Bharati S et al: Cardiac conduction system involvement in sudden death of obese young people. Am Heart J. 129(2):273-81, 1995
15. Michaëlsson M et al: Isolated congenital complete atrioventricular block in adult life. A prospective study. Circulation. 92(3):442-9, 1995
16. Bharati S et al: The conduction system findings in sudden cardiac death. J Cardiovasc Electrophysiol. 5(4):356-66, 1994
17. Gamache MC et al: Histopathological study following catheter guided radiofrequency current ablation of the slow pathway in a patient with atrioventricular nodal reentrant tachycardia. Pacing Clin Electrophysiol. 17(2):247-51, 1994
18. James TN: Congenital disorders of cardiac rhythm and conduction. J Cardiovasc Electrophysiol. 4(6):702-18, 1993
19. Bharati S et al: The conduction system in transplanted hearts. Chest. 102(4):1182-8, 1992
20. Kurosawa H et al: The conduction bundle at the atrioventricular junction. An anatomical study. Eur J Cardiothorac Surg. 3(4):283-7, 1989
21. Carter JB et al: Congenital heart block. Anatomic correlations and review of the literature. Arch Pathol. 97(1):51-7, 1974
22. Lev M et al: The pathogenesis of atrioventricular block in coronary disease. Circulation. 42(3):409-25, 1970
23. Lev M: The pathology of complete atrioventricular block. Prog Cardiovasc Dis. 6:317-26, 1964

Sinoatrial Block Removal

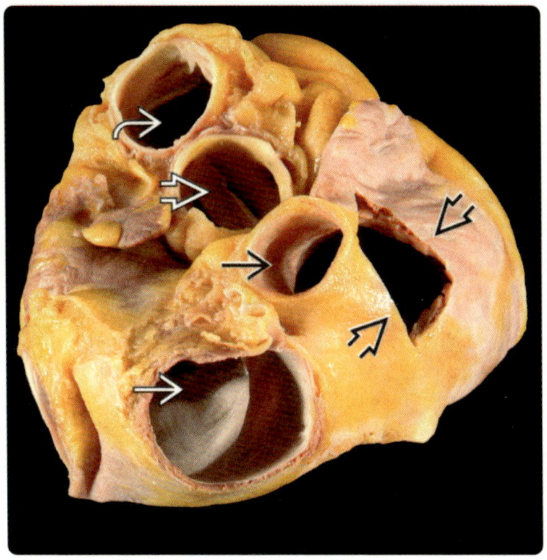

Sinoatrial Node Tissue Block (Prior to Sectioning)

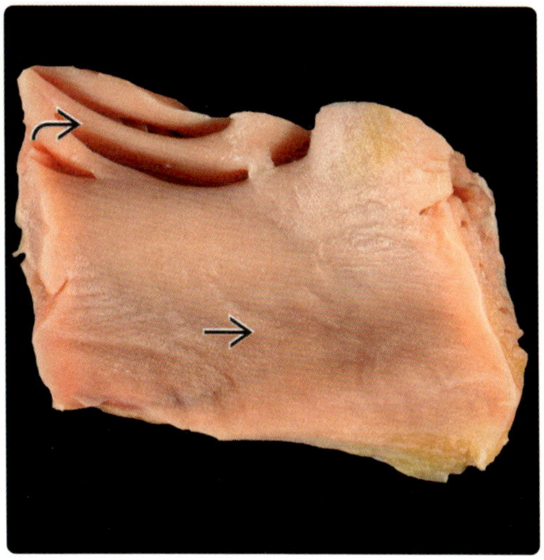

(Left) *This superior view of the heart shows the location of the tissue block removed for examination of the sinoatrial node. The pulmonary artery, aorta, superior vena cava, and left atrium are labeled for orientation.* **(Right)** *Viewed from the endocardial aspect, this sinoatrial node tissue block consists of a portion of terminal crest with a few pectinate muscles attached. The overlying epicardium (not seen, facing down) is intact.*

Sinoatrial Node: Serial Sections

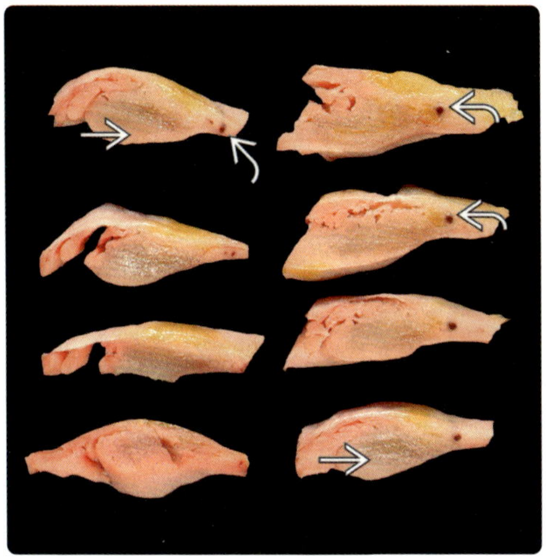

Sinoatrial Nodal Artery

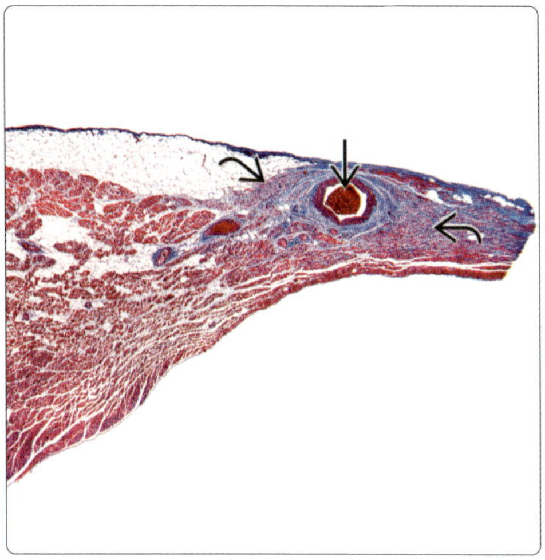

(Left) *After serial sectioning the tissue block, the belly of the terminal crest is now seen in cross section in each piece. The pinpoint sinus nodal artery can also be seen in many of the sections, identifying the location of the sinoatrial node.* **(Right)** *This cross section illustrates the dense, connective tissue-rich sinoatrial node tissue surrounding the sinus node artery.*

Sinoatrial Node: Fatty Infiltration

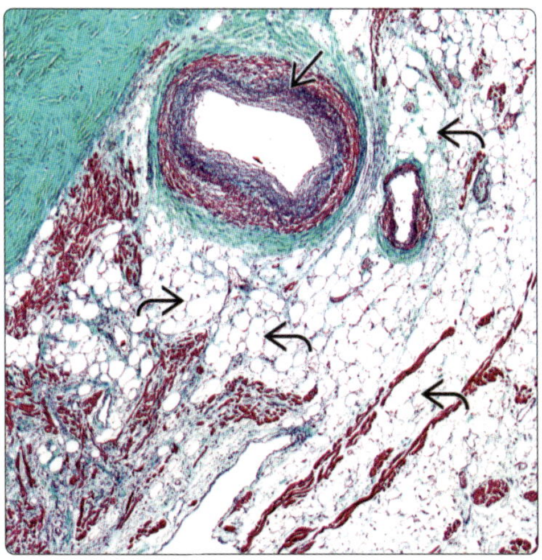

Sinoatrial Node: Fibrosis

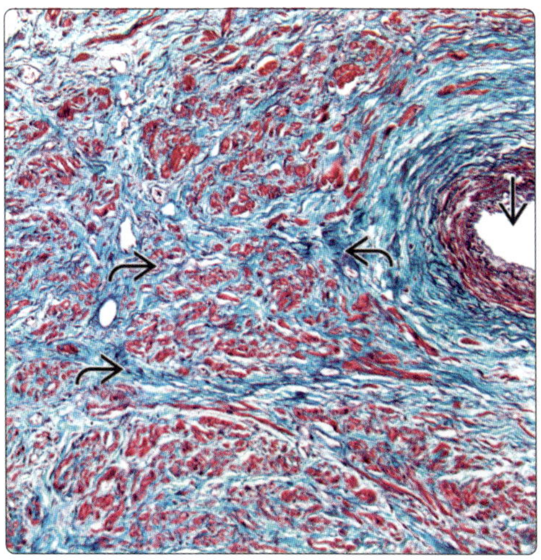

(Left) *This sinoatrial node from a 52-year-old man with sinus node dysfunction shows prominent fatty infiltration of the sinoatrial node. The sinus node artery is otherwise normal.* **(Right)** *This sinoatrial node from a patient with sick sinus syndrome shows increased interstitial fibrosis (blue green) within the sinoatrial node. The sinus node artery is otherwise normal. Clinical-pathologic correlation is essential in such cases.*

(**Left**) *This view of the opened right heart shows the defect after removing the tissue block containing the AV node (inside Koch triangle). The superior vena cava and pulmonary outflow tract are labeled for orientation.* (**Right**) *This view of the opened left heart demonstrates that the excised tissue block also includes a portion of anterior mitral valve leaflet (and aortomitral fibrous continuity).*

Atrioventricular Node: Removal (Right Side)

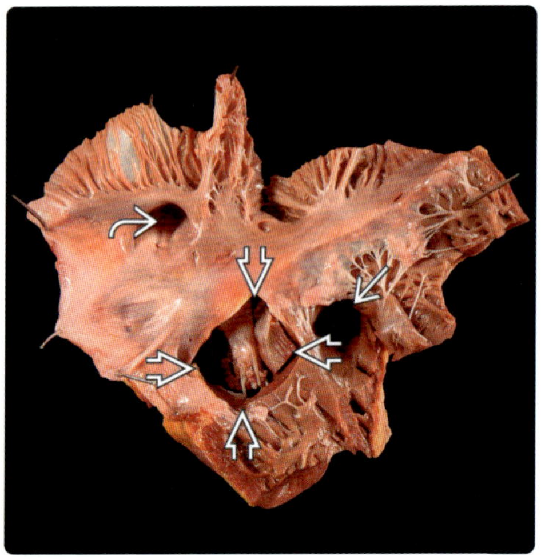

Atrioventricular Node: Removal (Left Side, Mitral)

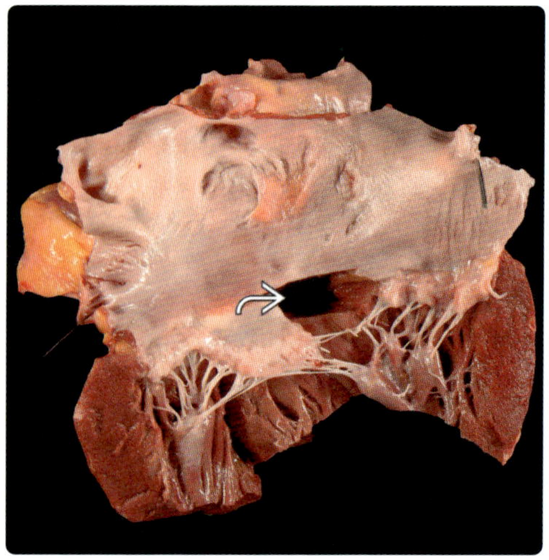

(**Left**) *The left-facing aspect of the AV node tissue block is shown here with membranous septum and pockets of 2 aortic valve cusps labeled for orientation.* (**Right**) *Serial cross sections through the excised AV node tissue block illustrate portions of tricuspid valve leaflet, membranous (AV) septum, and aortic valve cusp. Occasionally, the AV nodal artery may be seen grossly in the tricuspid annular fibrosa (not seen here).*

Atrioventricular Node Tissue Block (Prior to Sectioning)

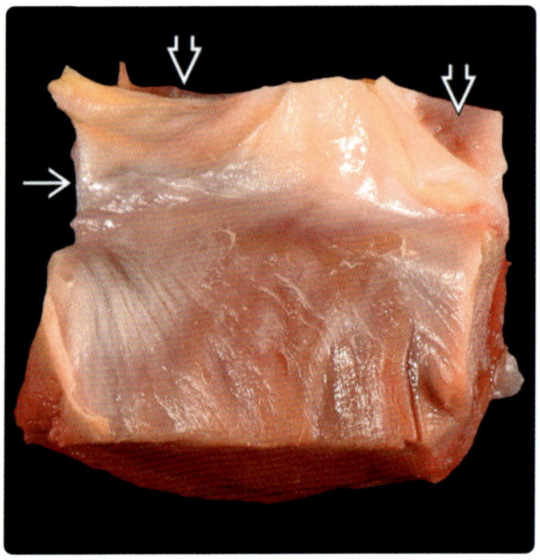

Atrioventricular Node: Serial Sections

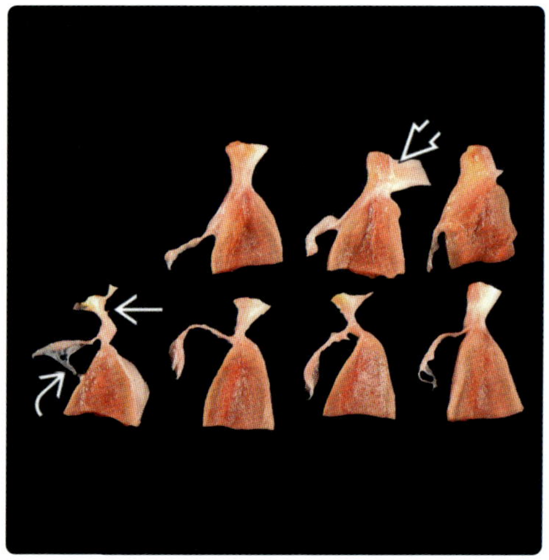

(**Left**) *The proximal bulbar portion of the AV node is shown here, seated within the annular fibrosa and insulated from the myocardium proper by dense collagen (blue). A portion of tricuspid valve leaflet is shown for orientation.* (**Right**) *This image shows the more distal bundle branches straddling the septal myocardium. The branches emanate from the His bundle. The right bundle is thin and cord-like. The left bundle is typically thicker and splays widely across the septum.*

Atrioventricular Node: Normal Histology

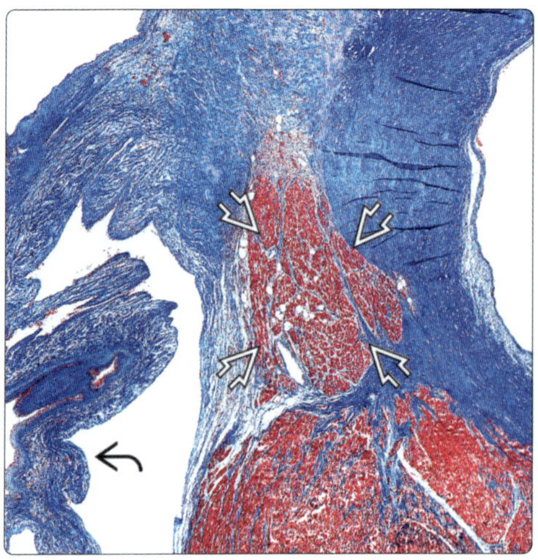

His Bundle and Bundle Branches: Normal Histology

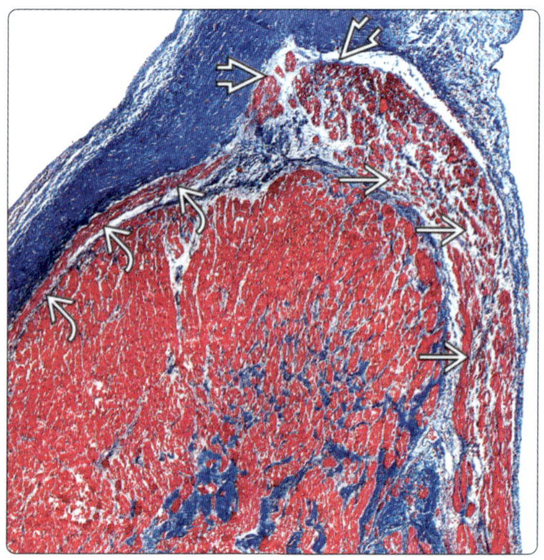

Low Magnification of Atrioventricular Node

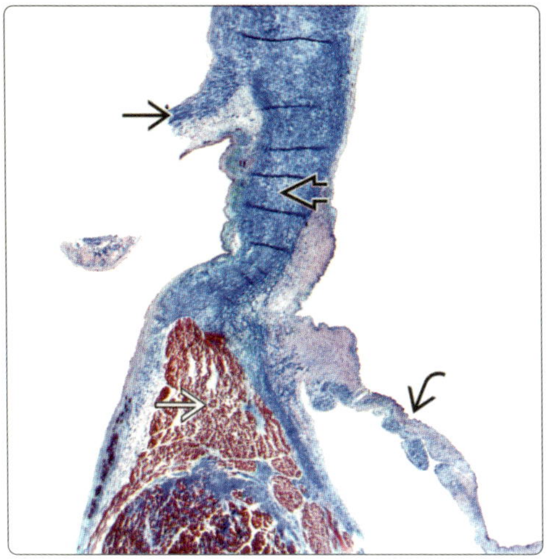

Left Bundle Branch

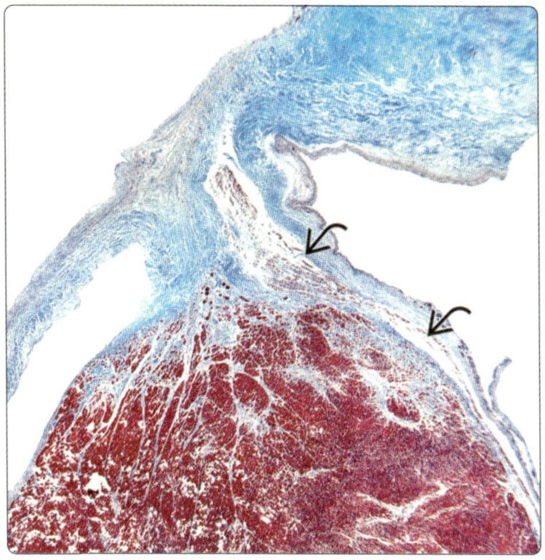

(Left) *This low-power photomicrograph shows the position of the AV node → just beneath the AV septum →, defined by the tricuspid valve septal leaflet → and the anterior mitral leaflet →.* **(Right)** *The left bundle branch → is larger and broadly splays out beneath the left ventricular outflow tract endocardium. The specialized myocytes are smaller than the adjacent normal myocardial myocytes and may also be more vacuolated.*

Atrioventricular Node: Normal Histology

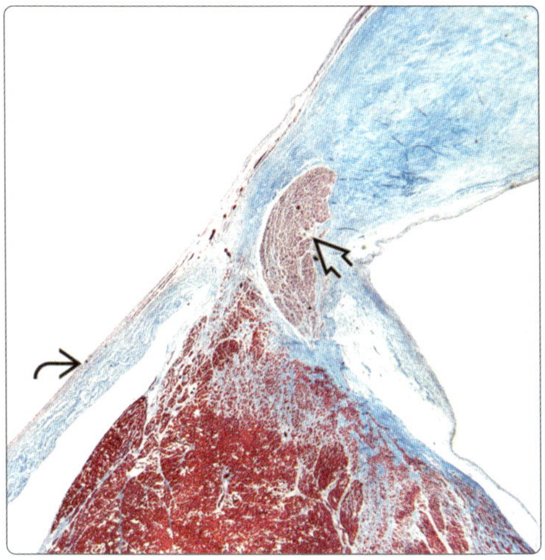

His Bundle and Right Bundle Branch: Normal Histology

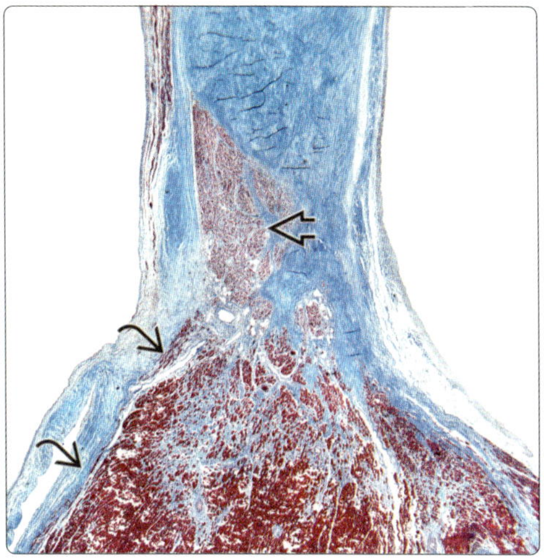

(Left) *Intermixed dense collagen and small myocytes comprise the AV node →, situated in the annular connective tissue, insulated from the atrial and ventricular myocardium. A portion of mitral valve leaflet → is also seen.* **(Right)** *The right bundle branch → consists of a thin, cord-like wisp of conduction system myocytes arising from the main His bundle →. Because of its small size, step sections through the paraffin block are typically required to see it well.*

Atrioventricular Node: High Magnification

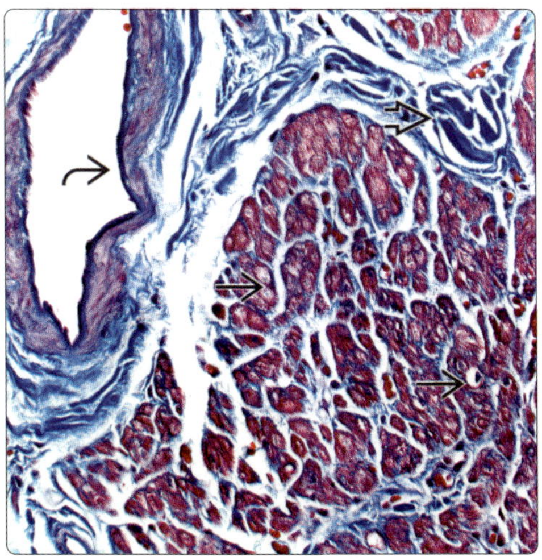

Atrioventricular Node: Medium Magnification

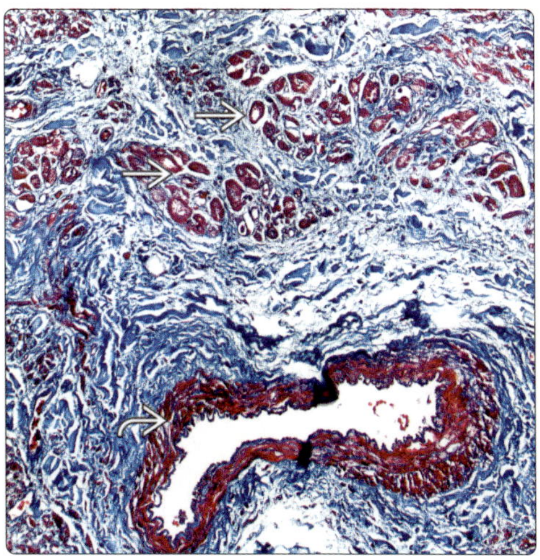

(Left) *This trichrome-stained section shows a portion of the AV node with accompanying AV nodal artery →. The conduction system myocytes are compact and show vacuolization of the sarcoplasm →. There is also dense collagenous connective tissue in the node →.* **(Right)** *This trichrome-stained section shows a portion of normal sinoatrial node with accompanying sinus node artery →. The nodal myocytes show prominent vacuolization →.*

(Left) *This image shows abundant fat in and around the specialized conducting cells of the AV node (note the landmark AV nodal artery). Determining how much fat is abnormal is somewhat subjective.* **(Right)** *This AV node section from a cardiac allograft in a patient with Mobitz type 2 heart block shows cardiac allograft vasculopathy affecting the AV nodal artery and mononuclear inflammation associated with the AV node myocytes.*

Fatty Infiltration Around Atrioventricular Node

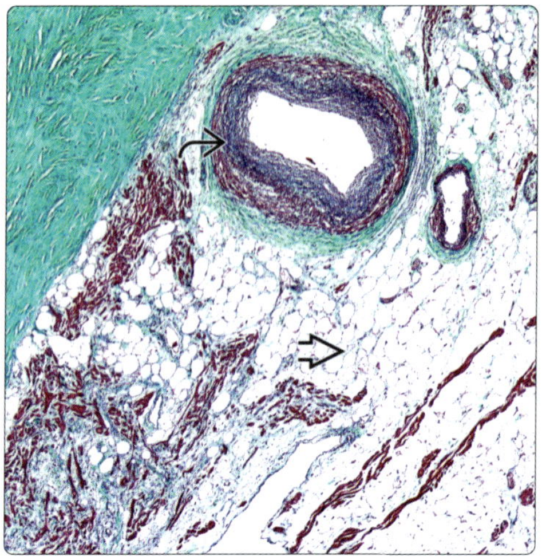

Atrioventricular Node in Allograft With Cardiac Allograft Vasculopathy

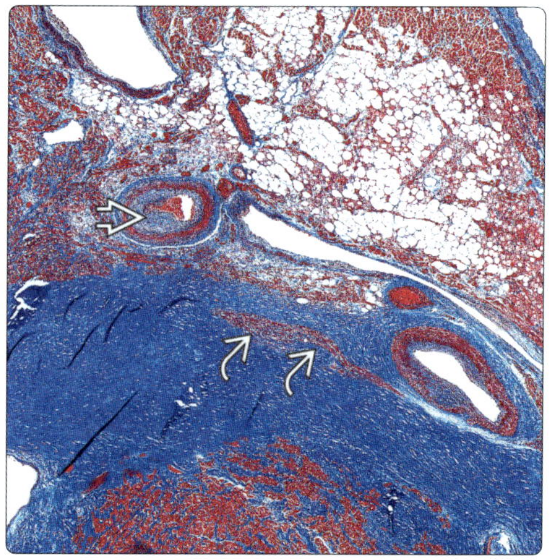

(Left) *This higher magnification view of the heart shows a mix of mononuclear cells with apparent injury to the AV nodal myocytes.* **(Right)** *This AV node tissue block section from a sudden cardiac death autopsy shows a grossly variegated, ill-defined mass lesion in the vicinity of the AV node. The aortic valve and tricuspid valve leaflets are labeled for orientation.*

Atrioventricular Node in Allograft With Rejection

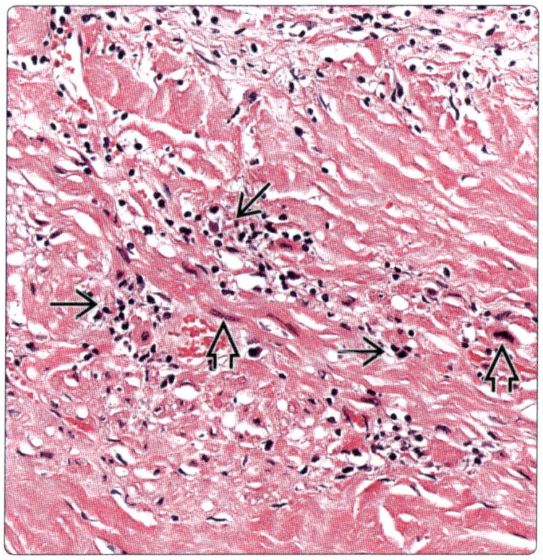

Cystic Tumor of Atrioventricular Node (Gross)

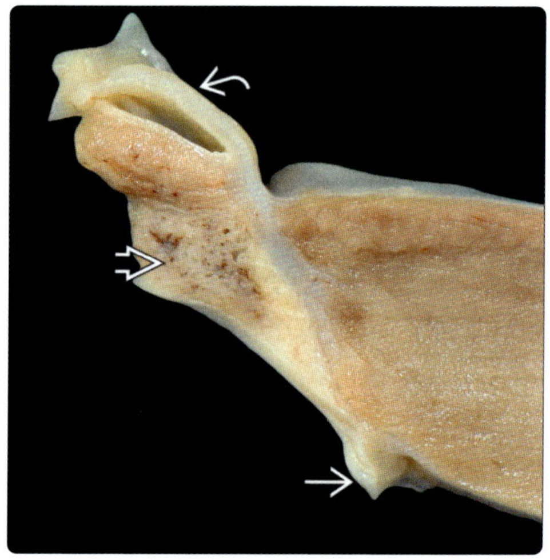

(Left) *Histologically, this mass shows multiple cystic structures lined by squamoid to cuboidal epithelium, features diagnostic of cystic tumor of the AV node.* **(Right)** *Higher magnification view of a cystic tumor of the AV node highlights the squamoid cyst lining and nests of mucinous cells.*

Cystic Tumor of Atrioventricular Node

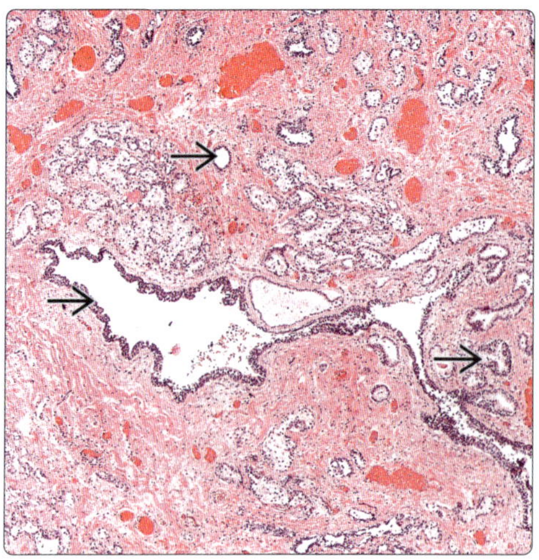

Cystic Tumor of Atrioventricular Node

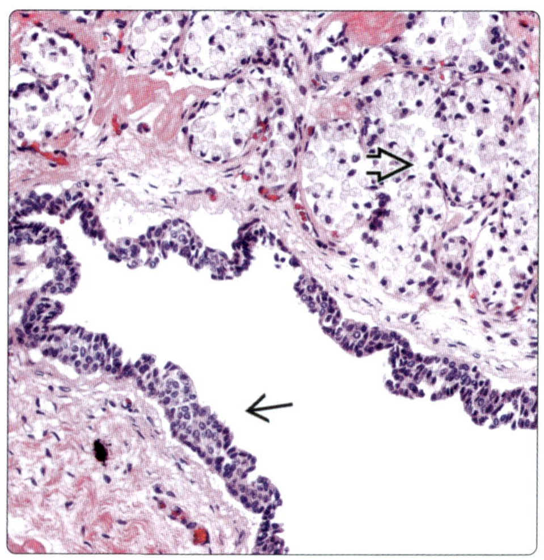

Amyloid Deposition in Atrioventricular Node: Trichrome Stain

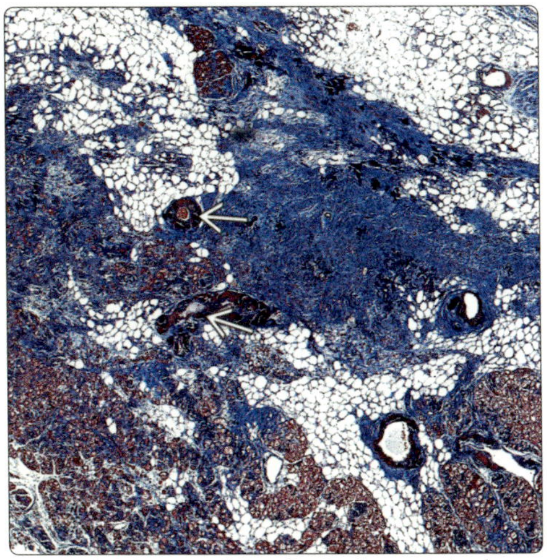

Amyloid Deposition in Atrioventricular Node: Sulfated Alcian Blue Stain

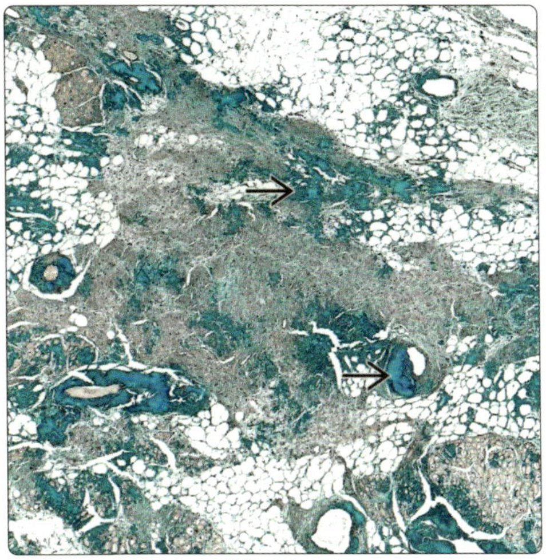

(Left) *Vascular deposition of amyloid → is apparent at low magnification within the vessel walls of the AV nodal tissue in this trichrome stain.* **(Right)** *Vascular deposition of amyloid → is apparent at low magnification around the AV nodal tissue in this sulfated alcian blue stain.*

Amyloid Deposition in Atrioventricular Node, Trichrome Stain: Higher Magnification

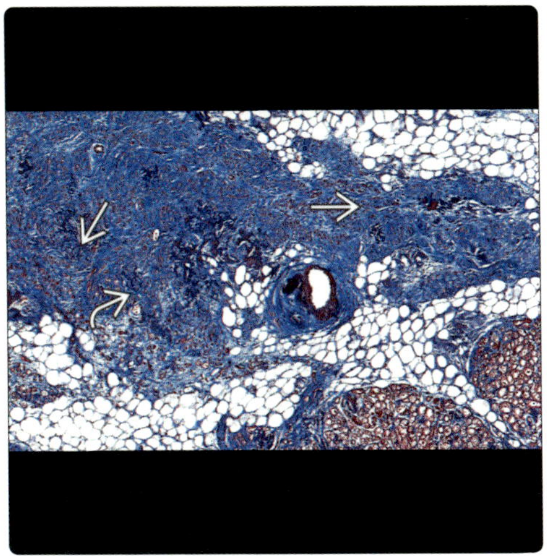

Amyloid Deposition in Atrioventricular Node: Sulfated Alcian Blue Stain, Higher Magnification

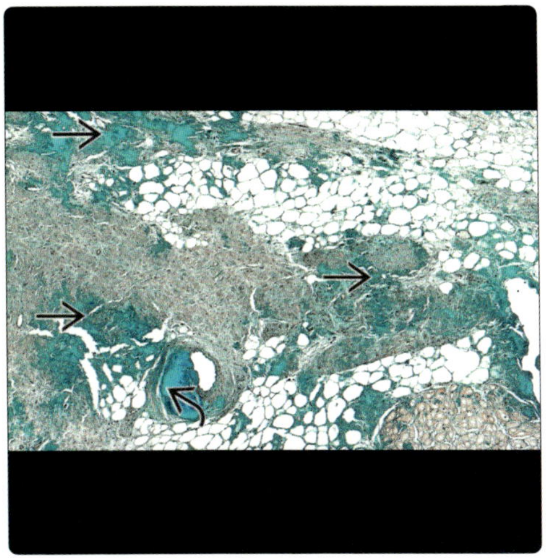

(Left) *This image shows deposits of amorphous and amphophilic material (amyloid) in the AV nodal artery ↪ and substance of the AV node →.* **(Right)** *This image shows deposits of amorphous and jade green (alcian blue-positive) material (amyloid) in the AV nodal artery ↪ and substance of the AV node →.*

Replacement Fibrosis in Atrioventricular Node

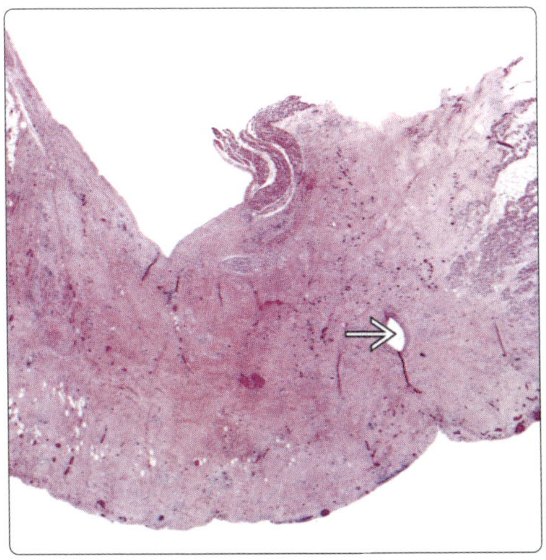

Replacement Fibrosis in Atrioventricular Node: Trichrome Stain

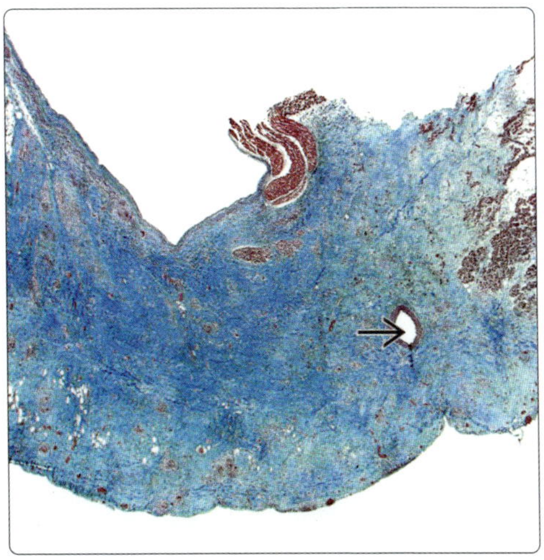

(Left) *The AV nodal artery → is apparent in this image, but no specialized conducting cells are present. Instead, there is fibrosis throughout the AV septal wall. This could be seen in Lenègre disease or when there has been prior surgery in this region.* **(Right)** *The AV nodal artery → is apparent in this image, but no specialized conducting cells are present. Instead, there is fibrosis throughout the AV septal wall.*

CLINICAL IMPLICATIONS

Ventricular Assist Devices in Clinical Practice

- Use of ventricular assist devices (VADs) has increased exponentially since USA FDA approval of HeartMate 2 in 2008
- Supports circulation during profound heart failure in 4 settings
  - Bridge to recovery: Temporary support until ventricular function is regained
    - For potentially reversible causes of heart failure (e.g., myocarditis)
    - Ventricular rest or unloading potentially allows for tissue healing
    - Recovery and pump removal is still rare event overall
  - Bridge to transplant: Support until donor heart is available
    - Duration may vary from weeks to years
  - Destination therapy: Provides support indefinitely (for patients who are not candidates for transplantation)
    - Increasingly becoming viable alternative to transplantation
    - Survival on VADs is expected to approach that of transplantation (average: 10-15 years) in future
    - Avoids expense and complications of immunosuppression and rejection monitoring
  - Bridge to decision: Support while determining candidacy for transplantation
    - Later transitioned to either destination therapy or transplantation

Left Ventricular Assist Device Applications

- Most common use of VAD
  - For profound systolic heart failure
  - Left ventricular dilatation must be present to allow adequate intake without "suction events"
  - Initial right-sided (pulmonary circulation) failure generally improves with unloading of left ventricle
- Other VAD uses
  - In profound right heart failure, right-sided VAD may be used
  - In biventricular failure, heart replacement with total artificial heart may be necessary

Left Ventricular Assist Device Complications

- Thrombosis
  - Continuous axial flow (HeartMate 2)
    - Rare, but typically seen around bearing at tip of axial impeller
  - Magnetically levitated rotary pumps (HeartWare)
    - Ring of thrombus is frequently seen around inflow cannula at polished, smooth-to-rough surface transition point
    - While there is potential to partially dislodge and enter pump, this seems rare
  - Embolic complications
  - Hemolytic complications
- Driveline site infection
  - Localized purulence, slow to heal
  - May track along driveline to pump pocket
- Conduit obstruction
  - Kinking, other external impingement by variety of processes
  - Extrinsic compression due to dependent settling of fibrin within bend relief (HeartMate 3)
- Driveline integrity failure
  - Externalized portion of driveline is subject to damage (cutting, scraping, melting, catching, chewing by pets, etc.)

INTERMACS

Interagency Registry for Mechanical Circulatory Support

- Postmarket monitoring of VAD use and outcomes
- > 36,000 patients followed
- Currently for continuous flow pumps, actuarial survival is 82-87% at 1 year and 74% at 2 years

HeartWare HVAD Device

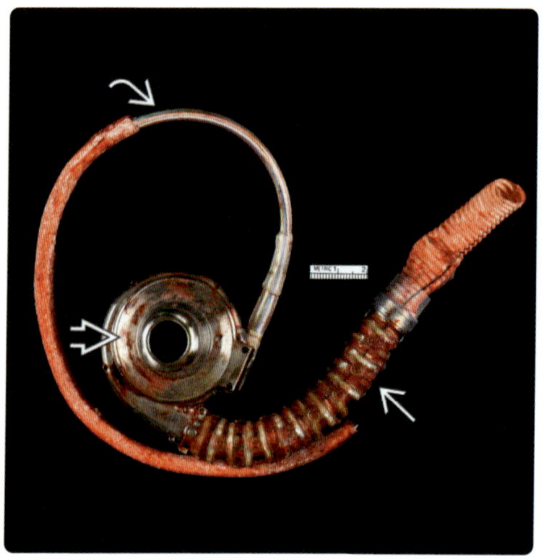

HeartMate 3 Device (Explanted Heart)

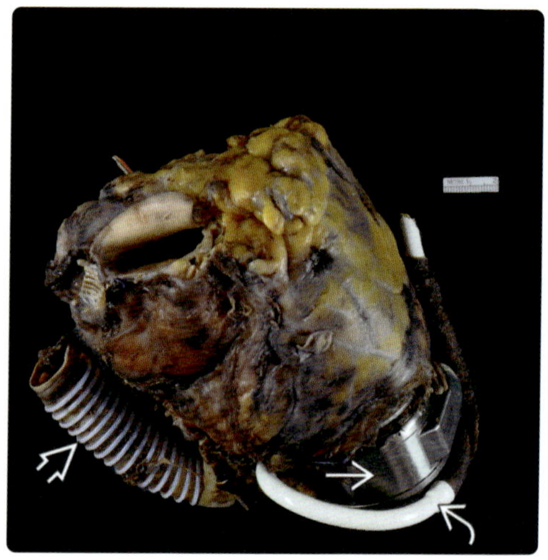

(Left) *This HeartWare HVAD device is implanted in the pericardial sac with the pump ➡ inserting directly into the left ventricle apex. The outflow conduit ➡ and driveline ➡ are also shown.* **(Right)** *A HeartMate 3 (intrapericardial) ventricular assist device ➡ with its outflow cannula ➡ and driveline ➡ is shown.*

Pulsatile Flow Pump Ventricular Assist Devices

Device Name	Manufacturer	Notes
EXCOR	Berlin Heart	Extracorporeal, pediatric applications
CardioWest	Syncardia Systems, Inc.	Total artificial heart
LVAD	Novacor	1st generation, now discontinued
BVS 5000	Abiomed	1st generation, now discontinued
HeartMate XVE	Thoratec	1st generation, now discontinued

Continuous Flow Pump Devices

Device Name	Manufacturer	Notes
HeartMate 2	Thoratec	1st FDA approval, now discontinued
HeartMate 3	Abbott	Similar to HVAD design but no smooth inflow cannula
HVAD	HeartWare, Inc.	Small size allows intrapericardial implantation
Heart Assist 5	MicroMed Cardiovascular, Inc.	Direct flow sensing and management
DuraHeart	Terumo Heart, Inc.	Centrifugal flow, magnetic levitation pump
2000 FlowMaker	Jarvik Heart, Inc.	Axial flow, magnetically driven pump
Impella	Abiomed	Axial flow, augments rather than replaces ventricle function

RESEARCH OPPORTUNITIES

Myocardial Recovery

- Multiple ongoing investigations exploring mechanisms of change during myocardial rest/unloading afforded by VAD support
  - Tissues obtained at time of VAD implantation and time of removal (recovery, transplant, autopsy)

TYPES OF VENTRICULAR ASSIST DEVICES

Extracorporeal

- Pump and controller external to body (EXCOR, BVS 5000)
- Easier to inspect circuit and replace components in event of clots
- More invasive, higher infection risk, less portable

Intracorporeal

- Intracardiac (HeartMate 3, HeartWare)
  - Direct cannulation of heart for inflow
  - Only driveline exits body, lower infection risk
  - Very portable with small battery packs and driver consoles
- Extracardiac (Tohuku EHAM)
  - Pneumatically driven sheath envelops ventricle
    - Sheath device compresses and relaxes similar to cardiac massage
  - Still in developmental testing phase

PATHOLOGIC EXAMINATION

Photographic Documentation

- External evaluation
  - Inflow cannula
  - Sewing ring
  - Outflow conduit
  - Driveline
- Internal examination
  - Open all conduits and examine for clots
  - Confirm cannula patency
  - Examine pump chamber (beam lighting and magnification or, if possible, pump disassembly)

Microscopy

- Any thrombus material
- Skin surrounding driveline exit site
- Any purulent material around device
- Aortic anastomosis

Additional Testing Modalities

- Scanning electron microscopy
  - Surface topography, biofilm, platelets, fibrin, abrasions, pitting, etc.
- Radiographs and CT scanning
  - Evaluate component integrity, mineralization, etc.

SELECTED REFERENCES

1. Jain SS et al: Outflow graft narrowing of the HeartMate 3 left ventricular assist device. Ann Thorac Surg. ePub, 2022
2. Molina EJ et al: The Society of Thoracic Surgeons Intermacs 2020 Annual Report. Ann Thorac Surg. 111(3):778-92, 2021
3. Duero Posada JG et al: Outflow graft occlusion of the HeartMate 3 left ventricular assist device. Circ Heart Fail. 10(9):e004275, 2017
4. Carpenter BA et al: A brief review of ventricular assist devices and a recommended protocol for pathology evaluations. Cardiovasc Pathol. 22(5):408-15, 2013
5. Garbade J et al: Heart transplantation and left ventricular assist device therapy: two comparable options in end-stage heart failure? Clin Cardiol. 36(7):378-82, 2013
6. Rose AG et al: Pathology in patients with ventricular assist devices: a study of 21 autopsies, 24 ventricular apical core biopsies and 24 explanted hearts. Cardiovasc Pathol. 14(1):19-23, 2005

(Left) *The HeartMate 2 device is implanted in the abdomen and connected to the heart by synthetic conduits. The pump body takes blood from the left ventricle apex and propels it into the ascending aorta. The pump is powered by an external battery pack via a Dacron-coated electric driveline.* **(Right)** *Clinical photograph shows the outflow cannula of a HeartMate 2 device with a nonocclusive thrombus. Thrombosis was thought to occur peritransplantation after reversing the patient's anticoagulation.*

HeartMate 2 Ventricular Assist Device

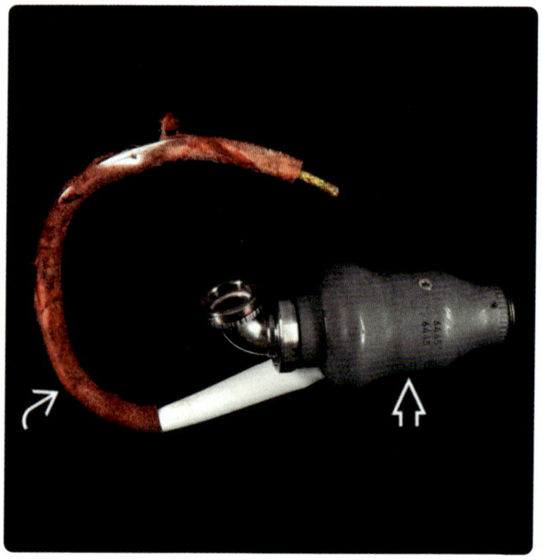

Outflow Cannula Thrombus (Recent)

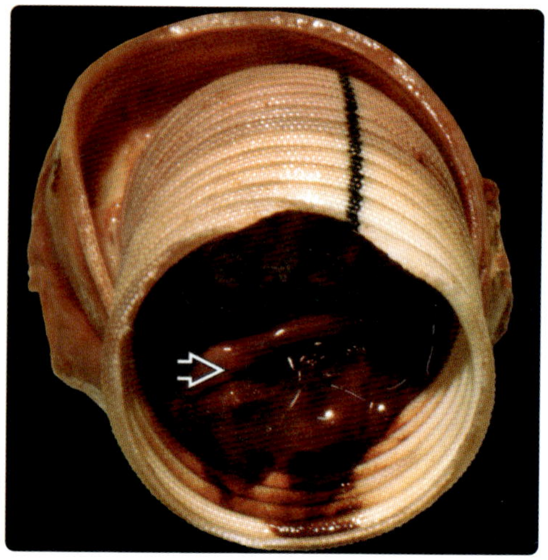

(Left) *This view into the pump chamber of a HeartMate 2 device demonstrates a white clot surrounding the driveshaft above the impeller. Thrombus formation is an important but infrequent complication of ventricular assist device therapy. Pathologic evaluation should include careful evaluation for clots.* **(Right)** *This view into the pump chamber of a HeartMate 2 device demonstrates a small circumferential clot surrounding the driveshaft above the impeller.*

White Clot Within HeartMate 2 Device

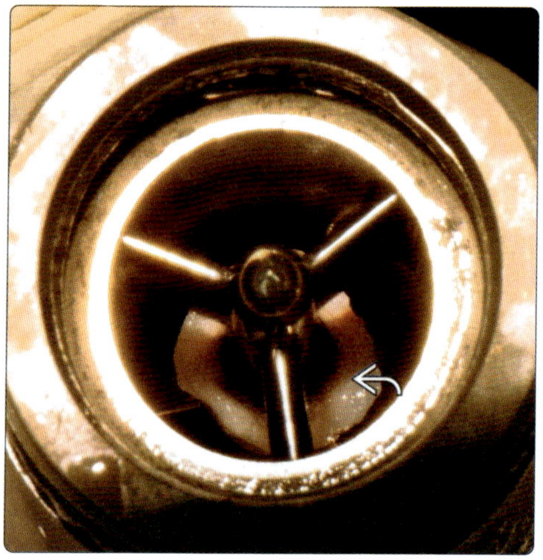

Clot Within HeartMate 2 Device

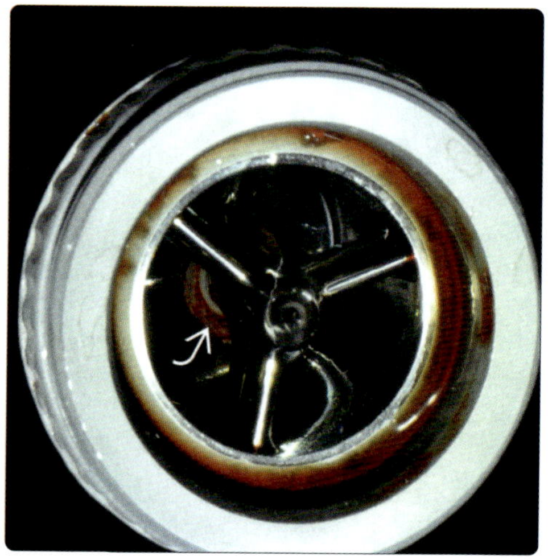

(Left) *After disassembly of a HeartMate 2 device, the driveshaft components are seen. A small, dark clot was present at the tip of the axial flow impeller.* **(Right)** *Histology of left ventricular assist device clots typically show prominent layering. The material is often amorphous and acellular (without identifiable platelets or recognizable structures), suggesting thermal coagulation change.*

HeartMate 2 Impeller

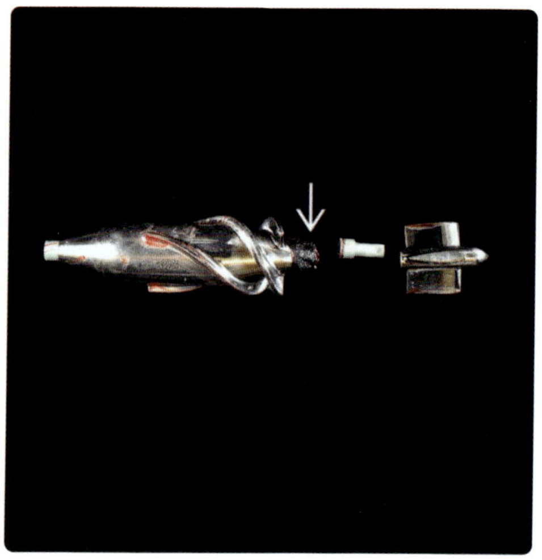

Histopathology of Left Ventricular Assist Device Clot

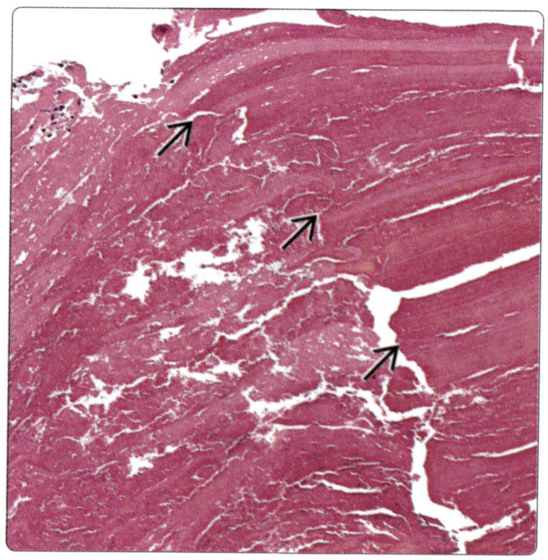

Shallow Thrombus (HeartWare HVAD Device)

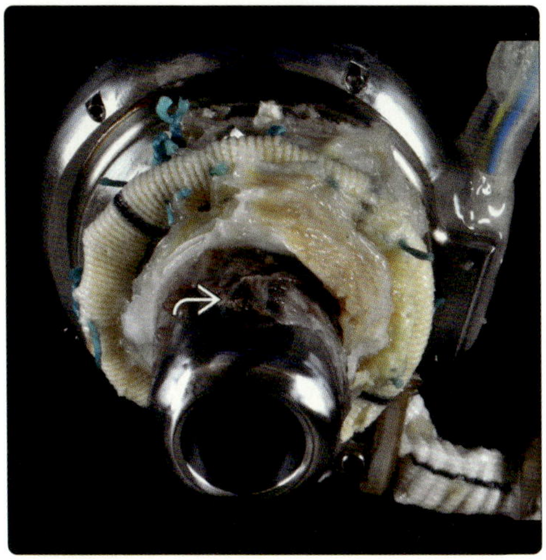

Device Thrombus (HeartWare HVAD Device)

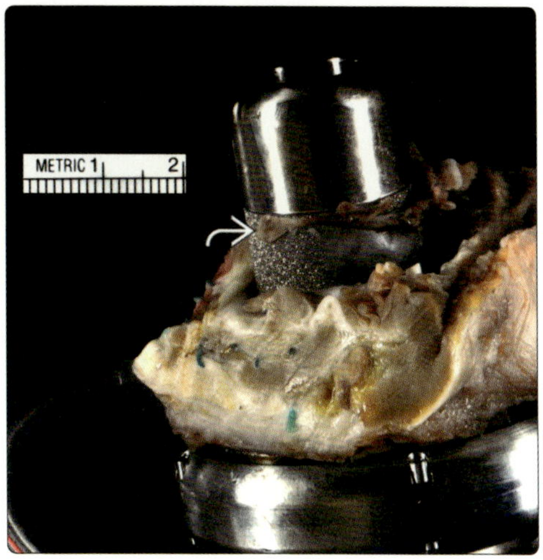

(Left) *This HeartWare HVAD device shows a small amount of thrombus near the base of the inflow port.* **(Right)** *This HeartWare HVAD device has a small, thread-like clot wrapping around the inflow port, centered on the smooth-to-rough transition point.*

HeartWare HVAD Device With Thrombus

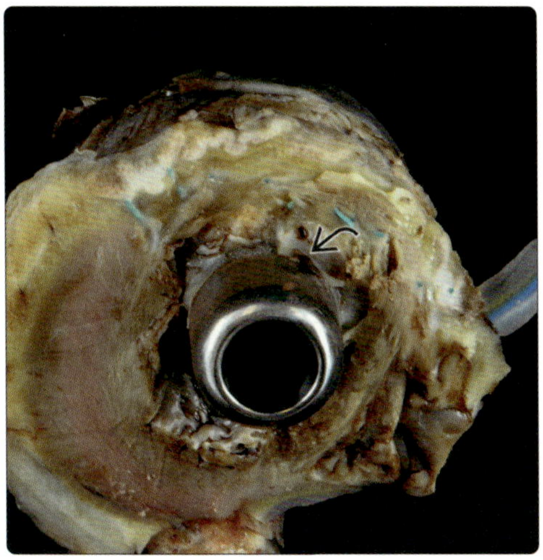

HeartWare HVAD Device With Inflow Cannula Clot

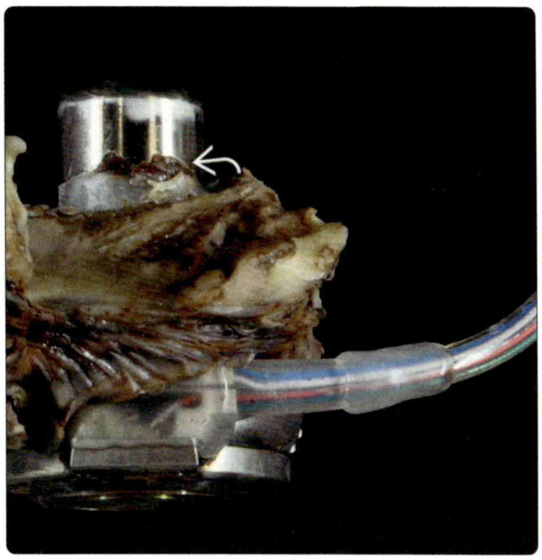

(Left) *This HeartWare HVAD device shows a recent-appearing clot at the rough-to-smooth interface of the inflow cannula port.* **(Right)** *This HeartWare HVAD device shows a recent clot wrapping around the inflow port, centered on the smooth-to-rough transition point.*

Thrombus Associated With HVAD Port

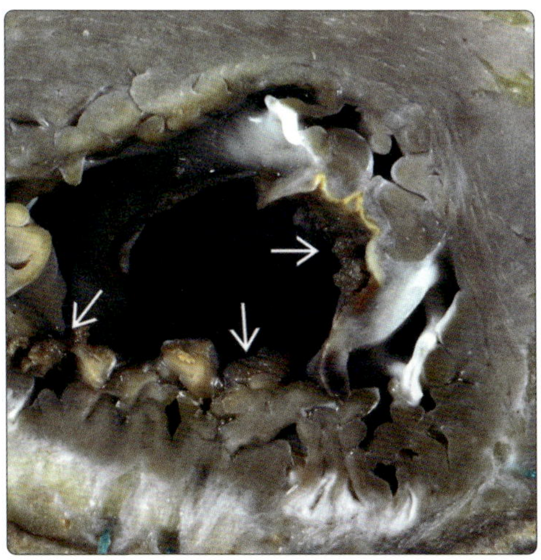

Histopathology of HVAD-Associated Thrombus

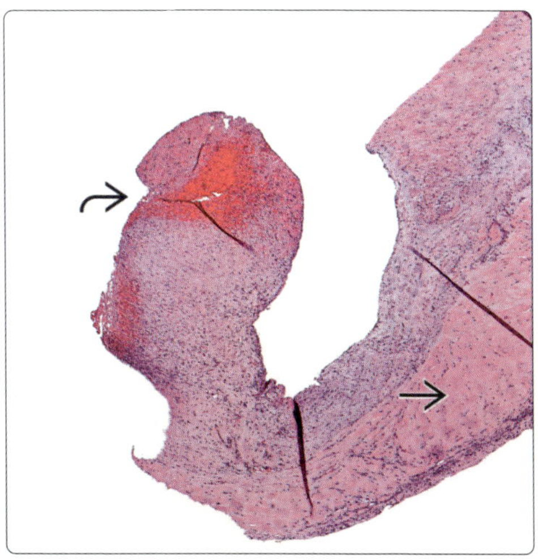

(Left) *This view of the left ventricle apex in short axis (after removal of the device) shows multiple shallow thrombi embedded in the trabeculae near the interface with the device.* **(Right)** *Thrombus removed from the inflow cannula of a HeartWare HVAD device shows the thrombus undergoing progressive organization. More recent thrombus transitions into areas of fibrotic organized thrombus.*

(Left) *The magnetically levitated impeller of this HeartWare HVAD device shows a translucent "gummy" deposit* ➡ *(degenerated clot) that led to increased power consumption detected in this pump.* **(Right)** *The same HeartWare HVAD device also showed a small amount of recent clot* ➡ *inside the pump. The impeller is still in place* ➡.

HeartWare HVAD Disassembled With Clot

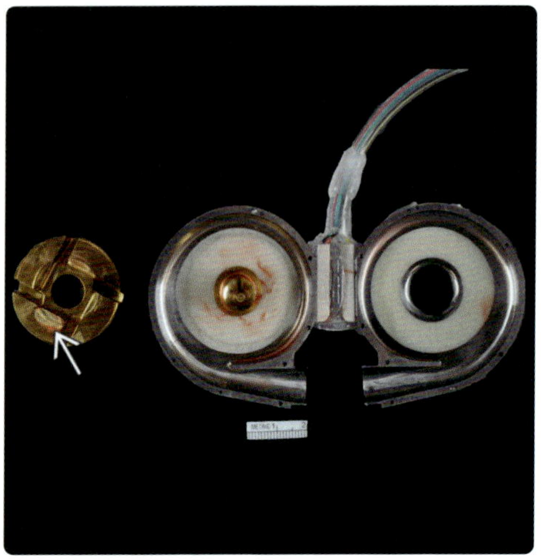

HeartWare HVAD Device: Internal Clot

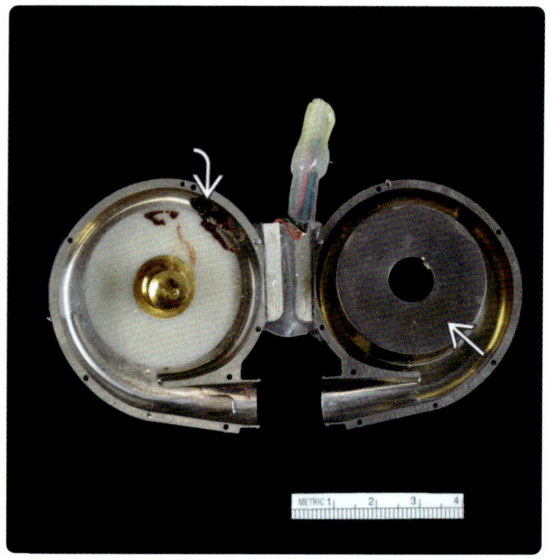

(Left) *The magnetically levitated impeller of this HeartWare HVAD device shows a translucent "gummy" deposit* ➡ *(degenerated clot).* **(Right)** *The impeller of this HeartWare HVAD device shows a translucent degenerated clot* ➡ *that led to increased power consumption detected in this pump in a patient that also showed evidence of intravascular hemolysis.*

HeartWare HVAD Impeller With Clot

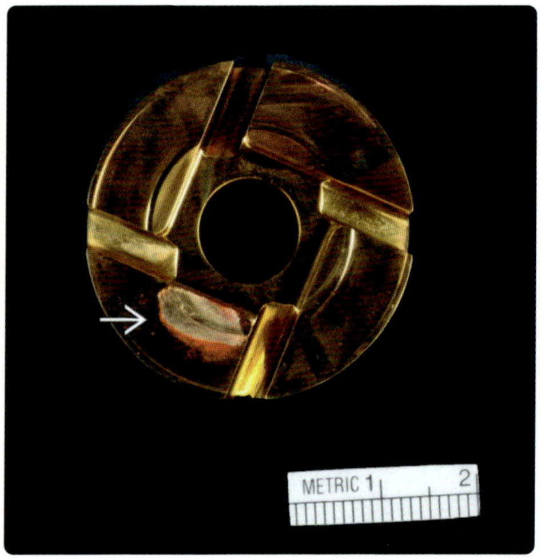

HeartWare HVAD Impeller With Clot

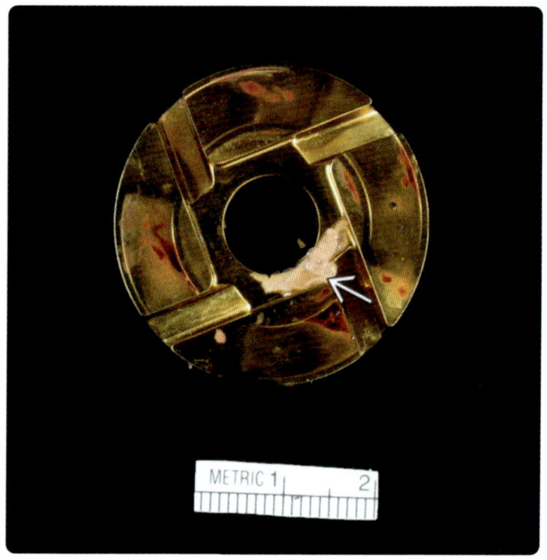

(Left) *After disassembly of this HeartWare HVAD device, a small, adherent, white translucent clot* ➡ *was present on the levitated rotary impeller.* **(Right)** *Photomicrograph shows the components making up a pump thrombus adherent to an HVAD impeller. There is mostly amorphous fibrin* ⇨ *with sparse, embedded leukocytes* →.

Clot Associated With HeartWare HVAD Pump Components

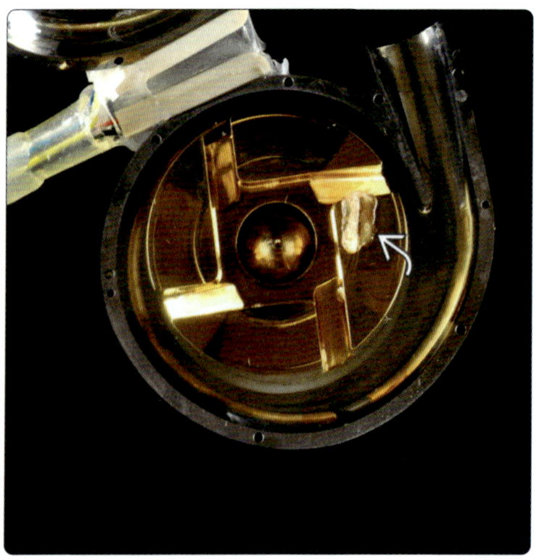

HVAD Pump Thrombus Histology

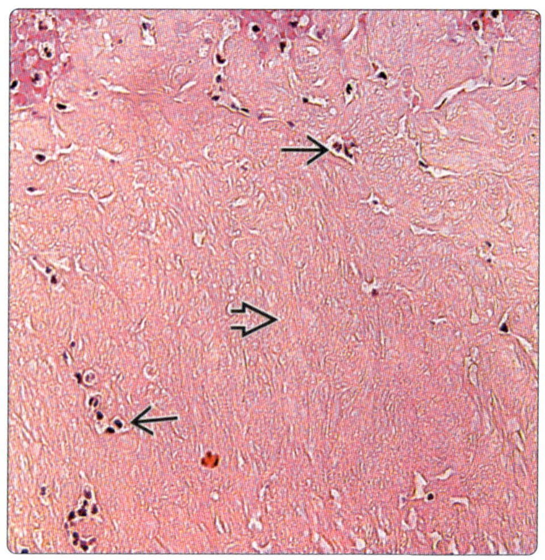

HeartMate 3 Inflow Cannula With Neointima

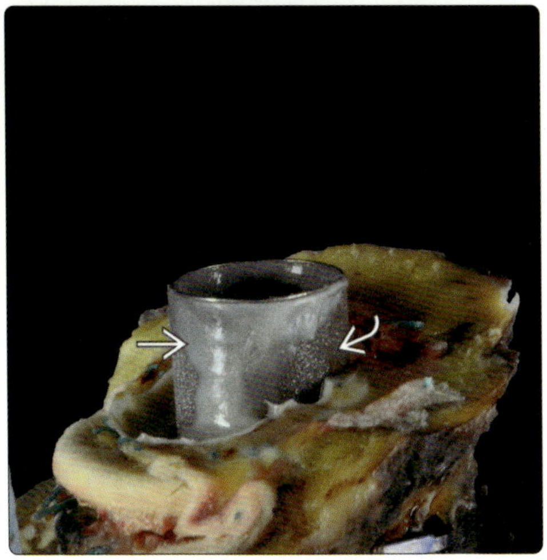

HeartMate 3 With Fibrin Compressing Outflow

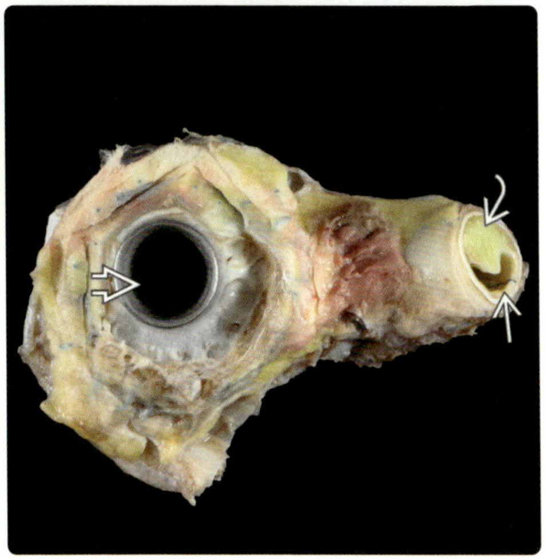

(Left) *The inflow cannula of the HeartMate 3 device lacks a smooth component. This is intended to help facilitate reendothelialization, as seen here (at least partially) →. An exposed "rough" surface → can also be seen.* **(Right)** *The inflow cannula → of this HeartMate 3 device is free from thrombus, but the outflow cannula shows some extrinsic compression due to fibrin → accumulating in the space between the open plastic bend relief and the inner tube graft →.*

HeartMate 3 Outflow Graft Compression

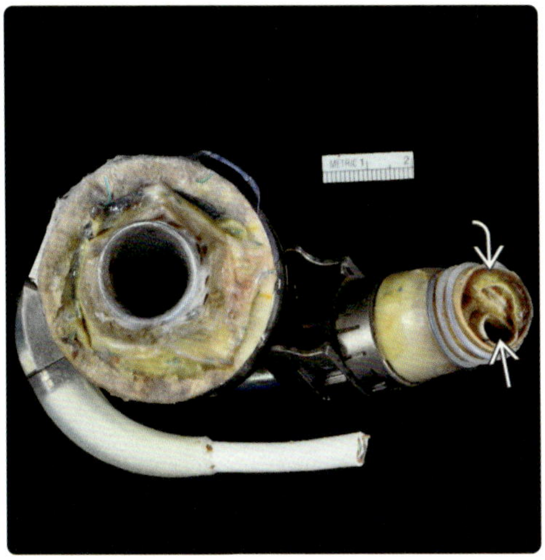

HeartMate 3 Outflow Compression

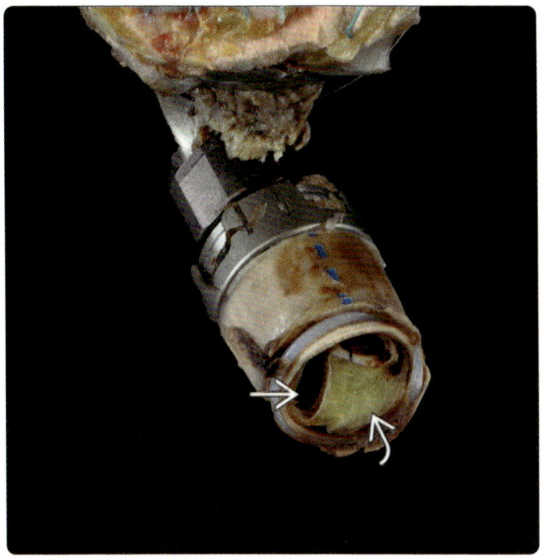

(Left) *The outflow of this HeartMate 3 device shows some extrinsic compression due to fibrin → accumulating in the space between the open plastic bend relief and the inner tube graft →.* **(Right)** *The outflow cannula of this HeartMate 3 device is free from thrombus, but the outflow graft shows some extrinsic compression due to fibrin → accumulating in the space between the plastic bend relief and the inner tube graft →.*

HeartMate 3 Outflow Cannular: Serially Sectioned

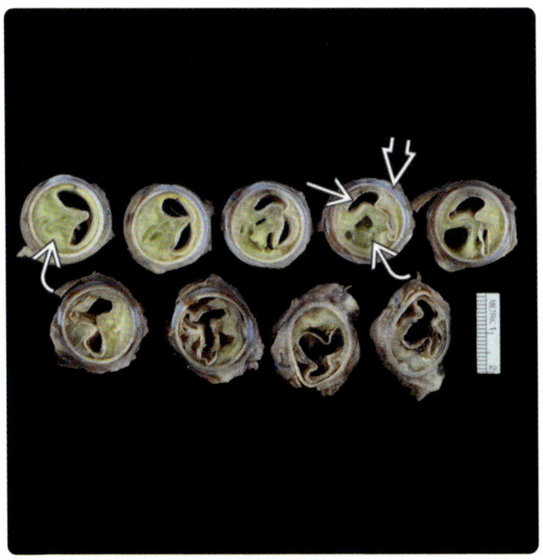

HeartMate 3 Outflow Cannular: Serially Sectioned

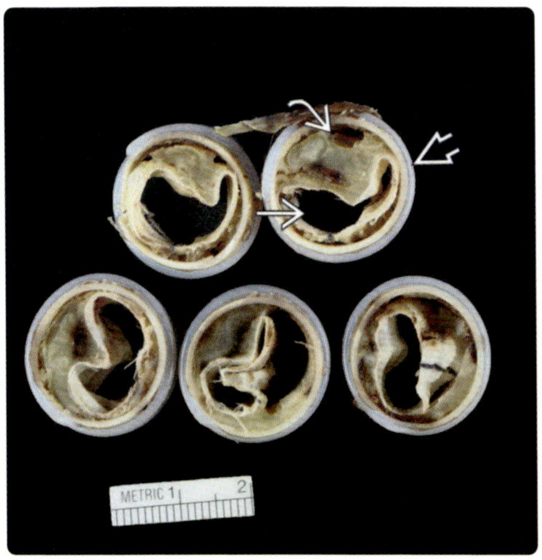

(Left) *Fibrin → accumulating in the potential space between the rigid plastic bend relief → and the inner synthetic tube graft → is shown, in this case leading to a degree of extrinsic compression.* **(Right)** *Fibrin → accumulating in the potential space between the rigid plastic bend relief → and the inner synthetic tube graft → is shown, in this case leading to a degree of extrinsic compression.*

Heart Weight (g)

Before Fixation	After Fixation	Normal Mean	Normal Range
____________	____________	____________	____________

Measurements (cm)

Left Ventricle	Right Ventricle	Aortic	Mitral	Pulmonary	Tricuspid	Other
Anterior ________	Anterior ________	________	________	________	________	________
Inferior ________	Inferior ________					
Lateral ________	Lateral ________					
Septum ________						

Valves

Valve	Notes
Aortic	
Mitral	
Pulmonary	
Tricuspid	

Chambers

Chamber	Hypertrophy	Dilation	Fibrosis	Other
Left ventricle	____________	____________	____________	____________
Right ventricle	____________	____________	____________	____________
Left atrium	____________	____________	____________	____________
Right atrium	____________	____________	____________	____________

Coronary Arteries

Parameter	Notes
Coronary dominance/ostia	
LMA	
LAD	
LCX	
RCA	

Coronary Artery/Bypass Graft

Location	Notes
Coronary Artery	
Stenosis proximal to anastomosis	
Stenosis distal to anastomosis	
Bypass Graft	
Aortic anastomosis	
Body of graft	
Coronary anastomosis	

This worksheet is intended to be photocopied and used as a practical aid in the evaluation of cardiac specimens. It is designed to help capture salient findings by marking up the diagrams and to facilitate report generation.

Coronary Arteries

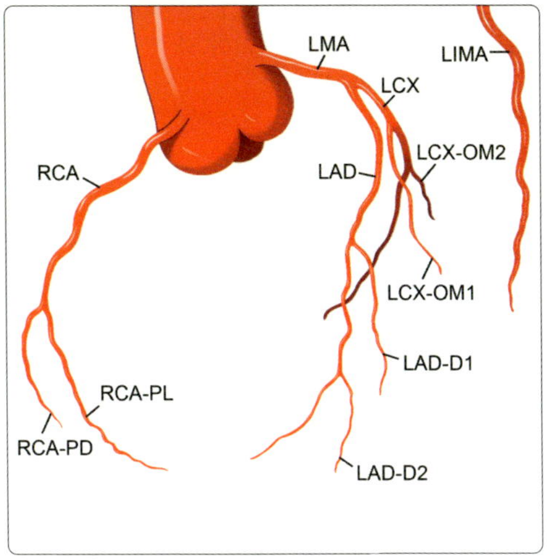

Basal Short Axis

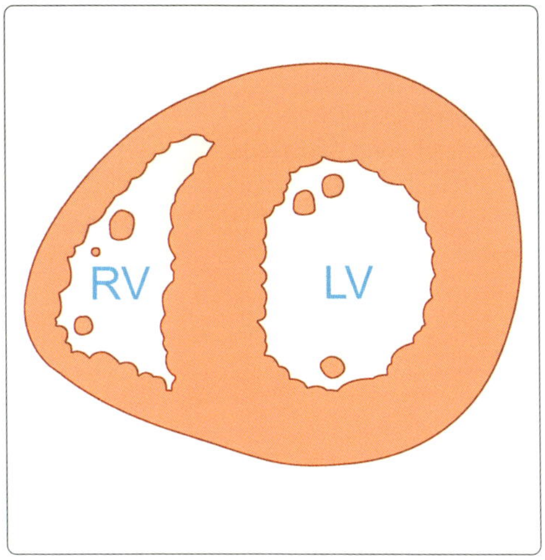

(Left) *Use coronary artery diagram to document findings.* **(Right)** *Use basal short-axis diagram to document findings.*

Basal Midshort Axis

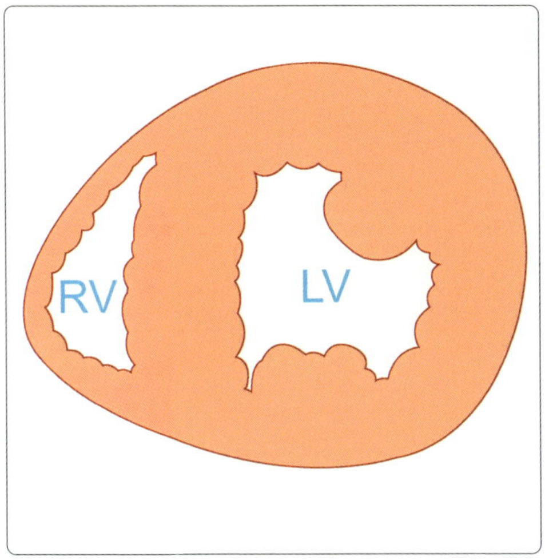

Midshort Axis

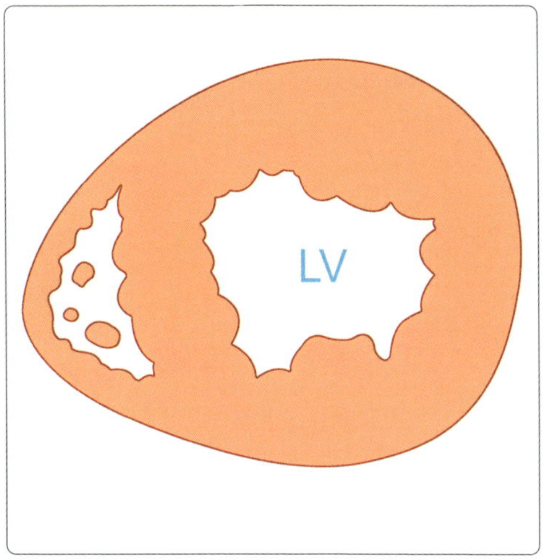

(Left) *Use basal midshort-axis diagram to document findings.* **(Right)** *Use midshort-axis diagram to document findings.*

Midapical Short Axis

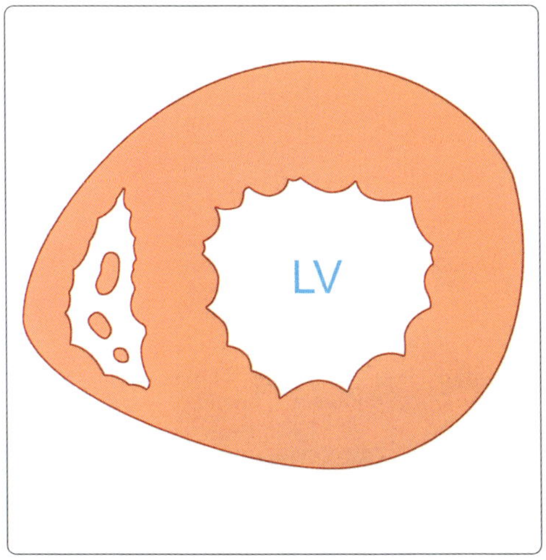

Apical Short Axis

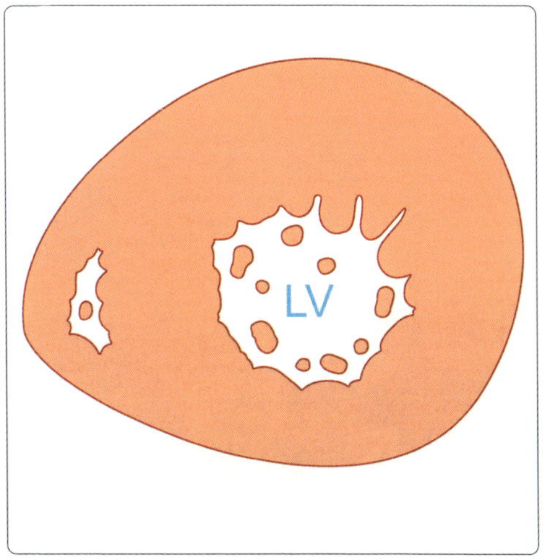

(Left) *Use midapical short-axis diagram to document findings.* **(Right)** *Use apical short-axis diagram to document findings.*

INTRODUCTION

Overview

- Cardiomyopathies are complex set of disorders often posing diagnostic challenges
- This document outlines systematic approach to cardiomyopathies, primarily on basis of gross pathologic features
- Main forms, classes, or "phenotypes" of cardiomyopathies are reviewed with attention to specific disease entities encompassed by each

ENDOMYOCARDIAL BIOPSY

Histopathologic Features

- Fibrosis and hypertrophy predominate
- Substantial overlap among classes and with secondary adaptive response to
  - Hypertension
  - Valvular disease
  - Ischemic heart disease
- Utility of biopsy in diagnosis and classification is limited
- Chronic changes (especially fibrosis) exclude reversible chamber dilatation (e.g., due to myocarditis)
- Biopsy can also rule out (or confirm)
  - Amyloidosis
  - Myocarditis
  - Hemochromatosis
  - Storage and infiltrative disease
  - Immune complex disease
- Myocyte disarray
  - Relatively specific for hypertrophic cardiomyopathy (HCM)
  - Cannot be reliably assessed in biopsies due to sampling and traumatic, disruptive nature of tissue tearing by bioptome
  - Better assessed on full-thickness (autopsy/explant) or septal myectomy specimens
  - Right ventricle shows comparatively minor changes in HCM, again limiting utility of biopsy

Complex Cardiac Autopsy Specimen

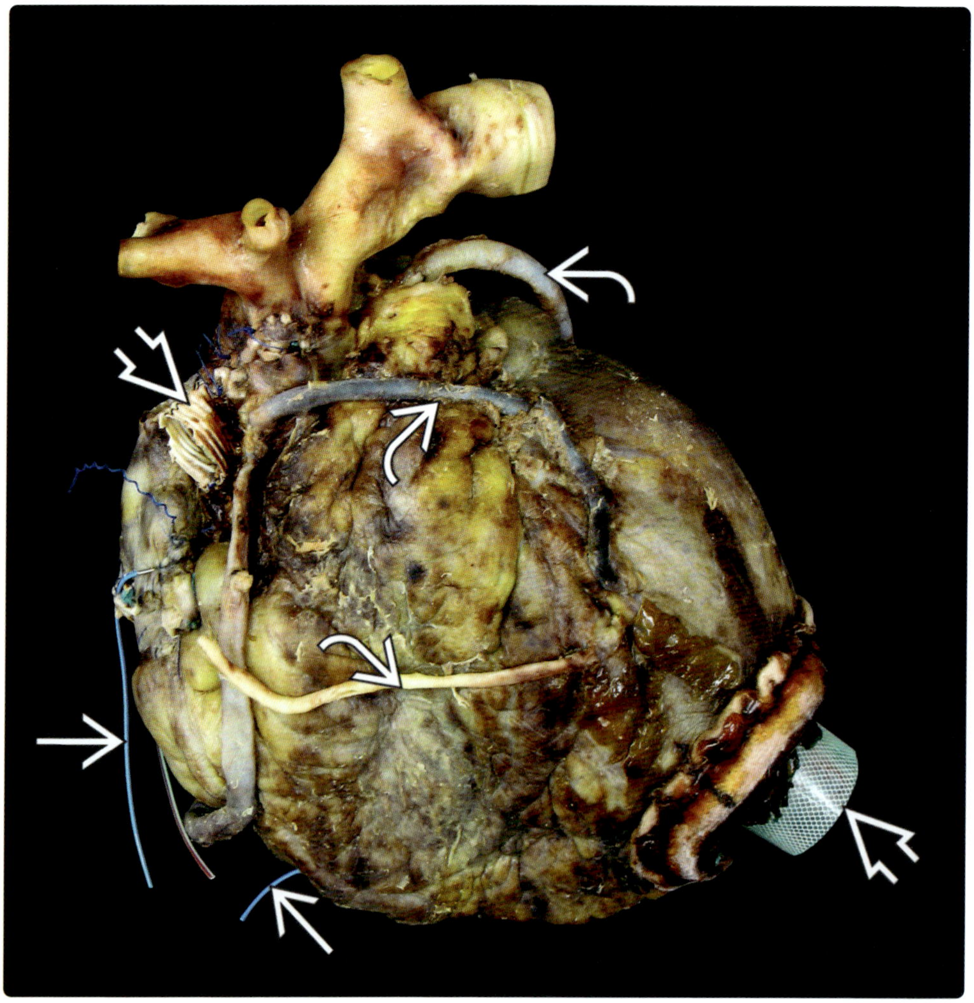

Autopsied heart specimen from a patient with ischemic heart disease and multiple interventions is representative of the challenges encountered in contemporary cardiomyopathy evaluation. There are multiple coronary bypass grafts ➡, epicardial leads ➡, and left ventricular assist device conduits ➡. Rather than having the normal tapered strawberry shape, the cardiac silhouette is rounded and globoid.

Ultrastructural Features

- Identification of
  - Deposited material
    - Fibrils in amyloidosis
    - Glycogen/lipids in storage diseases
    - Granular deposits in light/heavy chain deposition disease
    - Intermediate filaments
  - Mitochondrial abnormalities
  - Viral particles
  - Intracytoplasmic vacuoles (anthracycline toxicity)

AUTOPSY/EXPLANT SPECIMENS

Heart Weight

- Accurate heart weight (after removing great arteries and all parietal pericardium) is most reliable measure of left ventricular hypertrophy (LVH)
  - Mild LVH: 126-150% of expected heart weight
  - Moderate LVH: 151-200% of expected heart weight
  - Severe LVH: > 200% of expected heart weight

Chamber Morphology

- Cardiomyopathy evaluation depends on ventricle chamber size (internal short-axis diameter) and wall thickness; gross assessment of atrial enlargement is also key
  - Gross (Gestalt) assessment of atrial enlargement
  - Ventricle wall thickness
  - Left ventricle chamber size (internal diameter)
- Left ventricular internal short-axis diameter (LVISD) reliably gauges left ventricular dilatation (LVD)
  - Mild LVD: 3.5- to 4.0-cm LVISD
  - Moderate LVD: 4.0- to 5.0-cm LVISD
  - Severe LVD: > 5.0-cm LVISD
- Right ventricle geometry is too complex for reliable measurement of internal diameter
  - Instead, use relative comparison to left ventricle chamber size
- Due to rigor mortis, cardiac chambers in pathologic specimens approximate end-systolic appearance of in vivo imaging studies

Dissection Techniques

- Approaches vary, but short-axis sections through ventricles are most helpful in assessing chamber morphology
- Other sectioning planes simulating echocardiographic windows can also be demonstrative

Valve Assessment

- Significant valve disease should be absent in primary cardiomyopathy (age-related changes may be seen)
- Mitral annular dilatation (circumference > 10.5 cm) is relatively specific for dilated cardiomyopathy
- Tricuspid annular dilatation (circumference > 13.0 cm) is not specific (common in many cardiomyopathies)

Coronary Arteries

- Presence of significant obstructive coronary disease (and regional/territorial myocardial scarring) distinguishes idiopathic from ischemic dilated cardiomyopathy

CARDIOMYOPATHY CLASSIFICATION

Means of Classification

- Etiology
  - Primary
  - Secondary
    - Alcoholic
    - Peripartum
- Morphology
  - Dilated
  - Hypertrophic
  - Restrictive
  - Noncompaction/hypertrabeculation
  - Arrhythmogenic
- Physiology
  - Systolic heart failure
  - Diastolic heart failure (including "preserved ejection fraction" heart failure)

American Heart Association Classification (2006)

- Primary
  - Genetic
    - HCM
    - Arrhythmogenic cardiomyopathy
    - Left ventricular noncompaction/hypertrabeculation
    - Mitochondrial myopathies
    - Ion channel disorders
  - Mixed
    - Dilated cardiomyopathy
    - Restrictive cardiomyopathy
  - Acquired
    - Inflammatory (myocarditis)
    - Stress provoked (Takotsubo/apical ballooning)
    - Peripartum
    - Tachycardia induced
- Secondary (lists of common specific secondary disorders are not all inclusive; there are several other entities in each category)
  - Amyloidosis
    - Primary (light chain amyloidosis)
    - Familial
    - Wildtype *TTR*
  - Other infiltrative disease
    - Gaucher disease
    - Hurler syndrome
    - Hunter syndrome
  - Storage disease
    - Fabry disease
    - Hemochromatosis
  - Eosinophilic endomyocardial disease
  - Sarcoidosis
  - Endocrine
    - Diabetic cardiomyopathy
    - Thyroid dysfunction (hyper or hypo)
  - Cardiofacial
    - Noonan syndrome
    - Lentiginosis
  - Neuromuscular
    - Friedreich ataxia
    - Muscular dystrophies

- Nutritional deficiencies
  - Beriberi
  - Pellagra
- Autoimmune/collagen
  - Lupus
  - Rheumatoid
- Electrolyte imbalance
- Consequence of cancer therapy
  - Radiation
  - Anthracyclines

SPECIFIC CARDIOMYOPATHIES

Dilated Cardiomyopathy

- Features
  - Moderate to severe LVD (LVISD > 4.0 cm)
  - Moderate to severe LVH (heart weight > 150% of expected weight)
  - Usually 4-chamber enlargement developing over time due to congestion from impaired forward flow in left ventricle (systolic failure)
  - Ischemic form shows regional wall scarring and coronary obstruction(s)
  - Myocyte hypertrophy and interstitial fibrosis histologically
- Etiologies and clinicopathologic correlation
  - Idiopathic
    - Presumed to be late post myocarditis (viral or post viral) in most cases
    - Termed "idiopathic" due to lack of definitive causation
    - Wide age range (congenital to old age)
  - Ischemic
    - Regional wall scarring, but dilatation is caused by "remodeling" of entire ventricle
    - Ventricular aneurysms may develop in areas of transmural scar
    - Usually, diffuse coronary obstruction
  - Alcoholic
    - Clinical history of heavy alcohol consumption for many years
    - Potentially reversible with cessation of alcohol consumption
    - Pathologically indistinguishable from idiopathic
  - Hemochromatosis
    - Iron deposition within myocytes (positive iron stain)
    - Diabetes, liver failure, skin pigmentation
    - Genetic testing for *HFE* mutations (C282Y)
  - Anthracycline
    - History of previous exposure at sufficient dose and duration
    - Sarcoplasmic clearing and vacuolization evaluated on toluidine-stained plastic sections and by electron microscopy
  - Familial
    - Typically younger age at onset
    - Family history (unless index case)
    - Sarcomere gene mutations [especially *TTN* (20%)]
    - Otherwise indistinguishable from other dilated forms
  - Peripartum
    - Onset from 3rd trimester to 5 months post partum
    - Obesity, multiparity, age > 30, and preeclampsia are all risk factors
    - 50% of cases recover to normal function 6 months after diagnosis
  - Tachycardia induced
    - Prolonged ventricular tachycardia (weeks to months)
    - Potentially reversible with rate control
  - Sarcoidosis
    - Well-formed granulomas, most prevalent in leftward ventricular septum
    - Frequent involvement of atrioventricular node, His bundle, and bundle branches
    - May be part of systemic sarcoidosis or limited to heart
- Differential diagnosis
  - Mainly valvular heart disease
    - Chronic mitral &/or aortic regurgitation lead to "volume hypertrophy" with left ventricle dilatation

Hypertrophic Cardiomyopathy

- Features
  - Thick left ventricle walls, especially septum (septum:free wall ratio > 1.3)
  - Small left ventricle chamber volume
  - Moderate to severe LVH (heart weight > 150% of expected)
  - Focal anterior mitral leaflet and outflow septal fibrosis (mitral contact lesions) due to systolic anterior motion of mitral valve
  - Myocyte hypertrophy, interstitial fibrosis, myocyte disarray histologically
  - 4-chamber enlargement from impeded forward flow due to impaired left ventricular relaxation
  - Diastolic heart failure; preserved or hyperdynamic ejection fraction
- Etiologies and clinicopathologic correlation
  - Hereditary
    - Presumed due to genetic mutations in sarcomeric or sarcomere-associated gene products (though not all mutations are known)
    - Genetic testing for *MYH7*, *MBL2*, and many others
    - May manifest at any age
    - Electrocardiogram (EKG), echocardiography screening
    - Common cause of sudden death in young people
- Differential diagnosis
  - "Sigmoid" septum
    - Age-related acquired curvature of basal ventricular septum
    - Results in subaortic stenosis in older patients
  - Athlete's heart
    - Wall thickening and chamber volume reduction but not as severe as HCM
    - Younger elite athletes
  - Hypertensive heart disease
    - Concentric wall thickening (septum:free wall ratio < 1.3)
    - History of longstanding hypertension
  - Infiltrative/storage disease
    - Usually concentric wall thickening
    - Danon disease (*LAMP2* mutation) can show marked asymmetric septal hypertrophy

- Low-voltage EKG pattern (as opposed to high voltage in HCM)
- Special stains and ancillary tests
- Family history; other organs also involved
- Chronic aortic stenosis
  - Concentric wall thickening (septum:free wall ratio < 1.3) due to pressure hypertrophy
  - Concurrent aortic valve pathology

Restrictive Cardiomyopathy

- Features
  - Normal heart weight or mild hypertrophy (< 150% of expected heart weight)
  - Mild wall thickening, usually concentric
  - Left atrial enlargement with normal-sized left ventricle and normal valves
  - Right chamber enlargement (impeded forward flow due to inadequate left ventricular relaxation)
    - Diastolic heart failure
    - Preserved or hyperdynamic ejection fraction
- Etiologies and clinicopathologic correlation
  - Primary/idiopathic
    - Rare
    - Often familial (troponin I mutation implicated)
    - Onset in mid to late adulthood
  - Infiltrative diseases
    - Extrasarcoplasmic accumulation of abnormal deposit material
    - Amyloid, Gaucher, Hurler, Hunter diseases
  - Storage diseases
    - Intrasarcoplasmic accumulation of abnormal deposit material
    - Fabry, glycogen storage, Niemann-Pick diseases
- Differential diagnoses
  - Eosinophilic endomyocardial disease
    - Diffuse, thick, ventricular endocardial fibroelastosis with embedded eosinophils
    - Eosinophilic myocarditis
    - Often with peripheral eosinophilia due to protozoal infection or hypereosinophilic syndrome
  - Mitral stenosis
    - Left atrial enlargement ± right-sided chamber dilatation but normal left ventricle
    - Rheumatic mitral valve disease with fused and fibrotic cords and commissures
  - Constrictive pericarditis
    - Readily distinguished on clinical and imaging grounds
    - Left atrium not enlarged
    - Septal "bounce" and engorged inferior vena cava seen on echocardiogram

Arrhythmogenic Cardiomyopathy

- Features
  - Normal heart weight
  - Mild chamber dilatation (at most)
  - Fibrofatty transmural replacement of ventricular wall
  - Right ventricle is more often involved, but left ventricular and combined forms are also recognized
  - Diverticular outpouchings from ventricles
    - Seen in thinned, fibrofatty replaced portions of ventricle walls
- Etiologies and clinicopathologic correlation
  - Sudden cardiac death in young patients
    - F > M
  - Monomorphic ventricular tachycardia
  - Electrophysiologic studies; clinical detection on MR
  - Viral and genetic factors are implicated in pathogenesis (possibly complex interaction of environment and genetic predisposition)
  - Screening for cell junction protein defects (desmoplakin, plakoglobin, plakophilin) by frozen tissue immunofluorescence
  - Genetic testing for *DSG2*, *DSP*, *JUP*, *PKP2*, and others
- Differential diagnosis
  - Normal mural fat, especially in right ventricle wall
  - Fatty degeneration/replacement of myocardium in dilated cardiomyopathy

SELECTED REFERENCES

1. Verdonschot JAJ et al: Phenotypic clustering of dilated cardiomyopathy patients highlights important pathophysiological differences. Eur Heart J. 42(2):162-74, 2021
2. Yogasundaram H et al: Cardiomyopathies and genetic testing in heart failure: role in defining phenotype-targeted approaches and management. Can J Cardiol. 37(4):547-59, 2021
3. Musunuru K et al: Genetic testing for inherited cardiovascular diseases: a scientific statement from the American Heart Association. Circ Genom Precis Med. 13(4):e000067, 2020
4. Finsterer J et al: Left ventricular noncompaction cardiomyopathy: cardiac, neuromuscular, and genetic factors. Nat Rev Cardiol. 14(4):224-37, 2017
5. Schafer S et al: Titin-truncating variants affect heart function in disease cohorts and the general population. Nat Genet. 49(1):46-53, 2017
6. Burke MA et al: Clinical and mechanistic insights Into the genetics of cardiomyopathy. J Am Coll Cardiol. 68(25):2871-86, 2016
7. Richards S et al: Standards and guidelines for the interpretation of sequence variants: a joint consensus recommendation of the American College of Medical Genetics and Genomics and the Association for Molecular Pathology. Genet Med. 17(5):405-24, 2015
8. Towbin JA: Inherited cardiomyopathies. Circ J. 78(10):2347-56, 2014
9. Marcus FI et al: Genetics of arrhythmogenic right ventricular cardiomyopathy: a practical guide for physicians. J Am Coll Cardiol. 61(19):1945-8, 2013
10. Rapezzi C et al: Diagnostic work-up in cardiomyopathies: bridging the gap between clinical phenotypes and final diagnosis. A position statement from the ESC Working Group on Myocardial and Pericardial Diseases. Eur Heart J. 34(19):1448-58, 2013
11. Asimaki A et al: The role of endomyocardial biopsy in ARVC: looking beyond histology in search of new diagnostic markers. J Cardiovasc Electrophysiol. 22(1):111-7, 2011
12. Basso C et al: Pathophysiology of arrhythmogenic cardiomyopathy. Nat Rev Cardiol. 9(4):223-33, 2011
13. Maron BJ et al: How should hypertrophic cardiomyopathy be classified?: What's in a name? Dilemmas in nomenclature characterizing hypertrophic cardiomyopathy and left ventricular hypertrophy. Circ Cardiovasc Genet. 2(1):81-5; discussion 86, 2009
14. McLeod CJ et al: Histologic characterization of hypertrophic cardiomyopathy with and without myofilament mutations. Am Heart J. 158(5):799-805, 2009
15. Maron BJ et al: Contemporary definitions and classification of the cardiomyopathies: an American Heart Association Scientific Statement from the Council on Clinical Cardiology, Heart Failure and Transplantation Committee; Quality of Care and Outcomes Research and Functional Genomics and Translational Biology Interdisciplinary Working Groups; and Council on Epidemiology and Prevention. Circulation. 113(14):1807-16, 2006
16. Lamke GT et al: Surgical pathology of subaortic septal myectomy associated with hypertrophic cardiomyopathy. A study of 204 cases (1996-2000). Cardiovasc Pathol. 12(3):149-58, 2003

(Left) *Short-axis view of the ventricles demonstrates features of dilated cardiomyopathy. The internal short-axis diameter is > 3.5 cm. No regional ischemic changes are noted. The right ventricle is normal in size and shows fibrosis surrounding a pacer lead* ➡. **(Right)** *Short-axis view of the ventricles shows ischemic cardiomyopathy with massive transmural infarction of the anteroseptal wall with global left ventricle remodeling (dilatation and wall thinning).*

Dilated Cardiomyopathy: Short Axis

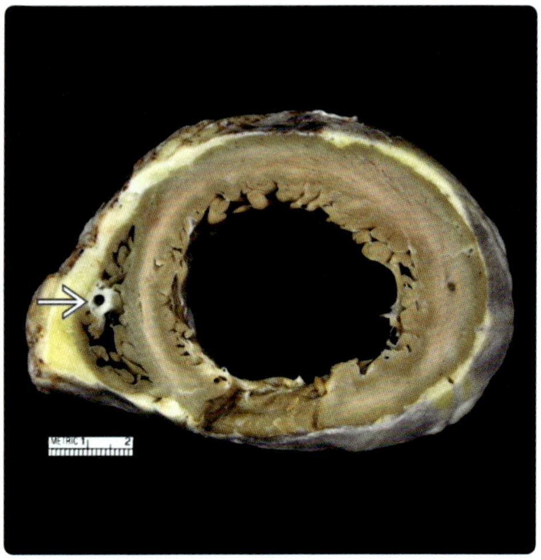

Ischemic (Dilated) Cardiomyopathy: Short Axis

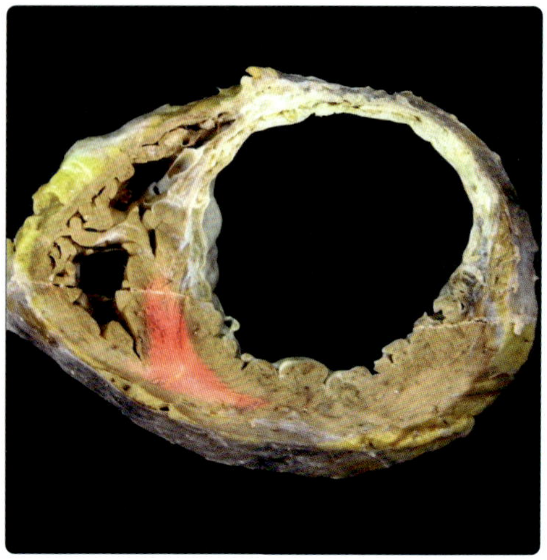

(Left) *Short-axis view of the ventricles shows transmural infarction in a left circumflex coronary artery territory distribution* ➡. *There is early mild chamber dilatation. The right ventricle also appears hypertrophic.* **(Right)** *The conventional regions, or "segments," assessed by echocardiography have been superimposed on these short-axis views of the ventricles. Yellow indicates the LAD territory, blue indicates the LCX territory, and red indicates the RCA territory (assuming right dominance).*

Ischemic Cardiomyopathy: Short Axis

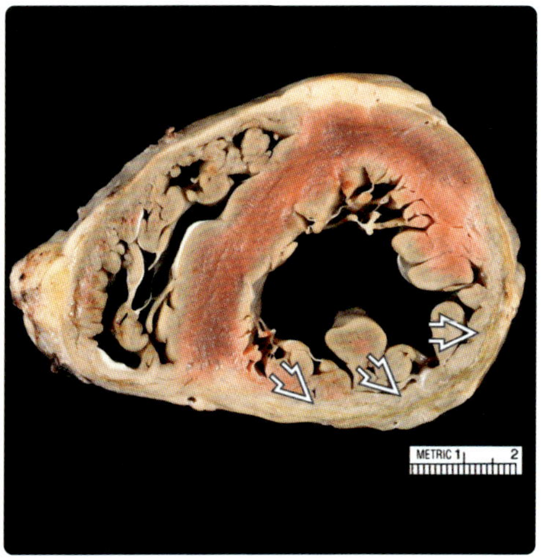

Short-Axis Cardiac "Segments"

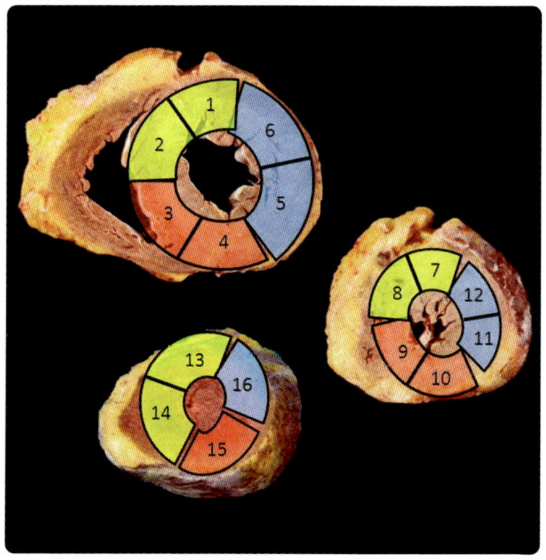

(Left) *Short-axis view of the left ventricle shows an unusual mix of gross morphologic patterns. Besides left ventricular dilatation, there are features of hypertrabeculation (noncompaction)* ➡ *and fibrofatty infiltration of the left ventricle myocardium* ➡, *illustrating that not all cardiomyopathies are readily classified by morphology.* **(Right)** *Short-axis view of the ventricles shows right ventricular hypertrophy* ➡ *due to pulmonary arterial hypertension. The left ventricle is D-shaped* ➡.

Mixed Cardiomyopathy Phenotype: Short Axis

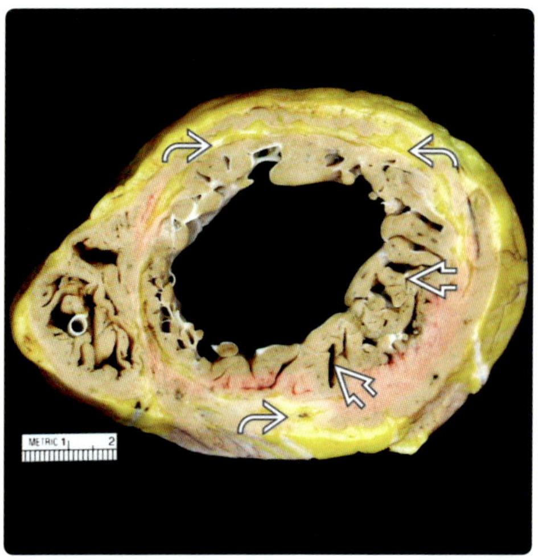

Right Ventricular Hypertrophy

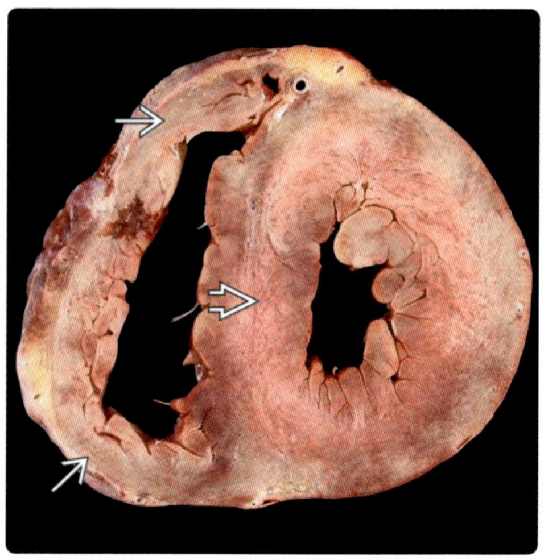

Ischemic Cardiomyopathy: 4 Chamber

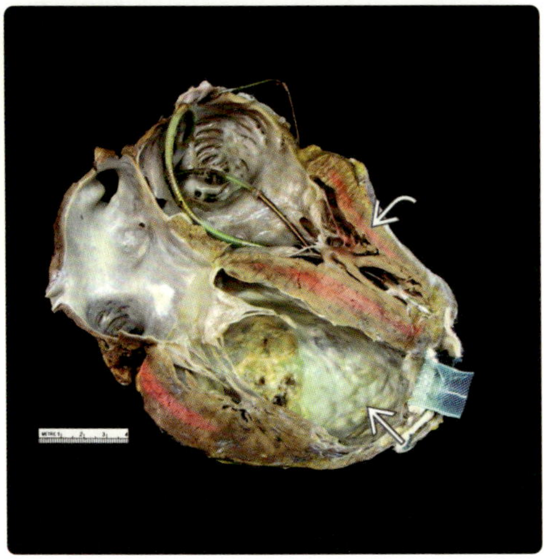

Myocardial Infarction: Long Axis

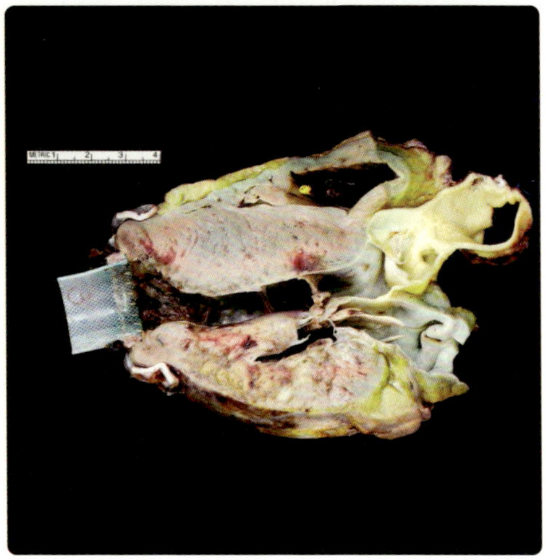

(Left) *4-chamber view shows marked left ventricular dilatation with apical aneurysm formation → from ischemic cardiomyopathy. The right ventricle is also hypertrophied →, suggesting high left-sided filling pressures. Both atria are also enlarged.* **(Right)** *This plane of section simulates the parasternal long-axis view by echocardiography in a patient with recent massive anterolateral wall infarction. The septum appears artificially thickened due to tangential sectioning.*

Hypertensive Heart Disease: 4 Chamber

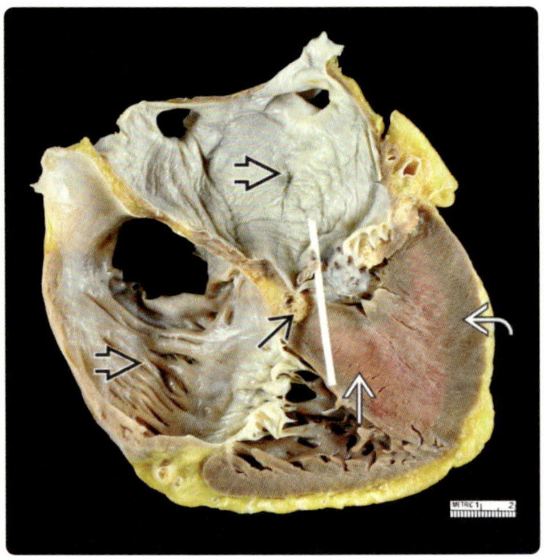

Dilated Cardiomyopathy: Laminated Mural Thrombus

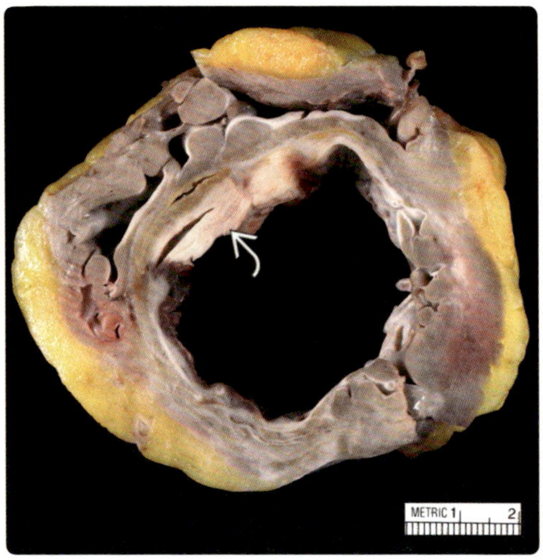

(Left) *This autopsy heart is from an older patient with hypertensive heart disease. The ventricular septal → thickness is slightly greater than the left ventricular free wall → thickness (excluding trabeculations), raising the possibility of hypertrophic cardiomyopathy. Both atria → are massively dilated. Mitral annular calcification is also seen →.* **(Right)** *Laminated mural thrombus → is present over the septum of this heart involved by ischemic dilated cardiomyopathy.*

Individual Myocyte Hypertrophy

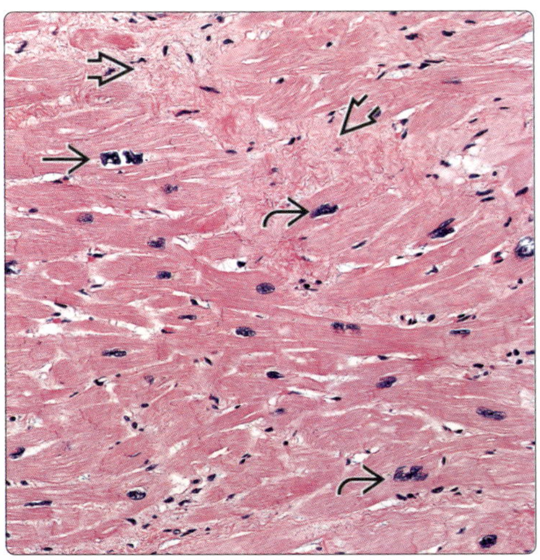

Myocyte Disarray

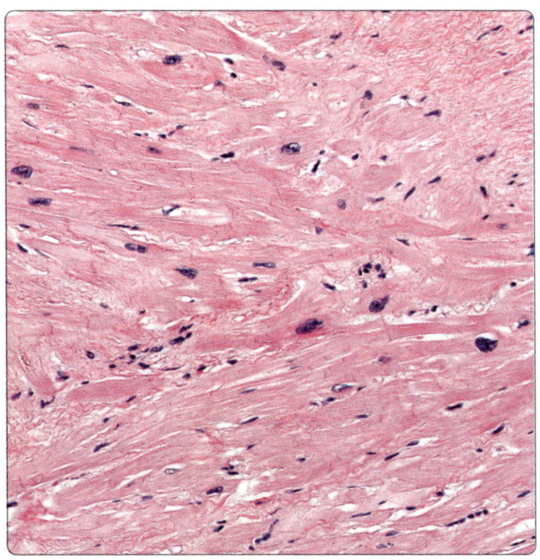

(Left) *The histologic features of many forms of cardiomyopathy overlap and are characterized by myocyte hypertrophy (nuclear enlargement → and binucleation →) with interstitial fibrosis →.* **(Right)** *The term "disarray" denotes myocytes intersecting at random angles, as seen here, and is fairly specific for hypertrophic cardiomyopathy. This should be interpreted with caution since this phenomenon is normal in some myocardial regions (e.g., union of septum and free wall).*

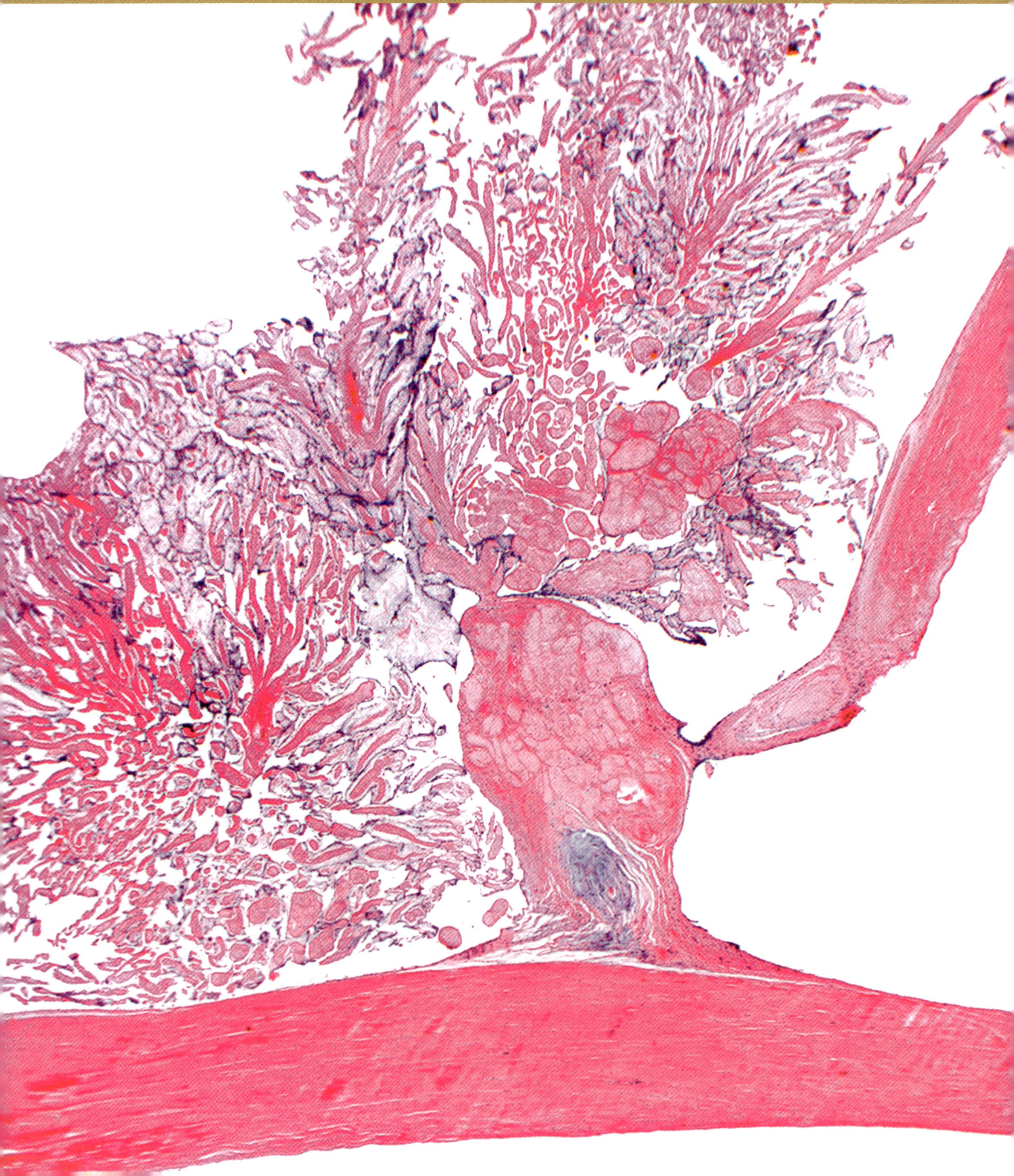

SECTION 3

Heart, Tumors

Benign

Malignant

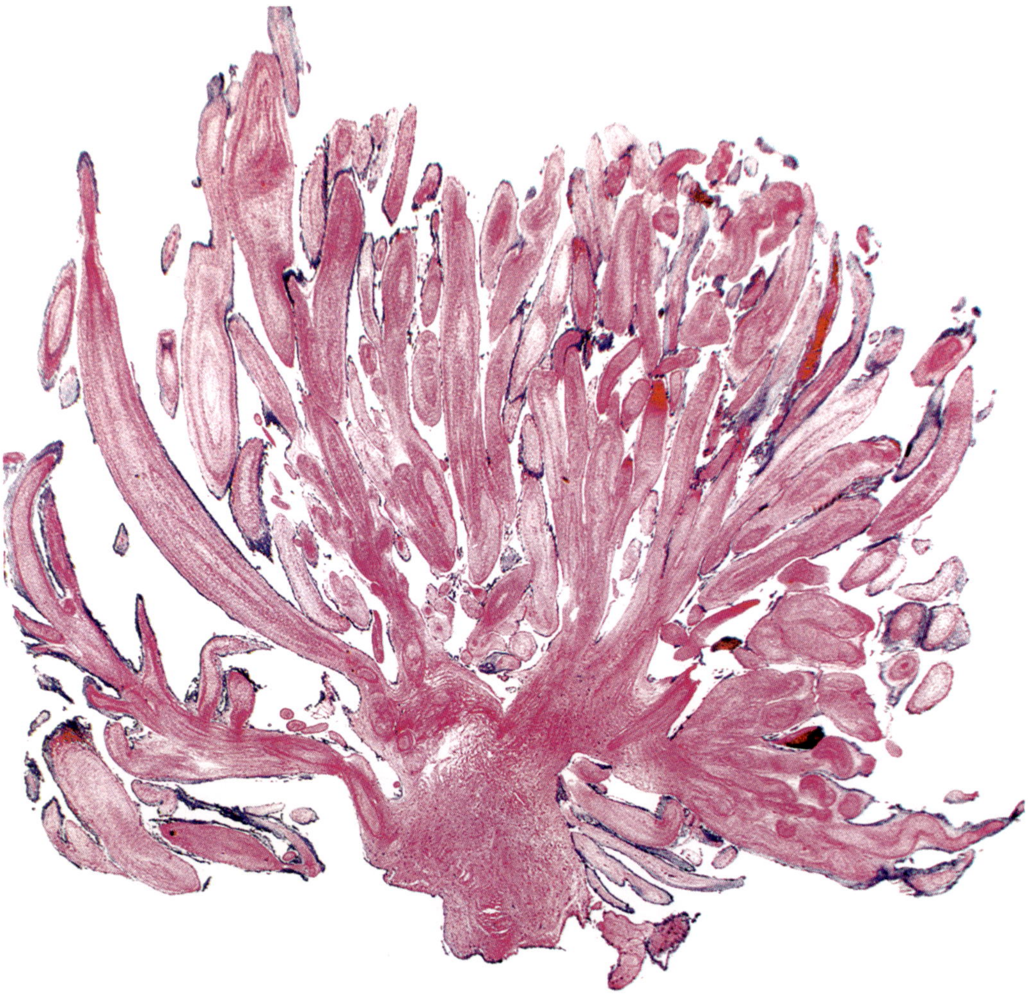

Cardiac Myxoma

KEY FACTS

TERMINOLOGY

- Cardiac myxoma: Neoplasm of uncertain histogenesis composed of bland, often polymorphous "myxoma cells" in myxoid matrix

ETIOLOGY/PATHOGENESIS

- Precise etiology unclear

CLINICAL ISSUES

- Most cardiac myxomas found in 3rd-6th decades of life
- Sporadic cardiac myxomas occur more commonly in women
- Familial cardiac myxomas occur more commonly in men

MACROSCOPIC

- Heterogeneous tumors with smooth or papillary surface (with latter being more likely to embolize)
- Typically arise in left atrium, near valve of fossa ovalis, but can be found anywhere in heart

MICROSCOPIC

- Diagnosis reliant on identification of "myxoma cells" (a.k.a. lepidic cells) usually seen in myxoid background
- Hemorrhage frequently identified, may manifest as Gamna-Gandy bodies
- Unusual features, such as gland-like structures, hematopoietic elements, calcification/ossification, heterotopic endocrine tissues, and thymic tissue, can be seen
- Myxoma cells identified individually, in nests, or arranged in single or multiple layers ("ring structure") around vascular channels

ANCILLARY TESTS

- Myxoma cells reactive with antibodies directed against calretinin (75%), S100 (60-85%), NSE (50%), CD34 (65%), and vimentin (50%)

Pedunculated Cardiac Myxoma

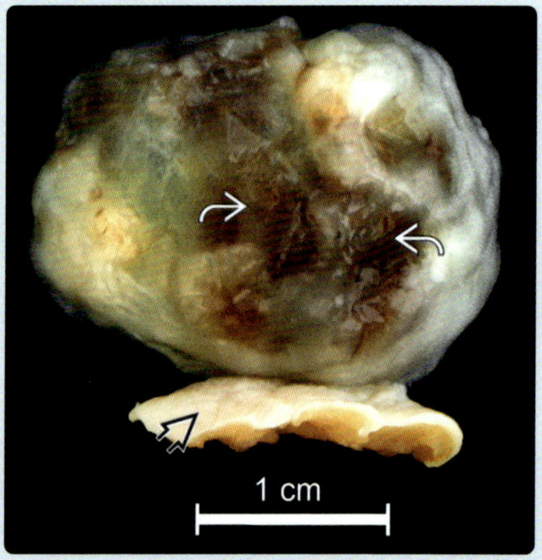

Classic Histologic Features of Cardiac Myxoma

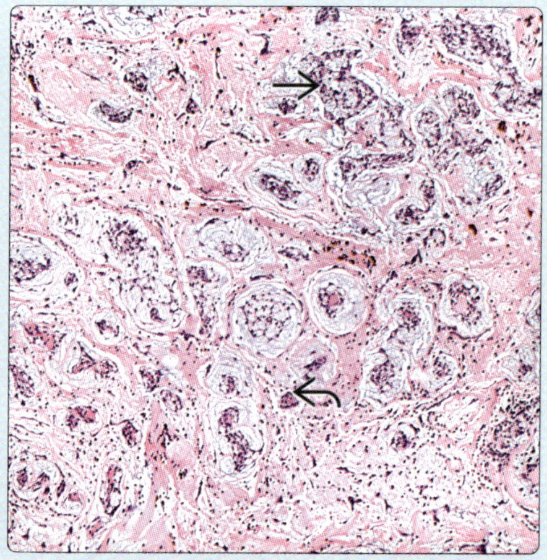

(Left) *Gross photograph of a surgically resected, pedunculated cardiac myxoma shows the tumor's smooth surface with focal red-brown discoloration. A segment of atrial septum is visible at the base.* **(Right)** *Low-power view of a cardiac myxoma shows classic proliferation of myxoma cells (individually and around thin-walled vessels) in a myxoid background.*

Smooth External Surface of Cardiac Myxoma

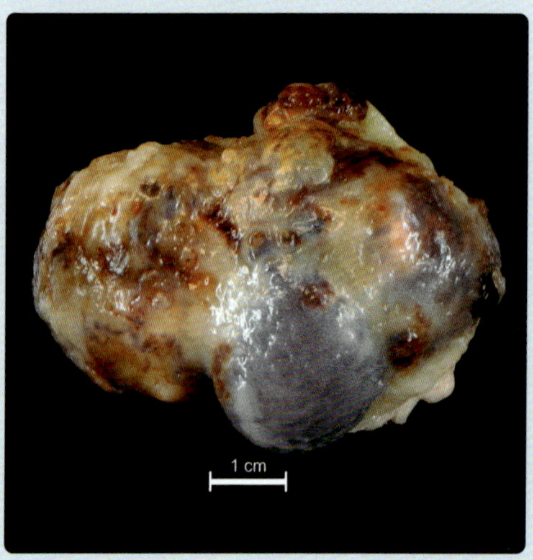

Cardiac Myxoma With Extensive Intratumoral Hemorrhage

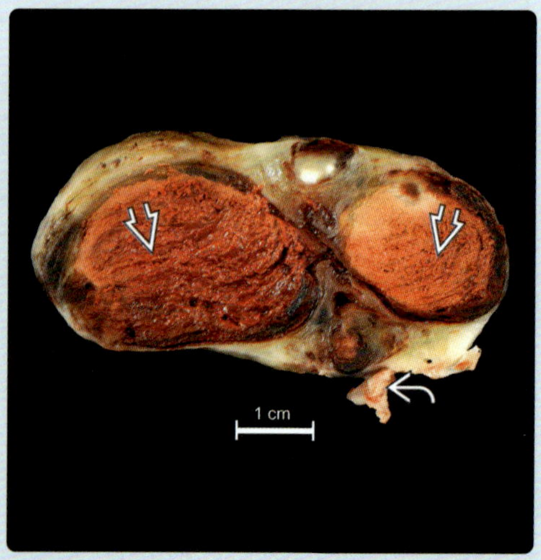

(Left) *Gross photograph shows a surgically resected cardiac myxoma exhibiting the relatively smooth surface and variegated appearance of the tumor. Lesions with such a smooth surface have lower embolic potential.* **(Right)** *Gross photograph of a longitudinally sectioned cardiac myxoma reveals that the bulk of the tumor mass consists of prominent intratumoral hemorrhage surrounded by gelatinous white-tan areas. The stalk of the myxoma can be seen on the lower right side.*

TERMINOLOGY

Definitions

- Neoplasm of uncertain histogenesis composed of bland, often polymorphous "myxoma cells" in myxoid matrix

ETIOLOGY/PATHOGENESIS

Etiology

- Precise etiology unclear
- Cyclic AMP-dependent protein kinase A (*PRKAR1A*) frequently mutated in familial cardiac myxomas

CLINICAL ISSUES

Epidemiology

- Incidence
  - Thought to be most common primary cardiac neoplasm, though exact frequency differs among series
    - Sporadic cardiac myxomas (~ 90%)
    - Familial cardiac myxomas (5-10%)
- Age
  - Most cardiac myxomas found in 3rd-6th decades of life
- Sex
  - Sporadic cardiac myxomas occur more commonly in women
  - Familial cardiac myxomas occur more commonly in men

Presentation

- Systemic symptoms include
  - Fatigue
  - Weight loss
  - Myalgia and muscle weakness
  - Arthralgia
  - Fever
  - Anemia
  - Leukocytosis
  - Hypergammaglobulinemia
- Symptoms related to mass effect and embolization
  - Syncope
  - Chest pain
  - Heart failure
  - Sudden death
  - Embolic events: 50% to brain, causing stroke or aneurysm; other arteries may be involved

Laboratory Tests

- Elevated IL-6
- Elevated erythrocyte sedimentation rate (ESR)

Treatment

- Surgical approaches
  - Surgical resection remains preferred treatment strategy
- Drugs
  - No effective chemotherapeutic treatments have been established

Prognosis

- Long-term prognosis excellent following surgical resection
- Higher rate of recurrence in familial myxomas (20%) than sporadic (1-2%)

Features of Myxoma Syndrome

- Myxomas, frequently multiple and recurrent, involving
  - Heart
  - Skin
  - Breast
- Mucocutaneous pigmentation (lentiginosis, blue nevi, or combination)
- Glandular abnormalities, including
  - Adrenocortical disease (Cushing syndrome)
  - Testicular neoplasms (Sertoli cell tumors)
  - Pituitary adenomas (often growth hormone-producing)
- Psammomatous melanocytic schwannoma

IMAGING

Radiographic Findings

- 2-dimensional echocardiography is imaging modality of choice
  - Variably sized, often mobile masses attached to endocardial surface
  - Hyperechoic appearance
  - Prolapse through mitral valve may be identified
  - Stalk often well visualized

CT Findings

- Tumor may not be visible without contrast
- Hypodense compared to blood
- Calcification seen in 50% of tumors
- 80% show low attenuation
- Generally no contrast enhancement
- Occasionally cystic
- May change position during cardiac cycle

MACROSCOPIC

General Features

- Heterogeneous tumors with soft gelatinous or friable consistency but may be firm
- Smooth or papillary surface (with latter being more likely to embolize)
- Pedunculated or sessile
- Mucoid and frequently variegated, particularly on sectioning, often with significant intratumoral hemorrhage
- Areas of calcification not uncommon
  - 50% in right-sided tumors
- Surface thrombus may be seen

Size

- Variable, ranging 1 mm to 15 cm
- Some can reach 450 g in weight

Location

- Typically arise in left atrium, near valve of fossa ovalis
- Right atrium 2nd most common site with ventricular origin uncommon
- Occasionally biatrial
- Rare sites
  - Inferior vena cava
  - Left ventricle
  - Right ventricle
  - Valve leaflets or cusps

- When identified outside of left atrium, strongly suggests myxoma (Carney) syndrome

MICROSCOPIC

Histologic Features

- Diagnosis reliant on identification of "myxoma cells" (a.k.a. lepidic cells) usually seen in myxoid background
- Myxoma cells typically elongated and fusiform, polyhedral or stellate with bland (usually oval) nuclei and slightly eosinophilic cytoplasm
- Myxoma cells identified individually, in nests, or arranged in single or multiple layers ("ring structure") around vascular channels
- Myxoid matrix composed of proteoglycans, elastin, fibrinogen, fibrin, and collagen
- Hemorrhage frequently identified, may manifest as Gamna-Gandy bodies
    - Sclerosiderotic granulomatous lesion; degenerated collagen fibers encrusted with iron and calcium
- Myxoid background typically infiltrated by varying numbers of inflammatory cells (plasma cells, lymphocytes, mast cells, histiocytes)
- Most vascular spaces thin-walled throughout lesion; vessels within stalk often thick-walled and sometimes rather atypical in appearance
- Unusual features, such as gland-like structures, hematopoietic elements, calcification/ossification, heterotopic endocrine tissues, and thymic tissue, can be seen
- Cases with extensive multinucleated giant cells have been reported
- Rarely, may exhibit invasion into subjacent myocardium, although significance of this finding unknown

ANCILLARY TESTS

Immunohistochemistry

- Myxoma cells reactive with antibodies directed against
    - Calretinin (75%)
    - S100 (60-85%)
    - NSE (50%)
    - CD34 (65%)
    - Vimentin (50%)
- PRKAR1 antibody expression may be useful to exclude myxoma syndrome

DIFFERENTIAL DIAGNOSIS

Thrombus

- Lacks myxoma cells
- Zonated appearance with prominent fibrin

Papillary Fibroelastoma

- Endothelial-lined, avascular papillary fronds without myxoma cells
- Usually valvular in location
- Most cases solitary
- Most have stalk
- Positive elastic stain

Myxoid Intimal Fibroplasia

- Lacks myxoma cells

Cardiac Lipoma

- Often localized in interatrial septum
- Histology demonstrates adipose tissue

Myxoid Sarcomas

- Highly pleomorphic spindle cells
- High mitotic rate
- Often exhibit tumoral necrosis

Metastatic Carcinoma

- Lacks myxoma cells
- Usually, patient has history of carcinoma
- Typically only problem when glandular or gland-like structures present
- Keratin immunohistochemical stain highlights epithelial cells

DIAGNOSTIC CHECKLIST

Clinically Relevant Pathologic Features

- Gross appearance
- Number of lesions identified

Pathologic Interpretation Pearls

- Myxoma cells in myxoid matrix
- Unusual features, such as gland-like structures, calcification/ossification, and heterotopic thymic tissue, can be seen

SELECTED REFERENCES

1. Nenna A et al: miRNAs in cardiac myxoma: new pathologic findings for potential therapeutic opportunities. Int J Mol Sci. 23(6):3309, 2022
2. WHO Classification of Tumours Editorial Board. Thoracic Tumours. 5th ed. IARC Press, 2021
3. Di Vito A et al: The mysterious pathways of cardiac myxomas: a review of histogenesis, pathogenesis and pathology. Histopathology. 66(3):321-32, 2015
4. Maleszewski JJ et al: PRKAR1A in the development of cardiac myxoma: a study of 110 cases including isolated and syndromic tumors. Am J Surg Pathol. 38(8):1079-87, 2014
5. Singhal P et al: Molecular basis of cardiac myxomas. Int J Mol Sci. 15(1):1315-37, 2014
6. Goševl et al: Cardiac myxoma the great imitators: comprehensive histopathological and molecular approach. Int J Cardiol. 164(1):7-20, 2013
7. Zheng JJ et al: Clinical and histopathological analysis of 66 cases with cardiac myxoma. Asian Pac J Cancer Prev. 14(3):1743-6, 2013
8. Garatti A et al: Surgical excision of cardiac myxomas: twenty years experience at a single institution. Ann Thorac Surg. 93(3):825-31, 2012
9. Edwards A et al: Carney's syndrome: complex myxomas. Report of four cases and review of the literature. Cardiovasc Surg. 10(3):264-75, 2002
10. Kirschner LS et al: Genetic heterogeneity and spectrum of mutations of the PRKAR1A gene in patients with the carney complex. Hum Mol Genet. 9(20):3037-46, 2000
11. Kirschner LS et al: Mutations of the gene encoding the protein kinase A type I-alpha regulatory subunit in patients with the Carney complex. Nat Genet. 26(1):89-92, 2000
12. Burke AP et al: Cardiac myxoma. A clinicopathologic study. Am J Clin Pathol. 100(6):671-80, 1993
13. Molina JE et al: Primary cardiac tumors: experience at the University of Minnesota. Thorac Cardiovasc Surg. 38 Suppl 2:183-91, 1990
14. Carney JA et al: The complex of myxomas, spotty pigmentation, and endocrine overactivity. Medicine (Baltimore). 64(4):270-83, 1985
15. Wold LE et al: Cardiac myxomas: a clinicopathologic profile. Am J Pathol. 101(1):219-40, 1980
16. Ferrans VJ et al: Structural features of cardiac myxomas. Histology, histochemistry, and electron microscopy. Hum Pathol. 4(1):111-46, 1973

Cut Surface of Cardiac Myxoma With Gelatinous Appearance

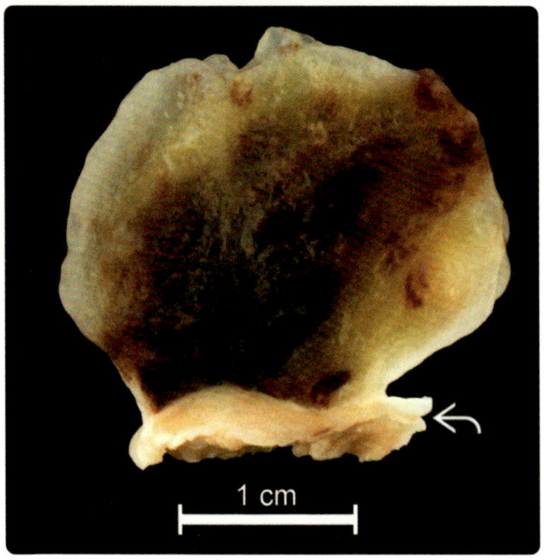

Cardiac Myxoma With Papillary Appearance

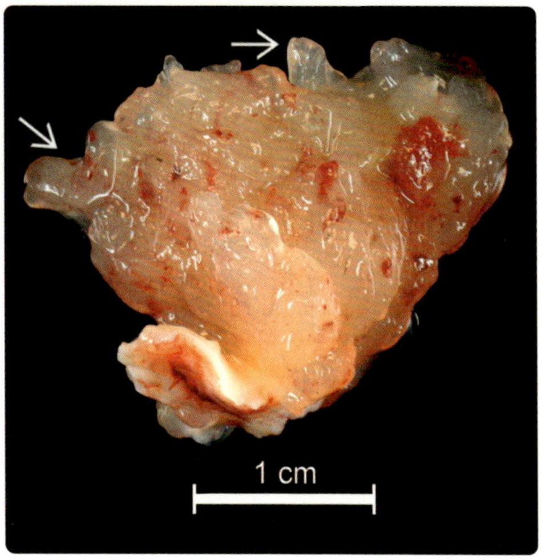

(Left) *Gross photograph of a sectioned, surgically resected myxoma reveals the somewhat gelatinous ("myxoid") appearance of the tumor; the dark areas correspond to highly vascular areas of the myxoma. A small portion of atrial septum (from where the myxoma arose) can be seen at the bottom of the tumor .* **(Right)** *Gross photograph shows a surgically resected, friable papillary myxoma. The gelatinous ("myxoid") tan-yellow appearance is readily apparent .*

Pedunculated Atrial Myxoma

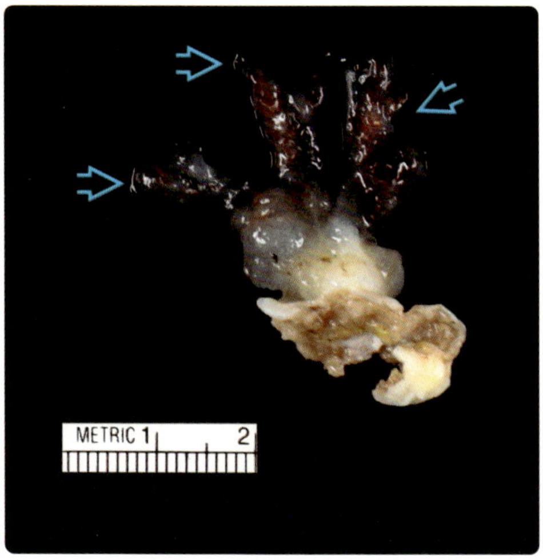

Myxoid Background Typical of Cardiac Myxoma

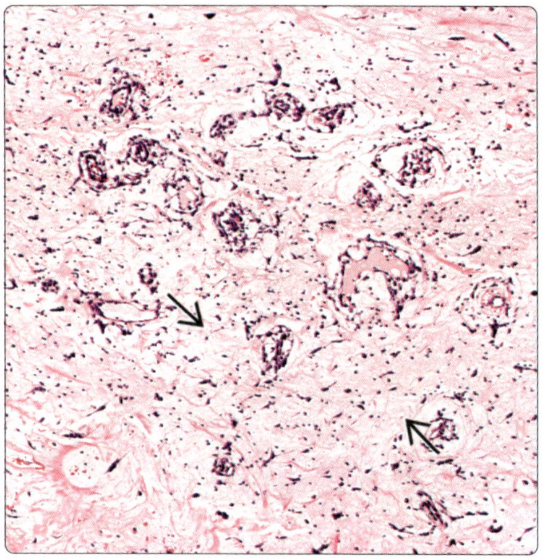

(Left) *This pedunculated myxoma arising from the atrial septum shows friable branches . Myxomas with this configuration can often produce embolic symptoms because of their propensity to detach from the tumor base.* **(Right)** *Proliferation of myxoma cells in a myxoid background is shown.*

Features of Myxoma Cells

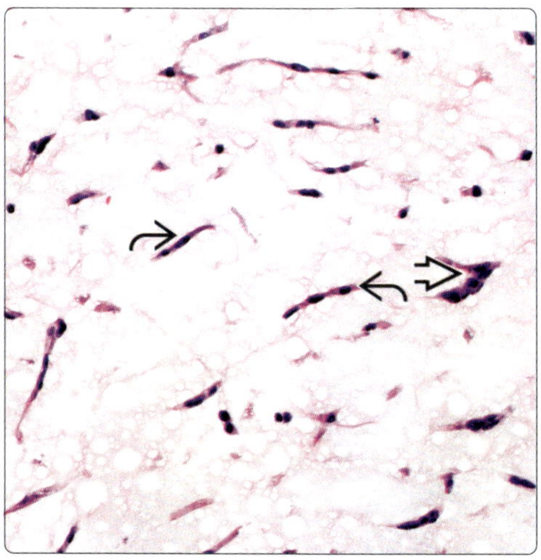

Perivascular Growth of Myxoma Cells

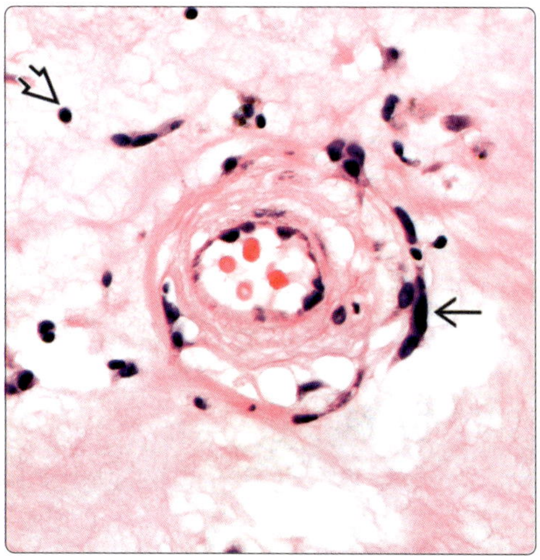

(Left) *High-power view exhibits numerous myxoma (lepidic) cells characterized by bland, elongated, and fusiform cells with oval nuclei and eosinophilic cytoplasm. Note the polymorphous nature of the cells, forming both cords and vague nests , in a pale myxoid background.* **(Right)** *Myxoma cells are often seen aggregating around small vessels . This perivascular ring phenomenon is very frequently identified in cardiac myxomas. Rare inflammatory cells are present.*

(Left) *Cardiac myxoma shows recent, prominent, intratumoral hemorrhage. The numerous small vessels throughout the tumor and the mechanical strain that these lesions experience are thought to contribute to the hemorrhage. Despite the many erythrocytes, myxoma cells* → *can still be identified.* **(Right)** *High-power view of a cardiac myxoma exhibits numerous hemosiderin-laden macrophages, serving as evidence of prior intratumoral hemorrhage.*

Cardiac Myxoma With Intratumoral Hemorrhage

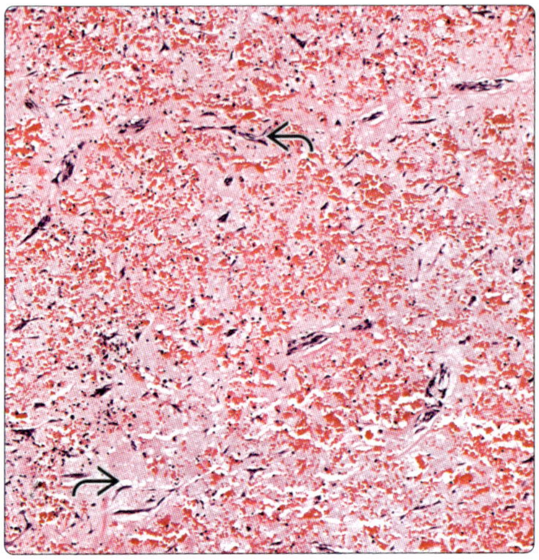

Hemosiderin-Laden Macrophages in Cardiac Myxoma

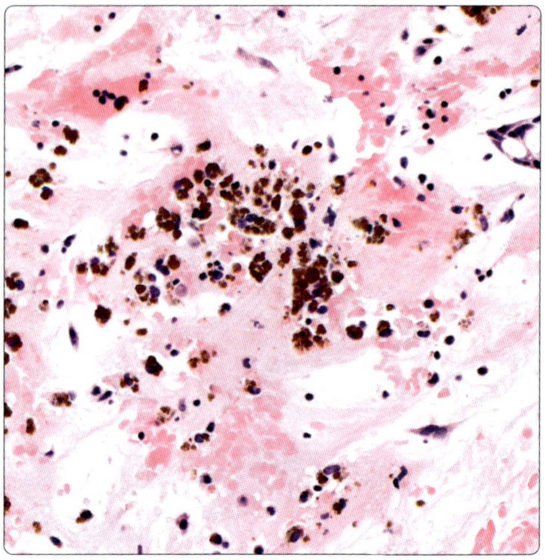

(Left) *Thick-walled small muscular arteries are frequently identified in the stalk of cardiac myxoma and often exhibit strikingly atypical changes, such as medial hypertrophy* → *and eccentric intimal fibroplasia* →. **(Right)** *Extensive Gamna-Gandy body formation* → *is frequently encountered in cardiac myxomas. These structures are the result of iron and calcium deposition on connective tissues (predominately collagen and elastin) and are often the result of intratumoral hemorrhage.*

Muscular Arteries With Atypical Features

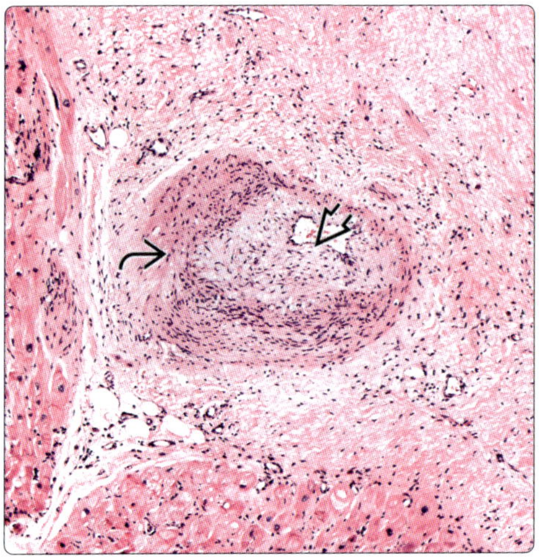

Gamna-Gandy Body Formation

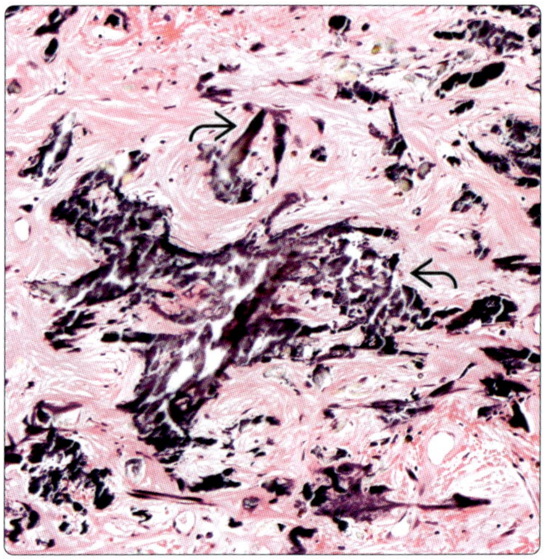

(Left) *Gland-like structures are identified in < 5% of cardiac myxomas and can exhibit frankly mucinous features that can be highlighted with a PAS stain. The cells within these structures may exhibit reactivity with cytokeratins and raise the possibility of metastatic carcinoma.* **(Right)** *Myxoma cells can form somewhat complex, cribriform-like structures. Morphologically, these structures may also raise the possibility of a metastatic carcinoma.*

Gland-Like Structures in Cardiac Myxoma

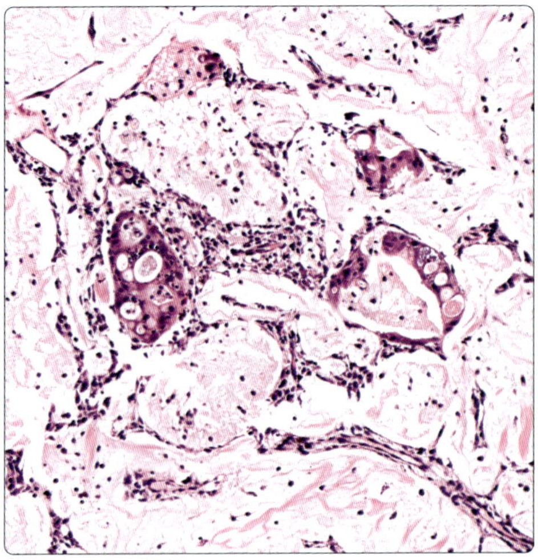

Cribriform-Like Structures in Cardiac Myxoma

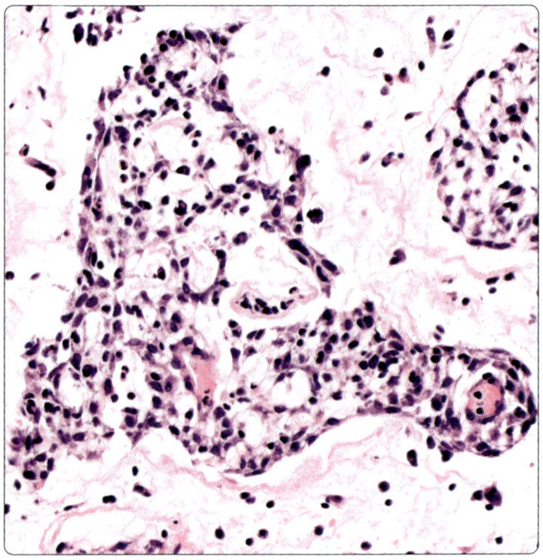

Cardiac Myxoma With Papillary Excrescences

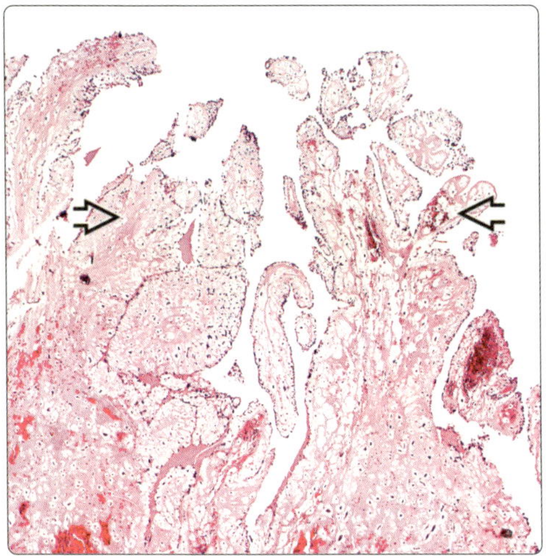

Cardiac Myxoma Embolization

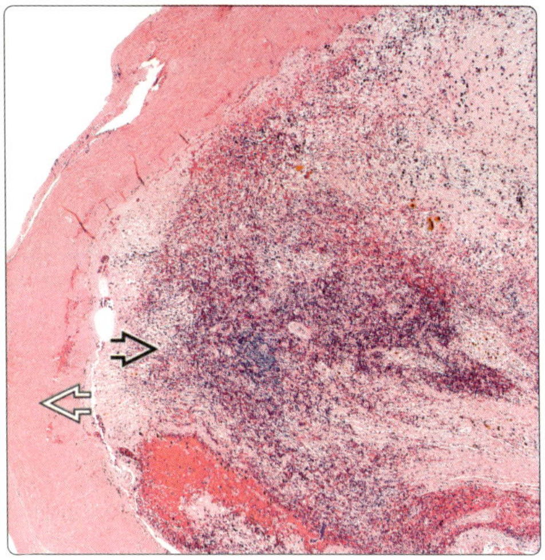

(Left) *Low-power view shows prominent papillary excrescences. Cardiac myxomas with this feature are more likely to embolize, owing to the somewhat friable nature of the excrescences.* **(Right)** *A myxoma embolus is seen within a medium-sized muscular artery (internal carotid in this instance). Systemic embolization (causing a large ischemic stroke in this case) can be one of the most devastating consequences of these tumors.*

Heterotopic Bone Formation in Cardiac Myxoma

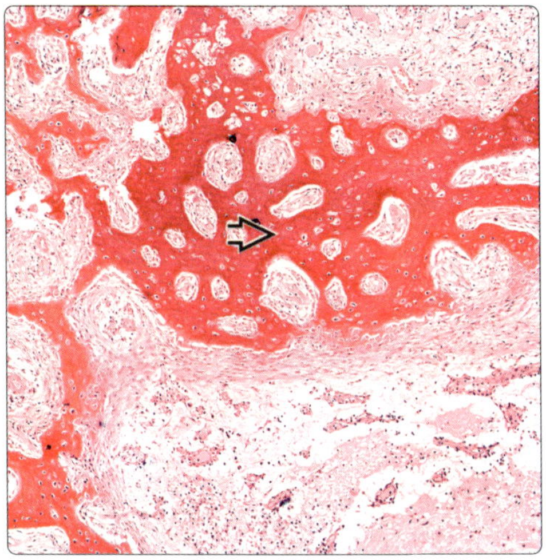

Positive Calretinin Stain of Myxoma Cells

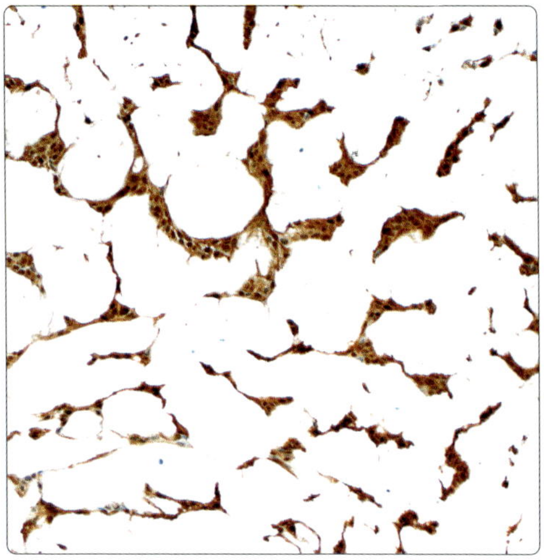

(Left) *Heterotopic bone formation, and even hematopoiesis, can sometimes be seen within myxomas. Dense bone formation (or calcification) can occasionally be appreciated on radiologic studies.* **(Right)** *75% of cardiac myxomas exhibit reactivity of the neoplastic cells with antibodies directed against calretinin. Typically, myxoma cells exhibit both nuclear and cytoplasmic reactivity.*

Endovascular Needle Biopsy of Myxoma

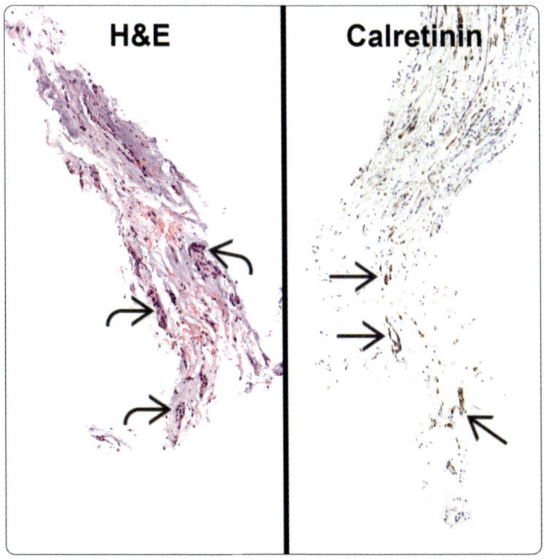

Loose Granulation Tissue in Thrombus

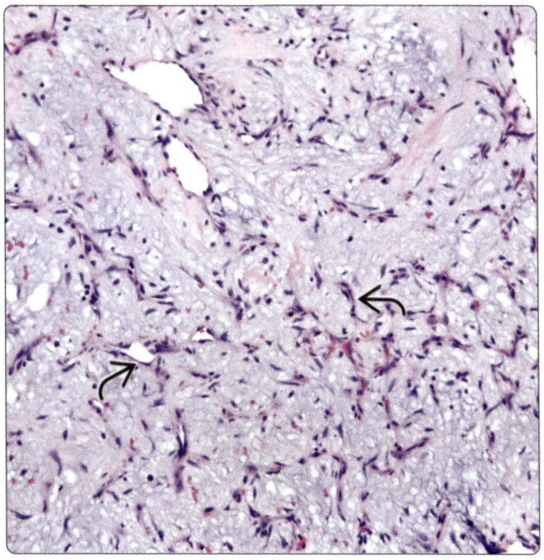

(Left) *Needle core biopsy illustrates that even limited samples can show diagnostic features of cardiac myxoma with perivascular rings of myxoma cells. Calretinin stain highlights myxoma cells, confirming the diagnosis.* **(Right)** *By way of comparison to myxoma, the proliferating vessels in this organizing thrombus lack a 2nd layer of myxoma cells.*

Papillary Fibroelastoma

KEY FACTS

TERMINOLOGY

- Papillary fibroelastoma (PFE): Benign lesion of uncertain histogenesis composed of avascular papillary fronds arising from common stalk

ETIOLOGY/PATHOGENESIS

- Unknown (reactive, hamartomatous, neoplastic, or congenital)

CLINICAL ISSUES

- Most common primary tumor of cardiac valves
- 4th and 8th decades of life
- Surgical removal usually curative with very low propensity for recurrence
- Most are found incidentally on imaging (echocardiography) or at time of surgery or autopsy
- Symptoms are usually consequence of embolization (of lesion or thrombus) but may also be related to in situ obstruction

IMAGING

- Peripheral "shimmer," most commonly seen on transesophageal echocardiogram, is very suggestive of lesion

MACROSCOPIC

- 1 mm to 7 cm
- Typically overtly papillary with identifiable stalk (sea anemone appearance)
  - Submerging in clear liquid makes fronds more apparent
- May have calcification (typically in larger PFEs)
- Occasionally, may occur in multiples
- Commonly arise at areas of trauma or previous instrumentation (secondary type)

MICROSCOPIC

- Avascular fronds consisting of collagen and elastic fibers with surface endothelial lining

Papillary Fibroelastoma (Gross)

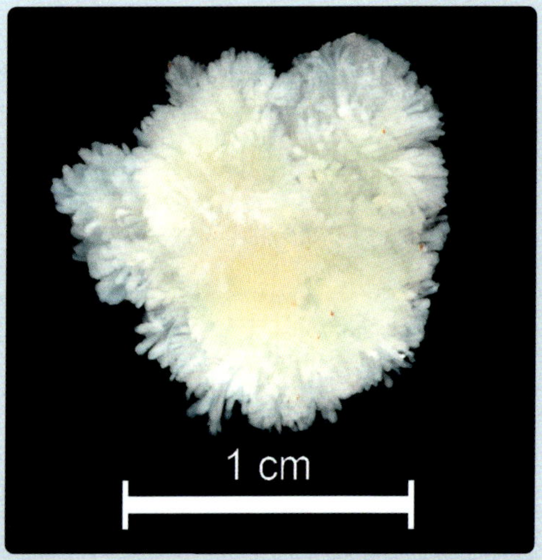

Papillary Fibroelastoma (Medium Magnification)

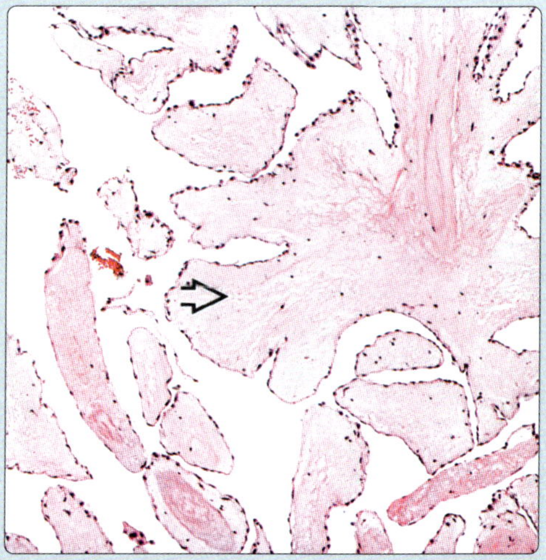

(Left) *Surgically excised papillary fibroelastoma (submerged in alcohol) exhibits the delicate fronds that give these lesions their sea anemone appearance.* **(Right)** *Branching, avascular, papillary fronds with surface layer of endothelium ➲ are noted histologically. The complex branching fronds help to differentiate papillary fibroelastoma from the more simple Lambl excrescence.*

Papillary Fibroelastoma (Dry vs. Floating)

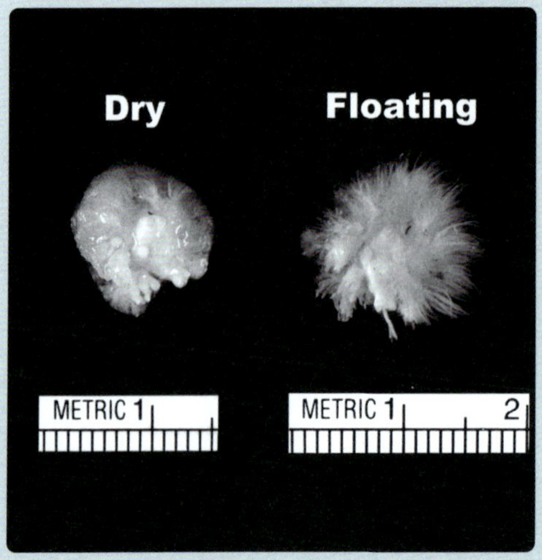

Papillary Fibroelastoma (Low and High Magnification)

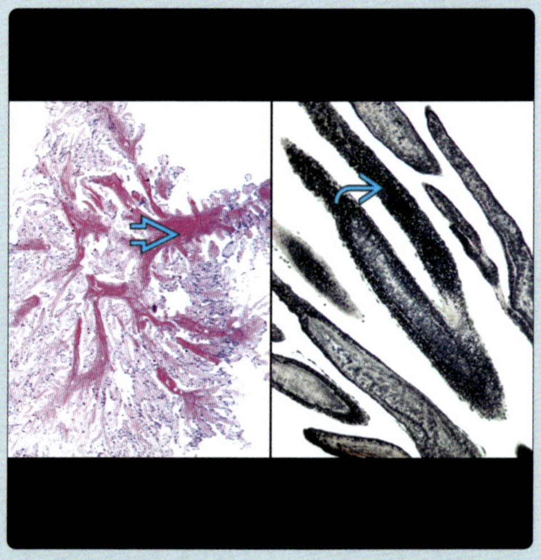

(Left) *Gross photographs of the same papillary fibroelastoma removed surgically demonstrate how suspending the tissue in clear liquid can help accentuate the papillary fronds.* **(Right)** *Low magnification shows the central stalk ➲ with branching, frond-like architecture. Elastic stain shows the elastin-rich fibrovascular cores ➦ comprising each frond.*

TERMINOLOGY

Abbreviations

- Papillary fibroelastoma (PFE)

Synonyms

- Papillary tumor of cardiac valve, giant Lambl excrescence

Definitions

- Benign lesion of uncertain histogenesis composed of avascular papillary fronds arising from common stalk

ETIOLOGY/PATHOGENESIS

Etiology

- True nature unknown
- Reactive, hamartomatous, neoplastic, congenital theories

CLINICAL ISSUES

Epidemiology

- Incidence
  - Most common primary tumor of cardiac valves
  - Thought to be 2nd most common primary cardiac tumor
- Age
  - Most are diagnosed between 4th and 8th decades of life
- Sex
  - Slightly more common in men

Presentation

- Most are found incidentally on imaging (echocardiography) or at time of surgery or autopsy
- Symptoms usually due to embolization (of lesion or thrombus) but may also be related to in situ obstruction
- Rare reports of fever and thrombocytopenia with resolution following removal

Treatment

- Surgical approaches
  - Surgical excision is treatment of choice given embolic potential of these lesions
  - Most amenable to valve-sparing resection

Prognosis

- Surgical removal is usually curative with very low propensity for recurrence in most large series

IMAGING

Radiographic Findings

- Echocardiographic characteristics include endocardial-based lesion with pedicle (stalk) attachment, high mobility, and refractive appearance
- Peripheral "shimmer," most commonly seen on transesophageal echocardiogram, is very suggestive of lesion

MACROSCOPIC

General Features

- Submerging in clear liquid makes fronds more apparent
- Typically overtly papillary with identifiable stalk (sea anemone appearance)
- May have adherent surface thrombus obscuring fronds
- May have calcification (typically in larger PFEs)
- Occasionally, may occur in multiples

Size

- 1 mm to 7 cm

Location

- Usually arises on cardiac valves (left sided > right sided) but may arise from any endocardial surface
- Commonly arises at areas of trauma or previous instrumentation (secondary type)
  - Rheumatic valve disease
  - Hypertrophic obstructive cardiomyopathy
  - Postseptal myectomy

MICROSCOPIC

Histologic Features

- Avascular fronds consisting of collagen and elastic fibers, lined on surface with endothelial cells

ANCILLARY TESTS

Histochemistry

- Elastic van Gieson
  - Staining pattern: Elastic fibers within papillary fronds

Immunohistochemistry

- Markers of endothelial differentiation (CD31, CD34, and factor VIII) highlight endothelial lining

DIFFERENTIAL DIAGNOSIS

Lambl Excrescence

- Located solely on closing surface of valves
- Simple architecture without complex branching papillae

Cardiac Myxoma

- Contains myxoma cells
- Typically lacks fine papillae

Vegetation

- Lacks elastic fibers seen in PFE
- Papillae are uncommon

DIAGNOSTIC CHECKLIST

Clinically Relevant Pathologic Features

- Gross appearance

Pathologic Interpretation Pearls

- Avascular papillary fronds lined by surface endothelium

SELECTED REFERENCES

1. Wittersheim M et al: KRAS mutation in papillary fibroelastoma: a true cardiac neoplasm? J Pathol Clin Res. 3(2):100-4, 2017
2. Tamin SS et al: Prognostic and bioepidemiologic implications of papillary fibroelastomas. J Am Coll Cardiol. 65(22):2420-9, 2015
3. Mariscalco G et al: Papillary fibroelastoma: insight to a primary cardiac valve tumor. J Card Surg. 25(2):198-205, 2010
4. Gowda RM et al: Cardiac papillary fibroelastoma: a comprehensive analysis of 725 cases. Am Heart J. 146(3):404-10, 2003
5. Klarich KW et al: Papillary fibroelastoma: echocardiographic characteristics for diagnosis and pathologic correlation. J Am Coll Cardiol. 30(3):784-90, 1997

(Left) *Papillary fibroelastoma ➡ can be seen arising from the free edge of an aortic valve cusp. A small Lambl excrescence ➡ can be seen to the left of the papillary fibroelastoma. Note the simple, nonbranching Lambl excrescence in comparison to the arborizing papillary fibroelastoma.* (Right) *Gross photograph shows a large papillary fibroelastoma excised from the aortic valve. This papillary fibroelastoma had a densely calcified core.*

Aortic Valve Fibroelastoma

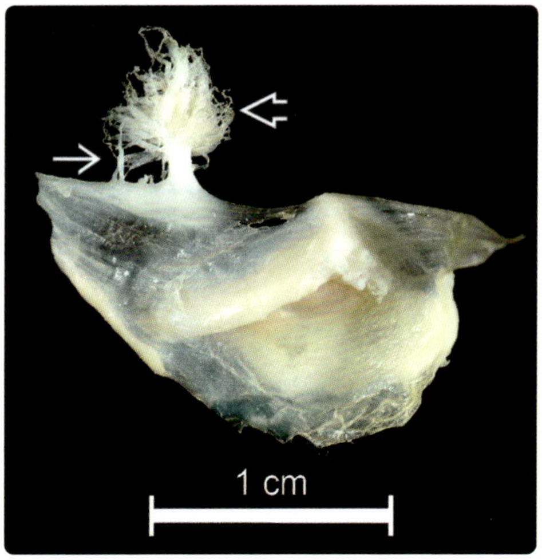

Massive Papillary Fibroelastoma

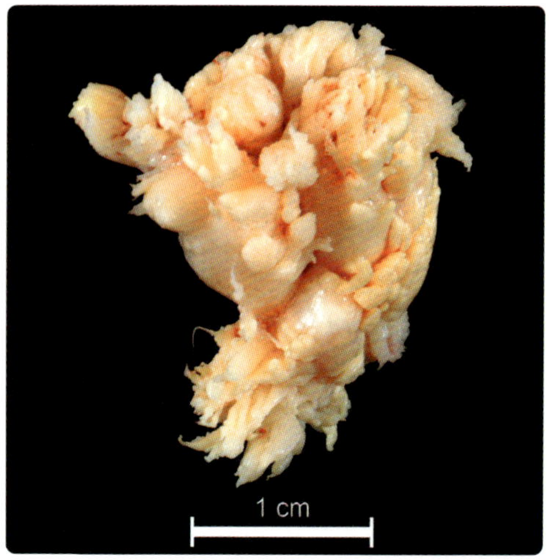

(Left) *Papillary fibroelastoma ➡ is seen arising on the surface of the aortic valve. Additionally, this case exemplifies the precarious location in which these lesions sometimes arise, in this case adjacent to a coronary ostium ➡. (Courtesy W. Edwards, MD.)* (Right) *Papillary fibroelastoma ⇨ is noted arising on the anterior leaflet of a postinflammatory (rheumatic) mitral valve.*

Papillary Fibroelastoma Near Coronary Artery Ostium

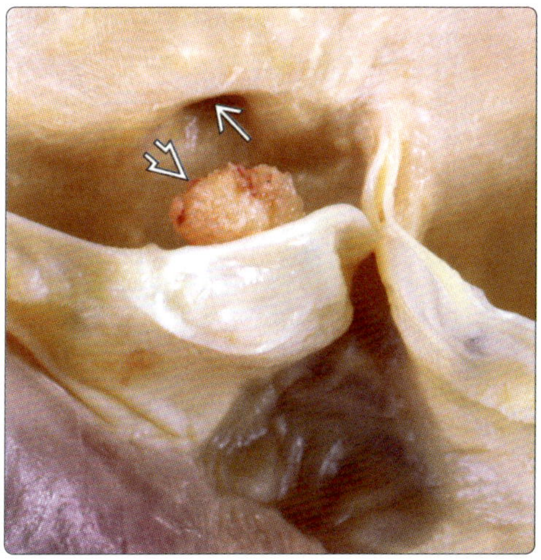

Mitral Valve Fibroelastoma

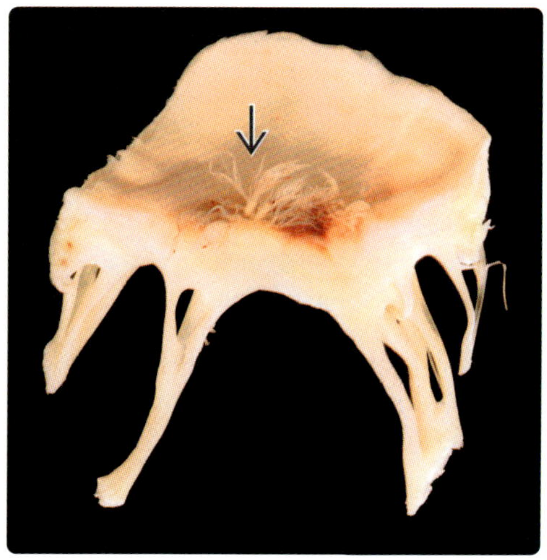

(Left) *Surgically excised papillary fibroelastoma shows numerous avascular papillary fronds ⇨ emanating from a common (central) stalk ⇨.* (Right) *High-power view of a single frond demonstrates the simple surface endothelial lining ⇨. The core contains proteoglycans, elastin, and occasionally smooth muscle myocytes. This basic structure is nearly identical to the microscopic appearance of Lambl excrescences with the primary difference being the architectural complexity of the papillary fibroelastoma.*

Papillary Fibroelastoma (Micro)

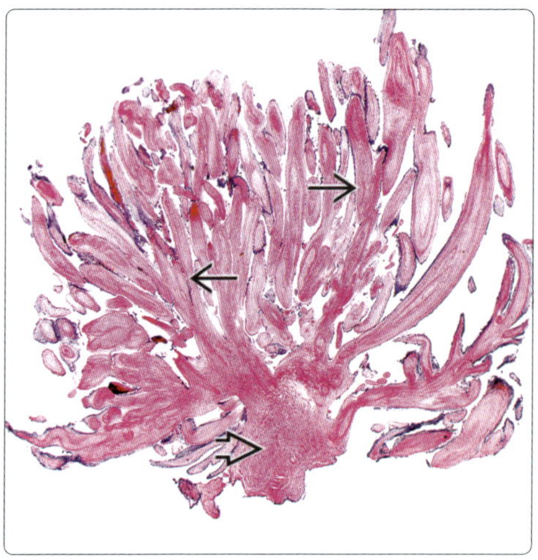

Single Frond of Papillary Fibroelastoma

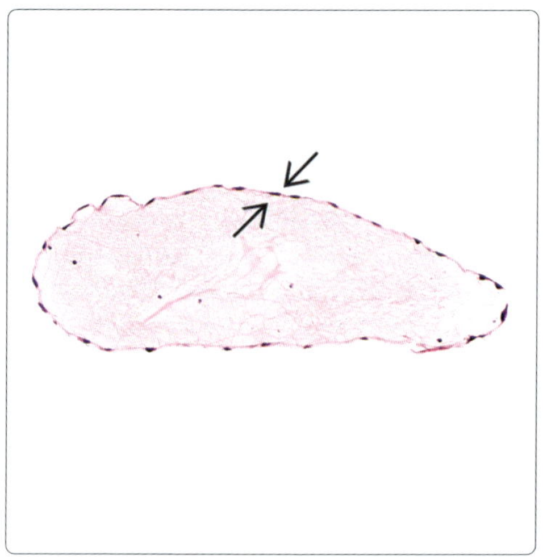

Papillary Fibroelastoma (High Magnification)

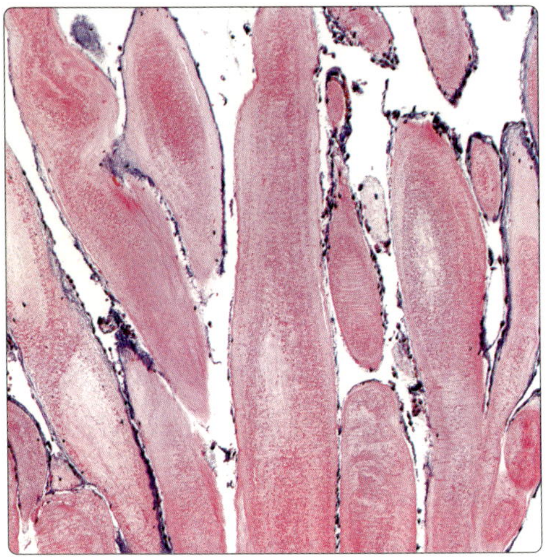

Papillary Fibroelastoma (Elastic Stain)

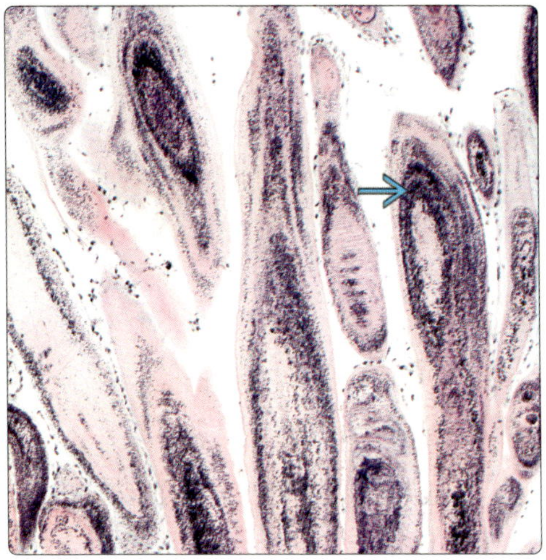

(Left) *Avascular papillary fronds are seen histologically and are composed largely of collagen and elastin with partially denuded surface endothelium.* **(Right)** *Elastic stain highlights the prominent elastic fibers → within the papillary fronds. The presence of the elastic fibers can be helpful in differentiating these lesions from cardiac myxomas with the latter typically not demonstrating such condensed elastic tissue.*

Incipient Papillary Fibroelastoma

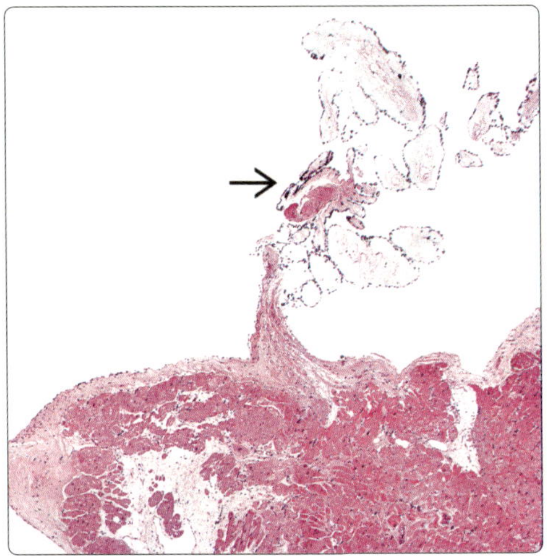

Tendinous Cord Papillary Fibroelastoma

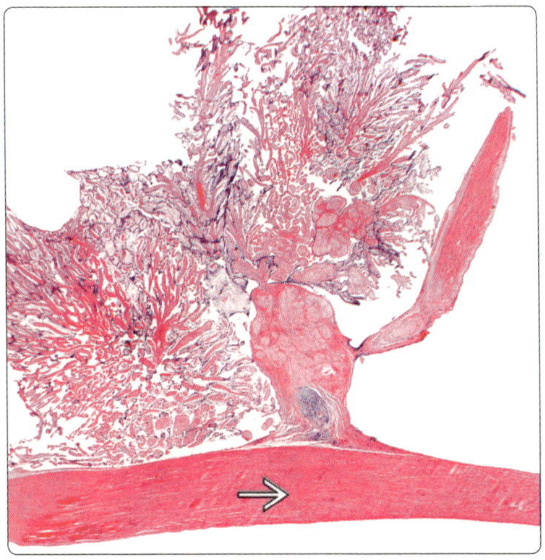

(Left) *A small, incipient, papillary fibroelastoma →, incidentally found at autopsy, is seen arising from the endocardium of the left ventricular outflow tract. Papillary fibroelastomas arising in this location are seen in the setting of hypertrophic obstructive cardiomyopathy or aortic stenosis (with basal septal bulge) where turbulent flow in an abnormally shaped outflow tract may be a factor.* **(Right)** *A papillary fibroelastoma was found at autopsy arising from a tendinous cord → of the mitral valve.*

Fused Fronds in Papillary Fibroelastoma

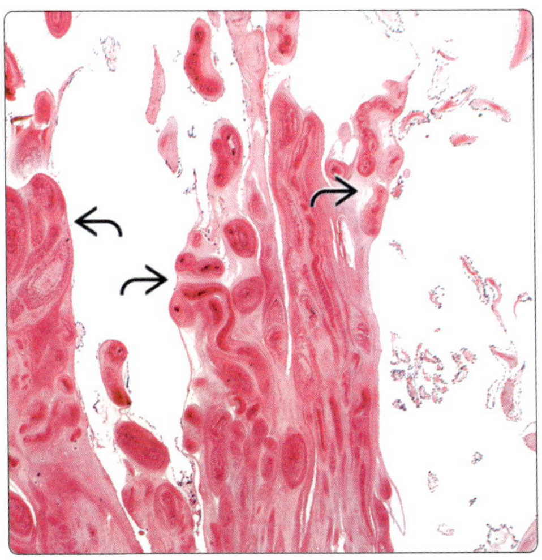

Calcification in Papillary Fibroelastoma

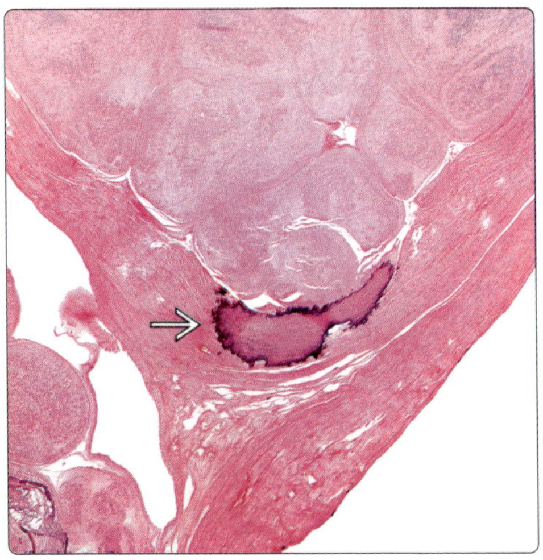

(Left) *Prominent fibrotic fusion ↗ of the papillary fronds can mask the gross papillary appearance of these lesions. Microscopy, however, will usually delineate the entrapped fronds. Elastic stains can also help to highlight the underlying architecture of these lesions.* **(Right)** *Focal calcification → is observed in this papillary fibroelastoma that also exhibits fibrotic fusion of the papillae. Calcification is more commonly encountered in larger lesions.*

Cardiac Rhabdomyoma

KEY FACTS

TERMINOLOGY

- Benign tumor of cardiac myocyte origin characterized by large vacuolated (glycogen-filled) polygonal cells
- Most frequently encountered congenital cardiac tumor

ETIOLOGY/PATHOGENESIS

- Poorly understood, but most evidence seems to suggest that these lesions are hamartomatous
- Most have clinical signs, radiologic signs, or family history of tuberous sclerosis complex (TSC)
- TSC is autosomal dominant neurocutaneous disorder characterized by benign hamartomatous lesions, often involving multiple organ systems
- *TSC1* and *TSC2* genes have been implicated

CLINICAL ISSUES

- Spontaneous regression in ~ 50% of cases (often in first 2-4 years of life)
- Cardiac rhabdomyomas not associated with TSC have generally good prognosis

MACROSCOPIC

- Often multiple (particularly in setting of TSC in which they may appear as numerous miliary nodules)
- Well-circumscribed, firm, tan-gray nodules
- Usually ventricular but may occur anywhere in heart

MICROSCOPIC

- Well-circumscribed lesions composed of distinctive vacuolated cells
- Cells often exhibit central nuclei with radial cytoplasmic extensions ("spider" cell)

ANCILLARY TESTS

- Periodic acid-Schiff
- Desmin
- Abundant glycogen with irregular myofilaments

Cardiac Rhabdomyomatosis: Gross

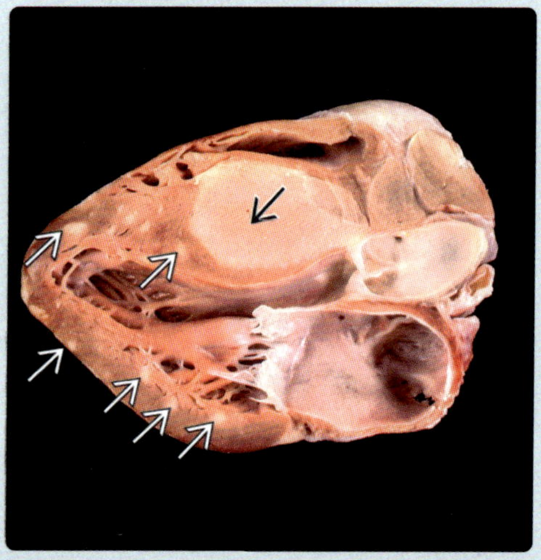

Cardiac Rhabdomyoma

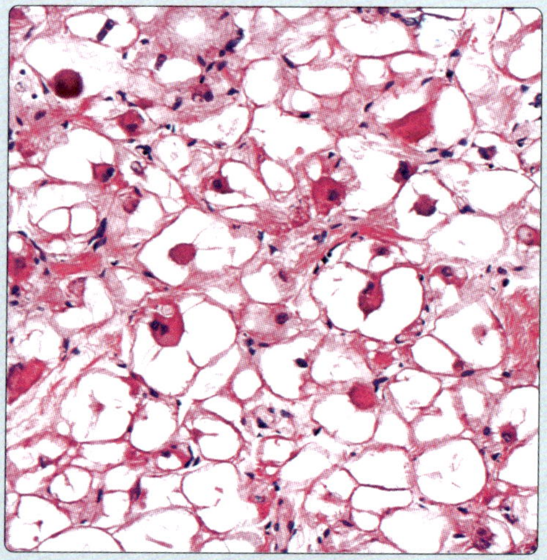

(Left) *A single large rhabdomyoma ⇨ within the ventricular septum narrows both the right and left ventricular outflow tracts. Numerous smaller rhabdomyomas ➡ are scattered throughout the myocardium.* **(Right)** *Photomicrograph shows large vacuolated cells that are characteristic of a cardiac rhabdomyoma. These modified myocytes can reach sizes of > 80 µm in diameter.*

"Spider" Cell in Cardiac Rhabdomyoma

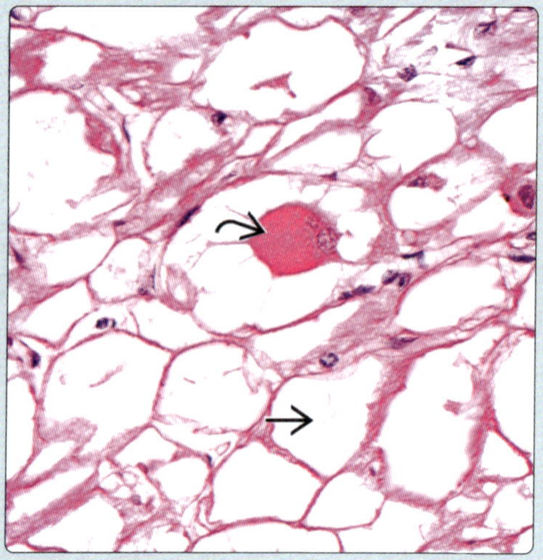

Myofibril Remnants in Rhabdomyoma

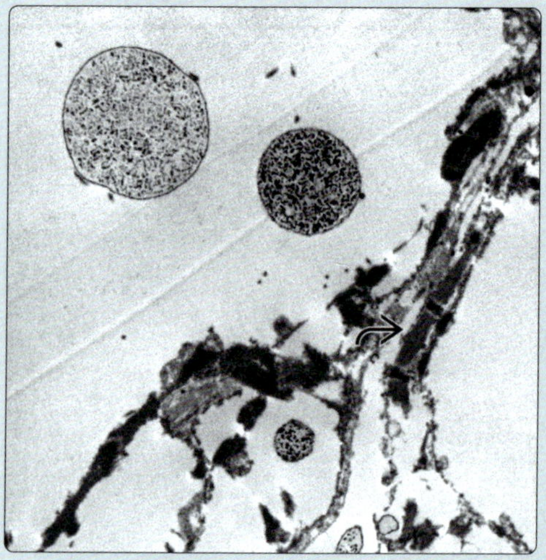

(Left) *Microscopically, most cells in rhabdomyoma show marked vacuolation ⇨, but the hallmark cell of this lesion ("spider" cell) shows a central eosinophilic globule ⇨, often associated with the nucleus. Wispy strands of sarcoplasm radiate from this central body.* **(Right)** *Transmission electron microscopy of cardiac rhabdomyoma shows contractile elements in sparse myofibrils ⇨. Much of the sarcoplasm is replaced (cleared) with glycogen.*

TERMINOLOGY

Definitions

- Benign tumor of cardiac myocytes (resembling fetal cardiomyocytes)
- Most common congenital cardiac tumor

ETIOLOGY/PATHOGENESIS

Etiology

- Most cases have clinical signs, radiologic signs, or family history of tuberous sclerosis complex (TSC)
    - TSC is autosomal dominant neurocutaneous disorder characterized by benign hamartomatous lesions, often involving multiple organ systems
    - *TSC1* and *TSC2* genes have been implicated
    - Cardiac rhabdomyomas found in 50-60% of cases
- Association with other congenital heart diseases (e.g., Ebstein anomaly, hypoplastic left heart syndrome, transposition of great arteries, ventricular septal defect) has been described

CLINICAL ISSUES

Epidemiology

- Age
    - Usually discovered in childhood
- Sex
    - No predilection

Presentation

- Often presents prenatally by fetal ultrasound
- Antenatally, may present with murmur, tachycardia, or other cardiac symptoms
- Discovered on screening after diagnosis of TSC

Treatment

- Options, risks, complications
    - Due to relatively high frequency of spontaneous regression, surgical excision reserved for cases with serious symptoms (intractable arrhythmias or obstruction)
    - Some evidence suggests mTOR inhibition (with everolimus) may induce regression in unresectable cases associated with TSC

Prognosis

- Cardiac rhabdomyomas not associated with TSC have generally good prognosis
- Spontaneous regression in ~ 50% of cases (often in first 2-4 years of life)

IMAGING

General Features

- Homogeneous, well-circumscribed masses within myocardium

Ultrasonographic Findings

- Multiple lobulated hyperechoic intramural masses

MR Findings

- Isointense on T1, hypointense on T2, minimal enhancement

MACROSCOPIC

General Features

- Well-circumscribed, firm, tan-gray nodules
- Often multiple (particularly in setting of TSC in which they may appear as numerous miliary nodules)

Size

- Wide range (< 1 mm to > 10 cm)

Location

- Usually ventricular but may occur anywhere in heart

MICROSCOPIC

Histologic Features

- Well-circumscribed lesions composed of distinctive vacuolated cells
- Cells often exhibit central nuclei with radial cytoplasmic extensions ("spider" cells)

ANCILLARY TESTS

Histochemistry

- Periodic acid-Schiff

Immunohistochemistry

- Positive for desmin, myoglobin; variable for HMB-45

Electron Microscopy

- Abundant glycogen with irregular myofilaments
- Leptomeric fibers adjacent to cell membrane

DIFFERENTIAL DIAGNOSIS

Fibroma

- Vacuolated ("spider") cells of rhabdomyoma absent
- Cardiac rhabdomyoma typically does not exhibit calcification seen in fibroma

Lipoma

- Absence of striations and "spider" cells

Glycogen Storage Disease

- Typically not mass forming
- Glycogen granules typically diastase resistant

Histiocytoid Cardiomyopathy

- Cells are granular rather than vacuolated

DIAGNOSTIC CHECKLIST

Clinically Relevant Pathologic Features

- Age distribution
- Gross appearance
- Symptom complex

SELECTED REFERENCES

1. Çetiner N et al: Rapid regression everolimus therapy in a neonate with cardiac rhabdomyoma. Pediatr Int. 64(1):e15188, 2022
2. Bielefeld KJ et al: Cardiac tumors in infants and children: study of 120 operated patients. Pediatr Cardiol. 34(1):125-8, 2013
3. Jain D et al: Benign cardiac tumors and tumorlike conditions. Ann Diagn Pathol. 14(3):215-30, 2010

Cardiac Rhabdomyoma

(**Left**) *Multiple large rhabdomyomas are seen in this autopsy specimen from a child with tuberous sclerosis. Both right atrial* ➡ *and right ventricular* ⇨ *tumors are identified. The right atrial tumor appears to involve the tricuspid valve and obstruct the valvular orifice. Several small mural tumors* ➡ *can also be seen throughout the ventricle.* (**Right**) *Autopsy specimen shows multiple rhabdomyomas* ➡ *involving the interventricular septum (viewed from the left ventricle).*

Cardiac Rhabdomyomas: Gross

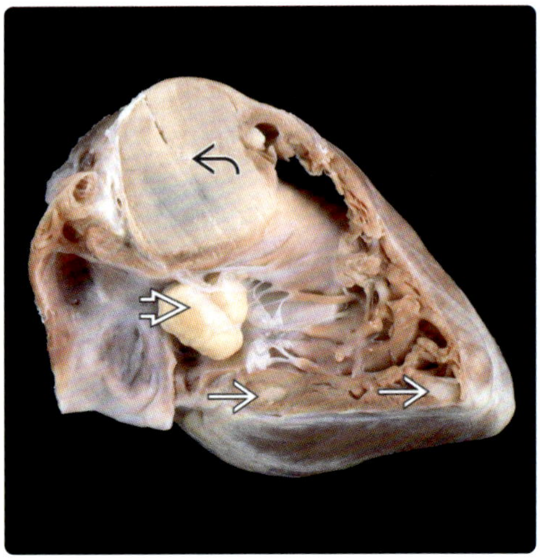

Subendocardial Rhabdomyomas: Gross

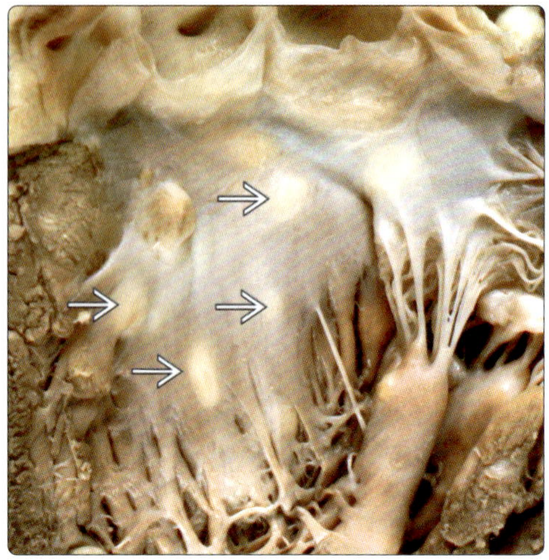

(**Left**) *High-power photomicrograph exhibits a classic cardiac rhabdomyoma "spider" cell. Note the numerous cytoplasmic extensions radiating from the perinuclear region to the cell membrane. Subtle sarcomeric elements can occasionally be identified within these extensions.* (**Right**) *Cardiac rhabdomyoma ("spider") cells can sometimes have multiple nuclei* ⇨ *in addition to their prominent cytoplasmic vacuolization. The foamy quality of the cytoplasm can mimic that of brown fat.*

"Spider" Cell in Rhabdomyoma

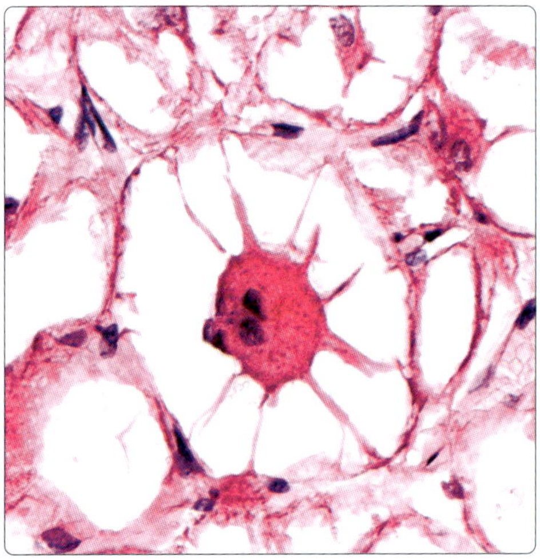

Cardiac Rhabdomyoma Cells

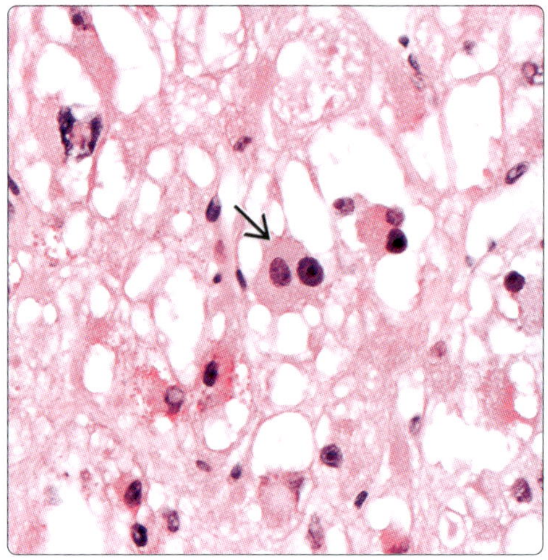

(**Left**) *At low power, cardiac rhabdomyoma* ⇨ *is usually very easily identified in comparison with the adjacent normal myocardium* ⇨*. High glycogen content imparts the vacuolated quality that is so characteristic of these tumor cells. The well-circumscribed border is also apparent in this photomicrograph.* (**Right**) *Photomicrograph exhibits a small intramural rhabdomyoma discovered incidentally at autopsy. The well-circumscribed border with the adjacent myocardium is evident.*

Cardiac Rhabdomyoma: Low Magnification

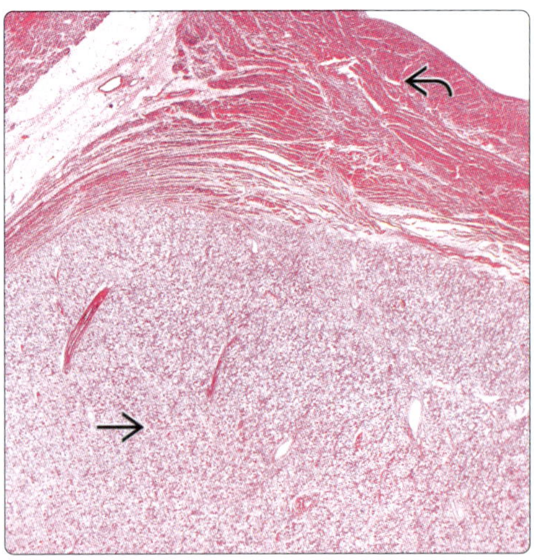

Intramural Rhabdomyoma

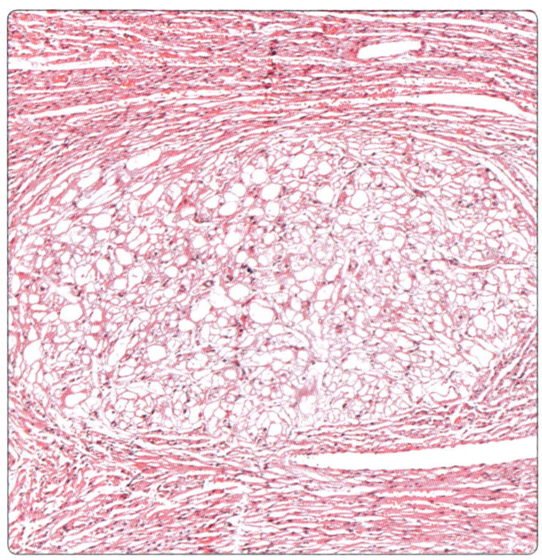

Lipoma-Like Changes in Cardiac Rhabdomyoma

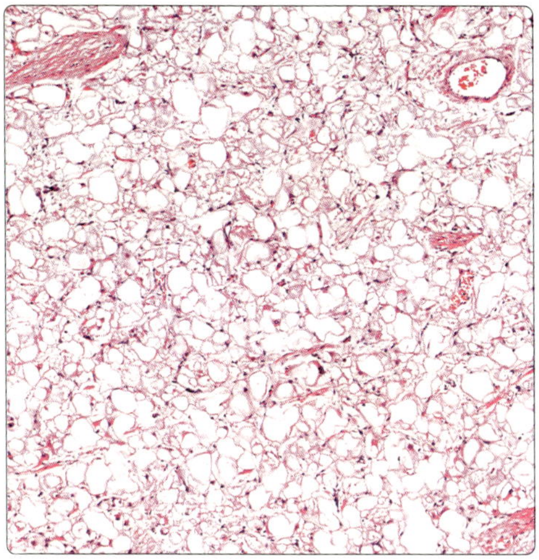

Involution in Cardiac Rhabdomyoma

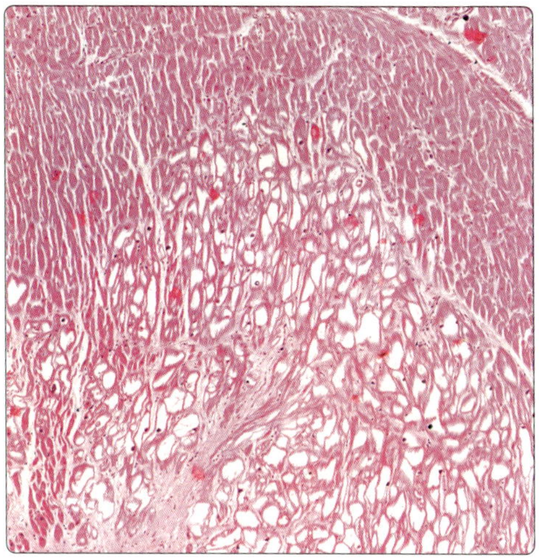

(Left) *Prominent vacuolization can cause cardiac lipoma to enter into the differential diagnosis of cardiac rhabdomyoma, but the central nuclei and occasional myofilaments will help confirm the diagnosis.* **(Right)** *Occasionally, rhabdomyomas will consist predominately of enlarged, anucleate myocytes. This finding is believed to be indicative of involutional change but can lead to misdiagnosis as lipoma; however, careful evaluation for striations will allow for appropriate classification.*

Glycogen in Cardiac Rhabdomyoma (PAS Stain)

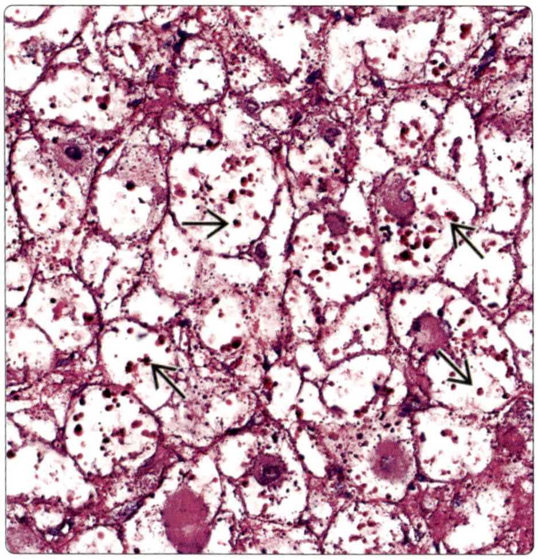

Glycogen in Cardiac Rhabdomyoma (Absent Staining on PAS-D)

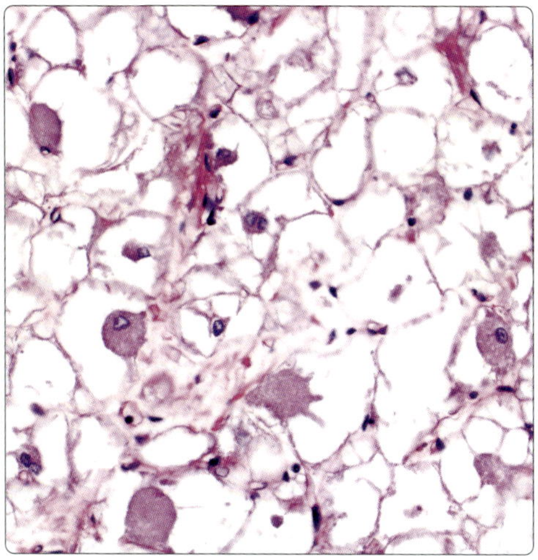

(Left) *The abundant glycogen contained within the enlarged, vacuolated myocytes can be readily demonstrated with a PAS stain. Best results are typically seen with alcohol-fixed or frozen tissue. Note the many magenta-colored granules ➔ contained within the cytoplasm of the "spider" cells.* **(Right)** *Enzymatic treatment with diastase will virtually eliminate the magenta-colored cytoplasmic granules seen with periodic acid-Schiff stain in a case of rhabdomyoma.*

Ultrastructure of Cardiac Rhabdomyoma

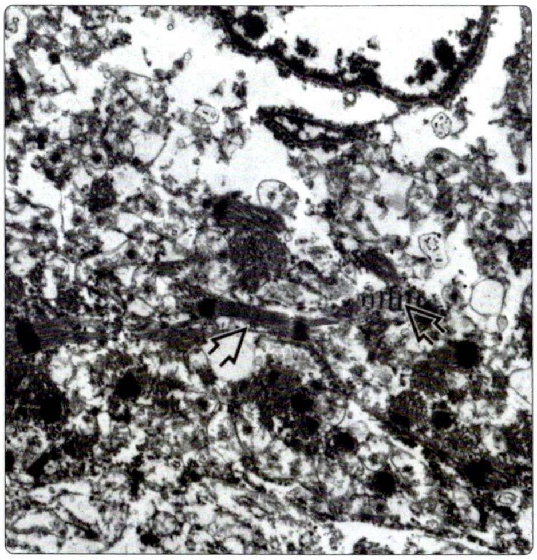

Desmin Staining in Cardiac Rhabdomyoma

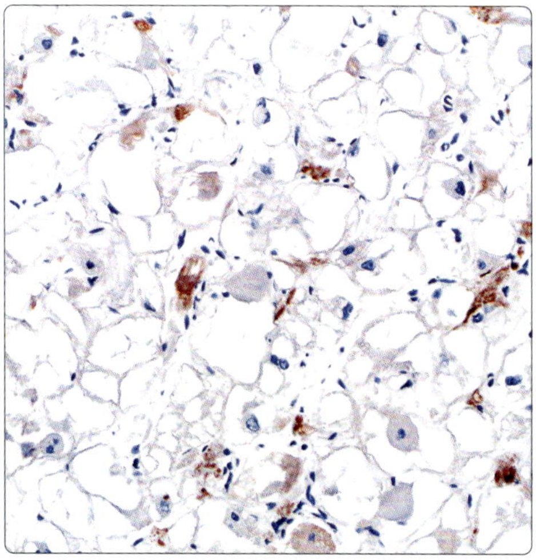

(Left) *Transmission electron microscopy shows scattered, fragmented myofilaments ➔ within the cytoplasm. Typically, abundant glycogen will accompany this finding; however, in a deparaffinized section (such as this), much of the glycogen may be lost during processing.* **(Right)** *The vacuolated cells exhibit focal reactivity with antibodies directed against desmin, helping to confirm their myogenic nature. This finding can be helpful in the differential diagnosis with cardiac lipomas.*

Cardiac Fibroma

KEY FACTS

TERMINOLOGY

- Benign fibroblastic/myofibroblastic cell proliferation within variably collagenous matrix

ETIOLOGY/PATHOGENESIS

- Frequently identified prenatally

CLINICAL ISSUES

- Ventricular septum is most common location
- Arrhythmias common
  - Up to 2/3 of patients having clinically significant arrhythmia
  - May result in syncope or sudden death
- Prognosis generally good
- Conservative management if asymptomatic; surgical if symptomatic
- Gorlin syndrome (a.k.a. nevoid basal cell carcinoma syndrome, Gorlin-Goltz syndrome)
  - Cardiac fibromas in < 20% of Gorlin syndrome patients

IMAGING

- Well-circumscribed mass within ventricular wall, sometimes calcified

MACROSCOPIC

- Typically well circumscribed, white-tan in color, and whorled in appearance
- Ragged interface with surrounding myocardium

MICROSCOPIC

- Not encapsulated and often interdigitate with adjacent myocardium, imparting infiltrative look (staining with Masson trichrome often highlights this finding)
- Cellularity is highly variable and often inversely related to age of patient (cellular lesions often seen in childhood; paucicellular lesions often seen in adults)

Gross Appearance of Cardiac Fibroma

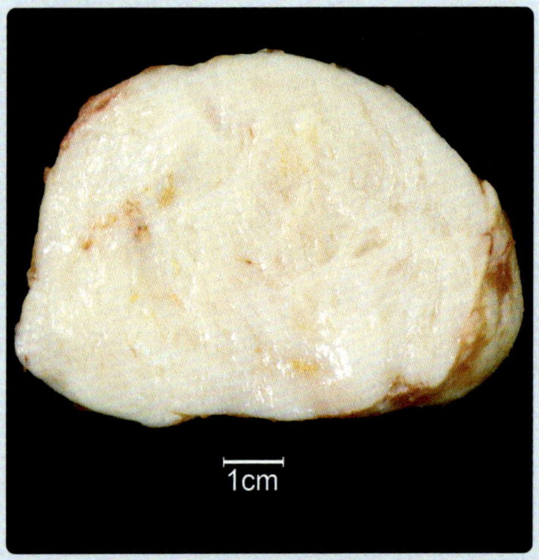

Dense Collagen Within Cardiac Fibroma

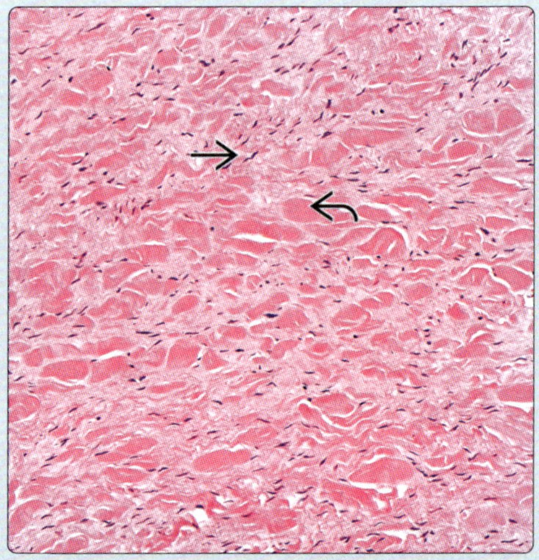

(Left) *Cardiac fibromas frequently exhibit a somewhat homogeneous cut surface with a white and whorled appearance. (Courtesy W. Edwards, MD.)* **(Right)** *A cardiac fibroma exhibits bland spindle cells → in an abundant collagenous stroma. The dense pink bundles of collagen ↶ are often the dominant feature of these lesions.*

Cardiac Fibroma: Extramedullary Hematopoiesis

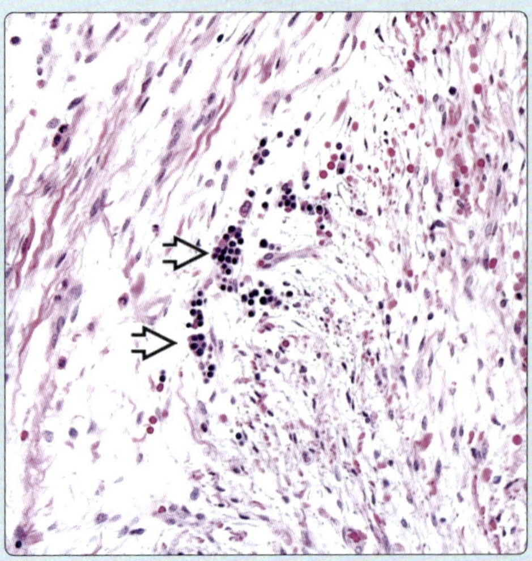

MR Appearance of Cardiac Fibroma

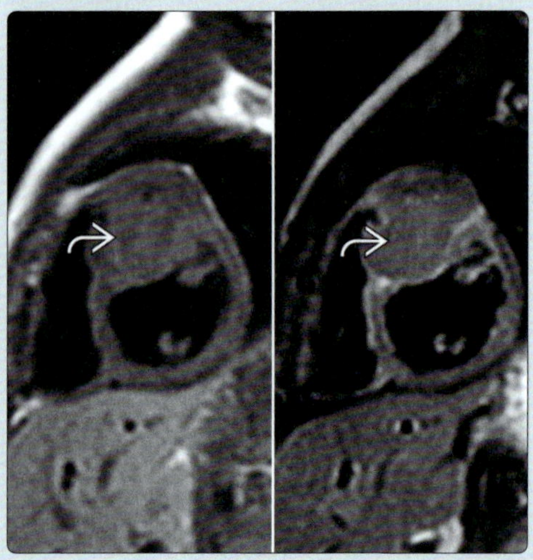

(Left) *Some cardiac fibromas, especially in neonates and infants, may show focal extramedullary hematopoiesis with clusters of nucleated erythrocyte ⇨ and other precursor cells.* **(Right)** *Short-axis T1 (left) and T2 (right) MR images of an anterior left ventricular fibroma ↱ in a 1-year-old infant are shown. The lesion is isointense on T1 and iso- to mildly hyperintense on T2 imaging. Fibromas in infants and young children may not show the T2 hypointensity commonly seen in adults.*

TERMINOLOGY

Synonyms

- Fibrous hamartoma, fibroelastic hamartoma

Definitions

- Benign fibroblastic/myofibroblastic cell proliferation within variably collagenous matrix

ETIOLOGY/PATHOGENESIS

Developmental Anomaly

- Frequently identified prenatally
  - Possibly all are congenital in origin (even if not detected until later)

CLINICAL ISSUES

Epidemiology

- Incidence
  - Very rare; precise incidence unknown
- Age
  - Presentation typically in childhood or prenatally
- Sex
  - No evident predilection

Site

- Ventricular septum most common
- May involve wall of any chamber, though atrial location is very uncommon
- May grow around coronary vasculature and compromise cardiac blood supply

Presentation

- Most present due to mass effect with some degree of hemodynamic compromise
- Arrhythmias are common (up to 2/3 of patients), may result in syncope or sudden death
- May also be asymptomatic

Treatment

- Options, risks, complications
  - Conservative management if asymptomatic; surgical if symptomatic
  - Rare reports of spontaneous regression
- Surgical approaches
  - Surgical resection (complete or incomplete) is treatment of choice when symptomatic with at least 1 study showing excellent arrhythmia abatement (100%)
  - Very large tumors sometimes necessitate cardiac transplantation

Prognosis

- Generally good, but worse outcomes with young age at presentation and septal involvement

Syndromic Associations

- Gorlin syndrome (a.k.a. nevoid basal cell carcinoma syndrome, Gorlin-Goltz syndrome)
  - Autosomal dominant disorder caused by germline mutation in *PTCH1* gene (chromosome 9q22.3)
  - Characterized by body overgrowth, odontogenic keratocysts of jaws, skeletal anomalies, and multiple neoplasms (including basal cell carcinomas)
  - Cardiac fibromas seen in < 20% of patients
- Sotos syndrome, hydrocephalus, cleft palate

IMAGING

Radiographic Findings

- Often appear as well-circumscribed masses within ventricular walls
- Reduced signal intensity compared to myocardium
- Calcifications, sometimes seen on CT scans

MACROSCOPIC

General Features

- Typically well circumscribed, white-tan in color, whorled

Size

- Mean reported size: 5 cm

MICROSCOPIC

Histologic Features

- Proliferation of bland spindle cells with abundant collagenous stroma
- Cellularity is highly variable and often inversely related to age of patient (cellular lesions often seen in childhood; paucicellular lesions often seen in adults)
- Calcification (macro- or microscopic) frequent
- Variable elastin fibers can be identified

Margins

- No capsule, interdigitates with myocardium
- Symptoms may abate even with residual tumor

DIFFERENTIAL DIAGNOSIS

Inflammatory Pseudotumor

- More prominent inflammatory infiltrate than what is seen in cardiac fibroma

Fibrosarcoma

- More mitotically active, often with cellular atypia, in contrast to bland proliferation in cardiac fibroma

Scar

- Usually associated with mural thinning instead of mass effect (and wall thickening) produced by cardiac fibroma

SELECTED REFERENCES

1. Ritter AL et al: Cardiac fibroma with ventricular tachycardia: an unusual clinical presentation of nevoid basal cell carcinoma syndrome. Mol Syndromol. 9(4):219-23, 2018
2. Delmo Walter EM et al: Primary cardiac tumors in infants and children: surgical strategy and long-term outcome. Ann Thorac Surg. 102(6):2062-9, 2016
3. Torimitsu S et al: Literature survey on epidemiology and pathology of cardiac fibroma. Eur J Med Res. 17(1):5, 2012
4. Miyake CY et al: Cardiac tumors and associated arrhythmias in pediatric patients, with observations on surgical therapy for ventricular tachycardia. J Am Coll Cardiol. 58(18):1903-9, 2011
5. Miller DV et al: Beta-catenin mutations do not contribute to cardiac fibroma pathogenesis. Pediatr Dev Pathol. 11(4):291-4, 2008
6. Scanlan D et al: Loss of the PTCH1 gene locus in cardiac fibroma. Cardiovasc Pathol. 17(2):93-7, 2008

(Left) *Gross photograph exhibits an incidental cardiac fibroma ➡ discovered at autopsy. It is located on the left ventricular free wall and has a grossly well-defined border with the adjacent myocardium. This well-circumscribed gross appearance is often discordant with the microscopic appearance. (Courtesy W. Edwards, MD.)* **(Right)** *Gross photograph exhibits a large cardiac fibroma → within the interventricular septum. (Courtesy W. Edwards, MD.)*

Cardiac Fibroma of Left Ventricular Free Wall

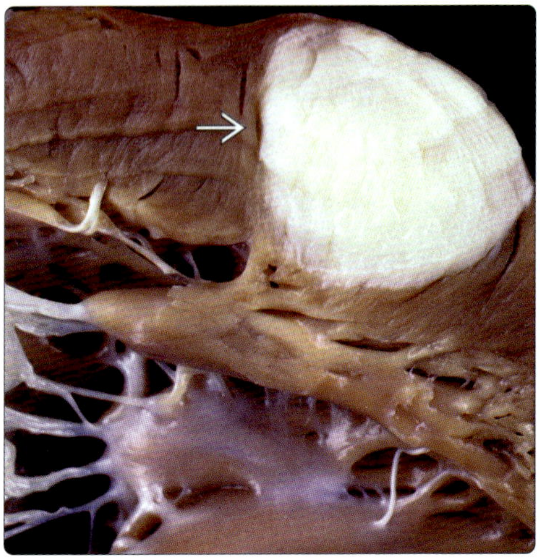

Cardiac Fibroma of Ventricular Septum

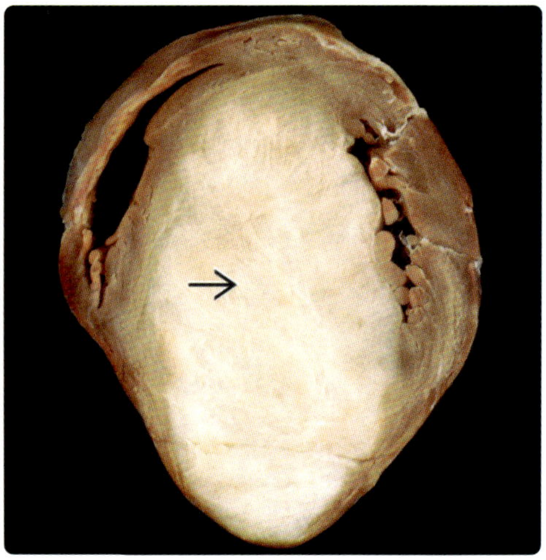

(Left) *Photomicrograph shows a cellular cardiac fibroma. These cellular lesions are typically identified in younger children and are thought to become less cellular with time (associated with increased collagen deposition). The example shown here is from a 3-month-old boy.* **(Right)** *Photomicrograph demonstrates a somewhat paucicellular proliferation of spindle cells → in an abundant, fibrillar, collagenous stroma ↪. The example shown here is a fibroma from a 57-year-old man.*

Cardiac Fibroma With High Cellularity

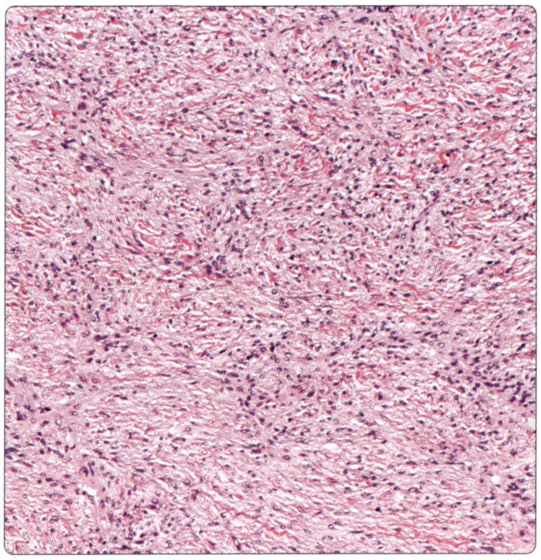

Cardiac Fibroma With Sparse Cellularity

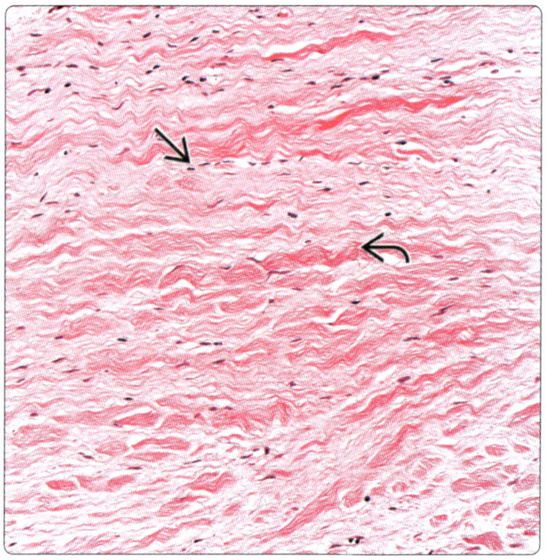

(Left) *Though cardiac fibromas may appear well circumscribed grossly, they often demonstrate remarkable interdigitation with the adjacent myocardium. This Masson trichrome-stained section exhibits this phenomenon. The mature collagen is blue, whereas the myocardium itself is red.* **(Right)** *Photomicrograph shows the interface between a fibroma → and myocardium ↪, demonstrating remarkable interdigitation of the tumor with the adjacent myocardium.*

Cardiac Fibroma: Trichrome Staining

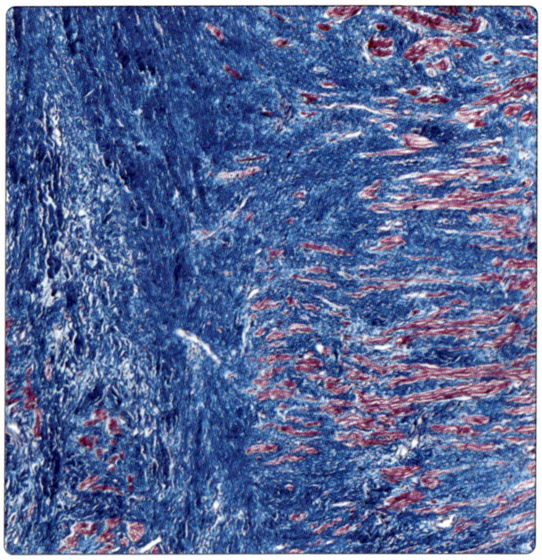

Cardiac Fibroma: Myocardium Interface

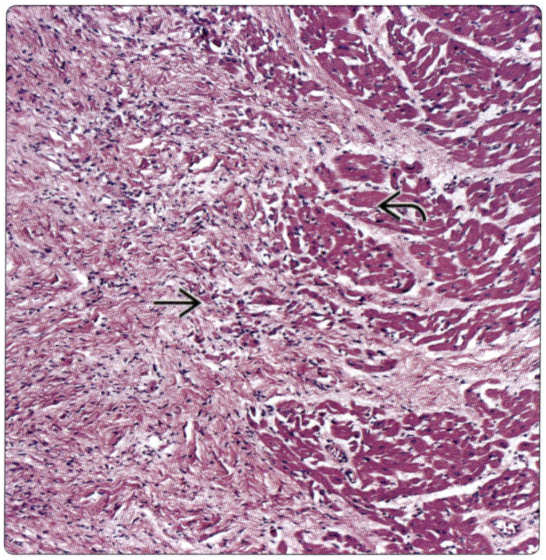

Bland Spindle Cells in Cardiac Fibroma

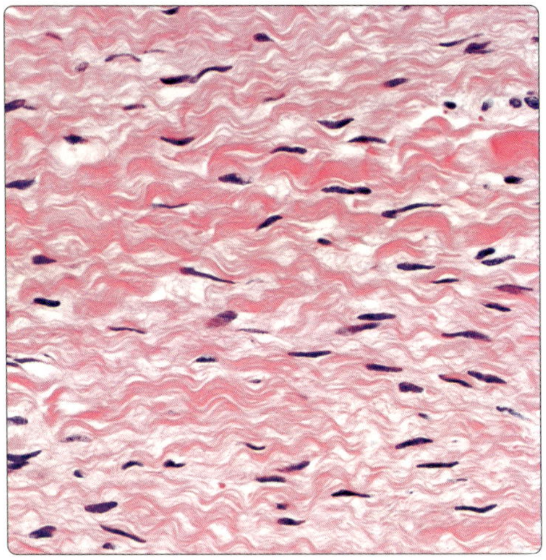

Inflammation in Cardiac Fibroma

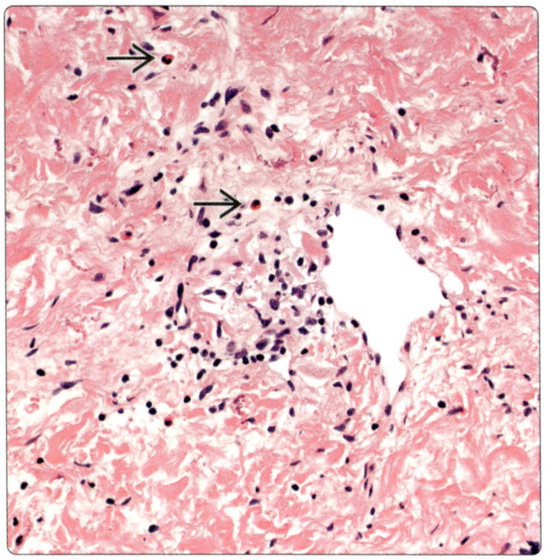

(Left) *Cardiac fibromas are composed of bland spindle cells in a densely collagenous stroma. The cells contain nuclei that are generally fusiform or oval in shape without apparent nucleoli. The cytoplasm of the cells is pale pink and somewhat indistinct.* **(Right)** *Mild, mixed inflammation is sometimes encountered in cardiac fibromas. Rare eosinophils → are identified in this case. Typically, the degree of inflammation is far less than that usually found in inflammatory pseudotumor.*

CT Appearance of Cardiac Fibroma

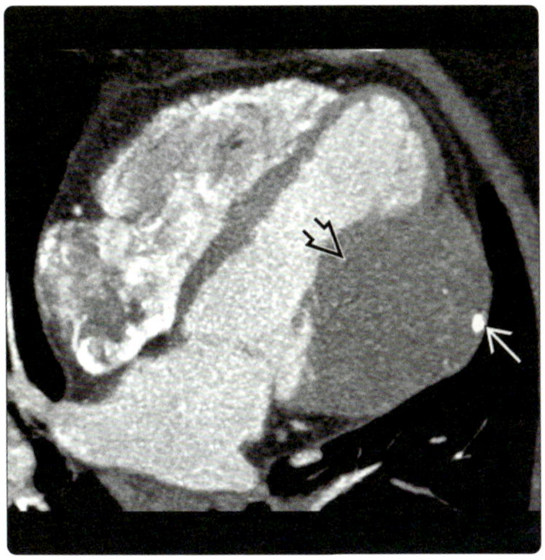

Calcification in Cardiac Fibroma

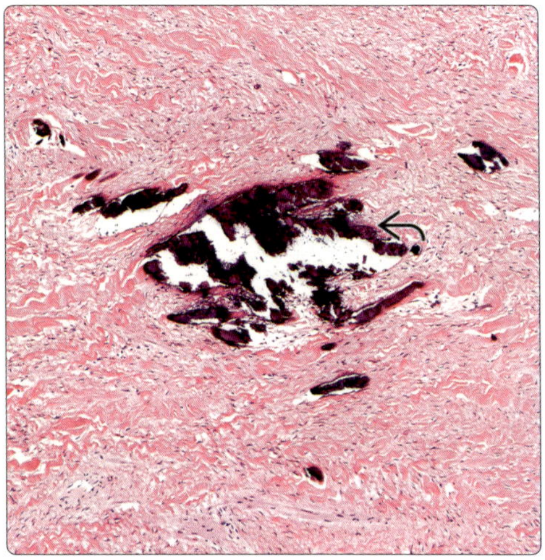

(Left) *Axial cardiac CT shows a large posterolateral left ventricular mass with relatively smooth borders ⇨. The small microcalcifications ➡ can be seen in the mass and are often a radiologic clue to the diagnosis of cardiac fibroma. This lesion abuts but does not invade the pericardium. (Courtesy C. White, MD.)* **(Right)** *Calcification is a common finding in cardiac fibromas and may be microscopic ↶ or grossly evident.*

Cardiac Fibroma: Trichrome Staining

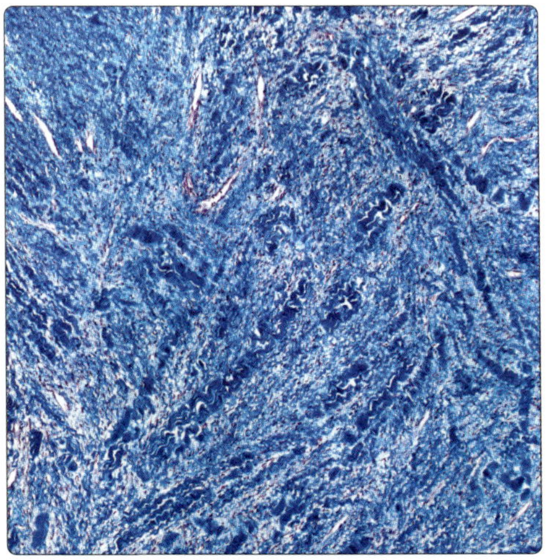

Blood Vessels in Cardiac Fibroma

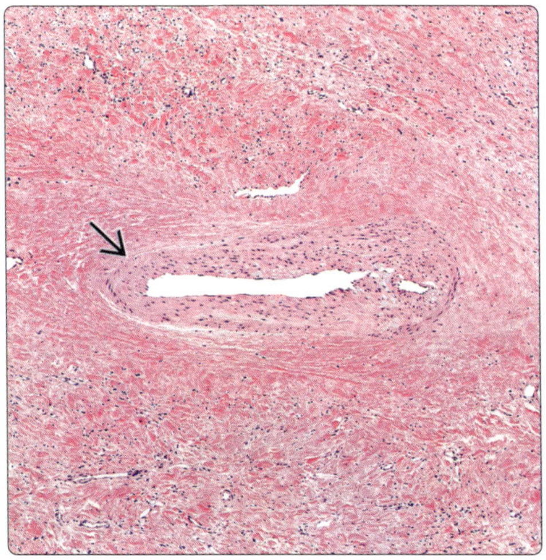

(Left) *The haphazard arrangement of the collagen fibers (seen here on this Masson trichrome stain) causes the cut surface of cardiac fibromas to have a whorled appearance grossly.* **(Right)** *Thick-walled blood vessels → can be identified throughout cardiac fibromas, but they are more frequently encountered at the periphery of the lesion, near the interface with the myocardium.*

Ectopic Tissues, Heart

KEY FACTS

TERMINOLOGY

- Structurally normal tissue found abnormally within heart
- Several different types of ectopic tissue have been described, including
  - Ultimobranchial heterotopia [cystic tumor of atrioventricular (AV) node]
  - Bronchogenic cysts
  - Thyroid, thymus, liver, breast
  - Teratoma

CLINICAL ISSUES

- Most symptomatic ectopias present in childhood; most found in adults are incidental
- Prognosis generally good

MACROSCOPIC

- Generally well circumscribed
- May be solid or cystic (depending on nature of ectopic tissue)

MICROSCOPIC

- Thyroid
  - Usually found in right ventricle (septum)
- Cystic tumor of AV node (ultimobranchial heterotopia)
  - Variably sized cysts, nests of cells with 2 populations
- Bronchogenic cysts
  - Cystic structure lined by respiratory epithelium
- Thymus
  - Benign thymic tissue
- Teratoma
  - Identical to teratomas found elsewhere in body

ANCILLARY TESTS

- Cystic tumor of AV node: Calretinin reactivity
- Ectopic thyroid: TTF-1 and thyroglobulin reactive

Pericardial Cyst

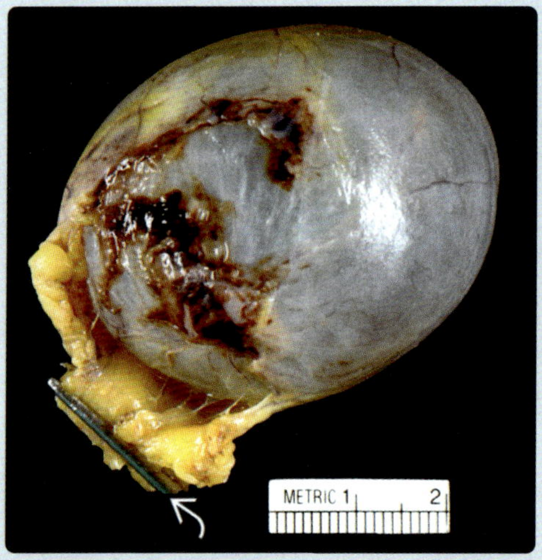

Myocardial Ectopic Thyroid

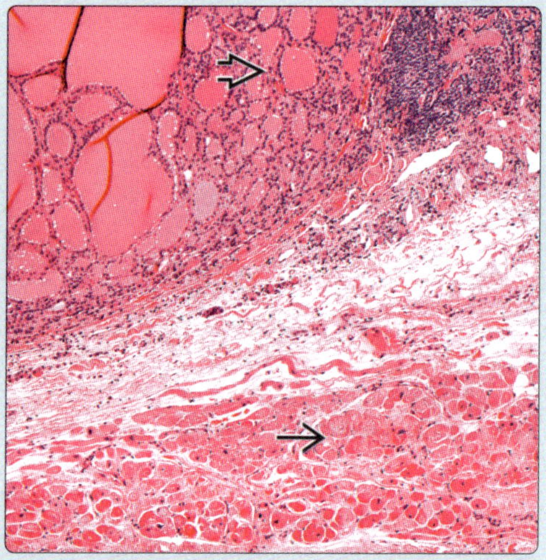

(Left) *This incidental (benign) pericardial cyst was encountered during open aortic valve replacement. The lining was mostly serous with focal bronchogenic features. A surgical clip helps with the image scale.* **(Right)** *Photomicrograph shows ectopic thyroid tissue surgically removed from the ventricular septum. The ectopic tissue has a relatively well-circumscribed interface with the adjacent myocardium.*

Ultimobranchial Heterotopia (Cystic Tumor of Atrioventricular Node)

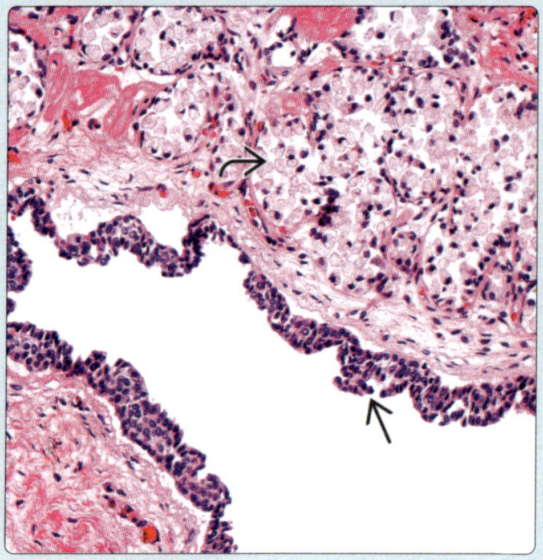

Cardiac Bronchogenic Cyst

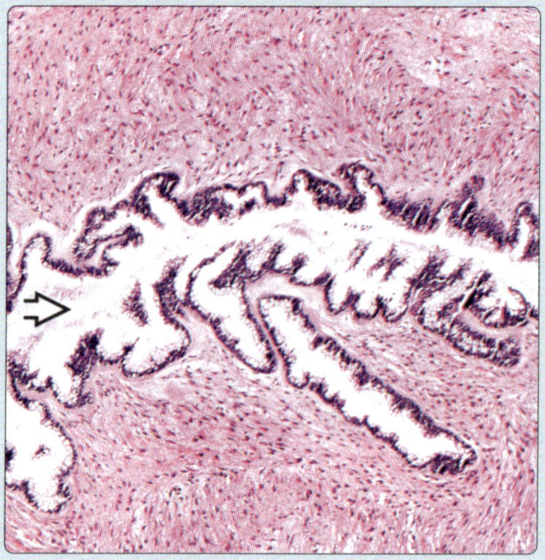

(Left) *High-power photomicrograph exhibits a cystic tumor of the atrioventricular node showing stratified epithelial surface cells with underlying sebaceous cells.* **(Right)** *Photomicrograph exhibits a bronchogenic cyst lined by respiratory epithelium.*

TERMINOLOGY

Synonyms

- Heterotopic tissue

Definitions

- Structurally normal tissue found abnormally within heart
- Several different types of ectopic tissue have been described, including
  - Thyroid
  - Ultimobranchial heterotopia [cystic tumor of atrioventricular (AV) node]
  - Bronchogenic cysts
  - Thymus
  - Teratoma
  - Liver
  - Breast

ETIOLOGY/PATHOGENESIS

Developmental Anomaly

- Generally result of abnormal persistent tissue that fails to involute during development or abnormal migration of tissue to developing heart
- Ectopic liver tissue may be result of hepatic embolization during instrumentation owing to proliferative capabilities of hepatocytes

CLINICAL ISSUES

Epidemiology

- Incidence: All ectopic tissues within heart are exceedingly rare
- Age: Believed to be present at birth (variably symptomatic)
- Sex: Female predilection for most types of ectopic tissues found within heart

Presentation

- Most symptomatic ectopias present in childhood; most found in adults are incidental
- Uncommonly, can present with symptoms of heart failure or cardiac tamponade
- Cystic tumors of AV node are thought to be smallest tumors associated with sudden cardiac death

Treatment

- Surgical approaches
  - Simple excision is warranted if symptomatic

Prognosis

- Generally good

IMAGING

General Features

- Location
  - Many ectopic tissues occur in ventricular septum or right ventricle

MACROSCOPIC

General Features

- Generally well circumscribed
- May be solid or cystic (depending on nature of ectopic tissue)

MICROSCOPIC

Histologic Features

- Thyroid
  - Usually found in right ventricle (septum)
  - Variably sized thyroid follicles
- Cystic tumor of AV node (ultimobranchial heterotopia)
  - Usually multiple variably sized cysts and nests of epithelioid (low cuboidal cells) (single or multiple layers)
  - Sebaceous cells may be present within lesions
  - Nests and cysts typically contained within fibrotic stroma
- Bronchogenic cysts
  - Cystic structure lined by respiratory epithelium
  - Cyst wall may contain smooth muscle, cartilage, lymphoid aggregates, and mucous glands
  - Pulmonary parenchyma is variably present
- Thymus
  - Benign thymic tissue within heart
  - Rarely may have thymoma contained therein
- Teratoma
  - May resemble bronchogenic cysts but usually contain ectodermal tissue (hair, teeth, or neural tissue)
  - Identical to teratomas found elsewhere in body
  - May have other germ cell tumor elements present, in which case tumors are malignant
- Liver
  - Benign hepatic parenchyma within heart
- Breast
  - Rare; only 1 reported case found in left atrium
  - Benign breast parenchyma within heart

ANCILLARY TESTS

Immunohistochemistry

- Cystic tumor of AV node: Calretinin reactivity
- Ectopic thyroid: TTF-1 and thyroglobulin reactive

DIFFERENTIAL DIAGNOSIS

Metastatic Neoplasms

- Carcinoma
  - Follicular thyroid carcinoma
  - Hepatocellular carcinoma
- Thymoma
  - Cardiac presentation is rare; clinical history of carcinoma or thymoma is helpful

SELECTED REFERENCES

1. Stewart BD et al: Benign lesions of the mediastinum: a review with emphasis on cytology and small biopsy specimens. Semin Diagn Pathol. 37(4):199-210, 2020
2. Cohle SD: Cystic tumour of the atrioventricular node: case report and literature review. Forensic Sci Res. 4(3):287-9, 2019
3. Nishida N et al: Intramyocardial bronchogenic cyst: histological appearance and a review of the literature. Cardiovasc Pathol. 28:64-7, 2017
4. Xu L et al: Ectopic hepatic tissue presenting as right atrial mass. Hum Pathol. 43(6):958-60, 2012
5. Sasaki K et al: Heterotopic breast epithelial inclusion of the heart: report of a case. Am J Surg Pathol. 34(10):1555-9, 2010
6. Miller DV et al: Cardiovascular tumor-like conditions. Semin Diagn Pathol. 25(1):54-64, 2008

Lipomatous Hypertrophy of Atrial Septum

KEY FACTS

CLINICAL ISSUES

- Most commonly asymptomatic
- Older age (> 50 years); F > M
- May mimic cardiac neoplasm by appearing as mass projecting into right atrium
- Weak association with obesity

IMAGING

- Echocardiography
  - Brightly echogenic enlargement of intraatrial septum with bilobed (dumbbell-shaped) appearance, usually with larger superior fat mass
- Cardiac CT
  - Nonenhancing, homogeneous thickening of intraatrial septum

MACROSCOPIC

- Thickening of intraatrial septum (limbus), usually ≥ 20 mm by nonencapsulated fatty tissue
- Valve of fossa ovalis spared (dumbbell appearance)
- Bulges toward right atrium, not left, because limbus is right-sided structure
- Rare reports of involvement of other areas (free wall of left atrium, intraventricular septum)

MICROSCOPIC

- Mature adipocytes
- Vacuolated adipocytes with central nuclei (brown fat)
- Interspersed hypertrophied myocytes,
- Fine fibrous septa
- Scattered chronic inflammation
- Nerve fibers and ganglion

TOP DIFFERENTIAL DIAGNOSES

- Lipoma and liposarcoma

Oval Fossa of Interatrial Septum (Normal)

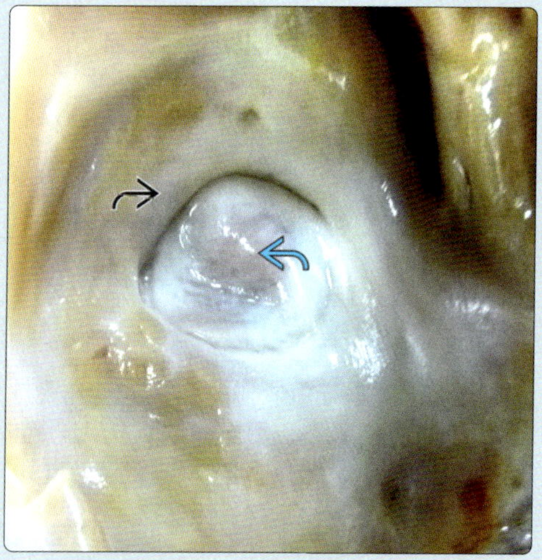

Bulging Limbus of Oval Fossa in Lipomatous Hypertrophy of Atrial Septum

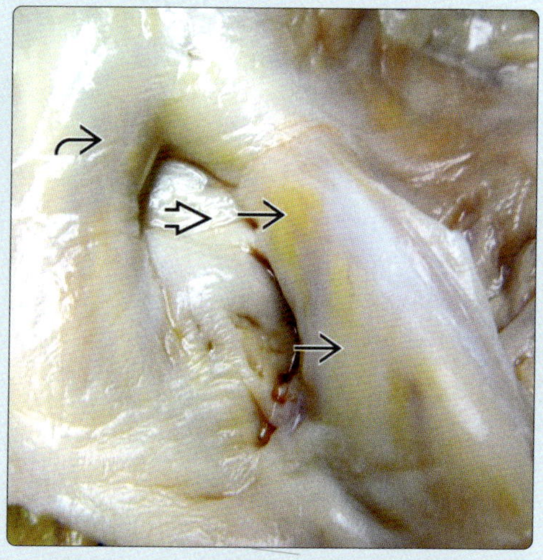

(Left) *The limbus of the fossa ovalis in a normal intraatrial septum represents the embryologic septum secundum as a right-sided structure. The valve of the fossa ovalis is noted.* **(Right)** *The limbus of the fossa ovalis is thickened to 3.0 cm by fatty tissue that can be seen through the endocardial surface. The valve of the fossa ovalis is spared.*

Section Through Oval Fossa in Lipomatous Hypertrophy of Atrial Septum

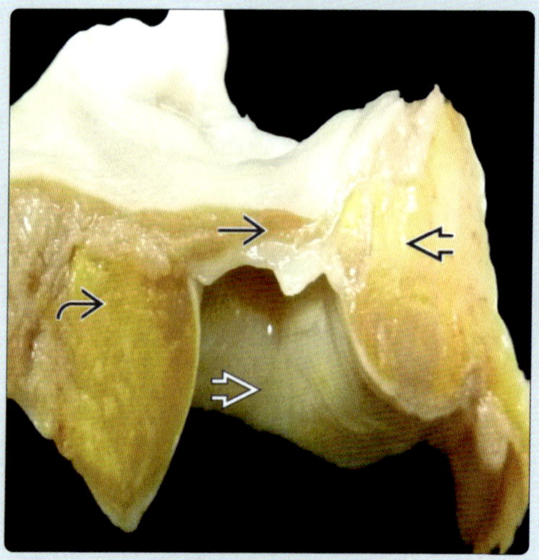

Mature and Brown Fat in Lipomatous Hypertrophy of Atrial Septum

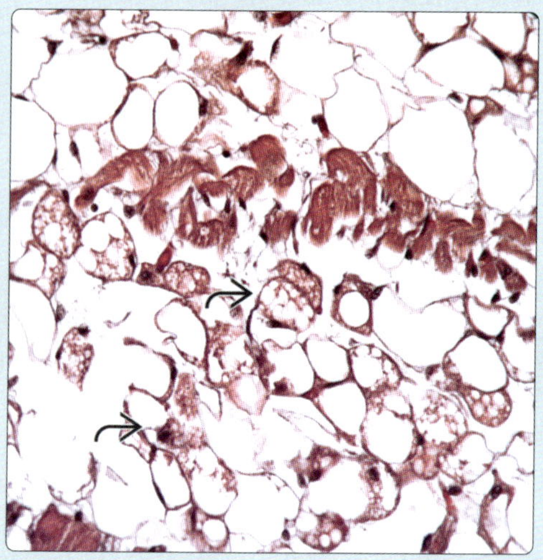

(Left) *Gross photograph shows lipomatous hypertrophy of the cephalad and caudal septum (3.0 cm) sparing the valve of the fossa, creating a dumbbell-shaped septum. The tissue bulges toward the right atrium.* **(Right)** *Lipomatous hypertrophy consists of mature fat, vacuolated adipocytes with central nuclei resembling brown fat, and scattered hypertrophied myocytes.*

TERMINOLOGY

Definitions

- Cardiac pseudoneoplasm characterized by enlargement of intraatrial septum (limbus of fossa ovalis) by nonencapsulated mass of mature adipose tissue with admixed hypertrophied myocytes and brown fat

ETIOLOGY/PATHOGENESIS

Developmental Aberrancy

- Expansion of fat cells that have been trapped within intraatrial septum during development as atrial walls form by progressive infolding
  - Trigger for expansion of entrapped adipocytes is unknown

CLINICAL ISSUES

Epidemiology

- Incidence
  - Seen in ~ 1% of autopsies
  - 2-8% of echocardiographic examinations
- Age
  - Older patients (> 50 years)
- Sex
  - F > M

Presentation

- Most commonly asymptomatic
- Rare sudden cardiac death, sustained supraventricular tachycardia, superior vena cava obstruction
- May mimic cardiac neoplasm by appearing as mass projecting into right atrium
- Weak association with obesity

IMAGING

Echocardiography

- Brightly echogenic enlargement of intraatrial septum with bilobed (dumbbell-shaped) appearance, usually with larger superior fat mass

Cardiac CT

- Nonenhancing, homogeneous thickening of intraatrial septum

PET

- May show increased uptake due to presence of hypermetabolic brown fat

MACROSCOPIC

General Features

- Thickening of intraatrial septum (limbus), usually ≥ 20 mm
- Valve of fossa ovalis spared
  - Gives dumbbell appearance of lesion
- Cephalad portion of septum usually thicker than caudal portion
- Bulges toward right atrium, not left, because limbus is right-sided structure
  - Rare reports of involvement of other areas (free wall of left atrium, intraventricular septum)
- Thickening caused by infiltrating, nonencapsulated, yellow adipose tissue that is often contiguous with epicardial adipose tissue
  - Usually increase in amount of epicardial adipose tissue, especially around atrioventricular sulcus (75% of patients)

MICROSCOPIC

Histologic Features

- No capsule identified
- Mature adipocytes
- Vacuolated adipocytes with central nuclei (brown fat)
- Interspersed hypertrophied myocytes
- Fine, fibrous septa
- Scattered chronic inflammation
- Other epicardial elements, such as ganglia, may be noted

DIFFERENTIAL DIAGNOSIS

Lipoma

- Encapsulated without interspersed hypertrophied myocytes or brown fat cells

Liposarcoma

- Look for lipoblasts
  - Confusing vacuolated adipocytes (brown fat) of lipomatous hypertrophy with lipoblasts may occur
    - Lipoblasts have clear cytoplasm with vacuoles indenting central hyperchromatic nucleus
  - Rarely, single hypertrophied myocytes may appear atypical, causing confusion with lipoblast
    - Usually, these cells retain enough sarcoplasmic elements to be recognized as myocytes

SELECTED REFERENCES

1. An KR et al: Lipomatous hypertrophy of the interatrial septum is a pathologic, not an anatomic diagnosis. J Card Surg. 35(5):1132-4, 2020
2. Rob D et al: A rare case of regressively changed lipomatous hypertrophy of the interatrial septum presenting with anemia and recurrent fever. Cardiovasc Pathol. 25(2):161-4, 2016
3. Sheikh M et al: Syncope as an initial manifestation of atypical lipomatous hypertrophy of the interatrial septum. J Card Surg. 27(4):454-7, 2012
4. Nezafati MH et al: Lipomatosis of interventricular septum and both ventricles: an extremely rare pattern. Interact Cardiovasc Thorac Surg. 12(3):511-2, 2011
5. Hsieh TC et al: Extensive lipomatous hypertrophy of the interatrial septum with involvement of the right atrium. Anesth Analg. 110(3):725-6; discussion 727, 2010
6. Klein MA et al: Intensely hypermetabolic lipomatous hypertrophy of the interatrial septum on 18-FDG PET with MRI and CT correlation. Clin Nucl Med. 35(12):972-3, 2010
7. Miller DV et al: Cardiovascular pseudoneoplasms. Arch Pathol Lab Med. 134(3):362-8, 2010
8. Silbiger JJ et al: Lipomatous hypertrophy of the interatrial septum revisited. J Am Soc Echocardiogr. 23(7):789-90, 2010
9. Dettrick AJ: Lipomatous hypertrophy of the interatrial septum: report of an unusual case. Histopathology. 54(6):777-9, 2009
10. Xanthos T et al: Lipomatous hypertrophy of the interatrial septum: a pathological and clinical approach. Int J Cardiol. 121(1):4-8, 2007
11. Abboud H et al: Lipomatous hypertrophy of the inter-atrial septum and stroke. Cerebrovasc Dis. 18(2):178, 2004
12. Salanitri JC et al: Cardiac lipoma and lipomatous hypertrophy of the interatrial septum: cardiac magnetic resonance imaging findings. J Comput Assist Tomogr. 28(6):852-6, 2004
13. Gay JD et al: Clinical and morphologic features of lipomatous hypertrophy ("massive fatty deposits") of the interatrial septum. Am J Forensic Med Pathol. 17(1):43-8, 1996

Cardiac Lymphoma

KEY FACTS

TERMINOLOGY

- Extranodal lymphoma primarily involving heart

CLINICAL ISSUES

- Primary cardiac lymphoma (PCL) represents 1-2% of primary cardiac tumors and only 0.5% of all lymphomas
- Usually presents after 5th decade (median age: 64 years)
- M:F ~ 3:1
- Symptoms vary by specific site of heart involvement
- More common in immunocompromised patients

IMAGING

- Echocardiography may detect pleural effusions or masses (hypoechoic, obstructive or infiltrative)
- Isointensity of tumor and normal myocardium on T1 and T2; heterogeneous gadolinium enhancement

MACROSCOPIC

- More often involves right atrium or ventricle
- Grossly white-tan "fish-flesh" cut surface

MICROSCOPIC

- > 80% of PCLs are non-Hodgkin diffuse large B-cell lymphomas (DLBCLs)
- Monomorphic lymphocytes with prominent nucleoli
- Predominantly centroblast or immunoblast types
- Histologic/immunophenotypic classification of DLBCL continuously evolving (refer to WHO or other system)

ANCILLARY TESTS

- DLBCLs are CD19(+), CD20(+), CD22(+), CD79-α(+), CD45(+), CD10(+), BCL6(+), BCL2(+/-), CD5(-)
- FISH for MYC, BCL2; ISH for EBV
- MYC/BCL2 coexpression ("double expressor") phenotype more aggressive
- p53, Ki-67 may also add prognostic data

Short-Axis View of Primary Cardiac Lymphoma

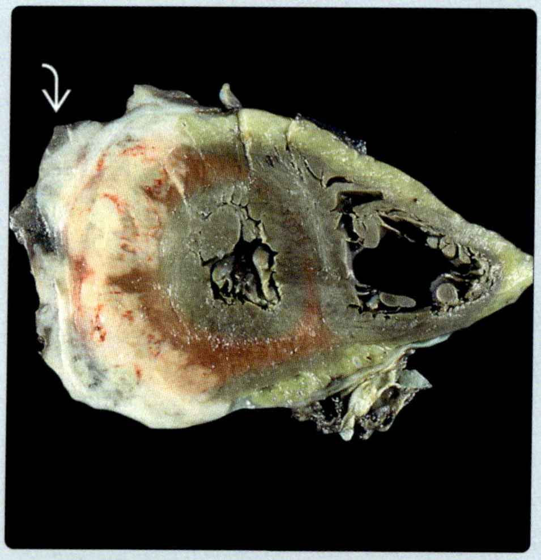

Histologic Section of Primary Cardiac Lymphoma

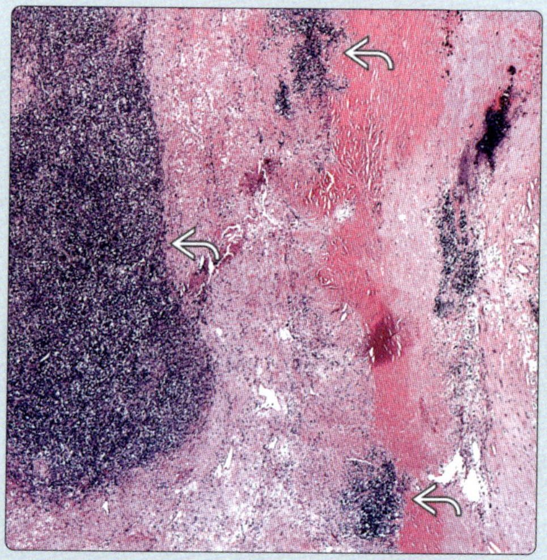

(Left) *Short-axis view of the heart demonstrates the left ventricle wall involved by a white-tan, fleshy tumor with a lobulated cut surface, characteristic of primary cardiac lymphoma (PCL). Involvement of the left ventricle is a feature of worse prognosis.* **(Right)** *Low-power view of PCL shows sheets of lymphocytes infiltrating through the myocardium.*

Histologic Section of Primary Cardiac Lymphoma

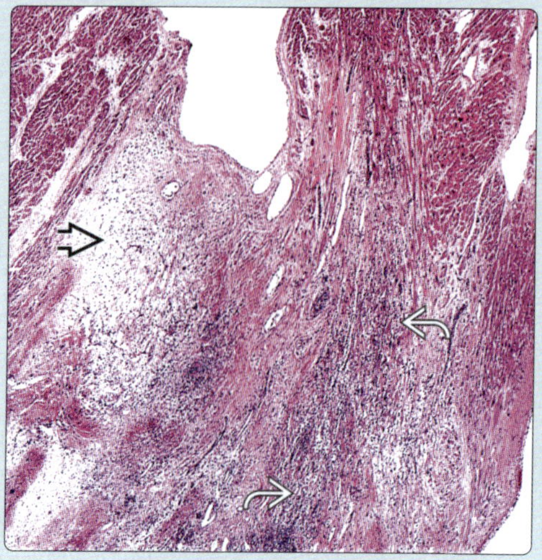

High-Power View of Primary Cardiac Lymphoma

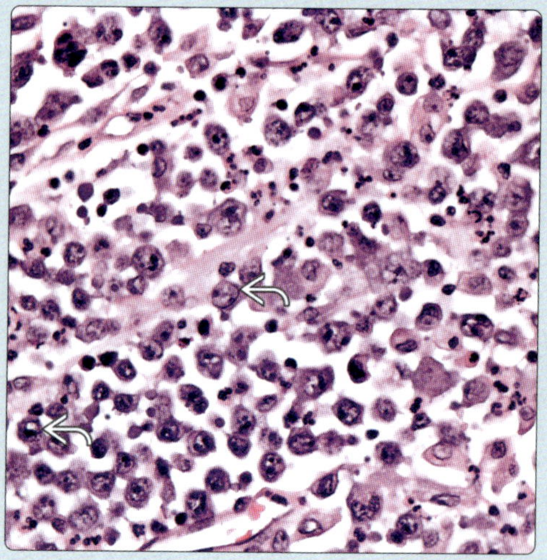

(Left) *Low-power view of PCL shows lymphocytes diffusely infiltrating myocytes. Areas of edema are present.* **(Right)** *High-power view demonstrates numerous large, atypical lymphocytes of diffuse large B-cell lymphomas. Most of these cells have a more centroblastic appearance with open chromatin and multiple large nucleoli that cling to the nuclear membrane.*

TERMINOLOGY

Definitions

- Extranodal lymphoma primarily involving heart

CLINICAL ISSUES

Epidemiology

- Incidence
  - Primary cardiac lymphoma (PCL) represents 1-2% of primary cardiac tumors and only 0.5% of all lymphomas
    - Cardiac involvement by thoracic or systemic lymphoma is much more common
  - Incidence ↑ in immunocompromised patients
- Age
  - Usually presents after 5th decade (median: 64 years)
  - Very rarely affects children
- Sex
  - M:F ~ 3:1

Presentation

- Symptoms vary by site of heart involvement
  - Pericardial effusion
  - Atrioventricular block
  - Heart failure
- More common in immunocompromised patients
  - HIV/AIDS, transplant patients

Treatment

- Surgical approaches
  - Generally discouraged; pericardiostomy recurrent pericardial effusions
- Drugs
  - Chemotherapy [e.g., CHOP ± rituximab (R-CHOP)]
- Radiation
  - Radiation therapy (only few cases in literature) does appear to further improve prognosis alone or in combination with chemotherapy

Prognosis

- PCL has poor prognosis with median survival of 7 months after 1st treatment and ≤ 1 month without treatment
- Left ventricle involvement, extracardiac extension, immunodeficiency, as well as arrhythmia at presentation impart worse prognosis

IMAGING

Radiographic Findings

- Chest x-ray may show enlarged heart ± pulmonary effusion &/or pulmonary vascular congestion

Ultrasonographic Findings

- Echocardiography may detect pleural effusions or masses (hypoechoic, obstructive or infiltrative)
  - Transesophageal more sensitive for right heart

MR Findings

- Isointensity of tumor and normal myocardium on T1 and T2; heterogeneous gadolinium enhancement

CT Findings

- Lymphomas show low attenuation, bright enhancement

MACROSCOPIC

General Features

- Often involves right atrium or ventricle
- Grossly white-tan "fish-flesh" cut surface

MICROSCOPIC

Histologic Features

- > 80% are diffuse large B-cell lymphoma (DLBCL)
  - Histologic/immunophenotypic classification of DLBCL continuously evolving (refer to WHO or other system)
  - Sheets of large, atypical B lymphocytes
  - Fibrin associated DLBCL [EBV(+)] shows no cardiac tissue infiltration

ANCILLARY TESTS

Immunohistochemistry

- DLBCLs are typically CD19(+), CD20(+), CD22(+), CD79-α(+), CD45(+), CD10(+), BCL6(+), BCL2(+/-), CD5(-)
- MYC/BCL2 coexpression ("double expressor") phenotype more aggressive
- p53, Ki-67 may also add prognostic data

In Situ Hybridization

- MYC, BCL2, EBV

PCR

- *IGH* and *IGL*, *BCL2*, *BCL6*, *MYC* rearrangements

DIFFERENTIAL DIAGNOSIS

Undifferentiated Carcinoma

- Cytokeratin positive, usually represents metastasis from known primary (most commonly lung)

Melanoma

- Positive for S100 and melanoma-specific antigens
- Patient usually has history of melanoma but not always

Seminoma/Dysgerminoma

- Usually associated lymphocytic infiltrate surrounding large sheets of PLAP(+), CD117(+), OCT4(+) monomorphous cells

Granulocytic (Myeloid) Sarcoma

- Very rare; usually associated with synchronous leukemia

SELECTED REFERENCES

1. Miller DV, Quintanilla-Martinez L: Cardiac Diffuse Large B-cell Lymphoma: In Thoracic Tumors: WHO Classification of Tumors series, 5th ed. 2021
2. Boyer DF et al: Cardiac Fibrin-Associated Diffuse Large B-cell Lymphoma: In Thoracic Tumors: WHO Classification of Tumors series, 5th ed. 2021
3. Shah K et al: A "low and slow" approach to successful medical treatment of primary cardiac lymphoma. Cardiovasc Diagn Ther. 4(3):270-3, 2014
4. Jeudy J et al: From the radiologic pathology archives: cardiac lymphoma: radiologic-pathologic correlation. Radiographics. 32(5):1369-80, 2012
5. Menke J et al: Diagnosis of a primary cardiac B-cell lymphoma. Am J Hematol. 87(4):426-7, 2012
6. Miguel CE et al: Primary cardiac lymphoma. Int J Cardiol. 149(3):358-63, 2011
7. Petrich A et al: Primary cardiac lymphoma: an analysis of presentation, treatment, and outcome patterns. Cancer. 117(3):581-9, 2011
8. Antoniades L et al: Primary cardiac lymphoma: case report and brief review of the literature. Echocardiography. 26(2):214-9, 2009

Cardiac Angiosarcoma

KEY FACTS

TERMINOLOGY

- Malignant neoplasm composed of cells with endothelial differentiation

CLINICAL ISSUES

- Primary cardiac sarcomas are very uncommon
- Angiosarcoma: Most common primary cardiac sarcoma with differentiation
- Occurs across entire age spectrum, from birth to 10th decade, with peak in 4th decade
- Symptoms usually related to location
  - Bleeding into pericardium may cause tamponade with its associated symptoms
- Poor prognosis with mean life expectancy of 3-6 months from diagnosis

MACROSCOPIC

- Usually arise in right atrium with distinct predilection for right atrioventricular groove
- Usually multilobated and highly vascular, imparting dark appearance to tumor

MICROSCOPIC

- May consist of epithelioid cells, spindle cells, or combination
- Malignant cells (of either type) often merge to form irregular anastomosing vascular sinusoids
- Vascular sinusoids or lumina may be absent, making immunohistochemical studies essential to demonstrate endothelial differentiation

ANCILLARY TESTS

- CD31, ERG most reliable markers

TOP DIFFERENTIAL DIAGNOSES

- Undifferentiated high-grade pleomorphic sarcoma
- Mesothelioma
- Hemangioma
- Kaposi sarcoma

(Left) *Basal short-axis section of an autopsied heart specimen shows an angiosarcoma arising from the right atrial groove with intraatrial growth as well as hemopericardium.* **(Right)** *Angiosarcoma characterized by malignant spindle cells forming overt and more subtle vascular spaces is shown. Numerous extravasated erythrocytes can also be identified throughout the neoplasm.*

Cardiac Angiosarcoma: Gross

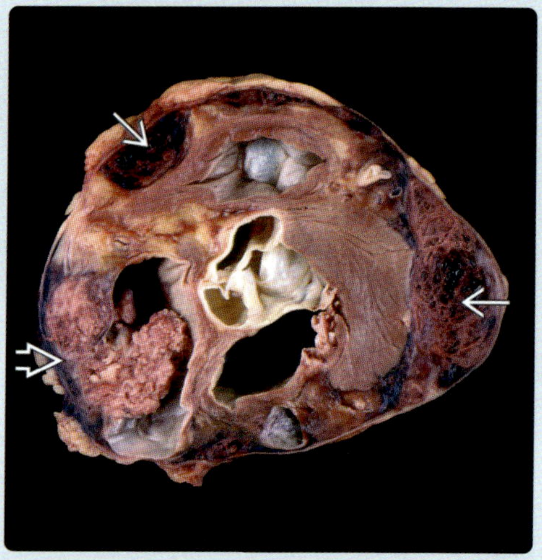

Angiosarcoma

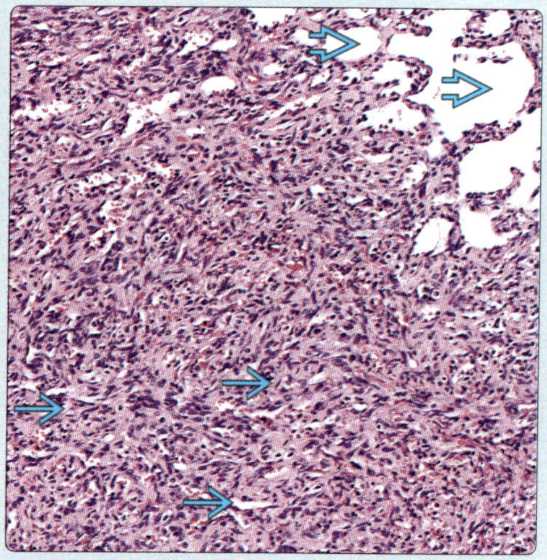

(Left) *This highly variegated cardiac tumor resection specimen shows areas of hemorrhage as well as more solid regions. Histology confirmed angiosarcoma.* **(Right)** *High-magnification view shows a malignant spindle cell process with only subtle interanastomosing vascular channels. Immunostaining would be needed to confirm endothelial differentiation.*

Cardiac Angiosarcoma: Gross

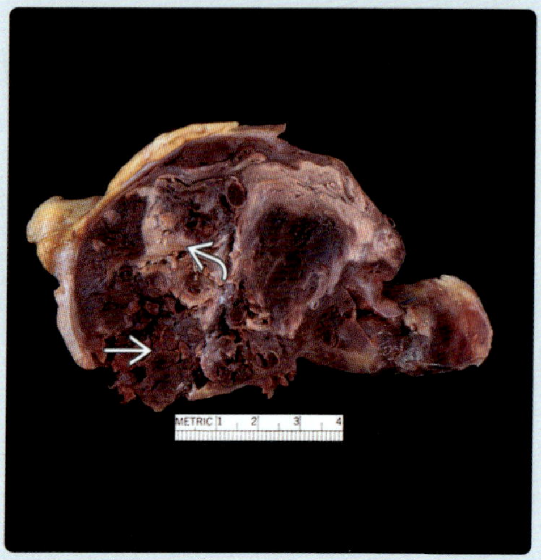

Angiosarcoma, Spindle Cells

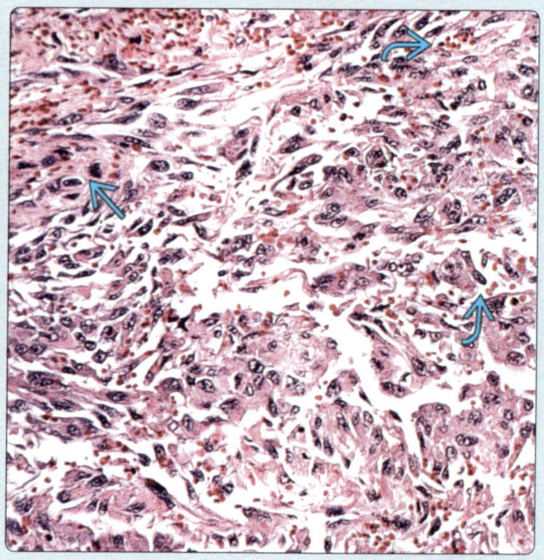

TERMINOLOGY

Synonyms

- Malignant hemangioma, hemangiosarcoma, endothelial sarcoma

Definitions

- Malignant neoplasm of endothelial differentiation

CLINICAL ISSUES

Epidemiology

- Incidence
  - Most common primary cardiac sarcoma
  - Primary cardiac sarcomas are very uncommon overall
- Age
  - Occurs across entire age spectrum, from birth to 10th decade, with peak in 4th decade
- Sex
  - Unclear sex predilection: Some studies report male predilection; others report equal distribution

Presentation

- Symptoms usually related to location, dissemination
  - Chest pain common
  - Right-sided heart failure
- Bleeding into pericardium may cause tamponade

Treatment

- Treatment is usually aimed at symptom palliation
- Surgical excision, radiotherapy, and chemotherapy (no evidence for decrease in mortality)

Prognosis

- Poor survival (5-13 months from diagnosis)
- Younger age, localized disease, and complete resection of primary tumor are favorable prognostic factors for longer survival

IMAGING

Ultrasonographic Findings

- Echogenic, lobulated mass (typically right atrial)
- Often associated with hemorrhagic pericardial effusion

MR Findings

- Often exhibit heterogeneous attenuation with evidence of hemorrhage (T1), bright contrast

CT Findings

- Similar to MR findings, may exhibit variable attenuation secondary to necrotic and hemorrhagic components

MACROSCOPIC

General Features

- Usually arises in right atrium with distinct predilection for right atrioventricular groove
- Pericardial location has also been described, along with all 3 other chambers
- Usually multilobated and highly vascular, imparting dark appearance to these tumors
- May show invasion of valvular or subvalvular apparatus when growing inside chambers

MICROSCOPIC

Histologic Features

- May consist of epithelioid cells, spindle cells, or combination
- Malignant cells (of either type) often merge to form irregular anastomosing vascular sinusoids
- Epithelioid angiosarcomas typically grow in papillary tufts, in solid sheets, or combination
- Spindle cell type can also form primitive vascular channels with pools of extravasated erythrocytes
- Vascular sinusoids or lumina may be absent, making immunohistochemical studies important in demonstrating endothelial differentiation
- May have supporting stroma (either hyalinized or myxoid)

ANCILLARY TESTS

Immunohistochemistry

- CD31 (most reliable), ERG (more sensitive marker in recent studies), CD34, FLI1, FVIIIR-Ag, cytokeratins (usually focal)

Genetic Testing

- Trisomy 4, 8, 11, 17 and 20 and gain of 1q are recurrent cytogenetic abnormalities recently described

DIFFERENTIAL DIAGNOSIS

Undifferentiated High-Grade Pleomorphic Sarcoma

- Undifferentiated spindle cell areas of angiosarcomas can be indistinguishable from undifferentiated high-grade pleomorphic sarcoma
- Unlikely that there is much prognostic significance given poor prognosis of both entities

Mesothelioma

- Angiosarcoma occasionally exhibits mesothelial antigenic profiles; mesotheliomas tend to exhibit more concentric pericardial involvement

Hemangioma

- Lacks marked cytologic atypia, mitotic rate usually low

Kaposi Sarcoma

- Highly unusual to have isolated cardiac involvement
- Usually only minimal invasion into myocardium
- Strong association with immunosuppression

DIAGNOSTIC CHECKLIST

Clinically Relevant Pathologic Features

- Tissue distribution
  - Right atrioventricular groove origin
- Histologic features
  - May consist of epithelioid cells, spindle cells, or combination; forming irregular anastomosing sinusoids

SELECTED REFERENCES

1. Chen TW et al: Optimal clinical management and the molecular biology of angiosarcomas. Cancers (Basel). 12(11), 2020
2. Chen Y et al: Clinical and imaging features of primary cardiac angiosarcoma. Diagnostics (Basel). 10(10), 2020
3. Leduc C et al: Cardiac angiosarcoma: histopathologic, immunohistochemical, and cytogenetic analysis of 10 cases. Hum Pathol. 60:199-207, 2017
4. Travis D et al: WHO Classification of Tumours of the Lung, Pleura, Thymus and Heart. 4th ed. IARC Press, 2015

Cardiac Angiosarcoma: Gross

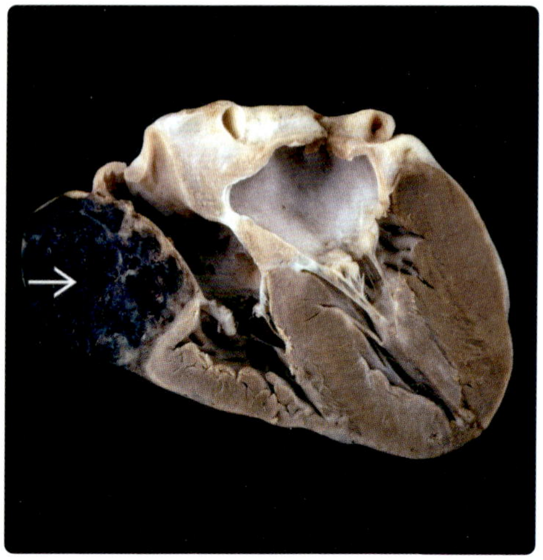

Cardiac Angiosarcoma: Gross

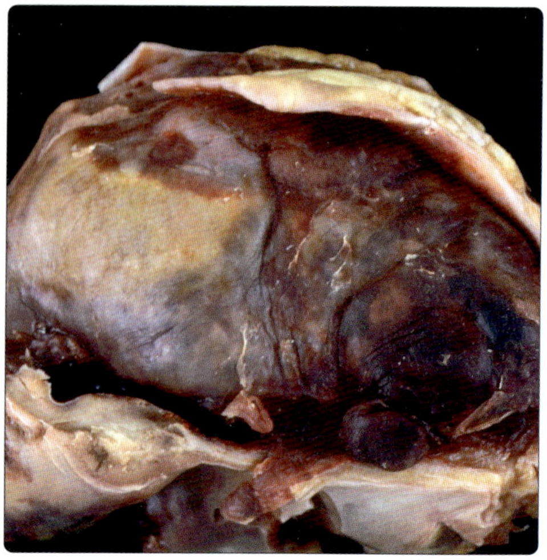

(Left) *Four-chamber view shows a dark, lobular mass ➡ arising from the right atrioventricular groove (the classic location for cardiac angiosarcoma). Note the apparent compressive effect that these tumors can have on the chambers. Growth into the chambers is not evident at this point.* **(Right)** *Surgically resected cardiac angiosarcoma demonstrates the variegated and lobular character of these tumors. In this example, prominent intraatrial growth is seen.*

Entrapped Myocytes in Cardiac Angiosarcoma

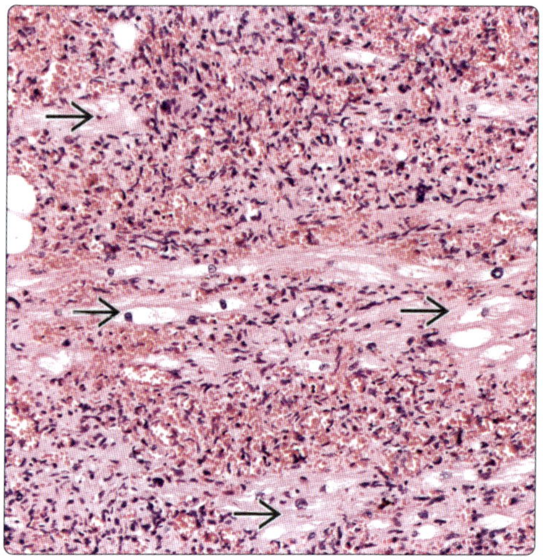

Cardiac Epithelioid Angiosarcoma

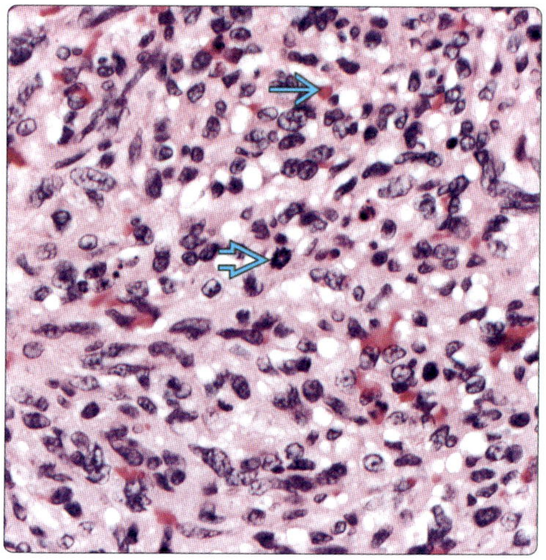

(Left) *H&E exhibits a spindle cell angiosarcoma with myocardial involvement. Entrapped, vacuolated, cardiac myocytes are present ➡. While vascular spaces or sinusoids are not immediately apparent, the abundant erythrocytes should raise the possibility of the diagnosis of cardiac angiosarcoma.* **(Right)** *The epithelioid cells comprising this angiosarcoma show increased mitotic activity ➡ and intracytoplasmic lumina that contain occasional erythrocytes ➡.*

Cardiac Epithelioid Angiosarcoma

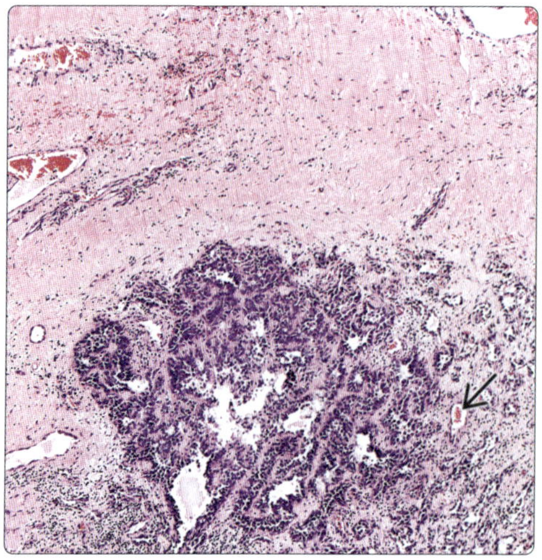

Papillary Projections in Cardiac Epithelioid Angiosarcoma

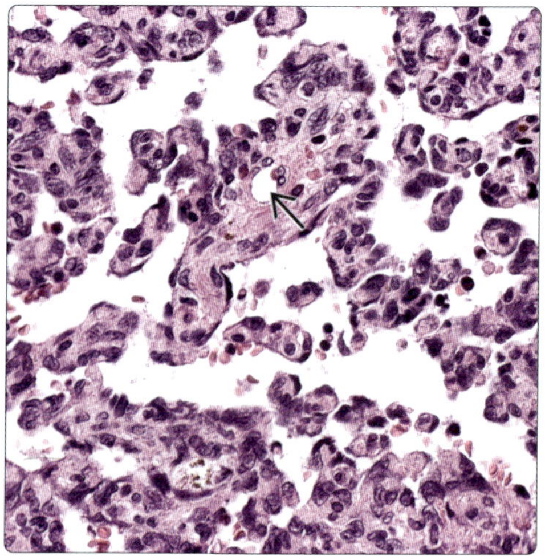

(Left) *Surgically resected cardiac angiosarcoma shows primarily epithelioid morphology with a vaguely papillary growth pattern and formation of vascular channels ➡.* **(Right)** *This epithelioid cardiac angiosarcoma consists of highly atypical papillary fronds that are lined by atypical endothelial cells. The endothelial cells exhibit hyperchromasia and an increased nuclear:cytoplasmic ratio. Vascular spaces can occasionally be found within the papillary fronds ➡.*

Cardiac Angiosarcoma

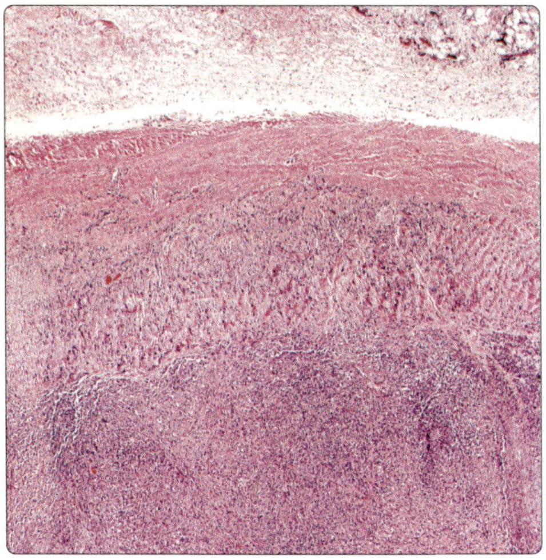

Spindle Cells in Cardiac Angiosarcoma

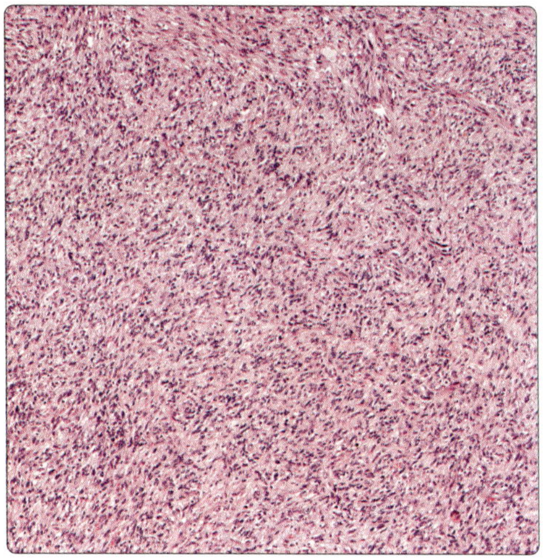

(Left) *Intramyocardial angiosarcoma demonstrates a relatively well-circumscribed border.* **(Right)** *In this cardiac angiosarcoma with primarily spindle cell morphology, vascular spaces are not readily apparent. Likewise, erythrocytes are not a striking feature in this example. In cases such as this, immunohistochemistry can be particularly helpful in showing endothelial differentiation and discriminating between angiosarcoma and other sarcomas.*

Cardiac Epithelioid Angiosarcoma

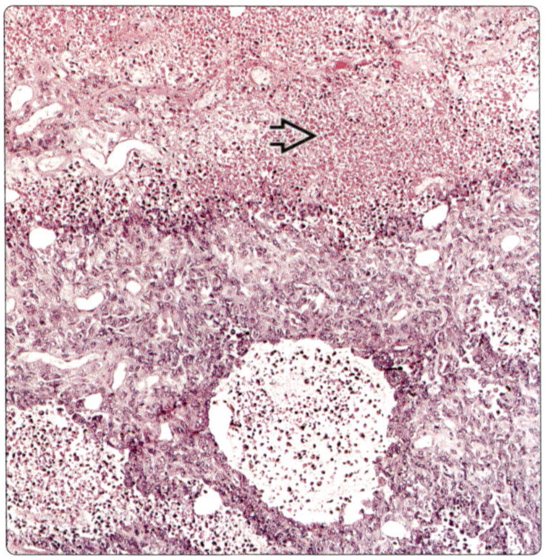

Myxoid Change in Spindle Cell Cardiac Angiosarcoma

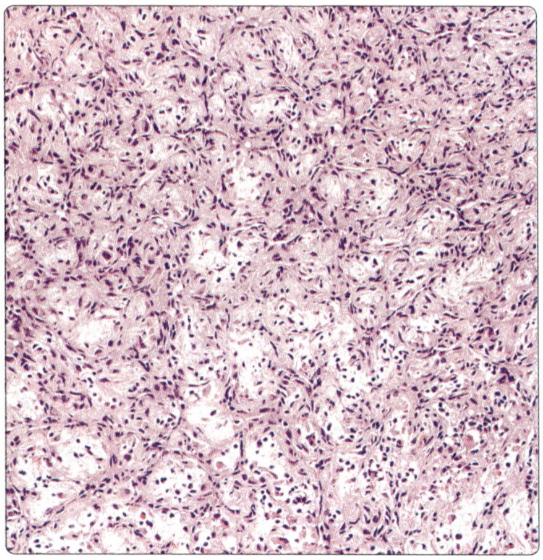

(Left) *This epithelioid cardiac angiosarcoma exhibits variably sized vascular spaces. The cells have a moderate amount of eosinophilic cytoplasm. Prominent tumoral necrosis ➡ is also present.* **(Right)** *This cardiac angiosarcoma of the spindle cell variety exhibits a myxoid stroma. Other diagnostic considerations would include myxoid sarcoma. The neoplastic cells, however, showed striking reactivity with markers of endothelial differentiation.*

CD31 in Cardiac Angiosarcoma

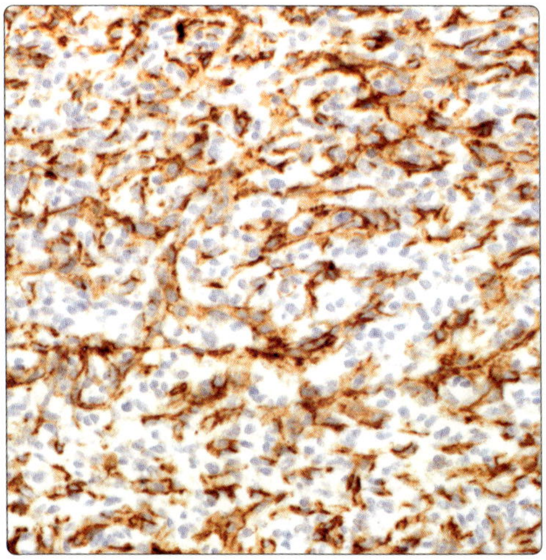

FLI-1 in Cardiac Angiosarcoma

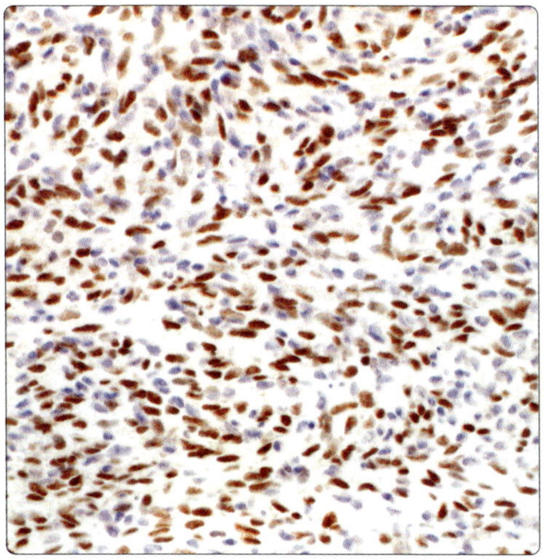

(Left) *The neoplastic cells of this surgically resected angiosarcoma demonstrate strong cytoplasmic reactivity with endothelial marker CD31. CD31 is typically regarded as providing both good sensitivity and specificity for endothelial neoplasms.* **(Right)** *The neoplastic spindle cells in this cardiac angiosarcoma demonstrate strong nuclear reactivity with FLI-1 (another endothelial marker). The lack of overt vascular spaces in this example makes this finding particularly useful.*

Cardiac Sarcoma, Other

KEY FACTS

TERMINOLOGY

- Undifferentiated pleomorphic sarcoma (UPS), fibrosarcoma, myxoid sarcoma, rhabdomyosarcoma, leiomyosarcoma, liposarcoma, synovial sarcoma, Kaposi sarcoma

CLINICAL ISSUES

- Very rare with < 400 case reports
- Symptoms include
  - Chest pain, arhythmia, heart failure
  - Ischemia related (secondary to embolism)
- Average survival: 6 months
- Metastatic sarcomas to heart are far more common (60x) than primary cardiac sarcomas
- Mean age: ~ 42 years
- Surgical excision, radiotherapy, and chemotherapy (no evidence for decreased mortality)

MACROSCOPIC

- Left atrium: UPS, fibrosarcomas, and leiomyosarcomas
- Parietal pericardium: Synovial sarcoma and Kaposi sarcoma
- No particular site: Rhabdomyosarcomas

MICROSCOPIC

- Other types: Virtually any sarcoma outside heart may occur within heart

ANCILLARY TESTS

- Synovial sarcoma: t(X;18)(p11.2;q11.2) (*SYT::SSX*)
- Many other tumor-associated translocations
- Whole-genome/exome (next-generation) sequencing

TOP DIFFERENTIAL DIAGNOSES

- Cardiac myxoma (grossly)
- Lipomatous hypertrophy of atrial septum
- Fibroma (grossly)
- Mesothelioma

(Left) *Short-axis section from an autopsy specimen shows an infiltrative tan mass involving the left ventricle in a transmural fashion. The mass exhibits some endocardial growth as well.* **(Right)** *While this cardiac sarcoma is largely undifferentiated (consisting predominately of highly atypical cells), focal areas of osseous differentiation, characterized by osteoid production, are identified.*

Primary Cardiac Sarcoma (Gross)

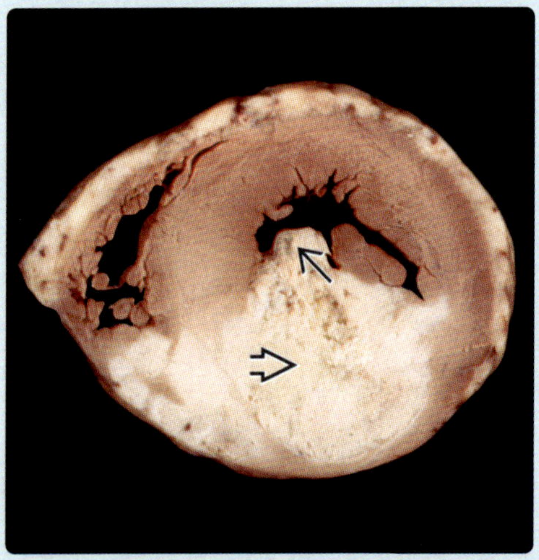

Focal Osteoid in Pleomorphic Sarcoma

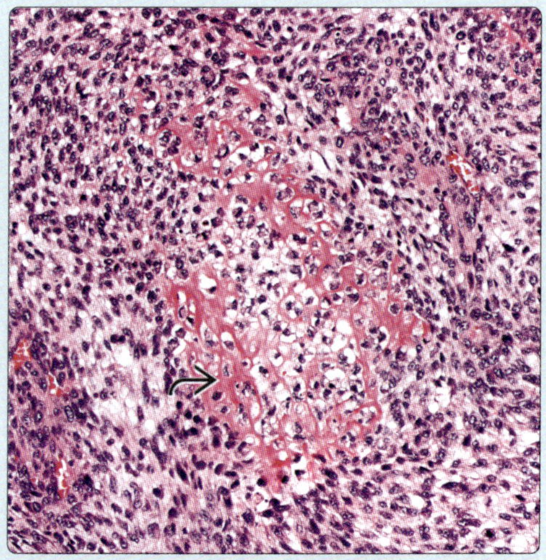

(Left) *Intraoperative transesophageal echocardiogram shows a large mass attached to the mitral valve in the left atrium. Clinically, it was associated with a "tumor plop" on auscultation.* **(Right)** *Ancillary tests, such as FISH testing for characteristic gene rearrangements, are a helpful adjunct in the diagnosis of cardiac sarcomas. This synovial sarcoma shows fused green and red FISH probe signals, indicating an SYT::SSX translocation.*

Echocardiogram of Left Atrial Mass

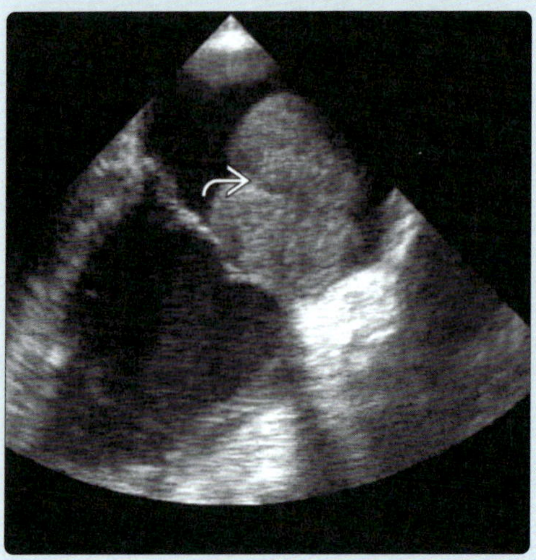

***SYT::SSX* FISH**

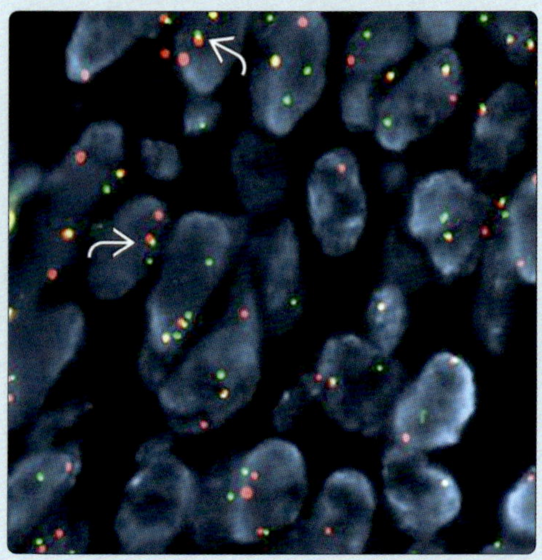

TERMINOLOGY

Synonyms

- Undifferentiated pleomorphic sarcoma (UPS), fibrosarcoma, myxoid sarcoma, rhabdomyosarcoma, leiomyosarcoma, liposarcoma, synovial sarcoma, Kaposi sarcoma

Definitions

- Malignant neoplasm of mesenchymal derivation arising from heart or pericardium

CLINICAL ISSUES

Epidemiology

- Incidence
  - Very rare with < 400 case reports
  - Metastatic sarcomas to heart are far more common (60x) than primary cardiac sarcomas
- Age
  - From birth to 10th decade
  - Mean age: ~ 42 years
- Sex
  - No definitive predilection

Presentation

- Mean duration of symptoms prior to presentation: 3-5 months
- Symptoms include
  - Chest pain, arrhythmia, heart failure
  - Ischemia related (secondary to embolism)

Treatment

- Usually aimed at symptom palliation
- Surgical excision, radiotherapy, and chemotherapy (no evidence for decreased mortality)

Prognosis

- Average survival: 6 months

IMAGING

General Features

- Dependent on type of sarcoma imaged
  - May have focal calcification/ossification
  - May show prominent areas of necrosis

MACROSCOPIC

General Features

- Typically firm masses with fleshy, gray-white surfaces
- May be sessile or pedunculated

Location

- Left atrium: UPS, fibrosarcomas, and leiomyosarcomas
- Parietal pericardium: Synovial sarcoma and Kaposi sarcoma
- No particular site: Rhabdomyosarcomas

MICROSCOPIC

Histologic Features

- UPS: Pleomorphic, storiform; myxoid, giant cell, inflammatory, and angiomatoid subtypes
- Fibrosarcoma: Fascicular arrangement, herringbone pattern
- Rhabdomyosarcoma: Typically embryonal type
- Synovial sarcoma: Biphasic or monophasic
- Liposarcoma: Usually myxoid type ± dedifferentiation
- Leiomyosarcoma: Oval nuclei, arranged in fascicles
- Myxosarcoma: Atypical cells within myxoid stroma
- Other types: Virtually any sarcoma outside heart may occur within heart

ANCILLARY TESTS

Immunohistochemistry

- Leiomyosarcomas: Desmin and actin (+)
- Rhabdomyosarcoma: Desmin and myogenin (+)
- Synovial sarcoma: Focal keratin and TLE1 (+)
- Liposarcoma: Lipoblasts S100(+)

Genetic Testing

- Whole-genome/exome (next-generation) sequencing

Fluorescence In Situ Hybridization

- Synovial sarcoma: t(X;18)(p11.2;q11.2) (*SYT::SSX*)
- Many other tumor-associated translocations

DIFFERENTIAL DIAGNOSIS

Cardiac Myxoma

- Myxoma gross features could simulate myxoid sarcoma, but is benign tumor composed of myxoma cells without atypia

Lipomatous Hypertrophy of Atrial Septum

- Mixture of atypical myocytes, brown fat, and mature fat

Fibroma

- Atypia, necrosis, and mitotic figures usually absent

Mesothelioma

- Epithelioid types express mesothelial markers, sarcomatoid types express keratin

GRADING

Primary Cardiac Sarcomas

- No universally accepted guidelines, but most agree that combination of histologic type, mitotic index, and presence of necrosis and cellularity should be factored into histologic grade
- Increased mitotic rate and presence of necrosis portend poor prognosis

SELECTED REFERENCES

1. Awad AK et al: Specific causes of death among patients with cardiac sarcoma in the United States-an analysis of the Surveillance, Epidemiology, and End Results (SEER) program. J Card Surg. 37(11):3961-3, 2022
2. WHO Classification of Tumours Editorial Board: Thoracic Tumors. In: WHO Classification of Tumors. 5th ed: vol 5. IARC Press, 2021
3. Hasan SM et al: Outcomes after resection of primary cardiac sarcoma. JTCVS Open. 8:384-90, 2021
4. Burke A et al: The 2015 WHO classification of tumors of the heart and pericardium. J Thorac Oncol. 11(4):441-52, 2016
5. Varma T et al: Primary cardiac synovial sarcoma. Arch Pathol Lab Med. 136(4):454-8, 2012
6. Orlandi A et al: Cardiac sarcomas: an update. J Thorac Oncol. 5(9):1483-9, 2010

Cardiac Sarcoma, Other

(Left) *Left ventricular long-axis section of a heart shows undifferentiated high-grade pleomorphic sarcoma involving the apical and midventricular myocardium. Typically, these tumors arise within left atrium but can arise anywhere in the heart. Regional wall motion abnormalities caused by infiltrating tumor replacing myocardium can allow mural thrombus to form.* **(Right)** *Gross photo shows a sarcoma surgically resected from left atrium with a fleshy, gray-white surface with focal degeneration/necrosis.*

Cardiac Undifferentiated Pleomorphic Sarcoma

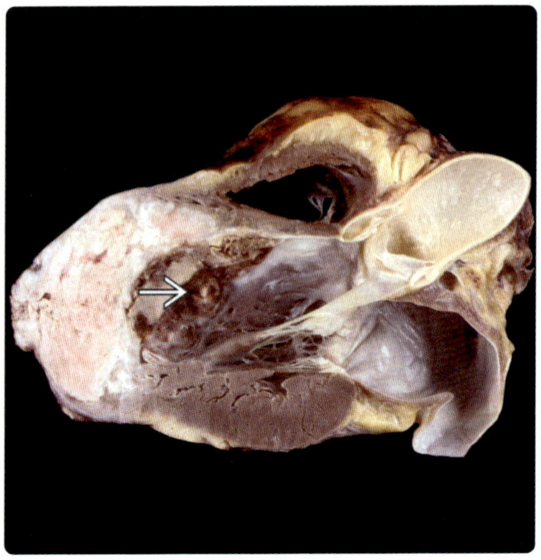

Cardiac Sarcoma: Surgically Resected

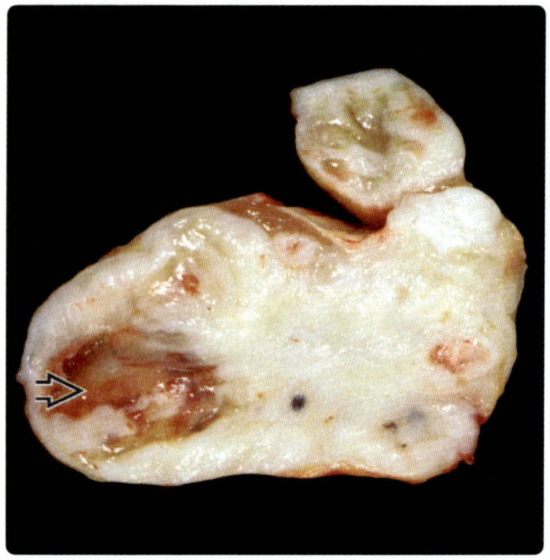

(Left) *H&E of an undifferentiated high-grade pleomorphic sarcoma shows a peculiar corded growth pattern. Cells of this sarcoma were nonreactive to all antibodies tested with the exception of vimentin.* **(Right)** *Focal osseous differentiation, characterized by osteoid production and lamellar bone formation, is seen in > 15% of cases of undifferentiated sarcomas. Whether these represent a type of extraskeletal osteosarcoma or a variant of undifferentiated sarcoma remains unclear.*

Cardiac Sarcoma With Corded Pattern

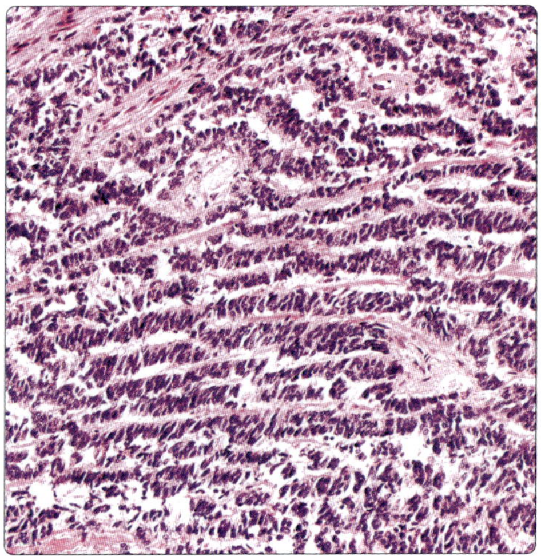

Osseous Differentiation in Cardiac Sarcoma

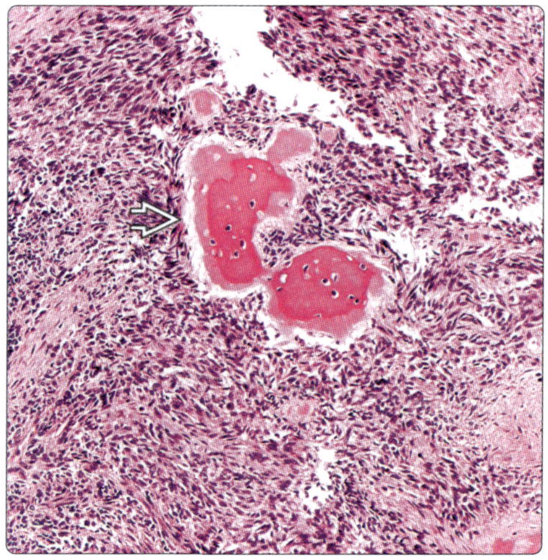

(Left) *H&E of an autopsy specimen exhibits a high-grade sarcoma infiltrating the ventricular myocardium.* **(Right)** *H&E shows a myxoid sarcoma characterized by spindle cells with a mild to moderate degree of atypia proliferating in a myxoid stroma. Unlike cardiac myxomas, "myxoma cells" are not identified within the lesion, and no perivascular ring structures are identified around small vessels.*

Cardiac Sarcoma: Infiltrative Growth

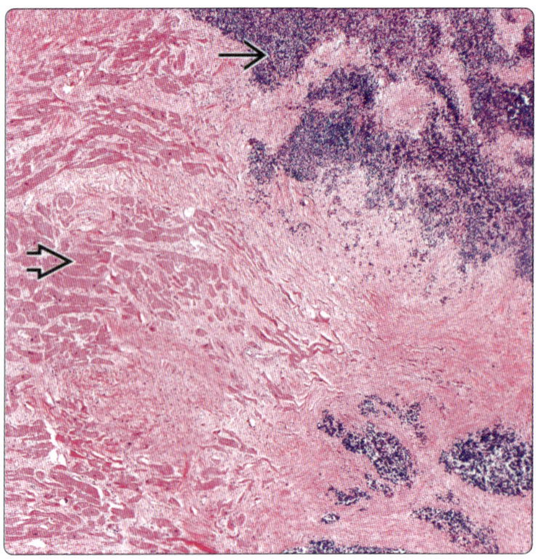

Cardiac Myxosarcoma

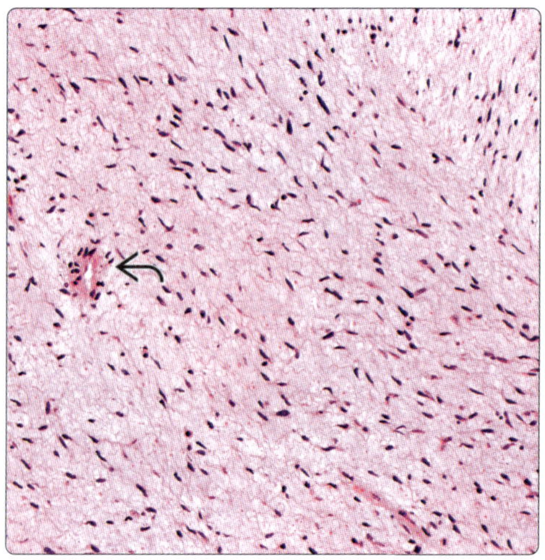

Primary Cardiac Leiomyosarcoma

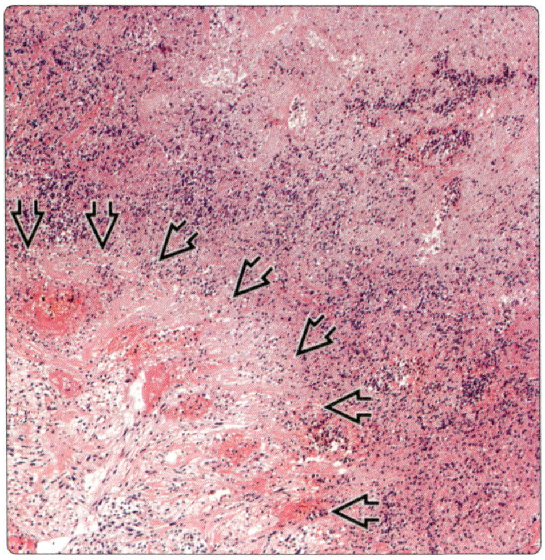

Cardiac Sarcoma Embolism

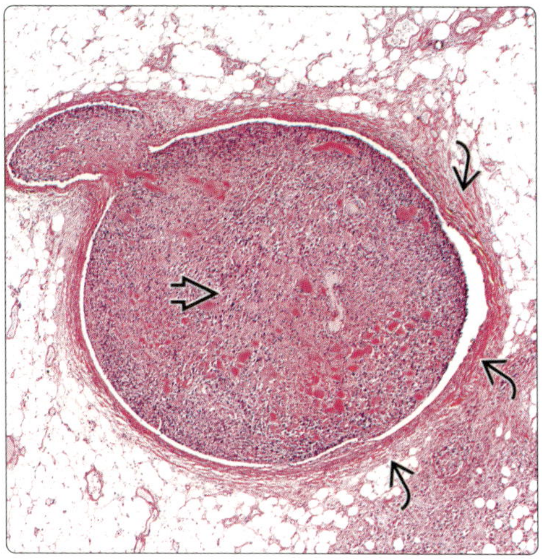

(Left) *H&E of a high-grade leiomyosarcoma resected from the left atrium (near one of the pulmonary vein ostia) shows abundant tumoral necrosis. Atrial myocardium can also be identified in this photomicrograph.* **(Right)** *H&E shows an undifferentiated high-grade pleomorphic sarcoma arising in the left atrium that was also noted within the small pericardial blood vessels at the time of autopsy. Primary cardiac sarcomas can embolize, particularly when they exhibit an endocardial growth pattern.*

Cardiac Monophasic Synovial Sarcoma

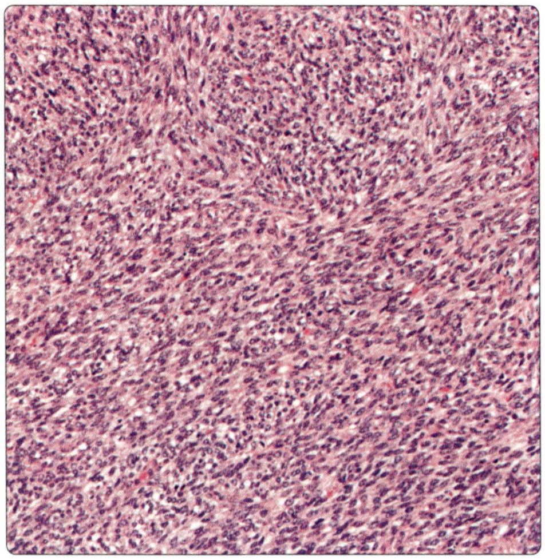

Cardiac Epithelioid Fibrosarcoma

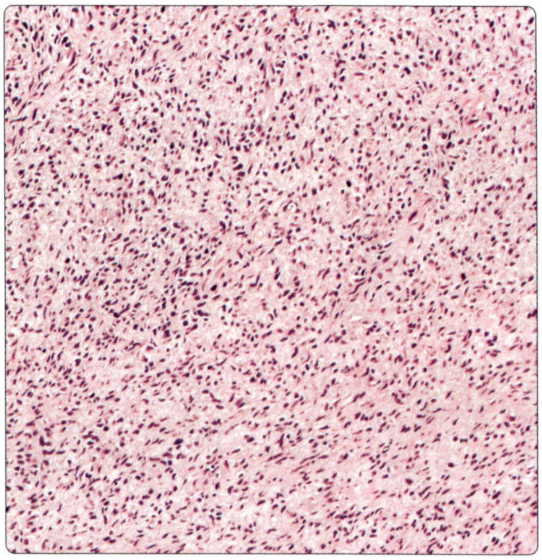

(Left) *H&E reveals a synovial sarcoma (monophasic type). The spindle cells of this neoplasm are small, compact, and arranged in a plump fascicular pattern. Scattered mononuclear cells are also usually identified.* **(Right)** *H&E shows an unusual variant of fibrosarcoma (epithelioid fibrosarcoma). Pleomorphism is typically minimal in all types of fibrosarcoma. Hemorrhage and necrosis are also uncommonly seen in fibrosarcomas.*

Cardiac Primary Leiomyosarcoma (Pleomorphic)

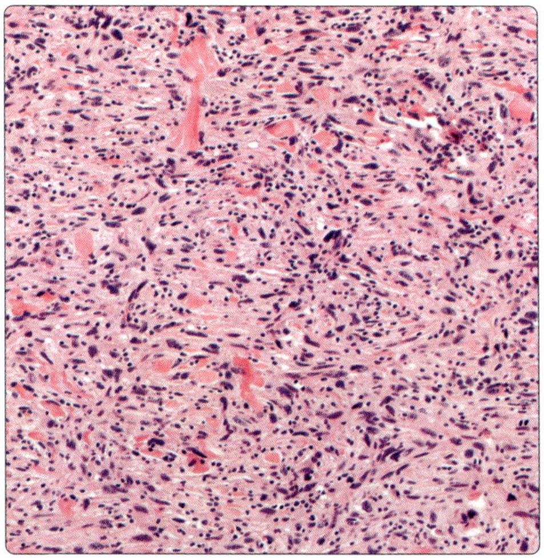

Smooth Muscle Actin Staining in Cardiac Leiomyosarcoma

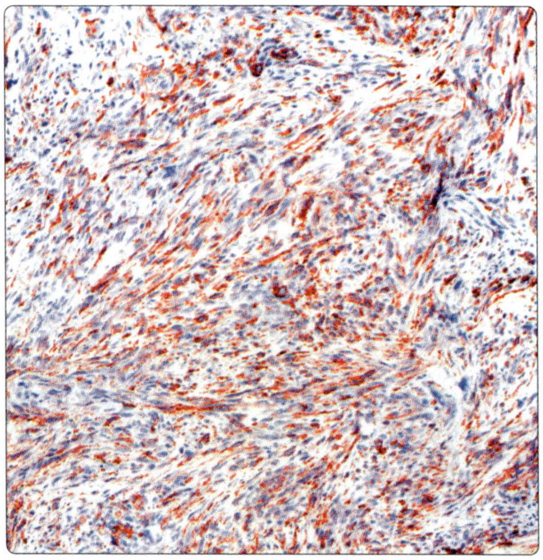

(Left) *H&E shows a high-grade pleomorphic leiomyosarcoma. The spindle cells that comprise this tumor usually contain features of smooth muscle myocytes, including blunt-ended oval nuclei and perinuclear vacuoles.* **(Right)** *Photomicrograph shows the spindle cells of a cardiac leiomyosarcoma exhibiting strong cytoplasmic reactivity with antibodies directed against smooth muscle actin. The fascicular arrangement of the cells is also apparent.*

Cardiac Metastases

KEY FACTS

TERMINOLOGY

- Cardiac metastases (CMs): Distant spread of malignant tumors to any heart structures, including intracavitary neoplastic masses

ETIOLOGY/PATHOGENESIS

- 4 routes of metastasis to heart: Lymphatic, hematogenous, direct extension, and intracavitary diffusion
- Predominant route is retrograde lymphatic spread
- Pericardium is commonly involved by direct extension of intrathoracic or mediastinal tumors, myocardium by lymphatic route, and endocardium by hematogenous route

CLINICAL ISSUES

- 30x more common than primary neoplasms
- Lung cancer is most common source, followed by hematologic malignancies
- Melanoma has highest frequency of CMs
- Metastasis to right side more common than to left side
- CMs most commonly involve pericardium (69%), epicardium (34%), myocardium (32%), endocardium (5%)
- Clinical manifestations depend on extent/location of CM
- ~ 90% are asymptomatic
- 2D echocardiography is gold standard for diagnosis
- Treatment is usually palliative

MACROSCOPIC

- Metastatic tumors of heart are usually multiple solid lesions producing myocardial or pericardial nodules
- Associated with pericardial adhesions and hemorrhagic pericardial effusion

MICROSCOPIC

- Similar to those of primary neoplasm

Metastatic Lung Carcinoma With Epicardial Involvement

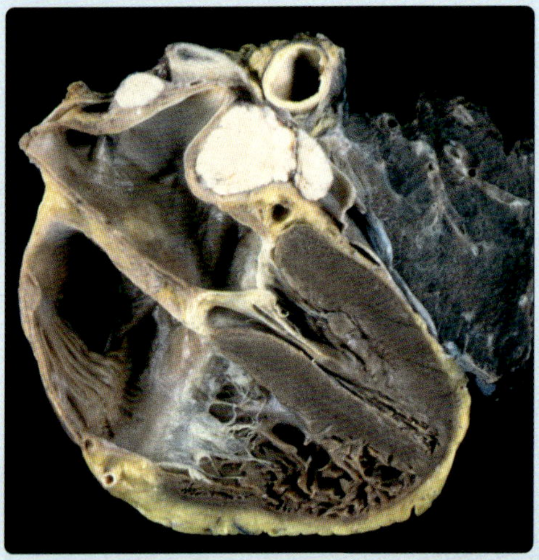

Multifocal Myocardial Involvement by Metastatic Breast Carcinoma

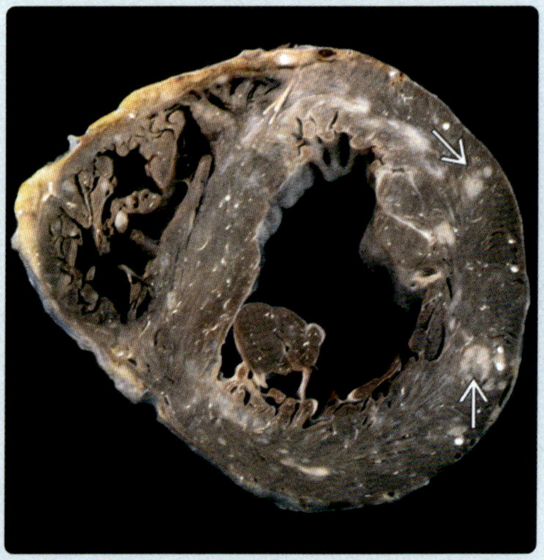

(Left) *Autopsy specimen shows primary lung carcinoma with metastatic tumor in lymph node, erosion of pericardium, and extension to epicardium.* **(Right)** *Short-axis section of heart shows metastatic carcinoma of the breast along with ischemic disease of the heart. Several mural white nodules ➡ are present.*

Gross Images of Epicardial Metastasis

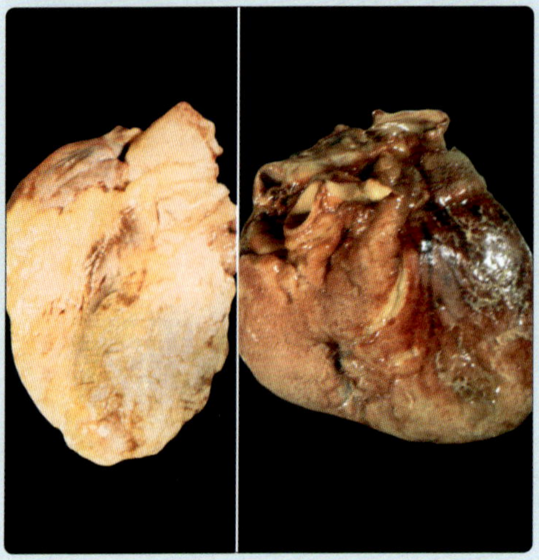

Epicardial Involvement by Metastatic Carcinoma

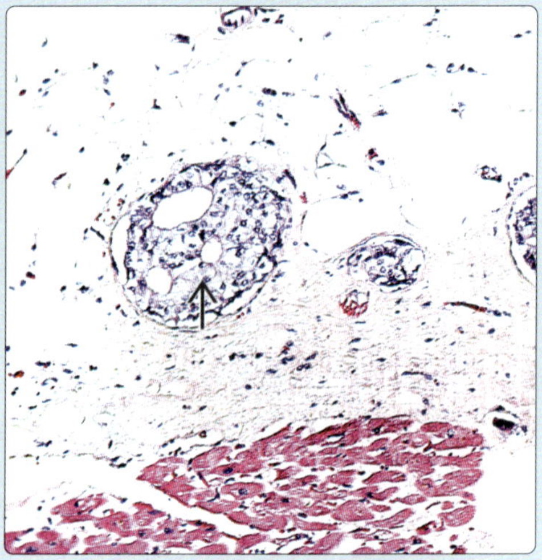

(Left) *Gross specimens show epicardial metastases. The primary malignancy has not been specified in either case.* **(Right)** *H&E-stained section shows epicardial metastases ➡ of a carcinoma in epicardial fat. The epicardium is the most common site of metastasis to the heart. Carcinomas from lung and breast and hematologic malignancies show preference for epicardial involvement.*

TERMINOLOGY

Abbreviations

- Cardiac metastases (CMs)

Synonyms

- Secondary tumors of heart

Definitions

- Distant spread of malignant tumors to any heart structures, and also tumors affecting heart cavities or producing intracavitary neoplastic masses

ETIOLOGY/PATHOGENESIS

Metastatic Pathways

- 4 routes of metastasis to heart
  - Lymphatic
  - Hematogenous
  - Direct extension from adjacent tumors
  - Intracavitary extension through inferior vena cava, superior vena cava, or pulmonary veins
- Predominant route is retrograde lymphatic spread producing pericardial nodules or effusion
- Pericardium is commonly involved through direct invasion by intrathoracic or mediastinal tumors
- Lymphatic spread preferentially involves pericardium, whereas hematogenous spread involves myocardium and endocardium

CLINICAL ISSUES

Epidemiology

- Incidence
  - ↑ in last 30 years
  - CMs are 30x more common than primary neoplasms
  - Autopsy incidence
    - 1.7-14% in cancer patients
    - 0.7-3.5% in general population
- Types of primary tumors metastasizing to heart
  - Rare tumors with ↑ rate of CMs (malignant melanoma, germ cell tumor, malignant thymoma)
  - Common tumors with intermediate rate of CMs (lung, stomach, ovary, colon, liver, or kidney)
  - Common tumors with rare metastasis to heart
- Most common tumors showing CMs are carcinomas of lung, pleura, breast, esophagus, kidney, malignant lymphoma, leukemia, sarcoma, and malignant melanoma
  - Bronchogenic carcinoma, hematologic malignancies, and breast cancer account for 2/3 of CMs
  - Melanoma has highest frequency of CMs
- In children, > 90% of metastases originate from lymphomas, leukemias, Wilms tumor, neuroblastoma, hepatoblastoma, and sarcomas
- CNS tumors; only tumors that do not form CMs
- Site
  - Metastases to right side of heart are more common than to left side
    - Low right systolic pressures favor anchorage of neoplastic cells
  - Most commonly involved is pericardium (69%) followed by epicardium (34%), myocardium (32%), and endocardium (5%)
  - Heart valves are rarely involved due to their constant motion and relatively poor vascularity
  - Tumors of lung and breast and hematologic malignancies mainly show pericardial involvement
  - Melanomas usually to myocardium and endocardium

Presentation

- Clinical presentation
  - Depends on extent and anatomic location of metastatic tumor in heart
  - Pericardial involvement may manifest as
    - Pericardial effusion
    - Cardiac tamponade
    - Constrictive pericarditis
    - Dyspnea, hypotension, and tachycardia
  - Myocardial involvement causes
    - Arrhythmias
    - Conduction disturbances
    - Complete atrioventricular block
  - Multifocal ventricular involvement can cause congestive heart failure
  - Tumors, such as renal cell carcinoma, reach right atrium by extension into renal veins and inferior vena cava, causing
    - Obstruction and damage to tricuspid and mitral valves
    - Myocardial restrictive disease
    - Cardiac tamponade
    - Distant metastasis due to systemic embolization
  - Neoplastic thrombi in coronary circulation can cause
    - Acute myocardial infarction
  - In child with history of cancer, development of heart failure, or rapid onset of cardiomegaly, arrhythmias, or chest pain, diagnosis of CM is indicated
- Symptoms
  - ~ 90% are asymptomatic
  - May present with shortness of breath, palpitation, chest pain, dizziness, hypotension, syncope, and edema
- Signs
  - Patients may present with
    - New systolic &/or diastolic murmurs
    - Gallop rhythm
    - Congestive cardiac failure
    - Pericardial friction sounds
    - Attenuated heart sounds due to pericardial effusion

Laboratory Tests

- Electrocardiogram can reveal
  - Conduction disorders
  - Atrial or ventricular arrhythmias
  - ST segment abnormalities
  - Localized and prolonged ST segment elevation without Q waves: Pathognomonic of myocardial tumor invasion

Treatment

- Options, risks, complications
  - Usually palliative because of advanced stage of disease
- Surgical approaches
  - Indications

- Solitary lesions
- Patients with complete resection of primary tumor without disseminated disease and having good prognosis
- In circumscribed lesions: Coil embolization of branch of coronary artery supplying lesion
- Surgery with postoperative chemotherapy &/or radiotherapy is indicated to prevent recurrence

- Adjuvant therapy
  - Indications
    - Chemosensitive tumors (e.g., lymphomas, leukemias, and germ cell tumors) may be treated with chemotherapy
- Radiation
  - Treatment of choice for patients with disseminated disease and chemotherapy-resistant CMs
- Malignant pericardial effusion can be treated with
  - Local irradiation
  - Systemic chemotherapy
  - Local infusion of tetracycline or radioactive phosphorous or chemotherapeutic agents, such as cisplatin
  - Drainage of effusion via subxiphoid pericardiotomy or pericardial window
- Orthotopic heart transplantation

Prognosis

- Median survival is 17-24 months for patients undergoing complete resection of tumor and 6-10 months for those who do not undergo complete resection
- 5-year survival rate is ~ 7%
- Patients with malignant pericardial effusion have median survival of 4 months

IMAGING

Radiographic Findings

- Chest x-ray may reveal enlarged cardiac silhouette, calcification, and pericardial effusion

Ultrasonographic Findings

- 2D echocardiography
  - Gold standard for diagnosing CMs, demonstrates
    - Shape, size, site, extent, and mobility of tumor
    - Tumor's relation to other cardiac structures
    - Myocardial wall mobility, pericardial thickening
- Transesophageal echocardiography (TEE)
  - Preferred over transthoracic echocardiography (TTE)
    - Can identify small tumor masses < 5 mm and tumors localized to posterior cardiac segment
- Contrast echocardiography
  - Differentiates between tumor and thrombus
    - Malignant tumors are highly vascular and show intense enhancement in contrast to thrombi
    - Benign tumors show medium enhancement of echocardiographic signals

MACROSCOPIC

General Features

- Usually multiple solid lesions producing myocardial or pericardial nodules associated with
  - Pericardial adhesions
  - Hemorrhagic pericardial effusion

MICROSCOPIC

Histologic Features

- Similar to those of primary neoplasm

ANCILLARY TESTS

Cytology

- Examination of pericardial fluid yields positive results in 80-90% of patients with malignant pericardial effusion

Immunohistochemistry

- Useful to characterize metastatic tumor of unknown primary

DIFFERENTIAL DIAGNOSIS

Benign or Malignant Primary Cardiac Tumors

- Metastatic lesions of heart are invariably malignant
- Cystic lesions are usually benign, whereas solid lesions are usually malignant
- Solitary mass in ventricular wall is usually primary benign cardiac tumor, whereas multiple myocardial &/or pericardial nodules are usually metastatic malignant neoplasms, except rhabdomyoma
- Pedunculated lesions are usually benign, whereas sessile lesions are mostly malignant
- Malignant lesions are more likely to produce pericardial adhesions and hemorrhagic pericardial effusion

DIAGNOSTIC CHECKLIST

Pathologic Interpretation Pearls

- Definitive diagnosis is made by pathologic examination of tumor tissue obtained by transthoracic or open biopsy

SELECTED REFERENCES

1. Balinski AM et al: Metastatic melanoma of the heart: retrospective cohort study and systematic review of prevalence, clinical characteristics, and outcomes. Cancer Med. ePub, 2022
2. Jain G et al: Cardiac metastasis after curative treatment of hepatocellular carcinoma: assessment of risk factors, treatment options, and prognosis. J Patient Cent Res Rev. 9(3):181-4, 2022
3. Nova-Camacho LM et al: Cardiac metastasis from solid cancers. Arch Pathol Lab Med. ePub, 2022
4. Hudzik B et al: Malignant tumors of the heart. Cancer Epidemiol. 39(5):665-72, 2015
5. Hoffmeier A et al: Cardiac tumors–diagnosis and surgical treatment. Dtsch Arztebl Int. 111(12):205-11, 2014
6. Kassop D et al: Cardiac masses on cardiac CT: a review. Curr Cardiovasc Imaging Rep. 7:9281, 2014
7. Kwekkeboom DJ: Myocardial metastases from neuroendocrine tumors: incidence and relevance. Endocrine. 47(1):5-6, 2014
8. Al-Mamgani A et al: Cardiac metastases. Int J Clin Oncol. 13(4):369-72, 2008
9. Simpson L et al: Malignant primary cardiac tumors: review of a single institution experience. Cancer. 112(11):2440-6, 2008
10. Bussani R et al: Cardiac metastases. J Clin Pathol. 60(1):27-34, 2007
11. Butany J et al: A 30-year analysis of cardiac neoplasms at autopsy. Can J Cardiol. 21(8):675-80, 2005
12. Kühl HP et al: The impact of transesophageal echocardiography on daily clinical practice. Eur J Echocardiogr. 5(6):455-68, 2004
13. Reynen K et al: Metastases to the heart. Ann Oncol. 15(3):375-81, 2004
14. Roberts WC: Primary and secondary neoplasms of the heart. Am J Cardiol. 80(5):671-82, 1997

Pericardial Metastasis From Ovarian Carcinoma

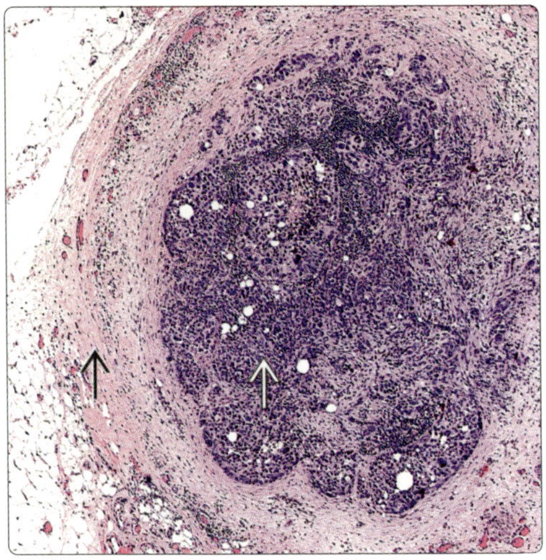

Movat Stain of Pericardial Section Involved by Metastatic Ovarian Carcinoma

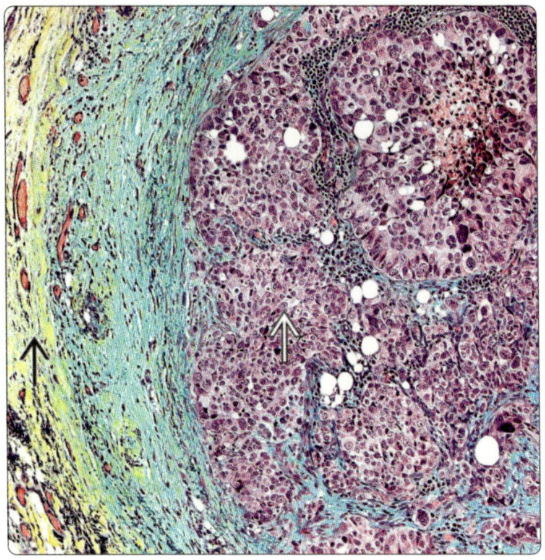

(Left) *Low-power view of an H&E-stained section shows a metastatic deposit of a high-grade ovarian carcinoma* ➡ *involving the pericardium* ⇨*. Carcinomas from different origins are common tumors that metastasize to the heart.* **(Right)** *Higher power view of a Movat-stained section shows a high-grade ovarian carcinoma* ➡ *involving the pericardium* ⇨*. Immunohistochemical stains are also contributory for identification of the type of neoplasm, especially when the primary malignancy is unknown.*

Histologic Section of Metastatic Melanoma in Pericardium

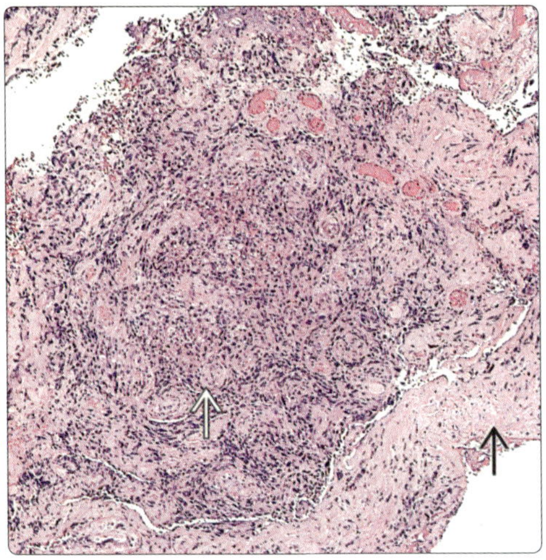

Movat Stain of Pericardial Section Involved by Metastatic Melanoma

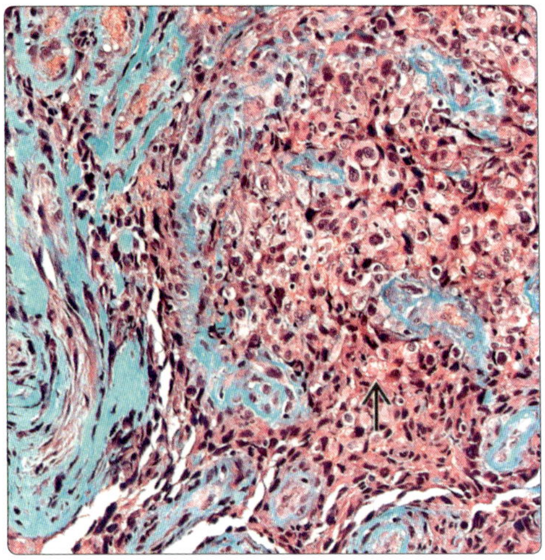

(Left) *Low-power view of an H&E-stained section shows a metastatic dedifferentiated malignant melanoma* ➡ *in the pericardium* ⇨*. Melanoma has the highest frequency of metastasis to the heart.* **(Right)** *Movat-stained section shows metastatic deposits of dedifferentiated malignant melanoma* ⇨*. Prior history of malignant melanoma was known in this case.*

Multiple Epicardial Metastases

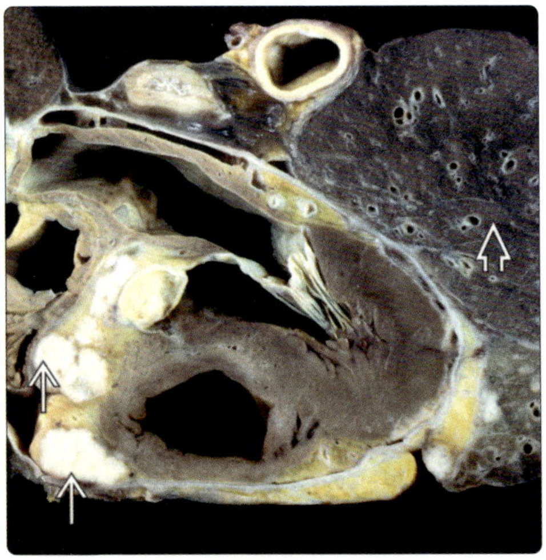

Metastatic Renal Cell Carcinoma With Septal Involvement

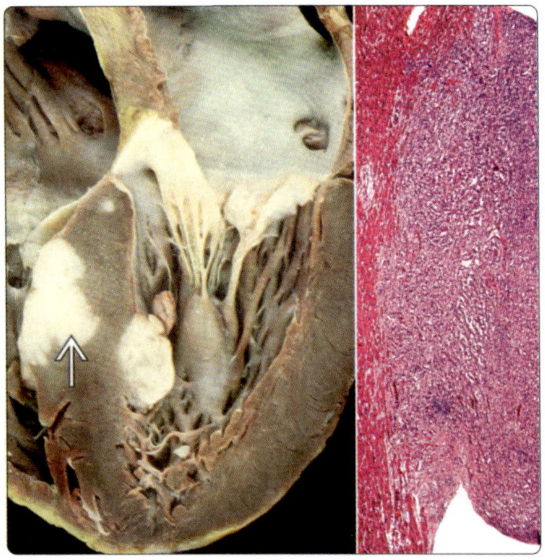

(Left) *Autopsy specimen shows epicardial metastases* ➡ *with adherence of the lung* ➡*. Site of primary malignancy was not known. Metastatic deposits are usually multiple and may be circumscribed.* **(Right)** *Autopsy specimen shows foci of metastatic renal cell carcinoma in intraventricular septum* ➡*. A low-power view of an H&E-stained section details the histologic features.*

(Left) *Sections of myocardium show metastatic deposits* → *from a primary malignant melanoma of the eye. The deposits have dark brown coloration, and, in histologic examination, melanin pigment can be identified, which is helpful for diagnosis.* (Right) *H&E-stained paraffin section shows malignant melanoma deposits in the myocardium* →*. Melanin pigment is seen* →*, which is helpful for diagnosis.*

Multifocal Myocardial Involvement by Metastatic Malignant Melanoma

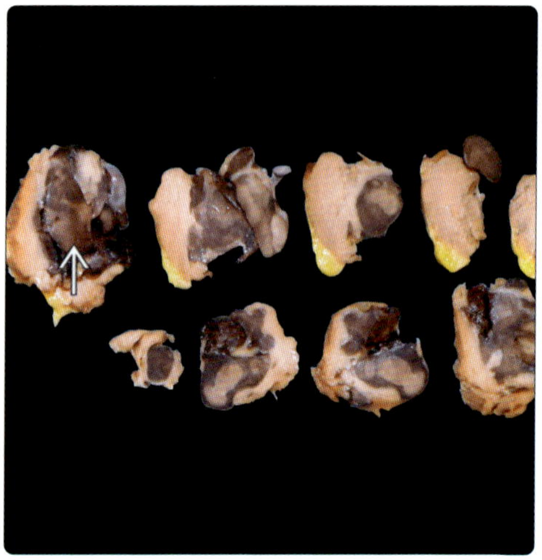

Metastatic Melanoma in Myocardium

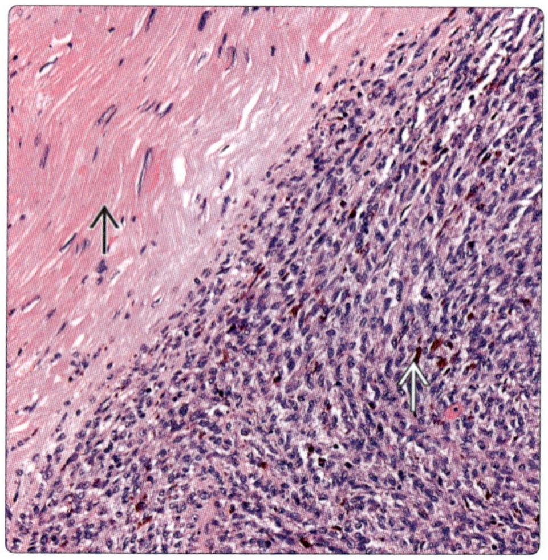

(Left) *Movat-stained section shows a malignant melanoma* → *with infiltration* → *in the myocardium* →*. When there is extensive involvement of the ventricular myocardium, congestive heart failure may be the clinical presentation.* (Right) *Short-axis section of heart shows extensive involvement of the right ventricle by metastatic thyroid carcinoma* →*. In the left ventricle free wall, an area of scarring* → *from a previous myocardial infarction can be appreciated.*

Movat Stain of Metastatic Melanoma in Myocardium

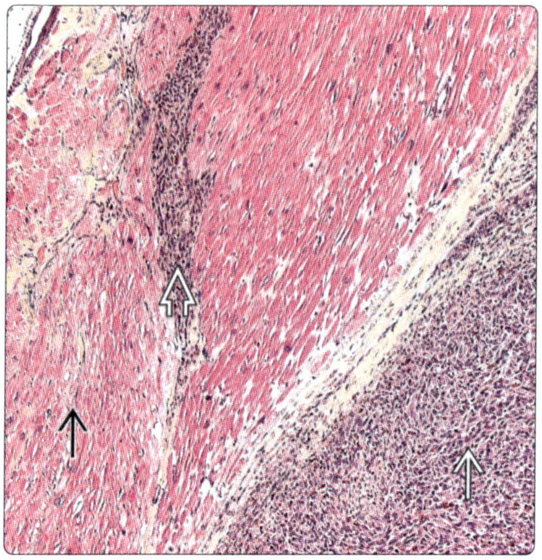

Right Ventricle Involvement by Metastatic Thyroid Carcinoma

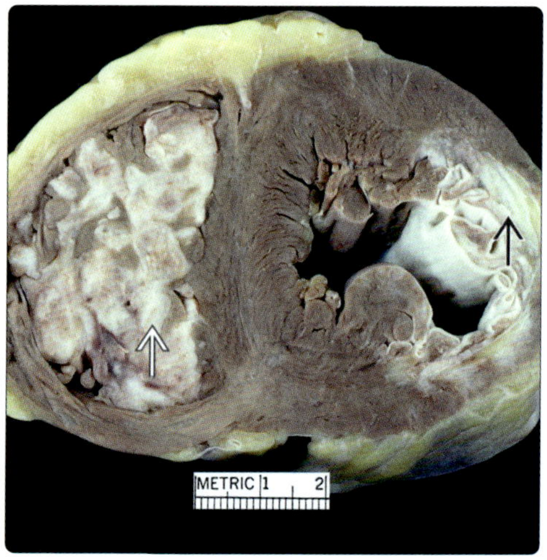

(Left) *H&E-stained section shows large cell lymphoma* → *forming a nodule in the pericardium* →*. There was adjacent mediastinal lymph node involvement.* (Right) *H&E section of left ventricle shows a nodule* → *composed of large atypical lymphocytes from a large cell lymphoma originating from the mediastinum in a patient with extensive involvement of abdominal lymph nodes and gastrointestinal organs. The adjacent myocytes appear vacuolated* → *and with hypertrophic changes.*

Pericardial Infiltration by Lymphoma

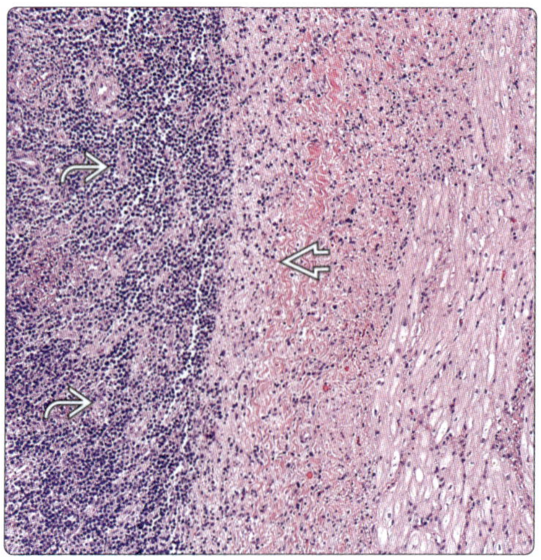

Nodular Myocardial Infiltration by Large Cell Lymphoma

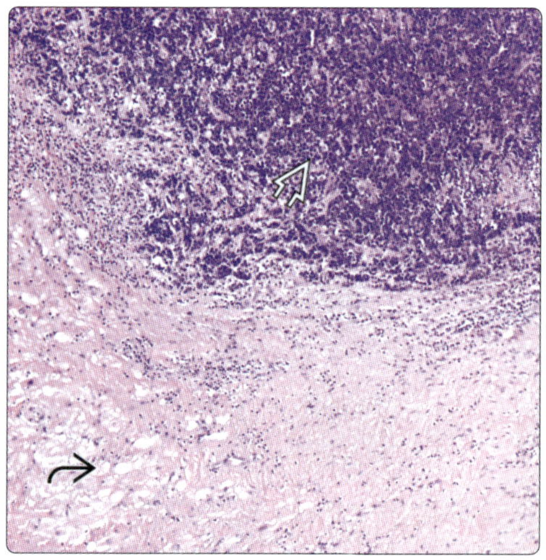

Myocardial Involvement by Metastatic Sarcoma

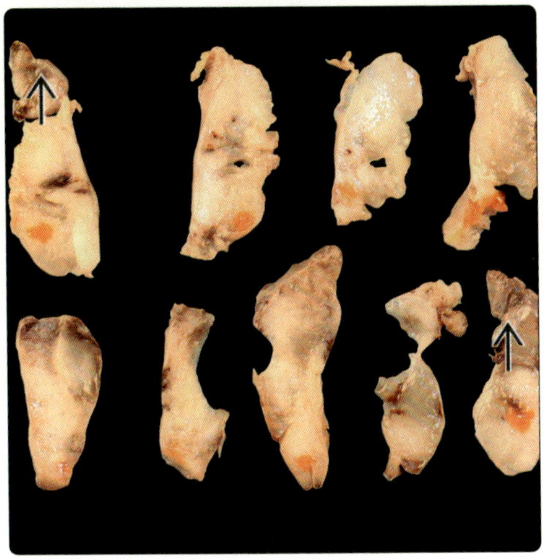

Histologic Section of Myocardium Involved by Metastatic Myxoid Liposarcoma

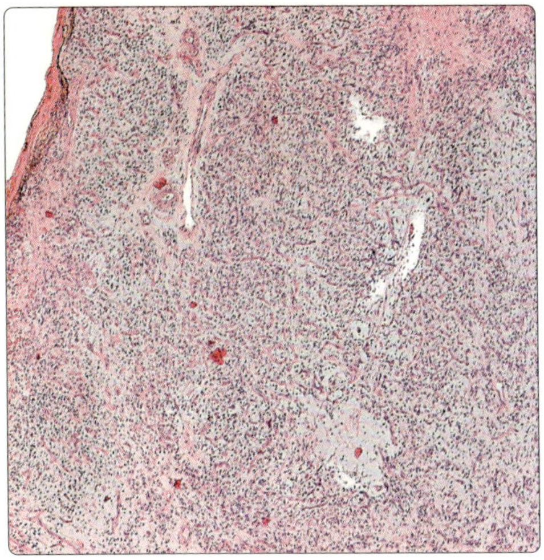

(Left) *Gross sections of myocardium show extensive involvement by a metastatic myxoid liposarcoma →. The neoplasm appears yellow-tan in color.* **(Right)** *Low-power view of an H&E-stained section shows a myxoid liposarcoma composed of malignant adipocytes surrounded by delicate arborizing vasculature.*

Movat Stain of Myocardium Involved by Metastatic Myxoid Liposarcoma

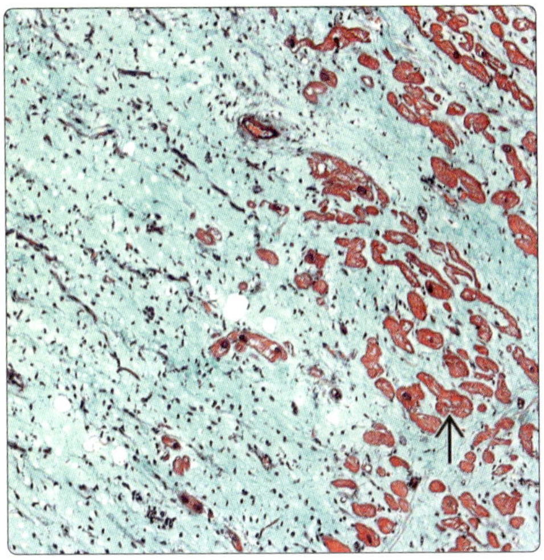

Myocardium Involved by Metastatic Sarcoma

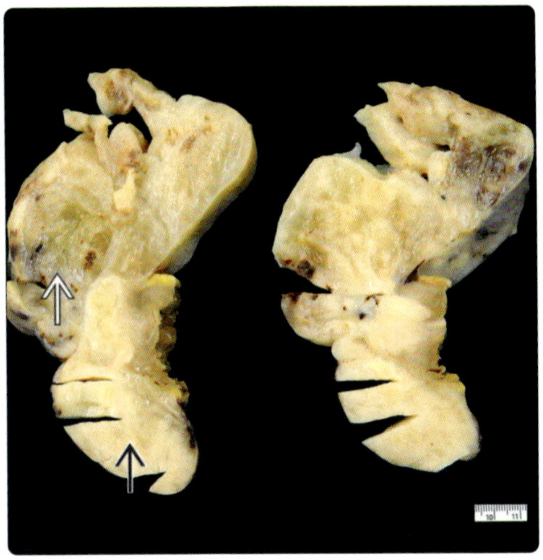

(Left) *High-power view of a Movat-stained section shows myxoid liposarcoma cells (green) infiltrating the myocardium →. Sarcomas may infiltrate diffusely into myocardial tissue and do not show well-defined borders.* **(Right)** *Gross specimens show metastatic deposits ➡ in myocardium → from a primary myxoid sarcoma of the thigh.*

Histologic Section of Myocardium Involved by Metastatic Myxoid Sarcoma

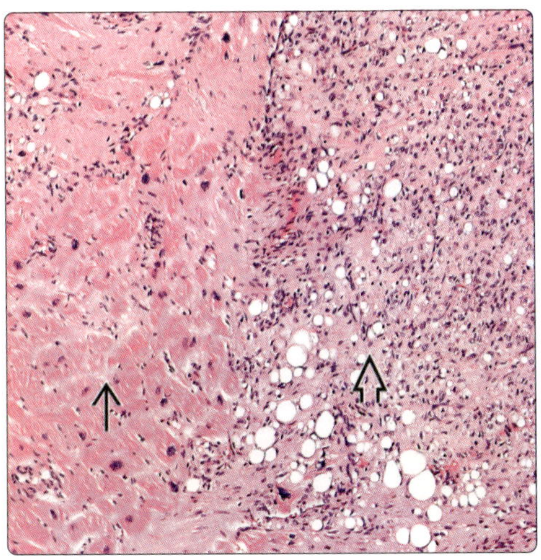

Movat Stain of Myocardium Involved by Metastatic Myxoid Sarcoma

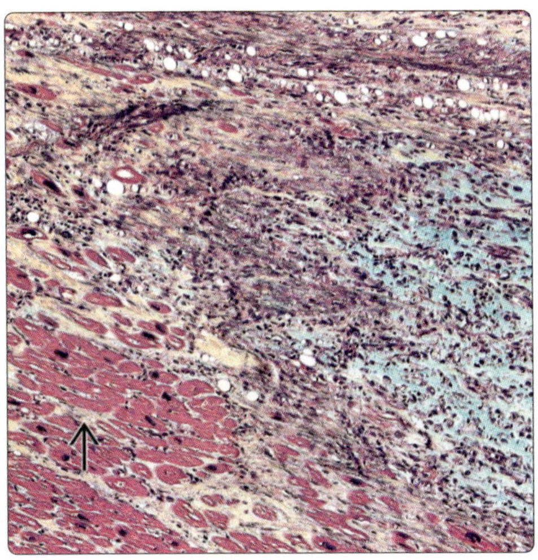

(Left) *Low-power view of an H&E-stained section shows a metastatic myxoid sarcoma ⇒ infiltrating the myocardium →. There is an ill-defined border between the myocytes and neoplasm.* **(Right)** *Low-power view of a Movat-stained section shows myxoid sarcoma (green) metastasizing into the myocardium →.*

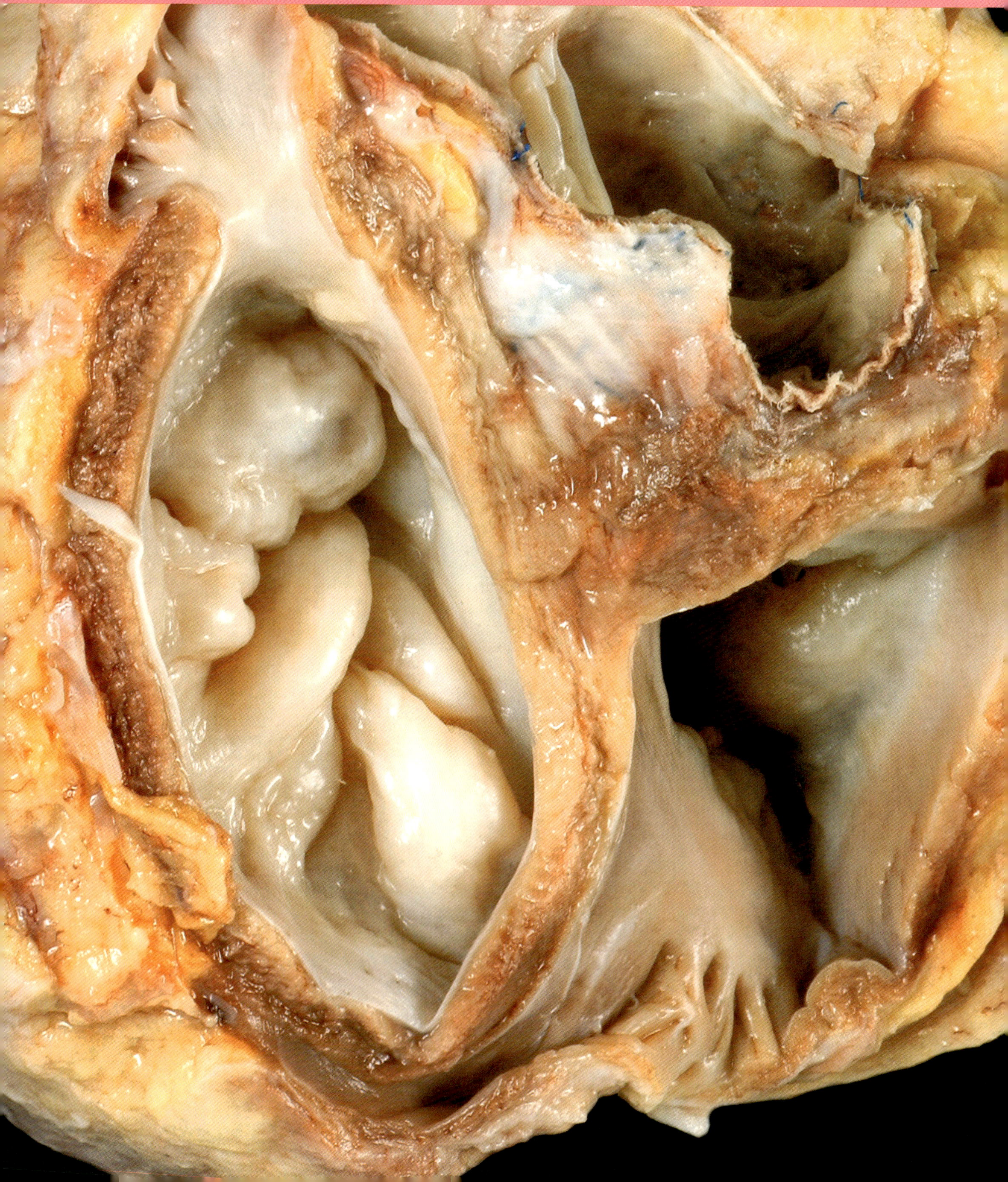

SECTION 4

Cardiac Valves, Native

Aortic

Mitral

Tricuspid

Pulmonary

Endocarditis

Unicommissural Aortic Valve

KEY FACTS

TERMINOLOGY

- Unicuspid aortic valve (UAV): Rare anomaly in which 2 of 3 commissures are congenitally abnormal and represented by raphe/raphae of varying size

ETIOLOGY/PATHOGENESIS

- UAV has 1 lateral attachment to aorta, at level of orifice, and 2 raphae, resulting in slit-like orifice that requires surgery later in adulthood

CLINICAL ISSUES

- Mean age of presentation is 28 years
- M:F = 2.2:1
- Presenting features: Aortic stenosis ± regurgitation
- UAV is associated with left ventricular hypertrophy and ascending aortic abnormalities
- Congenital anomalies associated with UAV include: Anomalous coronary arteries, patent ductus arteriosus, coarctation of aorta, ventricular septal defect
- Real-time 3D transesophageal echocardiography shows horseshoe-shaped unicuspid aortic valve with 1 posterior commissure and 2 raphae with eccentric orifice and thick, fibrotic, heavily calcified tissue
- Treatment is aortic valve replacement

MACROSCOPIC

- UAV has 1 cusp, 1 true commissure, and 2 raphae
- Cusp is thick and fibrotic with areas of calcification, ulceration, tears, and perforation
- Most common position of true commissure is left posterior

MICROSCOPIC

- UAV shows fibrous and fibroelastic thickening, ventricular and aortic surface pads, and zona spongiosa and zona fibrous layers
- Valve cusp shows areas of nodular calcification, often with foci of ossification, cartilaginous metaplasia, ulceration, neovascularization, and chronic inflammation around some calcific nodules

Gross Image of UAV, Flow Surface

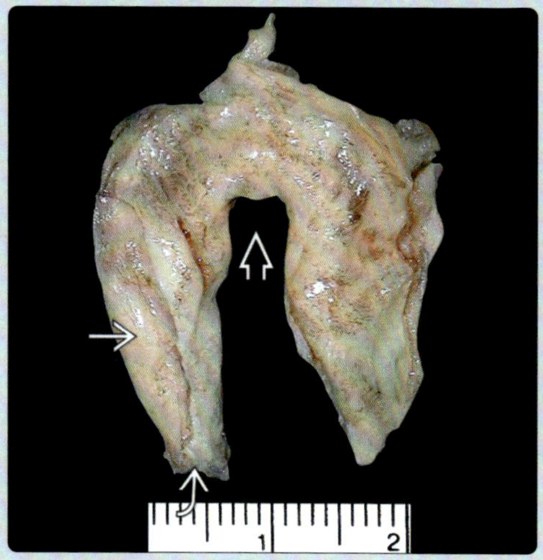

Gross Image of UAV, Nonflow Surface

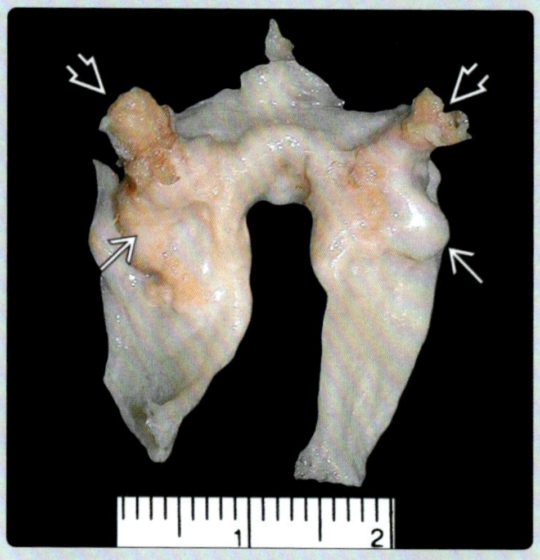

(Left) *Unicuspid aortic valve (UAV) shows an exclamation mark-like orifice. The flow surface of UAV shows a thick, fibrotic, single cusp with nodular calcification. The true commissure has been cut through, and the surrounding area is mildly distorted.* **(Right)** *The nonflow surface of the same valve shows 2 raphae and nodular calcifications. The tissue between and around the raphae shows the greatest degree of fibrosis, thickening, and nodular calcification.*

Histologic Features of UAV

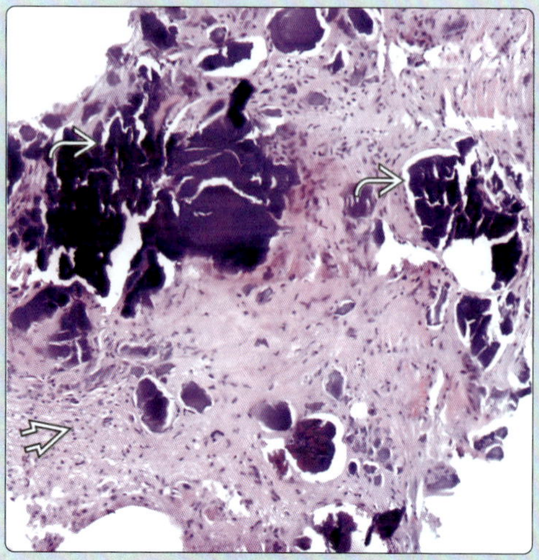

Histologic Changes of UAV

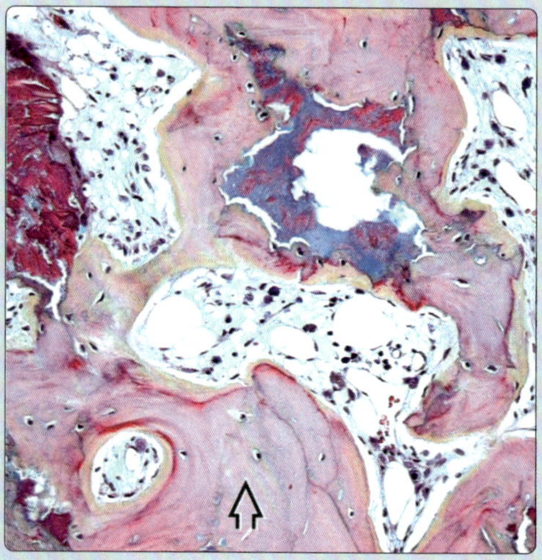

(Left) *H&E-stained section from a unicommissural aortic valve shows fibrous thickening of the cusp with irregular areas of calcification. Foci of ossification, cartilaginous metaplasia, and neovascularization may also be present.* **(Right)** *Movat elastic stain of the same unicommissural aortic valve shows metaplastic bone formation.*

TERMINOLOGY

Definitions

- Unicuspid aortic valve (UAV)
  - Rare anomaly in which 2 of 3 commissures are congenitally fused
  - Point(s) of fusion represented by raphe/raphae of varying sizes
    - 2 cusps are therefore prolapsed from birth, and valve is dysfunctional

ETIOLOGY/PATHOGENESIS

Development and Features

- Aortic valve develops from 3 tubercles, each of which forms cusp and sinus of Valsalva
- Unicuspid aortic valve has 1 fused cusp
- Unicuspid aortic valve has 2 forms: Acommissural and unicommissural
  - Both have dome shape
  - Acommissural form has no commissure or lateral attachment to aorta and has central stenotic orifice, of varying size, causing severe stenosis in early childhood
  - Unicommissural form has 1 lateral attachment to aorta, at level of orifice, and 2 raphae, resulting in slit-like or exclamation mark-like orifice that requires surgery later in adulthood
  - In adults, unicuspid aortic valves are mostly unicommissural

Pathogenesis

- UAV is associated with increased cusp flexion during systole and increased stretching of cusps during diastole with incomplete valve closure
- Altered hemodynamics and stress distribution cause early and ongoing structural damage to cusps, which leads to endothelial damage and fibrosis with calcification
- UAV is often associated with congenital changes in aorta and pulmonary artery

CLINICAL ISSUES

Epidemiology

- Incidence
  - Unicuspid aortic valve is seen in 0.02% of patients during echocardiographic evaluation
  - In adult population, UAV accounts for 3% of patients undergoing surgery for aortic valve disease
  - UAV accounts for 1-5% of congenital aortic valvar stenosis
- Age
  - Mean age of presentation is 28 years with bimodal distribution
    - 1st peak is in infancy and childhood (birth to 10 years of age)
    - 2nd peak occurs ~ 30-50 years of age, when premature calcific stenosis manifests
  - Younger patients have more aggressive form and also aortic dilatation
  - Older patients present with less aggressive form without aortic dilatation
- Sex
  - Males are more likely than females to have UAV
    - M:F = 2.2:1

Presentation

- Most UAVs present with features of aortic stenosis ± regurgitation
- Acquired cardiovascular diseases associated with UAV
  - Left ventricular hypertrophy
  - Ascending aortic abnormalities (dilation, aneurysm, dissection)
- Congenital anomalies associated with UAV
  - Anomalous coronary arteries
  - Patent ductus arteriosus
  - Coarctation of aorta
  - Ventricular septal defect
- UAV is uncommonly associated with infective endocarditis
- Patients with UAV develop severe calcification at younger age
  - UAV has higher rate of progression to aortic valve stenosis and requires aortic valve replacement 10-20 years earlier than bicuspid aortic valve and 20-30 years earlier than tricuspid valve
- Symptoms
  - Shortness of breath, angina, palpitation, fatigue, and presyncope, all of which are increased with exertion
- Signs
  - Systolic murmur at right upper sternal border radiating to carotid artery

Laboratory Tests

- Electrocardiogram
  - Lateral lead ST depression and T wave inversion that marks left ventricular hypertrophy
  - Occasional P waves, which show left atrial enlargement

Treatment

- Surgical approaches
  - Aortic valve replacement, often with replacement of ascending aorta, has shown better outcomes
  - Bicuspidization (either surgically or by balloon) of unicuspid aortic valve may provide short-term relief

IMAGING

Radiographic Findings

- Chest radiograph
  - Boot-shaped heart typical of concentric left ventricular hypertrophy
  - Enlarged left atrium
  - Aortic valve calcification
  - Poststenotic aortic dilatation

Ultrasonographic Findings

- Transthoracic echocardiography
  - Concentric left ventricular hypertrophy with normal systolic function
  - Severe aortic stenosis with calcified aortic valve
  - Valve dysfunction
    - 40% combined stenosis and regurgitation
    - 40% pure stenosis
    - 20% pure regurgitation
  - Commissure orientation

- 70% left posterior
- 20% right posterior
- 10% horizontal (right-left)

- Real-time 3D transesophageal echocardiography
  - Horseshoe-shaped unicuspid aortic valve with single posterior commissure and 2 raphe with eccentric orifice and thick, fibrotic, heavily calcified tissue

Angiography

- UAV shows orifice contiguous with posterior wall of aorta with no intervening valvular tissue
- Sinus of Valsalva is present anteriorly and on either side but absent posteriorly
- During systole, aortic leaflet tissue shows motion anteriorly but not posteriorly
- During diastole, sinus of Valsalva is deep anteriorly and shallow posteriorly

MACROSCOPIC

General Features

- UAV most often has 1 cusp, 1 true commissure, and 2 raphae
- Cusp is thick, fibrotic, and with areas of calcification, ulceration, tears, and perforation
- Occasionally, cusp may be myxoid, and valve is clinically incompetent
- Early thickening begins at raphe/raphae and then spreads laterally into cuspal tissues, significantly reducing aortic valve annulus
- Cuspal tissues around true commissure show least degree of fibrosis and calcification
- Calcification increases exponentially with patient age
- Leaflets may show dysplastic/malformed features grossly
- Valves with mild fibrosis or calcification have dome-shaped cusp with circular orifice
- Valves with severe fibrosis and calcification have fixed, rigid noncircular cusp with teardrop-shaped orifice
- Range of annular diameter: 2.1-3.7 cm
- Forme fruste leaflets/cusps (right, left, posterior) may be similar in size or show size disparity
  - 45% show dominant leaflet forming 1 side of commissure
  - 35% have equal sizes
  - 20% show small size of middle cusp
- Free margin of cusp also shows thickening
- Like other malformed valves, there is risk of endocarditis, and valves should be closely inspected for vegetations, perforations, etc.
- Aortopathy
  - Ascending aortic pathology frequently accompanies UAV
    - 40% dilatation/ectasia
    - 20% true aneurysm
    - 2% dissection

MICROSCOPIC

Histologic Features

- UAV shows fibrous and fibroelastic thickening, ventricular and aortic surface pads, and disrupted zona spongiosa and zona fibrosa layers
- Valve cusp shows areas of nodular calcification, often with foci of ossification, cartilaginous metaplasia, ulceration, neovascularization, and chronic inflammation around some calcific nodules
- Ulceration and thrombus may overlie ruptured calcific nodules
- Calcification often begins in valvular fibrosa and gradually reaches midportion of cusps without extending to valve edge
- Leaflets may show dysplastic/malformed valve layer architecture
- Macrophages, which are predominant inflammatory cells seen, cause degradation of extracellular matrix through matrix metalloproteinase
- Stenotic UAV
  - Shows increased expression of osteopontin, MMP-2, MMP-9, and MMP-14
  - Shows reduced expression of TIMP-1 and TIMP-2
- Aortopathy
  - Medial degeneration with accumulation of mucopolysaccharide

DIFFERENTIAL DIAGNOSIS

Bicuspid Aortic Valve With Acquired Fusion of True Commissure

- Angle between cusps in bicuspid aortic valve is acute, whereas it is obtuse in UAV
- Bicuspid aortic valve has 2 cusps, and free edge of cusp continues to opposite commissural attachment zone, which is distorted due to calcification

SELECTED REFERENCES

1. Chang HH et al: Assessment of unicuspid aortic valve stenosis using multimodality imaging, x-ray radiography and Raman analysis. Int Heart J. 60(2):482-8, 2019
2. Krepp JM et al: Bicuspid and unicuspid aortic valves: different phenotypes of the same disease? Insight from the GenTAC Registry. Congenit Heart Dis. 12(6):740-5, 2017
3. Noly PE et al: New insights into unicuspid aortic valve disease in adults: not just a subtype of bicuspid aortic valves. Can J Cardiol. 32(1):110-6, 2016
4. Zhu Y et al: Outcomes after operations for unicuspid aortic valve with or without ascending repair in adults. Ann Thorac Surg. 101(2):613-9, 2016
5. Singh S et al: Unicuspid unicommissural aortic valve: an extremely rare congenital anomaly. Tex Heart Inst J. 42(3):273-6, 2015
6. Fealey ME et al: Unicommissural aortic valves: gross, histological, and immunohistochemical analysis of 52 cases (1978-2008). Cardiovasc Pathol. 21(4):324-33, 2012
7. Mookadam F et al: Unicuspid aortic valve in adults: a systematic review. J Heart Valve Dis. 19(1):79-85, 2010
8. Butany J et al: Ascending aortic aneurysms in unicommissural aortic valve disease. Cardiovasc Pathol. 18(1):11-8, 2009
9. Collins MJ et al: Implications of a congenitally abnormal valve: a study of 1025 consecutively excised aortic valves. J Clin Pathol. 61(4):530-6, 2008
10. Agnihotri AK et al: Two distinct clinical presentations in adult unicuspid aortic valve. J Thorac Cardiovasc Surg. 131(5):1169-70, 2006
11. Butany J et al: Morphological and clinical findings in 247 surgically excised native aortic valves. Can J Cardiol. 21(9):747-55, 2005
12. Anderson RH: Understanding the structure of the unicuspid and unicommissural aortic valve. J Heart Valve Dis. 12(6):670-3, 2003
13. Novaro GM et al: Incidence and echocardiographic features of congenital unicuspid aortic valve in an adult population. J Heart Valve Dis. 12(6):674-8, 2003
14. Datta BN et al: Anatomically isolated aortic valve disease. Morphologic study of 100 cases at autopsy. Jpn Heart J. 29(5):661-70, 1988
15. Subramanian R et al: Surgical pathology of pure aortic stenosis: a study of 374 cases. Mayo Clin Proc. 59(10):683-90, 1984
16. Simon AL et al: The angiographic features of bicuspid and unicommissural aortic stenosis. Am J Cardiol. 28(3):353-8, 1971

Aortic Changes Associated With UAV

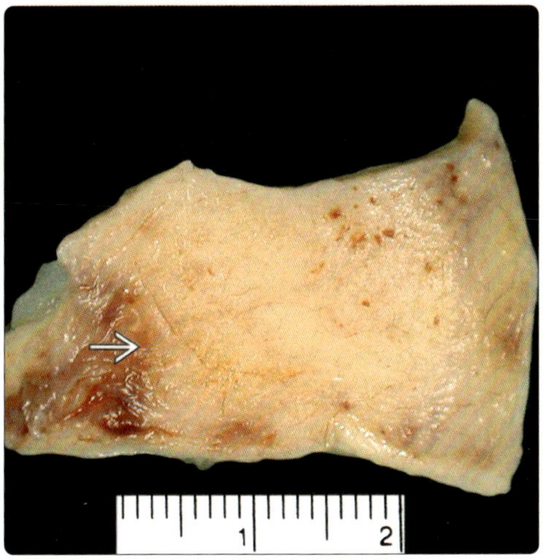

Cross Section of Aorta

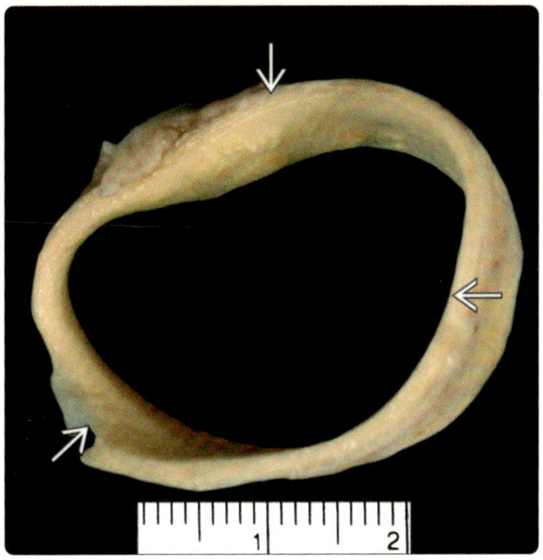

(Left) *Gross appearance of the aorta shows aneurysmal dilatation.* **(Right)** *Cross section of the same aorta shows aneurysmal dilatation. Most ascending aortic aneurysms are fusiform in shape. By size criteria, ascending aneurysms are dilatations > 3.5 cm. Aneurysms > 5.5 cm require surgical repair.*

Histologic Features of UAV

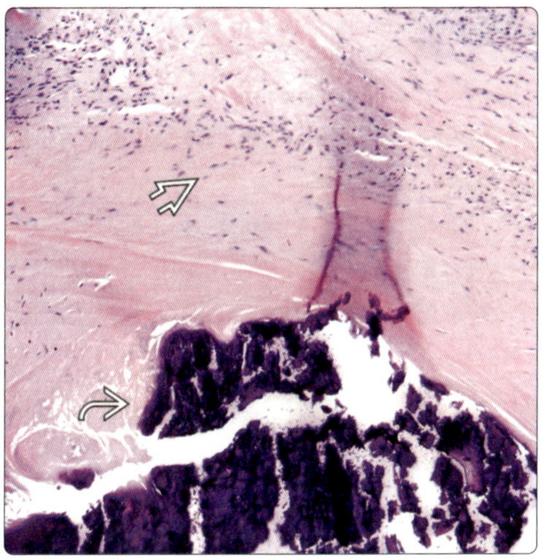

Transverse Section of UAV

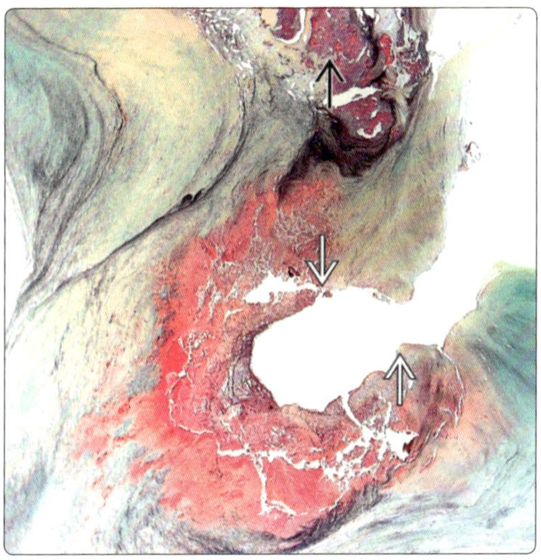

(Left) *H&E-stained section of a unicommissural aortic valve shows marked fibrous thickening of the cusp with nodular calcification. Calcification increases significantly with patient age.* **(Right)** *Movat elastic stain of a unicommissural aortic valve shows fibroelastic thickening, an area of calcification, and ulceration.*

Transverse Section of UAV

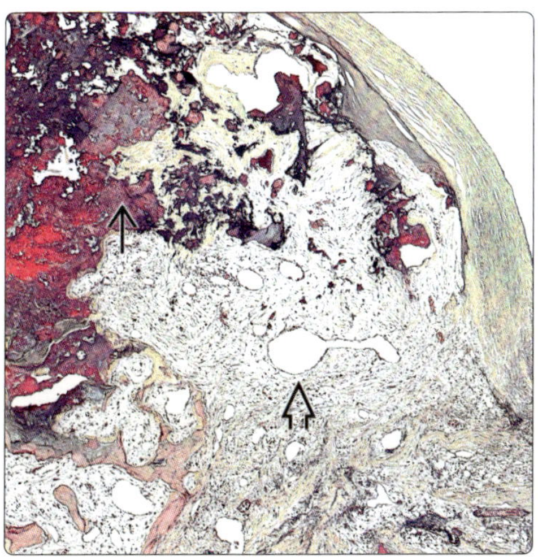

Histologic Changes of Aorta Wall Associated With UAV

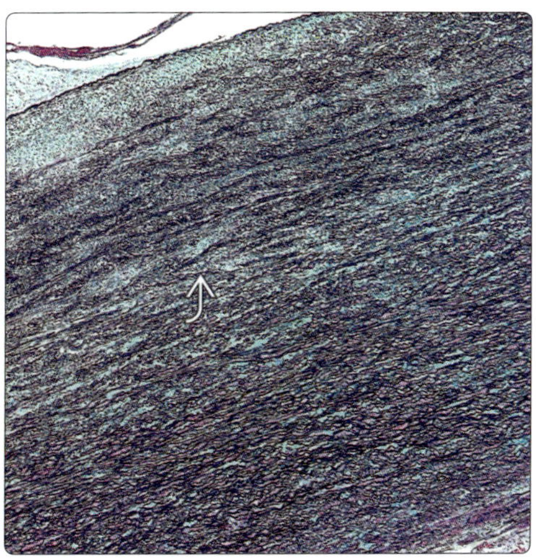

(Left) *Movat elastic stain of the same unicommissural aortic valve shows areas of neovascularization and extensive calcification.* **(Right)** *Movat elastic stain of the aorta in the same case shows increased mucopolysaccharides and loss of smooth muscle, consistent with aneurysmal dilatation.*

Bicuspid Aortic Valve

KEY FACTS

TERMINOLOGY

- Bicuspid aortic valve (BAV): Most common congenital heart abnormality; occurs isolated or associated with other structural abnormalities of heart and vessels

ETIOLOGY/PATHOGENESIS

- BAV has been noted to be inheritable
- Association between BAV and other structural abnormalities suggests developmental etiology

CLINICAL ISSUES

- Prevalence of BAV is 1-2% of general population
- 3x more common in males than females
- Clinical course is variable; ranges from severe aortic stenosis in childhood to asymptomatic in old age
- Severity of disease and course of illness depend on presence of other associated abnormalities
- Main factor affecting prognosis is aortic diameter
  - Estimated 15-year freedom from complications
    - 86% in patients with aortic diameter < 40 mm
    - 43% in patients with aortic diameter ≥ 45 mm
- Surgical treatment is considered most appropriate and definitive treatment for BAV
- Balloon valvuloplasty is management strategy of choice in children due to absence of valve calcification
- β-blockers considered 1st-line therapy in medical treatment of BAV

IMAGING

- Transthoracic or transesophageal echocardiography considered as mainstay of diagnosis

MACROSCOPIC

- Important gross finding of BAV is presence of raphe

MICROSCOPIC

- Valve cusp thickening, fibrosis, and calcification
  - Raphe is major site of calcification

Gross Image of Flow Surface of BAV

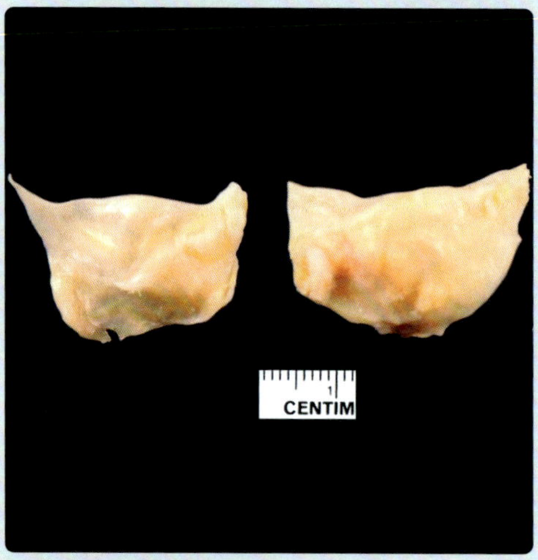

Gross Image of Nonflow Surface of BAV

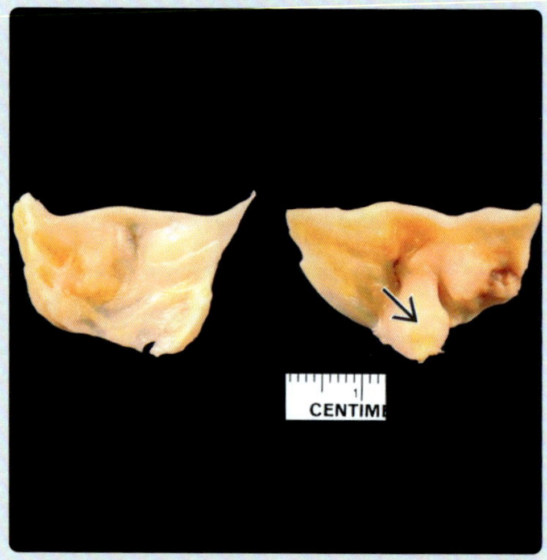

(Left) *This is the flow surface of a congenital bicuspid aortic valve (BAV). The cusps show diffuse fibrosis and nodular calcification.* **(Right)** *The nonflow surface of the valve cusps shows that one cusp is larger than the other. The larger cusp shows the raphe, which is seen as a large calcified ridge ⇨ on the inner (nonflow) side of the cusp.*

Histologic Features of BAV

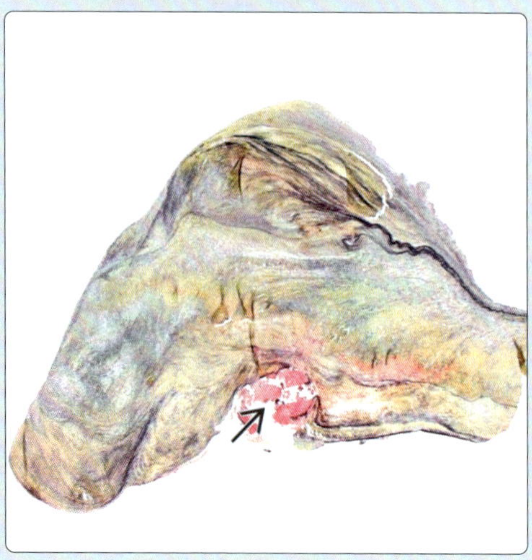

Histologic Features of BAV

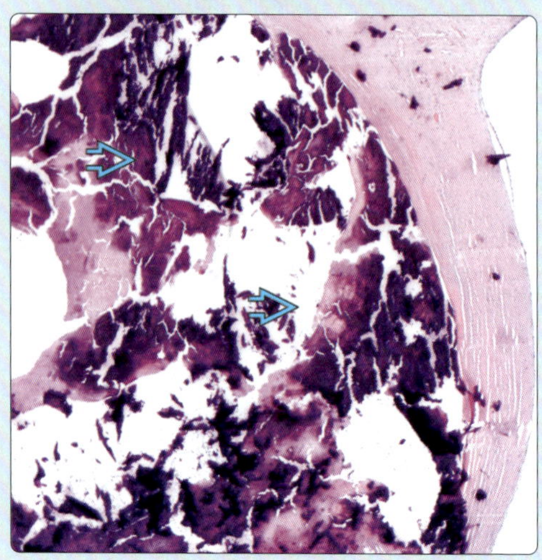

(Left) *Movat elastic stain of a longitudinal section of BAV shows extensive fibroelastic thickening, especially in the distal 2/3 of the cusp. A focal area of ulceration ⇨ is seen on the sinus (nonflow) surface of the cusp.* **(Right)** *H&E-stained section of aortic valve cusp shows thickening and marked calcification ⇨. This leads to progressive aortic stenosis and clinical symptoms.*

TERMINOLOGY

Abbreviations

- Bicuspid aortic valve (BAV)

Definitions

- Most common congenital heart abnormality; occurs isolated or associated with other structural abnormalities of heart and vessels, such as
  - Enlargement of ascending aorta (most common associated abnormality)
  - Coarctation
  - Interrupted aortic arch
  - Anomalous coronary ostium

ETIOLOGY/PATHOGENESIS

Familial

- BAV has been noted to be inheritable with autosomal dominant pattern with reduced penetrance and variable expressivity
- 10% chance of BAV in 1st-degree relatives of patient

Developmental

- Association between BAV and other structural abnormalities suggests developmental etiology

Genetic

- *NOTCH1* gene: Transmembrane receptor that has role in determining cell outcome in organogenesis
  - Mutations were noted in 2 families with BAV
- Other candidate genes include *GATA4*, *GATA5*, *GATA6*, *TBX5*, *SMAD6*, *FBN1*, *ROBO4*, *ACTA2*, and *ELN*

Pathogenesis

- Fusion of valve cushions at beginning of its development appears to be key factor in BAV formation
- BAVs with fused right or left and noncoronary leaflet are due to defects that occur before cardiac outflow tract septation
- BAVs with fused right and left leaflets are due to anomalous septation of proximal portion of cardiac outflow tract caused by dysfunctional neural crest cells

CLINICAL ISSUES

Epidemiology

- Incidence
  - Prevalence of BAV is 1-2% of general population
  - Some reports suggest prevalence of 4.6 cases per 1,000 live births
- Sex
  - 3x more common in males than females

Presentation

- Clinical course is variable; ranges from severe aortic stenosis in childhood to asymptomatic in old age
- Incidental findings of minimally calcified BAV in patients in their 70s have also been reported
- Severity of disease and course of illness depend on presence of other associated abnormalities

Treatment

- Surgical
  - Valve replacement is considered definitive treatment for BAV
  - Indications for valve surgery in patients with BAV are similar for those patients with 3-leaflet aortic valves
  - Valve replacement in children is usually avoided since they outgrow prosthetic valve
  - Balloon valvuloplasty is management strategy of choice in children due to absence of valve calcification
  - Surgical treatment also includes replacement of ascending aorta if > 45 mm in diameter
  - Valve repair in cases of aortic regurgitation is also surgical option
  - Transcatheter aortic valve implantation has also been used as method of treating BAV
- Medical treatment
  - Indicated for symptomatic relief and to slow progression of disease
  - Blood pressure should be aggressively controlled to slow progression of aortopathy
  - β-blockers are 1st-line therapy in medical treatment of BAV

Prognosis

- Main factor affecting prognosis is aortic diameter
  - Estimated 15-year freedom from complications
    - 86% in patients with aortic diameter < 40 mm
    - 81% in patients with aortic diameter 40-44 mm
    - 43% in patients with aortic diameter ≥ 45 mm

BAV-Associated Complications

- Aortic stenosis
  - Estimated incidence 15-75% in autopsy series, 5-50% in surgical specimens; most common in females
  - Commonly occurs due to progressive fibrocalcific stenosis of valve
  - Usually leads to presentation in middle age
  - Only ~ 2% of children have clinically significant BAV disease
  - Main symptoms
    - Exertional dyspnea
    - Syncope
    - Chest pain
    - Ejection systolic murmur heard loudest at apex in most patients
- Aortic incompetence
  - Estimated incidence 1.5-10%; most common in males
  - Caused by
    - Myxoid degeneration: Valve tissue is replaced by acid mucopolysaccharides affecting structural integrity of valve
    - Aging that leads to dilatation of ascending aorta, which further leads to functionally regurgitant valve
  - In children, incompetence is most common in males and usually caused by
    - Prolapsing cusps
    - Valve surgery
    - Endocarditis
- Aortopathy (progressive dilatation of aortic root, ascending aorta, and aortic arch)
  - Diameter of ascending aorta is larger in patients with BAV compared to those with normal valves

- Factors leading to increased incidence of aortic dissection, aneurysms, or aortopathy in BAV
  - Increased amount of mechanical stress in ascending aorta
  - Systemic endothelial dysfunction
  - Increased fragmentation of elastic tissue in aortic wall compared to people with normal aortic valve
  - Types I and III collagen and fibrillin are significantly decreased in dilated aortas of BAV patients
  - Fewer smooth muscle cells
  - Higher plasma levels of matrix metalloproteinases
- Aortic dissection
  - Matrix metalloproteinases have been implicated in formation of atherosclerotic aneurysms
  - Aortic wall usually shows cystic medial change or mucoid degeneration
  - Thinner elastic lamellae of media
  - Greater distances between elastic lamellae than in patients with normal valves
- Endocarditis
  - Estimated incidence 0.16% per year in unoperated children and adolescents
  - Outcomes in BAV patients with infective endocarditis tend to be worse than in those with normal valves
  - Patients with BAV are younger at presentation and have higher incidence of periaortic abscess

IMAGING

Echocardiography

- Transthoracic or transesophageal echocardiography
  - Considered as mainstay of diagnosis
  - Can provide definitive diagnosis in majority of patients
  - 92% sensitivity and 96% specificity when images are adequate
  - However, utility of echocardiography can be limited due to effects of severe calcification

Other Imaging Modalities

- CT/MR
  - Have been used to augment diagnostic process
  - MR especially allows valve assessment without interference from calcification
    - Also allows for excellent assessment of aorta
  - Combination of both imaging modalities makes them excellent surveillance tools for aortic assessment
  - Interval measurements should be performed with same image modality and compared side by side

MACROSCOPIC

General Features

- Asymmetric 2 leaflets
- Important gross finding of BAV is presence of raphe
  - Raphe: Incompletely formed commissure that extends to free margin of cusp
    - Because of this, cusp prolapses into aortic valve orifice

MICROSCOPIC

Histologic Features

- Valve cusp thickening, fibrosis, and calcification
  - Raphe is major site of calcification

DIFFERENTIAL DIAGNOSIS

Rheumatic Aortic Valve Stenosis

- Commissural fusion is characteristic of rheumatic valve disease
- Concomitant mitral valve involvement is universally present

SELECTED REFERENCES

1. Cheng C et al: Clinical outcomes of adults with bicuspid aortic valve: a European perspective. Mayo Clin Proc. 96(3):648-57, 2021
2. Della Corte A et al: Risk stratification in bicuspid aortic valve aortopathy: emerging evidence and future perspectives. Curr Probl Cardiol. 46(3):100428, 2021
3. Engel Gonzalez P et al: Treatment of bicuspid aortic valve stenosis using transcatheter heart valves. Interv Cardiol Clin. 10(4):541-52, 2021
4. Husso A et al: Transcatheter and surgical aortic valve replacement in patients with bicuspid aortic valve. Clin Res Cardiol. 110(3):429-39, 2021
5. Junco-Vicente A et al: Update in biomolecular and genetic bases of bicuspid aortopathy. Int J Mol Sci. 22(11), 2021
6. Michelena HI et al: International consensus statement on nomenclature and classification of the congenital bicuspid aortic valve and its aortopathy, for clinical, surgical, interventional and research purposes. J Thorac Cardiovasc Surg. 162(3):e383-414, 2021
7. Mozzini C et al: An exploratory look at bicuspid aortic valve (BAV) aortopathy: focus on molecular and cellular mechanisms. Curr Probl Cardiol. 46(3):100425, 2021
8. Roselli EE: Bicuspid valve repair. Ann Thorac Surg. 111(4):1232-3, 2021
9. Sievers HH: The bicuspid aortic valve complex: still a mystery. Eur J Cardiothorac Surg. 60(3):479-80, 2021
10. Bravo-Jaimes K et al: Genetics in bicuspid aortic valve disease: where are we? Prog Cardiovasc Dis. 63(4):398-406, 2020
11. Chim YH et al: Bicuspid valve aortopathy is associated with distinct patterns of matrix degradation. J Thorac Cardiovasc Surg. 160(6):e239-57, 2020
12. Kong WKF et al: Sex differences in bicuspid aortic valve disease. Prog Cardiovasc Dis. 63(4):452-6, 2020
13. Balistreri CR et al: An overview of the molecular mechanisms underlying development and progression of bicuspid aortic valve disease. J Mol Cell Cardiol. 132:146-53, 2019
14. Pasipoularides A: Clinical-pathological correlations of BAV and the attendant thoracic aortopathies. Part 2: pluridisciplinary perspective on their genetic and molecular origins. J Mol Cell Cardiol. 133:233-46, 2019
15. Ayad RF et al: Accuracy of two-dimensional echocardiography in determining aortic valve structure in patients >50 years of age having aortic valve replacement for aortic stenosis. Am J Cardiol. 108(11):1589-99, 2011
16. Michelena HI et al: Incidence of aortic complications in patients with bicuspid aortic valves. JAMA. 306(10):1104-12, 2011
17. Park CB et al: Should the proximal arch be routinely replaced in patients with bicuspid aortic valve disease and ascending aortic aneurysm? J Thorac Cardiovasc Surg. 142(3):602-7, 2011
18. Tanaka R et al: Diagnostic value of cardiac CT in the evaluation of bicuspid aortic stenosis: comparison with echocardiography and operative findings. AJR Am J Roentgenol. 195(4):895-9, 2010
19. Tzemos N et al: Endothelial function, carotid-femoral stiffness, and plasma matrix metalloproteinase-2 in men with bicuspid aortic valve and dilated aorta. J Am Coll Cardiol. 55(7):660-8, 2010
20. Fernández B et al: Bicuspid aortic valves with different spatial orientations of the leaflets are distinct etiological entities. J Am Coll Cardiol. 54(24):2312-8, 2009
21. Collins MJ et al: Variation in the histopathological features of patients with ascending aortic aneurysms: a study of 111 surgically excised cases. J Clin Pathol. 61(4):519-23, 2008
22. Michelena HI et al: Natural history of asymptomatic patients with normally functioning or minimally dysfunctional bicuspid aortic valve in the community. Circulation. 117(21):2776-84, 2008
23. Garg V et al: Mutations in NOTCH1 cause aortic valve disease. Nature. 437(7056):270-4, 2005
24. Cripe L et al: Bicuspid aortic valve is heritable. J Am Coll Cardiol. 44(1):138-43, 2004
25. Bauer M et al: Morphometric analysis of aortic media in patients with bicuspid and tricuspid aortic valve. Ann Thorac Surg. 74(1):58-62, 2002

Gross Image of Nonflow Surface of BAV

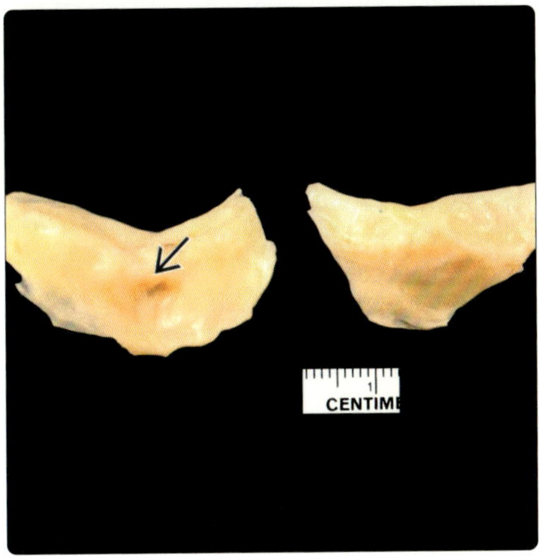

Gross Image of Flow Surface of BAV

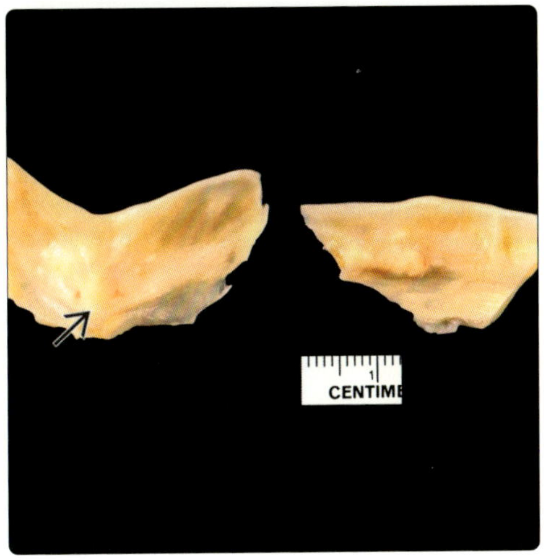

(Left) *The nonflow surface of congenital BAV shows features suggestive of fusion → or lack of separation of 2 cusps of the valve.* **(Right)** *The flow surface of congenital BAV shows the 2 unequally sized cusps with a raphe identified in the larger cusp →. The raphe appears less prominent but still is calcified.*

Histologic Features of Aortic Valve Cusp in BAV

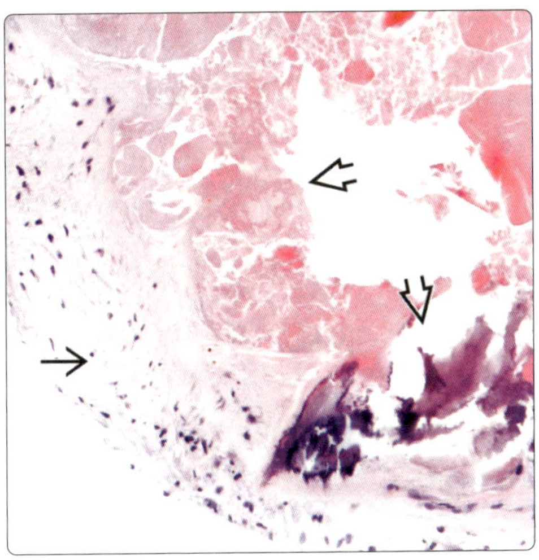

Movat Stain of BAV With Marked Calcification

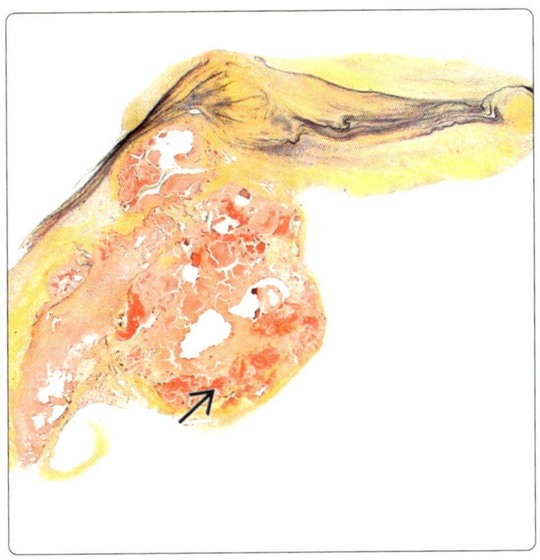

(Left) *H&E-stained section of aortic valve cusp shows thickening → and marked nodular calcification → in this case of BAV.* **(Right)** *Movat elastic stain of a longitudinal section of BAV shows fibroelastic thickening and an area of marked calcification → seen on the sinus (nonflow) surface of the cusp.*

Movat Stain of BAV Sectioned Across Raphe

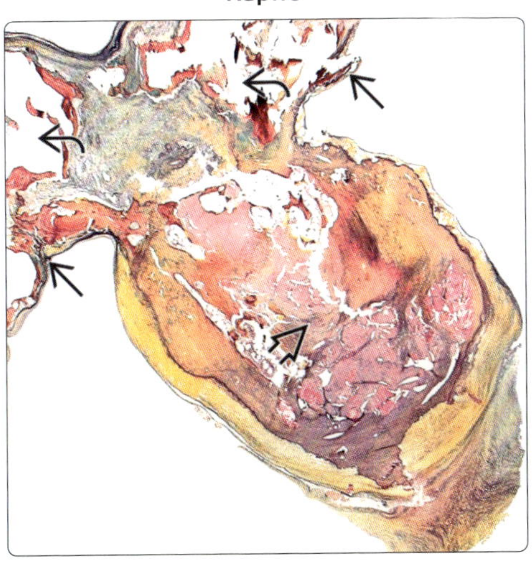

BAV With Calcification and Osteocartilaginous Metaplasia

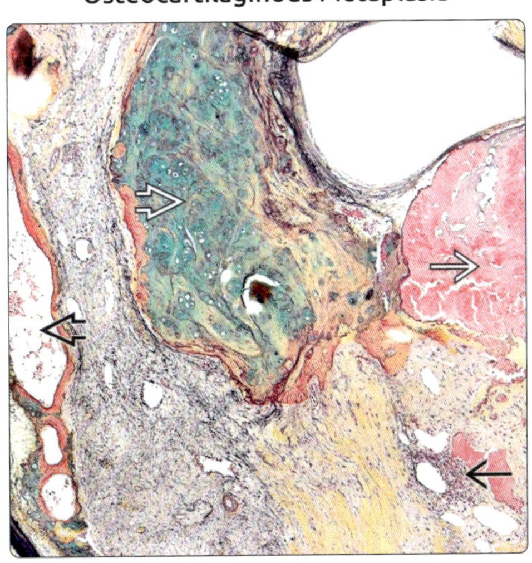

(Left) *Movat elastic stain of BAV in horizontal section across the raphe shows calcification of the cusps → and the raphe →. Ossification and fat cells (marrow elements) → are also seen.* **(Right)** *Movat-stained section of BAV shows an area of extensive calcification → and osteocartilaginous metaplasia → with marrow elements →. Areas of chronic inflammation → and a few neovessels are also seen.*

Senile Calcific Aortic Stenosis

KEY FACTS

TERMINOLOGY

- Degenerative age-related process involving trileaflet aortic valve with calcification and reduction of aortic valve orifice area

ETIOLOGY/PATHOGENESIS

- Risk factors include: Older age, male sex, increased serum low-density lipoprotein, hypertension, smoking, renal dysfunction, abnormalities in calcium/phosphate metabolism (primary hyperparathyroidism), shorter stature

CLINICAL ISSUES

- Most frequently acquired valve abnormality in developed countries
- Affects individuals ≥ 70 years of age
- M:F = 1.6:1.0
- Surgical treatment should be indicated in symptomatic patients
- Prognosis is good with surgical treatment
- Death may occur within 3 years in 50% of symptomatic patients without treatment

MACROSCOPIC

- Nodular calcification predominantly near base of cusp in aortic aspect of leaflet
- Calcium deposits appear as heaped-up masses protruding through outflow surface into sinus of Valsalva
- Calcification more prominent in noncoronary cusp
- Sparing of free margin of cusp
- Absent commisural fusion
- Fibrosis and retraction of cusps

MICROSCOPIC

- Subendothelial thickening and cusp fibrosis
- Intra-/extracellular neutral lipids
- Inflammatory infiltrate (macrophages and lymphocytes/T-helper cells)
- Large calcium deposits and bone metaplasia

Pathogenesis of Aortic Valve Calcification

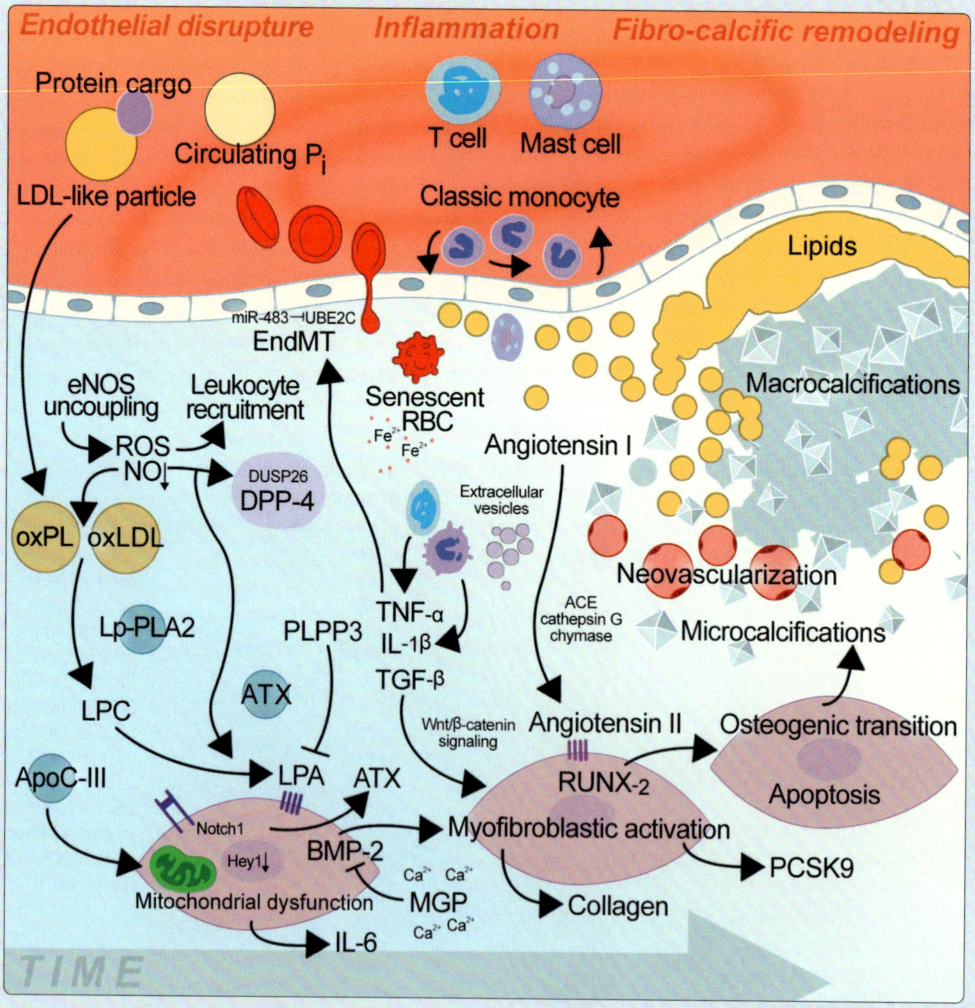

Endothelial disruption promotes the uptake of modified lipids along with the protein cargo they carry and passage of red blood cells, T cells, and macrophages into the fibrosa layer, promoting inflammation, differentiation of valvular interstitial cells to myofibroblasts with final transition to an osteogenic phenotype, leading to fibro-calcific remodeling. Complex molecular mechanisms are activated in this process.

TERMINOLOGY

Definitions

- Degenerative age-related process involving trileaflet aortic valve with calcification and reduction of aortic valve orifice area (AVA)
  - Mild: 1.5-2.0 cm^2
  - Moderate: 0.8-1.5 cm^2
  - Severe: < 0.8 cm^2

ETIOLOGY/PATHOGENESIS

Risk Factors

- Older age, male sex, increased serum low-density lipoprotein, hypertension, smoking, renal dysfunction, diabetes mellitus, abnormalities in calcium/phosphate metabolism (primary hyperparathyroidism)

CLINICAL ISSUES

Epidemiology

- Incidence
  - Most frequently acquired valve abnormality in developed countries
  - 2-3% of population > 65 years
- Age
  - ≥ 70 years
- Sex
  - M:F = 1.6:1.0

Presentation

- Decrease in exercise tolerance
- Syncope
- Angina
- Dyspnea
- Heart failure
- Left ventricle hypertrophy
- Systolic murmur crescendo/decrescendo over right 2nd intercostal space with radiation to carotids

Treatment

- Options, risks, complications
  - Clinical trials are undergoing with several targeted therapies in development
  - Surgical treatment should be indicated in symptomatic patients
- Surgical approaches
  - Valve replacement is considered definitive treatment
  - Transcatheter aortic valve implantation may be appropriate if valve replacement is not option due to secondary comorbidities
  - Balloon aortic valvuloplasty (complicated by early restenosis) palliative option or for high-risk patients in need of urgent intervention

Prognosis

- Good with surgical treatment
- Death may occur within 3 years in 50% of symptomatic patients without treatment

IMAGING

Ultrasonographic Findings

- Transthoracic echocardiogram is primary imaging modality for diagnosis and staging of disease severity
  - Calcified thickened valve leaflets
  - High systolic transvalvular pressure gradient
  - Assessment of left ventricular function, hypertrophy, and enlargement
- Color and pulsed Doppler
  - Increased transvalvular pressure gradient (> 40 mm Hg) and velocity (> 4 m/s)
  - Calculation of AVA

CT/MR Findings

- NECT: Quantification of aortic valve calcification (> 1,100 Agatston score units as cut-off for severe stenosis)
- Cardiac-gated CT allows planimetric measurement of AVA during mid-late systole
- Phase-contrast MR allows for calculation of peak systolic velocity and gradients

MACROSCOPIC

General Features

- Nodular calcification predominantly near bases of cusps in aortic aspect of leaflets
  - Calcium deposits appear as heaped-up masses protruding through outflow surface into sinus of Valsalva
- Calcification more prominent in noncoronary cusp
- Sparing of free margins of cusps
- Cusp retraction and absent commisural fusion

MICROSCOPIC

Histologic Features

- Subendothelial thickening and cusp fibrosis (more prominent in female valves)
- Intra-/extracellular neutral lipids
- Inflammatory infiltrate (macrophages and lymphocytes/T-helper cells)
- Large calcium deposits and bone metaplasia (more prominent in male valves)

DIFFERENTIAL DIAGNOSIS

Rheumatic Aortic Valve Stenosis

- Thickening predominantly along commisural edge with fusion
- Rheumatic mitral valve disease is universally present

SELECTED REFERENCES

1. Cionca C et al: Advanced cardiovascular multimodal imaging and aortic stenosis. Heart Fail Rev. 27(2):677-96, 2022
2. Kraler S et al: Calcific aortic valve disease: from molecular and cellular mechanisms to medical therapy. Eur Heart J. 43(7):683-97, 2022
3. Šteiner I et al: Calcific aortic valve stenosis - comparison of inflammatory lesions in the left, right, and non-coronary cusp. Pathol Res Pract. 227:153636, 2021
4. Fishbein GA et al: Pathology of the aortic valve: aortic valve stenosis/aortic regurgitation. Curr Cardiol Rep. 21(8):81, 2019
5. Ladich E et al: Pathology of calcific aortic stenosis. Future Cardiol. 7(5):629-42, 2011

(Left) *Autopsy specimen shows tricuspid aortic valve with nodular calcifications at the base of the cusps protruding in the flow surface and sinus of Valsalva. Thickening of the cusps is also seen. Commisural fusion is absent.* **(Right)** *Surgically removed aortic valve shows 3 cusps with nodular calcifications at the base of the cusps, which protrude into the flow surface and sinus of Valsalva. Thickening of the cusps is also seen. Commisural fusion is absent, and the free margins are largely uninvolved.*

Calcific Aortic Stenosis

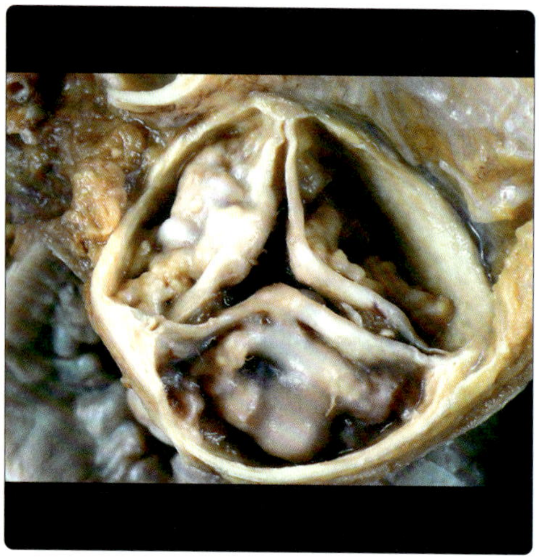

Aortic Valve

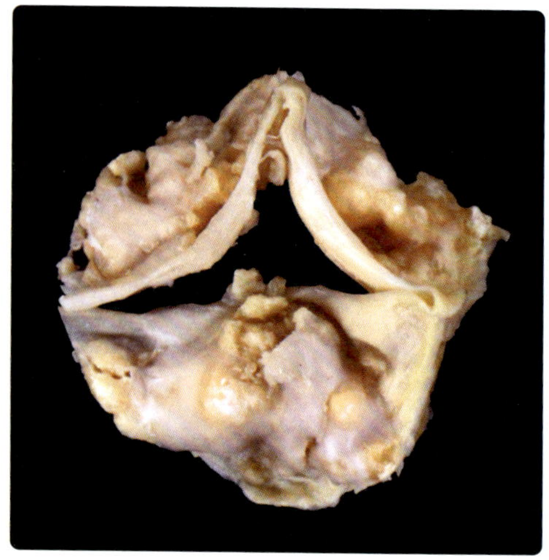

(Left) *Aortic valve flow surface seen from the left ventricle aspect in aortic stenosis shows thickened cusps with small yellow calcifications toward the base of the cusps.* **(Right)** *Aortic valve cusps seen from the aortic aspect in aortic stenosis show thickened cusps with large nodular calcifications toward the base of the cusps. The free cusp margin is still spared.*

Aortic Valve Cusps With Focal Calcifications

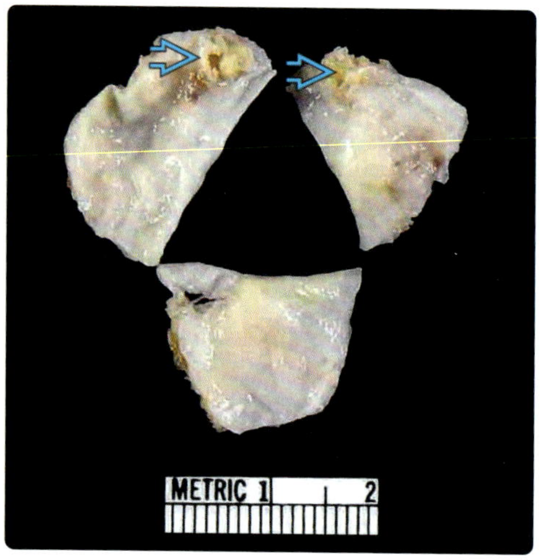

Aortic Valve Cusps With Marked Base Calcification

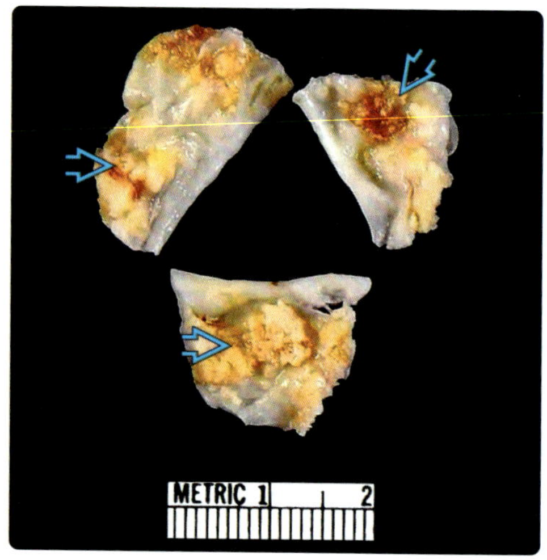

(Left) *H&E-stained section of an aortic valve shows thickening and fibrosis of the cusp with large deposits of calcium within the midportion.* **(Right)** *H&E-stained section of an aortic valve at higher magnification shows deposits of calcium and bone metaplasia. Inflammatory mononuclear cells and small capillaries are also seen.*

Histology of Calcified Aortic Cusp

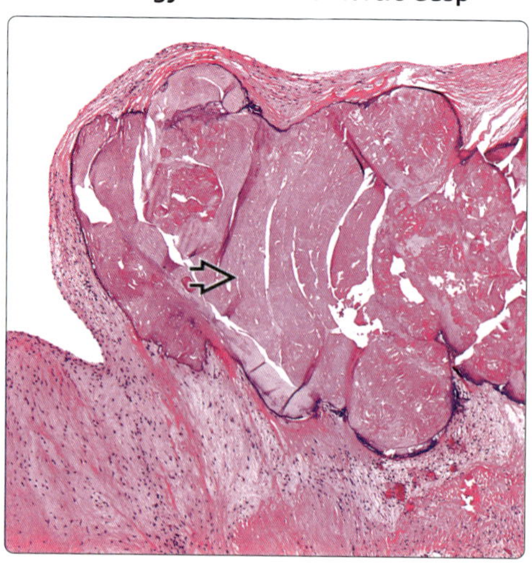

Bone Metaplasia in Aortic Cusp

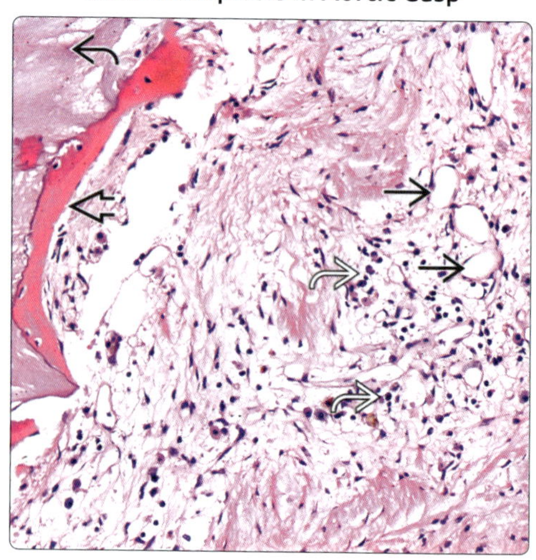

Axial Oblique Cardiac CT of Aortic Stenosis

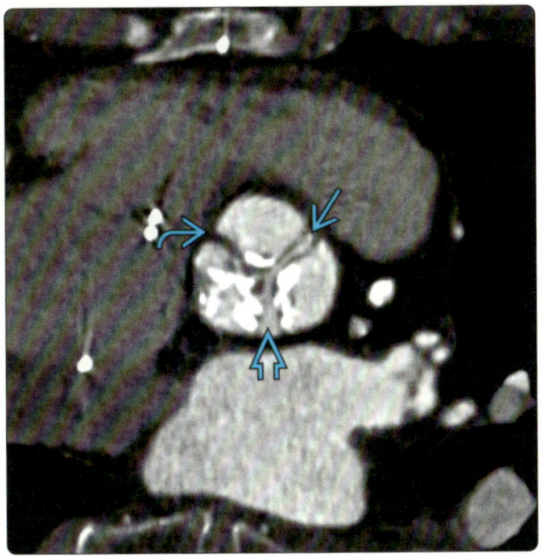

MR of Aortic Stenosis

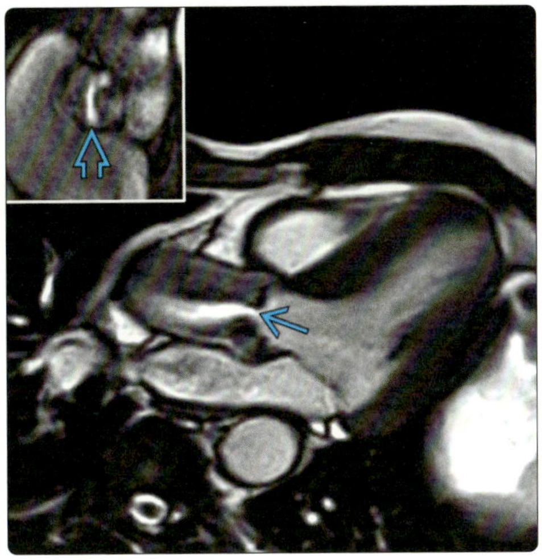

(Left) *Cardiac CT during systole in a patient with aortic stenosis shows thickening and fusion of noncoronary and right cusps ↪, narrow systolic orifice area between noncoronary and left coronary cusps ⇨, and left and right cusps →.* **(Right)** *Three-chamber view of severe aortic stenosis shows thickened aortic valve cusps resulting in restricted opening → and systolic flow acceleration. On inset, the aortic valve has a bicuspid appearance ⇨ due to fusion of the right and left cusps. (From CT and MR in Cardiology.)*

Radiologic Image of Calcified Aortic Valve

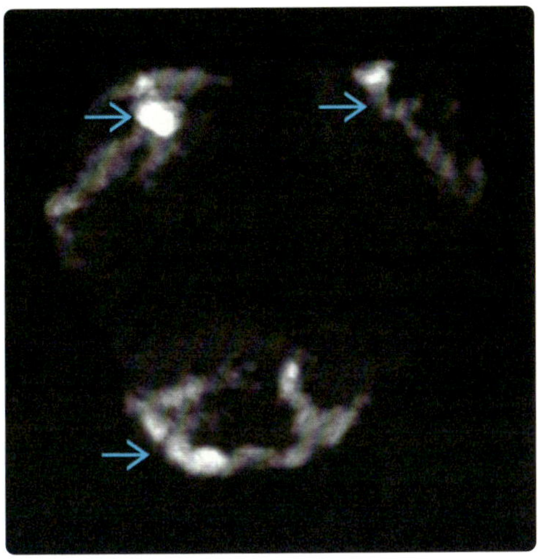

Aortic Valve Cusps With Calcifications

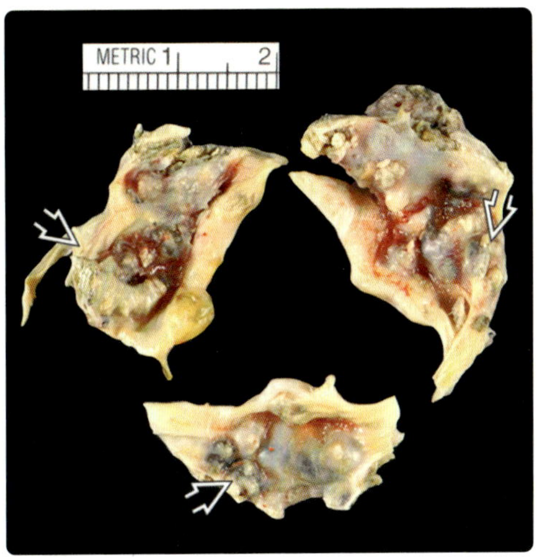

(Left) *Radiologic image shows areas of calcification at the base of the aortic valve cusps → with the free edges toward the orifice free of calcification.* **(Right)** *Aortic valve cusps seen from the aortic aspect in severe aortic stenosis show thickening with large nodular calcifications toward the base of the cusps ⇨. The free margin is still spared but appears retracted.*

History of Calcified Aortic Valve

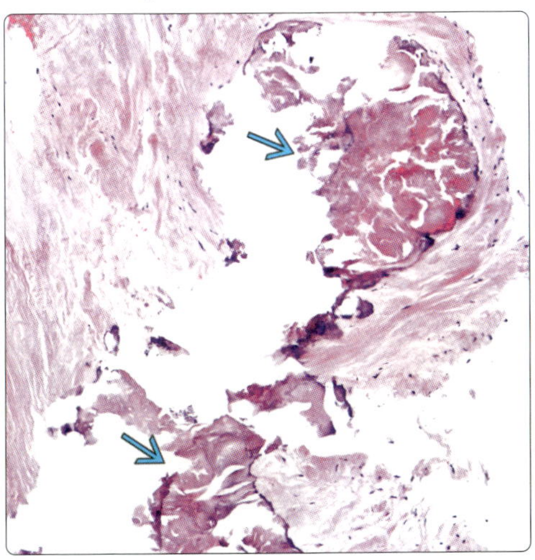

Histology of Calcified Aortic Valve

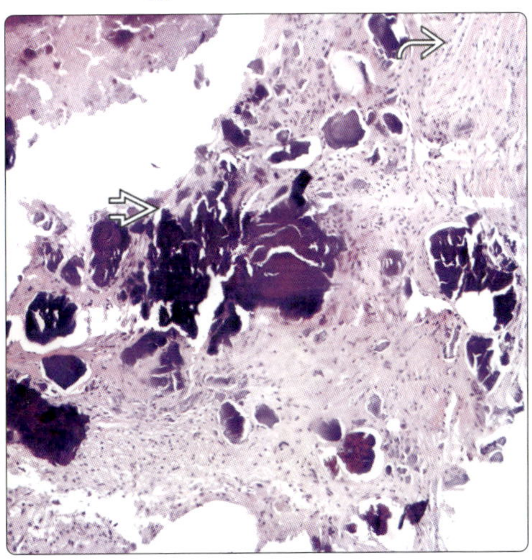

(Left) *H&E-stained section of an aortic valve shows thickening and fibrosis of the cusp with large deposits of calcium → within the midportion with basophilic coloration. In this case, no inflammatory reaction is seen, and the free edge of the cusp is not involved.* **(Right)** *H&E-stained section of an aortic valve shows thickening and fibrosis of the cusp with multiple deposits of calcium within the midportion ⇨. There are focal inflammatory cells and neovascularization ↪.*

Discrete Membranous Subaortic Stenosis

KEY FACTS

TERMINOLOGY

- Stenosis secondary to discrete crescent-shaped or circumferential membrane or fibromuscular band located at varying distances below aortic valve
- May extend onto aortic cusps and almost always contacts anterior mitral leaflet at base
- Does not appear to be associated with sarcomeric (cardiomyopathy) mutations

CLINICAL ISSUES

- 8-30% of congenital left ventricular outflow tract obstruction (LVOTO)
- Early intervention with aggressive resection of membrane is recommended
- Surgery indicated when gradient is > 30 mm Hg to avoid leaflet damage
- Substantial recurrence rate ~ 20%
- Transaortic surgical approaches
  - Membranectomy
  - Myomectomy
- Valve repair or replacement

MACROSCOPIC

- Crescent-shaped thin (type I) or thick (type II) translucent or opalescent tissue
- Abnormal geometry of LVOT
  - Steeper aortoseptal angle
  - Wider mitral/aortic separation

MICROSCOPIC

- Up to 5 layers have been identified
  - Endothelium
  - Subendothelial layer composed of acid mucopolysaccharides
  - Collagen-rich fibrous layer
  - Fibroelastic layer
  - Smooth muscle cell bundles

Discrete Subaortic Membrane (Echocardiography)

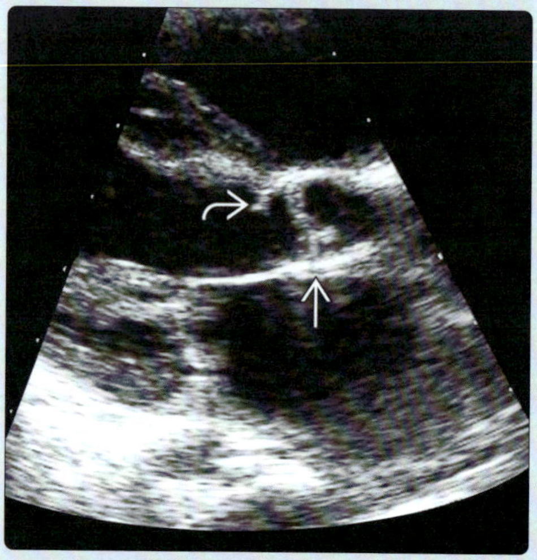

Subvalvular Aortic Stenosis (CT)

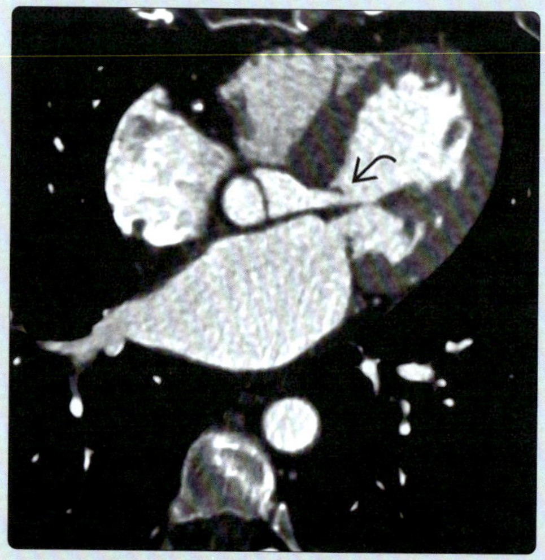

(Left) *This long-axis echocardiography image shows subvalvular aortic stenosis with a discrete fibrous ridge/membrane just below the level of the aortic leaflets.* **(Right)** *Three-chamber view cardiac CT from a patient with subvalvular aortic stenosis shows a thin membrane causing left ventricular outflow tract obstruction LVOTO). (From DI: Cardiovascular.)*

Subaortic Membrane Ring

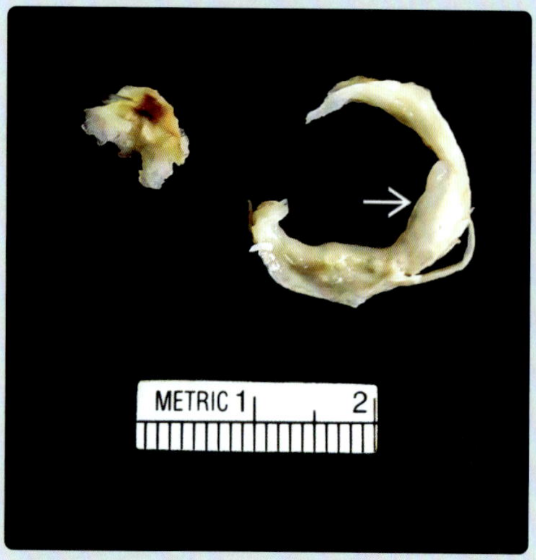

Subaortic Valvular Membrane Ring

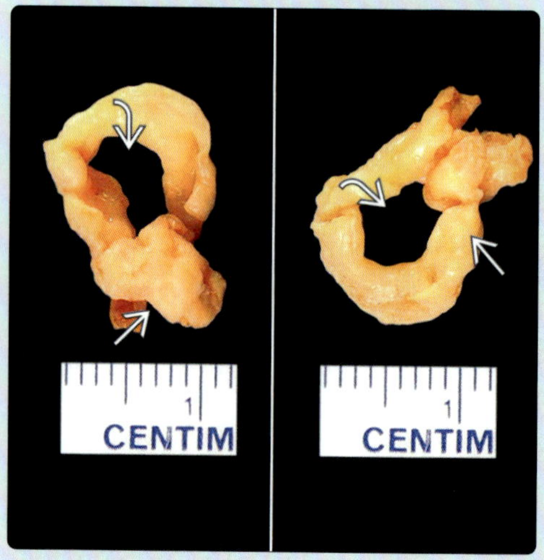

(Left) *This surgical specimen shows a complete membranous ring resected from below the aortic valve. The tissue is thickened and nodular.* **(Right)** *This surgical specimen shows a complete membranous ring resected from below the aortic valve. The tissue is thickened and nodular, and the lumen is restrictive.*

TERMINOLOGY

Definitions

- Stenosis secondary to discrete crescent-shaped or circumferential membrane or fibromuscular band located at varying distances below aortic valve
  - Process may extend onto aortic cusps and almost always contacts anterior mitral leaflet at base

ETIOLOGY/PATHOGENESIS

Developmental Anomaly

- Congenital
  - Embryologic failure of bulbus cordis regression theorized
  - Associated congenital abnormalities: Ventricular septal defect, aortic coarctation, atrioventricular septal defect, patent ductus arteriosus, bicuspid aortic valve
  - Isolated in 39% of cases
  - Higher incidence in related family members

Other Proposed Mechanisms

- Multifactorial: Interplay between genetic predisposition, altered septal shear stress, cellular proliferation, and signaling

CLINICAL ISSUES

Epidemiology

- Incidence
  - 8-30% of congenital left ventricular outflow tract obstruction (LVOTO)
- Age
  - Variable: Infants, children, younger and older adults all reported

Presentation

- Systolic murmur along lower left sternal border without ejection click
- Palpable thrill
- Chest pain
- Dyspnea
- Syncope
- Asymptomatic

Natural History

- Unpredictable
- Usually progression to LVOTO in childhood and adolescence
  - Progression depends on distance of membrane from aortic valve and degree of anterior mitral valve leaflet involvement

Treatment

- Options, risks, complications
  - Early intervention with aggressive resection of membrane
    - Surgery indicated when gradient is > 30 mm Hg to avoid leaflet damage
  - Complications post surgery include
    - Acute complete (3°) AV block
    - Iatrogenic ventricular septal defect
    - Mitral/aortic valve regurgitation
  - Substantial recurrence rate ~ 20%
- Surgical approaches
  - Transaortic
    - Membranectomy
    - Myomectomy
  - Valve repair or replacement

Prognosis

- Good if resection is successful
- Possible progression if untreated
  - Aortic valve injury (jet lesion) leading to mixed subvalvular stenosis and valvular regurgitation
    - Tethering of cusps by fibrous membrane
  - Infective endocarditis
  - Left ventricular hypertrophy and dynamic LVOTO

MACROSCOPIC

General Features

- Crescent-shaped thin (type I) or thick (type II) translucent or opalescent tissue
- Abnormal geometry of LVOT
  - Steeper aortoseptal angle
  - Wider mitral/aortic separation

MICROSCOPIC

Histologic Features

- Stratification similar to normal valve leaflet
  - Endothelium
  - Subendothelial mucopolysaccharides
  - Collagen-rich fibrous layer
  - Fibroelastic layer
  - Smooth muscle cell bundles

DIFFERENTIAL DIAGNOSIS

Tunnel-Type Subaortic Stenosis

- Long segment of fibromuscular narrowing of left ventricle vestibule
- More severe form of subaortic stenosis
- Not amenable to subaortic septal myectomy

SELECTED REFERENCES

1. Sharkey A et al: Sub-aortic membrane - a three-dimensional echocardiographic perspective. Echocardiography. 39(8):1146-8, 2022
2. Mun HS et al: Noninvasive evaluation of membranous subaortic stenosis: complimentary roles of echocardiography and computed tomographic angiography. Echocardiography. 27(3):E34-5, 2010
3. Butany J et al: Discrete subaortic membranes in adults–a clinicopathological analysis. Cardiovasc Pathol. 18(4):236-42, 2009
4. Allen RD et al: Surgical pathology of subaortic septal myectomy not associated with hypertrophic cardiomyopathy: a study of 98 cases (1996-2000). Cardiovasc Pathol. 12(4):207-15, 2003
5. Lamke GT et al: Surgical pathology of subaortic septal myectomy associated with hypertrophic cardiomyopathy. A study of 204 cases (1996-2000). Cardiovasc Pathol. 12(3):149-58, 2003
6. Marasini M et al: Discrete subaortic stenosis: incidence, morphology and surgical impact of associated subaortic anomalies. Ann Thorac Surg. 75(6):1763-8, 2003
7. Rayburn ST et al: Discrete membranous subaortic stenosis: improved results after resection and myectomy. Ann Thorac Surg. 64(1):105-9, 1997
8. Sigfússon G et al: Abnormalities of the left ventricular outflow tract associated with discrete subaortic stenosis in children: an echocardiographic study. J Am Coll Cardiol. 30(1):255-9, 1997

Myxomatous Mitral Valve Disease

KEY FACTS

TERMINOLOGY

- Presumed congenital myxomatous transformation of mitral valve, annulus, and subvalvular apparatus

ETIOLOGY/PATHOGENESIS

- Complex genetic disorder with autosomal dominant form of inheritance and highly variable penetrance
- Myxomatous mitral changes are also prominent in patients with underlying connective tissue disorder
- Some familial forms of myxomatous mitral valve prolapse (MMVP) described
  - MMVP1: Chromosome 16
  - MMVP2: Chromosome 11
  - MMVP3: Chromosome 13
  - X-linked MMVP: Chromosome Xq28

CLINICAL ISSUES

- Most common cause of primary mitral valve prolapse (MVP) and regurgitation in USA and Europe
- Associated with higher risk of valvular complication

MACROSCOPIC

- In surgical specimens, often only segments of valve leaflet are received, appearing diffusely thickened, rubbery, and edematous
- Whole specimen often shows diffuse involvement, redundancy, interchordal hooding, stretched cords
- Dilatation of mitral annulus, generally > 10.5 cm

MICROSCOPIC

- Thickening of spongiosa layer by loose myxoid tissue that extends into and disrupts underlying fibrosa layer

ANCILLARY TESTS

- Myxoid substance best highlighted with Alcian blue (pH 2.5), PAS-PASD, or colloidal iron

Myxomatous Mitral Valve: Base of Heart

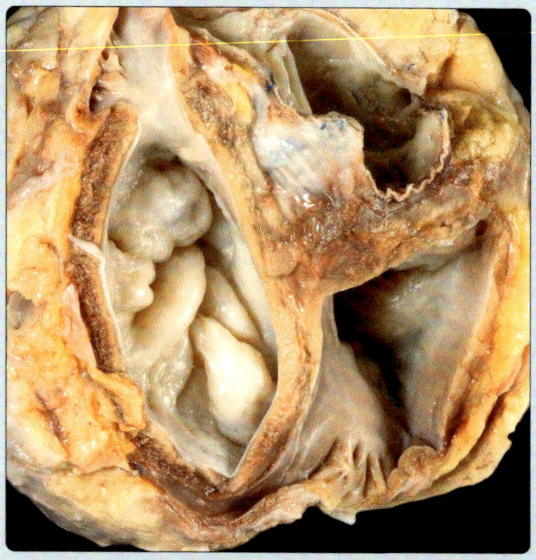

Myxomatous Mitral Valve Cut Section: Surgical Specimen

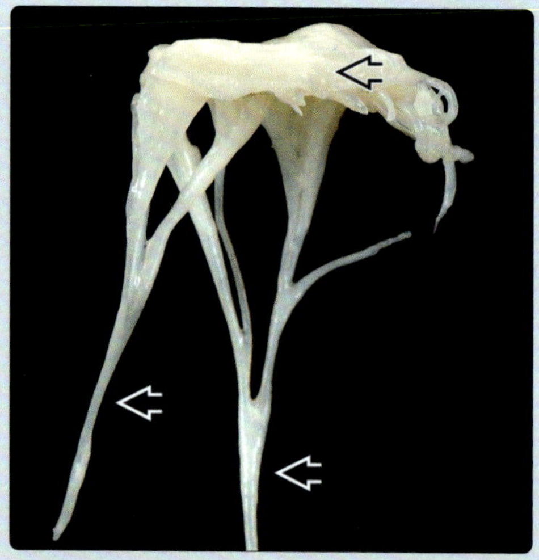

(Left) *Upper view of the mitral valve from the atria shows important redundancy of the thickened white leaflets. This myxomatous mitral valve (MMV) was found in an autopsy of a patient with Marfan syndrome.* **(Right)** *Surgical specimen of an MMV shows a thickened leaflet with a grayish edematous appearance of the spongiosa (middle) layer ⇨ and elongation of the chordae tendineae ➡.*

Myxomatous Mitral Valve: Atrial Surface

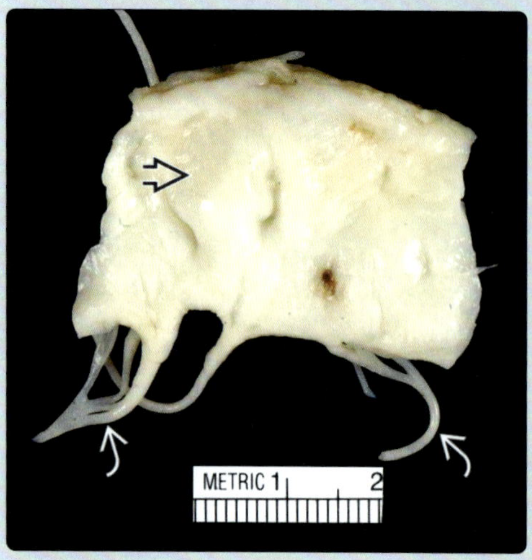

Myxomatous Mitral Valve: Ventricular Surface

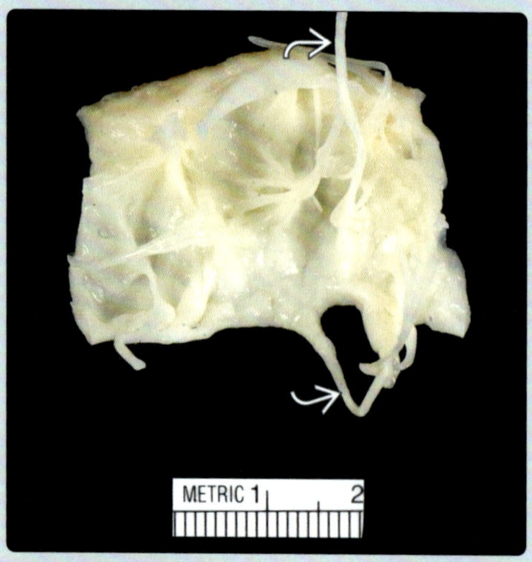

(Left) *This specimen shows diffuse rubbery thickening with a bulbous outpouching ⇨. The cords ➡ are slender and not fused (unlike in rheumatic mitral valve disease).* **(Right)** *Diffuse rubbery thickening is apparent from the under surface of this valve, and all of the tendinous cords ➡ are slender and unfused (unlike in rheumatic mitral valve disease).*

TERMINOLOGY

Abbreviations

- Myxomatous mitral valve (MMV)

Synonyms

- Mitral valve prolapse (MVP)
  - MMV is most common, but not sole cause of, MVP
- Myxomatous degeneration
  - This terminology is preferred by some to recognize general process and associated valvular changes rather than defining these features as specific disease entity
- Barlow syndrome
  - Diffuse myxomatous changes of mitral valve with extensive bileaflet redundancy and broad prolapse

Definitions

- Presumed congenital myxomatous transformation of mitral valve leaflets and subvalvular apparatus that causes their weakening and increases risk of secondary complications
- Cut surface of thickened leaflets appears gelatinous, similar to myxoma, hence term myxomatous
- Mitral prolapse
  - Dynamic excursion of mitral leaflet above plane of mitral annular ring during systole
  - MMV is commonest cause with deformed leaflets billowing up like sails into left atrium
  - Usually associated with mitral regurgitation ± torn tendinous cords

ETIOLOGY/PATHOGENESIS

Primary

- Classically, majority of cases were considered sporadic and idiopathic
- Actual data favor complex genetic disorder with autosomal dominant form of inheritance and highly variable penetrance, dependent on sex and age
  - Posttranslational and environmental factors also appear to affect penetrance in familial cases
- Some familial forms of MMV prolapse (MMVP) described

Secondary

- Myxomatous-type mitral valve changes are also prevalent in patients with underlying connective tissue disorders
  - Marfan syndrome
  - Ehlers-Danlos syndrome
  - Osteogenesis imperfecta
  - Pseudoxanthoma elasticum
- Often described in association with other miscellaneous diseases
  - Ebstein anomaly, Down syndrome, adult polycystic kidney disease, von Willebrand syndrome, Turner syndrome
  - Valvular myxomatous changes usually more subtle, focal, and less well defined in these settings

Pathophysiology

- Abnormal accumulation of proteoglycan in valvular leaflets associated with weakening of valve
- Exact cause remains unclear, although several hypotheses, not necessarily mutually exclusive, have been proposed
  - Abnormalities in production, distribution, architecture, &/or function matrix proteins, such as fibrillin, elastin, and collagen
  - Increased concentration of various proteolytic enzymes, such as metalloproteinase, produced by activated myofibroblasts
- Ultimately, these pathologic processes affect capacity to respond to mechanical stress and subsequent iterative repair cycles
- Eventually, as morphologic changes progress, coaptation of leaflets becomes compromised, and regurgitation follows, causing global cardiac adverse effects

CLINICAL ISSUES

Epidemiology

- Incidence
  - Most common cause of primary (nonischemic) MVP and regurgitation in USA and Europe
  - Newer data indicate that prevalence is ~ 1-3% in general population and equal in proportion between male and female patients

Presentation

- Often nonspecific, such as palpitation and atypical chest pain, especially in early phase
- Auscultatory findings, such as midsystolic click, classically associated with MMV/MVP
- Global cardiac adverse effects
  - Chronic mitral regurgitation
    - Atrial fibrillation
    - Cerebrovascular ischemic events
    - Congestive heart failure
  - Chordal rupture and acute mitral insufficiency
    - Acute hemodynamic instability
  - Infective endocarditis
  - Arrhythmias and sudden death

Natural History

- Can exist in stable form without symptoms or complications
- However, disease can progress and lead to worsening of mitral valve regurgitation and congestive heart failure
- Classic or diffuse form of MMV disease, such as Barlow syndrome, seems to be associated with higher risk of valvular complications

Treatment

- Medical treatment oriented toward mitral regurgitation, congestive heart failure, and anticoagulation for associated atrial fibrillation
- Surgical intervention indicated as regurgitation becomes severe, especially if
  - Symptomatic heart failure
  - Left ventricular enlargement or reduced systolic function
  - Acute onset (i.e., ruptured chordae)
  - Atrial fibrillation, pulmonary hypertension
- Mitral valve repair is preferred over replacement when possible
  - Better long-term survival, similar to general population
- Classic mitral valve repair consists of

- Segmental resection of redundant or flail leaflet (often P2) and closing resultant defect
- Placement of annuloplasty ring to prevent further annular dilatation
- Percutaneous mitral valve intervention with MitraClip device is being developed at some centers

IMAGING

Ultrasonographic Findings

- Visualize and quantify degree of prolapse, regurgitation, thickening of leaflets, involvement of subvalvular apparatus, and ventricular function

MACROSCOPIC

Surgical Specimens

- Most commonly, only segment (often P2) of valve leaflet is excised for repair
  - Enlarged, thickened, rubbery, and white
  - Grayish, moist, glistening, gelatinous, or edematous cut surface appearance of spongiosa layer

Autopsy and Explant Specimens

- Examination of valve in entirety as well as cardiac chambers usually shows
  - Diffuse involvement of valve (frequent) though severity varies from segment to segment
    - P2 segment more commonly and more severely diseased
    - Involvement of whole leaflet length is characteristic, including at least 1/2 of anterior or 2/3 of posterior leaflet
  - Redundancy of leaflets (excessively disproportionate leaflet surface area relative to annulus)
  - Interchordal hooding or billowing toward left atrium
    - > 0.4 cm in height often used as criteria
  - Elongation and stretching of chordae with mild irregular thickening or thinning
    - Chordae rupture can also be observed
  - Dilatation of mitral annulus, generally > 10.5 cm
    - Annular calcification is sometimes found
- Tricuspid, aortic, and pulmonary valves can also be involved although much less frequently
- Other complications and secondary cardiac changes can be described
  - Endocardial friction lesion under subvalvular chordae
  - Cardiomegaly, left atrial &/or ventricular dilatation, and, eventually, right heart alterations

MICROSCOPIC

Histologic Features

- Primary changes
  - Marked thickening of spongiosa layer caused by increase in loose myxomatous tissue
  - Extension of myxomatous tissue in underlying fibrous layer causing collagen disruption and elastic fiber fragmentation
    - Similar changes observed in subvalvular chordae tendineae
  - Overall trilaminar architecture of valve becomes disorganized and interfaces blurred
  - Eventually, all layers becoming more fibrotic
- Secondary changes
  - Endocardial fibrosis with elastic fiber increase and disorganization on both sides of leaflet and cords
  - Particularly prominent on valve edges

ANCILLARY TESTS

Histochemistry

- Myxoid substance best highlighted with Alcian blue (pH 2.5), PAS-PASD, or colloidal iron
- Collagen fragmentation more evident on connective tissue stains, such as trichrome
- Movat pentachrome is very useful to demonstrate entire spectrum of changes on single slide

DIFFERENTIAL DIAGNOSIS

Mitral Valve Prolapse

- Although most cases of primary MVP are thought to be myxomatous in nature, other valvular alterations can appear similar clinically and by imaging
- Non-MMV-associated MVP includes
  - Ventricular wall or papillary motion anomalies
  - Primary ventricular or mitral annular dilatation
    - Failure of leaflet edges to appose due to increased annular diameter

Reactional Degenerative Myxomatous Changes

- Mild myxomatous changes are often found on leaflet of older adults or those affected by abnormal stress, secondary regurgitation, or other influences
- Leaflet changes are usually milder and more focal; characterized by
  - Limited and focal increase in myxomatous tissue, essentially only in prolapsing segment, mostly P2
  - Less impressive thickening of leaflet
  - Relative preservation of 3-layer architecture
  - Less annular dilatation

Fibroelastic Tissue Deficiency

- Probably same mechanism as reactional degenerative myxomatous changes
  - Identical macroscopic and histologic characteristics

Postinflammatory Mitral Valve Disease

- Can also cause mitral regurgitation and severe leaflet thickening
- Usually shows more rigidity, calcification, and fusion of commissures and cords
- Although some myxomatous changes can be seen, fibrosis predominates, and there is clear destruction evident in trilaminar architecture

SELECTED REFERENCES

1. Fishbein GA et al: Mitral valve pathology. Curr Cardiol Rep. 21(7):61, 2019
2. Guy TS et al: Mitral valve prolapse. Annu Rev Med. 63:277-92, 2012
3. Grau JB et al: The genetics of mitral valve prolapse. Clin Genet. 72(4):288-95, 2007

Endocarditis Complicating Myxomatous Mitral Valve: Base of Heart

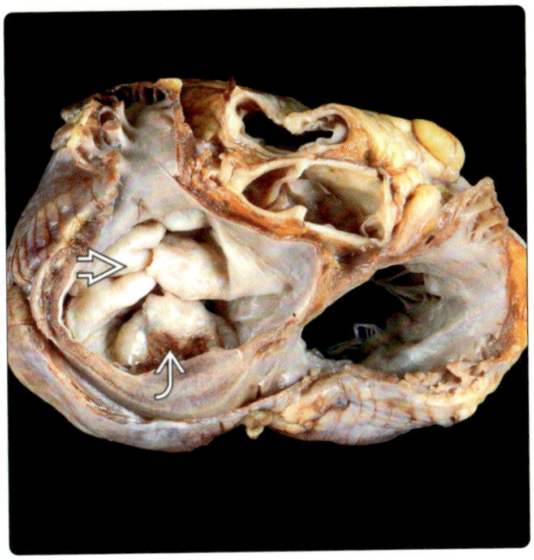

Endocarditis Complicating Myxomatous Mitral Valve: Annular View

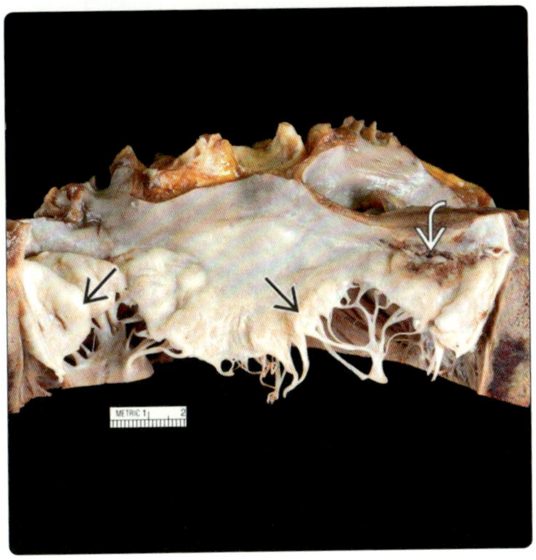

(Left) *Superior view of the mitral valve shows severe redundancy of the leaflets* ➡ *and an area of endocarditis* ↪*, a common complication of MMV, in this case associated with annular abscess.* **(Right)** *In addition to endocarditis* ↪*, this opened view of the mitral valve from the same patient shows annular dilatation, thickened elongated leaflets, and some interchordal hooding* ⇨*. There is no commissural fibrosis or fusion, calcification, or significant retraction.*

Segmental Resection Specimen From Myxomatous Mitral Valve Repair

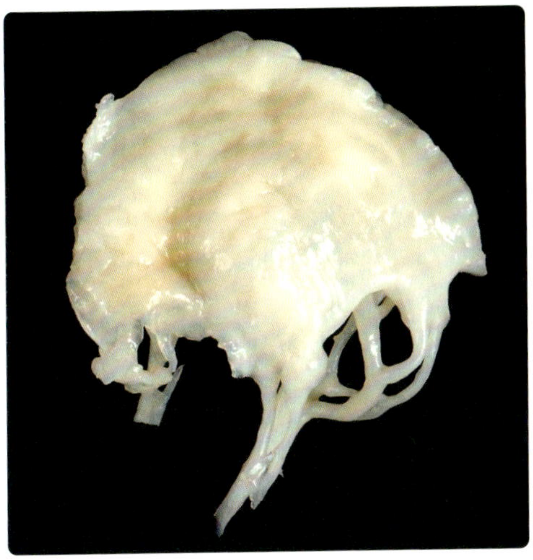

Thickened Leaflet Tissue in Myxomatous Mitral Valve

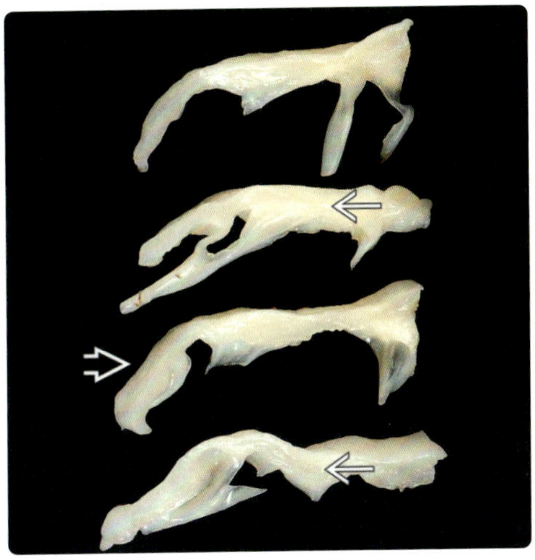

(Left) *This segment of posterior leaflet (P2) was removed during surgical repair of the mitral valve. This upper atrial view shows some billowing of the thickened leaflet with an impression of mingled subvalvular chordae, which can be thickened or thinned.* **(Right)** *Cut sections from an MMV surgical specimen show a gelatinous thickening of the spongiosa layer* ➡*, giving a rubbery consistency to the specimen. Fibrous thickening of the surfaces* ➡ *can also be appreciated.*

Myxomatous Mitral Valve Histology: Movat Stain

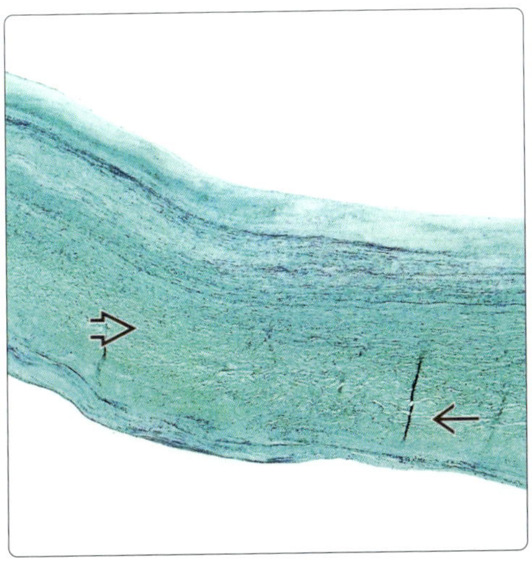

Myxomatous Expansion of Spongiosa Layer: Movat Stain

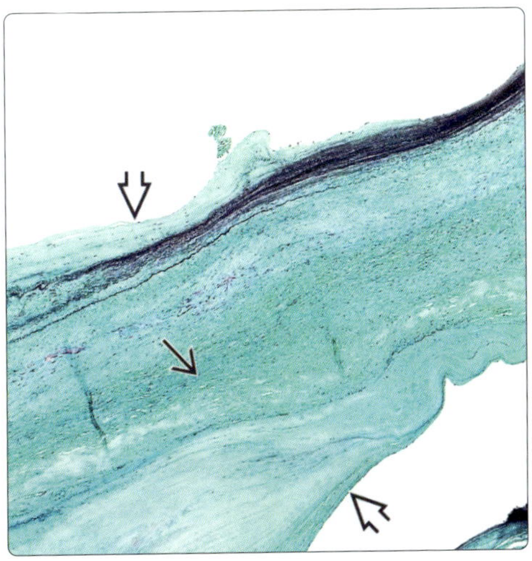

(Left) *Movat stain shows accumulation of proteoglycan in the spongiosa layer* ⇨*, imparting a myxomatous/edematous appearance and causing leaflet thickening. The proteoglycan also extends into the fibrosa layer* ⇨*, causing homogenization of the various layers.* **(Right)** *Movat-stained section from the same specimen also shows reactive fibroelastic endocardial thickening* ⇨*. The expanding myxomatous spongiosa can also be seen disrupting collagen fibers of the fibrous layer* ⇨*.*

Rheumatic Heart Disease

KEY FACTS

TERMINOLOGY

- Chronic valvular scarring and deformity as sequela of acute rheumatic fever (ARF)

ETIOLOGY/PATHOGENESIS

- ARF: Noninfectious postinflammatory autoimmune response related to group A *Streptococcus* M protein antigens
- Rheumatic heart disease (RHD): Chronic progressive fibrosing process in patients with antecedent (usually remote) ARF

CLINICAL ISSUES

- RHD latency averages 20-25 years but may be > 40 years

IMAGING

- Hockey stick/bent knee appearance of anterior leaflet
- Transvalvular gradient and valve area (typically, area ≤ 1 cm^2 is considered severe)

MACROSCOPIC

- All valves can be involved in following order of frequency
    - Mitral > aortic > tricuspid > pulmonary
- Dipped in candle wax appearance
- Mitral commissural fusion, bridging fibrosis, and calcification
- Chordae shortened, retracted, fused
- "Fish mouth" deformity when viewed from ventricular aspect up into atrium
- Left ventricle typically normal size unless there is significant mitral regurgitation

MICROSCOPIC

- Neovascularization with thick-walled irregular blood vessels

TOP DIFFERENTIAL DIAGNOSES

- Postinflammatory valve disease
- Carcinoid valvular disease
- Mitral annular calcification

(Left) *Gross photograph of the heart removed at autopsy shows classic rheumatic mitral stenosis with leaflet thickening and fusion of the mitral commissures ⇒ ("fish mouth" deformity).* **(Right)** *This mitral valve section shows neovascularization with thick-walled vessels ⇒ within the valve. This finding is always abnormal, indicating a postinflammatory etiology, such as rheumatic disease.*

Rheumatic Mitral Stenosis (Atrial View)

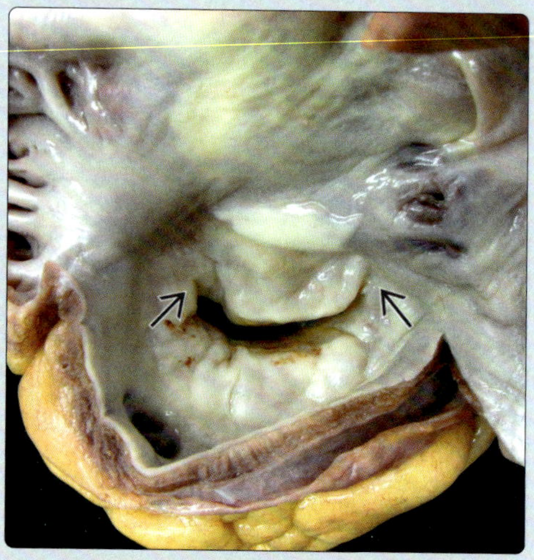

Vessels Within Valve Tissue (Rheumatic)

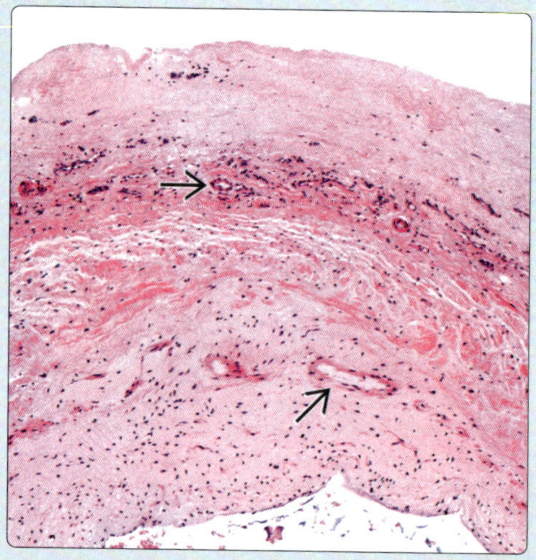

(Left) *Gross photograph shows the undersurface of a rheumatic mitral valve resembles the mouth of a catfish ⇒ with the thickened fused cords resembling barbels. There is fusion of both commissures (above the papillary muscles ➡).* **(Right)** *Gross photograph shows diffuse thickening and fusion of the 3 commissures of this aortic valve are characteristic of aortic valve rheumatic disease.*

"Fish Mouth" Deformity in Rheumatic Mitral Disease

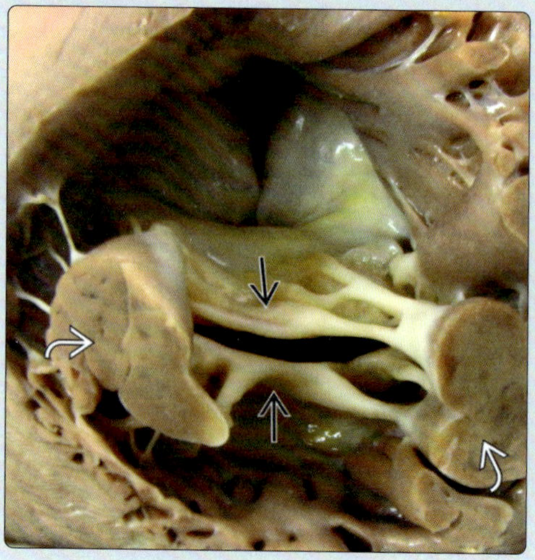

Rheumatic Aortic Valve

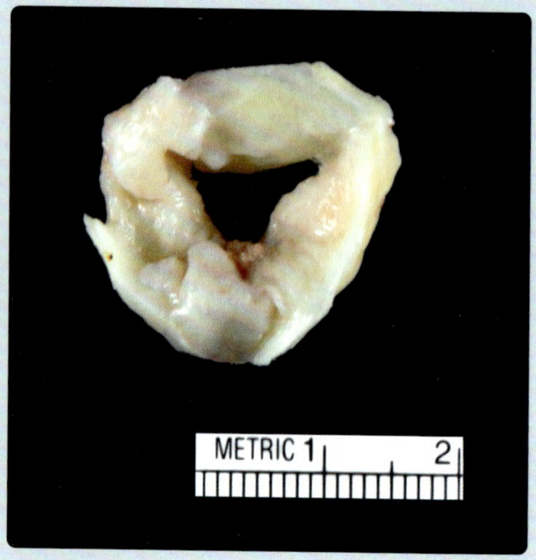

TERMINOLOGY

Abbreviations

- Rheumatic heart disease (RHD)

Definitions

- Chronic valvular scarring and deformity as sequela of acute rheumatic fever (ARF)

ETIOLOGY/PATHOGENESIS

Etiology

- ARF: Noninfectious postinflammatory autoimmune response related to group A *Streptococcus* M protein antigens
  - Postpharyngitis (or less often, skin infection)
- RHD: Chronic progressive fibrosing process in patients with antecedent (usually remote) ARF

Pathogenesis

- Cross-reactive anti-M protein group antibodies bind to myosin, laminin, and vimentin in connective tissue and heart
- Antibody-dependent cytotoxicity mechanisms (complement activation and Fc recognition by cytotoxic cells) lead to tissue injury
- Repetitive cycles of injury and repair lead to progressive fibrosis

CLINICAL ISSUES

Epidemiology

- Incidence
  - Incidence and prevalence vary among countries (proportionate to antibiotic scarcity for treating primary streptococcal pharyngitis)
  - RHD remains public health issue worldwide but has and likely will continue to decrease significantly in developed nations
  - Because group A streptococcal infections can be asymptomatic, there will likely always be cases of ARF and RHD

Presentation

- Modified Jones criteria for ARF (required criteria + 2 major criteria or 1 major and 2 minor criteria)
  - Required criteria
    - Evidence of group A streptococcal infection (culture, immunoassay, or positive serologic tests)
  - Major criteria
    - Carditis
    - Polyarthritis
    - Chorea
    - Erythema marginatum
    - Subcutaneous nodules
  - Minor criteria
    - Fever
    - Arthralgias
    - Previous ARF/RHD
    - Acute-phase reactants elevated
    - Prolonged PR interval (EKG)
- RHD
  - Mitral stenosis is universal (± combined insufficiency)
  - Aortic valve is also affected in 20-30% of cases
  - Tricuspid and pulmonary valves are less often involved and are rarely as significant clinically when involved
- Secondary complications of rheumatic mitral stenosis include
  - Left atrial enlargement with chronic atrial fibrillation
  - Secondary pulmonary venous congestion, pulmonary hypertension, right ventricular pressure overload, and right heart failure
  - Atrial thrombus and embolization
  - Infective endocarditis

Natural History

- Clinical manifestations of RHD appear years to decades after initial episode of ARF
  - RHD latency averages 20-25 years but may be > 40 years
  - Most cases become symptomatic in 4th-5th decades but can manifest during childhood and adolescence as well (especially in resource-poor nations)

Treatment

- Surgical commissurotomy
  - Indications include
    - Moderate to severe mitral stenosis with maximal medical therapy for symptom relief
    - Pulmonary (venous) hypertension
- Percutaneous mitral balloon valvulotomy should be considered 1st if
  - Favorable valve morphology: Pliable leaflets and minimal calcification
  - No or only mild mitral regurgitation
  - Mild subvalvular chordal fusion
  - No atrial thrombus
- Valve replacement
  - Last resort but more permanent outcomes
  - Resection of valve often limited to anterior leaflet (keeping subvalvular elements intact and thereby decreasing risk of ventricular rupture or dilatation)

Prognosis

- Most patients are followed observantly without progression
- Survival is excellent for patient with NYHA functional class II or lower at time of diagnosis
- Survival for patients with NYHA class > II at diagnosis is poor (~ 15% at 10 years) without intervention

IMAGING

Ultrasonographic Findings

- Evaluation of valvular morphology and subvalvular apparatus
  - Degree of fibrosis, thickening, and calcification
- Evaluation of valvular motion
  - Immobility of the posterior leaflet
  - Hockey stick/bent knee appearance of anterior leaflet
- Evaluation of hemodynamic effects
  - Transvalvular gradient and valve area (typically, area ≤ 1 cm^2 is considered severe)
- Evaluation of regurgitation, atrial and ventricular enlargement, and presence of atrial thrombus

MACROSCOPIC

General Features

- All valves can be involved in following order of frequency
  - Mitral > aortic > tricuspid > pulmonary
- Order of frequency mirrors closing pressure for each valve
  - Mitral: 120 mm Hg
  - Aortic: 80 mm Hg
  - Tricuspid: 25 mm Hg
  - Pulmonary: 10 mm Hg

Acute Rheumatic Fever

- Macroscopic features
  - Multiple small vegetations on closing surfaces on mitral valve (valvulitis)

Surgical Specimen: Rheumatic Heart Disease

- Leaflet fibrosis, often more irregular at edges
- Tendinous cord fusion and thickening
- Commissural fusion (if sample includes commissures)
- Leaflets are usually rubbery to rigid on manipulation
- Calcification may be present, particularly at annulus and along fused commissures
- Ulceration of leaflet surface may be seen

Autopsy/Explant Specimens: Rheumatic Heart Disease

- Mitral commissural fusion, bridging fibrosis, and calcification
  - "Fish mouth" deformity when viewed from ventricular aspect up into atrium
  - Mitral orifice reduced with oval or slit-like configuration
  - Funnel-shaped orifice results from chordal retraction with leaflet extension to papillary muscles
- Chordae shortened, retracted, fused
  - Dipped in candle wax appearance
- Left atrial dilatation
  - Mural or left atrial appendage thrombus
  - Focal endocardial thickening (MacCallum patch) represents regurgitant jet lesion
- Aortic and other valves show similar fibrosis and commissure fusion
- Secondary effects on other chambers (right ventricular and right atrial dilatation)
  - Left ventricle is typically normal unless there is significant mitral regurgitation

MICROSCOPIC

Histologic Features

- ARF
  - Aschoff nodules in myocardium, pericardium, &/or valve tissue
    - Granuloma-like, histocyte-rich nodules with characteristic Anitschkow cells showing dense central chromatin bar ("owl's eye" in cross section and "caterpillar" longitudinally)
- RHD
  - Diffuse fibrous and fibroelastic thickening with gradual loss of valve layers
  - Neovascularization with thick-walled, irregular blood vessels
  - Chronic inflammation, lymphocyte rich
  - Aschoff nodules are not seen in chronic stage of RHD
    - Aschoff nodules may rarely be seen in excised atrial appendages (11%) and papillary muscles (1%)
  - Calcifications may erode/ulcerate through endocardium

DIFFERENTIAL DIAGNOSIS

Postinflammatory Valve Disease

- Post irradiation
  - History of radiation treatment
  - Diffuse cusp and leaflet fibrosis not as severe as in RHD
- Healed endocarditis
  - Leaflets and cusps may show extensive deformity
- Autoimmune disease
  - In chronic stage, differentiation from RHD may be difficult
  - Clinical systemic manifestations and serologic studies are necessary for diagnosis
- Ergotamine or fenfluramine/phentermine (fen-phen) valve disease
  - Morphologic features similar to carcinoid valvular disease
  - Valve regurgitation is more common than stenosis
  - Left-side valve involvement is more common than right

Carcinoid Valvular Disease

- Similar gross appearance but lacking neovascularization and disruption of valve layers
- Right-sided valves > left-sided valves [unless patent foramen ovale or gonadal (nonportal drainage) carcinoid]
- Carcinoid valve plaques consist of smooth muscle cells within proteoglycan matrix deposited upon unremarkable valve endothelium

Mitral Annular Calcification

- May extend into leaflets with associated commissural fusion
- May also extend into myocardium and show liquefactive "caseous" degeneration
- More common in older patients with risk factors, including hypertension, mitral stenosis, radiation exposure, and dialysis

SELECTED REFERENCES

1. Fishbein GA et al: Mitral valve pathology. Curr Cardiol Rep. 21(7):61, 2019
2. Cunningham MW: Streptococcus and rheumatic fever. Curr Opin Rheumatol. 24(4):408-16, 2012
3. Sliwa K et al: Rheumatic heart disease: the tip of the iceberg. Circulation. 125(25):3060-2, 2012
4. Guilherme L et al: Rheumatic fever and rheumatic heart disease: cellular mechanisms leading autoimmune reactivity and disease. J Clin Immunol. 30(1):17-23, 2010
5. Zakkar M et al: Rheumatic mitral valve disease: current surgical status. Prog Cardiovasc Dis. 51(6):478-81, 2009
6. Guilherme L et al: Molecular mimicry in the autoimmune pathogenesis of rheumatic heart disease. Autoimmunity. 39(1):31-9, 2006
7. Veinot JP: Pathology of inflammatory native valvular heart disease. Cardiovasc Pathol. 15(5):243-51, 2006
8. Redfield MM et al: Valve disease associated with ergot alkaloid use: echocardiographic and pathologic correlations. Ann Intern Med. 117(1):50-2, 1992
9. Horstkotte D et al: Pathomorphological aspects, aetiology and natural history of acquired mitral valve stenosis. Eur Heart J. 12 Suppl B:55-60, 1991

Subacute Rheumatic Valvulitis

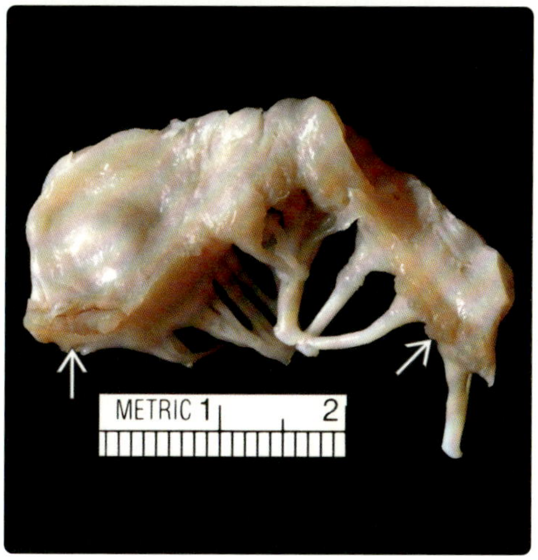

Aschoff Body in Rheumatic Valvulitis

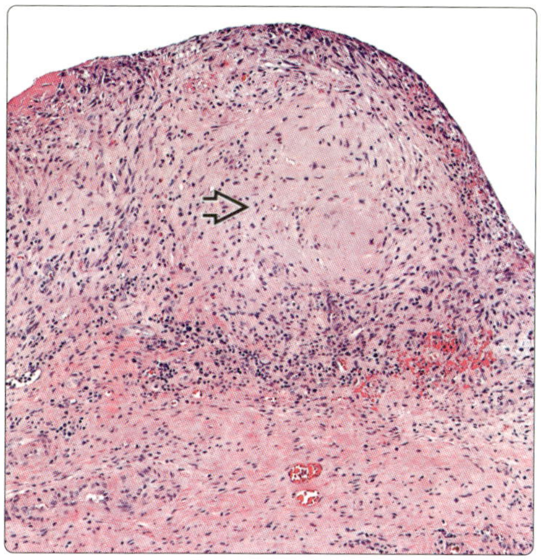

(Left) *Gross photograph shows valve resection in a 15-year-old patient with not only leaflet and cord thickening but also fleshy, pearl-like vegetations ➡ along the closing surfaces, consistent with acute rheumatic valvulitis.* **(Right)** *H&E-stained section of mitral leaflet shows an Aschoff body ⇨, characterized by granuloma-like lymphohistiocytic inflammation with central eosinophilic collagen change typical of acute rheumatic fever (ARF).*

Anitschkow Cells in Rheumatic Valvulitis

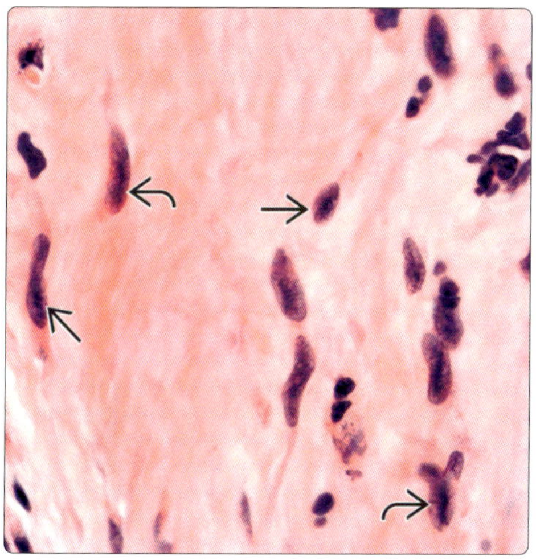

"Fish Mouth" Rheumatic Mitral Deformity

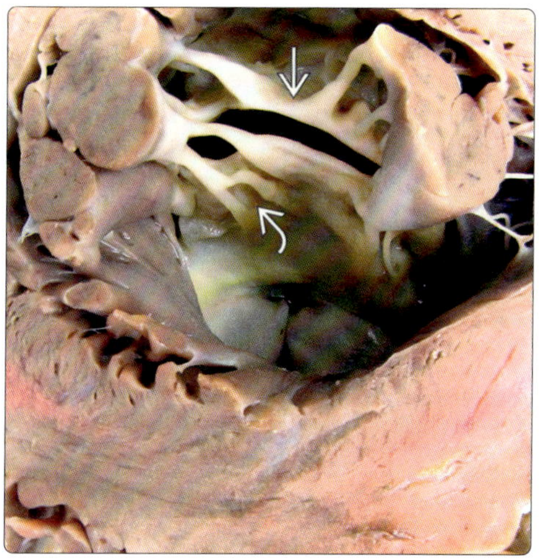

(Left) *Several Anitschkow cells can be seen within and surrounding an Aschoff body in acute rheumatic carditis. Within the nuclei of these cells is a central bar of condensed chromatin that, when seen in cross section, resembles an owl's eye* ⇨ *and, when seen longitudinally, resembles a caterpillar* ⇨. **(Right)** *Gross specimen shows another rheumatic mitral valve resembling a fish mouth* ➡ *when viewed from the ventricular side is shown. Cordal fusion and thickening can also be seen* ➡.

Rheumatic Mitral Valve

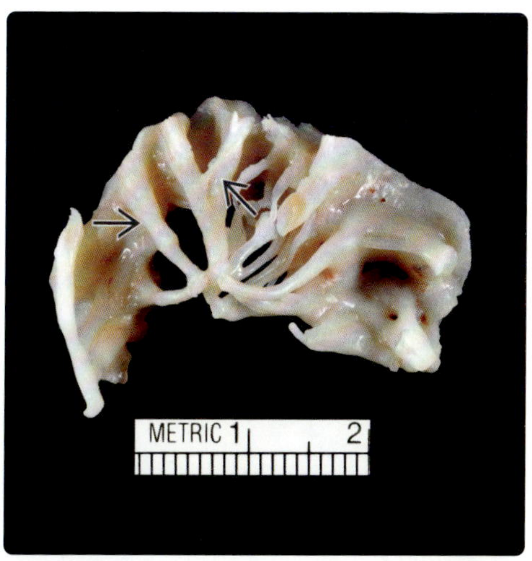

Rheumatic Aortic Valve

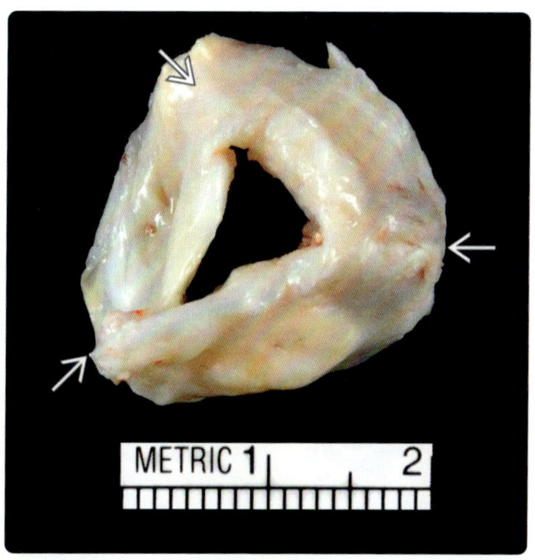

(Left) *Resected posterior mitral leaflet is shown from the ventricular aspect and displays significant cordal fusion and thickening* ⇨, *characteristic of rheumatic valve disease.* **(Right)** *This aortic valve was removed during valve replacement surgery in a patient who also had severe rheumatic mitral stenosis and rheumatic fever as a child. The overall appearance fits the dipped in candle wax description, and there is fusion of all 3 commissures* ➡.

KEY FACTS

TERMINOLOGY

- Endocardial and heart valve abnormalities likely related to vasoactive agents produced by carcinoid tumor

ETIOLOGY/PATHOGENESIS

- Small bowel and other gastrointestinal carcinoids with metastasis to liver are responsible for > 90% of cases
- Carcinoid heart disease (CHD) develops in > 50% of individuals with carcinoid syndrome and is associated with increased morbidity and mortality
- Typically affects right-sided cardiac structures, though may affect left-sided structures when right-to-left shunt is present, pulmonary carcinoid tumor is present, and very high levels of 5-hydroxytryptamine overwhelm metabolic capabilities of liver/lungs

CLINICAL ISSUES

- Tricuspid valve regurgitation (sometimes with stenosis)
- Pulmonary valve stenosis (usually with regurgitation)
- If untreated, survival of patients with CHD is typically 1 year
- Valve surgery is excellent option for individuals with well-controlled systemic disease but marked cardiac involvement

MACROSCOPIC

- Thickening (often with retraction) of valve cusps/leaflets and tendinous cords
- Chamber dilatation (owing to volume hypertrophy) may be apparent on autopsy specimens
- Valve thickening may range from smooth and porcelain-like to nodular and irregular
- Patchy endocardial plaque formation may also be present

MICROSCOPIC

- Carcinoid plaques consist of bland fibrous tissue with variable numbers of myofibroblastic cells contained therein
- Underlying architecture of valvular apparatus is typically undamaged

Atrioventricular Valve With Carcinoid Plaque

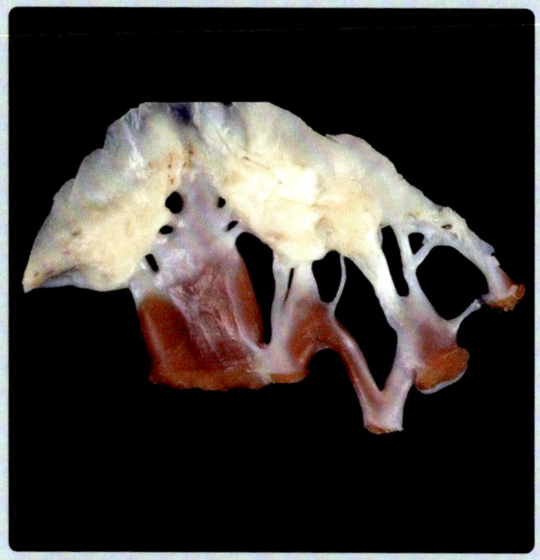

Pulmonary Cusp With Carcinoid Plaque

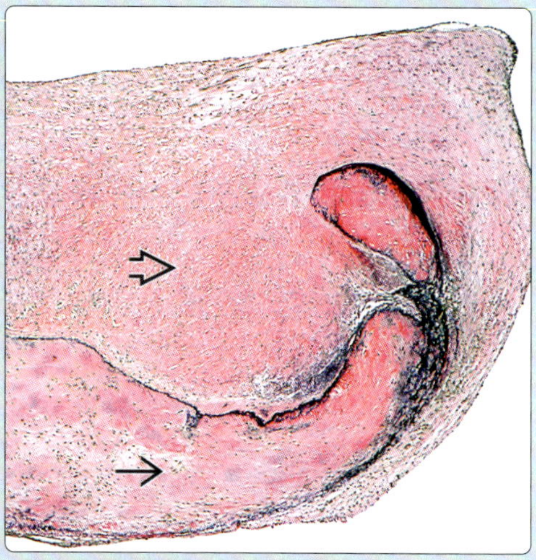

(Left) *Gross photograph of an atrioventricular valve shows thickening of both the leaflet and cordal apparatus due to the presence of carcinoid plaque on the endocardial surface.* **(Right)** *Verhoeff van Gieson stain shows a pulmonary valve cusp ⇨ with a bland, thick, adherent endocardial plaque →, primarily on the arterial (outflow) aspect of the cusp.*

Right- and Left-Sided Carcinoid Heart Disease

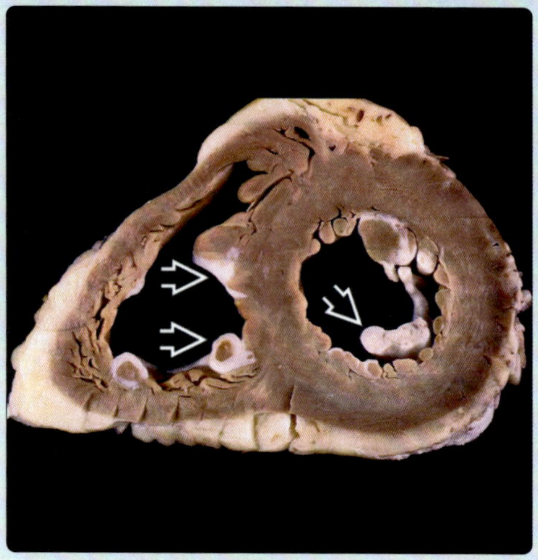

Metastatic Carcinoid in Liver

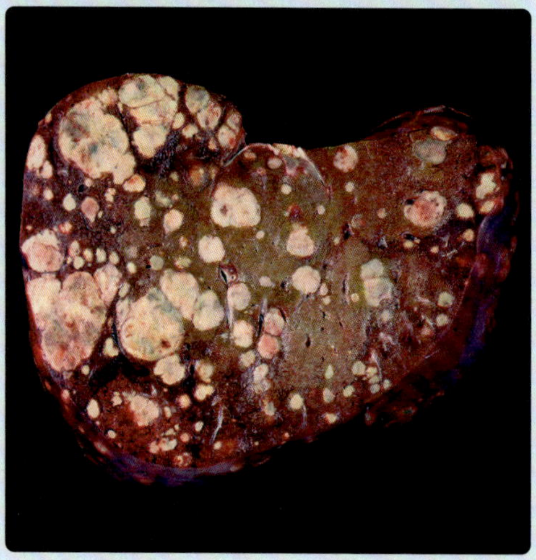

(Left) *Gross photograph shows a midventricular, short-axis section of a heart with both right- and left-sided carcinoid heart disease (CHD) ⇨, characterized by plaques located on the tendinous cords of both the tricuspid and the mitral valve. In this case, the bilateral involvement is due to very high serum serotonin levels.* **(Right)** *This liver exhibits numerous metastases from a small bowel carcinoid tumor. Metastatic disease is usually present in cases of right-sided CHD.*

TERMINOLOGY

Abbreviations

- Carcinoid heart disease (CHD)

Definitions

- Endocardial and heart valve abnormalities likely related to vasoactive agents produced by neuroendocrine tumor

ETIOLOGY/PATHOGENESIS

Pathogenesis

- Small bowel and other gastrointestinal carcinoids with metastasis to liver are responsible for > 90% of cases
- Neuroendocrine tumors (enterochromaffin cells) release vasoactive substances [5-hydroxytryptamine (5-HT), histamine, bradykinins, tachykinins, and prostaglandins] in circulation
- Rarely, primary tumor could not be found or is located in lung, testis, or ovary (gonads drain directly into systemic venous circuit, bypassing liver)
- CHD develops in 20-40% of individuals with carcinoid syndrome and is associated with increased morbidity and mortality
- Precise mechanism for development of CHD is unknown but likely arises from vasoactive substances eliciting mitogenic response on fibroblasts
- Typically affects right-sided cardiac structures though may affect left-sided structures when right-to-left shunt is present, pulmonary carcinoid tumor is present, and very high levels of 5-HT overwhelm metabolic capabilities of liver/lungs

CLINICAL ISSUES

Presentation

- Right-sided heart failure with normal angiogram
- Tricuspid valve regurgitation (sometimes with stenosis)
- Pulmonary valve stenosis (usually with regurgitation)
- Left-sided valves are typically regurgitant when involved (only rarely with stenosis)

Treatment

- Surgical approaches
  - Valve replacement is only effective intervention for advanced CHD
- Drugs
  - Somatostatin analogs

Prognosis

- Time from onset of symptoms of carcinoid syndrome to diagnosis of CHD is typically 2 years
- If untreated, survival of patients with CHD is typically 1 year
- Valve surgery is excellent option for individuals with well-controlled systemic disease but marked cardiac involvement
- Elevated levels of 5-HIAA (hydroxy indoleacetic acid) primary metabolite of 5-HT are associated with CHD diagnosis, disease progression and mortality

IMAGING

Echocardiographic Findings

- Tricuspid valve leaflets and cords thickened and retracted with decreased mobility
- Pulmonary valve cusps thickened and retracted, also with reduced mobility
- With decreased cusp/leaflet mobility, regurgitation often ensues as they are often fixed in open position
- Chronic regurgitation often causes volume overload of right-sided chambers and dilatation

MACROSCOPIC

General Features

- Thickening (often with retraction) of valve cusps/leaflets and tendinous cords with focal commisural fusion
- Valve thickening may range from smooth and porcelain-like to nodular and irregular
- Patchy endocardial plaque formation may also be present
- Chamber dilatation (owing to volume overload) may be apparent on autopsy specimens

MICROSCOPIC

Histologic Features

- Carcinoid plaques consist of bland fibrous tissue with variable numbers of myofibroblastic cells
- Severe fibrosis may be encountered on tricuspid valve but only rarely so in semilunar valves
- Mild chronic inflammation and delicate neovascularization may be seen within carcinoid plaques
- Underlying architecture of valvular apparatus is typically undamaged
- Plaques tend to occur on either ventricular or atrial aspect of tricuspid valve and arterial (outflow) aspect of pulmonary valve

ANCILLARY TESTS

Histochemistry

- Verhoeff van Gieson
  - Elastic stains often aid in identification of plaque and its relationship to underlying undamaged valvular apparatus

DIFFERENTIAL DIAGNOSIS

Drug-Induced Valvulopathy

- Drug molecules, such as fenfluramine and ergot agents, cause disease similar to CHD and have similarities in structure and receptor affinity with 5-HT
- History of exposure to methysergide, ergot derivatives, or fenfluramine and phentermine

SELECTED REFERENCES

1. Jin C et al: Carcinoid heart disease: pathophysiology, pathology, clinical manifestations, and management. Cardiology. 146(1):65-73, 2021
2. Oleinikov K et al: Update in carcinoid heart disease - the heart of the matter. Rev Endocr Metab Disord. 22(3):553-61, 2021
3. Perry D et al: Carcinoid heart disease: a guide for clinicians. Cardiol Clin. 37(4):497-503, 2019
4. Ram P et al: Carcinoid heart disease: review of current knowledge. Tex Heart Inst J. 46(1):21-7, 2019

(Left) *Gross photograph (taken at autopsy) shows an aortic semilunar valve with marked cusp thickening and cusp retraction resulting from the deposition of carcinoid plaque. The patient was noted to have marked aortic insufficiency as a result of the carcinoid valvulopathy.* **(Right)** *Gross photograph shows the ventricular aspect of the tricuspid valve. The extent of cordal thickening and fusion resulting from the plaque is readily apparent.*

Aortic Valve Changes Secondary to Carcinoid Heart Disease

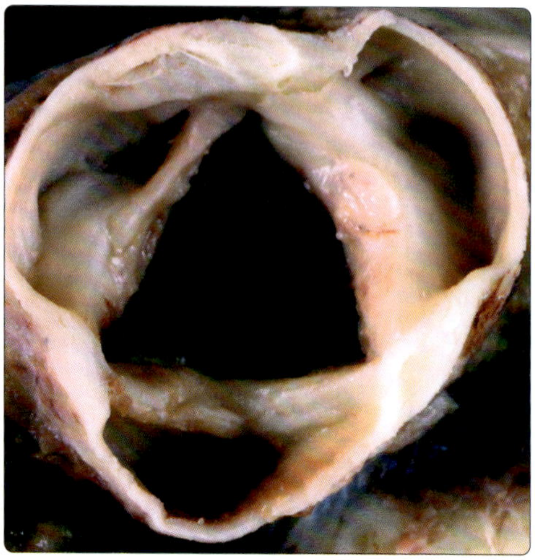

Ventricular Aspect of Tricuspid Valve With Carcinoid Plaque

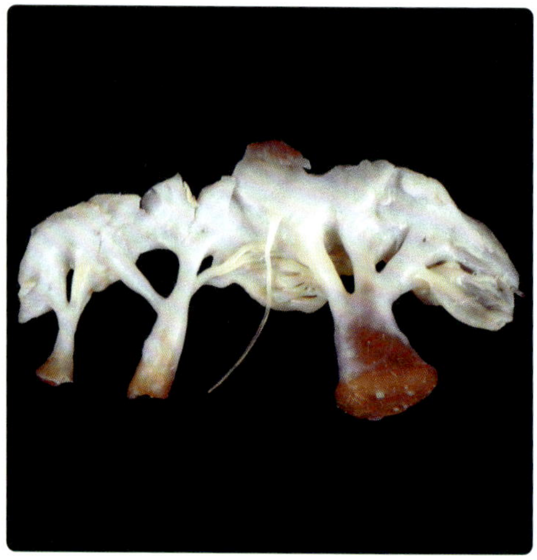

(Left) *Gross photograph of a tricuspid valve shows the atrial aspect of the leaflets with thickening caused by a white-yellow plaque adhering to the endocardial surface. Thickening of the cordal apparatus as well as the endocardium of the papillary muscle can also be appreciated.* **(Right)** *Gross photograph of a surgically resected pulmonary valve shows variable thickening of the 3 cusps due to the presence of carcinoid plaque.*

Tricuspid Valve With Carcinoid Plaque

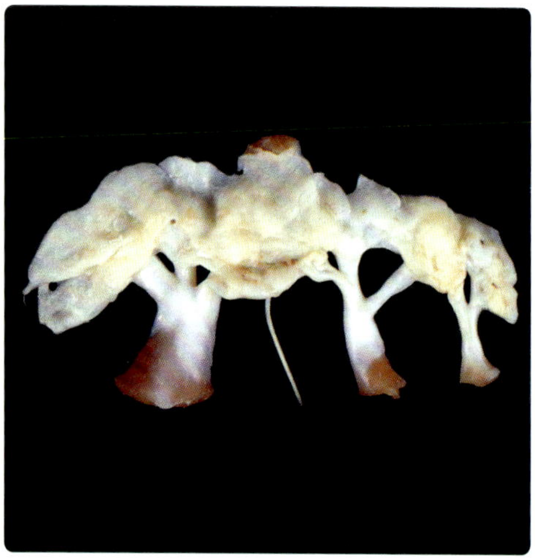

Pulmonary Cusps With Carcinoid Plaque

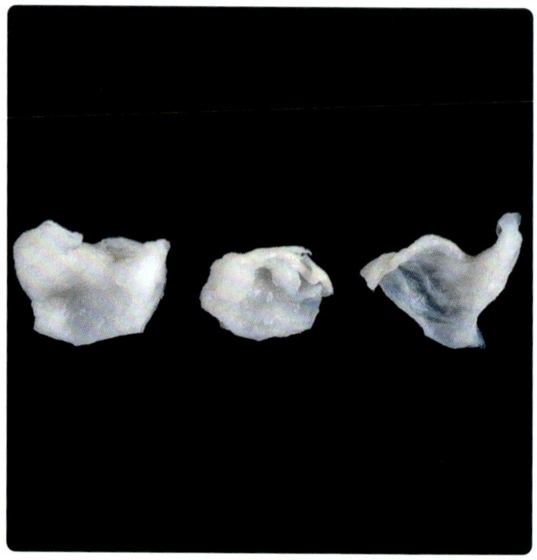

(Left) *H&E shows a bland carcinoid plaque ⇨ causing apparent endocardial thickening within the coarse trabeculations of the right ventricle. Grossly, this would manifest as a thick white plaque on the endocardium of the right ventricular wall.* **(Right)** *Masson trichrome stain exhibits the light blue staining quality of the endocardial carcinoid plaque on the right ventricular endocardium. Note that the subjacent myocardium is uninvolved by the process.*

Histology of Carcinoid Plaque

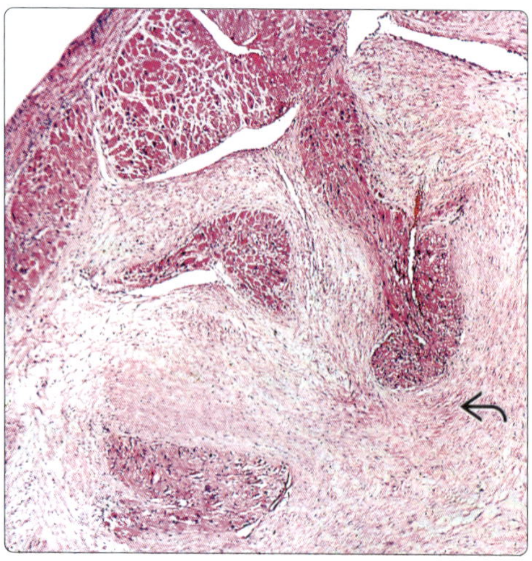

Trichrome Stain of Endocardial Carcinoid Plaque

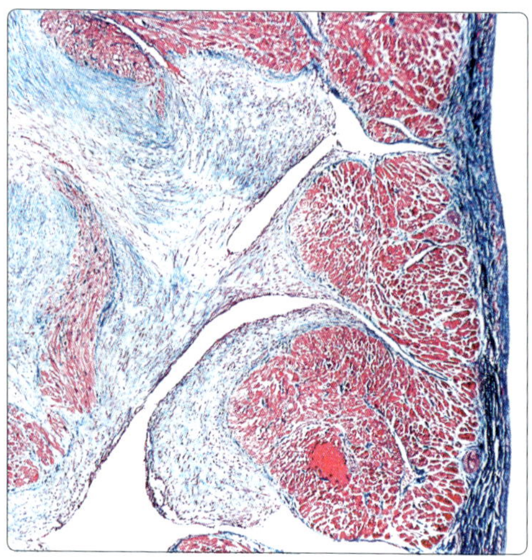

Tricuspid Valve With Carcinoid Plaque

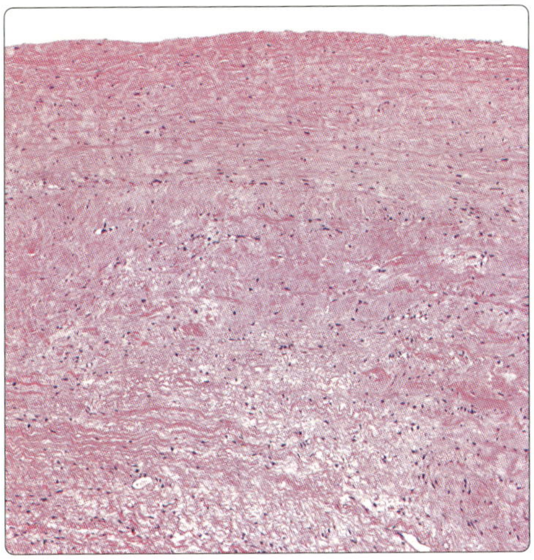

Elastic Stain of Carcinoid Plaque

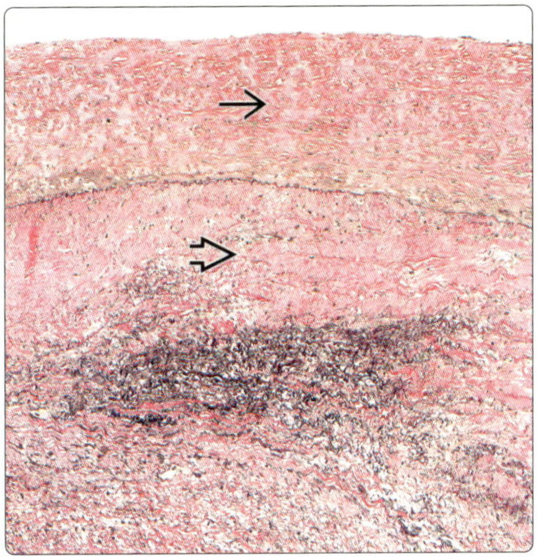

(Left) *Surgically resected tricuspid valve shows that, occasionally, the carcinoid plaque may be difficult to distinguish from the underlying valve by routine H&E staining.* **(Right)** *Verhoeff van Gieson stain of a tricuspid valve shows clear distinction between the underlying valve ⇨ and the endocardial carcinoid plaque →. Use of elastic stain can help to assess the valve and plaque.*

Histology of Carcinoid Plaque

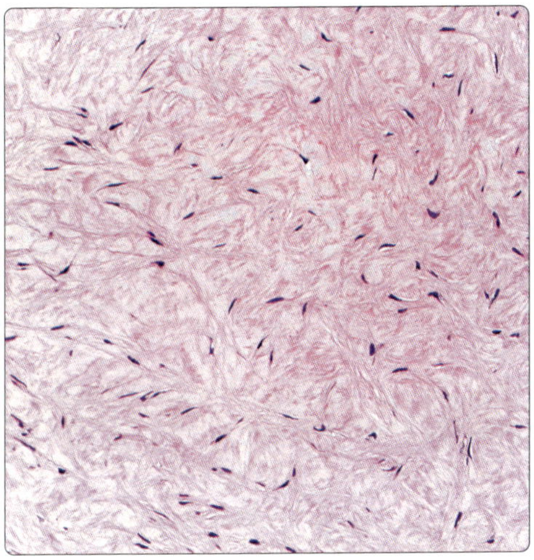

Myocardium With Metastatic Carcinoid Implant

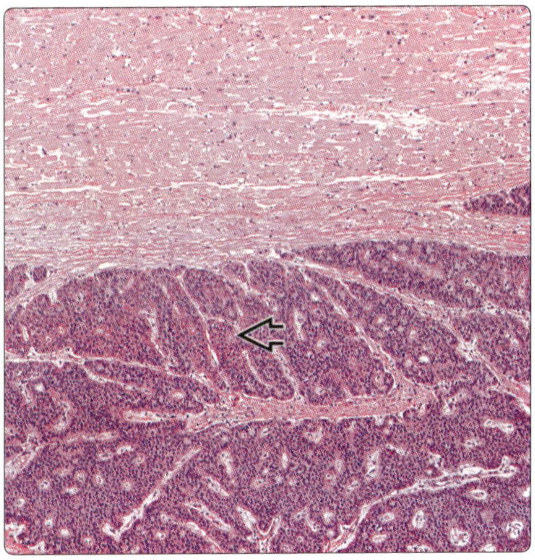

(Left) *High-power H&E shows the bland proliferation of myofibroblastic cells that are so characteristic of carcinoid plaques. These can be variably cellular with some areas exhibiting more paucicellular fibrosis.* **(Right)** *Plaque-like deposits are not the only effect of carcinoid tumor on the heart. Rarely, carcinoid tumors themselves may metastasize to the heart, as in this case, where a metastatic implant is noted within the myocardium ⇨.*

Pulmonary Valve With Myxoid Degeneration

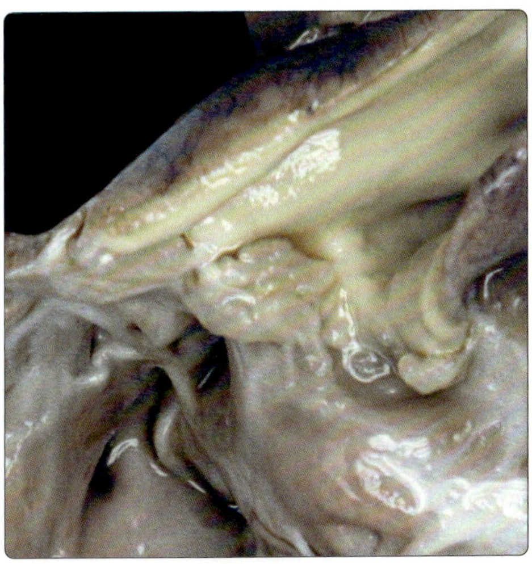

Myxoid Degeneration in Pulmonary Valve Cusp

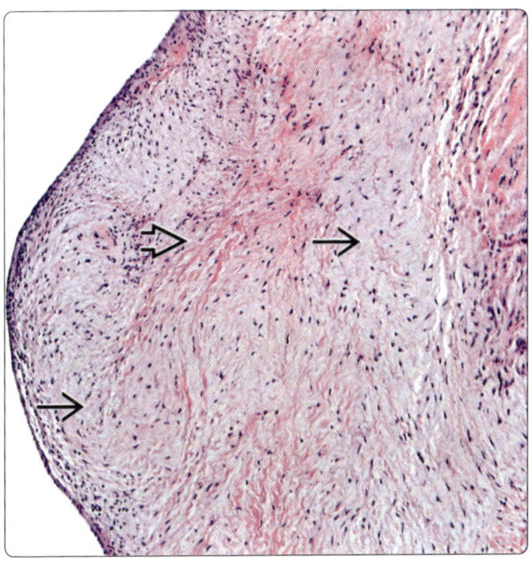

(Left) *Myxomatous valve disease may be confused with CHD. The myxomatous valve is more rubbery than the carcinoid plaque.* **(Right)** *Pulmonary valve cusp shows myxoid change → involving the whole thickness of the cusp with associated collagen disruption ⇨ and abnormal valve architecture.*

Ebstein Anomaly

KEY FACTS

TERMINOLOGY

- Congenital malformation of tricuspid valve (TV) characterized by downward displacement and leaflet adherence to right ventricular wall [so-called atrialization of right ventricle (RV)]

CLINICAL ISSUES

- ~ 2.5 per 100,000 live births
- ~ 1% of congenital heart diseases overall
- Valve repair: Success depends on morphology; techniques include
  - Plication of atrialized RV
  - Tricuspid annuloplasty
  - Reduction of right atrium
- Valve replacement (when repair not possible)
- Natural history
  - Milder forms may manifest as progressive exercise intolerance during childhood or early adulthood
  - Severe malformations present early and, without surgical intervention, lead to heart failure and death

MACROSCOPIC

- Adherence of septal and posterior tricuspid leaflets to underlying myocardium
- Downward (apical) displacement of coaptation point
- Few, short, or sometimes absent tendinous cords
- Frequent interatrial communication as either secundum atrial septal defect or patent foramen ovale
- Variable degrees of attachment to ventricle wall (complete to rare, tethering strands)

TOP DIFFERENTIAL DIAGNOSES

- Uhl anomaly (parchment RV): Dilated RV with diffuse severe thinning of wall
- TV dysplasia: Cords may also be dysplastic but delamination complete; absence of downward displacement of valve
- Pulmonary hypertension: Right-chamber dilatation and hypertrophy

Ebstein Anomaly (Graphic)

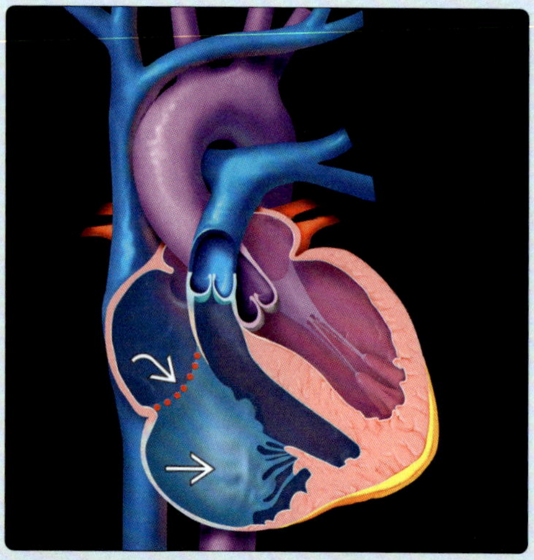

Ebstein Anomaly (MR)

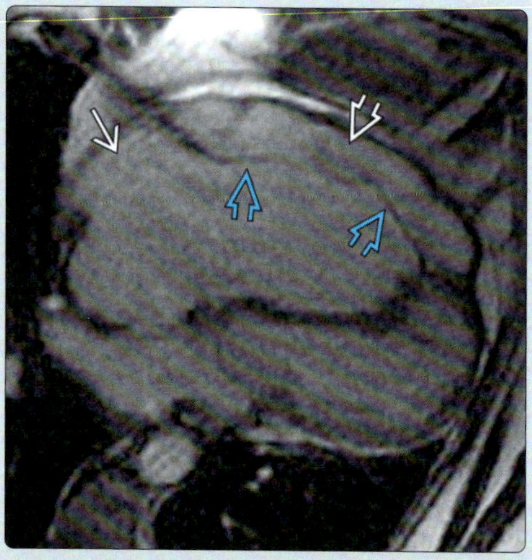

(Left) *Graphic illustrates Ebstein anomaly or "atrialization" of the right ventricle (RV) due to adherence of the tricuspid leaflets. The anatomic valve annulus is marked by red dots.* **(Right)** *Short-axis, 4-chamber FIESTA cine MR shows massive dilation of the RV and right atrium. The tricuspid valve (TV) leaflets are apically displaced, resulting in atrialization of the RV, diagnostic of Ebstein anomaly.*

Ebstein Anomaly (Gross)

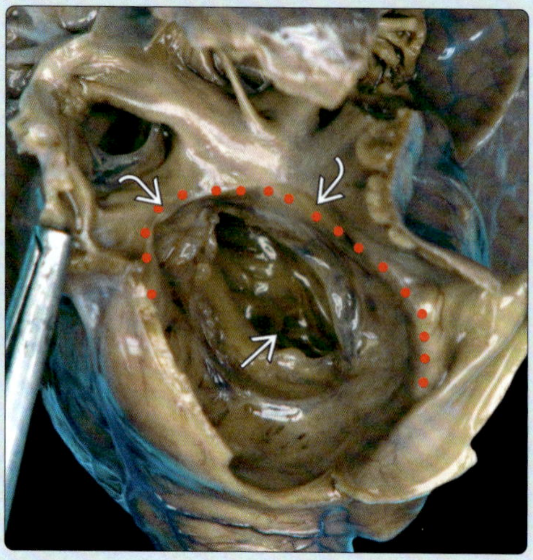

Ebstein Anomaly (Autopsy)

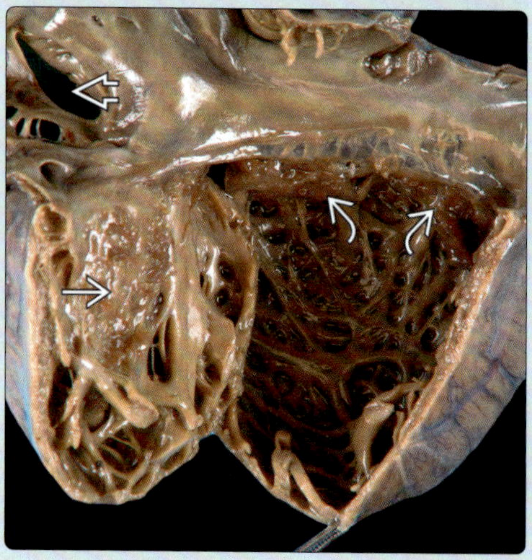

(Left) *The valve orifice in this heart with Ebstein anomaly is well below the annulus (red dots).* **(Right)** *This autopsy specimen from an infant with Ebstein anomaly shows an enlarged, malformed septal tricuspid leaflet adhering to the ventricular wall. The other leaflets are also adhered. An atrial septal defect is present.*

TERMINOLOGY

Definitions

- Congenital malformation of tricuspid valve (TV) characterized by downward displacement and leaflet adherence to right ventricular wall [so-called atrialization of right ventricle (RV)]

ETIOLOGY/PATHOGENESIS

Developmental Anomaly

- Incomplete delamination or failure of undermining during development of septal and posterior leaflets from ventricular myocardium
  - Tricuspid leaflets originate from ventricle but separate through process of tissue undermining or delamination
  - Cordal and papillary muscles also underdeveloped

CLINICAL ISSUES

Epidemiology

- Incidence
  - ~ 1% of congenital heart diseases overall
  - ~ 2.5 per 100,000 live births
  - Most common cause of congenital tricuspid regurgitation

Presentation

- Highly variable, depending on severity of abnormalities
  - From heart failure to progressive exercise intolerance
- Cardiomegaly with massive right atrial/ventricular dilatation
- Tricuspid regurgitation, chronic venous congestion, hepatomegaly, and splenomegaly
- Wolff-Parkinson-White syndrome common (accessory conduction pathways through tricuspid annulus)

Natural History

- Severe malformations present early and, without surgical intervention, lead to heart failure and death
- Milder forms may manifest as progressive exercise intolerance during childhood or early adulthood

Treatment

- Surgical approaches
  - Valve repair: Success depends on morphology; techniques include
    - Plication of atrialized RV
    - Tricuspid annuloplasty
    - Reduction of right atrium
  - Valve replacement (when repair not possible)
  - Bidirectional (Glenn) cavopulmonary shunt used in cases with severely dilated and dysfunctional RV

IMAGING

Ultrasonographic Findings

- 4-chamber view with Doppler most helpful
  - Apical displacement of TV septal leaflet compared to anterior mitral leaflet
  - Right heart volume and possible paradoxical interventricular septal motion
  - Atrial septal defects (secundum type) common

MACROSCOPIC

General Features

- Adherence of septal and posterior tricuspid leaflets to underlying myocardium
  - Any leaflet mobility is well below anatomic valve annulus
  - Downward (apical) displacement of coaptation point
- Dilatation of right atrioventricular junction at true tricuspid annulus
- Elongation, redundancy, and possible fenestration of anterior leaflet
  - May obstruct blood flow to pulmonary artery

Leaflets

- Often irregular, dysplastic
- Few, short, or sometimes absent tendinous cords
- Variable degrees of attachment to ventricle wall (complete to rare tethering strands)

Associated Cardiac Anomalies

- Frequent interatrial communication as either secundum atrial septal defect or patent foramen ovale
- Pulmonary atresia or stenosis (rare)

Right Ventricle

- Dilated, may distort ventricular septum
- Thin wall, may be fibrotic or aneurysmal
- Atrialized portion of RV shows
  - Endocardial fibrosis
  - Poorly developed myocardial trabeculations

MICROSCOPIC

Histologic Features

- Hypertrophy and fibrosis, nonspecific

DIFFERENTIAL DIAGNOSIS

Uhl Anomaly (Parchment Right Ventricle)

- Rare, usually < 1 year of age
- Dilated RV with diffuse severe thinning of wall
- TV regurgitant but with complete delamination

Tricuspid Valve Dysplasia

- Irregular leaflet thickening ± annular dilatation
- Cords may also be dysplastic, but delamination complete
- Absence of downward displacement of valve

Pulmonary Hypertension

- Right-chamber dilatation and hypertrophy
- TV often regurgitant but with complete delamination

SELECTED REFERENCES

1. Stephens EH et al: The congenital tricuspid valve spectrum: from Ebstein to dysplasia. World J Pediatr Congenit Heart Surg. 11(6):783-91, 2020
2. Barbara DW et al: Surgical pathology of 104 tricuspid valves (2000-2005) with classic right-sided Ebstein's malformation. Cardiovasc Pathol. 17(3):166-71, 2008
3. Brown ML et al: The outcomes of operations for 539 patients with Ebstein anomaly. J Thorac Cardiovasc Surg. 135(5):1120-36, 1136, 2008
4. Paranon S et al: Ebstein's anomaly of the tricuspid valve: from fetus to adult: congenital heart disease. Heart. 94(2):237-43, 2008

Congenital Pulmonary Stenosis

KEY FACTS

TERMINOLOGY

- Rare congenital malformation (acommisural, dome shape, bicuspid or "dysplastic") causing pulmonary stenosis and usually associated with other congenital heart defects

ETIOLOGY/PATHOGENESIS

- Multifactorial in origin although familial forms have been described
- Association with other congenital defects
  - Noonan syndrome
  - Pulmonary atresia with intact ventricular septum
  - Atrial/ventricular septal defects
  - Congenital rubella

CLINICAL ISSUES

- M = F
- Clinical manifestations depend on severity of stenosis and age at presentation
- Mild stenosis does not usually progress
- Moderate stenosis progresses in ~ 20% of untreated patients
- Severe stenosis will progress and should be treated
- Endovascular balloon valvuloplasty currently most common surgical approach
- Open commisurectomy/partial valvectomy
- Valve replacement (most common in TOF)

MACROSCOPIC

- Acommisural dome shape, bicuspid or dysplastic

MICROSCOPIC

- Myxoid change in cusps
- Increase of collagen and elastic fibers

TOP DIFFERENTIAL DIAGNOSES

- Acquired pulmonic stenosis
- Postinflammatory
- Carcinoid heart disease

(Left) *Graphic illustrates pulmonary valve leaflet thickening with right ventricle hypertrophy. The inset shows a dome-shaped valvular deformity with marked valvular orifice reduction.* **(Right)** *Autopsy heart specimen from a child with congenital pulmonary stenosis shows 3 dysplastic pulmonary valve leaflets with marked fleshy thickening. Right ventricle hypertrophy is noted.*

Congenital Pulmonary Stenosis (Graphic)

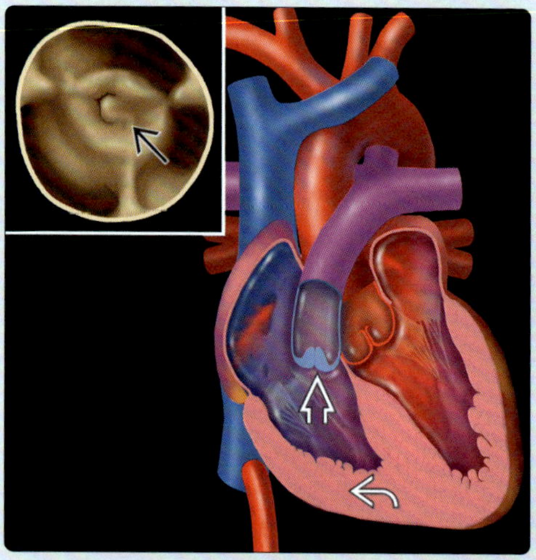

Dysplastic Pulmonary Valve Leaflets (Autopsy)

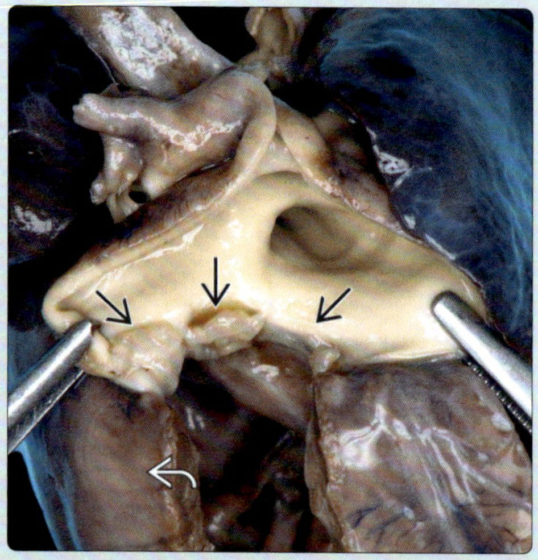

(Left) *Autopsy heart specimen from a child with congenital pulmonary stenosis shows a disproportionately small pulmonary trunk in comparison to the aorta. A large patent ductus arteriosus is seen.* **(Right)** *Autopsy heart specimen shows the great arteries from above. There is congenital pulmonary stenosis with 3 fused dysplastic and thickened pulmonary valve leaflets with retraction of the annular ring. The aortic root is of normal size (for comparison).*

Congenital Pulmonary Stenosis (Autopsy)

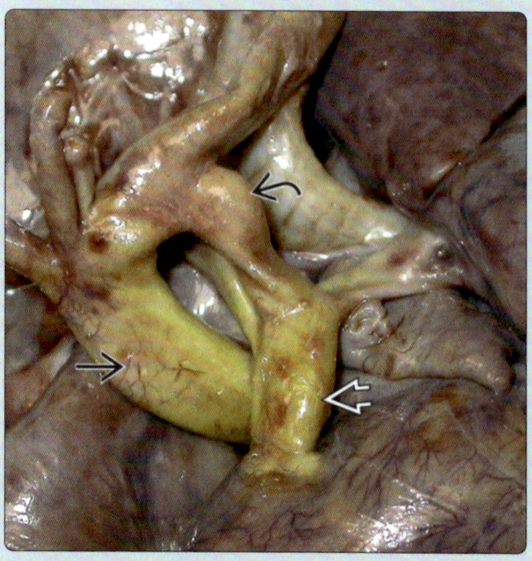

En-Face View of Congenital Pulmonary Stenosis

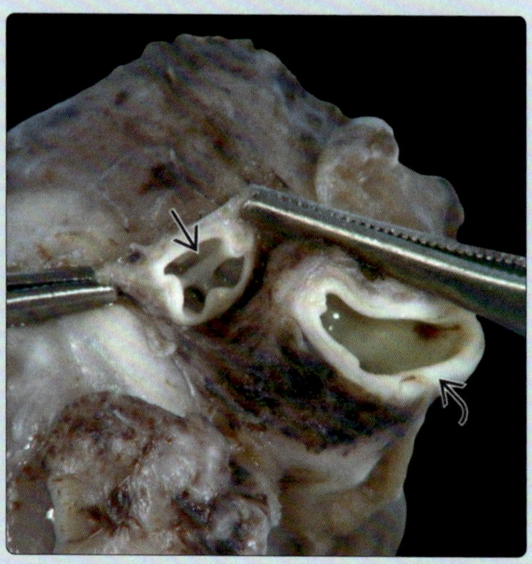

TERMINOLOGY

Definitions

- Rare congenital pulmonary valve malformation, usually associated with other congenital heart defects

ETIOLOGY/PATHOGENESIS

Congenital

- Multifactorial in origin, although familial forms have been described
- Association with other congenital defects
  - Noonan syndrome
  - Tetralogy of Fallot
  - Atrial/ventricular septal defects
  - Congenital rubella

CLINICAL ISSUES

Epidemiology

- Incidence
  - 7.5-9% of congenital malformations
- Sex
  - M = F

Presentation

- Clinical manifestations depend on severity of stenosis and age at presentation
  - Neonatal
    - Associated with pathology of tricuspid valve, right ventricle, &/or coronaries
    - Central cyanosis
    - Single 2nd heart sound
    - No ejection click
  - Beyond neonatal period
    - Usually isolated pulmonary valve defect
    - Systolic murmur on upper left sternal border
    - Cyanosis may be present if associated with atrial septal defect
  - Adult
    - Asymptomatic
    - If severe, signs of right ventricle failure present
- If associated with Noonan syndrome, hypertrophic cardiomyopathy may also be present

Natural History

- Mild stenosis does not usually progress
- Moderate stenosis progresses in ~ 20% if untreated
- Severe stenosis will progress and should be treated

Treatment

- Options, risks, complications
  - In neonates, prostaglandin E is given to maintain ductal patency until surgical procedure can be performed
  - Intervention indicated in adults when gradient > 50 mm Hg and symptoms present at rest
- Surgical approaches
  - Endovascular balloon valvuloplasty currently most common
    - May be complicated with restenosis ~ 10% of time
  - Open commisurectomy/partial valvectomy
  - Valve replacement (most common in TOF)

Prognosis

- Postrepair survival rates similar to general population

IMAGING

Radiographic Findings

- Chest x-ray
  - Neonate: Pulmonary oligemia &/or prominent right heart border
  - Infant/child/adult
    - Normal heart size
    - Normal pulmonary vasculature
    - Poststenotic dilatation of main and left pulmonary arteries
    - Right atrial and ventricular enlargement

Echocardiographic Findings

- Dysplastic valve appears thickened, fleshy
- Poststenotic dilatation of pulmonary artery
- Doppler demonstrating increased flow velocity and pressure gradient across stenotic valve

MACROSCOPIC

General Features

- Variable morphologies
  - 1 cusp without commissure (dome shaped, most common abnormality; 42% of cases)
  - Unicuspid/unicommissural valve
  - 2 cusps and 2 commissures (bicuspid valve)
  - 3 normally placed commissures with dysplastic cusps
    - Thickened and deformed
    - No commissural fusion
    - Small annulus
    - Outflow tract narrowing may be present
- Right ventricle
  - Infundibular hypertrophy proportional to degree of stenosis

MICROSCOPIC

Histologic Features

- Cusps show myxoid change &/or increase of collagen and elastic fibers

DIFFERENTIAL DIAGNOSIS

Acquired Pulmonic Stenosis

- Postinflammatory
  - Commissural fusion
  - Involvement of other heart valves (mitral and aortic)
  - Etiologies: Rheumatic, postirradiation, healed endocarditis
- Carcinoid heart disease
  - Metastatic carcinoid in liver (or ovary/testis)
  - Plaques of proteoglycan matrix and smooth muscle cells
  - Tricuspid valve also involved

SELECTED REFERENCES

1. Altrichter PM et al: Surgical pathology of the pulmonary valve: a study of 116 cases spanning 15 years. Mayo Clin Proc. 64(11):1352-60, 1989

Endocarditis, Native Valve

KEY FACTS

TERMINOLOGY

- Infective endocarditis is defined as inflammation of endocardium and typically refers to infection on valve surfaces

ETIOLOGY/PATHOGENESIS

- *Staphylococcus aureus* (31%), *Streptococcus viridans* (17%)
- Risk factors
  - Hemodialysis (7.9%)
  - Intravenous drug abuse (9.8%)
  - Degenerative valvular disease

CLINICAL ISSUES

- 3-10 episodes per 100,000 person-years
- Mean age: 51-65 years
- Fever > 38 °C
- Tissue and blood cultures necessary for diagnosis
- Hospital in-house mortality rates vary from 9.6-26%

IMAGING

- Oscillating intracardiac mass located at sites where vegetations typically occur, such as leaflets and chordae tendineae

MACROSCOPIC

- Vegetations measuring 3-4 mm in diameter
- Ulceration, rupture, and perforation of cusps; perivalvular abscess
- Necrosis of chordae tendineae and perivalvular apparatus
- Ruptured chordae tendineae

MICROSCOPIC

- Vegetations composed of matrix of fibrin, platelets, acute inflammatory infiltrate, and bacterial microcolonies
- Necrosis of cusps
- Intramyocardial abscess formation
- Special stains for Gram, GMS, and Steiner are contributory for diagnosis

(Left) *Gross photograph of mitral valve shows gray-tan vegetations placed at the atrial aspect of the valve leaflets.* **(Right)** *H&E shows the characteristic features of a valve vegetation composed of fibrin thrombus with acute inflammatory infiltrate and bacterial colonies. Vegetations are loaded with bacteria at very high densities that promote bacteremia and further growth of the vegetation, increasing friability and risk of embolization.*

Mitral Valve Involved by Infective Endocarditis

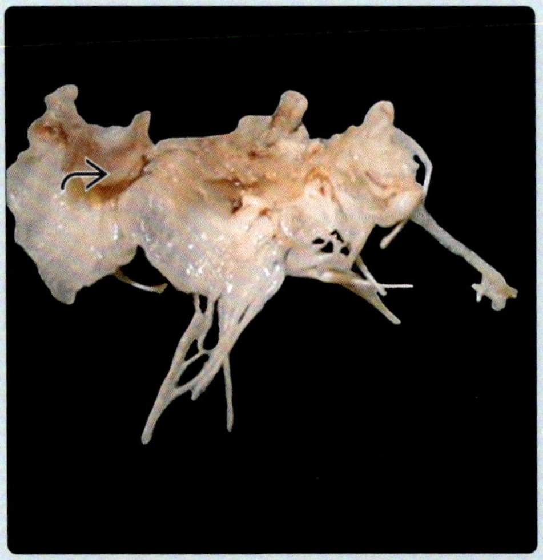

Microscopic Features of Infective Endocarditis

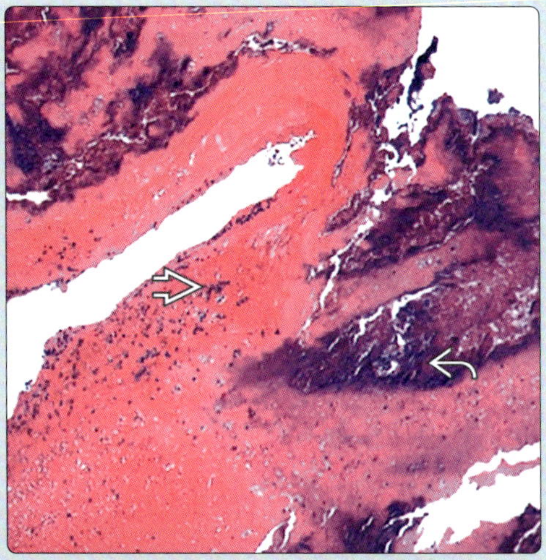

(Left) *Gross photograph shows an aortic valve cusp with destruction and aneurysmal thinning. Perforation of the cusp is noted.* **(Right)** *Gross photograph shows a surgically resected mitral valve with gray-tan vegetations. There is a perforation at the base of the valve. In the case of severe valve destruction and resultant regurgitation, valve replacement becomes necessary.*

Aortic Valve Involved by Infective Endocarditis

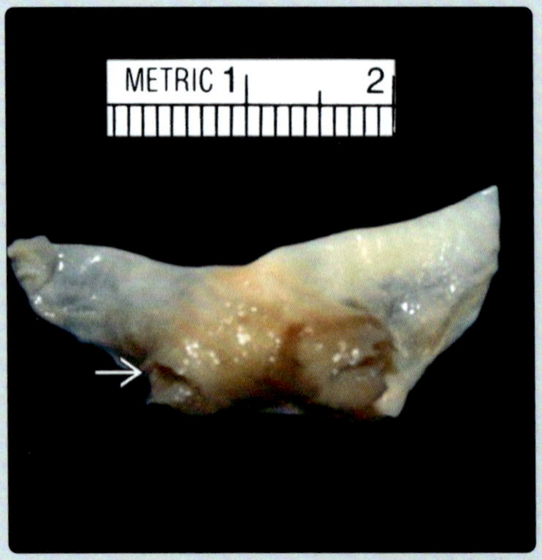

Mitral Valve Involved by Infective Endocarditis

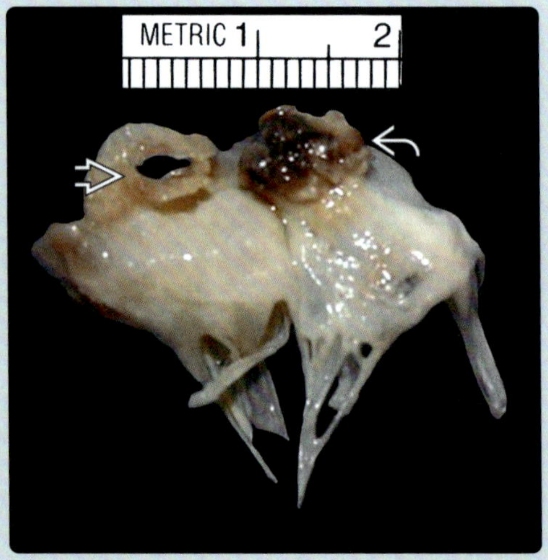

TERMINOLOGY

Abbreviations

- Native valve endocarditis (NVE)

Definitions

- Infective endocarditis is defined as inflammation of endocardium and typically refers to infection on valve surfaces

ETIOLOGY/PATHOGENESIS

Infectious Agents

- Gram-positive bacteria: *Staphylococcus aureus* (43%), *Streptococcus viridans* (9%), Coagulase-negative staphylococci (12%), *Enterococci* (13%), *Streptococcus gallolyticus* (2%)/other *Streptococci* (6%)
- Gram-negative bacteria: HACEK (*Haemophilus* species, *Aggregatibacter actinomycetemcomitans, Cardiobacterium hominis, Eikenella corrodens*, and *Kingella kingae*) (2%)/non-HACEK (2%)
- Fungi (3%)

Risk Factors

- Degenerative valvular disease: Mitral regurgitation (43.4%), aortic regurgitation (26.3%), rheumatic heart disease (5%)
- Congenital heart disease
- Intravenous drug abuse (9.8%)
- Long-term intravenous lines (9%)/indwelling cardiac devices (11%)
- Hemodialysis (7.9%)

CLINICAL ISSUES

Epidemiology

- Incidence
  - 3-10 episodes per 100,000 person-years
- Age
  - Range: 51-65 years
- Sex
  - M:F = 1.2-2.5:1

Presentation

- Fever > 38 °C (90%)
- Heart murmur (75%)
- Vascular phenomena: Arterial emboli, mycotic aneurysm, central nervous system and conjunctival hemorrhages, Janeway lesions
- Immunologic phenomena: Glomerulonephritis, Osler node, Roth spot, false-positive ANCA antibodies, rheumatoid factor or syphilis tests

Laboratory Tests

- Tissue and blood cultures are critical for diagnosis and management
- Serologic testing in culture-negative endocarditis

Treatment

- Surgical approaches
  - Valve replacement, valve-sparing surgery, vegetectomy
- Drugs
  - Antibiotics tailored to specific type of microorganism for 4-6 weeks duration

Prognosis

- Hospital in-house mortality rates vary from 9.6-26%; 5-year mortality rate 40%

MACROSCOPIC

General Features

- Cardiac
  - Vegetations measuring 3-4 mm in diameter
    - Located in atrial aspect of atrioventricular valves and on ventricular aspect of semilunar valves
  - Necrosis of chordae tendineae and perivalvular apparatus
  - Ruptured chordae tendineae
  - Ulceration, rupture, and perforation of cusps; perivalvular abscess
  - Satellite left atrial vegetations (MacCallum patches)
  - Intracardiac fistula
  - Myocardial infarction
- Systemic due to arterial embolization
  - Infarcts: Spleen, kidneys, lungs, mesentery, brain
  - Abscess: Kidneys, lungs, liver, spleen, brain
  - Septic spleen
  - Mycotic aneurysms

MICROSCOPIC

Histologic Features

- Vegetations composed of matrix of fibrin, platelets, acute inflammatory infiltrate, and bacterial microcolonies
- Necrosis of chordae tendineae and perivalvular apparatus
- Intramyocardial abscess formation

ANCILLARY TESTS

Histochemistry

- Gram, GMS, and Steiner stains can contribute to identify microorganism in valve

In Situ Hybridization

- May identify microorganisms in case of negative cultures

PCR

- Bacterial DNA sequencing to identify microorganisms in vegetations

DIFFERENTIAL DIAGNOSIS

Nonbacterial Thrombotic Endocarditis

- Vegetations typically along line of closure with no underlying valve destruction
- Vegetations vary in size, are friable, and easily embolize
- Histologically, composed of fibrin and platelets, devoid of bacteria and significant inflammation

SELECTED REFERENCES

1. Roberts WC et al: Morphologic findings in native mitral valves replaced for isolated acute infective endocarditis. Am J Cardiol. 162:136-42, 2022
2. Witten JC et al: Invasive aortic valve endocarditis: clinical and tissue findings from a prospective investigation. Ann Thorac Surg. 113(2):535-43, 2022
3. Chambers HF et al: Native-valve infective endocarditis. N Engl J Med. 383(6):567-76, 2020

(Left) *H&E shows a fibrin thrombus with evidence of organization with granulation tissue. Relatively little acute inflammation and absence of bacterial colonies may be noted because of antibiotic treatment.* **(Right)** *Gram stain shows numerous gram-positive cocci. Identification of bacteria in sampled valvular tissue is important for diagnosis and management of patients with infective endocarditis.*

Microscopic Features of Infective Endocarditis

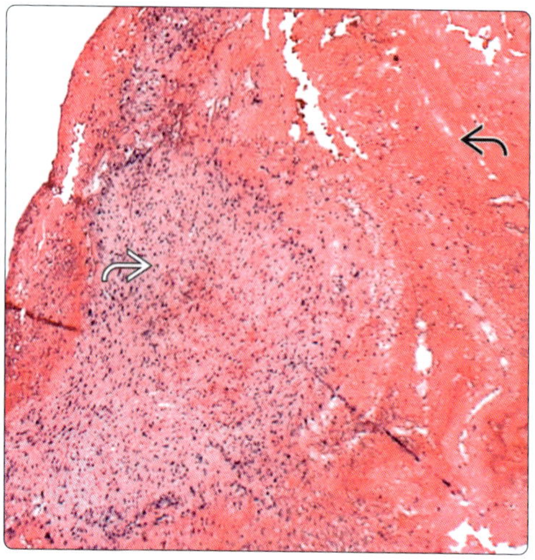

Microscopic Features of Infective Endocarditis: Gram Stain

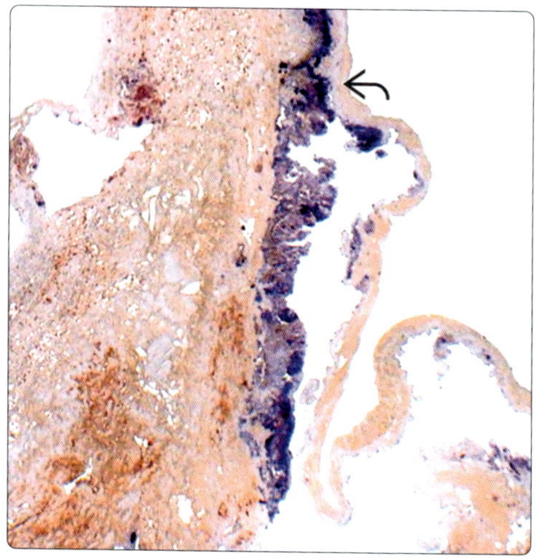

(Left) *H&E shows recent thrombus admixed with numerous fungal elements.* **(Right)** *GMS shows numerous fungal elements. In a case of fungal endocarditis, fungi are uncommon microorganisms causing endocarditis but can occur in immunosuppressed patients.*

Microscopic Features of Fungal Endocarditis

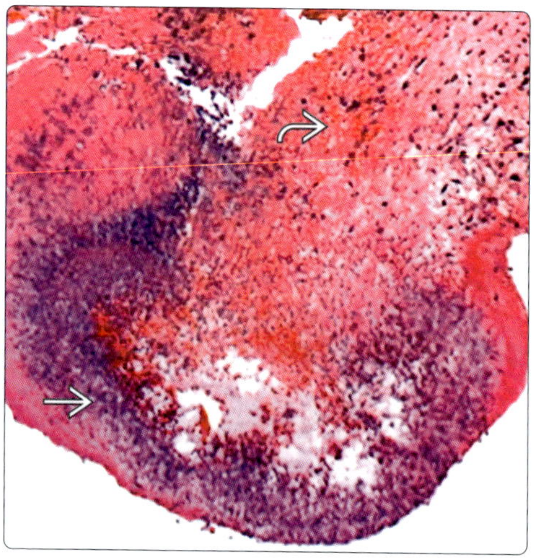

Microscopic Features of Fungal Endocarditis

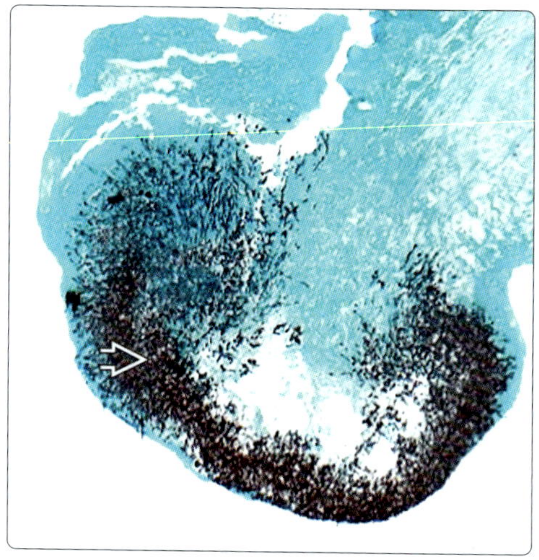

(Left) *Gross photograph of mitral leaflet shows severe preexisting rheumatic disease with superimposed infective endocarditis (vegetation and perforation). Damaged valves are a risk factor for development of endocarditis.* **(Right)** *Gross photograph of aortic valve shows changes consistent with "healed" endocarditis. There is marked rubbery thickening, cusp perforation, and erosion of remaining leaflets. No fleshy vegetations are seen.*

Mitral Valve Involved by Infective Endocarditis

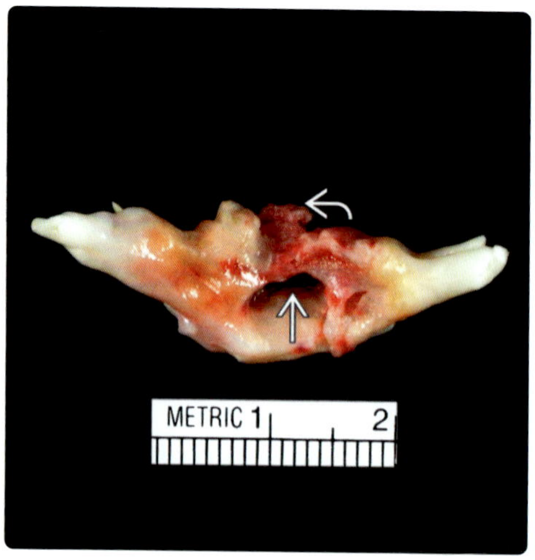

Aortic Valve Involved by Infective Endocarditis

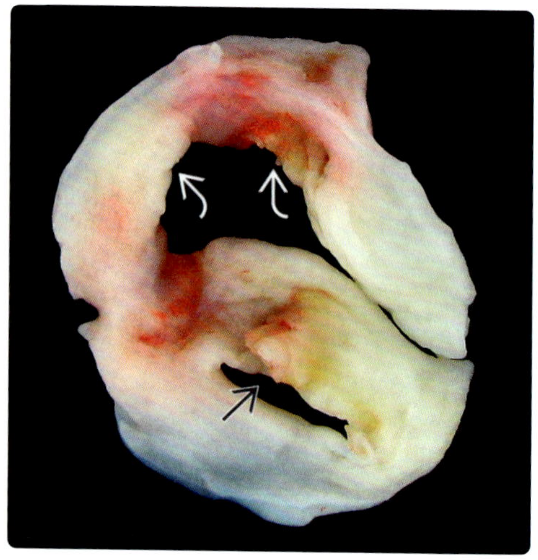

Mitral Valve Endocarditis

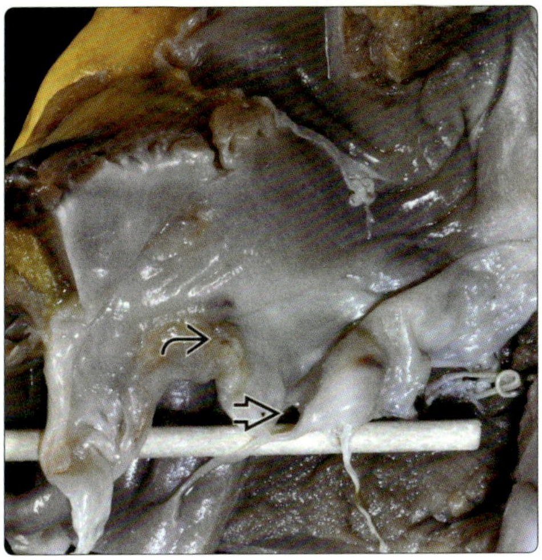

Aortic Valve Endocarditis

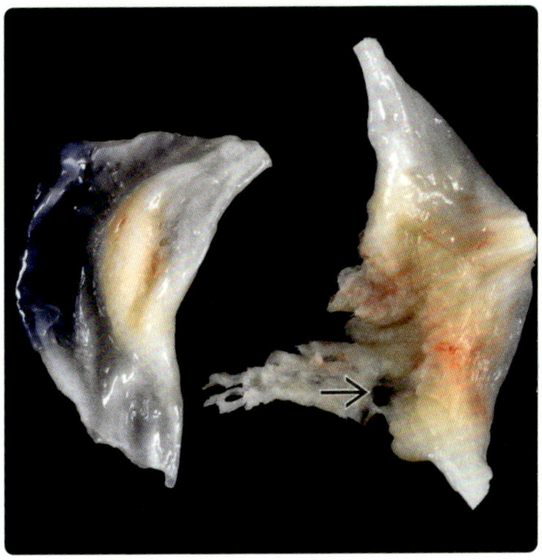

(Left) *Autopsy specimen shows mitral valve with thickened and shortened leaflets with vegetation ⇨ placed at the edge of the retracted leaflet on atrial surface. Prior valve damage is a risk factor for endocarditis. One leaflet shows a perforation ➩.* **(Right)** *Gross photograph of aortic valve shows cusp involved by bacterial endocarditis causing destruction of the tissue with cusp perforation →.*

Tricuspid Valve Involved by Infective Endocarditis

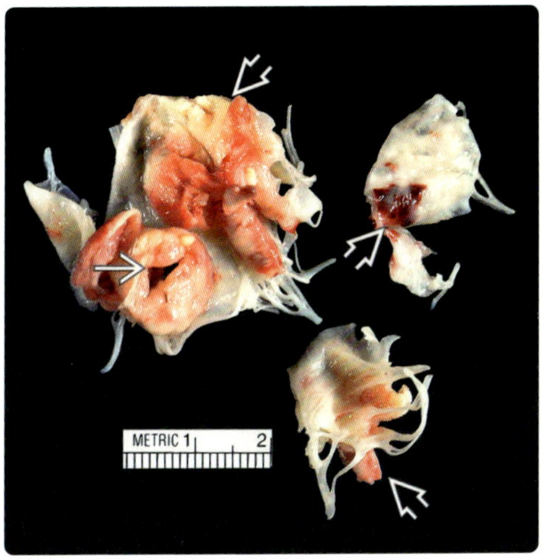

Tricuspid Valve Involved by Infective Endocarditis

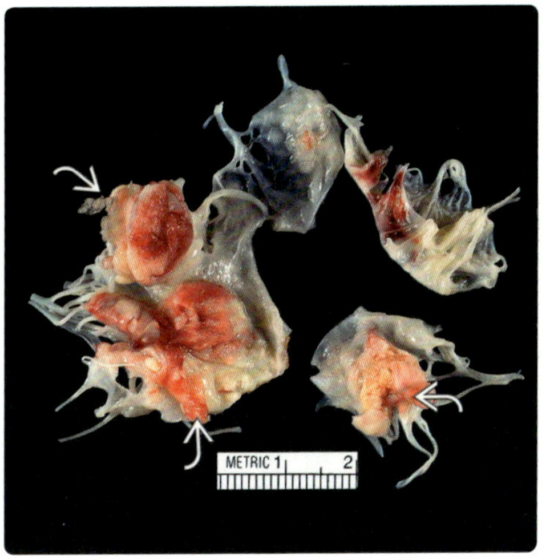

(Left) *Gross photograph of tricuspid valve shows vegetations involving multiple leaflets ➩ and one with associated cusp perforation →.* **(Right)** *Gross photograph of tricuspid leaflet shows large bulky exophytic vegetations → in a case of Candida endocarditis. Right-sided endocarditis is most commonly seen in intravenous drug abusers.*

Aortic Valve Involved by Infective Endocarditis

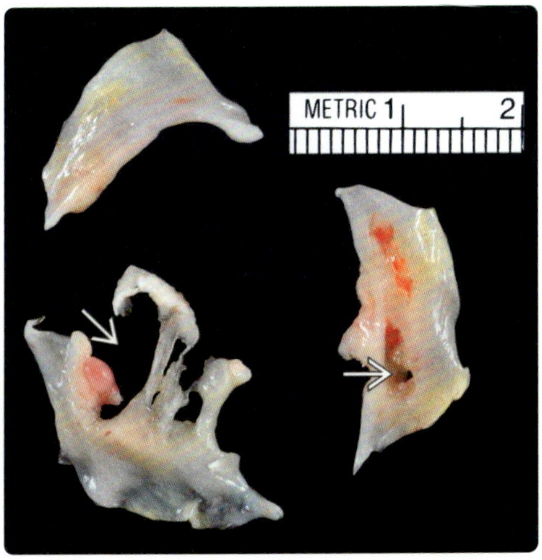

Special Stain of Vegetation

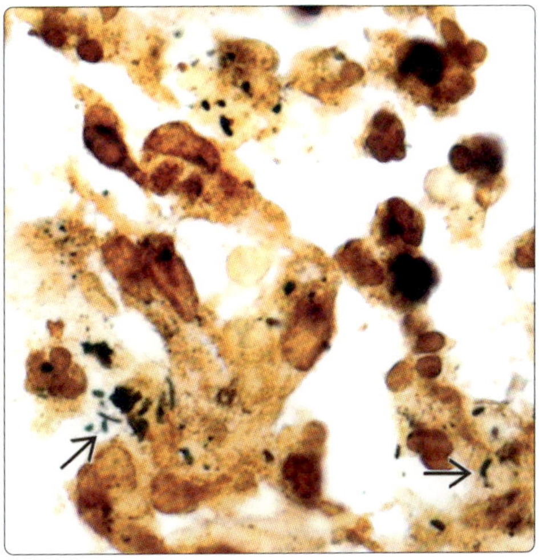

(Left) *Gross photograph of native aortic valve shows subacute infective endocarditis, without vegetations, but with several cusp perforations →.* **(Right)** *In some cases, a silver stain (such as Warthin-Starry or Steiner) may reveal the presence of microbes → when other techniques (Gram and GMS) are negative. This is especially true for syphilis and HACEK organisms.*

Nonbacterial Thrombotic Endocarditis

KEY FACTS

TERMINOLOGY

- Disease characterized by presence of vegetations on cardiac valves, which consist of fibrin and platelet aggregates and are devoid of inflammation or bacteria

ETIOLOGY/PATHOGENESIS

- Association with
  - Neoplastic diseases
  - Autoimmune diseases
  - Valvular diseases

CLINICAL ISSUES

- In ~ 1.2% of all autopsies, vegetations caused by nonbacterial thrombotic endocarditis (NBTE) may be found, although reported incidence of NBTE ranges 0.3-9.3%
- Most commonly affects patients from 4th-8th decades, though all age groups can be affected

MACROSCOPIC

- Lesions usually affect mitral and aortic valves, although all valves can be involved
- Vegetations occur on contact margins of valve leaflets, which can be normal or previously damaged
- Classification
  - Type 1: Small (< 3 mm), univerrucal, firmly attached to valve
  - Type 2: Large (> 3 mm), univerrucal, adherent to valve
  - Type 3: Small (< 3 mm), multiverrucal, friable
  - Type 4: Large (> 3 mm), multiverrucal, friable
- Type 5: Healed type, similar in consistency to attached valve

MICROSCOPIC

- Lesions are described as agglutinated blood and platelet thrombi with absence of inflammatory reaction
- Superficial and underlying valve tissue may be normal or show histologic evidence of abnormal collagen and elastic fibers

Gross Photograph of Nonbacterial Thrombotic Vegetations

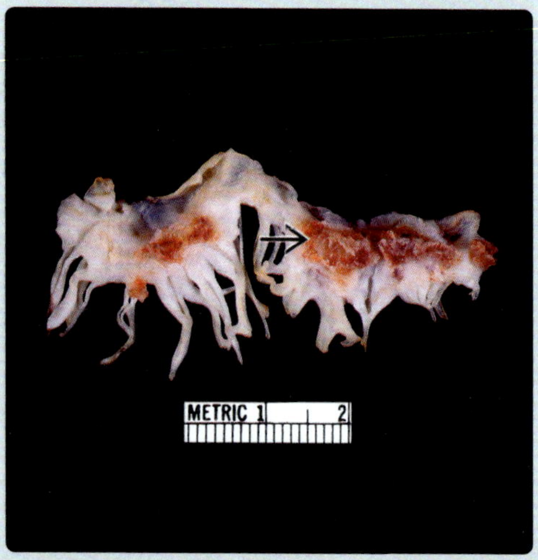

Histology of Nonbacterial Thrombotic Vegetations

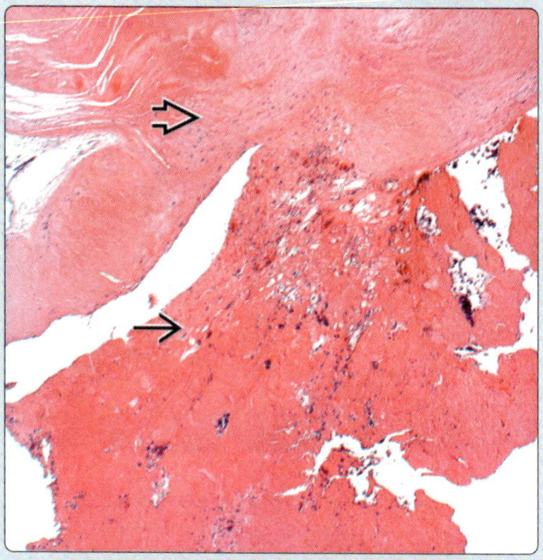

(Left) *Gross photograph shows nonbacterial thrombotic vegetations on the atrial surface of the mitral valve. They appear as small, granular, red lesions; significant abnormalities are not seen in the leaflets.* **(Right)** *H&E of a mitral valve shows superficial vegetations composed of platelets and fibrin with an underlying normal valve leaflet. Inflammatory cells are not prominent.*

Gross Photograph of Mitral Valve Involved by Nonbacterial Thrombotic Endocarditis

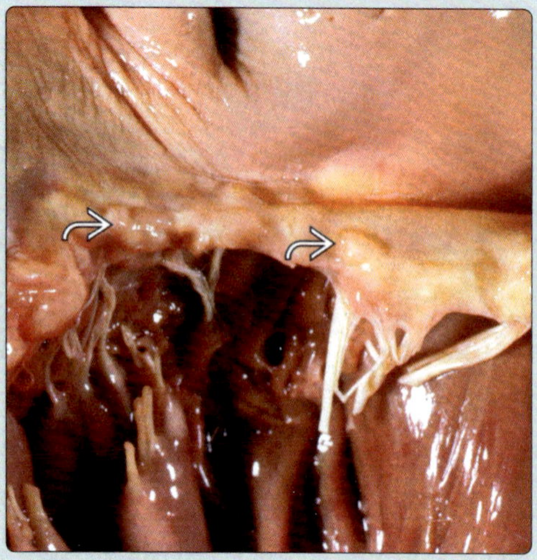

Histology of Nonbacterial Thrombotic Vegetations

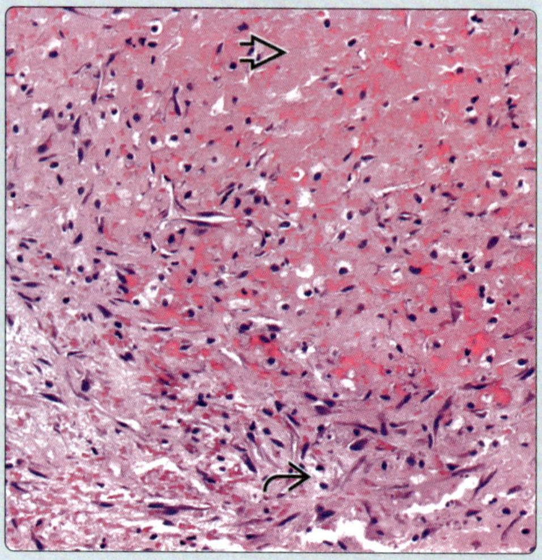

(Left) *Gross photograph of an autopsy specimen shows nonbacterial thrombotic vegetations on the atrial surface of the mitral valve. They appear as small, granular lesions; the leaflets are thickened and shortened due to prior rheumatic heart disease.* **(Right)** *H&E at higher magnification shows vegetation composed predominantly of fibrin without significant inflammatory cell reaction. There is evidence of early organization toward the vegetation base.*

Nonbacterial Thrombotic Endocarditis

TERMINOLOGY

Abbreviations

- Nonbacterial thrombotic endocarditis (NBTE)

Synonyms

- Marantic endocarditis, terminal endocarditis, Libman-Sacks endocarditis

Definitions

- Disease characterized by presence of vegetations on cardiac valves, which consist of fibrin and platelet aggregates and are devoid of inflammation or bacteria

ETIOLOGY/PATHOGENESIS

Associations

- Neoplastic diseases
  - Malignancies of lung, ovary, biliary system, pancreas, and stomach
- Autoimmune diseases
  - Systemic lupus erythematosus (SLE), antiphospholipid syndrome (APS)
- Hypercoagulable state
  - Sepsis, burns

CLINICAL ISSUES

Epidemiology

- Incidence
  - Vegetations caused by NBTE may be found in ~ 1.2% of all autopsies, although reported incidence of NBTE ranges 0.3-9.3%
    - 4% of all end-stage cancer patients
    - 11% in SLE patients
- Age
  - Most commonly affects patients from 4th-8th decades, though all age groups can be affected

Presentation

- No typical presentation; however, usually contains triad of
  - Disease processes known to be associated with NBTE
  - Presence of heart murmur
  - Evidence of multiple systemic emboli
- Also helpful in establishing diagnosis of NBTE
  - Venous thrombosis
  - Laboratory diagnosis of disseminated intravascular coagulation
    - Serial negative blood cultures (to exclude infective endocarditis)

Laboratory Tests

- Full blood count, prothrombin time, partial thromboplastin time, fibrinogen, thrombin time, D-dimers and cross-linked fibrin degradation products

Treatment

- Surgical approaches
  - Recommended in following settings
    - Presence of severe valvular dysfunction and large vegetations
    - Recurrence of embolic events despite adequate anticoagulation
    - Uncertainty regarding diagnosis and etiology
- Drugs
  - Anticoagulants: Low-molecular-weight heparin or warfarin to reduce risk of systemic embolism

Prognosis

- Even with established diagnosis, treatment is difficult
- Correction of underlying cause is important

IMAGING

MR Findings

- Head: Stroke pattern is multiple lesions that are small, medium, or large as well as disseminated lesions
- Cardiac: In case of aortic valve, delineated vegetations appear as areas of low signal at valve leaflets in contrast to bright, flowing blood in case of mitral valve vegetations

Echocardiography

- Vegetations are typically small (< 1 cm in diameter), broad based, and irregular in shape
- Usually localized in coaptation lines of valve without destruction of valvular tissue

MACROSCOPIC

General Features

- Lesions usually affect mitral and aortic valves, although all valves can be involved
- Vegetations occur on contact margins of valve leaflets, which can be normal or previously damaged
- Classification
  - Type 1: Small (< 3 mm), univerrucal, firmly attached to valve
  - Type 2: Large (> 3 mm), univerrucal, adherent to valve
  - Type 3: Small (< 3 mm), multiverrucal, friable
  - Type 4: Large (> 3 mm), multiverrucal, friable
  - Type 5: Healed, similar in consistency to attached valve

MICROSCOPIC

Histologic Features

- Lesions are described as agglutinated blood, fibrin, and platelet thrombi with absence of inflammatory reaction
- Superficial and underlying valve tissue may be normal or show histologic evidence of abnormal collagen and elastic fibers

DIFFERENTIAL DIAGNOSIS

Infective Endocarditis

- Presence of clinical signs of infection
- Vegetations with underlying leaflet destruction
- Histologically, composed of thrombus mixed with acute inflammatory cells and bacterial colonies

SELECTED REFERENCES

1. Quintero-Martinez JA et al: Contemporary demographics, diagnostics and outcomes in non-bacterial thrombotic endocarditis. Heart. ePub, 2022
2. Zmaili MA et al: A contemporary 20-year Cleveland Clinic experience of nonbacterial thrombotic endocarditis: etiology, echocardiographic imaging, management, and outcomes. Am J Med. 134(3):361-9, 2021
3. Hurrell H et al: Non-infective endocarditis. Heart. 106(13):1023-9, 2020

(Left) *Gross photograph of the aortic valve examined from the ventricular surface demonstrates small vegetations localized on the anterior aspect of valve cusps toward contact margins. The vegetations show a red, granular appearance. There is neither significant thickening of the valve cusps nor calcification.* **(Right)** *Gross photograph of a mitral valve shows multiple small vegetations along the free margin of the valve leaflets. The chordae are shortened and thickened, indicating a postinflammatory state.*

Gross Photograph of Aortic Valve With Nonbacterial Thrombotic Vegetations

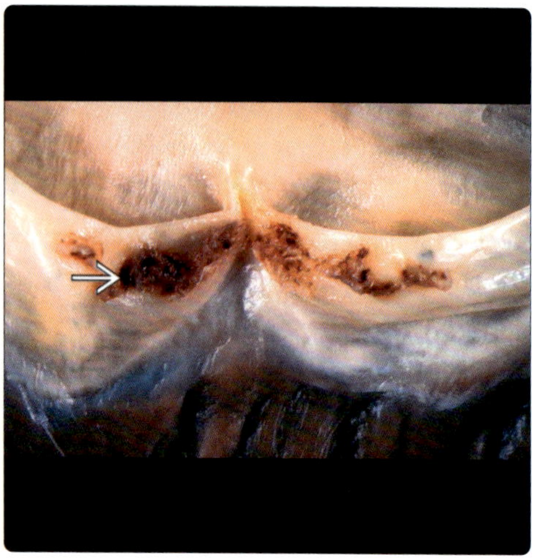

Gross Photograph of Mitral Valve With Nonbacterial Thrombotic Vegetations

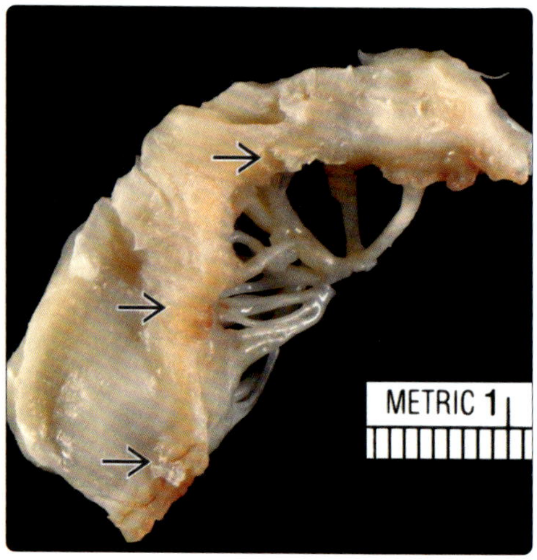

(Left) *H&E of an aortic valve leaflet shows vegetations composed predominantly of fibrin localized on the surface. Embolization to the brain is one of the most common complications in these patients with nonbacterial thrombotic endocarditis (NBTE).* **(Right)** *H&E of an aortic valve at higher magnification shows vegetations composed of fibrin and platelets with evidence of organization with underlying fibrosis.*

Histology of Nonbacterial Thrombotic Vegetations

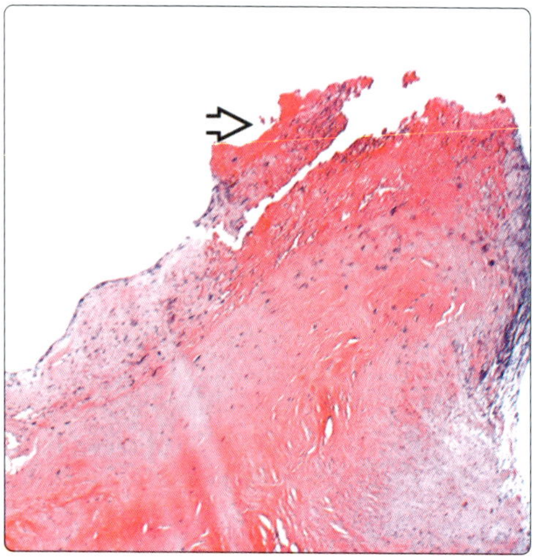

Histology of Aortic Valve With Nonbacterial Thrombotic Vegetations

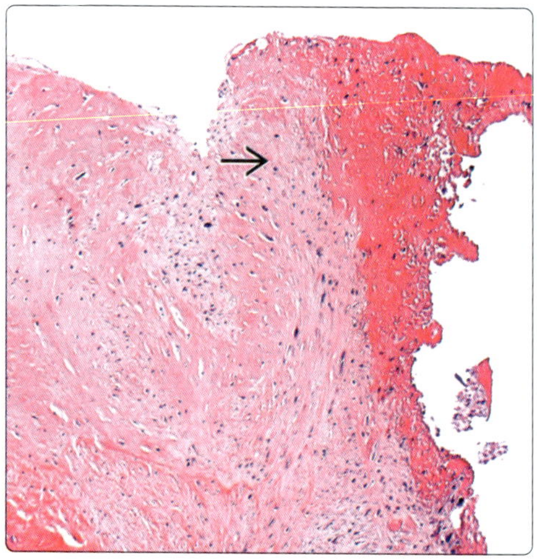

(Left) *H&E of a mitral valve shows a large, bland vegetation composed of fibrin and red cells attached to an intact underlying valve leaflet. At this power, it is not possible to identify inflammatory cells, but fibrosis or calcification in the valve leaflet is not noted.* **(Right)** *Trichrome stain of a mitral valve shows a bland thrombus composed of fibrin and red cells attached to an intact underlying valve leaflet.*

Histology of Mitral Valve With Nonbacterial Thrombotic Vegetations

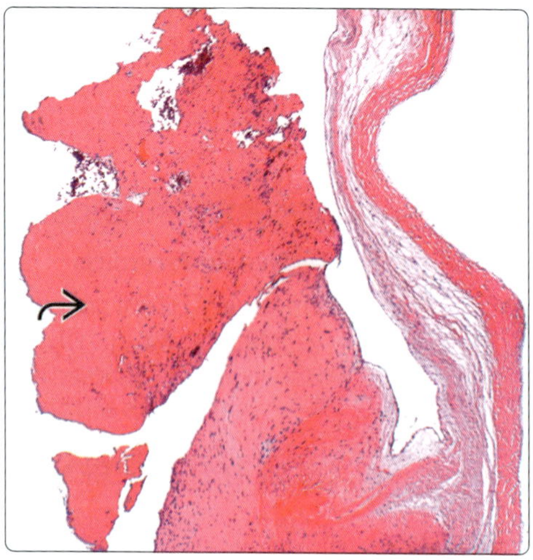

Trichrome Stain of Nonbacterial Thrombotic Vegetations

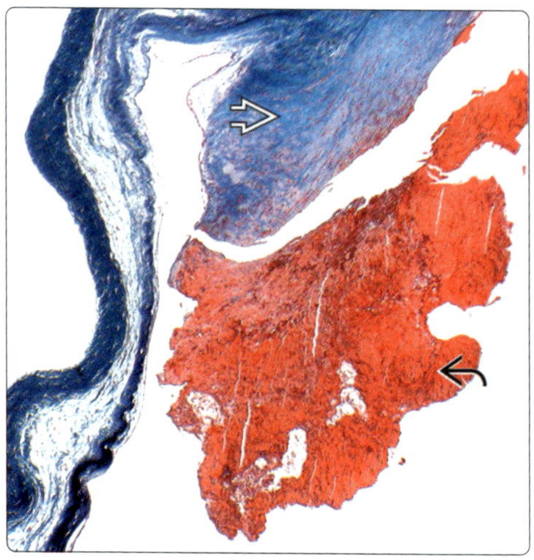

Trichrome Stain of Nonbacterial Thrombotic Vegetations

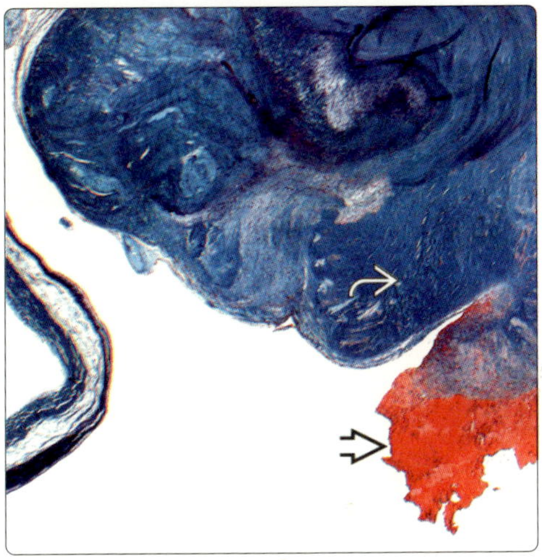

Trichrome Stain of Nonbacterial Thrombotic Vegetations

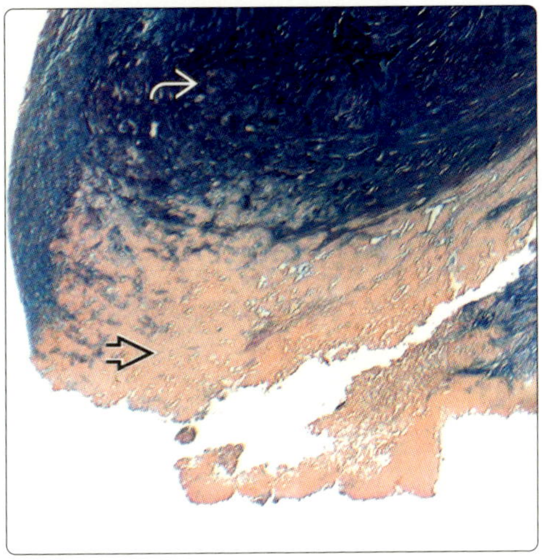

(Left) *Trichrome stain of a mitral valve shows a bland thrombus ⇨ composed of fibrin and red cells attached to an underlying valve leaflet ↪. There is thickening and fibrosis of the leaflet, which indicates a prior inflammatory process. Abnormal valves are at increased risk of developing NBTE.* **(Right)** *Trichrome stain of a heart valve at high magnification shows a thrombus ⇨ composed of fibrin and red cells attached to an underlying valve leaflet ↪.*

Histology of Nonbacterial Thrombotic Vegetations

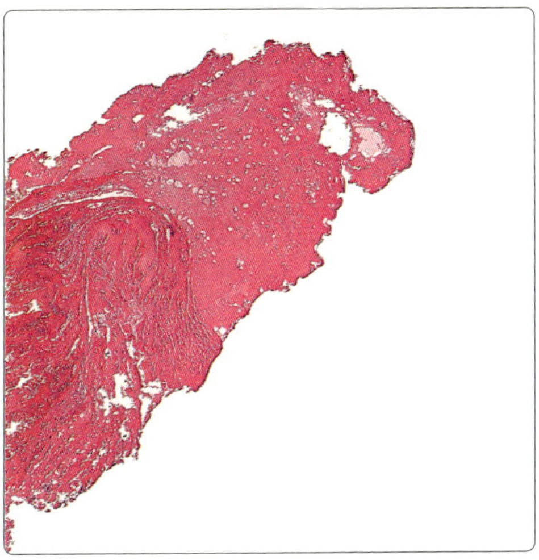

Elastic Stain of Nonbacterial Thrombotic Vegetations

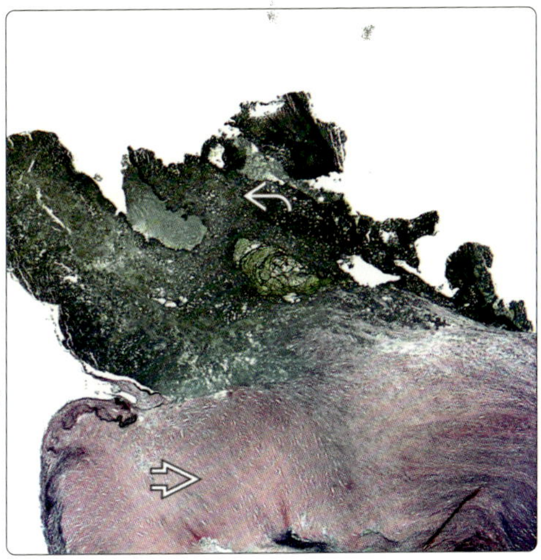

(Left) *H&E shows a bland vegetation composed predominantly of fibrin and platelets with the absence of inflammatory cells.* **(Right)** *Elastic stain of a heart valve shows a vegetation ↪ attached to the valve surface composed of fibrin and red cells, which is in turn attached to an intact underlying valve leaflet ⇨. Changes in elastic fibers are not seen.*

Histology of Nonbacterial Thrombotic Vegetations

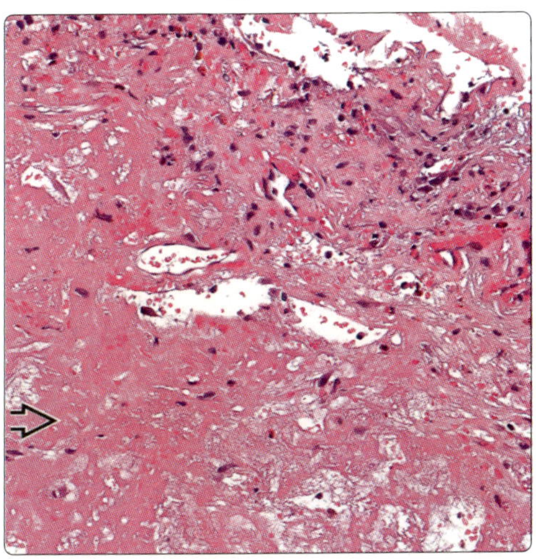

Gram Stain of Nonbacterial Thrombotic Vegetations

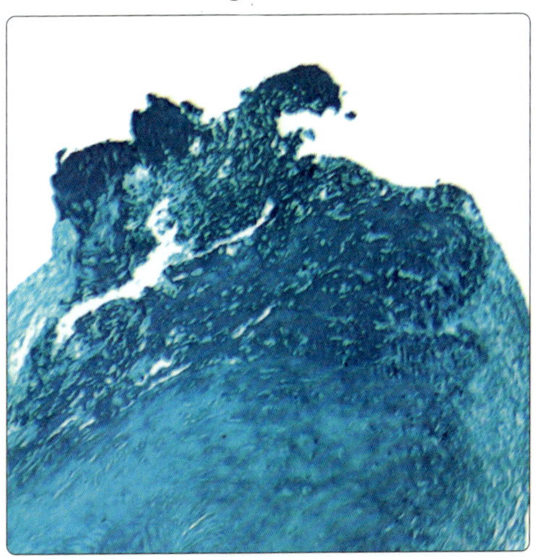

(Left) *H&E at higher magnification shows vegetation composed predominantly of fibrin ⇨ without significant inflammatory cell reaction in a case of NBTE.* **(Right)** *Gram stain should be used as an ancillary test in cases of NBTE to rule out bacterial infection. In this section, no bacteria are identified, which supports noninfectious etiology.*

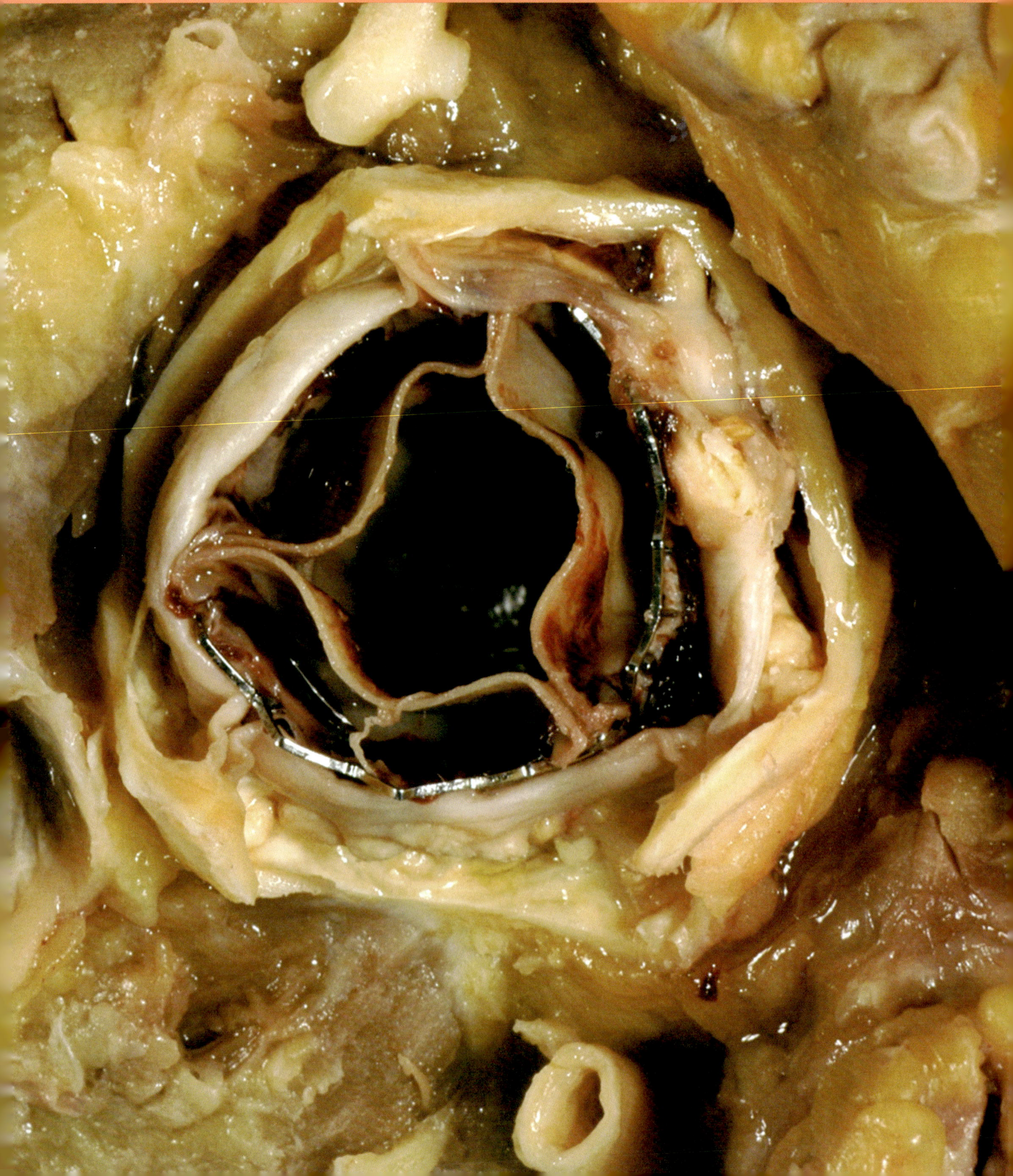

SECTION 5

Cardiac Valves

Prosthetic

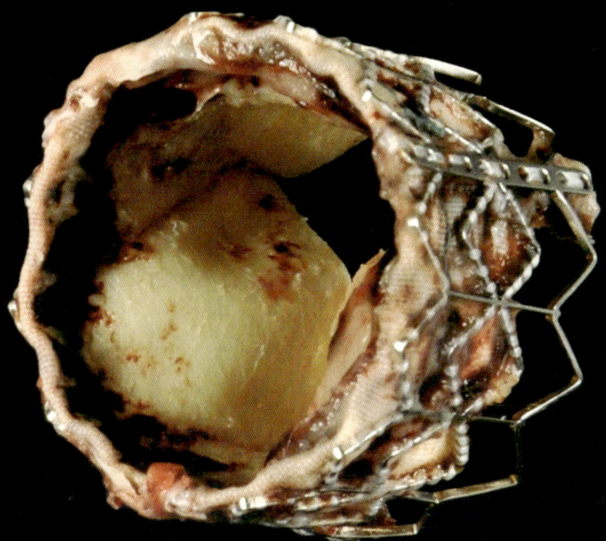

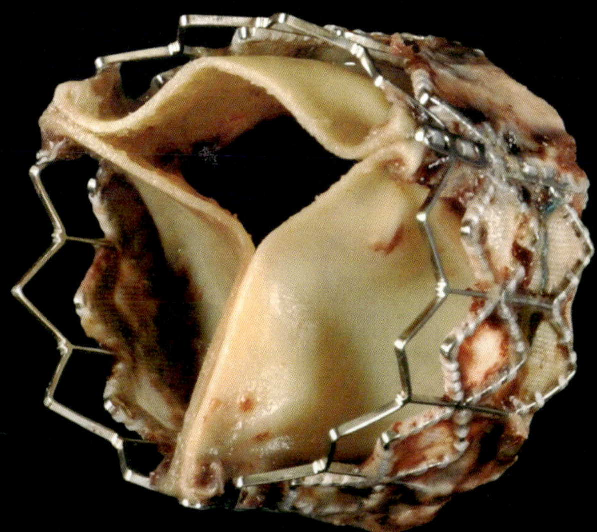

Leaflet Degeneration, Prosthetic Valves

KEY FACTS

TERMINOLOGY

- Major complication affecting bioprosthetic valves with calcification &/or tearing causing secondary valve dysfunction

ETIOLOGY/PATHOGENESIS

- Patient age
- Mechanical stress risk factors: Mitral position, hypertension

CLINICAL ISSUES

- Gradual onset of shortness of breath and other symptoms of heart failure is usual presentation
- Symptoms are related to valve dysfunction; stenosis or incompetence
- Reoperation and surgical replacement with another prosthetic valve is only effective treatment in patients with structural valve deterioration (SVD)
- Children and adolescents have highest rate of early primary tissue failure

IMAGING

- Severity of valve dysfunction can be evaluated by echocardiography or cardiac catheterization

MACROSCOPIC

- Thickening and disruption of cuspal tissue, sometimes associated with tears
- Calcification or calcified nodules can be felt when palpating cusps

MICROSCOPIC

- Cuspal tissue disruption
- Areas of calcification
- Pannus

DIAGNOSTIC CHECKLIST

- SVD is common complication occurring in bioprosthetic valves
- SVD more frequent when bioprosthesis is implanted in mitral, not aortic, position

Pericardial Bioprosthesis With Degenerative Changes (Flow Surface)

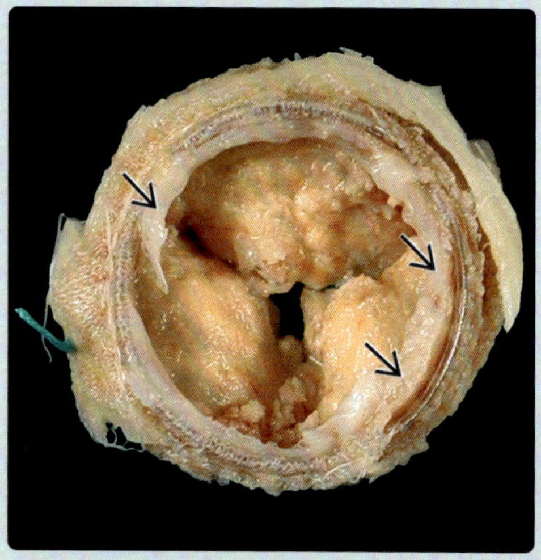

Pericardial Bioprosthesis With Degenerative Changes (Nonflow Surface)

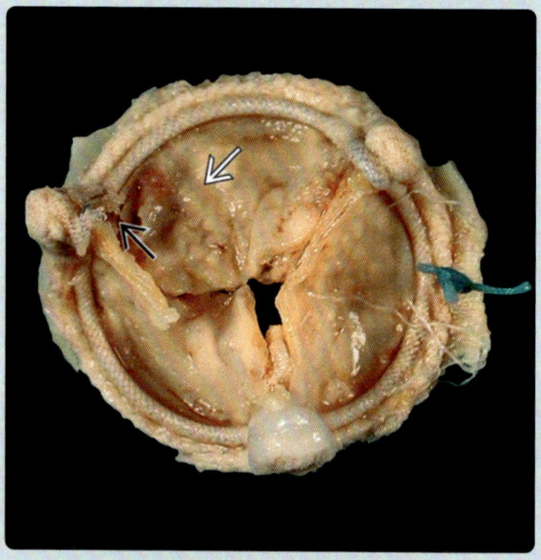

(Left) *Pericardial bioprosthesis 12 years post implantation shows severe tissue degeneration and pannus ⇨ on the flow surface of the sewing cuff and cusps.* **(Right)** *Pericardial bioprosthesis 12 years post implantation shows marked degenerative change with cusp calcification ➡ and cusp tears ⇨ on the nonflow surface, causing valve dysfunction.*

Degenerative Changes in Bioprosthetic Aorta Valve

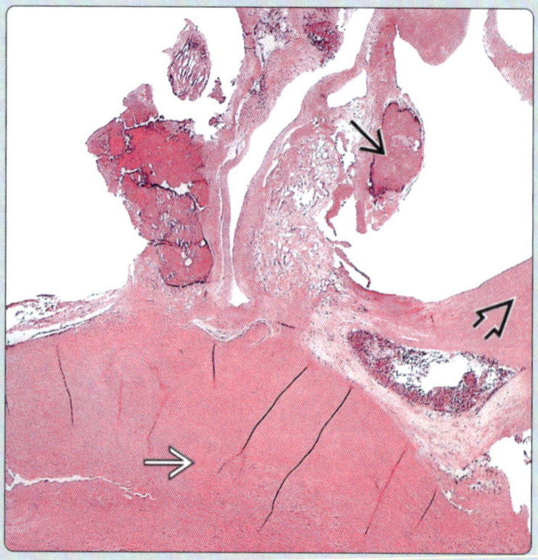

Bioprosthetic Aorta Valve With Degenerative Changes

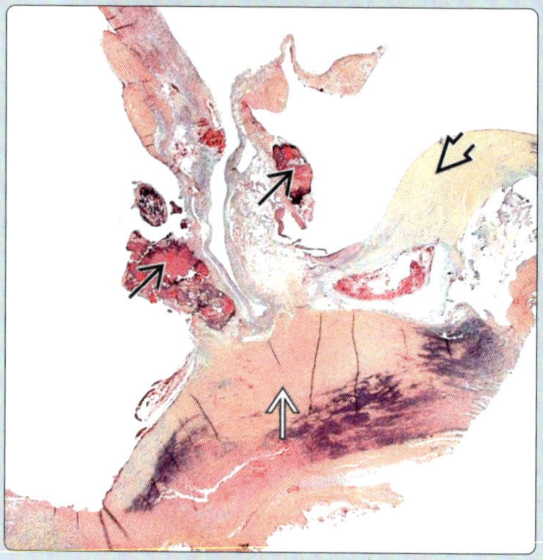

(Left) *H&E-stained section of a porcine prosthetic aortic valve ➡ at the commissure shows severe tissue degeneration and areas of cusp calcification ⇨ and pannus ⇨.* **(Right)** *Movat elastic-stained section of a porcine bioprosthesis removed from a stent shows porcine aorta ➡, commissural end of the 2 cusps with tissue degeneration, areas of calcification ⇨, and pannus ⇨.*

TERMINOLOGY

Synonyms

- Structural valve deterioration (SVD)

Definitions

- Major complication affecting bioprosthetic valves with calcification &/or tearing causing secondary valve dysfunction
  - All bioprosthetic valves regardless of method of implantation are susceptible to SVD

ETIOLOGY/PATHOGENESIS

Risk Factors

- Patient age
  - Younger patient is more likely to develop SVD
  - Likely related to more active immune system in young, causing more rapid tissue degeneration
- Comorbid illnesses
  - Atherosclerosis
    - Patients with diabetes, smoking, metabolic syndrome, and hypercholesterolemia more likely to develop SVD
    - Low-density lipoprotein oxidation may trigger inflammatory process
    - Inflammatory cytokines may induce osteoblastic differentiation of stem/progenitor cells that have colonized bioprosthetic tissue
  - Hypertension
    - Systemic hypertension accelerates tissue degeneration of aortic bioprosthesis
    - Due to chronically increased diastolic closure stress
  - Poor left ventricular function or left ventricular hypertrophy
  - Renal insufficiency
  - Hyperparathyroidism
- Mechanical stress
  - Mitral position
    - SVD is more frequent when bioprosthesis implanted in mitral, not aortic, position
    - Could be related to higher mechanical stress and closing pressures on leaflets during systole
  - Systemic hypertension
    - Causes chronic increase in diastolic closure stress of aortic bioprosthesis, thereby accelerating SVD
- Exposure to chemicals
  - Glutaraldehyde
    - Causes cell membrane damage in bioprosthetic tissue
    - Damaged tissue induces
      - Intracellular calcium influx
      - Residual phospholipids provide environment that leads to calcium crystal nucleation
      - Crystal growth leading to tearing or valve stenosis
- Size of bioprosthesis, especially when implanted in aortic position
  - Smaller valves are at higher risk of SVD
- Type of bioprosthesis
  - Newer generation of bioprostheses are more durable than older generation of models
  - Some reports suggest that pericardial valves might be more durable than porcine valves

CLINICAL ISSUES

Epidemiology

- Incidence
  - Rate of bioprosthesis failure
    - < 10% at 10 years in patients > 70 years of age
    - ~ 20-30% at 10 years in patients < 40 years of age
  - For porcine bioprostheses implanted in patients > 55 years of age
    - < 1% fail due to SVD within 5 years
    - 20-30% show degenerative changes within 10 years
    - > 50% fail because of primary tissue degeneration within 12-15 years post implantation

Presentation

- Gradual onset of shortness of breath and other symptoms of heart failure is usual presentation
- Very rarely, may be acute onset of heart failure symptoms
- Symptoms are related to valve dysfunction
  - Stenosis
  - Incompetence
- Valve regurgitation or stenosis can be detected by appropriate murmur on auscultation

Treatment

- Reoperation and surgical replacement with another prosthetic valve is only effective treatment for patients with SVD
- In pulmonary position, some patients may get short-term relief from endovascular deployment of stent within prosthetic valve
  - Likely followed by implantation of stentless bioprosthesis

Prognosis

- Children and adolescents have highest rate of early primary tissue failure
- Bioprosthetic heart valve failure occurs by 5 years in patients < 35 years old
- Only 10% of bioprosthetic heart valves fail within 10 years in patients > 65 years old

Complications

- Dehiscence of commissural insertion from strut
- Endocarditis
- Thrombosis

IMAGING

General Features

- Severity of valve dysfunction can be evaluated by echocardiography or cardiac catheterization

Radiographic Findings

- Chest radiography may show calcification of prosthetic valve cusps

CT Findings

- Abnormal mobility of prosthetic valve cusps can be detected
- CT density
  - Thrombus shows lower CT density
  - Pannus shows higher CT density

- Disruption of prosthetic valve leaflets can be identified
- Dehiscence can be seen
- Coexisting valvular regurgitation or stenosis

Echocardiographic Findings

- Transesophageal echocardiogram is better than transthoracic for evaluation of etiology of valve dysfunction, particularly for mitral valve prosthesis
- Presence of thrombus or pannus
  - Eccentric inflow pattern may be seen due to leaflet motion impairment
  - Thrombus shows low echogenicity
  - Pannus shows higher echogenicity
- Regurgitation or stenosis may be identified
- Paravalvular leakage
  - Eccentric Doppler jet (half-moon or sickle-shaped)

MACROSCOPIC

General Features

- Thickening and disruption of cuspal tissue, sometimes associated with tears
- Cuspal tissue disruption (tears) may occur at
  - Free margin
  - Crescentic tears at bases of sinus
  - Irregular tears in center of valve cusp
  - Multiple small perforations
- Calcification or calcified nodules can be felt when palpating cusps
- Leaflets can appear firm and stiff with little or no mobility
- Tissue overgrowth (pannus) may be seen around sewing ring or leaflets base
- Thrombi and vegetations can complicate SVD

MICROSCOPIC

Histologic Features

- Areas of calcification can be seen
  - In leaflets along tears or away from these areas
- Few macrophages can be identified, particularly around calcified areas
- Pannus
- Lipid insudation

DIFFERENTIAL DIAGNOSIS

Prosthetic Valve Thrombosis

- Often clinically asymptomatic
- Thrombi are composed of platelets, red blood cells, white blood cells, and fibrin in variable proportions
- SVD may predispose to thrombus formation

Prosthetic Valve Endocarditis

- Fever and thromboembolic episodes common initial clinical presentation
- Prosthesis-tissue interface is site most frequently involved
- Endocarditis may complicate SVD
- Ring abscess may occur

DIAGNOSTIC CHECKLIST

Clinically Relevant Pathologic Features

- SVD is common complication occurring in bioprosthetic valves
- Children and adolescents have highest rate of early primary tissue failure
- SVD more frequent when bioprosthesis is implanted in mitral, not aortic, position

Pathologic Interpretation Pearls

- SVD is most common complication occurring in bioprosthetic valves; characterized by
  - Tissue disruption
  - Calcification
  - Pannus

SELECTED REFERENCES

1. Cahill TJ et al: Valve thrombosis after transcatheter and surgical aortic valve replacement: incidence and outcomes. J Thorac Cardiovasc Surg. 163(4):1309-15, 2022
2. Carlson S et al: Multimodality imaging for prosthetic valves evaluation: current understanding and future directions. Prog Cardiovasc Dis. 72:66-77, 2022
3. Case BC et al: Early leaflet thickening, durability and bioprosthetic valve failure in TAVR. Interv Cardiol Clin. 10(4):531-9, 2021
4. Khan JM et al: Anatomical characteristics associated with hypoattenuated leaflet thickening in low-risk patients undergoing transcatheter aortic valve replacement. Cardiovasc Revasc Med. 27:1-6, 2021
5. Kwiecinski J et al: Native aortic valve disease progression and bioprosthetic valve degeneration in patients with transcatheter aortic valve implantation. Circulation. 144(17):1396-408, 2021
6. Marro M et al: Noncalcific mechanisms of bioprosthetic structural valve degeneration. J Am Heart Assoc. 10(3):e018921, 2021
7. Sellers SL et al: Transcatheter aortic heart valves: histological analysis providing insight to leaflet thickening and structural valve degeneration. JACC Cardiovasc Imaging. 12(1):135-45, 2019
8. Cremer PC et al: Early bioprosthetic valve failure: a pictorial review of rare causes. JACC Cardiovasc Imaging. 8(6):737-40, 2015
9. Cremer PC et al: Early bioprosthetic valve failure: mechanistic insights via correlation between echocardiographic and operative findings. J Am Soc Echocardiogr. 28(10):1131-48, 2015
10. Luk A et al: Pathologic evaluation of 28 mitroflow pericardial valves: a 12-year experience. Ann Thorac Surg. 99(1):48-54, 2015
11. Joshi V et al: Early prosthetic valve degeneration with Mitroflow aortic valves: determination of incidence and risk factors†. Interact Cardiovasc Thorac Surg. 19(1):36-40, 2014
12. Saleeb SF et al: Accelerated degeneration of a bovine pericardial bioprosthetic aortic valve in children and young adults. Circulation. 130(1):51-60, 2014
13. Grunkemeier GL et al: Durability of pericardial versus porcine bioprosthetic heart valves. J Thorac Cardiovasc Surg. 144(6):1381-6, 2012
14. Nair V et al: Characterizing the inflammatory reaction in explanted Medtronic Freestyle stentless porcine aortic bioprosthesis over a 6-year period. Cardiovasc Pathol. 21(3):158-68, 2012
15. Butany J et al: Modes of failure in explanted mitroflow pericardial valves. Ann Thorac Surg. 92(5):1621-7, 2011
16. Khan NA et al: Morphological changes in porcine bioprosthetic valves of a HeartMate left ventricular assist device. Can J Cardiol. 26(7):e270-2, 2010
17. Khan NA et al: Mitral valve-sparing procedures and prosthetic heart valve failure: a case report. Can J Cardiol. 25(3):e86-8, 2009
18. Pibarot P et al: Prosthetic heart valves: selection of the optimal prosthesis and long-term management. Circulation. 119(7):1034-48, 2009
19. Shetty R et al: Lipid-mediated inflammation and degeneration of bioprosthetic heart valves. Eur J Clin Invest. 39(6):471-80, 2009
20. Siddiqui RF et al: Bioprosthetic heart valves: modes of failure. Histopathology. 55(2):135-44, 2009
21. Butany J et al: Early changes in bioprosthetic heart valves following ventricular assist device implantation. Int J Cardiol. 117(1):e20-3, 2007
22. Butany JW et al: The role of pannus in the longevity of an Ionescu-Shiley pericardial bioprosthesis. J Card Surg. 21(5):505-7, 2006
23. Butany J et al: Analysis of prosthetic cardiac devices: a guide for the practising pathologist. J Clin Pathol. 58(2):113-24, 2005

Flow Surface of Porcine Bioprosthesis With Degenerative Changes

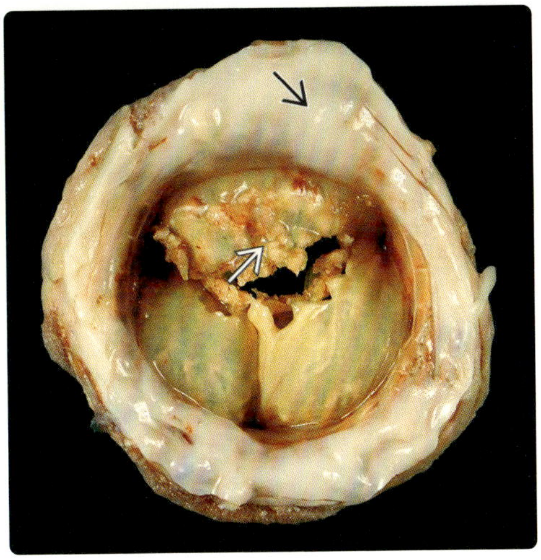

Nonflow Surface of Porcine Bioprosthesis With Degenerative Changes

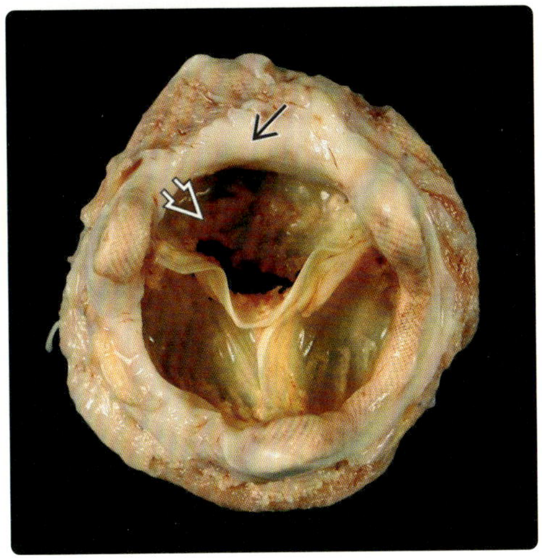

(Left) *Porcine bioprosthesis (flow surface) shows tissue degeneration with cusp tears, calcification ➡, and pannus ⇨. These changes made the valve significantly dysfunctional, likely both stenotic and incompetent.* **(Right)** *Porcine bioprosthesis (nonflow surface) 9 years post implantation shows significant degenerative changes with cusp tears and pannus ⇨. Extensive calcification is also present ➡, especially involving the valve cusps.*

Flow Surface of Porcine Bioprosthesis With Degenerative Changes

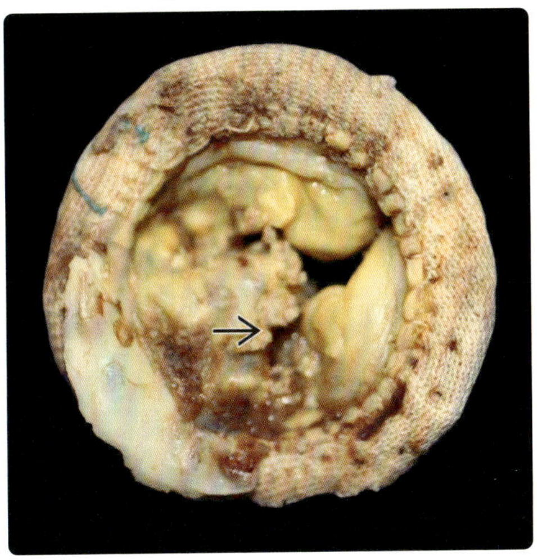

Nonflow Surface of Porcine Bioprosthesis With Degenerative Changes

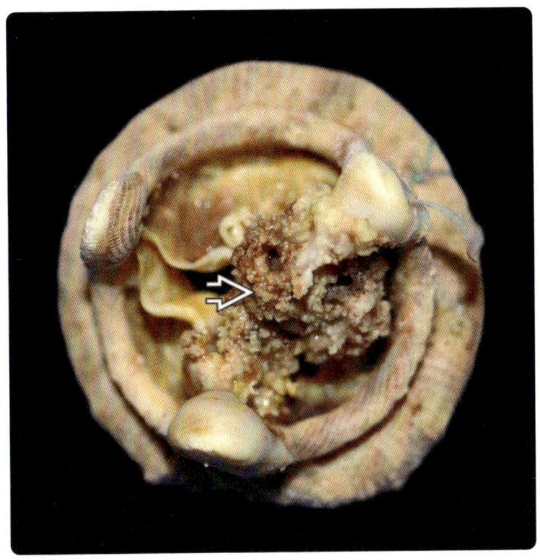

(Left) *Porcine bioprosthesis (flow surface) 12 years post implantation shows tissue degeneration with cusps calcification ⇨. These changes made the valve significantly dysfunctional.* **(Right)** *Porcine bioprosthesis (nonflow surface) 12 years post implantation shows significant degenerative changes with extensive calcification, especially involving the valve cusps and stents with cusps fusion ➡.*

Bioprosthetic Valve With Degenerative Changes

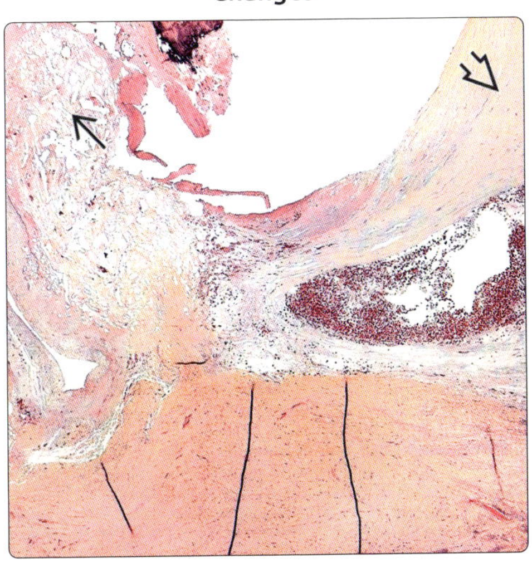

Bioprosthetic Valve With Degenerative Changes

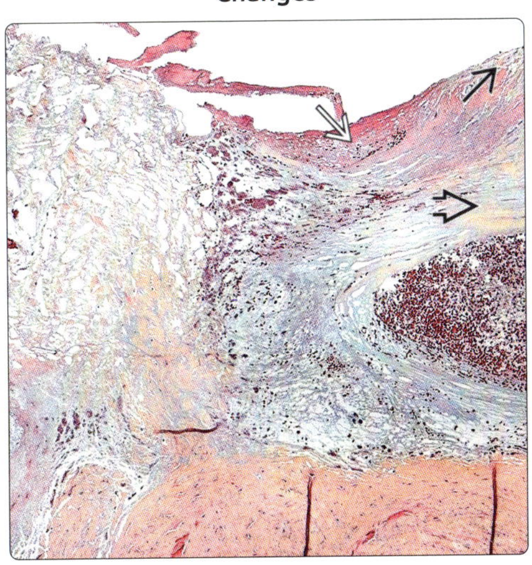

(Left) *High-magnification of porcine prosthetic valve cusp at the commissure shows tissue degeneration ⇨, calcification, organized thrombus, and pannus ⇨.* **(Right)** *Higher magnification elastin stain of porcine bioprosthetic valve cusp shows degeneration, areas of organized thrombus ⇨, recent thrombus with capillaries ➡, and pannus ⇨.*

Thrombosis of Prosthetic Valves

KEY FACTS

TERMINOLOGY

- Complication occurring after prosthetic valve placement, most commonly caused by inadequate anticoagulation

ETIOLOGY/PATHOGENESIS

- Inadequate anticoagulation therapy, especially during first 3 months post implantation
- Hemodynamic factors
  - Thrombosis is associated with altered blood flow in otherwise normal individual
  - Mitral location of prosthesis
  - Some porcine bioprosthetic valves have 1 cusp smaller than other 2
- Tissue degeneration of bioprosthetic valve

CLINICAL ISSUES

- Asymptomatic (typical presentation)
- Heparin IV should start immediately following confirmation by echocardiogram
- Surgical therapy for valve obstruction is associated with ~ 15% mortality
- Thrombolytic therapy should be assigned mainly to patients whose operative risk is high

IMAGING

- Doppler echocardiogram may demonstrate
  - Increased transvalvular pressure gradient
  - Reduced orifice area
  - Valvular regurgitation

MACROSCOPIC

- Laminated thrombi indicate rapid arterial blood flow at site of thrombus

MICROSCOPIC

- Laminated appearance; characterized by
  - Pale areas containing degranulated platelets and fibrin
  - Darker areas containing red blood cells, white blood cells, platelets, and fibrin

Mechanical Prosthetic Valve Thrombosis

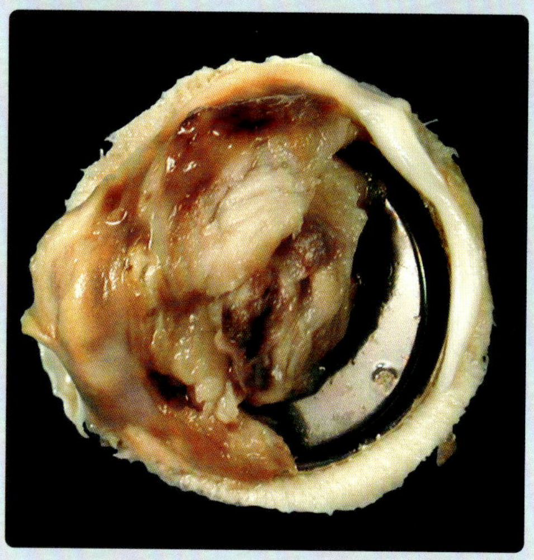

Thrombus: Histology

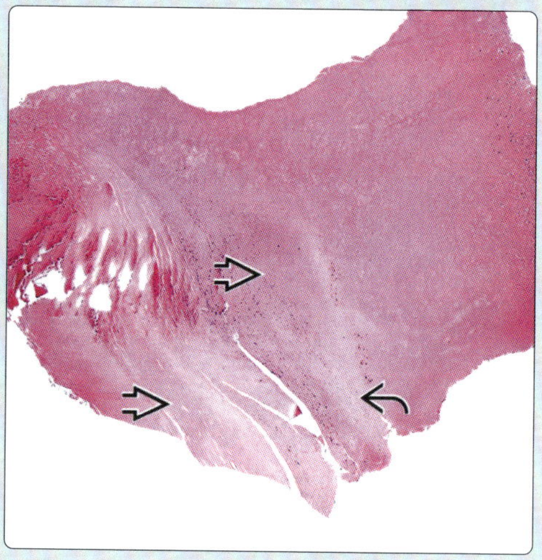

(Left) *Gross photograph of a single-leaflet mechanical valve, 18 years post implantation, shows a large thrombus with layered yellow to brown to black areas, which has "frozen" the disc in a partially open position.* **(Right)** *H&E-stained section shows a large laminated thrombus obtained from a prosthetic heart valve, showing pale areas (fibrin rich) ➔ alternating with other darker areas (red cell rich) ➔.*

Early Thrombus: Movat Stain

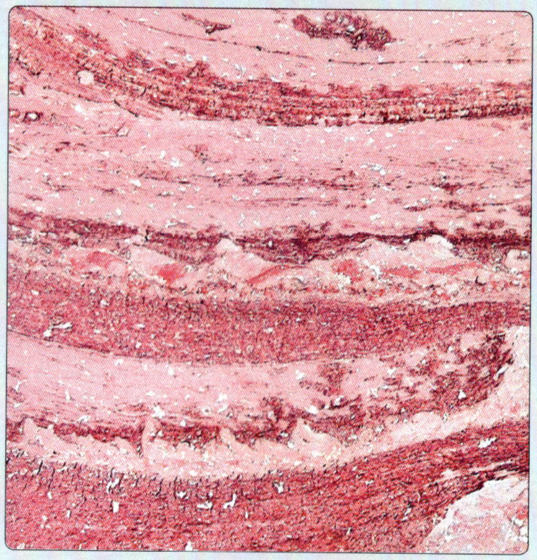

Organized Thrombus: Movat Stain

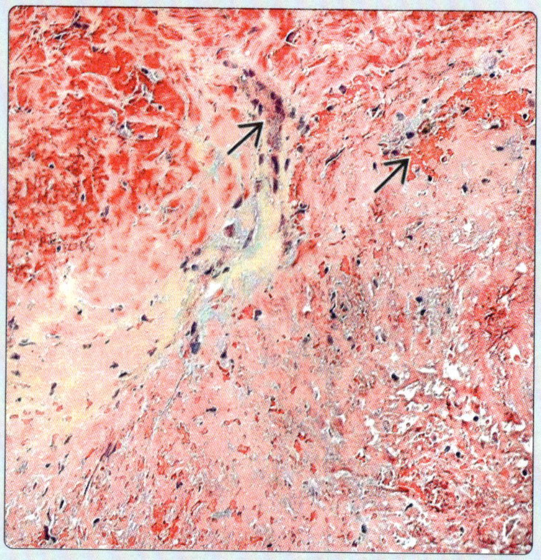

(Left) *Movat stain shows pale and dark areas of a laminated thrombus that was attached to a mechanical valve. This morphology indicates rapid arterial flow at the thrombus site.* **(Right)** *Movat stain shows the formation of capillaries ➔ containing red blood cells within the thrombus, indicating a late stage of thrombus organization.*

TERMINOLOGY

Definitions

- Complication occurring after prosthetic valve placement, most commonly caused by inadequate anticoagulation

ETIOLOGY/PATHOGENESIS

Predisposing Factors

- Increased blood viscosity
  - Inadequate anticoagulation therapy, especially during first 3 months post implantation
- Hemodynamic factors
  - Thrombosis is associated with altered blood flow in otherwise normal individual
  - Mitral (2-3x > aortic) location of prosthesis
  - Some porcine bioprosthetic valves have 1 cusp smaller than other 2
    - Leads to higher incidence of thrombosis in small cusp, particularly when bioprosthesis is implanted in mitral position with small cusp placed posteriorly
- Tissue degeneration of bioprosthetic valve
- Comorbid conditions
  - Large left atrial appendage
  - Atrial fibrillation
  - Severe left ventricular dysfunction
  - Bioprosthetic tissue infection (infective endocarditis)
  - Previous systemic embolization
- Type of bioprosthesis
  - Stented bioprosthetic valves and mechanical caged ball valve have higher incidence of thrombosis

CLINICAL ISSUES

Epidemiology

- Incidence
  - 0.1-5.7% per patient/year
  - Thrombosis equally affects bioprosthetic valves and mechanical valves in patients with adequate anticoagulant therapy

Presentation

- Asymptomatic (typical presentation)
- When thrombus is large, it may obstruct valve, causing pulmonary congestion and poor peripheral circulation
- When thrombus is dislodged, it causes systemic embolization
- Symptoms either progress gradually (weeks to months) or less commonly, rapidly, causing acute hemodynamic deterioration (shock)

Treatment

- Heparin IV should start immediately once diagnosis has been confirmed by echocardiogram
- Depends on size of thrombus seen by echocardiogram
  - Thrombus < 5 mm in diameter and not obstructing valve: Treatment includes anticoagulation treatment only
  - Thrombus ≥ 5 mm diameter: More aggressive therapy required (valve replacement or fibrinolysis)
- Thrombolytic therapy should be assigned mainly to patients whose operative risk is high

Prognosis

- Surgical therapy for valve obstruction is associated with ~ 15% mortality
  - Mortality can be considerably higher in patients with hemodynamic instability and emergency operations
- Thrombolytic therapy is more effective in patients who have had symptoms for < 2 weeks
  - Success rate: 81% in patients in New York Heart Association (NYHA) classes I-II and 74% in NYHA classes III-IV
  - Mortality rate: 9-10%

IMAGING

Ultrasonographic Findings

- New murmur may be detected by Doppler echocardiogram
- Doppler echocardiogram or catheterization may demonstrate
  - Increased transvalvular pressure gradient
  - Reduced orifice area
  - Valvular regurgitation

MACROSCOPIC

General Features

- Laminated thrombi may show alternating white and red bands (lines of Zahn)
  - Indicate rapid arterial blood flow at site of thrombus
  - Produced by successive deposition of platelets and fibrin forming light-colored areas, alternating with red blood cells (RBCs) and fibrin forming dark-colored areas
- Nonlaminated thrombi are usually found in large blood vessels

MICROSCOPIC

Histologic Features

- Laminated appearance; characterized by
  - Pale areas containing degranulated platelets and fibrin
  - Darker areas containing RBCs, white blood cells, platelets, and fibrin

DIFFERENTIAL DIAGNOSIS

Prosthetic Valve Endocarditis

- Most commonly involves prosthesis-tissue interface
- Ring abscess may occur
- Vegetations on cusps may facilitate thromboembolic events

SELECTED REFERENCES

1. Schaff HV: Progress in management of mechanical valve thrombosis. J Am Coll Cardiol. 79(10):990-2, 2022
2. Lim WY et al: Mechanical and surgical bioprosthetic valve thrombosis. Heart. 103(24):1934-41, 2017
3. Dangas GD et al: Prosthetic heart valve thrombosis. J Am Coll Cardiol. 68(24):2670-89, 2016
4. Gürsoy MO et al: A global perspective on mechanical prosthetic heart valve thrombosis: diagnostic and therapeutic challenges. Anatol J Cardiol. 16(12):980-9, 2016
5. Salamon J et al: Mechanical valve obstruction: review of diagnostic and treatment strategies. World J Cardiol. 7(12):875-81, 2015
6. Siddiqui RF et al: Bioprosthetic heart valves: modes of failure. Histopathology. 55(2):135-44, 2009

Endocarditis, Prosthetic Valve

KEY FACTS

ETIOLOGY/PATHOGENESIS

- Prosthetic valve endocarditis (PVE) is commonly caused by
  - *Staphylococcus epidermidis*, *Staphylococcus aureus*, streptococci

CLINICAL ISSUES

- More common in people whose native valves were damaged by previous infective endocarditis
- Early PVE is associated with 30-80% mortality
- Unexplained fever in patient with prosthetic valve (most common)
- New murmur or change in already existing murmur
- Congestive cardiac failure (30-70% of patients)
- Systemic emboli
- Valve replacement is main treatment for PVE
- Streptococcal PVE is cured by parenteral antibiotics in 50% of patients
- Use of warfarin in treatment of PVE is controversial

IMAGING

- Both transthoracic echocardiography and transesophageal echocardiography should be performed in PVE

MACROSCOPIC

- Ring abscess
- Valvular incompetence due to cusp destruction and tears
- Valvular stenosis due to large vegetations

MICROSCOPIC

- Intensity of inflammation and presence of vegetations and microorganisms should be considered when making diagnosis
- Cusp tears, perforation, and calcification; some mononuclear cell infiltrate
- Inflammatory reaction is greatest at site of attachment and base of vegetation
- Structural valve deterioration (SVD) may be associated with and mimic PVE; SVD and PVE should be differentiated

(Left) *Gross photograph of a porcine bioprosthetic heart valve, 13 years post implantation, shows tissue degeneration, tears, and prolapse. Thrombotic vegetations were noted on flow and nonflow surfaces of the cusps.* **(Right)** *H&E of porcine bioprosthetic tissue, detached from the stent, shows the porcine aorta →, cuspal tissue degeneration, tears →, and pannus →.*

Bioprosthetic Heart Valve With Endocarditis

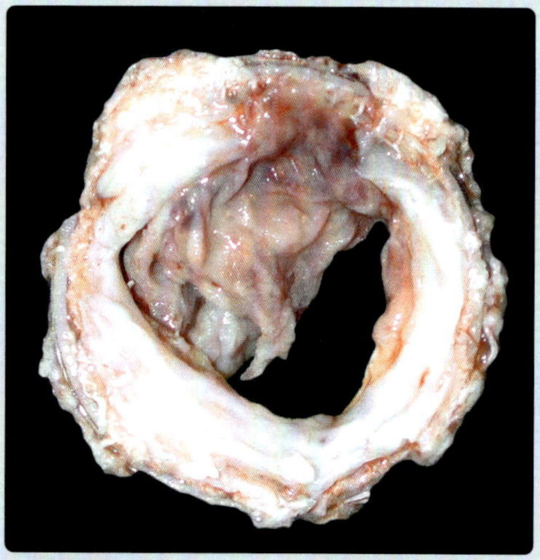

Histologic Findings in Bioprosthetic Heart Valve Endocarditis

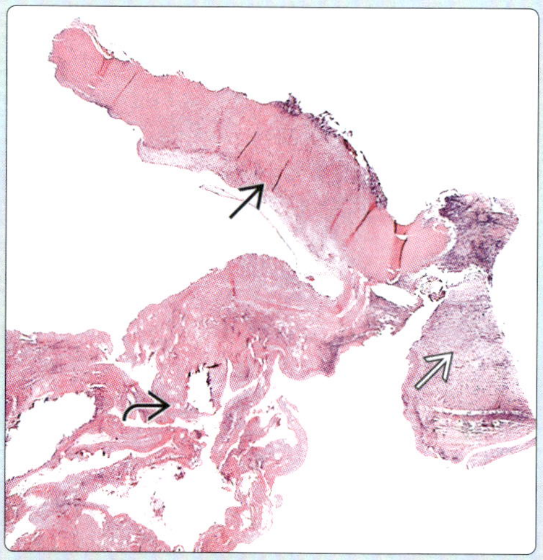

(Left) *Gross photograph of a bioprosthetic aortic valve involved by endocarditis shows vegetations → and fusion of 1 commissure →.* **(Right)** *Gross photograph of the same valve, viewed from the ventricular aspect, also shows fibrinous vegetation material on the inner sewing ring →.*

Bioprosthetic Aortic Valve With Vegetations and Commissure Fusion

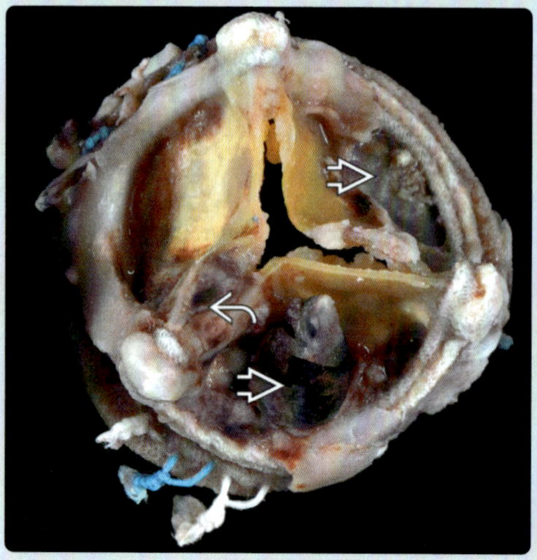

Ventricular Aspect of Bioprosthetic Heart Valve With Fibrinous Vegetation

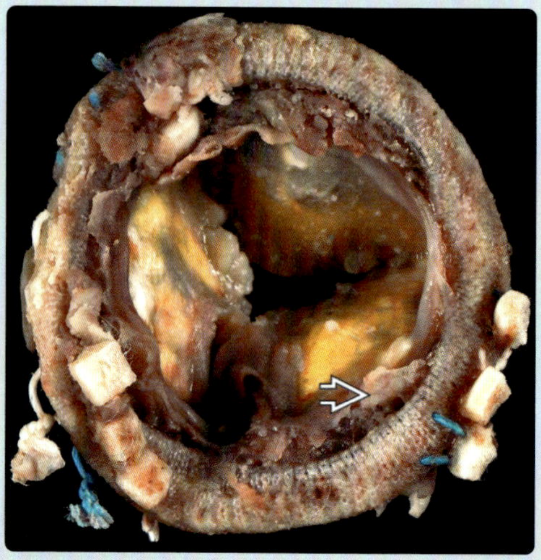

TERMINOLOGY

Abbreviations

- Prosthetic valve endocarditis (PVE)

ETIOLOGY/PATHOGENESIS

Infectious Agents

- *Staphylococcus epidermidis*
- *Staphylococcus aureus*
- Streptococci
- Gram-negative bacilli
- Fungi
- *Gemella morbillorum* (formerly *Streptococcus morbillorum*); affects bioprosthetic valves implanted in mitral position, intravenous drug users
- Early PVE occurs within 60 days of valve replacement due to perioperative bacteremia
  - Microorganisms involved include: *S. epidermidis*, *S. aureus*, gram-negative bacteria, diphtheroids, fungi, mycobacteria, and *Legionella*
- Late PVE occurs > 60 days following operation
  - Most common infectious agent: Streptococci
  - *S. epidermidis*: May cause PVE 12 months or more following valve surgery

CLINICAL ISSUES

Epidemiology

- Incidence
  - Commonly occurs within first 2 years following valve replacement with incidence of 1-6%
  - More common in people whose native valves were damaged by previous infective endocarditis
    - Native valve endocarditis is caused by same organism causing infection of implanted prosthetic valves

Presentation

- Unexplained fever in patient with prosthetic valve (most common)
- New murmur or change in already existing murmur
- Congestive cardiac failure (30-70% of patients)
- Systemic embolization
- Bacteremia (causative organism is detected by blood culture in > 90% of patients)
  - Blood culture results can be negative as result of
    - Recent use of antibiotics
    - Infection by fastidious organisms (HACEK group: *Haemophilus*, *Actinobacillus*, *Cardiobacterium*, *Eikenella*, *Kingella*)
    - Fungal infection
    - Infection with organisms that require special culture techniques (*Rickettsia*, fungi, mycobacteria, *Legionella*)
- Appropriate serologic or culture techniques should be used if organism is not identified initially
- Peripheral signs (Janeway lesions, Osler nodes, Roth spots) are rare in PVE
- Early PVE may present with
  - Poor peripheral perfusion
  - Rapid hemodynamic deterioration
  - New conduction abnormalities

Treatment

- Antibiotics
  - Streptococcal PVE is cured by parenteral antibiotics in 50% of patients
  - Blood culture: Ordered weekly following antimicrobial therapy until 1 month after completion of therapy
- Warfarin
  - Controversial
- Valve replacement
  - Main treatment for PVE
  - Indicated immediately in cases of
    - Heart failure
    - Valve obstruction
    - Recurrent embolization
    - Myocardial abscess
    - Fungal infection
    - New EKG conduction abnormalities
    - Persistent bacteremia despite antimicrobial therapy
    - Blood culture results that are positive after 3-5 days of antimicrobial therapy
    - Recurrent infection after cessation of antibiotic therapy
    - Infection with organism that requires valve replacement for cure
- Prophylaxis
  - Regular dental care
  - Patient education on role of antibiotics in prevention of morbidity/mortality with PVE

Prognosis

- Early PVE is associated with 30-80% mortality
- Late PVE is associated with 20-40% mortality
- Factors leading to increased mortality in PVE
  - Congestive heart failure (most common)
  - Persistent fever
  - New/changing murmur
  - Systemic emboli (due to valve vegetations)
  - Paravalvular abscess (associated with valve incompetence)
  - New conduction abnormality
  - Mycotic aneurysm
  - Neurologic complication
  - Deterioration in renal function

IMAGING

Ultrasonographic Findings

- Transthoracic echocardiography (TTE)
  - Provides assessment of valvular function
  - Provides assessment of chamber dimensions
  - However, TTE has limited ability to detect PVE due to intense reverberations from metallic structures, especially in mitral position
- Transesophageal echocardiography (TEE)
  - Far superior to TTE in detecting
    - Paravalvular abscess
    - Paravalvular leak
    - Valve dehiscence
    - Small vegetations (1-2 mm in diameter)
  - However

    - TEE may not allow complete valve function assessment
    - TEE may not allow complete visualization of anterior aspect of prosthetic aortic valve
  - Therefore, both TTE and TEE should be performed in PVE
  - Negative TEE makes PVE unlikely; however, repeat test when clinical suspicion is high

MACROSCOPIC

Gross Features

- PVE may present as
  - Ring abscess
  - Valvular incompetence due to cusp destruction and tears
  - Valvular stenosis due to large vegetations
- Therefore, careful assessment is given to
  - Sewing ring, as infection usually starts around it
  - Valve vegetations
  - Perforation and tears
  - Calcification

MICROSCOPIC

Histologic Features

- Cusp tears, perforation, and calcification; some mononuclear cell infiltrate
- Foreign body giant cell granulomas near sewing ring
- Inflammatory reaction is greatest at
  - Site of attachment
  - Base of vegetation
- Structural valve deterioration (SVD) may be associated with and mimic PVE; therefore, SVD and PVE should be differentiated
- Defining PVE only on basis of degree of inflammation is impossible as SVD may present similarly and be confused with PVE
- Therefore, it is recommended that
  - Intensity of inflammation described in terms of relative number and distribution of
    - Neutrophils
    - Histiocytes
    - Lymphocytes
  - Other criteria should be considered when making diagnosis of PVE, such as presence of
    - Vegetations
    - Microorganisms
    - Prosthetic tissue necrosis
    - Prosthetic tissue fibrosis
    - Prosthetic cusp tissue calcification

ANCILLARY TESTS

Histochemistry

- Gram, AFB, and GMS stains contribute to identify microorganisms

DIFFERENTIAL DIAGNOSIS

Conditions That Can Mimic Prosthetic Valve Infection

- Thrombotic obstruction
- Embolism
- Paravalvular leak
- Tissue degeneration
- Marantic endocarditis (extremely rare)

SELECTED REFERENCES

1. Romeo MG et al: Sars-Cov-2 infection as a possible risk factor for prosthesis endocarditis: a challenging redo-Bentall for subvalvular abscess. J Card Surg. 37(9):2845-8, 2022
2. Saha S et al: Surgery for aortic prosthetic valve endocarditis in the transcatheter era. J Clin Med. 11(12):3418, 2022
3. Latib A et al: TAVR-associated prosthetic valve infective endocarditis: results of a large, multicenter registry. J Am Coll Cardiol. 64(20):2176-8, 2014
4. Luk A et al: Pathologic evaluation of 28 mitroflow pericardial valves: a 12-Year experience. Ann Thorac Surg. 99(1):48-54, 2014
5. Riddell J 4th et al: Histoplasma capsulatum endocarditis: multicenter case series with review of current diagnostic techniques and treatment. Medicine (Baltimore). 93(5):186-93, 2014
6. Thuny F et al: Infective endocarditis: prevention, diagnosis, and management. Can J Cardiol. 30(9):1046-57, 2014
7. Castonguay MC et al: Surgical pathology of native valve endocarditis in 310 specimens from 287 patients (1985-2004). Cardiovasc Pathol. 22(1):19-27, 2013
8. Alkhatib B et al: Viridans streptococcal (Streptococcus mitis) biosynthetic aortic prosthetic valve endocarditis (PVE) complicated by complete heart block and paravalvular abscess. Heart Lung. 41(6):610-2, 2012
9. Fukuta Y et al: Legionella micdadei prosthetic valve endocarditis complicated by brain abscess: case report and review of the literature. Scand J Infect Dis. 44(6):414-8, 2012
10. Manne MB et al: Outcomes after surgical treatment of native and prosthetic valve infective endocarditis. Ann Thorac Surg. 93(2):489-93, 2012
11. Muraki S et al: [Bioprosthetic valve endocarditis associated with rapid progression of valvular stenosis;report of a case.] Kyobu Geka. 65(6):500-2, 2012
12. Boland JM et al: Fungal prosthetic valve endocarditis: Mayo Clinic experience with a clinicopathological analysis. Mycoses. 54(4):354-60, 2011
13. Lee JH et al: Prosthetic valve endocarditis: clinicopathological correlates in 122 surgical specimens from 116 patients (1985-2004). Cardiovasc Pathol. 20(1):26-35, 2011
14. Tornos P et al: Infective endocarditis: the European viewpoint. Curr Probl Cardiol. 36(5):175-222, 2011
15. Imazio M et al: Blood culture-negative early prosthetic valve endocarditis: be aware of fungi! Heart. 96(10):733-4, 2010
16. Wang HL et al: A clinical analysis of 25 cases of prosthetic valve endocarditis. Zhonghua Nei Ke Za Zhi. 49(9):758-61, 2010
17. Siddiqui RF et al: Bioprosthetic heart valves: modes of failure. Histopathology. 55(2):135-44, 2009
18. Butany J et al: Inflammation and infection in nine surgically explanted Medtronic Freestyle stentless aortic valves. Cardiovasc Pathol. 2007 Sep-Oct;16(5):258-67. Epub 2007 Apr 2. Erratum in: Cardiovasc Pathol. 17(2):128, 2008
19. Wang A et al: Contemporary clinical profile and outcome of prosthetic valve endocarditis. JAMA. 297(12):1354-61, 2007
20. Jegatheeswaran A et al: Pathology of infectious and inflammatory diseases in prosthetic heart valves. Cardiovasc Pathol. 15(5):252-5, 2006
21. Butany JW et al: Infective endocarditis in a hancock bioprosthetic heart valve. J Card Surg. 20(4):389-92, 2005
22. Mahesh B et al: Prosthetic valve endocarditis. Ann Thorac Surg. 80(3):1151-8, 2005

Prosthetic Aortic Valve With Outflow Obstruction and Endocarditis

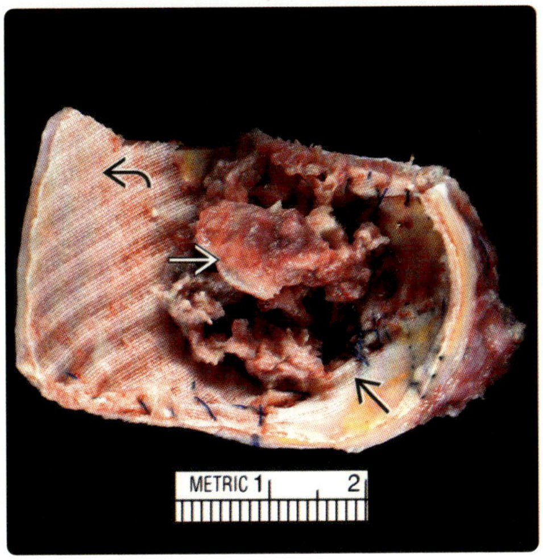

GMS Staining of Aortic Valve Vegetation

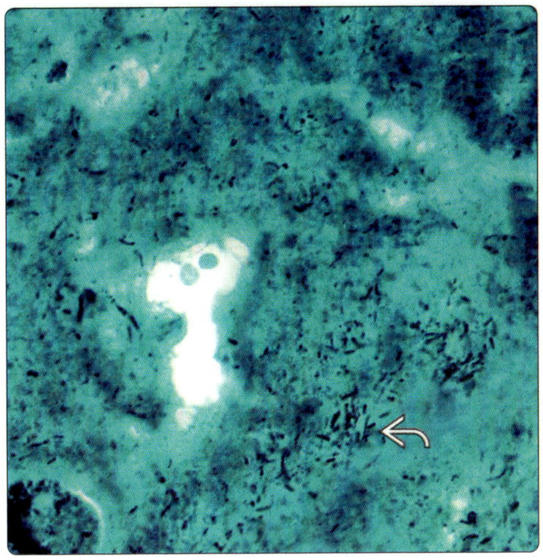

(Left) *Gross photograph shows that endocarditis involves a composite prosthetic aortic valve* ➾ *with an aortic tube graft* ↶. *A large and fleshy vegetation is seen obstructing the outflow* ➡. **(Right)** *Microorganism (diphtheroids)* ↶ *could be seen only on staining with GMS in sections from this vegetation.*

Bioprosthetic Heart Valve With Vegetations

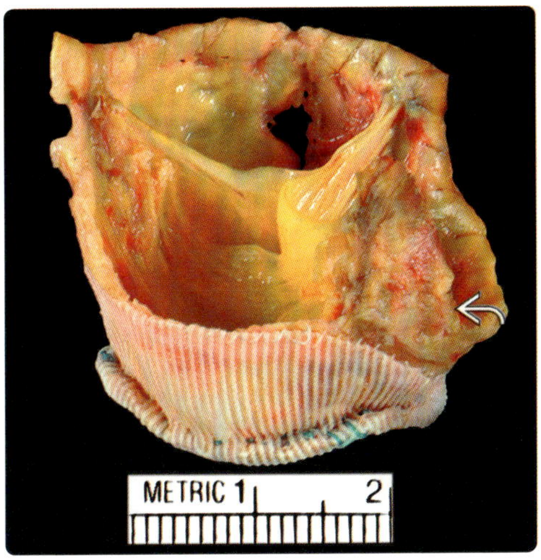

Prosthetic Heart Valve Vegetation: Gram Staining

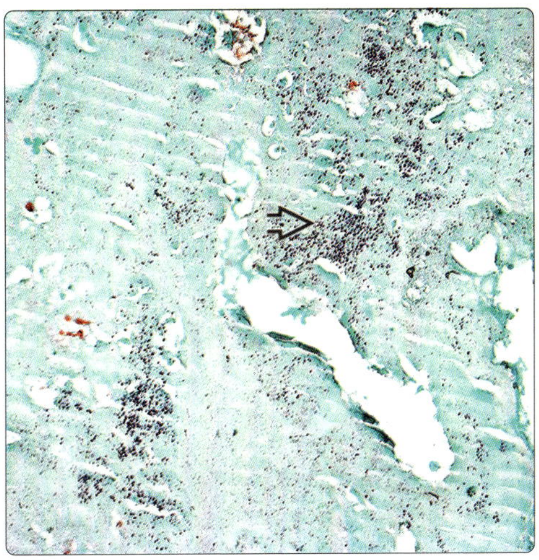

(Left) *Gross photograph of a stentless porcine prosthetic aortic valve shows large vegetations* ↶. **(Right)** *Gram staining of tissue from this vegetation shows sparse gram-positive cocci* ⇨. *After antibiotic treatment, it may be difficult to identify microbes by Gram staining.*

Aortic Bioprosthetic Prosthetic Valve Endocarditis

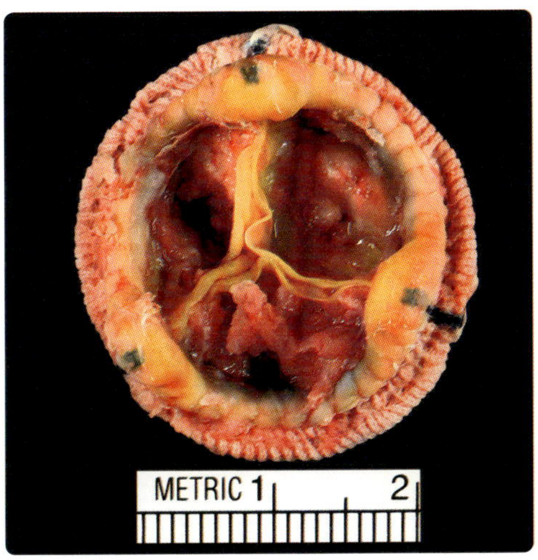

Bioprosthetic Heart Valve Endocarditis With Cusp Perforation

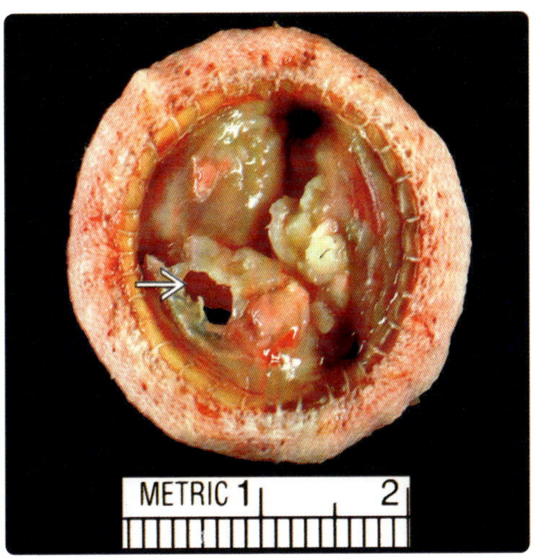

(Left) *Gross photograph of a bioprosthetic porcine aortic prosthetic valve shows vegetation in all 3 cusp pockets, which limits the opening orifice of the valve.* **(Right)** *Gross photograph of the undersurface of a valve reveals a perforation in 1 of the porcine cusps* ➡.

(Left) *Gross photograph of porcine leaflets resected from an infected bioprosthesis shows multiple cusp tears/perforations resulting from endocarditis-related tissue destruction.* **(Right)** *Sections from the resected valve leaflets did not show any viable microbes on special staining, but prominent, destructive lymphoplasmacytic inflammation was present.*

Bioprosthetic Valve Cusps With Vegetations

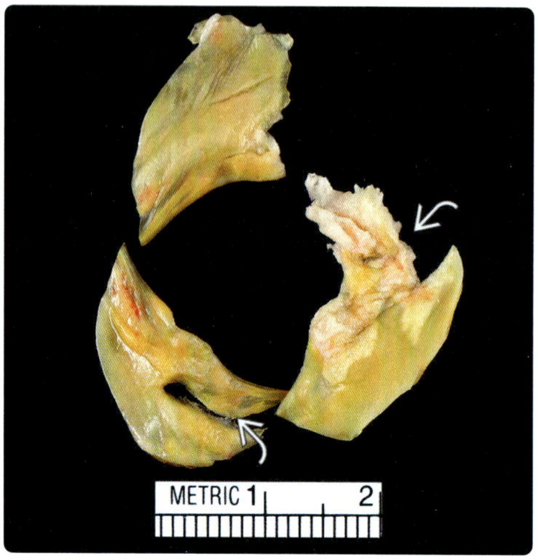

Prosthetic Heart Valve Endocarditis

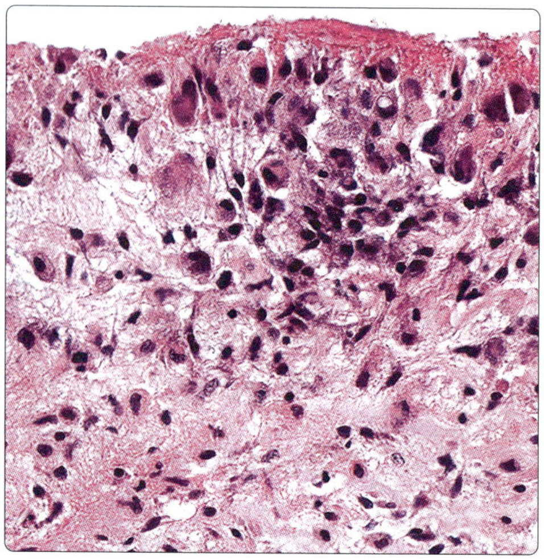

(Left) *Gross photograph of bileaflet prosthesis shows large fleshy vegetation encroaching on the hinge point and impairing mobility of the leaflets.* **(Right)** *The vegetation from this case contained yeast forms that were morphologically consistent with Candida species. Candidal endocarditis is typically associated with bulky obstructive vegetations like this.*

Prosthetic Heart Valve With Large Vegetation

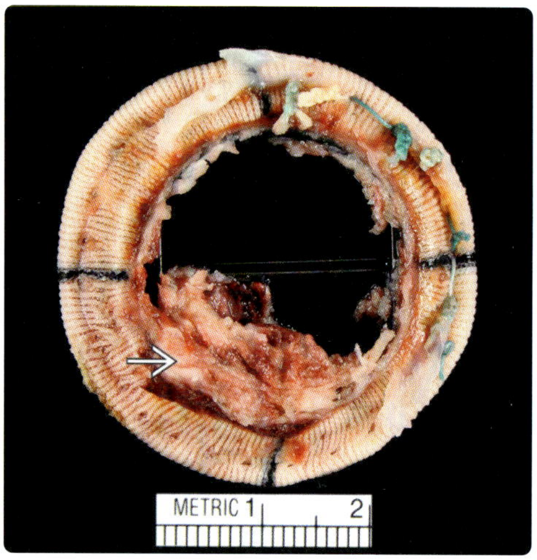

GMS Staining in Prosthetic Heart Valve Vegetation

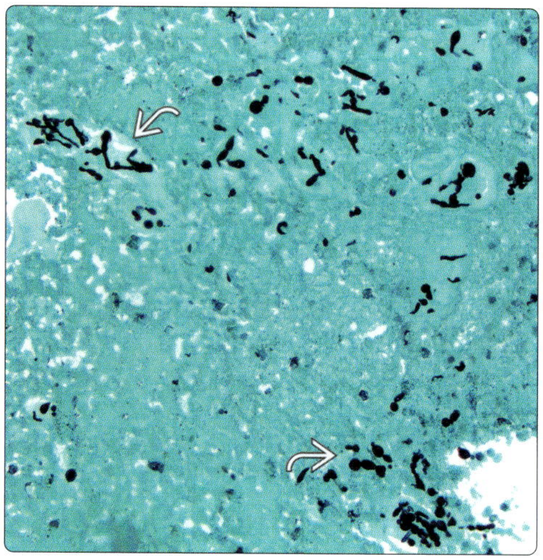

(Left) *H&E of porcine bioprosthetic tissue, detached from stent, shows tissue degeneration, thrombotic vegetations, and inflamed pannus.* **(Right)** *The porcine aortic tissue has been detached from the stent. Sections show tissue degeneration and tears with thrombotic vegetations, calcification, and pannus.*

Histologic Findings in Prosthetic Heart Valve Endocarditis

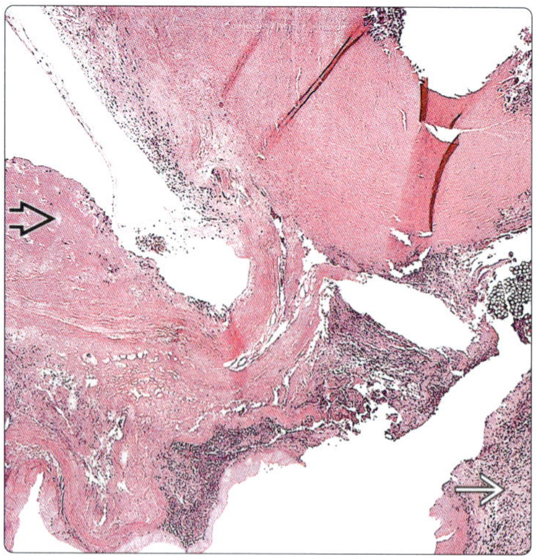

Prosthetic Valve Endocarditis: Elastic Stain

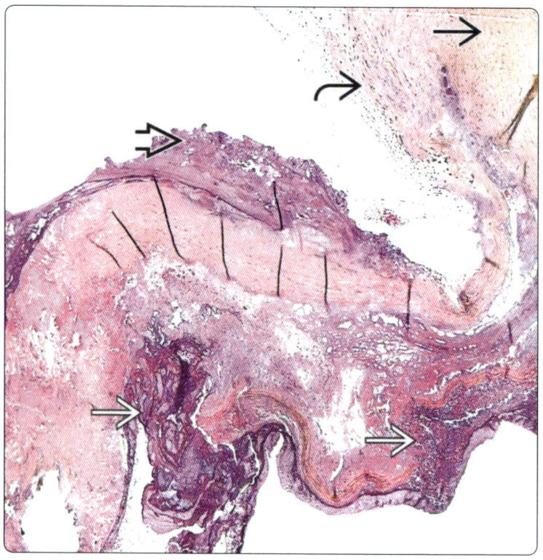

Prosthetic Heart Valve Endocarditis

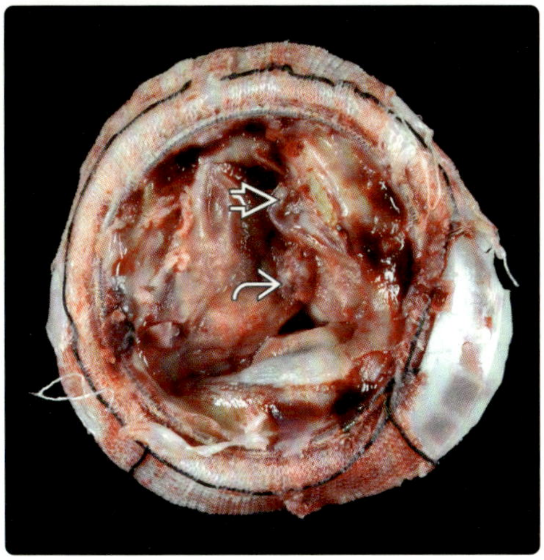

Prosthetic Heart Valve Endocarditis

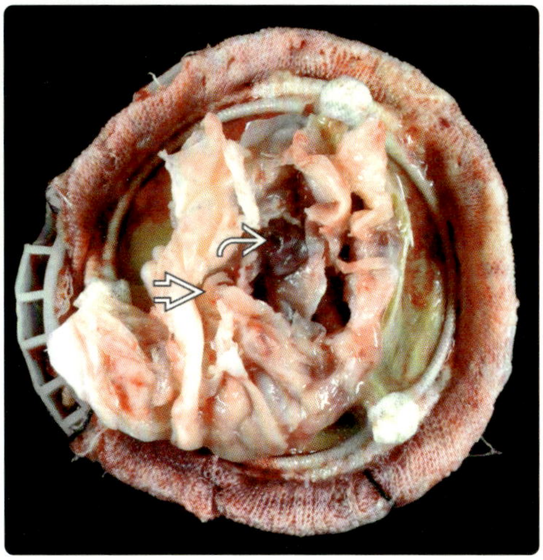

(Left) *Flow surface view from bioprosthetic valve shows cusp thickening and commisural fusion* ➲. *There is vegetation on the cusp* ➲ *with focal hemorrhage and a granular appearance.* **(Right)** *Gross photograph of the undersurface from this bioprosthetic valve shows cusp degenerative changes, thickening, and fusion* ➲. *There is a vegetation on the flow surface of the cusp* ➲ *with focal hemorrhage.*

Cusp From Bioprosthetic Valve With Calcification and Vegetation

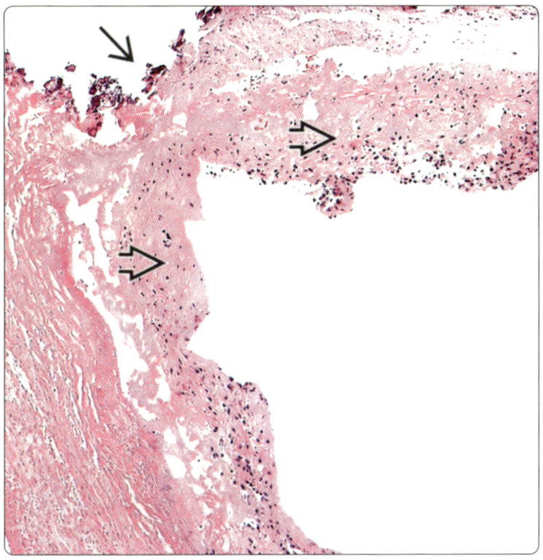

Bioprosthetic Valve With Endocarditis: Elastic Stain

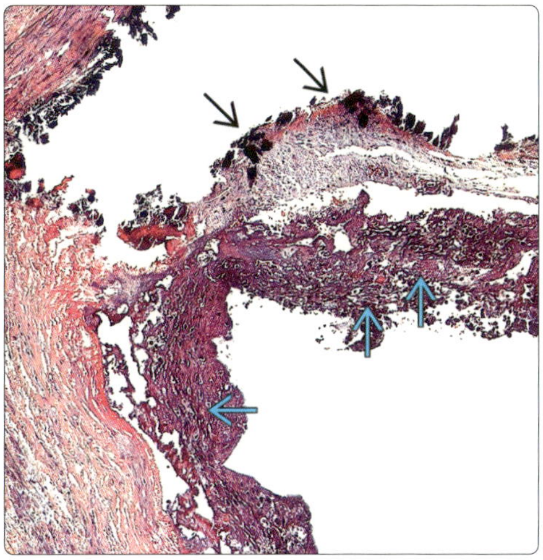

(Left) *H&E of another area of cusp tissue shows severe tissue degeneration, a calcified area that has become detached* ➲, *and thrombotic vegetation* ➲. **(Right)** *The same tissue section shows tissue degeneration, calcification* ➲, *and thrombotic vegetation* ➲.

Thrombotic Vegetation With Bacterial Colonies

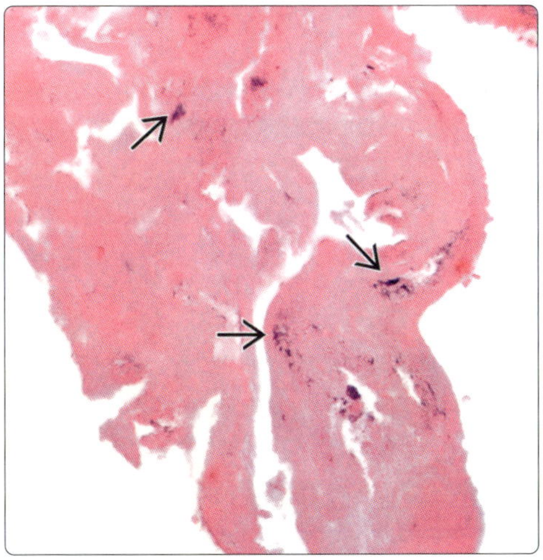

Valve Vegetation: Gram Stain

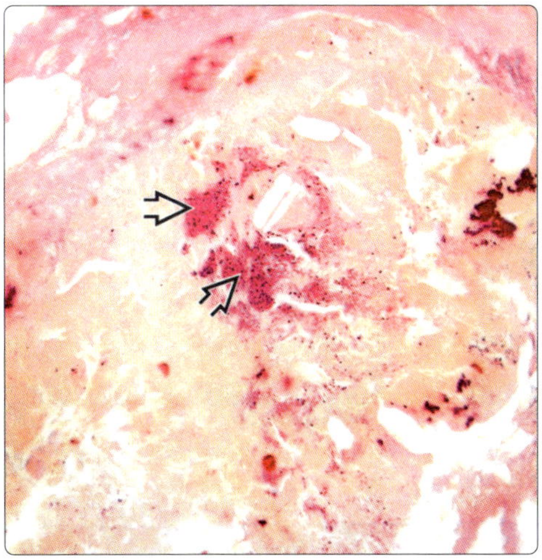

(Left) *H&E shows thrombotic vegetation containing scattered bacterial colonies in this case of endocarditis with gram-positive microorganisms* ➲. **(Right)** *Thrombotic vegetation shows gram-positive microorganisms* ➲.

Mechanical Heart Valve Prostheses: Modes of Failure

KEY FACTS

ETIOLOGY/PATHOGENESIS

- Mechanisms include
  - Failure of mechanical heart valve prostheses (MHVPs) can occur due to several causes
  - Pannus (increasingly common cause of failure)
  - Paravalvular leak
  - Break or separation of valve components leading to embolization and acute valve regurgitation
    - Although rare, affects mechanical valves more than bioprosthetic valves
  - Prosthetic valve endocarditis (PVE)

CLINICAL ISSUES

- Mechanical prostheses have excellent durability, and their degeneration is extremely rare with contemporary valves
- Mechanical valves less prone to structural valve deterioration than bioprosthetic valves
- Mortality for PVE may be as high as 80% in patients with early PVE
- Low-grade hemolytic anemia occurs in 70% of prosthetic heart valve recipients, and severe hemolytic anemia occurs in 3%
- Sudden death (within minutes) can occur in patients with strut fracture of aortic mechanical valve prosthesis
- Patients with strut fracture of mitral prosthesis may survive long enough to undergo valve replacement

MACROSCOPIC

- Examination of prosthetic valves at autopsy should specifically include search for
  - Paravalvular leaks
  - Annular abscess
  - Obstruction of coronary ostia (aortic prostheses)
  - Long suture knots or chordal remnants
  - Endocarditis

Starr-Edwards Valve

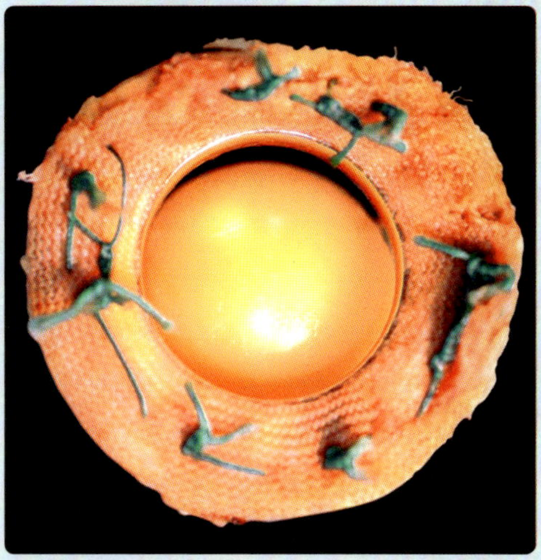

St. Jude Valve With Thrombosis

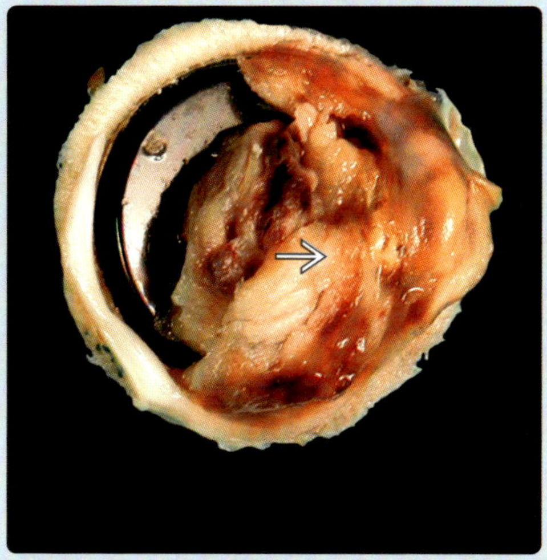

(Left) *Gross photograph of Starr-Edwards mechanical valve shows a yellow-colored poppet instead of pearly white, as it should be, due to lipid absorption. Mechanical failure was caused by a thrombus on the nonflow surface.* **(Right)** *A large thrombus* ➡ *has "frozen" the disc of a single leaflet mechanical valve in a partially open position. This led to mechanical failure of the valve.*

Pannus Formation: Medtronic Hall Valve

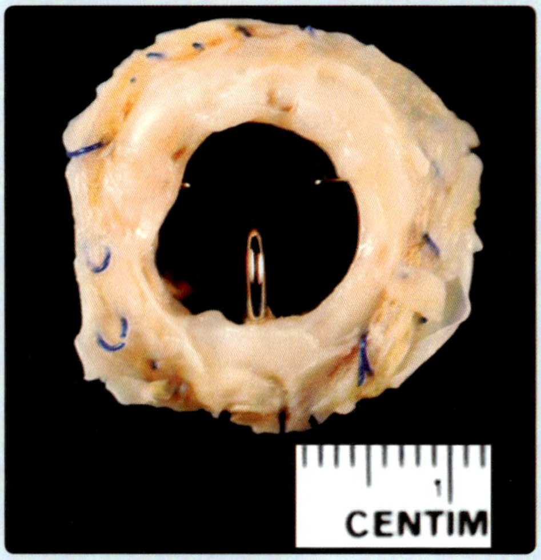

Early Pannus Formation on St. Jude Valve

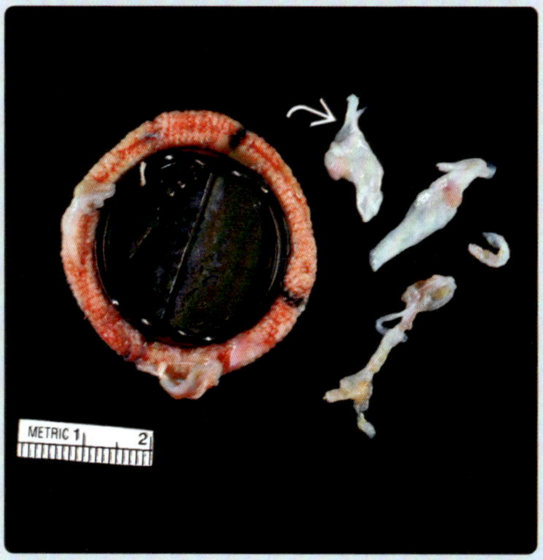

(Left) *Gross photograph of the flow surface of this single-disc mechanical aortic valve explanted from a 43-year-old woman shows a significant degree of pannus that narrowed the valve orifice, leading to valve stenosis and failure.* **(Right)** *Gross photograph of a surgically replaced mechanical valve showed early ingrowth of fibrous pannus* ➡ *(stripped from the sewing ring before this photo was taken).*

TERMINOLOGY

Definitions

- Mechanical heart valve prostheses (MHVPs) fail in ways resulting in both stenosis and regurgitation
  - Failure may be due to stenosis, incompetence of orifice, infections, or paravalvular leaks

ETIOLOGY/PATHOGENESIS

Etiology

- Failure of MHVPs can occur due to several causes
  - Pannus (increasingly common cause of failure)
  - Paravalvular leak
  - Break or separation of valve components leading to embolization and acute valve regurgitation
  - Thrombosis
    - Although rare, affects mechanical valves more than bioprosthetic valves
    - More common in mitral position
    - Mechanical valves require lifelong anticoagulation
  - Prosthetic valve endocarditis (PVE)
    - Mechanical and bioprosthetic valves equally susceptible to infection
    - PVE occurs in 2-4% of patients; incidence 3% in 1st postoperative year, then 0.5% in subsequent years
    - Early PVE: Occurs within 60 days of implantation; usually caused by perioperative contamination or hematogenous spread
    - Late PVE: Occurs > 60 days after implantation; usually caused by hematogenous spread
    - Incidence of PVE higher in mitral than other valves
  - Suture line dehiscence

Important Factors Related to Failure of MHVP

- Material used in manufacture of mechanical valve
  - Prior to 1966, Starr Edwards mechanical valve prostheses were reported to show poppet damage (cracks) and, occasionally, embolization
  - This was believed to be due to lipid imbibition
- Shape and design of mechanical valve
  - Single-tilting disc valve was withdrawn from market in 1986 due to very rare fractures of ring struts causing embolization of disc and sudden death
    - Estimated incidence of fracture of single-tilting disc valve < 0.5% per patient-year with 60° opening angle
    - Estimated incidence of fracture of single-tilting disc valve ≤ 2% per patient-year for model with 70° opening angle
- Patient age
  - Failure or fracture of single-tilting disc valve occurred more frequently in patients < 50 years old
- Size of mechanical prosthetic valve
  - Failure of single-tilting disc valve occurred more commonly in patients having large prosthetic valves (at least 29 mm in diameter)

CLINICAL ISSUES

Epidemiology

- Incidence
  - Mechanical prostheses have excellent durability, and degeneration is rare with contemporary valves

Presentation

- Clinical presentation
  - Embolization of poppet or fractured strut or leaflet usually results in
    - Sudden onset of dyspnea
    - Loss of consciousness
    - Shock or cardiovascular collapse, which may also result from acute, severe valvular regurgitation
    - Sudden death (within minutes)
    - No opening/closing click sounds on auscultation

Treatment

- Valve re-replacement surgery essential for survival
  - Immediate surgery indicated in patients with
    - Strut fracture
    - Embolization of part of mechanical valve

Prognosis

- Facts related to prognosis of mechanical valves
  - Most mechanical valves remain functional 20-30 years, compared to bioprosthetic valves where 30-35% fail within 10-15 years
  - Mechanical valves less prone to structural valve deterioration than bioprosthetic valves
  - Mortality for prosthetic endocarditis may be as high as 80% in patients with early (< 60 days from operative date) PVE
  - Sudden death (within minutes) can occur in patients with strut fracture of aortic mechanical valve prosthesis
  - Patients with strut fracture of mitral prosthesis may survive long enough to undergo valve replacement
  - Low-grade hemolytic anemia occurs in 70% of prosthetic heart valve recipients, and severe hemolytic anemia occurs in 3%

IMAGING

Ultrasonographic Findings

- Transesophageal echocardiography can provide high-quality image for evaluation of leaflet mobility

Fluoroscopy or Cinefluoroscopy

- May reveal absence of strut or radiopaque disc within valve ring or base of valve

MACROSCOPIC

General Features

- Examination of prosthetic valves at autopsy should specifically include search for
  - Paravalvular leaks
  - Annular abscess
  - Obstruction of coronary ostia (aortic prostheses)
  - Long suture knots or chordal remnants
  - Endocarditis

SELECTED REFERENCES

1. Butany J et al: Mechanical heart valve prostheses: identification and evaluation (erratum). Cardiovasc Pathol. 12(6):322-44, 2003

Catheter-Deployed Valve Therapies

KEY FACTS

TERMINOLOGY

- New technology for treating cardiac valve disease without sternotomy and cardiopulmonary bypass

CLINICAL ISSUES

- Research trials
  - PARTNER
  - SURTAVI
  - EVEREST
- Types of valves
  - Edwards SAPIEN
  - Medtronic CoreValve
  - Medtronic Melody

MACROSCOPIC

- MitraClip placement through venous access and atrial septostomy
- Transcatheter aortic valve replacement (TAVR) can be performed via
  - Femoral artery access (retrograde through aorta)
  - Transapically through small left thoracotomy incision (antegrade through left ventricle outflow tract)
- Complications include
  - Incomplete expansion
    - Proper leaflet coaptation requires full expansion to predesigned functional circumference
  - Degenerative changes and endocarditis
    - Calcification and tears
    - Thrombi and infective vegetations may also form on leaflets or around stent ring
  - Suboptimal seating and attachment failure
    - Improperly seated valves become loose and embolize distally
  - Overexpansion (rare, given calcification and sclerosis of aortic anulus in aortic stenosis)
  - Paravalvular leak
  - Calcific plaque embolization

Gross Photograph of Deployed Aortic Valve

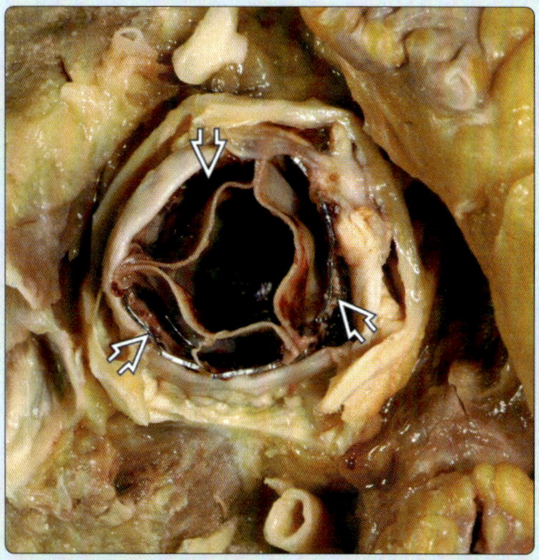

Gross Photograph of Deployed Aortic Valve

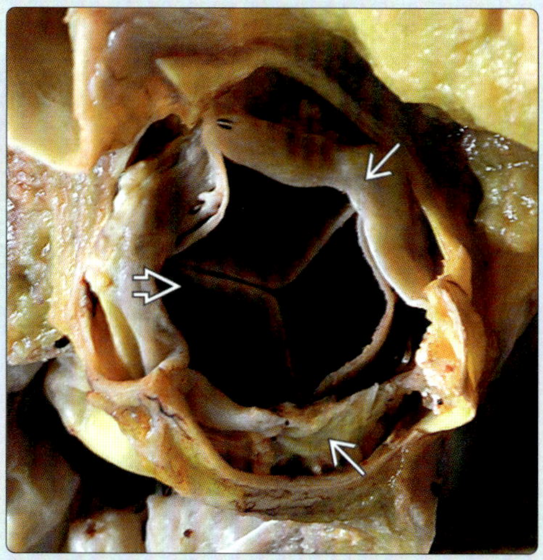

(Left) *Gross photograph of an autopsied heart shows a catheter-deployed aortic valve prosthesis ➡ seated within a markedly calcified and sclerotic native aortic valve.* **(Right)** *Gross photograph of an aortic valve prosthesis ➡ deployed using transcatheter aortic valve replacement (TAVR) shows sclerotic native leaflets ➡ that are pushed back but remain in place after this procedure.*

Edwards SAPIEN Prosthetic Aortic Valve

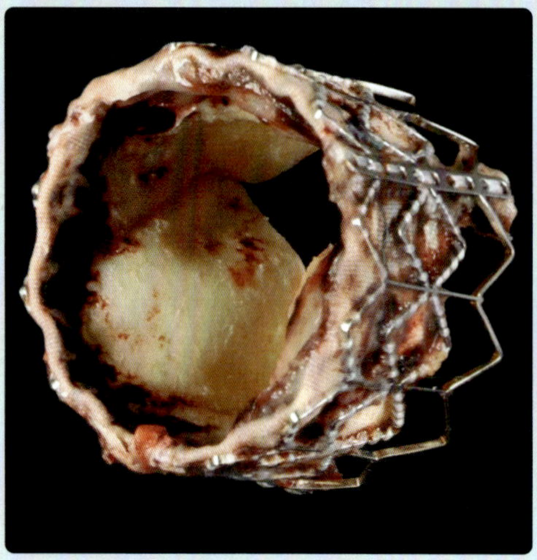

Edwards SAPIEN Prosthetic Aortic Valve

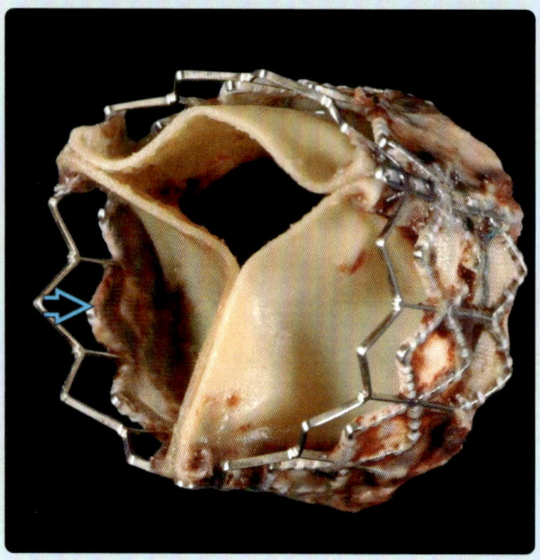

(Left) *Gross photograph shows a SAPIEN valve seen from the left ventricular aspect. The valve contains a metallic anulus and bioprosthetic bovine pericardial leaflets. Pathologic evaluation should include assessment of complete expansion and leaflet coaptation, as well as presence of degenerative changes or vegetations.* **(Right)** *Gross photograph shows a SAPIEN valve seen from the aortic aspect. One of the leaflets is detached from the anulus ➡.*

TERMINOLOGY

Definitions

- New technology for treating cardiac valve disease without sternotomy and cardiopulmonary bypass
  - Catheter-deployed bioprosthetic valve inserted in aortic position
  - Catheter-deployed bioprosthetic valve inserted in mitral position
  - Coated metallic clip devices applied to mitral leaflets

CLINICAL ISSUES

Presentation

- New technologies are currently being developed in patients who are too high risk to undergo open-heart surgery with cardiopulmonary bypass
  - Mostly in older adult patients since degenerative valve disease is most common in older adults, and they often have high-risk comorbidities
- Heart failure symptoms [New York Heart Association (NYHA) classes III-IV] and echocardiographic evidence of severe valve dysfunction

Treatment

- Clinical trials (aortic valve)
  - **P**lacement of **a**o**r**tic **t**ra**n**scathet**er** valve (PARTNER)
    - Randomized controlled trial (RCT) in high-surgical-risk aortic stenosis patients
    - SAPIEN vs. open-valve replacement vs. medical management
  - PARTNER II
    - RCT for intermediate-surgical-risk aortic stenosis patients
    - SAPIEN XT vs. open-valve replacement
  - PARTNER III
    - RCT for low-surgical-risk aortic stenosis patients
    - SAPIEN 3 vs. open-valve replacement
  - **Su**rgical **r**eplacement and **t**ranscatheter **a**ortic **v**alve **i**mplantation (SURTAVI)
    - Randomized trial for intermediate-surgical-risk aortic stenosis patients comparing transcatheter aortic valve replacement (TAVR) (Medtronic CoreValve) to open-valve replacement
- "Valve in valve" applications
  - Placing 2nd TAVR valve within another failed TAVR prosthesis
  - TAVR therapy is amenable to placement within both native and prosthetic valves
  - Successive rounds of TAVR are also reported
- Clinical trials (mitral valve)
  - **E**ndovascular **v**alve **e**dge-to-edge **re**pair **st**udy (EVEREST)
    - RCT for high-surgical-risk mitral regurgitation
    - MitraClip vs. open-valve replacement
  - EVEREST II
    - RCT for intermediate-surgical-risk mitral regurgitation
    - MitraClip vs. open-valve replacement
  - COAPT/COAPT CAS
    - RCT for mitral regurgitation not eligible for surgery
    - MitraClip vs. medical management
  - CLASP
    - Single-arm study of Edwards PASCAL clip valve repair system
  - ENCIRCLE
    - Single-arm study of Edwards SAPIEN M3 valve replacement system

Implantation Procedure

- Typically in hybrid catheterization laboratory/operating room with surgery support immediately available
- Under fluoroscopic and echocardiographic (2D or 3D) guidance
- Rapid ventricular pacing to reduce ventricular motion and valvular flow during certain steps of procedure

MACROSCOPIC

Catheter Access Sites

- TAVR can be performed via
  - Femoral artery access
    - Retrograde through aorta
  - Transapically through small left thoracotomy incision
    - Antegrade through left ventricle outflow tract
- Mitral valve repair/replacement can be performed via
  - Femoral venous access and atrial septostomy (transseptal)
  - Small left lateral chest incision (transapical) for replacement systems
- Tricuspid/pulmonary repair/replacement can be performed via
  - Femoral or jugular venous access

Types of Valves

- Aortic position (TAVR)
  - SAPIEN series
    - Heavy-gauge, metallic, self-expanding stent with bovine pericardial bioprosthetic leaflets
    - Slightly shorter than anulus, so no obstruction of coronary ostia when properly seated
  - CoreValve
    - Finer gauge, metallic, self-expanding stent support with bovine pericardial bioprosthetic leaflets
    - Much longer than native anulus, but supravalvular portion narrows to allow flow through stent interspaces to coronary ostia
  - Portico
    - Also consists of finer gauge, metallic, self-expanding stent support with bovine pericardial bioprosthetic leaflets
    - Longer than anulus with large spacing gaps in wire to allow coronary flow
    - More tapered at base
  - Lotus Edge
    - Metallic stent (more closely spaced than others) with bovine pericardial bioprosthetic leaflets
    - Not self-expanding, requires manual expanding, but this allows for easy repositioning and removal
- Mitral position (transcatheter mitral valve replacement)
  - SAPIEN M3
    - Similar to other SAPIEN (aortic) valves with fabric ring around base to facilitate seating in dock
    - Additional catheter-deployed docking system to ensure proper seating

- Many others in development (Cephea, EVOQUE, HighLife)
- Clip-type devices (repair not replacement; simulates "Alfieri stitch" approach to reducing regurgitant orifice)
  - MitraClip
  - Pascal
- AccuCinch (annuloplasty-type repair)
  - Several posts are inserted at intervals around mitral anulus
  - Wire is threaded through posts and then cinched to bring them closer together, thus reducing annular diameter
- Pulmonary
  - Melody
    - Fine-gauge, metallic, expandable stent with bovine jugular venous valve sutured to struts
    - Longer than native anulus and fully coated; intended for pulmonary, not aortic, valve replacement
  - Harmony
    - Also fully coated; flared at both ends to allow better seating
  - Alterra Adaptive
    - Also fully coated; shorter, even more flared at both ends to allow better seating
- Tricuspid
  - Clip-type devices (MitraClip, Pascal)
  - SAPIEN M3, EVOQUE (experimental)
  - Others in development (Navigate, Trisol, Lux)

Catheter Diameters

- 1st-generation devices were deployed on very large-gauge catheters (22 or 24 French; 0.73 or 0.8 cm, respectively)
  - Required femoral artery anatomy was conducive to such large introducer sheath
  - Large catheter size also presented significant risk of disruption to atherosclerotic plaques and distal embolization
- Newer versions of these devices have smaller catheters (18 or 19 French; 0.6 or 0.63 cm, respectively)

Valve Complications

- Incomplete expansion
  - Proper leaflet coaptation requires full expansion to predesigned functional circumference
  - Incomplete expansion may cause "tenting" of leaflets and fixed regurgitation
  - Overexpansion is potential problem but rarely seen given usual calcification and sclerosis of aortic anulus in aortic stenosis
- Leaflet degeneration and endocarditis
  - Like other bioprostheses, tissue leaflets are susceptible to degenerative changes (calcification and tears)
  - Thrombi and infective vegetations may also form on leaflets or around stent ring
- Suboptimal seating and attachment failure
  - Proper function requires alignment at level of anatomic anulus
  - Improperly seated valves become loose and embolize distally
- Paravalvular leak
  - Incomplete expansion or native wall adaptation response may lead to paravalvular leak and regurgitation
- Calcific plaque embolization
  - Debris from valve leaflets dislodged during balloon expansion prior to valve deployment
  - Debris from femoral, iliac, or aortic plaque dislodged by introducing large-diameter catheter
- Concentric fibrotic ingrowth, commissural fusion
  - Development of "pannus" impeding flow or movement of leaflets
  - May be chronic complication of shallow thrombosis

SELECTED REFERENCES

1. Geis NA et al: One-year results following PASCAL-based or MitraClip-based mitral valve transcatheter edge-to-edge repair. ESC Heart Fail. 9(2):853-65, 2022
2. Inci EK et al: Transcatheter electrosurgical laceration and stabilization of failed MitraClip[s]/SAPIEN M3 for treatment of failed MitraClip. Circ Cardiovasc Interv. 15(5):e012014, 2022
3. Mahmaljy H et al: Transcatheter aortic valve replacement. StatPearls, 2022
4. Flint N et al: State of the art: transcatheter edge-to-edge repair for complex mitral regurgitation. J Am Soc Echocardiogr. 34(10):1025-37, 2021
5. Ovcharenko EA et al: Mechanism of vascular injury in transcatheter aortic valve replacement. Sovrem Tekhnologii Med. 13(3):6-13, 2021
6. Rawish E et al: Current status of catheter-based mitral valve replacement. Curr Cardiol Rep. 23(8):95, 2021
7. Szerlip M et al: 2-year outcomes for transcatheter repair in patients with mitral regurgitation from the CLASP study. JACC Cardiovasc Interv. 14(14):1538-48, 2021
8. Salaun E et al: Transcatheter aortic valve replacement: procedure and outcomes. Cardiol Clin. 38(1):115-28, 2020
9. Ailawadi G et al: One-year outcomes after MitraClip for functional mitral regurgitation. Circulation. 139(1):37-47, 2019
10. Testa L et al: Transcatheter mitral valve replacement in the transcatheter aortic valve replacement era. J Am Heart Assoc. 8(22):e013352, 2019
11. De Carlo C et al: Mitral valve repair versus MitraClip. J Cardiovasc Med (Hagerstown). 19 Suppl 1:e80-3, 2018
12. Bourantas CV et al: Evolution of transcatheter aortic valve replacement. Circ Res. 114(6):1037-51, 2014
13. Rozeik MM et al: Percutaneous heart valves; past, present and future. Perfusion. 29(5):397-410, 2014

SAPIEN Valve With Adequate Placement

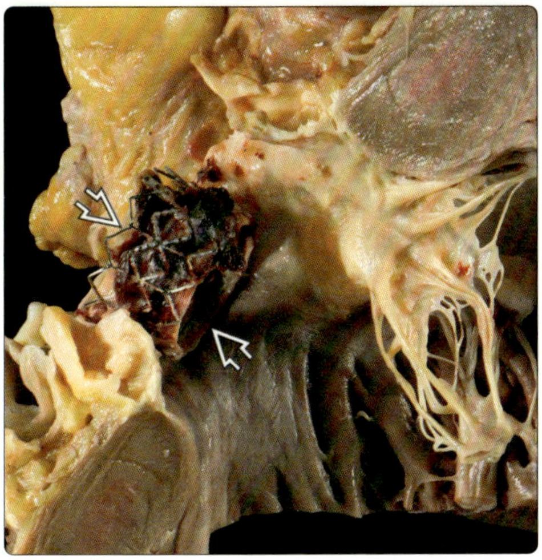

SAPIEN Valve With Adequate Placement

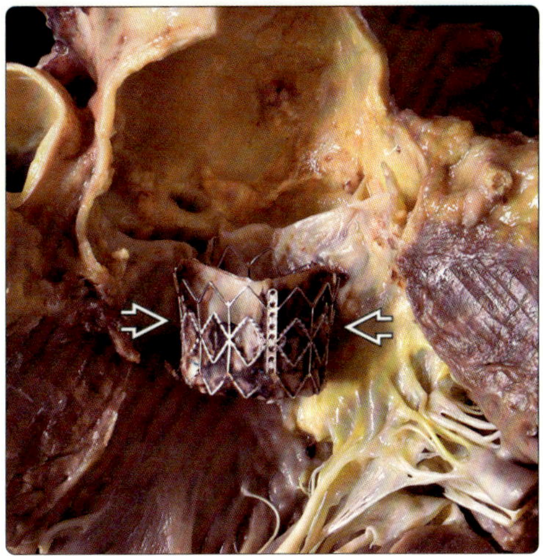

(Left) *Gross photograph of an autopsy specimen shows a SAPIEN valve properly seated in the aortic anulus. Evaluation at autopsy should include assessment of complete expansion and leaflet coaptation and any potential for paravalvular leak.* **(Right)** *Another appropriately placed TAVR aortic valve prosthesis is seen in this autopsied heart. Improper seating can lead to dislodgement and distal embolization of the valve.*

SAPIEN Valve With Incomplete Expansion

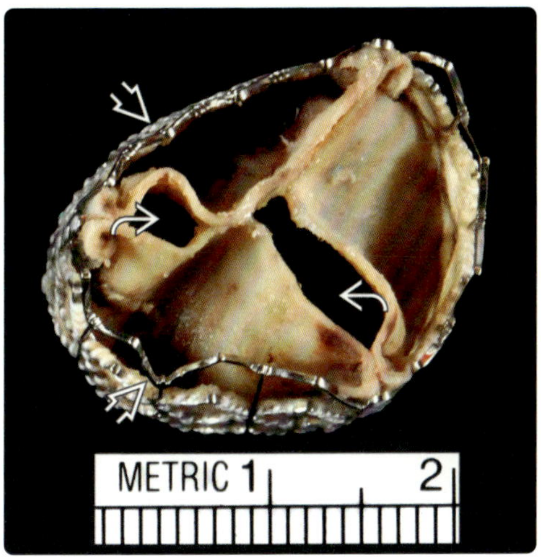

SAPIEN Valve With Incomplete Expansion

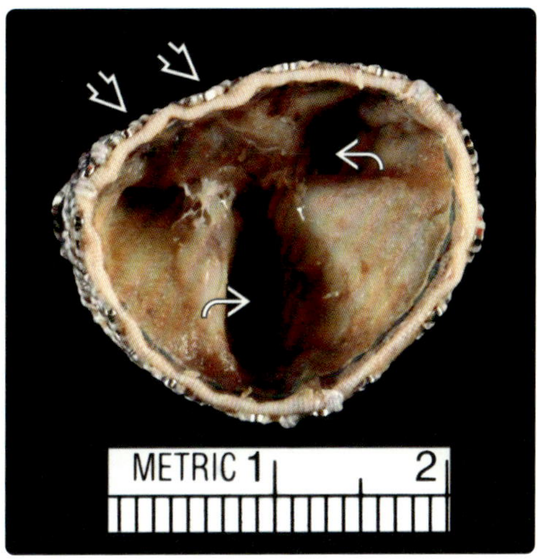

(Left) *Gross photograph of a SAPIEN valve shows incomplete expansion. Rather than a perfect circular circumference, there is deformation of the stent ring. Leaflet coaptation is impaired since the leaflet edges were predesigned to meet when the valve is fully expanded. As a result, there are fixed coaptation defects, leading to regurgitation.* **(Right)** *Viewed from the ventricular aspect, this SAPIEN valve has circumferential deformation and failure of the leaflets to coapt.*

SAPIEN Valve With Incomplete Expansion

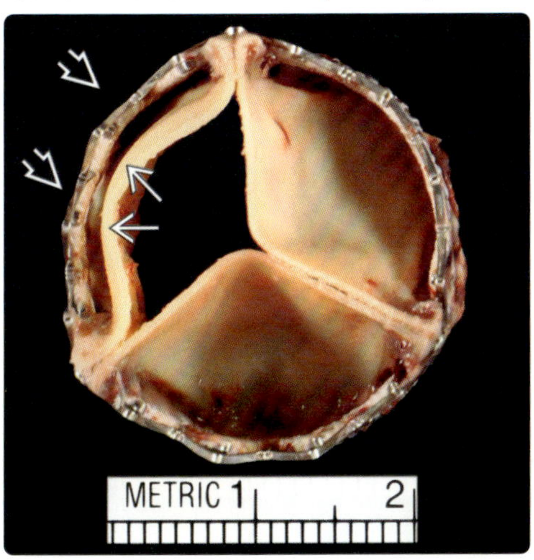

SAPIEN Valve With Tenting

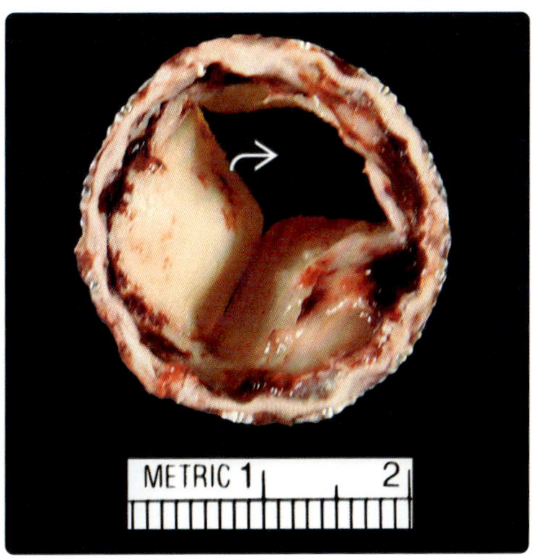

(Left) *This much more subtle example of incomplete expansion of a SAPIEN TAVR valve shows only slight inward bowing of a segment of the stent circumference. There is a resulting "tenting" deformity of the leaflet. The valve could manually be pushed down to coapt appropriately but recoiled when released.* **(Right)** *Viewed from the ventricular aspect, the tented leaflet is again apparent. The expansion seems to be more complete at this aspect of the prosthesis.*

(Left) *Gross photograph of a Medtronic Melody valve shows marked obstruction due to pannus and vegetation material* ➡ *on the leaflets, which are common degenerative changes and a complication of these bioprostheses.* **(Right)** *The Melody valve has been opened and splayed out to highlight destruction of the 3 leaflets* ⇨ *due to bulky vegetations. Endocarditis is an important complication occurring in these bioprostheses.*

Medtronic Melody Valve With Degenerative Changes and Vegetations

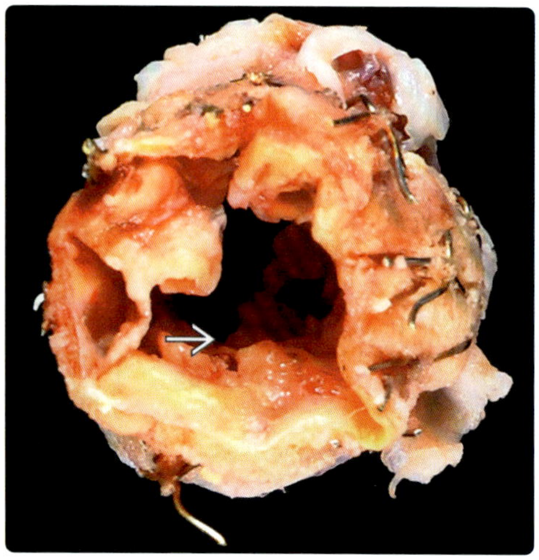

Melody Valve Complicated With Endocarditis

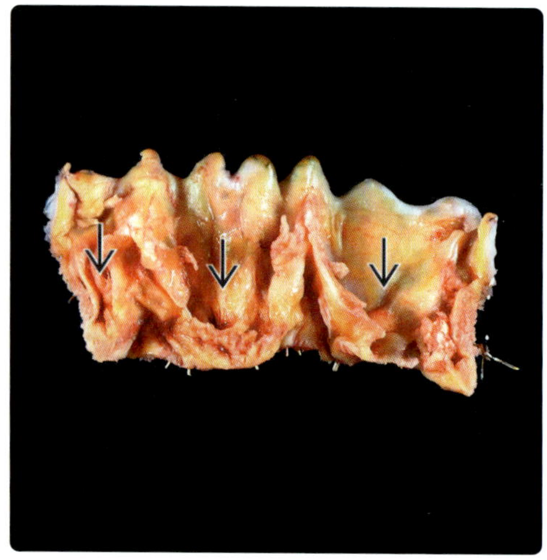

(Left) *This mitral valve is shown from the ventricular aspect. Two MitraClip devices* ➡ *are visible and fix the anterior leaflet to segments of the posterior leaflet. Typically, only 1 clip is placed, but additional clips may be added to help reduce regurgitation. For orientation (of the anterior leaflet), the aortic valve* ➡ *and aortomitral continuity are attached.* **(Right)** *A swab tip has been inserted into this valve to demonstrate the residual mitral orifice* ➡ *after MitraClip placement.*

2 MitraClip Devices Applied to Mitral Leaflets

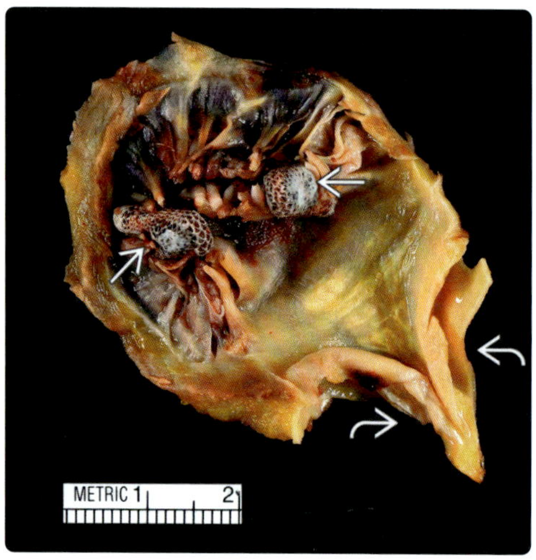

MitraClip Device Applied to Mitral Leaflets

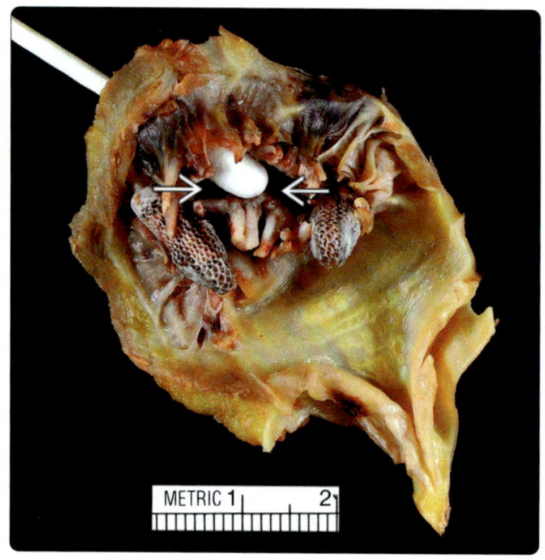

(Left) *Gross photograph of a surgically resected valve shows a healed reendothelialized MitraClip device* ➡ *placed at the midpoint of the closing edge of the anterior mitral leaflet.* **(Right)** *Gross photograph of a surgically resected mitral valve with healed reendothelialized MitraClip device is viewed on edge. The MitraClip device* ➡ *became detached from the posterior segment.*

MitraClip Device With Reendothelialization

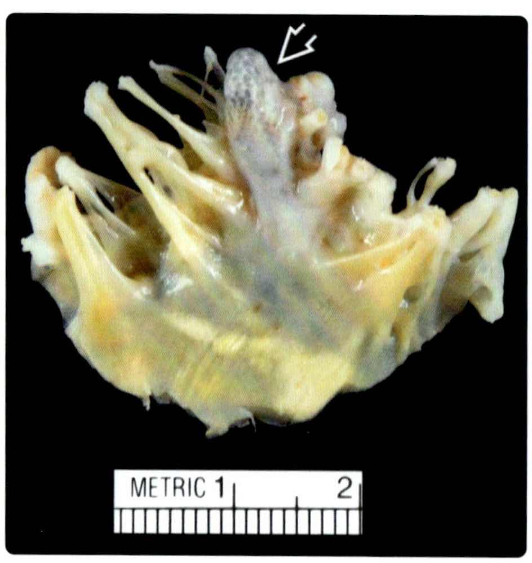

MitraClip Detached From Posterior Segment

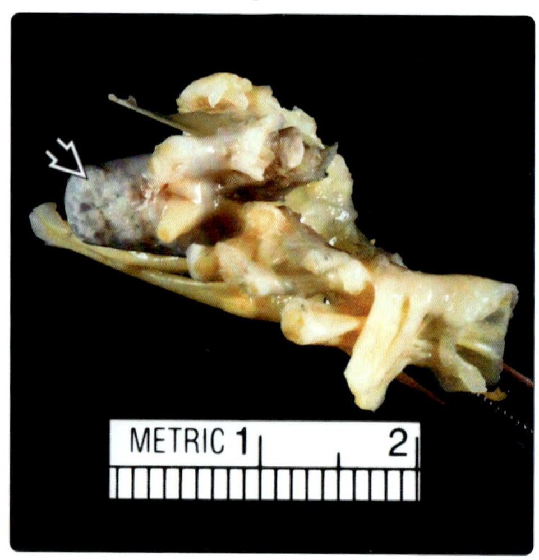

SAPIEN M3 Mitral Valve (Atrial View)

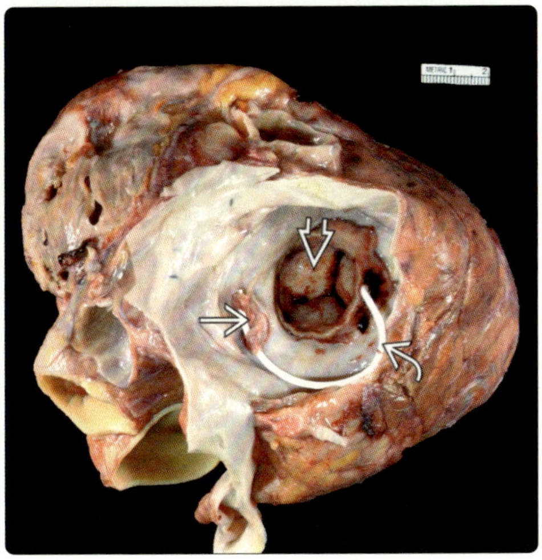

SAPIEN M3 Mitral Valve (Ventricular View)

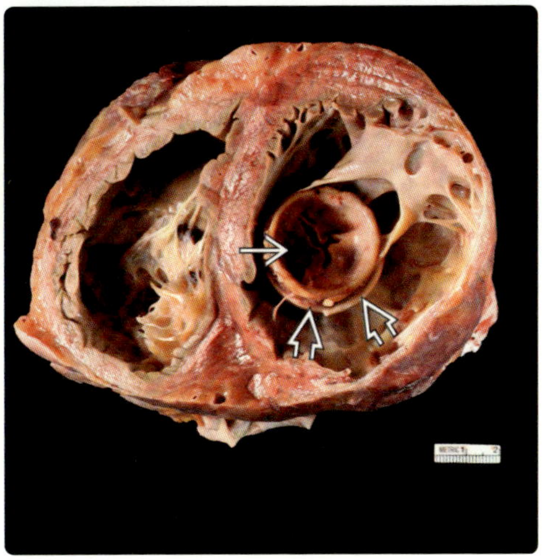

(Left) *Gross photograph of a heart removed at autopsy from a patient who had TAVR using the SAPIEN M3 system shows the expanded valve in place within the coiled dock (not seen). The dock "tail" extends into the left atrium and shows a small recent thrombus at the tip.* **(Right)** *Gross photograph of a heart removed at autopsy from a patient who had TAVR using the SAPIEN M3 system shows the expanded valve in place within the coiled dock (not seen).*

MitraClip Device (Anterior Leaflet)

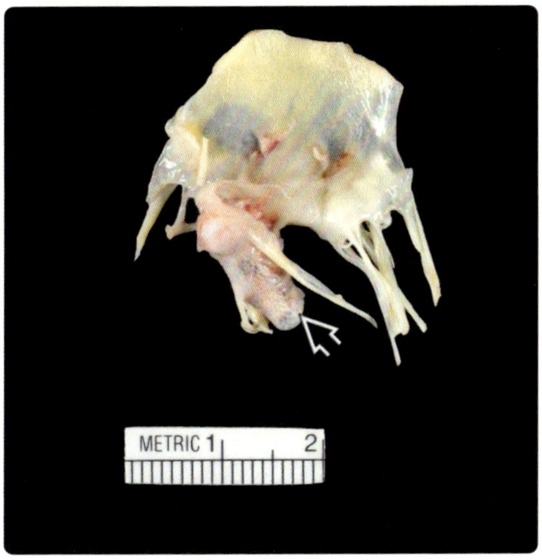

MitraClip Devices (In Situ)

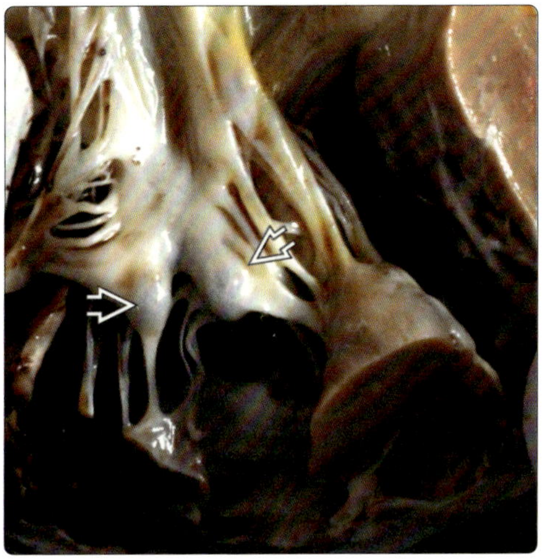

(Left) *Gross photograph of a surgically excised anterior mitral leaflet shows a MitraClip device attached to the closing edge, entrapping some of the tendinous cords.* **(Right)** *Gross photograph of the mitral valve in this explanted heart specimen shows 2 separate MitraClip devices that have been well incorporated by a layer of neointimal fibrous tissue.*

CoreValve Transcatheter Aortic Valve

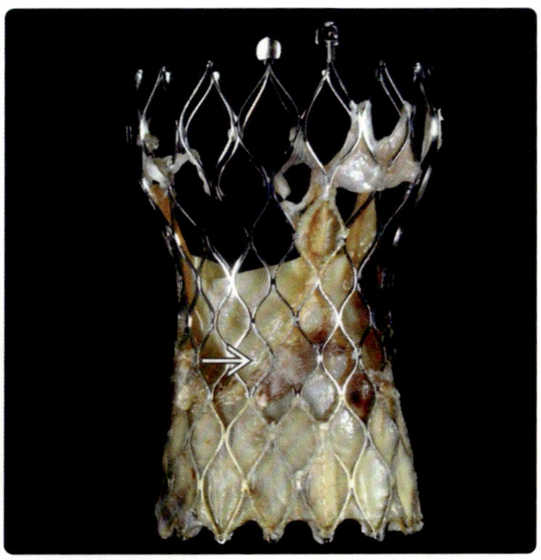

Fibrous Overgrowth of Transcatheter Aortic Valve

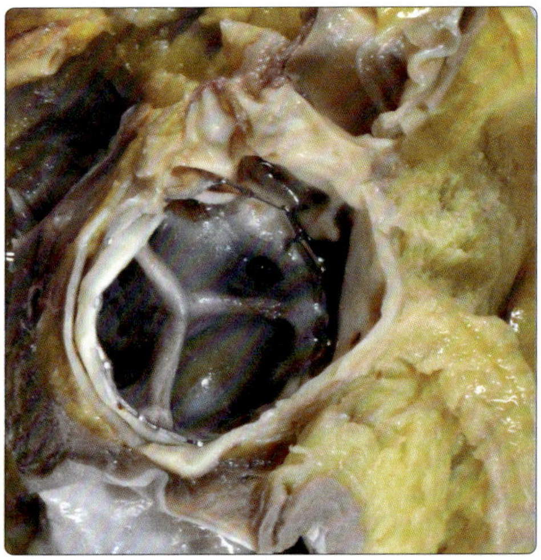

(Left) *This TAVR valve was removed surgically. Overall, the valve is longer than native anulus, but supravalvular portion is uncoated to allow flow through stent interspaces to coronary ostia.* **(Right)** *Gross photograph of an autopsied heart specimen from a patient on long-term left ventricular assist device (LVAD) support shows fibrous overgrowth causing fusion of the prosthetic leaflets. With continuous flow circulation from the LVAD, the leaflets stopped opening and closing, allowing this change.*

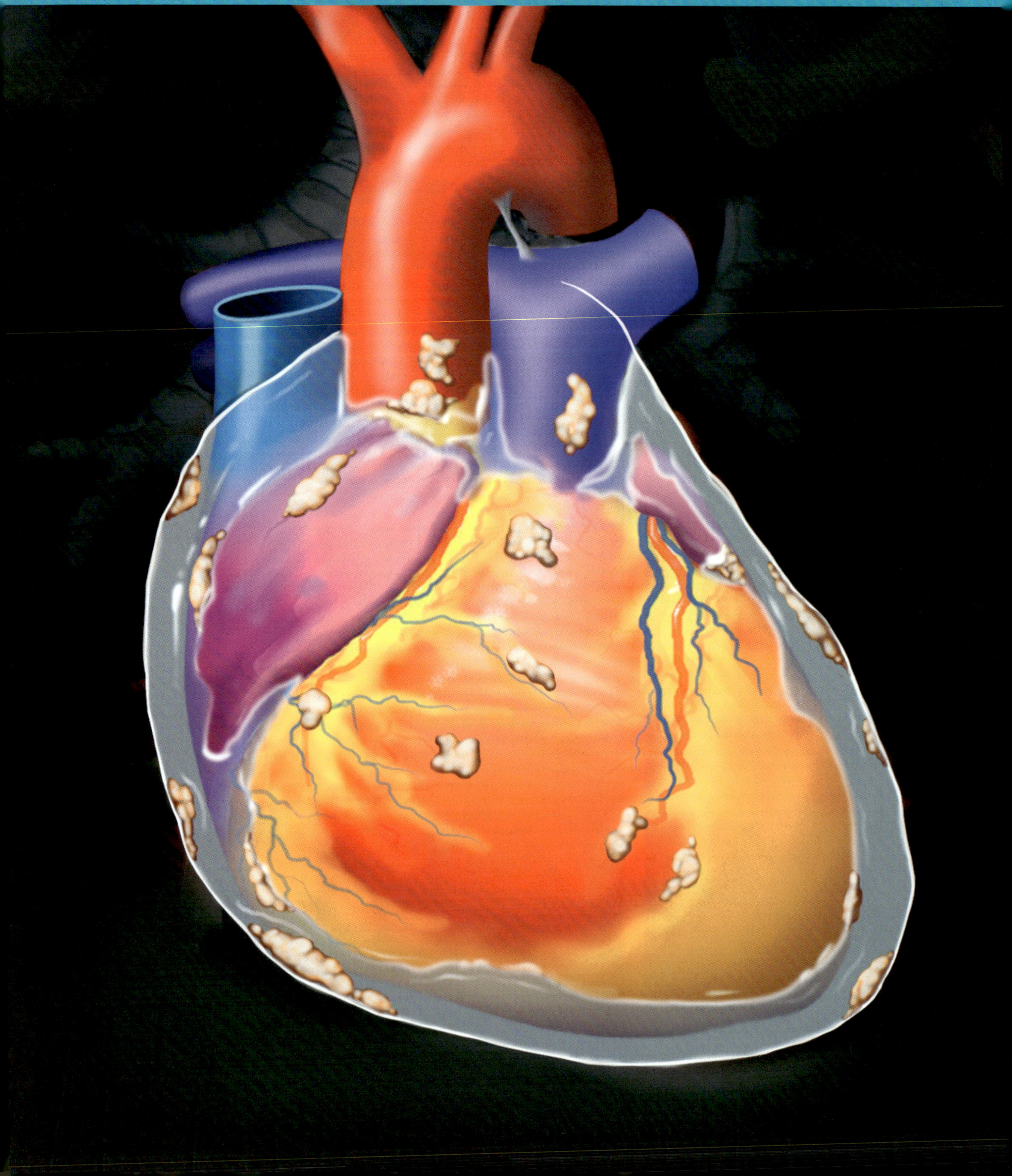

SECTION 6

Pericardium

Inflammatory

Tumors

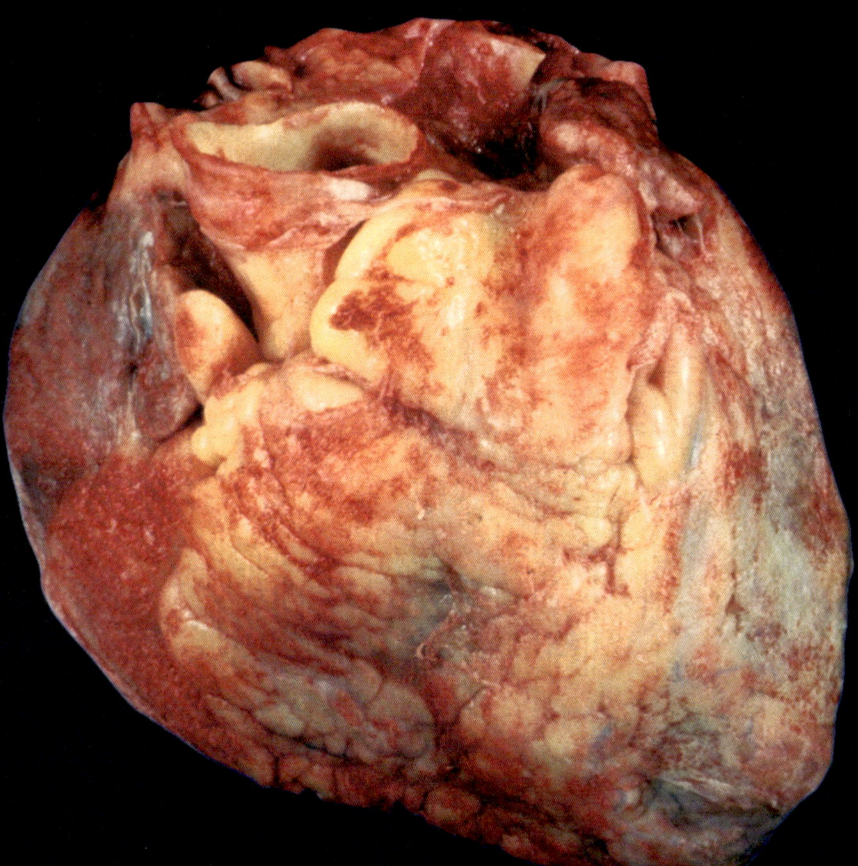

KEY FACTS

TERMINOLOGY

- Pericardial inflammation secondary to wide variety of diseases with duration of no more than 1-2 weeks
  - In majority of cases, etiology cannot be determined, and it is considered idiopathic

ETIOLOGY/PATHOGENESIS

- Idiopathic
- Infectious: Bacterial, viral, fungal
- Immune-inflammatory: Connective tissue disease
- Neoplastic
- Radiation
- Device or procedure related

CLINICAL ISSUES

- True incidence is unknown because great number of cases are undiagnosed
- Most common in children and older adults in bacterial pericarditis
- Precordial chest pain, fever, pericardial rub
- Culture, chemical analysis, and microbiologic evaluation of pericardial fluid are essential for specific diagnosis
- Complications include large pericardial effusion with tamponade, recurrent/constrictive pericarditis, aortic mycotic aneurysm in bacterial pericarditis, and death

MACROSCOPIC

- Pericardial thickening with shaggy exudate coating
- Variable types of pericardial fluid: Serous, fibrinous, serosanguineous, hemorrhagic, purulent

MICROSCOPIC

- Nonspecific inflammatory infiltrate with numerous neutrophils or predominantly mononuclear cells
- Abundant fibrin deposits
- Intracytoplasmic bacteria on Gram stain, fungal microorganisms identified on special stains
- Granulation tissue
- Fibrosis in resolving phase

Gross Image of Fibrinous Pericarditis

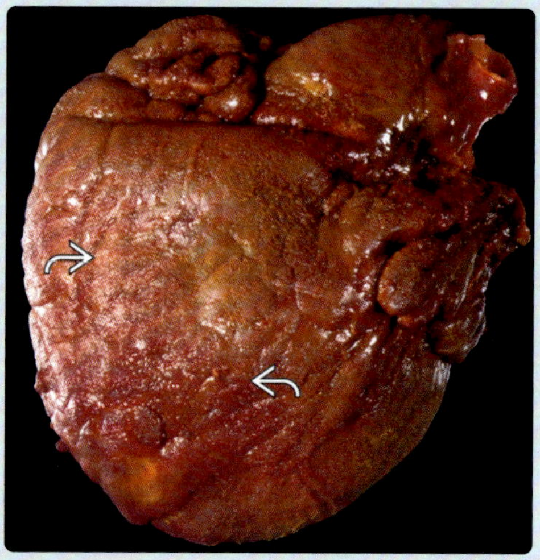

Histologic Features of Fibrinous Pericarditis

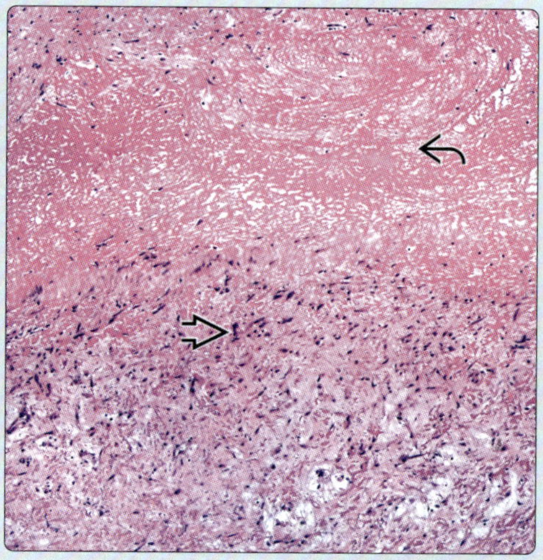

(Left) *Autopsy gross specimen shows anterior heart surface coated by fibrinous deposits, giving a shaggy irregular appearance ➔ characteristic of fibrinous pericarditis, which may be seen in viral infections.* **(Right)** *H&E-stained section shows pericardial thickening with an extensive deposit of fibrin ➔ on the surface and scant vascular proliferation ➔. These features are most commonly seen in viral pericarditis.*

Acute Bacterial Pericarditis

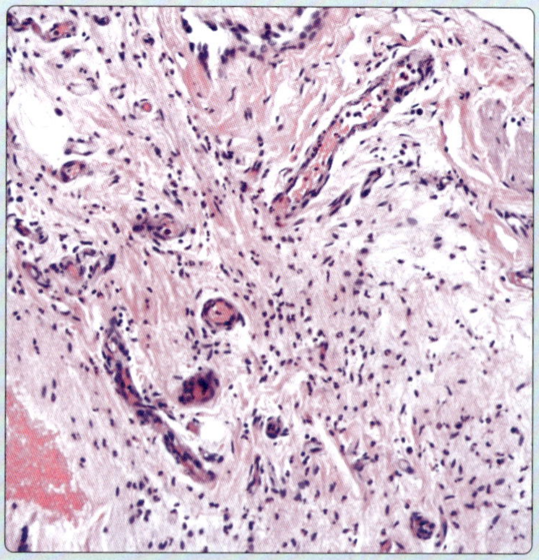

Histologic Features of Resolving Pericarditis

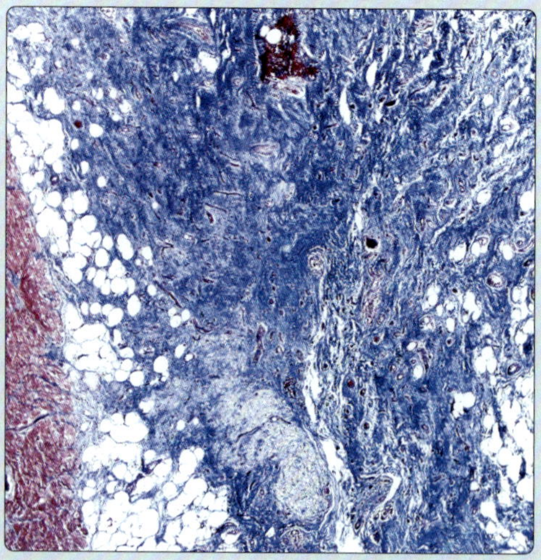

(Left) *H&E-stained section shows pericardium with edema, vascular proliferation, and diffuse neutrophilic inflammatory infiltrate. These features are nonspecific and may be seen in any type of acute infectious pericarditis.* **(Right)** *Trichrome-stained section shows pericardium with marked fibrosis and scant lymphocytic inflammatory infiltrate. These features are nonspecific and may be seen in any type of resolving pericarditis. Progression to constrictive pericarditis is unusually seen in cases of idiopathic/viral pericarditis.*

TERMINOLOGY

Definitions

- Pericardial inflammation secondary to wide variety of diseases with duration of no more than 1-2 weeks
  - In majority of cases, etiology cannot be determined, and it is considered idiopathic

ETIOLOGY/PATHOGENESIS

Infectious Agents

- Bacterial
  - Aerobic: *Staphylococcus aureus*, pneumococcus, *Streptococcus pyogenes*, *Haemophilus influenzae*, gram-negative rods
  - Anaerobic bacteria: *Prevotella*, *Peptostreptococcus*, *Propionibacterium acnes*, *Bacteroides fragilis*
- Viral: Echovirus, coxsackievirus, Adenovirus, Cytomegalovirus, hepatitis B, EBV, HIV, Parvovirus B19, Epstein-Barr virus
- Fungal: Histoplasmosis, coccidioidomycosis, *Candida*

Other Etiologies

- Idiopathic: Unknown etiology probably of viral origin
- Immune-inflammatory: Connective tissue diseases, early/late postmyocardial infarction, drug induced, chronic kidney disease, sarcoidosis, autoinflammatory disease
- Neoplastic disease: Primary or secondary
- Radiation induced
- Post cardiac surgery
- Trauma

Mechanisms of Bacterial Pericardial Infection

- Direct extension from lung focus (e.g., pneumonia, empyema)
- Hematogenous spread (e.g., bacteremia)
- Contiguous spread after thoracic surgery or trauma
- Rupture of perivalvular abscess
- Spread along fascial plains from oral cavity

Risk Factors for Pericardial Infection

- Chronic illness
- Immunocompromised state: Malignancies, diabetes mellitus, renal failure
- Postoperative infection

CLINICAL ISSUES

Epidemiology

- Incidence
  - Unknown because many cases are undiagnosed, but it is most common disorder involving pericardium
  - ~ 5% of emergency department visits for chest pain
  - Idiopathic is most common type
- Age
  - Most common in children and older adults in bacterial pericarditis
- Sex
  - M > F

Presentation

- Precordial chest pain (pleuritic/nonpleuritic)
  - Irradiation to trapezius ridge and over scapula
  - Commonly relieved by sitting forward
  - Worsens by lying down
- Pericardial friction rub
- Sinus tachycardia
- Fever
- Dyspnea/cough

Laboratory Tests

- Microbiologic evaluation of pericardial fluid with Gram, acid-fast bacilli (AFB), and silver stains
- Culture of pericardial fluid or blood for aerobic/anaerobic bacteria and fungi
- Viral cultures of pericardial fluid may not be diagnostic; PCR for viral identification is more effective
- Chemical analysis of pericardial fluid: Low glucose, high protein concentration, lactate dehydrogenase elevated
- CBC demonstrates variable elevation of white cells
- Sedimentation rate and C-reactive protein usually elevated
- Troponin and CK-MB isoenzyme can be elevated in association with myopericarditis
- Viral serologies for HIV/hepatitis C
- Specific panels of antibodies (ANA, anti-dsDNA) in case of connective tissue disease-associated pericarditis

Treatment

- Surgical approaches
  - Pericardiocentesis
  - Pericardial window
  - Pericardiectomy recommended in constrictive pericarditis or patients with multiple recurrences unresponsive to medical therapy
- Drugs
  - IV-specific antibiotics or antifungal agents
  - Antiinflammatories: NSAIDs, colchicine (recurrence prevention)
  - Steroids when no response to antiinflammatories
  - Failing to obtain remission with 1st- and 2nd-line medications, azathioprine, intravenous immunoglobulin or IL-1B antagonist are recommended
  - Intrapericardial fibrinolytic therapy in bacterial pericarditis is recommended

Prognosis

- Depends on etiology
  - Viral pericarditis is self-limited and generally resolves in 1-3 weeks, rarely progressing to constrictive pericarditis
  - Purulent pericarditis may progress to constrictive pericarditis, and prognosis is poor if delay in treatment
  - Pericarditis in connective tissue disease or idiopathic pericarditis may be recurrent
  - Patients with idiopathic pericarditis more likely fail treatment

Complications

- Large pericardial effusion with tamponade can occur in ~ 15% in idiopathic pericarditis
- Recurrent pericarditis occurs in ~ 20-30% of cases, over 18 months after 1st episode
- Constrictive pericarditis
- Aortic mycotic aneurysm in bacterial pericarditis
- Death

IMAGING

Radiographic Findings

- Cardiac silhouette in most cases is normal but will be enlarged in cases of large effusions
- Mediastinal widening or mass effect occurs in neoplasia-associated pericarditis
- Pulmonary infiltrates/pleural effusions may be seen in cases of bacterial pericarditis

Ultrasonographic Findings

- Pericardial effusion is identified as sonolucent space between pericardial layers, usually in small amount
- Pericardial thickening
- Intrapericardial fibrinous strands

EKG

- ST segment elevation, except in aV and often V1 leads
- PR segment depression
- In late stages, ST segment depression and T wave inversions

MACROSCOPIC

General Features

- Pericardial thickening
- Shaggy exudate coating epicardium
- Pericardial fluid varies in appearance: Serous, fibrinous, serosanguineous, hemorrhagic, purulent viscous

MICROSCOPIC

Histologic Features

- Viral pericarditis
    - Nonspecific mononuclear inflammation
    - Perivascular inflammation
    - Fibrinous exudate
- Bacterial pericarditis
    - Nonspecific inflammatory infiltrate with numerous neutrophils
    - In later stages, infiltrate turns lymphocytic or shows numerous plasma cells
    - Abundant fibrin deposits
    - Intracytoplasmic bacteria on Gram stain
    - Granulation tissue formation
    - Fibrosis in chronic phase
- Fungal pericarditis
    - Granulomatous or nonspecific inflammation
    - Necrotizing pericarditis may be seen
    - Fungal microorganisms can be identified with special stains
- Pericarditis secondary to connective tissue disease
    - Lupus pericarditis
        - Focal fibrinoid necrosis and hematoxylin bodies
        - Vessel wall necrosis and obstruction by granular hyaline material
        - Initial neutrophilic inflammation occurs
        - In later stages, mononuclear infiltrates predominate
        - Fibrosis and pericardial thickening
    - Rheumatoid arthritis
        - Rheumatoid granulomas are rarely found
        - Nonspecific mononuclear inflammation
        - In late stage, fibrosis is predominant finding
        - Cholesterol crystals may be prominent
- Pericarditis in acute rheumatic fever
    - Aschoff nodules are rarely identified
    - Histiocyte and mononuclear inflammation
    - Fibrinous exudate
- Sarcoidosis
    - Noncaseating granulomas
    - Nonspecific fibrosis
- Pericarditis following myocardial infarction
    - Postinfarction pericarditis
        - Acute inflammation associated with area of myocardial infarction
        - Hemorrhage can be seen
    - Dressler syndrome
        - Fibrinous exudate
        - Nonspecific inflammatory infiltrate
- Pericarditis in malignancy
    - Nonspecific inflammation
    - Carcinoma cells, especially from breast and lung origin, may infiltrate pericardium
    - Malignant mesothelial cells in primary or secondary mesothelioma
    - Sheets of atypical lymphocytes in cases of lymphoma

ANCILLARY TESTS

Histochemistry

- Gram stain
    - Reactivity: Positive/negative
- Gomori methenamine silver (GMS)
    - Reactivity: Positive in fungal microorganisms

Immunohistochemistry

- Epithelial, mesenchymal, and hematologic markers contribute to identification of lineage of malignant cells in malignancy-associated pericarditis

Immunofluorescence

- Immune complex deposits demonstrated in vessel wall in cases of connective tissue disease-associated pericarditis

DIFFERENTIAL DIAGNOSIS

Tuberculous Pericarditis

- Granulomatous inflammation
- AFB-positive bacteria
- Positive culture for AFB
- Clinical presentation is subacute with several weeks of symptoms prior to diagnosis

SELECTED REFERENCES

1. Bouriche F et al: Acute pericarditis: aetiologic diagnosis and practical aspect of the management. Curr Probl Cardiol. 46(4):100769, 2021
2. Chiabrando JG et al: Management of acute and recurrent pericarditis: JACC state-of-the-art review. J Am Coll Cardiol. 75(1):76-92, 2020
3. Ismail TF: Acute pericarditis: update on diagnosis and management. Clin Med (Lond). 20(1):48-51, 2020
4. Vecchié A et al: Clinical presentation and outcomes of acute pericarditis in a large urban hospital in the United States of America. Chest. 158(6):2556-67, 2020
5. Blank N et al: Idiopathic pericarditis-an autoinflammatory disease? Curr Rheumatol Rep. 21(5):18, 2019
6. Doctor NS et al: Acute pericarditis. Prog Cardiovasc Dis. 59(4):349-59, 2017

Histologic Features of Fibrinous Pericarditis

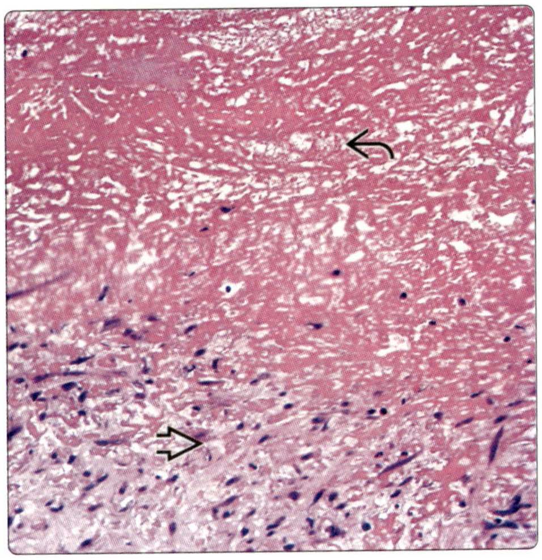

Viral Pericarditis in Resolving Phase

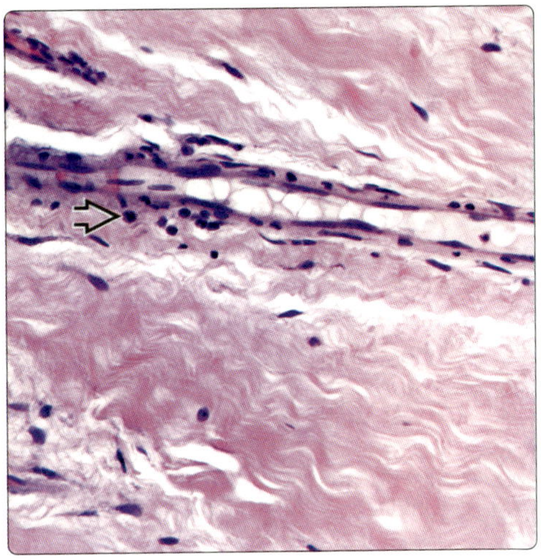

(Left) *H&E-stained section shows an extensive deposit of fibrin ⇨ on the pericardial surface and scant fibrovascular proliferation ⇨ in an early phase of viral pericarditis. Fibrinous pericarditis may also be a manifestation of acute rheumatic fever and lupus pericarditis.* **(Right)** *H&E-stained section shows pericardial fibrosis and scant mononuclear perivascular inflammatory infiltrate ⇨. Although not specific, these features are seen in cases of viral pericarditis in resolving phase.*

Histologic Features in Viral Pericarditis

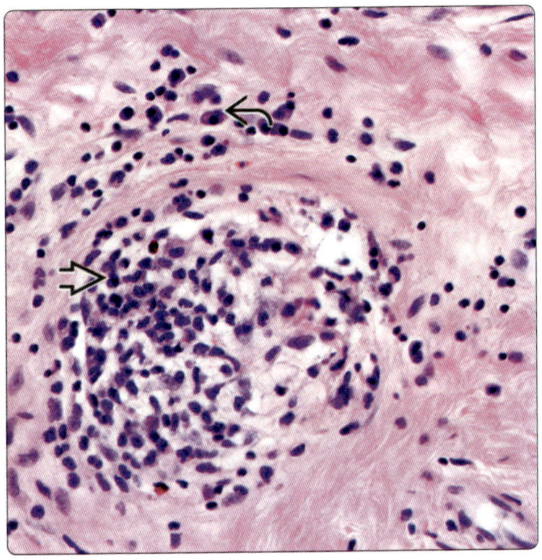

Pericarditis in Resolving/Chronic Phase

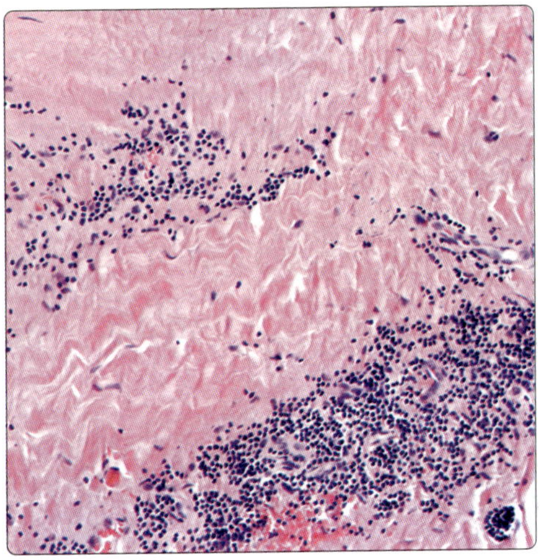

(Left) *H&E-stained section shows pericardium with focal aggregates of inflammatory cells, including lymphocytes ⇨ and frequent plasma cells ⇨, in a case of viral pericarditis. In most cases, this process will resolve without significant scarring.* **(Right)** *H&E-stained section shows pericardium with fibrosis and aggregates of lymphocytic inflammatory infiltrate. These features are nonspecific and may be seen in any type of pericarditis in resolving phase.*

Histologic Features in Bacterial Pericarditis

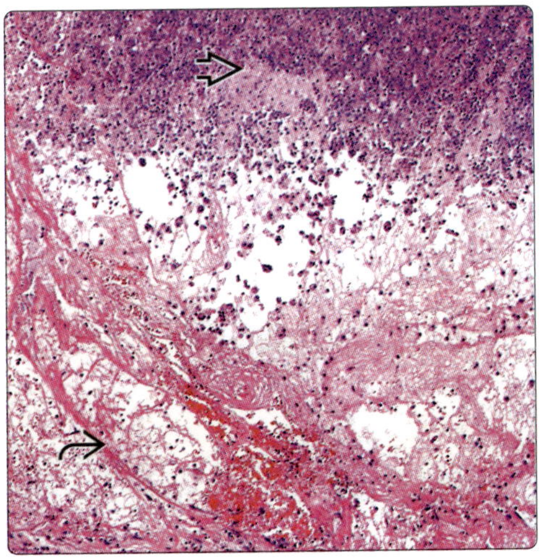

Pericarditis Associated With Myocardial Infarct

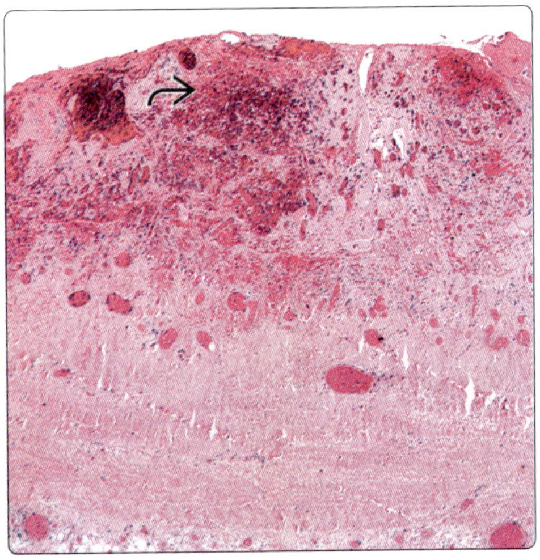

(Left) *H&E-stained section shows an extensive deposit of fibrin ⇨ on the pericardial surface, focal hemorrhage, and marked neutrophilic infiltrate ⇨ in a case of bacterial pericarditis. These features may be seen with any type of bacterial agent.* **(Right)** *H&E-stained section shows hemorrhage ⇨ on the pericardial surface and scant mononuclear inflammation in a case of pericarditis following myocardial infarction. This may occur on the 2nd or 3rd day following a transmural infarct.*

Constrictive Pericarditis

KEY FACTS

TERMINOLOGY

- End stage of inflammatory process involving pericardium; characterized by dense pericardial fibrosis, often calcification with obliteration of pericardial space, and restriction of diastolic filling

ETIOLOGY/PATHOGENESIS

- Any type of infectious pericarditis
- Early in this century, tuberculous pericarditis was most common cause of constrictive pericarditis and still remains so in nonindustrialized countries
- Others causes: Idiopathic, post radiation, post cardiac surgery, neoplasms, sarcoidosis, uremia

CLINICAL ISSUES

- Constrictive pericarditis is uncommon in children
- Clinical manifestations include
    - Right-sided heart failure with systemic venous congestion
    - Reduced cardiac index
    - Preserved myocardial contractile function
    - Tricuspid valve regurgitation
    - Marked elevation of jugular venous pressure
    - Paradoxical pulse
- Worse prognosis in radiation-induced constrictive pericarditis

MACROSCOPIC

- Marked pericardial thickening
- Obliteration of pericardial space
- Heart size may be within normal limits
- Rare cases show normal pericardial thickness

MICROSCOPIC

- Pericardial dense fibrosis
- Nonspecific chronic inflammation
- Granulomatous inflammation in cases associated with tuberculosis

Contrast-Enhanced CT Findings in Constrictive Pericarditis

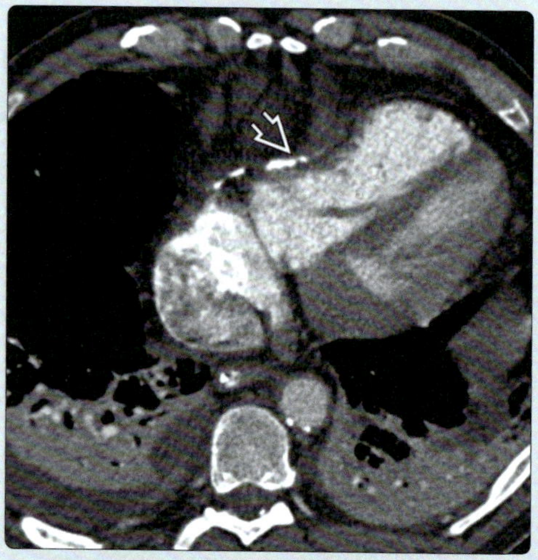

Pericardial Specimen From Case of Constrictive Pericarditis

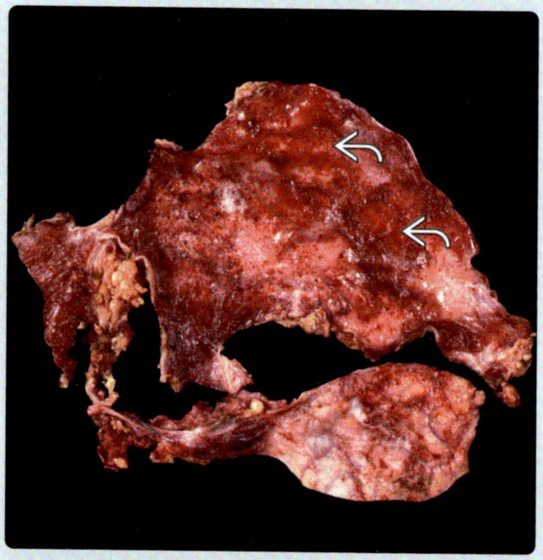

(Left) *Axial CECT through the inferior aspect of the heart shows thickening and linear calcification of the anterior pericardium ➔ with mass effect and tubular configuration of the right ventricle in this case of constrictive pericarditis. (Courtesy M. Rosado de Christenson, MD, FACR.)* **(Right)** *Surgically removed pericardiectomy specimen from a patient with constrictive pericarditis shows fibrotic thickening and hyperemic granulation tissue ➔.*

Histologic Features of Constrictive Pericarditis

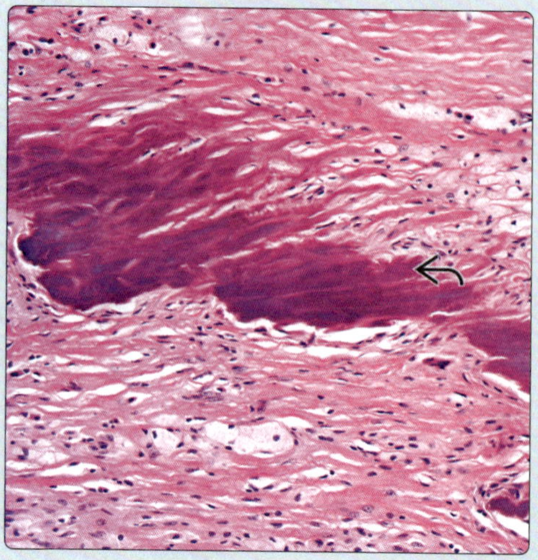

Histologic Features of Constrictive Pericarditis

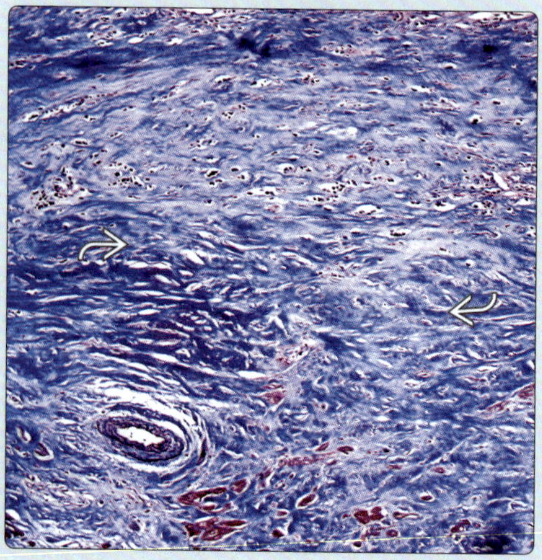

(Left) *H&E-stained section of pericardium shows marked fibrosis, scant nonspecific mononuclear inflammation, and focal calcification ➔.* **(Right)** *Trichrome-stained section highlights dense fibrosis ➔ associated with scant inflammatory infiltrate and vascular proliferation in this case of constrictive pericarditis.*

TERMINOLOGY

Definitions

- End stage of inflammatory process involving pericardium; characterized by dense pericardial fibrosis, often calcification with obliteration of pericardial space, and restriction of diastolic filling

ETIOLOGY/PATHOGENESIS

Infectious Agents

- Any type of infectious pericarditis may result in pericardial scarring and, eventually (~ 1.8%), constrictive pericarditis
- Early in this century, tuberculous pericarditis was most common cause of constrictive pericarditis and still remains so in nonindustrialized countries

Others

- Idiopathic (42%)
- Post cardiac surgery (11-37%)
- Post radiation (9-31%)
- Uremia (10%)
- Connective tissue disorders (3-7%)
- Posttraumatic
- Neoplasms (3%)
- Sarcoidosis
- Drug toxicity

CLINICAL ISSUES

Presentation

- Right-sided heart failure with systemic venous congestion
- Reduced cardiac index and ejection fraction
- Preserved myocardial contractile function
- Tricuspid valve regurgitation
- Marked elevation of jugular venous pressure
- Kussmaul sign: Inspiratory increase in systemic venous pressure
- Paradoxical pulse

Laboratory Tests

- B-type natriuretic peptide and N-terminal pro B-type natriuretic peptide levels are normal or mildly elevated

Treatment

- Surgical approaches
    - Pericardiectomy is most effective therapy
        - Partial or complete (improved long-term outcome)
- Drugs
    - Diuretics
    - Antibiotics if infectious etiology

Prognosis

- Worse prognosis in radiation-induced constrictive pericarditis

IMAGING

Ultrasonographic Findings

- Pericardial thickening
- Abrupt displacement of interventricular septum during early diastole (septal bounce)
- Systemic congestion: Hepatic congestion, distention of inferior vena cava
- Exaggerated septal shifting during respiration

MR Findings

- Pericardial thickening (> 4 mm), most prominent at base of ventricles
- Pericardium with late gadolinium enhancement
- Tubular morphology of ventricles and biatrial enlargement
- Septal bouncing and abnormal ventricular interdependence
- Increased ventricular coupling on real-time cine CMR

CT Findings

- Pericardial thickening (> 4 mm), calcifications, &/or adhesions
- Tubular deformity of ventricles (especially right) with decreased volume
- Flat or sigmoid intraventricular septum

Cardiac Catheterization and Angiography

- Right ventricular diastolic, pulmonary capillary wedge, and pre-A wave left ventricular diastolic pressure is elevated and equal or nearly so
- Right and left ventricular pressures show marked diastolic dip followed by plateau
- Pulmonary artery and right ventricular systolic pressures are modestly elevated

MACROSCOPIC

General Features

- Marked pericardial thickening (diffuse/focal)
- Obliteration of pericardial space
- Heart size may be within normal limits
- Rare cases show normal pericardial thickness (~ 20%)

MICROSCOPIC

Histologic Features

- Pericardial dense fibrosis
- Nonspecific chronic inflammation
- Calcification
- Necrotizing granulomatous inflammation in cases associated with tuberculosis

DIFFERENTIAL DIAGNOSIS

Restrictive Cardiomyopathy

- Pericardial thickening not present
- Thickened ventricular walls and biatrial enlargement
- Demonstration of amyloid deposits in cases of amyloidosis

SELECTED REFERENCES

1. Diaz-Arocutipa C et al: Natriuretic peptides to differentiate constrictive pericarditis and restrictive cardiomyopathy: a systematic review and meta-analysis. Clin Cardiol. 45(3):251-7, 2022
2. Liu VC et al: Pericardiectomy for constrictive pericarditis: analysis of outcomes. J Cardiothorac Vasc Anesth. 35(12):3797-805, 2021
3. Goldstein JA et al: Hemodynamics of constrictive pericarditis and restrictive cardiomyopathy. Catheter Cardiovasc Interv. 95(6):1240-8, 2020
4. Garcia MJ: Constrictive pericarditis versus restrictive cardiomyopathy? J Am Coll Cardiol. 67(17):2061-76, 2016
5. Porta-Sánchez A et al: Constrictive pericarditis: etiologic spectrum, patterns of clinical presentation, prognostic factors, and long-term follow-up. Rev Esp Cardiol (Engl Ed). 68(12):1092-100, 2015

Tuberculous Pericarditis

TERMINOLOGY

Definitions

- Necrotizing granulomatous pericardial inflammation due to infection with *Mycobacterium tuberculosis*

ETIOLOGY/PATHOGENESIS

Infectious Agents

- *M. tuberculosis* complex
  - *Mycobacterium tuberculosis*
  - *Mycobacterium africanum*
  - *Mycobacterium bovis*
  - *Mycobacterium microti*
  - *Mycobacterium mungi*

Risk Factors

- Immunosuppression (AIDS/corticosteroid use)
- Poor nutritional status
- Chronic noncommunicable diseases
- Black race

Mechanism of Pericardial Infection

- Retrograde lymphatic spread from regional lymph nodes (tracheobronchial, mediastinal, or hilar)
- Direct extension from pulmonary or lymph node focus
- Hematogenous spread from lung, genitourinary tract, or skeletal system

CLINICAL IMPLICATIONS

Epidemiology

- Incidence
  - Pericarditis occurs in 1-2% of patients with active pulmonary tuberculosis in endemic areas
  - 4% of acute pericarditis cases in developed countries
  - 7% of cardiac tamponade cases
  - > 90% of pericardial effusion in HIV-infected patients
  - 50-70% of pericardial effusions in individuals from developing countries, where tuberculosis is endemic
  - Most common cause of constrictive pericarditis in endemic areas
- Age
  - 3rd-5th decades
- Sex
  - 3-4x more common in males
- Ethnicity
  - Most frequent in developing countries
  - Black patients have 10-12x increased incidence

Presentation

- Heart-related symptoms
  - Chest pain/dyspnea
  - Cardiomegaly
  - Pericardial friction rub
  - Distant heart sounds when large effusion present
  - Right heart failure symptoms: Elevated jugular vein pressure, pulsus paradoxus
- Constitutional symptoms
  - Weight loss
  - Fever
  - Night sweats

Laboratory Tests

- Culture of pericardial fluid for *M. tuberculosis* positive in 53-75%
- Adenosine deaminase activity
- Lysozyme and unstimulated interferon-γ levels
- PCR amplification of mycobacterial DNA in tissue sample
- Rapid nucleic acid amplification test (Xpert MTB/RIF)

Treatment

- Surgical/interventional approaches
  - Early pericardiectomy if constrictive pericarditis develops
  - Pericardiocentesis if cardiac tamponade or for diagnosis
- Drugs
  - Standard antituberculosis therapy: Isoniazid, rifampicin, ethambutol, pyrazinamide
  - Corticosteroid use decreases incidence of death from pericarditis and development of constrictive pericarditis

Histologic Features of Tuberculous Pericarditis

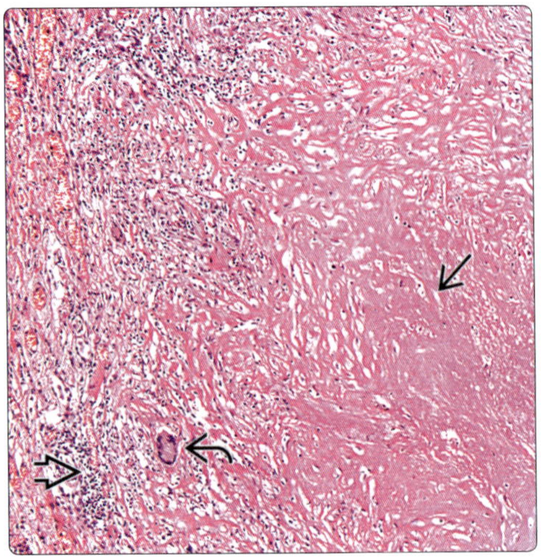

Positive Acid-Fast Stain in Tuberculous Pericarditis

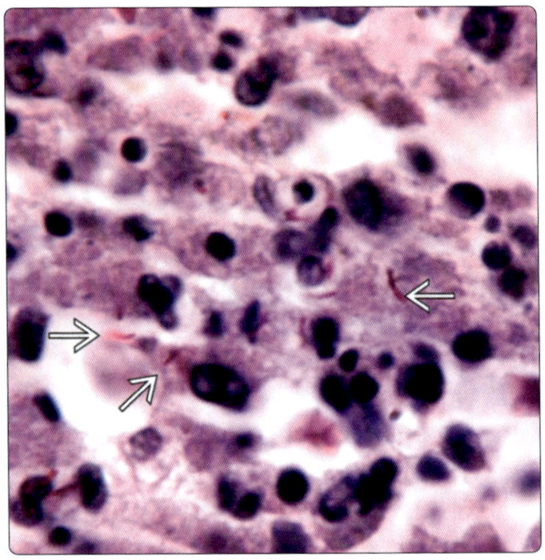

(Left) *H&E shows pericarditis with a granulomatous component showing a prominent multinucleated giant cell ➙, scattered mononuclear cells ➙, and central caseating necrosis ➙.* **(Right)** *Oil-immersion magnification field of an acid-fast stain shows positive acid-fast bacilli ➙ within macrophage cytoplasm. Identification of the mycobacterium in pericardial fluid or tissue is critical for definitive diagnosis of tuberculous pericarditis; however, they have a very poor yield.*

- Immunotherapy is controversial

Prognosis

- Without treatment, 50% of cases progress to constrictive pericarditis
- Mortality in ~ 8-17%, higher (34%) in AIDS patients

IMAGE FINDINGS

Radiographic Findings

- Cardiomegaly
- Evidence of lung involvement with interstitial infiltrates or pleural thickening/effusion

Ultrasonographic Findings

- Detects pericardial effusion
- Abnormalities in pericardium: Thickening, stranding, adhesions

MR/CT Findings

- Pericardial thickening (> 4 mm)
- Variable amount of pericardial effusion
- Pericardial late gadolinium enhancement (MR)
- Mediastinal/tracheobronchial lymphadenopathy

EKG

- Nonspecific ST-T waves
- Low voltage when large effusion is present

MACROSCOPIC

General Features

- Pericardial thickening
- Pericardial effusion with bloody appearance

MICROSCOPIC

Histologic Features

- Acute phase ("dry stage")
  - Fibrin deposit on pericardium admixed with neutrophils and lymphocytes
  - Abundant mycobacteria
- Subacute phase ("effusive stage")
  - Pericardium with necrotizing granulomatous inflammation
  - Low density of mycobacteria
  - Pericardial effusion
- Chronic adhesive phase ("absorptive stage")
  - Thickening of visceral and parietal pericardium
  - Fibroblastic proliferation
- Constrictive phase
  - Markedly fibrosed visceral and parietal pericardium
  - Calcification encasing heart

ANCILLARY TESTS

Histochemistry

- Acid-fast bacilli rarely positive (0-42%)
  - Reactivity
    - Bacilli appear bright red

PCR

- Amplification of mycobacterial DNA in tissue sample may be helpful for diagnosis

DIFFERENTIAL DIAGNOSIS

Sarcoidosis

- Rare cause of pericarditis
- Pericardium, myocardium, and endocardium involvement
- Presence of nonnecrotizing granulomas is necessary for diagnosis
- Caseous necrosis is not present
- Negative AFB stain and PCR studies for tuberculosis

Necrobiotic Rheumatoid Granuloma

- History of rheumatoid arthritis
- Granulomas show palisading histiocytes
- Caseous necrosis is not present
- Positive serologic tests for rheumatoid arthritis

Radiation Pericarditis

- History of prior radiation
- Fibrosis with atypical fibroblasts affecting predominantly parietal pericardium
- Scant inflammatory infiltrate of mononuclear cells

Idiopathic Constrictive Pericarditis

- Most common cause of constrictive pericarditis in developed countries
- Mesothelial hyperplasia
- Nonspecific fibrous pericardial thickening
- Hemosiderin deposits and cholesterol crystals
- Absence of caseating granulomatous inflammation

SELECTED REFERENCES

1. Alshoabi SA et al: The diagnostic deceiver: radiological pictorial review of tuberculosis. Diagnostics (Basel). 12(2), 2022
2. Dybowska M et al: Tuberculous pericarditis-Own experiences and recent recommendations. Diagnostics (Basel). 12(3), 2022
3. Fang L et al: The optimal duration of anti-tuberculous therapy before pericardiectomy in constrictive tuberculous pericarditis. J Cardiothorac Surg. 16(1):313, 2021
4. López-López JP et al: Tuberculosis and the heart. J Am Heart Assoc. 10(7):e019435, 2021
5. Tzani A et al: Meta-analysis of population characteristics and outcomes of patients undergoing pericardiectomy for constrictive pericarditis. Am J Cardiol. 146:120-7, 2021
6. Yadav S et al: Pericardiectomy for constrictive tuberculous pericarditis: a systematic review and meta-analysis on the etiology, patients' characteristics, and the outcomes. Cureus. 13(9):e18252, 2021
7. Howlett P et al: The immunopathogenesis of tuberculous pericarditis. Microbes Infect. 22(4-5):172-81, 2020
8. Kim MS et al: The clinical course of tuberculous pericarditis in immunocompetent hosts based on serial echocardiography. Korean Circ J. 50(7):599-609, 2020
9. Naicker K et al: Tuberculous pericardial disease: a focused update on diagnosis, therapy and prevention of complications. Cardiovasc Diagn Ther. 10(2):289-95, 2020
10. Chang SA: Tuberculous and infectious pericarditis. Cardiol Clin. 35(4):615-22, 2017
11. Adler Y et al: 2015 ESC Guidelines for the diagnosis and management of pericardial diseases: the Task Force for the Diagnosis and Management of Pericardial Diseases of the European Society of Cardiology (ESC) endorsed by: the European Association for Cardio-Thoracic Surgery (EACTS). Eur Heart J. 36(42):2921-64, 2015
12. Groves R et al: MR imaging evaluation of pericardial constriction. Magn Reson Imaging Clin N Am. 23(1):81-7, 2015
13. Lin HC et al: Tuberculous pericarditis. Circulation. 132(12):1154-6, 2015
14. Zumla A et al: Host-directed therapies for tuberculous pericarditis. Int J Infect Dis. 32:30-1, 2015
15. Mayosi BM et al: Prednisolone and Mycobacterium indicus pranii in tuberculous pericarditis. N Engl J Med. 371(12):1121-30, 2014
16. Hayase N et al: Sudden cardiac arrest caused by tuberculous pericarditis with hemorrhagic pericardial effusion. Intern Med. 51(22):3197-201, 2012

Lymphoma, Pericardium

KEY FACTS

CLINICAL ISSUES

- Rare entity, but incidence has increased in recent decades due to immunosuppression (AIDS, transplant recipient-related lymphoproliferative disorders)
- Treatment varies according to lymphoma type and stage
  - Chemotherapy and radiation
  - Surgical resection usually not indicated

MACROSCOPIC

- Lymphoma can involve pericardium in several ways
  - Widespread (systemic) advanced-stage lymphoma
  - Lymphatics course through/around pericardium
  - Direct extension from mediastinal nodal/extranodal lymphoma
  - Direct extension from primary cardiac or pleural lymphoma
  - Primary involvement of pericardium
  - Effusion lymphoma
- Generally soft, "fish-fleshed" cut surface grossly

MICROSCOPIC

- Several entities
  - Hodgkin lymphoma
  - Diffuse large B-cell lymphoma (DLBCL)
  - Mediastinal DLBCL
  - Primary effusion lymphoma
  - DLBCL associated with chronic inflammation

TOP DIFFERENTIAL DIAGNOSES

- Germ cell tumor
- Pericardial (ectopic) thymic epithelial tumor
- Castleman disease
- Mesothelial/monocytic incidental cardiac excrescence

(Left) *Short-axis SSFP MR in a patient with lymphoma shows a markedly thickened pericardium and right ventricle. A small pericardial effusion is also present. There are no intracavitary mass lesions.* **(Right)** *Cell block preparation from a pericardial fluid sample from a patient with diffuse large B-cell lymphoma (DLBCL) of the pericardium shows pleomorphic and enlarged neoplastic lymphocytes.*

Cardiac MR Appearance of Pericardial Lymphoma

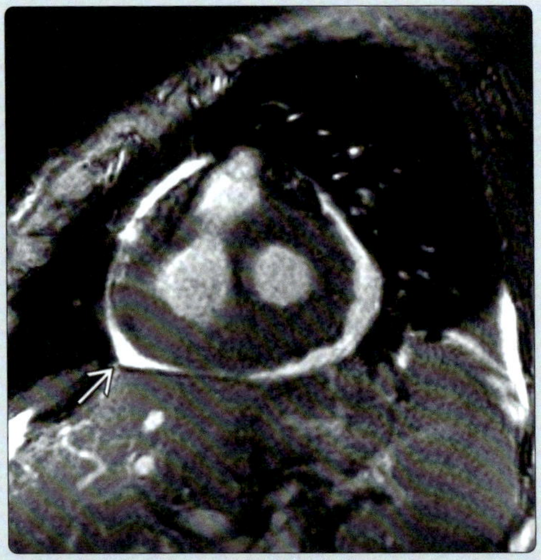

Large Atypical Lymphocytes

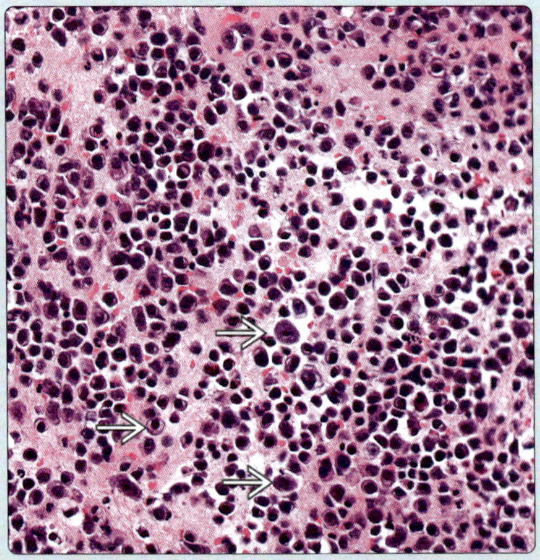

(Left) *Nodular sclerosis-type Hodgkin lymphoma shows broad fibrous septa dividing lymphoid aggregates containing prominent Hodgkin cells.* **(Right)** *Higher magnification of Hodgkin lymphoma shows large Hodgkin and Reed-Sternberg cells with macronucleoli in a reactive polymorphous background that includes eosinophils.*

Pericardial Nodular Sclerosis-Type Hodgkin Lymphoma

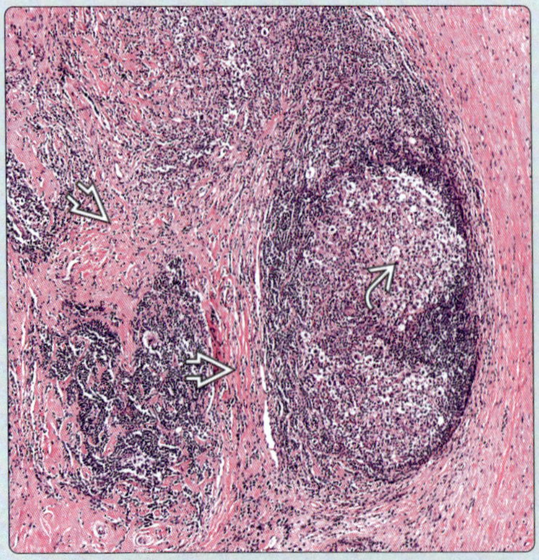

Hodgkin and Reed-Sternberg Cells

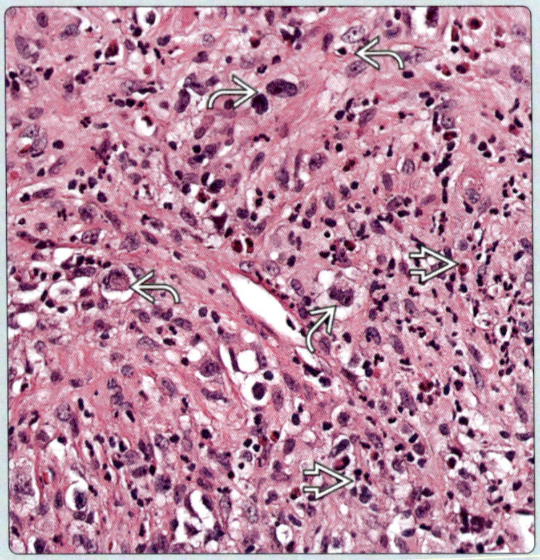

TERMINOLOGY

Definitions

- Malignant lymphoid neoplasm primarily or secondarily involving pericardium

CLINICAL ISSUES

Epidemiology

- Incidence
  - Rare entity, but incidence has increased in recent decades due to immunosuppression (AIDS, transplant recipient-related lymphoproliferative disorders)

Presentation

- Chest pain, dyspnea
- Pericardial effusion
  - ± tamponade, depending on volume and rapidity of accumulation
- Constitutional symptoms
- Mass: ± chamber compression, constriction of epicardial coronary arteries (rare)

Treatment

- Varies according to lymphoma type and stage
- Chemotherapy and radiation
- Surgical resection usually not indicated
  - May be curative in localized disease
  - Primary lymphoma diagnosis may be made on resected pericardial mass

Prognosis

- Varies according to lymphoma type and stage

MACROSCOPIC

General Features

- Lymphoma can involve pericardium in several ways
  - Widespread (systemic) advanced-stage lymphoma
    - Lymphatics course through/around pericardium
  - Direct extension from mediastinal nodal/extranodal lymphoma
  - Direct extension from primary cardiac or pleural lymphoma
  - Primary involvement of pericardium
  - Effusion lymphoma
- Generally soft, "fish-fleshed" cut surface grossly

Sections to Be Submitted

- Triaging tissue for flow cytometry and molecular studies should be considered if lymphoma enters gross differential with pericardial specimens

MICROSCOPIC

Hodgkin Lymphoma

- Hodgkin &/or Reed-Sternberg cells
  - Large cells with lobated nuclei and macronucleoli
  - Immunophenotype: CD20(-), CD45(-), CD30(+), CD15(+)
- Reactive inflammatory background with frequent eosinophils and plasma cells
- Coarse bands/fascicles of bland fibrosis prominent in nodular sclerosis type

Diffuse Large B-Cell Lymphoma

- Large "activated" CD20(+) B cells

Mediastinal Diffuse Large B-Cell Lymphoma

- Typically bulky lesion in anterior-superior mediastinum (postulated thymic origin)
- Middle-aged female patients most common
- Better prognosis compared to conventional diffuse large B-cell lymphoma (DLBCL)
- Histologically, characteristic pattern of delicate fibrosis interweaving among malignant lymphocytes is seen

Primary Effusion Lymphoma

- Effusions without discernible tissue mass
- Immunocompromised patients (especially AIDS)
- Invariably human herpesvirus 8 (HHV-8) positive
- Frequently Epstein-Barr virus (EBV) positive
- "Null" phenotype (negative B- and T-cell markers) or weak CD3 expression (despite putative B-cell origin)
- Poor prognosis: Median survival < 6 months

Diffuse Large B-Cell Lymphoma Associated With Chronic Inflammation (Pyothorax-Associated Lymphoma)

- EBV-driven chronic inflammation-associated lymphoproliferative disorder in patients with chronic pyothorax
- Immunosuppressed patients
- Diffusely thickened pleura, replete with malignant lymphoma
- HHV-8 negative

Other B-Cell Lymphomas

- Marginal zone B-cell lymphoma, mantle cell lymphoma, follicular lymphoma, small lymphocytic lymphoma, and Burkitt lymphoma have all been described in pericardium

Posttransplant Lymphoproliferative Disorder

- Varies from polymorphic to monomorphic type

DIFFERENTIAL DIAGNOSIS

Germ Cell Tumor

- Germinoma in particular may have prominent associated lymphocytic infiltrate and granulomas

Pericardial (Ectopic) Thymic Epithelial Tumor

- Similar morphology to thymic thymoma/carcinoma
- Keratin staining highlights diffuse dendritic process permeating tumor

SELECTED REFERENCES

1. Thoracic Tumors. WHO Classification of Tumors series. 5th ed. IARC Press, 2021
2. Guastafierro S et al: Pericardial effusion due to pericardium involvement by Hodgkin's lymphoma. Ann Hematol. 92(6):853-4, 2013
3. Attanoos R: Lymphoproliferative conditions of the serosa. Arch Pathol Lab Med. 136(3):268-76, 2012

KEY FACTS

ETIOLOGY/PATHOGENESIS

- Virtually all types of malignancy have been noted to involve pericardium
- Autopsy series reveal that tumors most frequently metastasizing to heart with primary pericardial pattern include lung carcinoma and mesothelioma, as well as ovary, stomach, and prostate carcinomas
- Pericardium is most common site of involvement of heart with metastatic disease followed by myocardium and endocardium

CLINICAL ISSUES

- Patients with metastatic pericardial disease are more likely to be symptomatic than patients with isolated myocardial metastatic disease due to propensity to develop malignant pericardial effusion
- 1/3 of patients with pericardial metastatic disease will eventually die of tamponade
- Direct extension of thoracic tumors into pericardium affects primary tumor staging

MACROSCOPIC

- Often small and multiple nodules but may cause diffuse pericardial thickening with obliteration of pericardial space

MICROSCOPIC

- Malignant neoplasm invading pericardium with histologic features of primary tumor

TOP DIFFERENTIAL DIAGNOSES

- Radiation pericarditis
- Drug-induced pericarditis
- Idiopathic pericardial effusion in patients with cancer
- Primary pericardial malignancy
- Rare but must consider primary pericardial mesothelioma and angiosarcoma in differential diagnosis of metastatic pericardial disease

Hemopericardium in Pericardial Metastasis

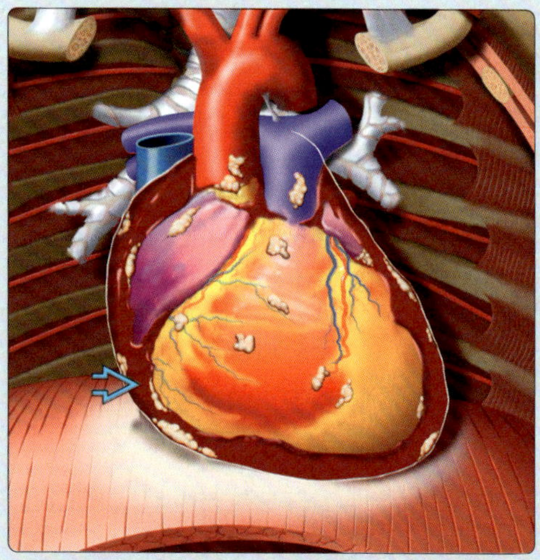

Hemopericardium in Pericardial Metastasis

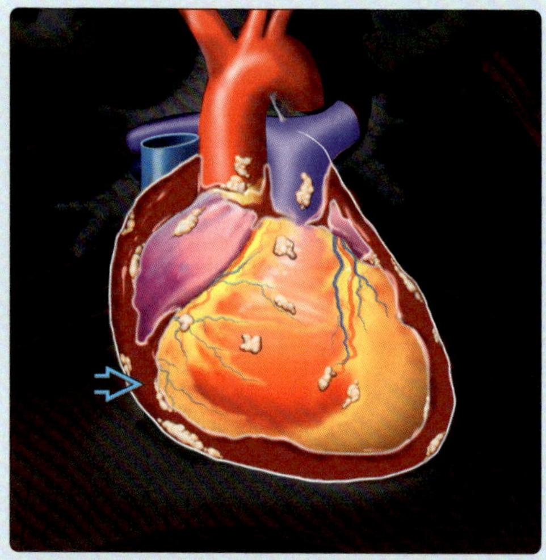

(Left) *Graphic shows hemopericardium in a patient with pericardial metastatic disease. These patients may expire secondary to cardiac tamponade. Malignancy must be considered in the evaluation of all hemorrhagic pericardial effusions* ➪. **(Right)** *Graphic shows hemopericardium in a patient with pericardial metastatic disease. These patients may expire secondary to cardiac tamponade. Malignancy must be considered in the evaluation of all hemorrhagic pericardial effusions* ➪.

Pericardial Disease Secondary to Epicardial Metastasis

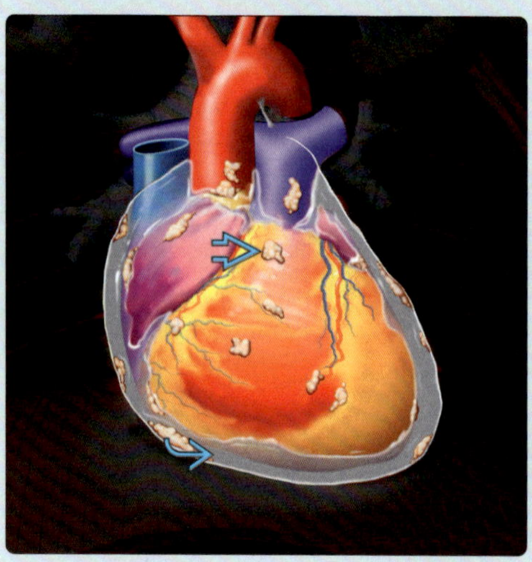

Pericarditis Secondary to Metastatic Carcinoma

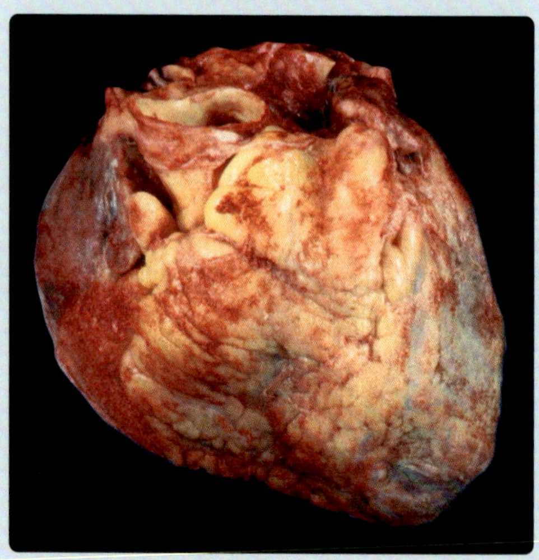

(Left) *Graphic shows pericardial disease secondary to epicardial metastasis* ➪. *There is associated pericardial effusion* ➪, *a common manifestation of malignant involvement of pericardium.* **(Right)** *Gross photograph of an autopsy case shows fibrinous pericarditis secondary to metastatic squamous cell carcinoma of the lung involving the pericardial space.*

TERMINOLOGY

Definitions

- Metastatic malignancy involving pericardium
  - Pericardium is defined as conical fibrous sac surrounding heart and root of great vessels

ETIOLOGY/PATHOGENESIS

Mechanism of Spread

- Metastases involve pericardium either by
  - Lymphatic/hematogenous spread
  - Direct extension by intrathoracic or mediastinal tumors
  - Secondarily through spread from myocardial/epicardial metastases

Types of Tumors That Spread to Pericardium

- Virtually all types of malignancy have been noted to involve pericardium
  - In autopsy studies, most frequently noted are lung carcinoma, mesothelioma, ovarian, gastric, and prostate carcinomas

CLINICAL ISSUES

Epidemiology

- Incidence
  - Pericardium most common site of cardiac metastatic disease followed by myocardium and endocardium
  - Reported autopsy rates of cardiac metastases are variable (1-25%)

Presentation

- Malignant pericardial effusion
  - Malignant pericardial disease blocks venous and lymphatic circulation of pericardial fluid
  - Cardiac tamponade may develop and may be primary presentation of patients with malignancy
    - Patients with metastatic pericardial disease are more likely to be symptomatic than patients with isolated myocardial metastatic disease due to propensity to develop malignant pericardial effusion
  - Less frequent but possible mechanisms of cardiac dysfunction related to malignant metastatic pericardial disease
    - Tumor compression of, embolization to, or direct invasion of coronary arteries leading to ischemic injury
    - Tumor may encase heart causing constrictive pericardial disease
    - Tumor may invade and injure cardiac nerves leading to dysrhythmias

Prognosis

- 1/3 of patients with pericardial metastatic disease will eventually die of tamponade
- Direct extension of thoracic tumors into pericardium affects primary tumor staging
  - Lung cancer with pericardial extension is T3 lesion
  - Thymoma with direct pericardial extension is modified Masaoka clinical stage III lesion
  - Esophageal carcinoma with direct pericardial extension is stage IIIC lesion
- Involvement of heart by distant metastatic disease represents advanced (T4) stage of malignancy

IMAGING

General Features

- CT and MR provide information of extent and mass effect of metastatic pericardial involvement
  - Pericardial effusion, prepericardial lymph nodes, pericardial thickening, enhancement, and nodules
    - Most frequent sites of pericardial nodules in imaging studies are free wall of right ventricle and right atrioventricular groove

MACROSCOPIC

General Features

- Pericardial effusion, often hemorrhagic (normal amount of pericardial fluid is 15-50 mL)
- Often small and multiple nodules, but may cause diffuse pericardial thickening with obliteration of pericardial space
  - With primary hematologic malignancy, lymphoma is more likely to form mass than leukemia
- Often have associated fibrinous pericarditis

MICROSCOPIC

Histologic Features

- Malignant neoplasm invading pericardium with histologic features of primary tumor
- May secondarily invade underlying epicardial adipose tissue and myocardium and show perineural and lymphatic invasion

Cytologic Features

- Pericardial effusion cytology is 80-90% accurate in diagnosis of malignant pericardial effusion
- Look for cytologic features of malignancy related to primary malignancy

ANCILLARY TESTS

Gene Expression Profiling

- Cytology specimens including pericardial fluid have been analyzed for tumor of origin using commercially available microarray-based gene expression tests

DIFFERENTIAL DIAGNOSIS

Other Causes of Pericardial Effusions in Patients With Malignancy

- Radiation and drug-induced pericarditis
  - Doxorubicin, cyclophosphamide, gemcitabine
- Idiopathic pericardial effusion in patients with cancer
- Primary pericardial malignancy
  - Rare primary pericardial mesothelioma and angiosarcoma

SELECTED REFERENCES

1. Shartouni R et al: The value of cytology in the evaluation of malignant pericardial effusions: a systematic review. Diagnostics (Basel). 12(2), 2022
2. Chahine J et al: Pericardial involvement in cancer. Am J Cardiol. 145:151-9, 2021

(Left) *Gross photograph of an autopsy case shows clear cell sarcoma metastatic to pericardium and lung. Yellow-tan nodules on the pericardial surface are visible.* **(Right)** *Opened pericardium demonstrates pericardial metastatic disease involving the free wall of the right ventricle in a patient with metastatic malignant melanoma.*

Pericardial Involvement by Metastatic Sarcoma

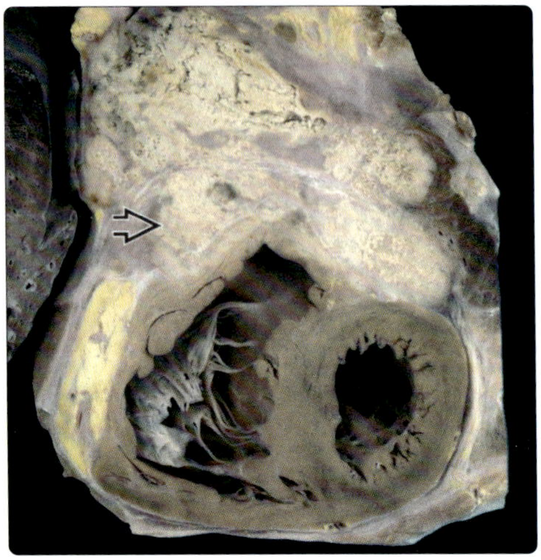

Pericardial Metastasis From Melanoma

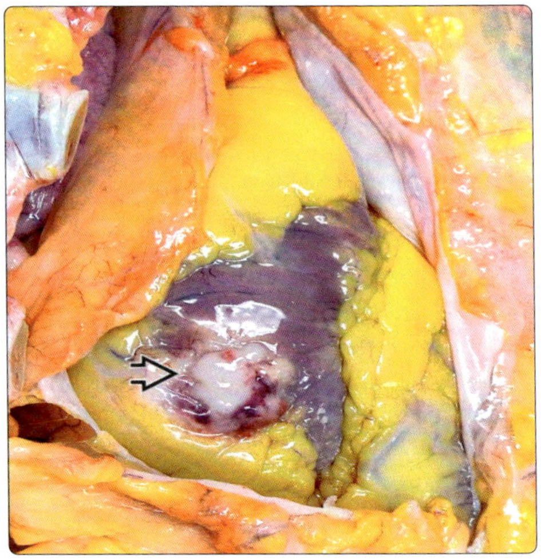

(Left) *Horizontal section through a heart specimen in the area of epipericardial metastatic disease reveals that it was a consequence of direct extension from a myocardial metastasis of malignant melanoma.* **(Right)** *In situ view shows a transplanted heart with metastatic epithelioid sarcoma involving the pericardium. There is also marked pericardial fibrosis related to the transplant procedure.*

Pericardial Metastasis From Melanoma

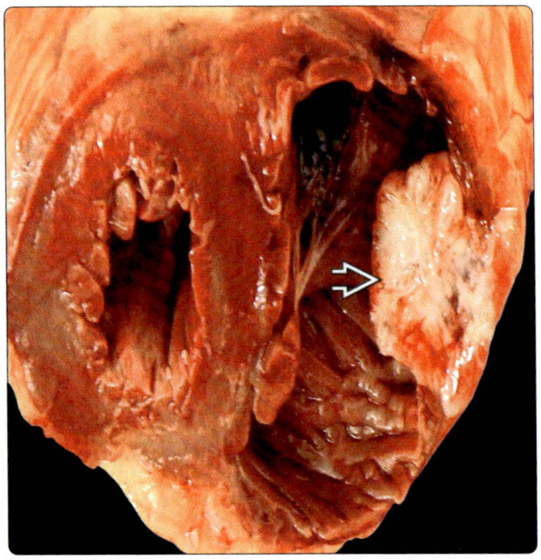

Pericardial Metastasis From Epithelioid Sarcoma

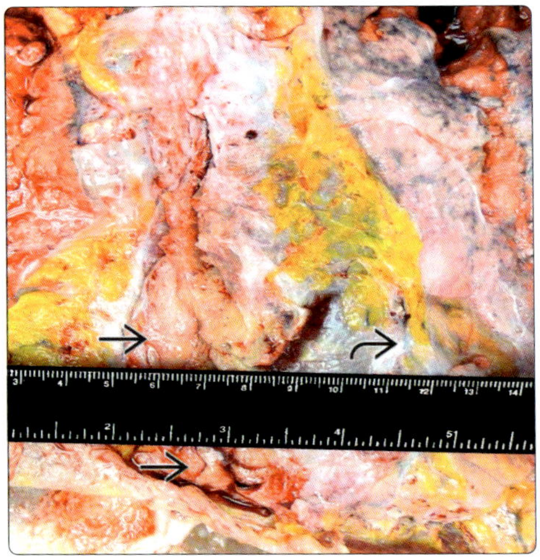

(Left) *Gross photograph shows small white nodules of metastatic tumor and fibrinous pericarditis in a patient with primary lung carcinoma.* **(Right)** *H&E shows metastatic mucinous adenocarcinoma involving the pericardium. Most metastatic carcinomas to the pericardium are adenocarcinomas. Note the lymphatic invasion by tumor cells.*

Pericardial Metastasis From Lung Carcinoma

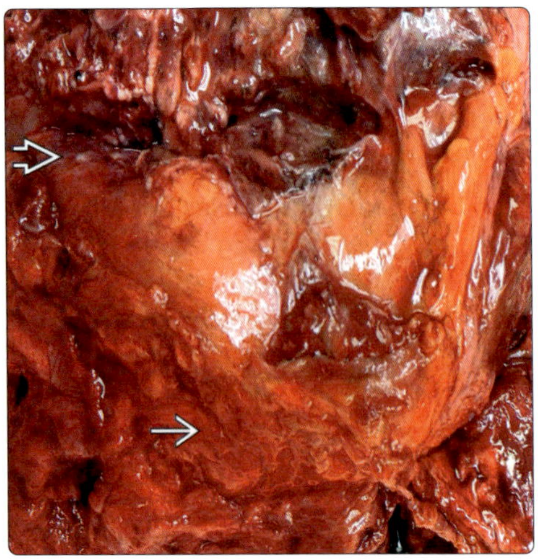

Histologic Findings of Pericardial Metastasis

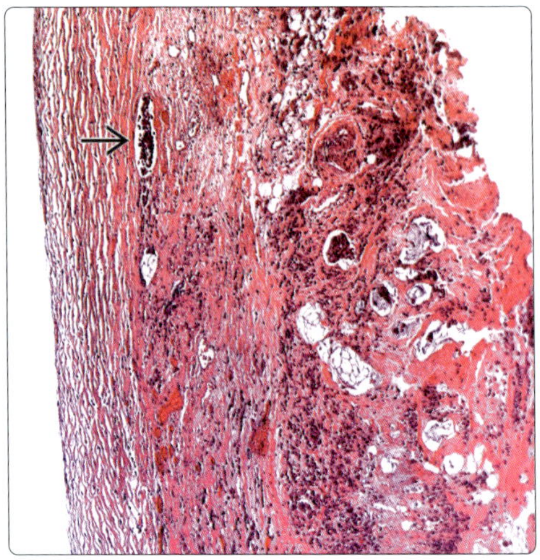

Histologic Findings of Pericardial Metastasis From Malignant Melanoma

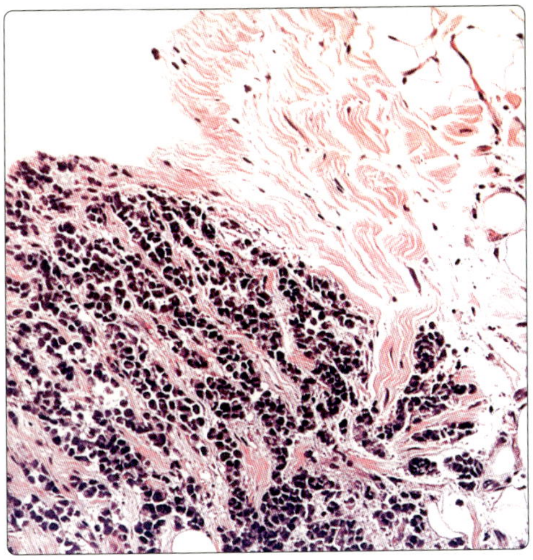

Histologic Findings of Pericardial Metastasis From Thymic Carcinoma

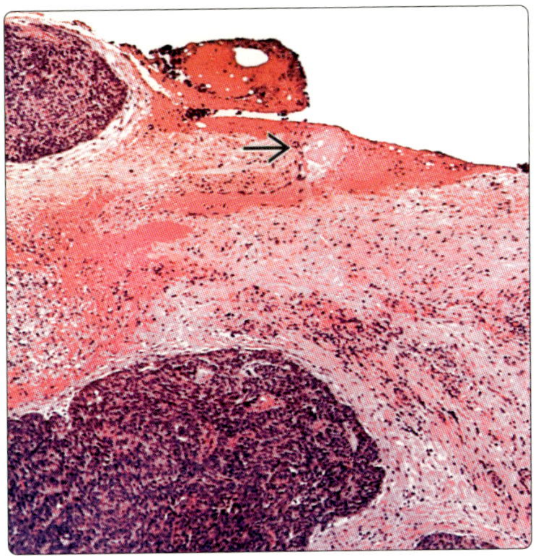

(Left) *H&E shows malignant melanoma infiltrating the pericardium from underlying epicardium. This tumor began as a myocardial metastasis. Melanoma has a high frequency of cardiac metastases and is one of the tumors that also has a high frequency of involving the myocardial tissue.* **(Right)** *H&E shows thymic carcinoma directly invading the pericardium. Note the overlying fibrinous and hemorrhagic pericarditis* ➔.

Pericardial Metastasis From Pleural Mesothelioma

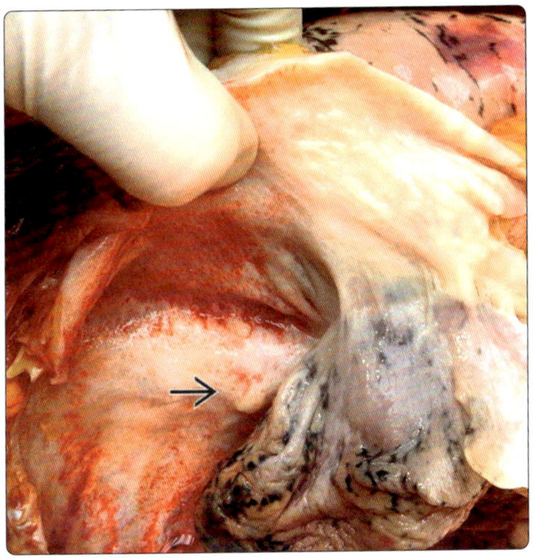

Angiosarcoma Involving Pericardium

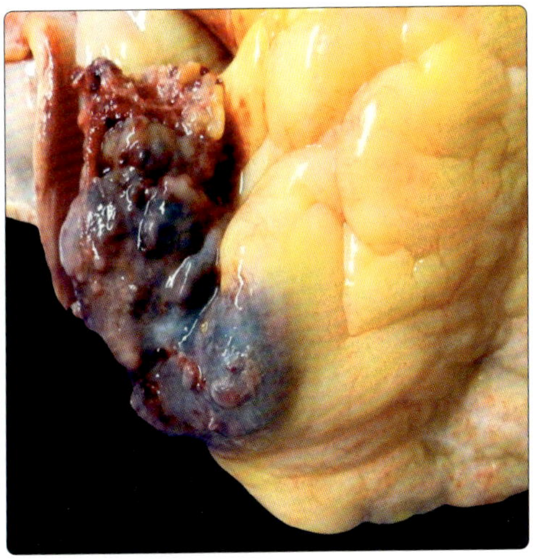

(Left) *Gross photograph shows malignant mesothelioma extending from the pleura into the pericardial sac (unopened)* ➔. **(Right)** *This epipericardial tumor on the surface of the heart is a primary cardiac angiosarcoma. Note the hemorrhagic appearance. This patient presented with recurrent pericardial effusions and expired secondary to cardiac tamponade. A more diffuse pericardial pattern of this tumor may occur but will appear grossly similar.*

Histologic Findings of Pericardial Metastasis From Angiosarcoma

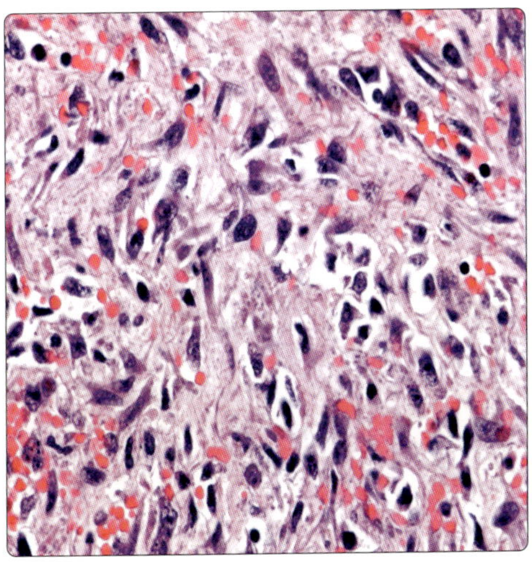

Cytologic Findings of Pericardial Metastasis From Adenocarcinoma

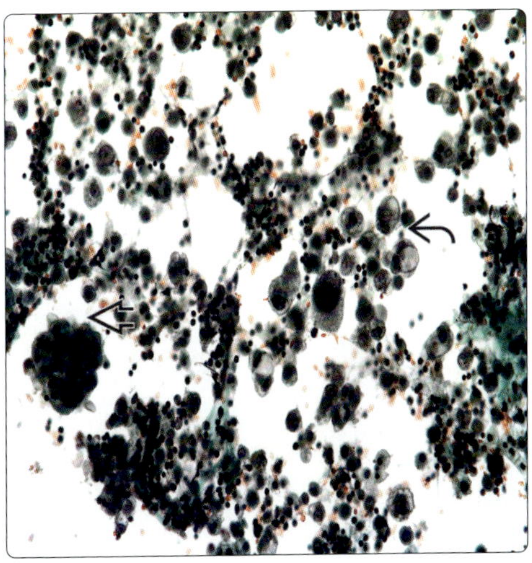

(Left) *Angiosarcoma involving the pericardium exhibits vessels lined by malignant spindled cells. These cells would stain positively with factor VIII antibody on immunohistochemical analysis.* **(Right)** *This malignant pericardial effusion demonstrates 3D clusters of cells* ⇨ *and individual large malignant epithelial cells focally with intracytoplasmic mucin* ↩. *This patient had a primary adenocarcinoma of the lung. Note the acute inflammatory cells in the background.*

Mesothelioma, Pericardium

KEY FACTS

TERMINOLOGY

- Malignant neoplasm arising primarily from pericardium
- Some definitions of pericardial mesothelioma preclude any pleural involvement

ETIOLOGY/PATHOGENESIS

- Association with asbestos exposure has been shown, but not as definitive as that between asbestos exposure and pleural mesotheliomas

CLINICAL ISSUES

- Very rare; < 300 reported cases in literature
- Mean age at presentation is 45 years, but cases from both children and older adult patients have been reported
- M:F ~ 2:1; lower than that seen in pleural mesothelioma
- Generally poor prognosis
- Radiation and chemotherapy have been attempted with little success

MACROSCOPIC

- Typically exhibits pericardium-centered growth pattern
- Can form bulky intrapericardial nodules
- May exhibit gross (usually superficial) invasion into myocardium

MICROSCOPIC

- Atypical, usually infiltrative, growth of neoplastic cells within pericardium, sometimes extending into superficial myocardium
- Morphologic types of pericardial mesothelioma are similar to those seen in other locations
- Broad immunohistochemical panel often assists with diagnosis

TOP DIFFERENTIAL DIAGNOSES

- Metastatic adenocarcinoma

(Left) *Basal short-axis section from an autopsy specimen shows a mesothelioma involving both the parietal and visceral pericardium with focal extension into the superficial myocardium ➯.* **(Right)** *H&E exhibits an epithelioid mesothelioma with invasive nests of tumor cells growing into a fibroblastic stroma. By morphology alone, it is difficult to distinguish this from a carcinoma.*

Pericardial Mesothelioma (Gross, Short Axis)

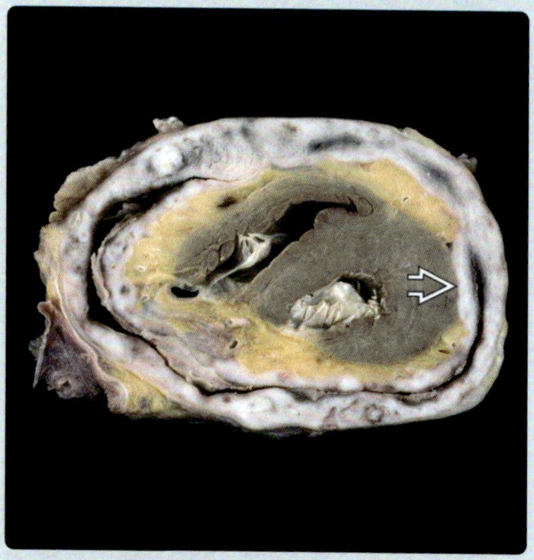

Pericardial Mesothelioma (Epithelioid, Low Magnification)

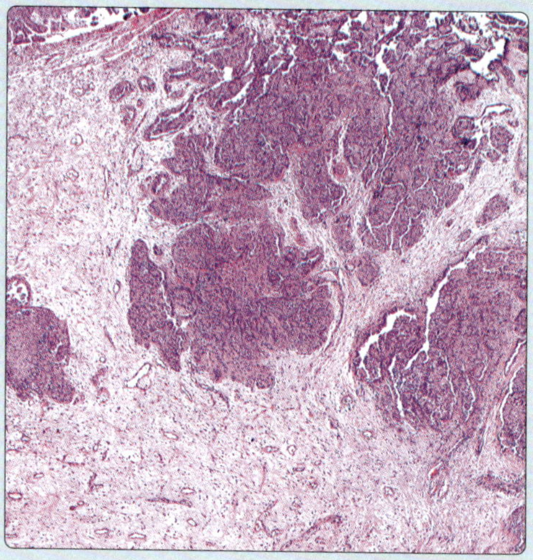

(Left) *Gross photograph shows mesothelioma creating constrictive changes in the pericardium.* **(Right)** *Keratin expression is not specific for mesothelioma but helps to highlight the infiltration into fat and beyond the pericardium.*

Pericardial Mesothelioma (Gross, Long Axis)

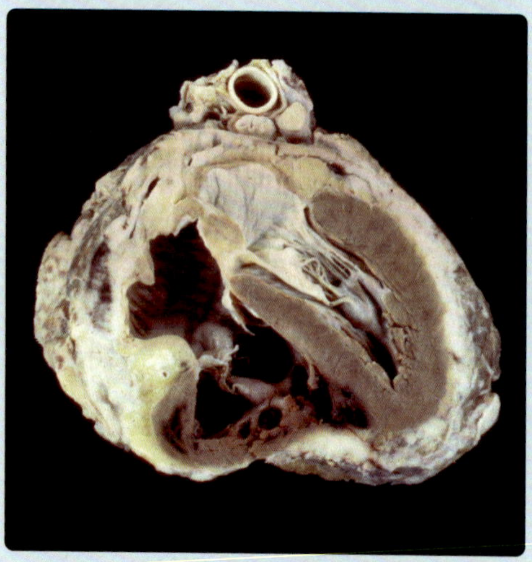

Keratin Staining in Mesothelioma

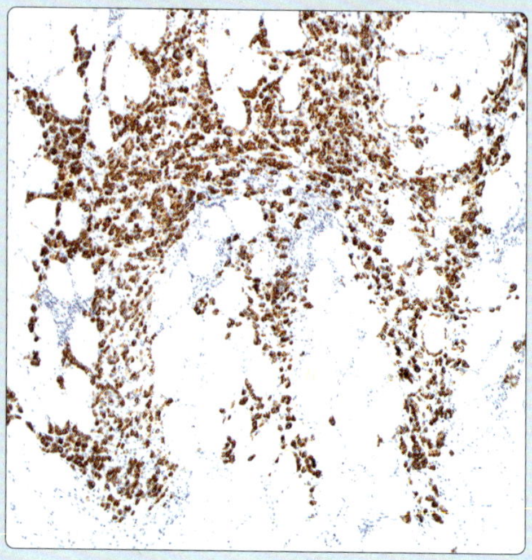

TERMINOLOGY

Definitions

- Malignant neoplasm arising primarily from pericardium
- Some definitions of pericardial mesothelioma preclude pleural involvement

ETIOLOGY/PATHOGENESIS

Environmental Exposure

- Association with asbestos exposure has been shown, but link is not as definitive as that between asbestos exposure and pleural mesotheliomas
- Possible association with radiotherapy

CLINICAL ISSUES

Epidemiology

- Incidence
  - Very rare; < 300 reported cases in literature
- Age
  - Mean at presentation is 45 years, but cases from both children and older adult patients have been reported
- Sex
  - M:F ~ 2:1; lower than that seen in pleural mesothelioma

Presentation

- Dyspnea, pericardial effusion, cardiac tamponade

Treatment

- Surgical approaches
  - Pericardiectomy or sclerotherapy may be performed to ameliorate constrictive symptoms
- Radiation and chemotherapy have been attempted with little success

Prognosis

- Generally poor

IMAGING

Radiographic Findings

- Pericardial effusion (hemorrhagic or serous)
- Pericardial thickening (often best demonstrated on CT or MR)

MACROSCOPIC

General Features

- Typically exhibits pericardium-centered growth pattern
- Can form bulky intrapericardial nodules
- May exhibit gross (usually superficial) invasion into myocardium
- Often encircles great vessels and may cause obstruction of vena cavae

MICROSCOPIC

Histologic Features

- Atypical, usually infiltrative, growth of neoplastic cells within pericardium, sometimes extending into superficial myocardium
- Morphologic types of pericardial mesothelioma are similar to those seen in other locations
- Broad immunohistochemical panel often assists with diagnosis

Morphologic Types

- Epithelioid
- Sarcomatoid
- Mixed (usually biphasic, epithelioid, and sarcomatoid)
- Desmoplastic
- Other variants (clear cell, adenomatoid, deciduoid) have also been described

ANCILLARY TESTS

Immunohistochemistry

- Positive: Calretinin, CK5/6, D2-40, WT1
- Loss of expression of MTAP and BAP1 in malignant mesothelial tumors

Electron Microscopy

- Long branched microvilli (typically seen in epithelioid type)
- Cytoplasmic perinuclear tonofibrils
- Long desmosomes

DIFFERENTIAL DIAGNOSIS

Pleural Mesothelioma

- Gross or radiologic evidence of pleural involvement (or involvement of other serosal surface)

Metastatic Adenocarcinoma

- Nonreactivity with mesothelial markers (calretinin, CK5/6, D2-40, WT1) and reactivity with carcinoma markers (mCEA, MOC31, BER-EP4)
- History of carcinoma

Primary Cardiac Sarcoma

- e.g., angiosarcoma
- Immunohistochemistry may be helpful in demonstrating different patterns of differentiation
- Secondary mesothelial reaction caused by sarcoma may make distinction difficult

Metastatic Sarcoma

- History of sarcoma

Reactive Mesothelial Proliferations

- Distinction can be difficult
- Lack tumefactive growth and frank invasion

SELECTED REFERENCES

1. Berg KB et al: Utility of methylthioadenosine phosphorylase compared with BAP1 immunohistochemistry, and CDKN2A and NF2 fluorescence in situ hybridization in separating reactive mesothelial proliferations from epithelioid malignant mesotheliomas. Arch Pathol Lab Med. 142(12):1549-53, 2018
2. Churg A et al: New markers for separating benign from malignant mesothelial proliferations: are we there yet? Arch Pathol Lab Med. 140(4):318-21, 2016
3. Mensi C et al: Pericardial mesothelioma and asbestos exposure. Int J Hyg Environ Health. 214(3):276-9, 2011
4. Patel J et al: Primary malignant mesothelioma of the pericardium. Cardiovasc Pathol. 20(2):107-9, 2011
5. Nilsson A et al: Primary pericardial mesothelioma: report of a patient and literature review. Case Rep Oncol. 2(2):125-32, 2009
6. Santos C et al: Primary pericardial mesothelioma. Lung Cancer. 60(2):291-3, 2008

(**Left**) *High-power H&E exhibits the plump, pleomorphic cells → of an epithelioid malignant mesothelioma. The cells exhibit an invasive pattern into dense collagen →.* (**Right**) *High-power H&E exhibits spindle-shaped cells with marked cellular atypia and scattered mitotic figures →. The cellular morphology can resemble sarcomas (of either the primary or metastatic variety). Pericardial growth can help in the distinction of these processes.*

Pericardial Mesothelioma (Epithelioid, High Magnification)

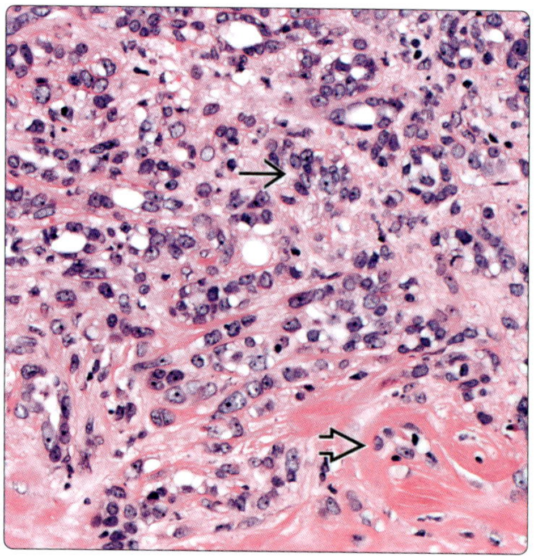

Pericardial Mesothelioma (Spindle Cell, High Magnification)

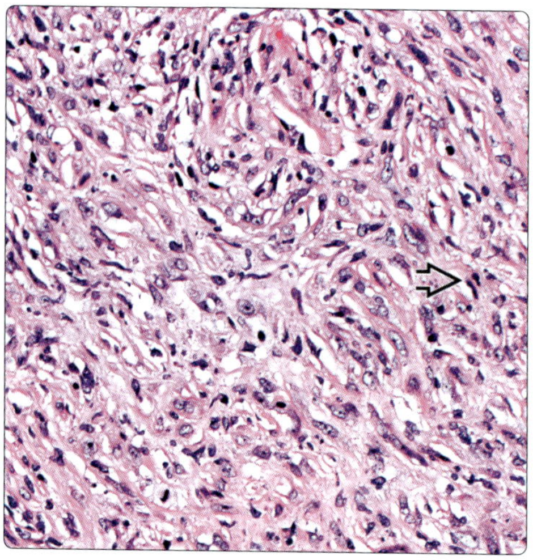

(**Left**) *High-power H&E shows an epithelioid malignant mesothelioma with prominent papillary growth pattern. The cells are rather monomorphic without striking atypia.* (**Right**) *H&E exhibits an epithelioid malignant mesothelioma forming pseudoglandular structures → within a desmoplastic background. Cases such as this can be difficult to differentiate from metastatic adenocarcinoma by morphologic features alone, making immunohistochemistry almost essential.*

Pericardial Mesothelioma With Papillary Growth Pattern

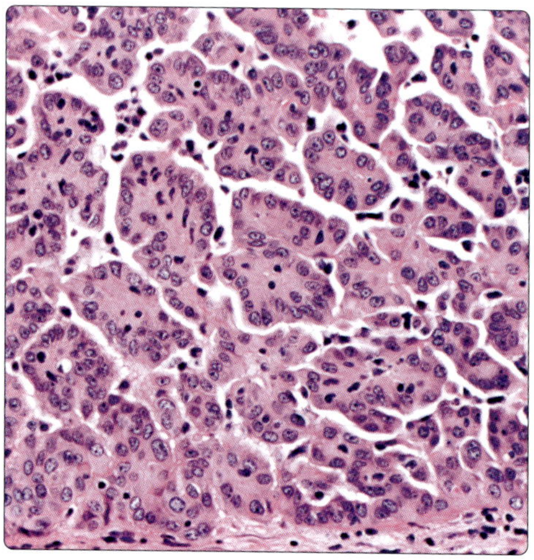

Pericardial Mesothelioma With Pseudoglandular Pattern

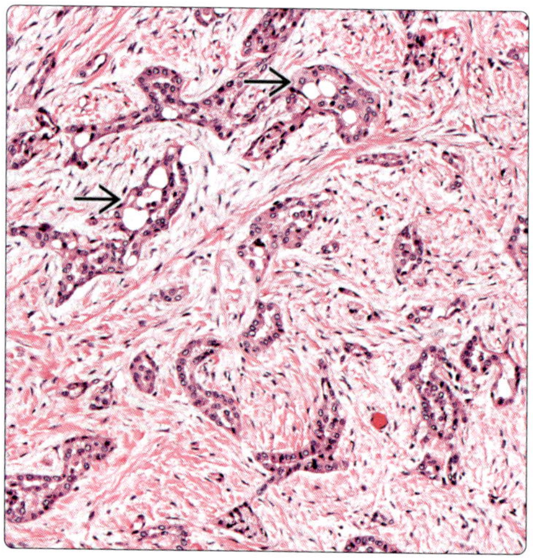

(**Left**) *Intermediate-power H&E exhibits a biphasic malignant pericardial mesothelioma. The epithelioid component → is seen alongside pleomorphic spindle cell infiltrate →.* (**Right**) *H&E exhibits a desmoplastic malignant pericardial mesothelioma. The tumor consists of deceptively bland spindle cells proliferating in a dense collagenous stroma, often in a storiform pattern. These tumors also typically exhibit variable cellularity throughout.*

Pericardial Mesothelioma (Biphasic)

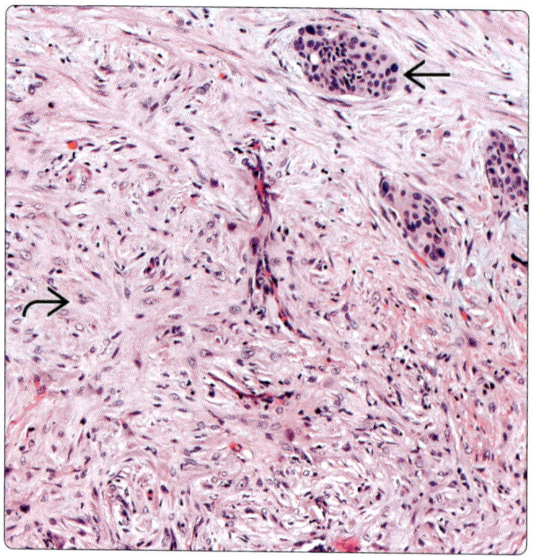

Pericardial Mesothelioma (Desmoplastic)

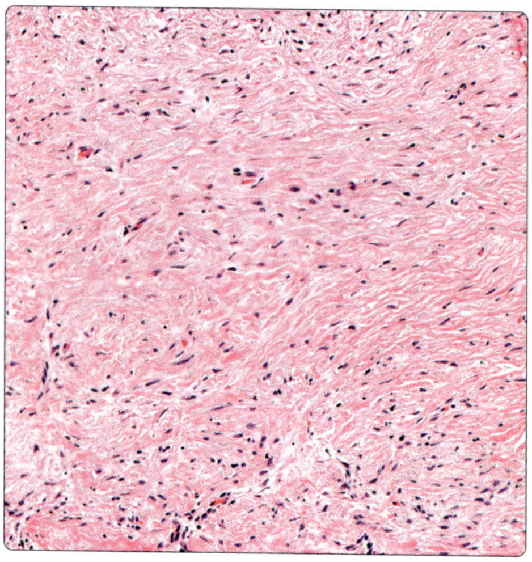

Pericardial Mesothelioma (Calretinin Stain, Low Magnification)

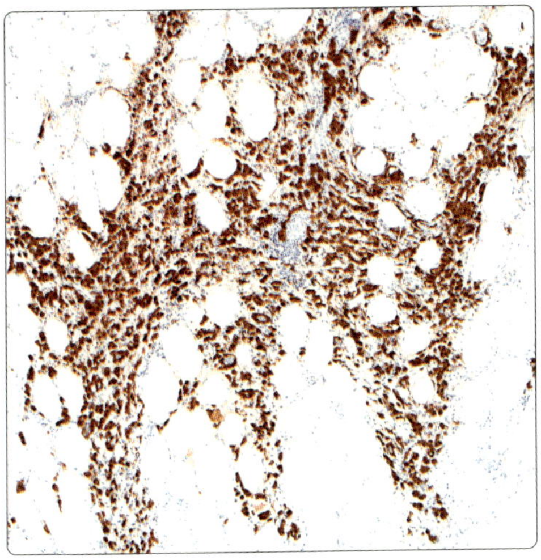

Reactive Mesothelial Proliferation in Pericarditis (Keratin Stain)

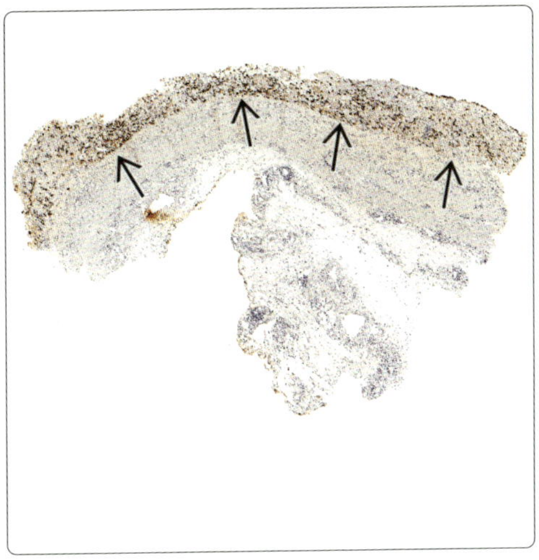

(Left) *Calretinin stain demonstrates extensive neoplastic mesothelial infiltration into the adjacent fibroadipose tissue. Note that reactivity with calretinin is not as consistently identified with sarcomatoid mesotheliomas.* **(Right)** *Keratin stain shows a distinct boundary* ⇨ *between the positive-staining mesothelium cells and the underlying fibrous pericardium.*

Pericardial Mesothelioma (CK5 Stain, High Magnification)

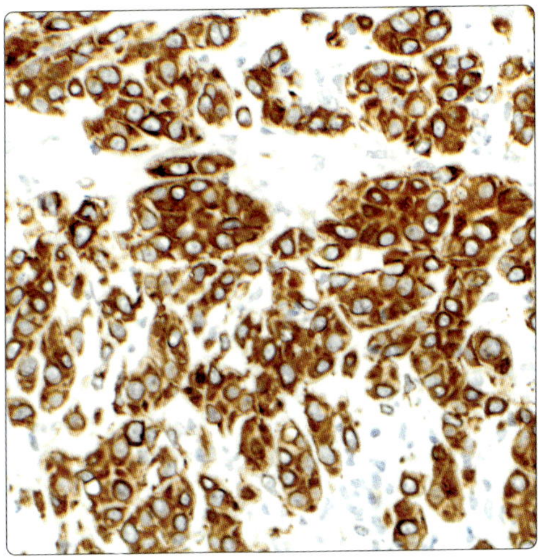

Pericardial Mesothelioma (Calretinin Stain, High Magnification)

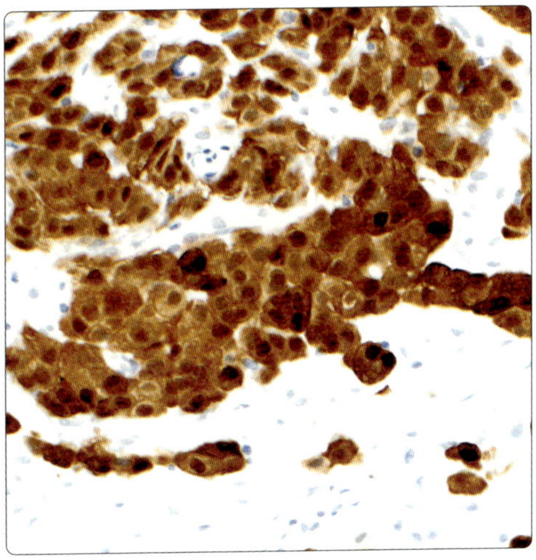

(Left) *Strong membranous reactivity with antibodies directed against CK5/6 is often observed, particularly in epithelioid-type malignant mesotheliomas.* **(Right)** *The reactivity with calretinin in malignant mesothelioma is usually strong and both nuclear and cytoplasmic in location.*

Pericardial Mesothelioma (WT1 Stain, High Magnification)

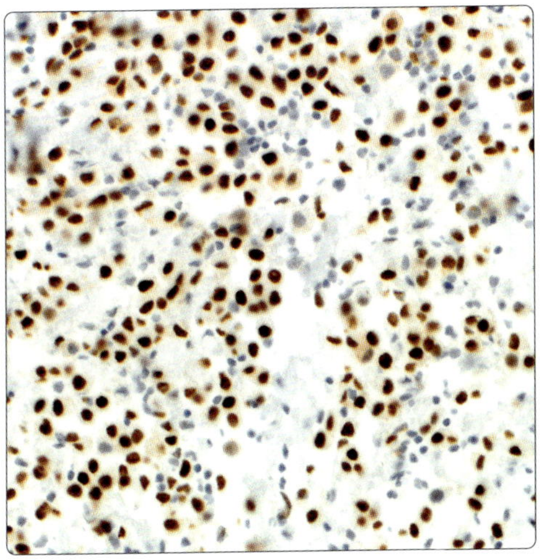

Pericardial Mesothelioma (BAP1 Stain)

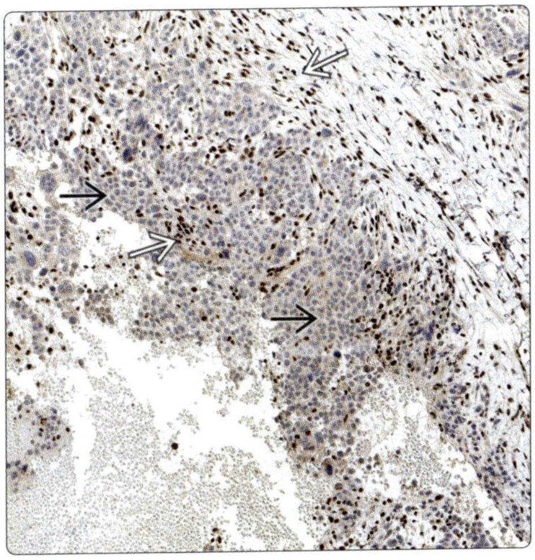

(Left) *Reactivity of the neoplastic epithelioid cells with antibodies directed against WT1 is shown in a case of malignant mesothelioma. This finding is not specific for mesothelial differentiation and can be seen in a variety of carcinomas.* **(Right)** *This mesothelioma shows loss of BAP1 expression in the malignant cells* ⇨*. Expression is preserved in benign stromal and inflammatory cells* ➡*. This is an immunophenotypic hallmark of mesothelioma.*

Mesothelial/Monocytic Incidental Cardiac Excrescence

KEY FACTS

TERMINOLOGY

- Mass-like aggregates of benign mesothelial cells, histiocytes (macrophages), and fibrin with entrapped blood and fat
- Histiocytic nodular mesothelial hyperplasia (HNMH)
- Clinically, both MICE/HNMH are often encountered incidentally during cardiac procedures and mistaken for neoplastic masses

ETIOLOGY/PATHOGENESIS

- Produced iatrogenically when mesothelial-lined cavity is entered

CLINICAL ISSUES

- Usually identified incidentally (rather than being reason for procedure)
- Clinical significance lies in potential for confusion with metastatic carcinoma or primary tumor of heart
- Reported to occur in
  - Cardiac chambers
  - Pericardial sac
  - Ascending aorta
  - Mediastinum
  - Endomyocardial biopsies
  - Transbronchial biopsies
  - Lymph nodes for lung cancer staging

MICROSCOPIC

- 2 predominant cell types: Histiocytoid and mesothelial
  - Admixed entrapped fat and blood
  - Overall pattern reminiscent of pleural fluid cell block preparation
  - Absent blood vessels, including capillaries, with no supporting stroma

ANCILLARY TESTS

- CD68, CD163, and lysozyme staining for monocytic cells
- CK5, calretinin, and WT1 staining for mesothelial cells

MICE

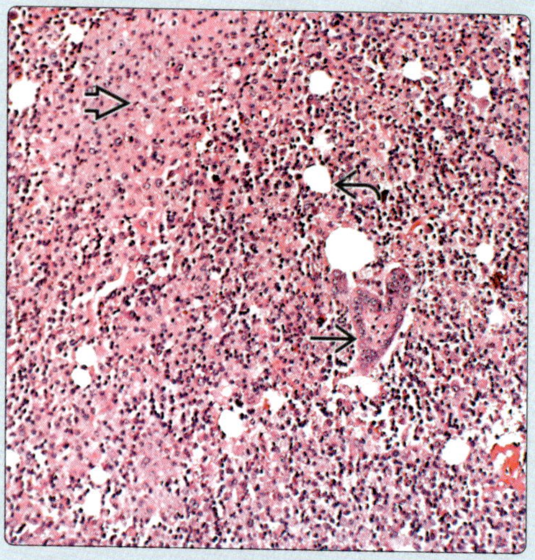

Mesothelial Atypia (Reactive) in MICE

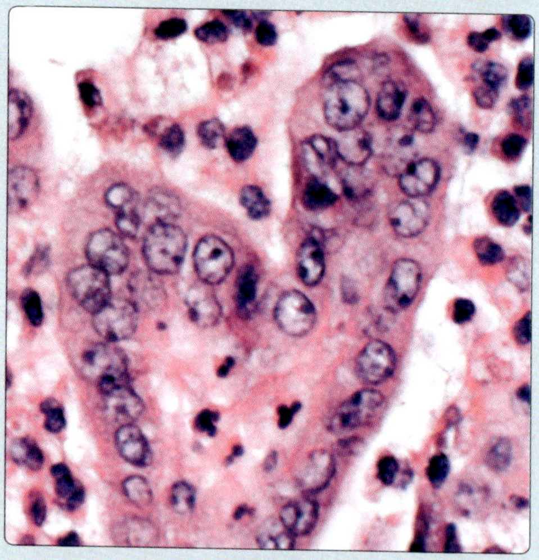

(Left) *This example of mesothelial/monocytic incidental cardiac excrescence (MICE) shows aggregates of histiocytes ⇨, cohesive groups of mesothelial cells →, and lipid-like inclusions ↪. Vessels and stroma are absent.* **(Right)** *Higher magnification view of a mesothelial cell cluster in MICE shows definite cohesion and papillary-like architecture. However, unlike true papillae, there is no defined fibrovascular core.*

CK5 Staining of Mesothelial Cells in MICE

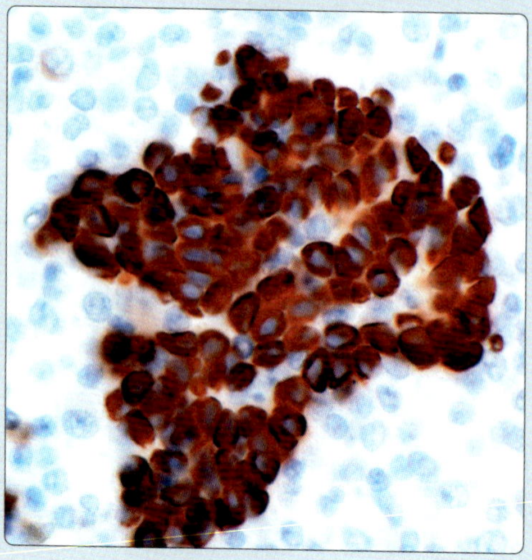

CD68 Staining of Macrophages in MICE

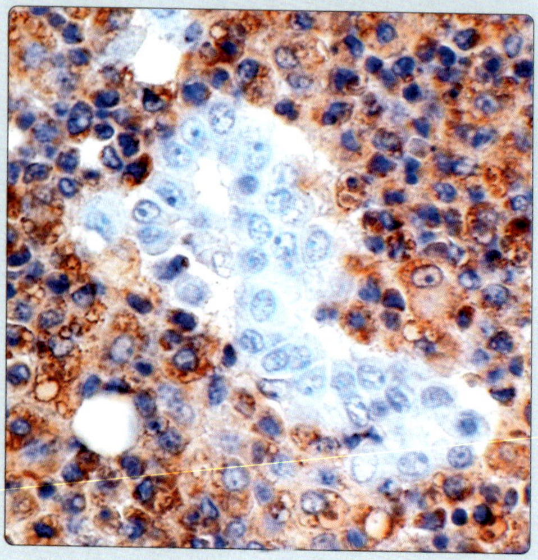

(Left) *High-magnification view of a mesothelial cell cluster in MICE shows strong reactivity for CK5. The surrounding histiocytic cells are negative.* **(Right)** *High-magnification view of MICE shows a mesothelial cell cluster stained for CD68. The mesothelial cells are clearly negative, but the surrounding histiocytic cells are positive.*

TERMINOLOGY

Abbreviations

- Mesothelial/monocytic incidental cardial excrescence (MICE)

Synonyms

- Histiocytic nodular mesothelial hyperplasia (HNMH)

Definitions

- Mass-like aggregates of mesothelial cells, histiocytes (macrophages), and fibrin with entrapped fat
  - Clinically, both MICE/HNMH are often encountered incidentally during cardiac procedures and mistaken for neoplastic masses

ETIOLOGY/PATHOGENESIS

Endogenous Artifact

- Produced iatrogenically when mesothelial-lined cavity is entered
  - Open thoracic surgery
  - Endomyocardial biopsy with right ventricle perforation
- Studies have demonstrated absence of well-developed cell junctions and no defined stroma, making it apparent that these represent artifactual aggregates of formerly free-floating cells
  - Similar to conglomeration that occurs when preparing cell block from cytology fluid specimen

CLINICAL ISSUES

Presentation

- Usually identified incidentally (rather than being reason for procedure)
  - Often found free-floating in pleural/pericardial fluid
- MICE has been identified in
  - Cardiac chambers
  - Cardiac valves
  - Pericardial sac
  - Ascending aorta
  - Mediastinum
  - Pleural space
  - Endomyocardial biopsies
  - Transbronchial biopsies
  - Lymph nodes for lung cancer staging

Prognosis

- Benign and incidental
  - Clinical significance lies in potential for confusion with metastatic carcinoma or heart primary tumor

MACROSCOPIC

General Features

- Range in size from < 1 mm up to 3 cm in diameter
- Vary from gray-white to dark red to brown in color
- Frequently associated with obvious thrombus but usually grossly distinct from other recognizable tissue submitted (valves, myocardium, aorta)

MICROSCOPIC

Histologic Features

- 2 predominant cell types
  - Histiocytoid cell
    - Round to oval with pale pink cytoplasm
    - Well-defined nuclei with prominent nuclear grooves
    - Cytoplasm rich in reticulin
    - Surface pseudopodia
  - Mesothelial cells
    - Cells present in small groups, strips, or tubular arrangements
    - Focally papillary structures occasionally seen
    - Less abundant eosinophilic cytoplasm
    - Small, round, noncleaved nuclei; inconspicuous nucleoli
- Admixed entrapped fat and blood
- Ropey and clumped acellular fibrin
- Overall pattern reminiscent of cell block preparation
- Absent blood vessels, including capillaries, with no supporting stroma

ANCILLARY TESTS

Immunohistochemistry

- Histiocytoid cells
  - CD68, CD163, lysozyme
- Mesothelial cells
  - CK5, calretinin, WT1, keratin

Electron Microscopy

- Histiocytes
  - Phagosomes, pseudopodia
- Mesothelial cells
  - Haphazardly arranged intermediate filaments and surface microvilli with well-developed desmosomes
- Adipocyte-like vacuoles
- Foreign material occasionally seen

DIFFERENTIAL DIAGNOSIS

Mesothelial Hyperplasia

- Can also form incidentally detected excrescences with mesothelial cells, macrophages, and fibrin
- Distinguished from MICE by presence of vessels and stroma
- Papillary architecture (with fibrovascular cores) common

Histiocytoid Epithelioid Hemangioma

- Presence of vessels and supporting stroma
- Hemosiderin is usually abundant
- Immunophenotype
  - Positive for endothelial markers
  - Negative for macrophage and mesothelial markers

SELECTED REFERENCES

1. Abboud S et al: Mesothelial or monocytic incidental cardiac excrescence on anterior leaflet of mitral valve. J Card Surg. 35(9):2418-21, 2020
2. Girolami I et al: Mesothelial/monocytic incidental cardiac excrescences (MICE): report of a case and review of literature with focus on pathogenesis. Cardiovasc Pathol. 36:25-9, 2018
3. Grossi VGR et al: Occurrence of mesothelial/monocytic incidental cardiac excrescences in material from open-heart procedures: case reports and literature review. Autops Case Rep. 8(1):e2018002, 2018

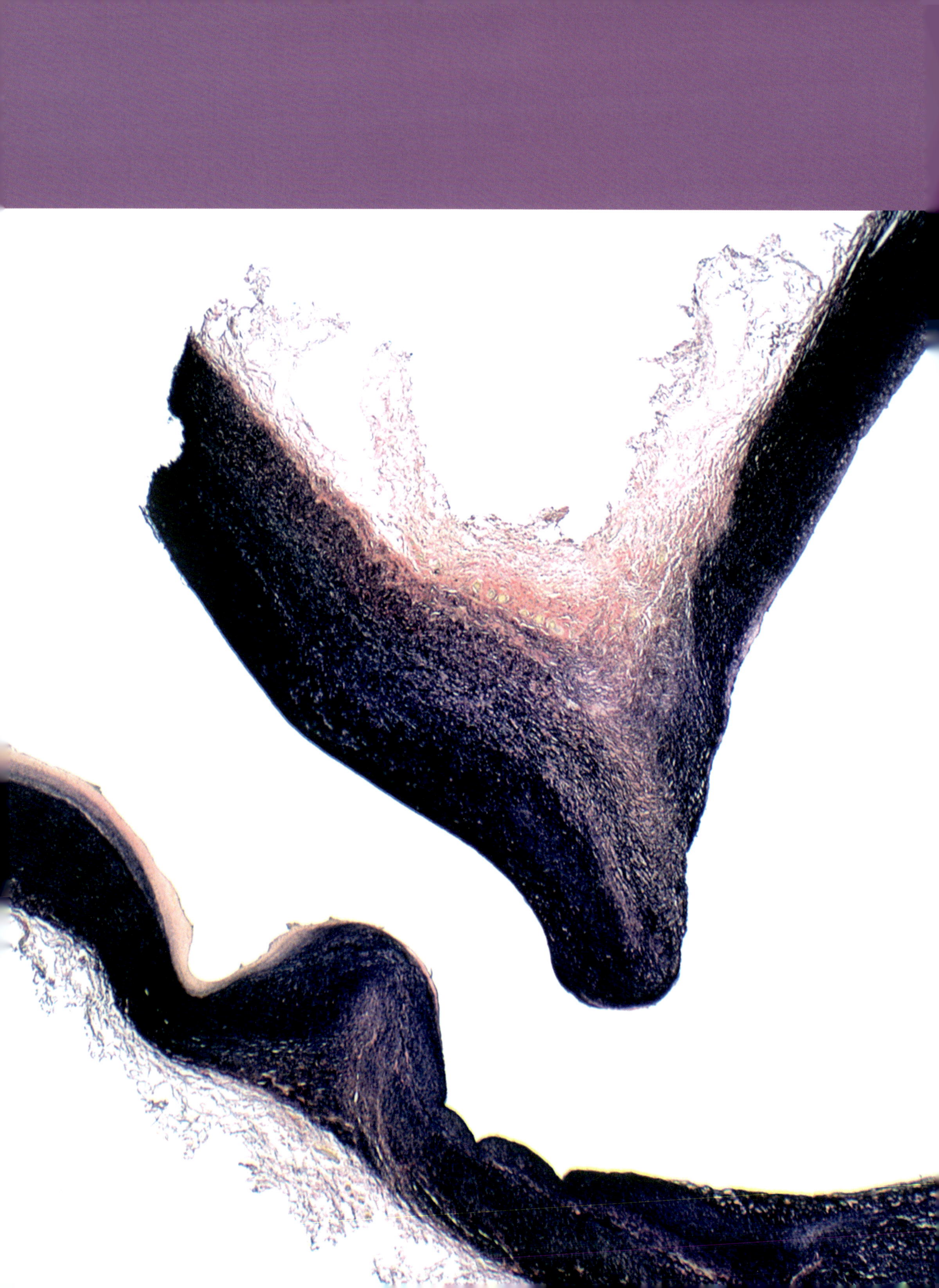

SECTION 7

Vascular Disease

Endarterectomy/Atherectomy/Thrombectomy

Thoracic Aorta

Abdominal Aorta

Coronary Arteries

Temporal Arteries

Peripheral Vessels

Vascular Tissue Grafts

Overview of Peripheral Vascular Specimens

TERMINOLOGY

Abbreviations

- Peripheral vascular disease (PVD)
- Peripheral arterial disease (PAD)

Definitions

- Pathology specimens related to disease entities that result in obstruction to blood flow in vascular beds
  - Obstruction of intracranial and coronary circulation especially relevant
  - Most commonly refers to atherosclerotic disease of extremities, usually lower
  - Amputation specimens of lower extremity are most frequent of these specimens; rare to see upper extremity
    - Lower extremity: Ray, transmetatarsal, above and below knee
    - Upper extremity (rare): Ray, wrist disarticulation, above and below elbow
  - Atherectomy specimens (usually carotid)
  - Thrombectomy specimens (any major vessel)
  - Aneurysm specimens (usually popliteal artery)
- Hypothenar hammer syndrome (repetitive vascular traumatic injury)
  - Affects arteries in hand supplying little finger
  - Intimal thickening and fibromuscular dysplasia-type changes present in vessel wall
  - ± superimposed thrombosis, usually with less prominent inflammation
  - Veins typically not involved

EPIDEMIOLOGY

Age Range

- PVD is generally disease of older adults
  - Intermittent claudication incidence, which is used as measure of PVD, increases with advancing age
    - 1% at < 55 years to 10-15% at > 70 years
- In younger patients, consider unusual causes
  - Vasculitis
  - Hypercoagulability (antiphospholipid antibody, etc.)
  - Cystic adventitial disease of popliteal artery
  - Raynaud phenomenon
  - Emboli
  - Systemic shock

Sex

- M > F (1.6-3:1)

CLINICAL IMPLICATIONS

Clinical Risk Factors

- Similar to those for atherosclerosis elsewhere
  - Age, sex
  - Diabetes mellitus
  - Smoking
  - Hypertension
  - Hyperlipidemia, hypertriglyceridemia, elevated lipoprotein A
  - Hyperhomocysteinemia
  - Elevated systemic inflammatory markers (ESR, CRP)
  - Increasing number of risk factors increases risk for PVD
- ESRD
  - Patients with ESRD at increased risk for PVD have high rate of traditional risk factors + additive risk from uremia/dialysis
  - Very high rate of vascular calcification
    - Associated with elevated serum phosphorous levels, elevated calcium phosphorous product, hyperparathyroidism

Clinical Presentation

- Intermittent claudication progressing to ischemic extremity pain at rest to ischemic ulceration and gangrene (critical limb ischemia)
  - Rutherford classification of PAD: 7 stages
    - Stage 0: Asymptomatic
    - Stages 1, 2, 3: Mild, moderate, severe intermittent claudication
    - Stage 4: Ischemic rest pain
    - Stage 5: Minor tissue loss

Ischemic Lower Extremity (Amputation)

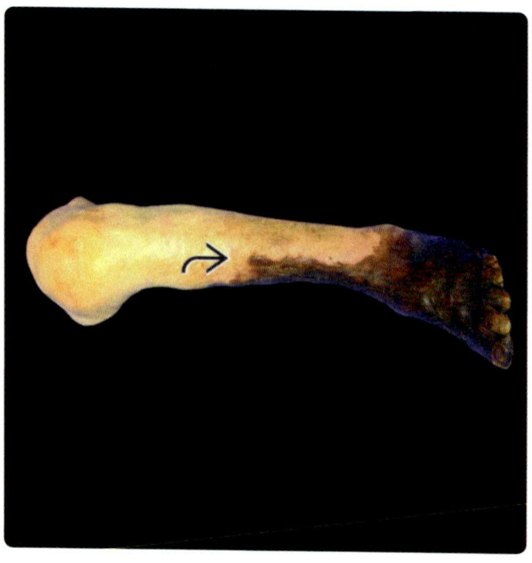

Heavily Calcified Arterial Plaque

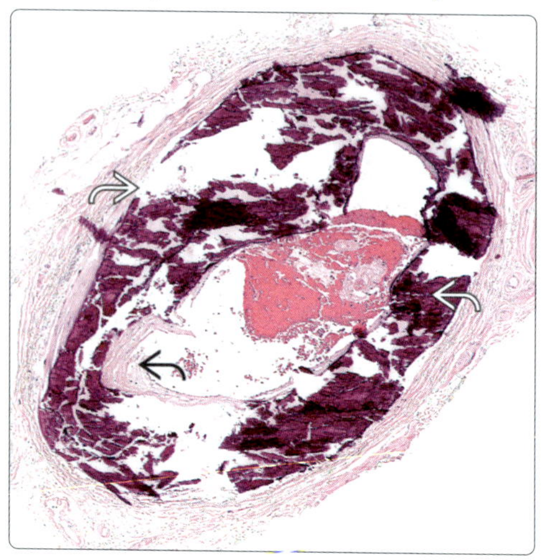

(Left) *Left above-knee amputation specimen shows dry gangrene extending midway up the medial shin. Marked atrophy of skeletal muscle is noted by the small calf circumference.* **(Right)** *Extremity vessels, particularly in older, diabetic, and ESRD patients, often demonstrate medial calcific sclerosis. The calcification extensively replaces the media in this example, and there is overlying intimal hyperplasia.*

- Stage 6: Ulceration or gangrene
- Many patients with PVD are asymptomatic (Rutherford stage 0), so noninvasive measure of ankle brachial index (ABI) used to screen for hemodynamically significant PVD
  - ABI: Ankle systolic pressure/brachial systolic pressure; ≤ 0.90 considered indicative of PVD
  - False readings due to arterial calcification in anterior tibial artery leading to markedly elevated readings
  - False-negative readings in patients with arterial disease distal to ankle
- Increased risk for amputation in critical limb ischemia patients with decreased microvascular flow or with complications that demand increased microvascular flow
  - Decreased microvascular flow in diabetes mellitus, severe renal failure, severe heart failure, smoking
  - Increased microvascular flow need in infection (cellulitis/osteomyelitis), skin breakdown
- Patients with PVD have very high rate of comorbidities
  - Age-adjusted mortality for claudication patients is ~ 4x higher than for nonclaudicants
    - Cardiovascular disease most common cause of death
- Patients with popliteal artery aneurysms may be asymptomatic or present with embolic phenomena or popliteal artery occlusion
  - With angiographic popliteal occlusion, thrombosed aneurysm likely cause
  - May have abdominal aortic aneurysm (AAA) (16-20% of AAA patients have popliteal aneurysm)
  - Differential diagnosis for popliteal occlusion in young patient includes cystic adventitial disease
    - Cystic adventitial disease is formation of uni- or multilocular cysts that contain mucinous material within adventitial layer of vessel wall
    - Usually seen in men 20-50 years of age

MACROSCOPIC

General Features

- Amputation specimens most commonly demonstrate features of critical limb ischemia
  - Critical limb ischemia, most severe manifestation of PVD, defined as patients with ischemic limb pain at rest and ischemic ulcers &/or gangrene
    - Wet gangrene has moist purulent necrosis, dry gangrene has eschar formation and mummification of necrotic tissue
    - Appearance related to ratio of coagulative necrosis (due to ischemia) to liquefactive necrosis (due to superimposed infection)
  - Diabetic ulcers, cellulitis, venous stasis changes may also be seen
    - Neuropathic diabetic ulcers due to repetitive mechanical forces affect plantar aspect of foot at metatarsal head or toes; ulcer usually surrounded by callus
    - Ischemic diabetic ulcers often at medial aspect of 1st metatarsophalangeal joint, lateral aspect of 5th metatarsophalangeal joint, or at tips of toes; usually superficial ulcers
    - Many diabetic patients with new foot ulcer will be shown to have significant PVD
  - Amputation specimens have bony resection margin that extends beyond soft tissue margin; disarticulation specimens (usually for tumor, not PVD) have articular cartilage at resection margin
  - Atherosclerosis of major vessels, usually diffusely distributed; may see thrombosis; medial calcific sclerosis also common
    - Prior grafting or stenting of major vessels may have been performed
    - Preferential sites for thrombi in leg are femoral and popliteal arteries
    - Angiographic studies of distribution of PVD reveal common diffuse bilateral disease, similar in men and women
  - Prior ray, transmetatarsal, or below-knee amputation wounds may be noted and may be poorly healed
- Amputation specimens in younger patients
  - Look for features of more unusual causes of peripheral ischemia and check clinical history
    - Vasospasm, septic shock, nonatherosclerotic emboli, vasopressor therapy, cystic adventitial disease of popliteal artery
- Atherectomy specimens (when intact) are tubular resections of inner portion of atherosclerotic vessel
  - Directional atherectomy
    - Removes lesional tissue by excising intact portions of vessel intima with some inner media
    - Often calcified; may have plaque erosion, rupture, and thrombosis
  - Rotational atherectomy
    - Ablates lesional tissue, fragmented specimen
- Thrombectomy specimens will contain thrombus in various states of organization
  - Occasionally, specimens labeled "thrombectomy" may represent unusual obstructive masses, such as embolic vegetations, neoplasms, etc.; always submit microscopic sections
- Peripheral arterial aneurysm specimens will vary depending on surgical repair (interposed graft or aneurysm ligation)
  - Atherosclerosis is common cause, and popliteal is most common location; often bilateral

Sections to Be Submitted

- Amputation specimens
  - Demonstrate gangrenous necrosis/ischemic ulcers, including intersection with viable tissue and underlying bone if osteomyelitis is suspected
  - Demonstrate any nonhealing wounds from prior surgical intervention
  - Dissect and identify major vessels in specimen and document areas of atherosclerosis, thrombosis
    - Identify any prior surgical revascularization attempts (grafts, stents) and inspect and section those areas
  - Dissect major venous vessels and assess for thrombosis, perivenous fibrosis; submit representative section
  - Sample peripheral nerve and skeletal muscle (most often performed as part of proximal soft tissue resection margin)
  - Proximal soft tissue resection margin
- Atherectomy specimens

- Serial cross sections of specimen following decalcification if needed; submit any areas of acute plaque changes, such as ulceration, rupture, thrombosis
- Thrombectomy specimens
  - Submit representative section or complete specimen if small
- Peripheral vessel aneurysms
  - Try to identify aneurysm wall from aneurysm content (thrombus) if possible and submit from wall and content

MICROSCOPIC

General Features

- Necrotic tissue shows varying amounts of coagulative and liquefactive necrosis
  - Often see bacteria or yeast/fungi that infiltrate skin to underlying subcutaneous tissue
  - Necrosis and acute inflammation of vessels under ulcers may be noted
    - Check proximal vessel margins for suppurative vasculitis/thrombophlebitis
  - Assess bone underneath deep ulcers for osteomyelitis
    - Acute inflammation, dead bone
    - Fat necrosis in marrow may often be seen as manifestation of ischemia, does not necessarily indicate osteomyelitis
- Major vessels demonstrate typical atherosclerosis ± overlying thrombus
- Calcification of media of arteries is commonly seen (medial calcific sclerosis)
- Calcification of smaller vessels extending up to dermis; consider calciphylaxis
  - Should be noted if present, as patients should be assessed for secondary hyperparathyroidism
  - Usually noted in specimens from patients with chronic renal failure
- Assess for unusual causes of ischemic disease
  - Vasculitis, antiphospholipid antibody syndrome, thromboangiitis obliterans (TAO) (Buerger disease, especially in young smokers)
    - TAO: Nonatherosclerotic inflammatory disorder of small to medium-sized arteries, veins, and nerves
    - TAO characterized by cellular thrombi with acute inflammation and occasional giant cells that undergoes organization with progressive fibrosis of vessel wall
    - Suspect TAO if marked perivascular, perivenular, and perineural fibrosis noted
    - Giant cell arteritis and polyarteritis nodosa have been noted to cause peripheral gangrene and would be evident on histologic analysis
  - Paraneoplastic gangrene
    - Rare presentation of underlying malignancy, usually underlying carcinoma (adenocarcinoma) or hematolymphoid malignancy; often advanced disease present; usually older patients
    - Usually digital gangrene (fingers and toes)
    - Unknown pathogenesis (putative: Tumor-derived vasospastic substance, microemboli, immunologic factors)
- Atherectomy specimens
  - Deep wall components (media > adventitia) may be seen
  - Atherosclerotic plaque, thrombus, intimal hyperplasia common

SELECTED REFERENCES

1. Estíbaliz AT et al: Bilateral hypothenar hammer syndrome case presentation and literature review. Case Rep Vasc Med. 2022:2078772, 2022
2. Gardiner GA Jr et al: Repetitive blunt trauma and arterial injury in the hand. Cardiovasc Intervent Radiol. 40(11):1659-68, 2017
3. Hai A et al: Symmetrical peripheral gangrene: a rare presentation of antiphospholipid syndrome. Intern Emerg Med. 7 Suppl 1:S71-3, 2012
4. Onitilo AA et al: Digital ischemia as a paraneoplastic consequence of squamous cell lung carcinoma. WMJ. 111(3):138-41; quiz 142, 2012
5. Williams VL et al: Distal extremity necrosis as a manifestation of cutaneous polyarteritis nodosa: case report and review of the acute management of a pediatric patient. Pediatr Dermatol. 29(4):473-8, 2012
6. Dattilo PB et al: Critical limb ischemia: endovascular strategies for limb salvage. Prog Cardiovasc Dis. 54(1):47-60, 2011
7. Kermani TA et al: Lower extremity vasculitis in polymyalgia rheumatica and giant cell arteritis. Curr Opin Rheumatol. 23(1):38-42, 2011
8. Moon JS et al: A controlled study of medial arterial calcification of legs: implications for diabetic polyneuropathy. Arch Neurol. 68(10):1290-4, 2011
9. Morris-Stiff G et al: Variations in the anatomical distribution of peripheral vascular disease according to gender. Ann R Coll Surg Engl. 93(4):306-9, 2011
10. Lutchman D et al: Phaeochromocytoma-associated critical peripheral ischaemia. Intern Med J. 40(2):150-3, 2010
11. Piazza G et al: Thromboangiitis obliterans. Circulation. 121(16):1858-61, 2010
12. Aronow WS: Peripheral arterial disease in women. Maturitas. 64(4):204-11, 2009
13. Wain RA et al: A contemporary review of popliteal artery aneurysms. Cardiol Rev. 15(2):102-7, 2007
14. Edmonds ME et al: Diabetic foot ulcers. BMJ. 332(7538):407-10, 2006
15. Poszepczynska-Guigné E et al: Paraneoplastic acral vascular syndrome: epidemiologic features, clinical manifestations, and disease sequelae. J Am Acad Dermatol. 47(1):47-52, 2002
16. O'Hare A et al: Lower-extremity peripheral arterial disease among patients with end-stage renal disease. J Am Soc Nephrol. 12(12):2838-47, 2001
17. Ouriel K: Peripheral arterial disease. Lancet. 358(9289):1257-64, 2001
18. Schnitt SJ et al: Histologic findings in specimens obtained by percutaneous directional coronary atherectomy. Hum Pathol. 23(4):415-20, 1992
19. Conn J Jr et al: Calciphylaxis: etiology of progressive vascular calcification and gangrene? Ann Surg. 177(2):206-10, 1973
20. Wessler S et al: Studies in peripheral arterial occlusive disease. I. Methods and pathologic findings in amputated limbs. Circulation. 7(5):641-55, 1953

Overview of Peripheral Vascular Specimens

Nonhealing Ischemic Wound (Gross)

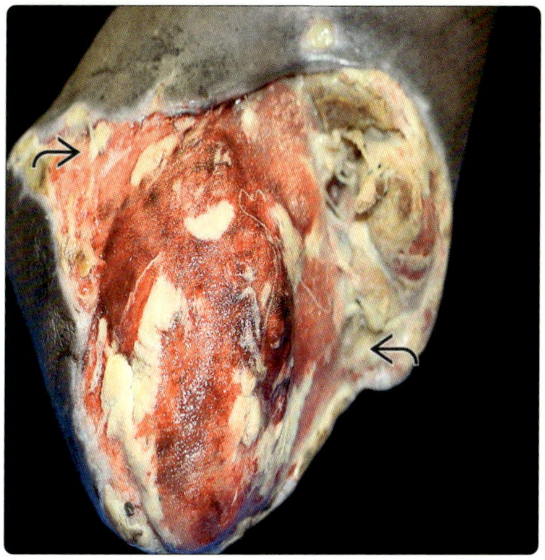

Wet Gangrene in Lower Extremity Ulcer

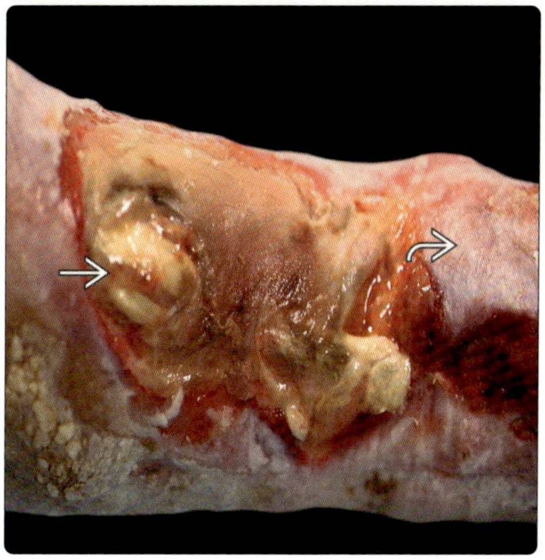

(Left) *Amputation specimens are often revisions of prior procedures. This is a revised below-knee to above-knee amputation specimen with a nonhealing distal wound ↪ that was infected.* **(Right)** *This specimen shows wet gangrene with moist purulent exudate, necrosis, and exposure of the extensor tendons of the foot →. Ascending cellulitis ↪ is also present.*

Popliteal Artery Aneurysm (Angiogram)

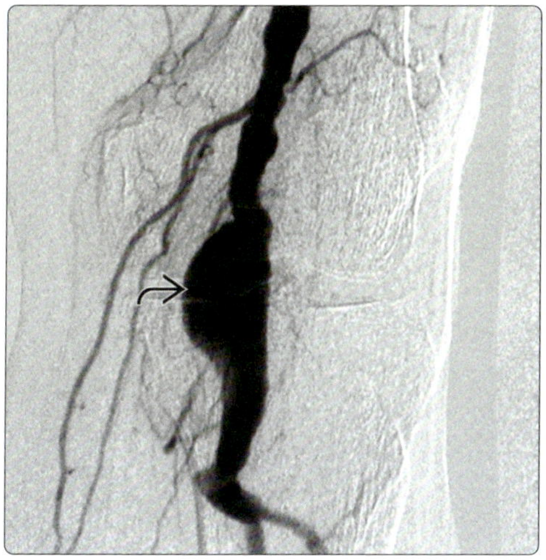

Necrosis of Digits

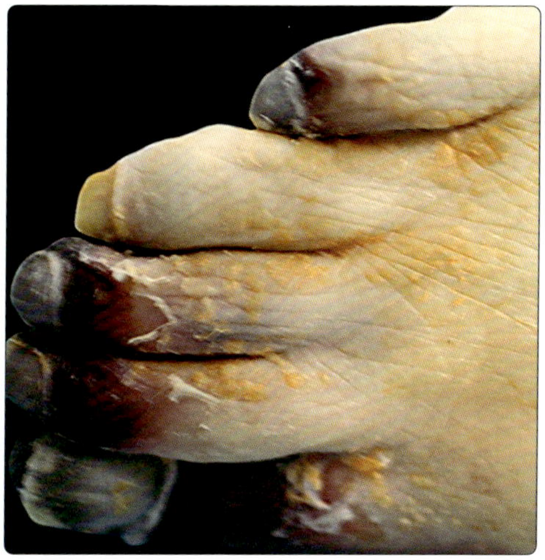

(Left) *DSA shows a fusiform popliteal artery aneurysm ↪. Popliteal artery is the most frequent location of peripheral vessel aneurysms. They are often thrombosed and may present as distal vessel embolization or limb ischemia. Patients may have abdominal aortic aneurysm.* **(Right)** *Necrosis of digits is frequent in PVD specimens and can be due to emboli, small vessel disease, or severe large vessel disease. Less common causes include vasopressor therapy, septic shock, pheochromocytoma, paraneoplastic disease, and Raynaud phenomenon.*

Dissecting Lower Extremity Vascular Bundles

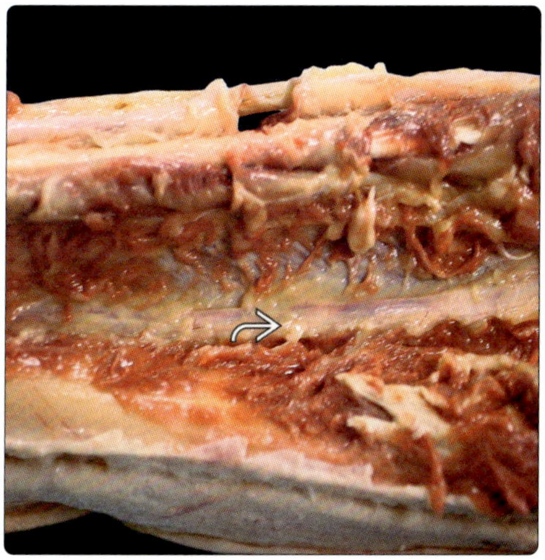

Anterior Tibial Artery Dissection

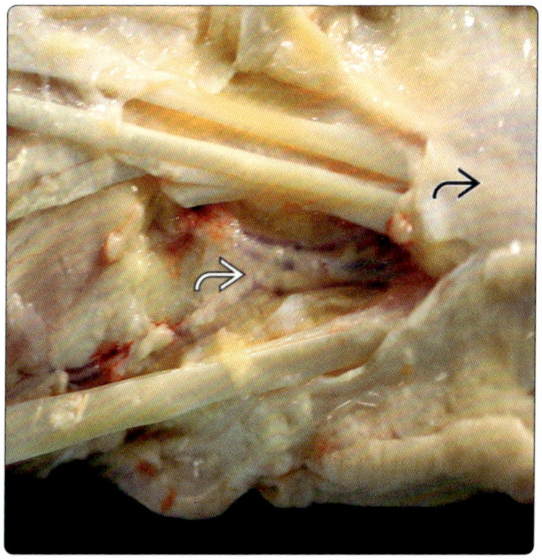

(Left) *Anatomic dissection of lower extremities entails identification of major vessels, such as the anterior tibial artery →, shown here coursing along the interosseous membrane between the tibia and fibula.* **(Right)** *The anterior tibial artery extends distally under the extensor retinaculum ↪ continuing as the dorsalis pedis artery →. False-negative ankle brachial index screening for PVD may be seen with distal arterial disease not affecting the anterior tibial artery at the ankle.*

(Left) *Atherosclerosis of distal extremity vessels is generally diffuse, but thrombosis tends to affect the femoral and popliteal vessels. This popliteal artery contains a small nonocclusive thrombus. This may present as claudication or critical limb ischemia.* **(Right)** *H&E-stained cross section through a popliteal artery reveals calcification in atherosclerotic plaque and media layer with nonobstructive thin mural thrombus.*

Atherosclerosis and Mural Thrombus (Nonocclusive)

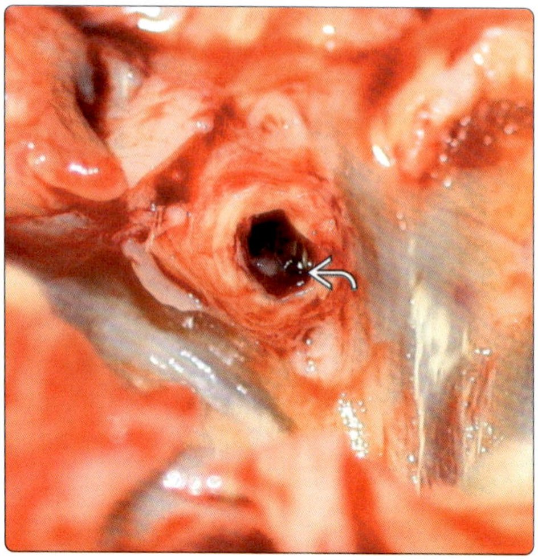

Calcified Arteriosclerosis/Atherosclerosis

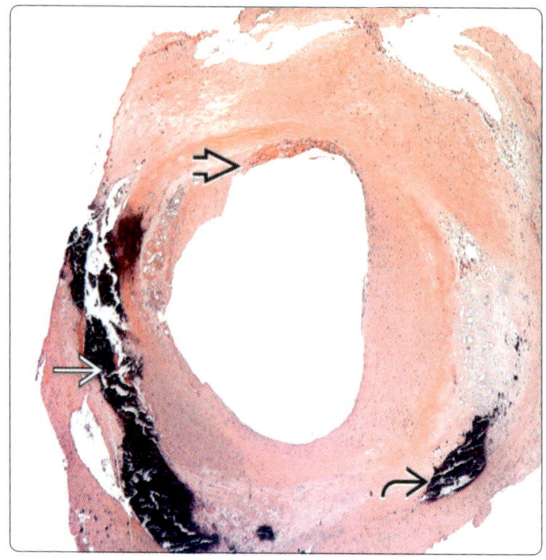

(Left) *Gross specimen, including anterior tibial artery, demonstrates severe obstruction with only a pinpoint lumen remaining and atherosclerotic plaque with overlying white tissue, suggestive of organized thrombus.* **(Right)** *H&E-stained cross section through the anterior tibial artery shows rupture of atherosclerotic plaque with extrusion of cholesterol crystals and necrotic contents into lumen and associated thrombosis.*

Anterior Tibial Artery Occlusion

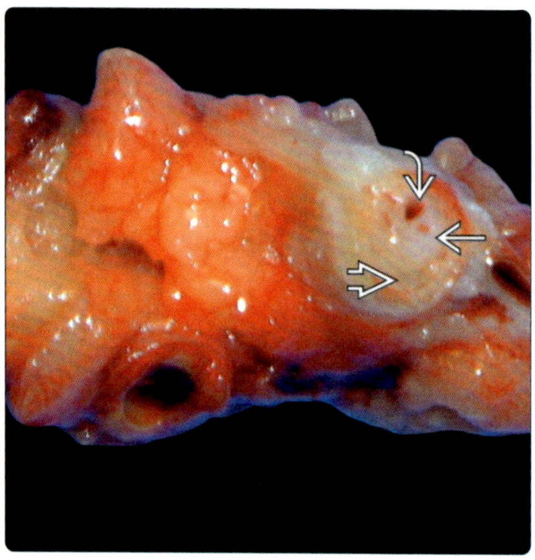

Lipid-Rich Atheroma

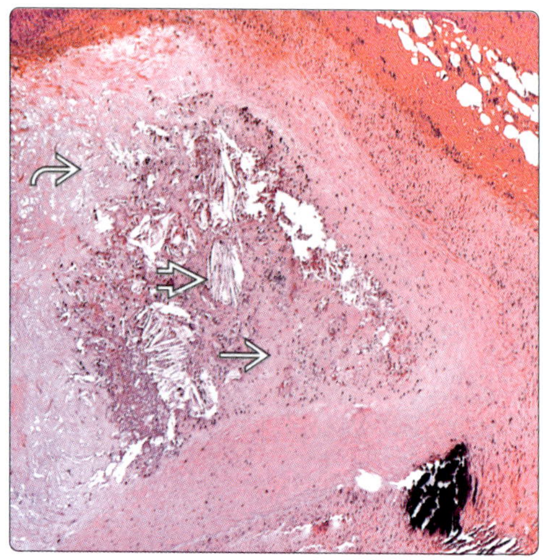

(Left) *Calciphylaxis is calcification of the media of small to medium-sized arteries of subcutaneous tissue and dermis. The calcified vessels may have thrombus or overlying intimal hyperplasia.* **(Right)** *Atherectomy specimens are resections of the intima and inner media of arteries. The intima contains atherosclerotic plaque with calcification.*

Calciphylaxis of Media

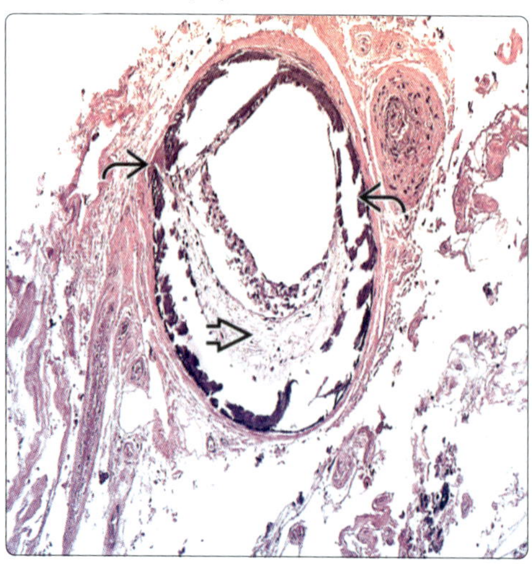

Endarterectomy Histology

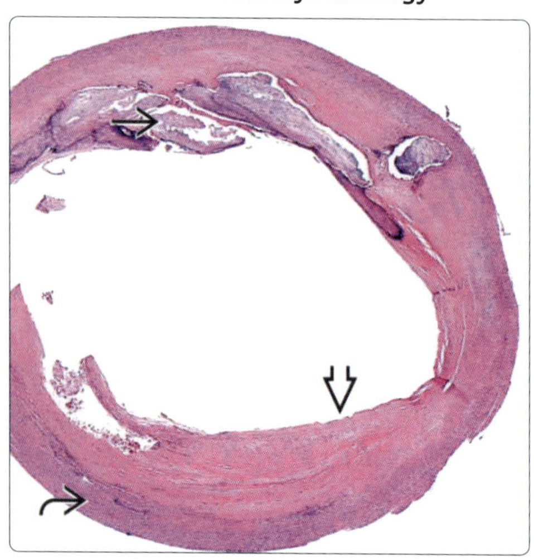

Ischemic Ulcer Histology (Dry Gangrene)

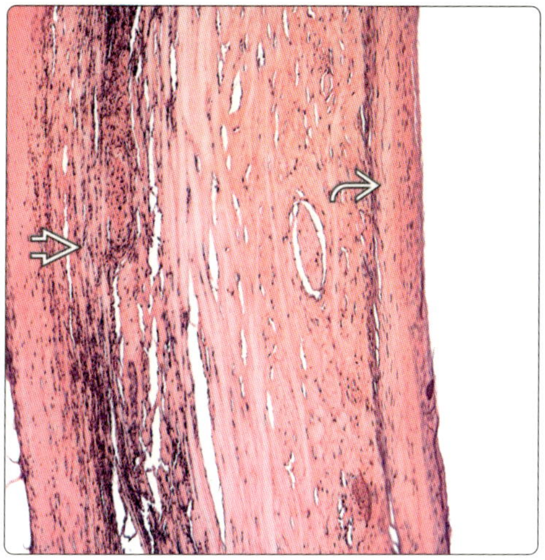

Ischemic Ulcer With Underlying Bone

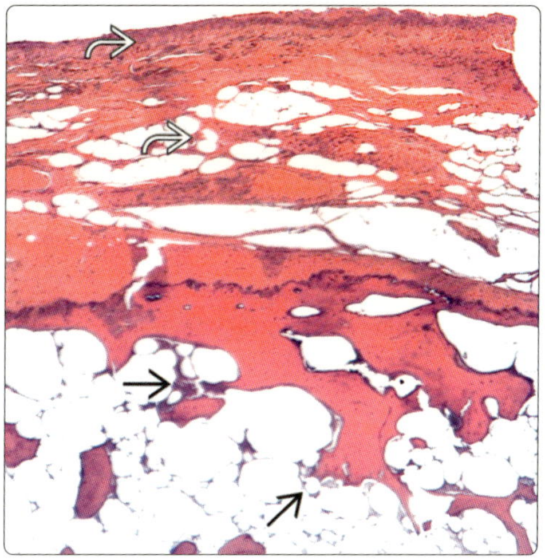

(Left) *Histologically, gangrenous necrosis is a combination of coagulative and liquefactive necrosis. In this section, the epidermis* → *is demonstrating predominantly coagulative necrosis, while there is acute suppurative inflammation in the dermis* →. **(Right)** *This cross section through an ischemic digit shows ischemic necrosis of skin and subcutaneous tissue* → *and also ischemic necrosis of the marrow in the underlying bone* →. *These are good sections to screen for osteomyelitis.*

Thrombectomy Histology

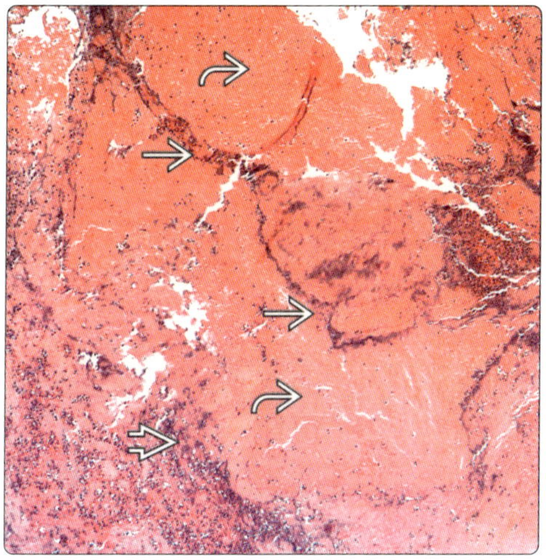

Hypothenar Hammer Syndrome

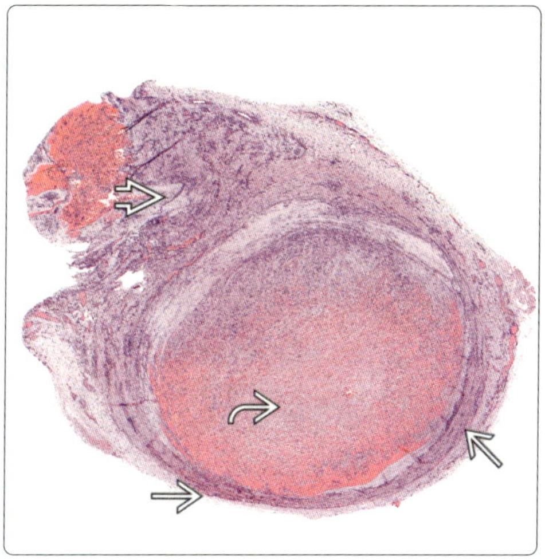

(Left) *This popliteal artery "thrombectomy" specimen is an embolized fragment of vegetation. Note the fibrin* →, *acute inflammatory cells* →, *and blue-staining bacterial colonies* →. *A history of aortic valve endocarditis and positive Gram stain helped confirm the diagnosis.* **(Right)** *This H&E-stained photomicrograph shows arterial injury due to repetitive trauma (hypothenar hammer syndrome). There is transmural chronic inflammation* → *and adventitial fibrosis and inflammation* →. *The lumen is occluded by thrombus* →.

Hypothenar Hammer Syndrome: Elastic Stain

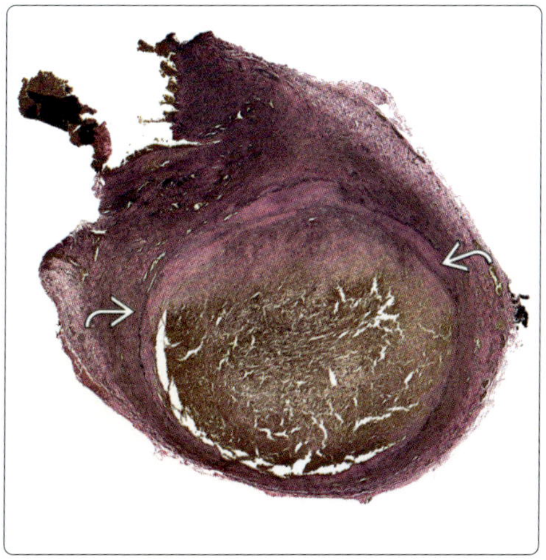

Hypothenar Hammer Syndrome: Trichrome

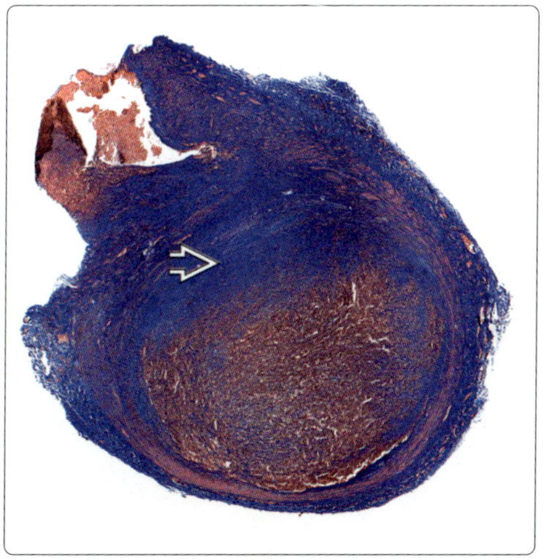

(Left) *This elastic van-Gieson stained photomicrograph shows arterial injury due to repetitive trauma (hypothenar hammer syndrome). There is attenuation of the internal elastic lamina* → *segmentally due to scarring in the artery wall.* **(Right)** *This trichrome stained photomicrograph shows arterial injury due to repetitive trauma (hypothenar hammer syndrome). There is transmural scarring/fibrous replacement of medial smooth muscle* → *segmentally.*

Thromboembolus, Vascular

KEY FACTS

TERMINOLOGY

- Embolus: Solid, gaseous, or liquid mass that travels in circulation from point of origin to distal location
- Thromboembolus: Embolus composed of thrombus material
- Pulmonary thromboembolism (PTE): Thromboemboli within pulmonary arterial circulation, virtually all arising from venous thrombi of lower extremities; thus, venous thromboemboli (VTE) is another term for this entity
- Systemic thromboembolism: Thromboemboli involving systemic arterial circulation generally arising from cardiac or aortic thrombi

CLINICAL ISSUES

- Sudden death when ≥ 60% of blood flow obstructed (2% of PTE)
- Primary hypercoagulable states
- Multiple risk factors for thrombophilia have additive effect on risk for VTE (multiple-hit hypothesis)
- Other risk factors
  - Obesity, immobilization, smoking, pregnancy, recent surgery, underlying malignancy, oral contraceptive use

MACROSCOPIC

- Paradoxical emboli arise in venous circulation and lodge in systemic arterial circulation
- Thromboemboli features
  - Red and rubbery with shaggy periphery from fibrin
  - May organize into delicate, intravascular web-like structure
- Pulmonary infarcts: Hemorrhagic, wedge-shaped area with base toward pleura and apex toward hilum
- Solid organ infarcts: Wedge-shaped areas of necrosis with base toward capsule and apex toward hilum

MICROSCOPIC

- Red blood cell-rich layers alternating with fibrin- and platelet-rich areas (lines of Zahn) indicate thrombus formed in setting of pulsatile blood flow

Saddle Thromboembolus at Pulmonary Artery Bifurcation

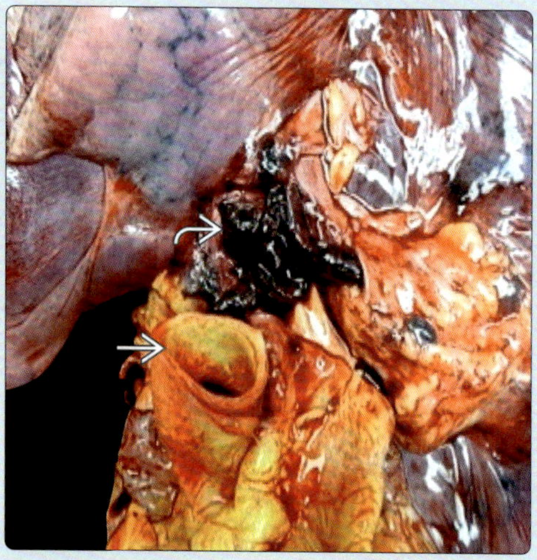

Thromboembolus, Histology

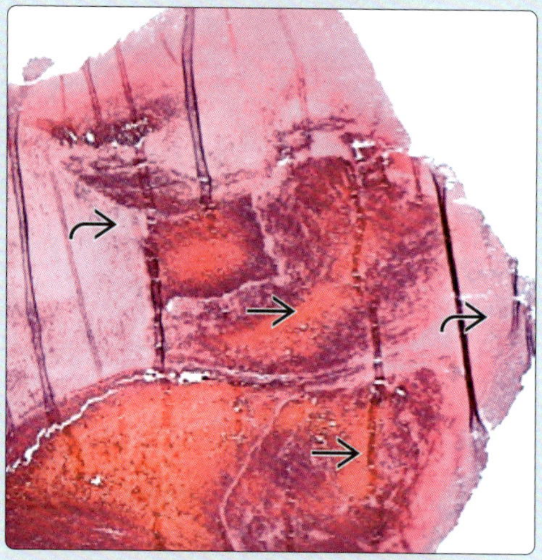

(Left) *A large, serpiginous, dark red thromboembolus ➡ is present at the bifurcation of the main pulmonary artery (saddle embolus) of this thoracic organ block. Note the cut end of the aorta ➡.* **(Right)** *Alternating areas rich in fibrin and platelets ➡ and red blood cells ➡ (lines of Zahn) in a thromboembolus indicate that it arose from a thrombus that formed in flowing blood (i.e., antemortem).*

Venous Thromboemboli

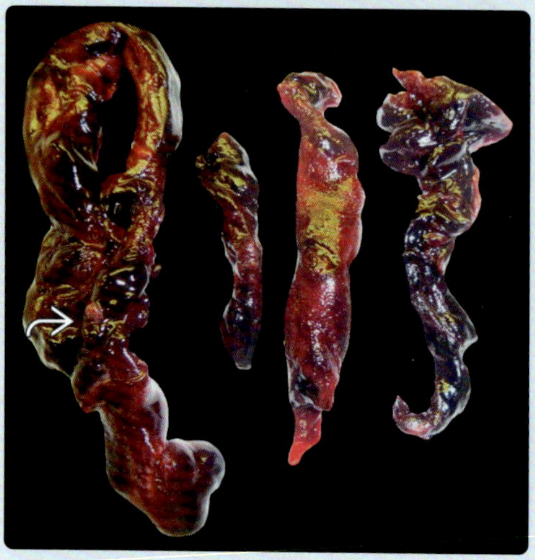

Thromboembolus, Histology

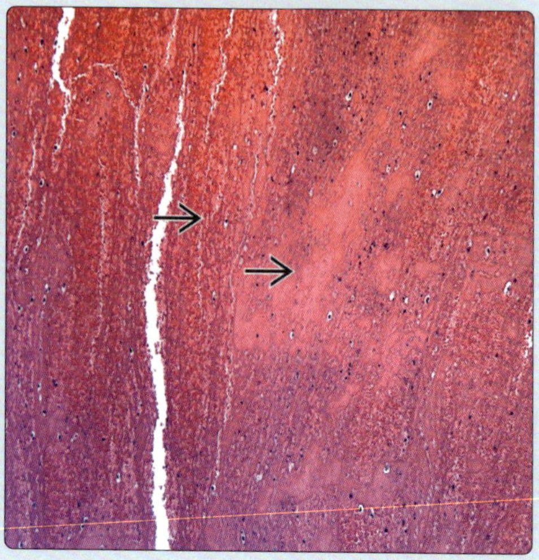

(Left) *These venous thromboemboli (VTE) were removed from a pulmonary artery at autopsy. Their shape is a cast of the vein in which they formed. Often, thromboemboli are coiled like the one on the left ➡. The shaggy external surface is due to fibrin formation, and on occasion, venous valve markings may be seen.* **(Right)** *The lines of Zahn are not prominent in this thromboembolus but are still recognizable ➡. Lines of Zahn are generally more prominent in arterial vs. venous thrombi.*

TERMINOLOGY

Definitions

- Embolus: Solid, gaseous, or liquid mass that travels in circulation from its point of origin to distal location
- Thromboembolus: Embolus composed of thrombus material
- Pulmonary thromboembolism (PTE): Thromboemboli within pulmonary arterial circulation, virtually all arising from venous thrombi of lower extremities
  - Venous thromboemboli (VTE) is another term for this entity
- Systemic thromboembolism: Thromboemboli involving systemic arterial circulation, generally arising from cardiac or aortic thrombi

CLINICAL ISSUES

Presentation

- PTE: Depends on size, number of thromboemboli, underlying cardiovascular status
  - Respiratory decompensation: Ventilation perfusion mismatch in area distal to embolus
  - Hemodynamic decompensation due to increased pulmonary vascular resistance
    - Sudden death when ≥ 60% of blood flow obstructed (2% of PTE)
  - Pulmonary infarction uncommon (~ 10%); usually seen in patients with severe underlying cardiopulmonary disease
  - Symptoms include shortness of breath, chest pain, cough, hemoptysis, syncope
  - Often, PTE is clinically silent; if chronic and recurrent (risk: 30%), may cause chronic thromboembolic pulmonary hypertension
- Systemic thromboembolism
  - Central nervous system (CNS) = embolic stroke; extremities = ischemia; solid organ = clinically silent or pain in area; intestine = abdominal pain/shock

Risk Factors

- Primary hypercoagulable states
  - Inherited thrombophilia has annual incidence of PTE 2-20x that of normal population
  - Recurrent VTE increased in antithrombin, proteins C and S defects, mild hyperhomocysteinemia, antiphospholipid antibody and homozygous or double heterozygote factor V Leiden, and prothrombin mutation
  - Multiple risk factors for thrombophilia have additive effect on risk for VTE (multiple-hit hypothesis)
- Other risk factors
  - Obesity, immobilization, smoking, pregnancy, recent surgery, underlying malignancy, oral contraceptive use, COVID-19 infection

MACROSCOPIC

General Features

- Most are VTE that arise from lower extremities and lodge in pulmonary arteries
  - Saddle pulmonary thromboembolus is within pulmonary artery bifurcation
- Systemic thromboemboli usually arise from cardiac source (80%); aortic aneurysm and thrombi overlying ulcerated aortic atherosclerotic plaques are other common origins
  - Most cardiac thrombi form in dilated left atria associated with atrial fibrillation, and remainder are in left ventricle over areas of infarction or in diseased/prosthetic valves
  - Can lodge in any arterial bed: Common sites include lower extremity and brain; less common sites include kidney, spleen, intestine, and upper extremity
    - Often associated with involved organ/tissue infarction
- Paradoxical emboli arise in venous circulation and lodge in systemic arterial circulation
  - Due to intracardiac communication with right to left shunting (usually patent foramen ovale)
- Thromboemboli features
  - Maintains shape of vessel of origin as opposed to distal vessel it lodges in
  - Red and rubbery with shaggy periphery from fibrin
    - Venous valve markings
    - Alternating fibrin- and platelet-rich areas and red blood cell-rich areas (lines of Zahn)
  - Acutely not attached to vessel wall; become attached with organization
- Pulmonary infarcts
  - Hemorrhagic, wedge-shaped area with base toward pleura and apex toward hilum
    - Often multiple and affecting lower lobes
- Solid organ infarcts
  - Wedge-shaped areas of necrosis with base toward capsule and apex toward hilum

MICROSCOPIC

Histologic Features

- Red blood cell-rich layers alternating with fibrin- and platelet-rich areas (lines of Zahn) indicate thrombus formed in setting of pulsatile blood flow
- With organization, fibroblastic ingrowth and recanalization with formation of small vascular channels within thromboembolus
- Infarction morphology depends on organ involved
  - Pulmonary: Hemorrhagic
  - Solid organ: Pale
- All infarcts (red or pale) associated with coagulative necrosis of parenchyma except CNS
  - CNS associated with liquefactive necrosis
  - May see thromboembolus in affected vessel leading to infarct

DIFFERENTIAL DIAGNOSIS

Postmortem Clots

- Gravity-induced layering of serum and red blood cells resembles "chicken fat and currant jelly"
- No gross or microscopic lines of Zahn

SELECTED REFERENCES

1. Yamashita Y et al: Venous thromboembolism: recent advancement and future perspective. J Cardiol. 79(1):79-89, 2022
2. Zuin M et al: Prevalence of acute pulmonary embolism at autopsy in patients with COVID-19. Am J Cardiol. 171:159-64, 2022
3. Lyaker MR et al: Arterial embolism. Int J Crit Illn Inj Sci. 3(1):77-87, 2013

(Left) *This lung contains multiple wedge-shaped, hemorrhagic pulmonary infarcts . The wide base is located at the pleura, and often there is overlying fibrin. Lower lobe infarcts are more common. Pulmonary infarcts generally only occur in patients with significant underlying cardiopulmonary disease.* **(Right)** *Pulmonary infarcts are hemorrhagic, but coagulative necrosis of the alveolar septa and vessels confirms that this hemorrhage is related to an infarct.*

Multiple Lung Infarcts

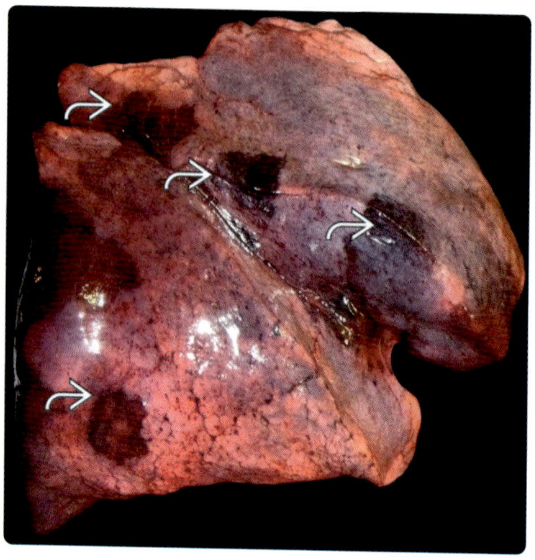

Lung Infarct, Histology

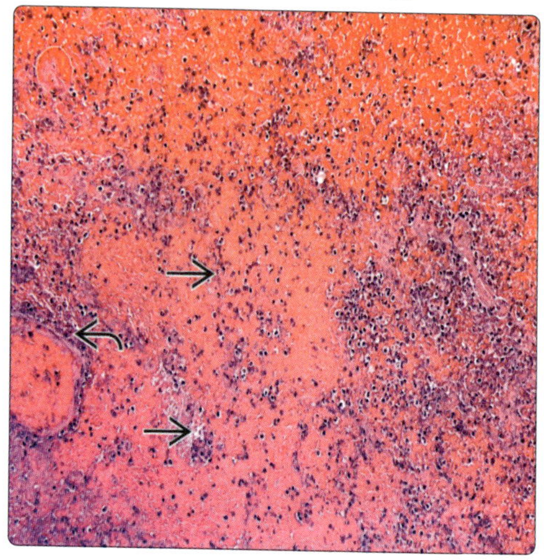

(Left) *Solid organ infarcts, such as splenic infarcts, are wedge-shaped with the base toward the capsule, and they are ischemic. This spleen has a yellow, wedge-shaped infarct that was the result of thromboembolic disease from a cardiac source.* **(Right)** *The spleen is an organ that can be involved in systemic thromboembolism arising from the heart or large vessels. The infarcted area is in subcapsular location and shows a wedge shape with the apex toward the hilum and the base toward the capsule.*

Splenic Infarct

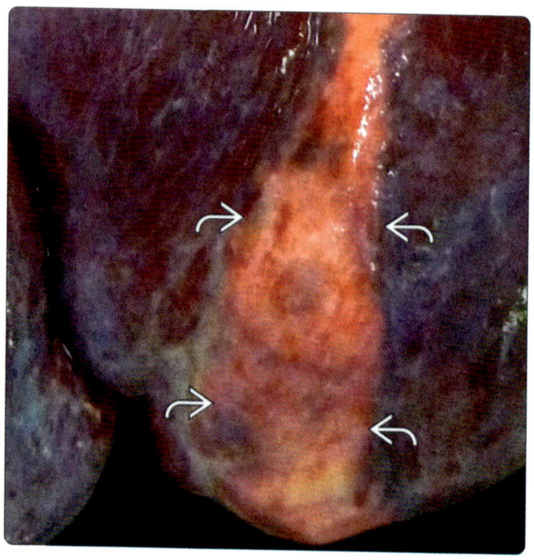

Splenic Infarct, Histology

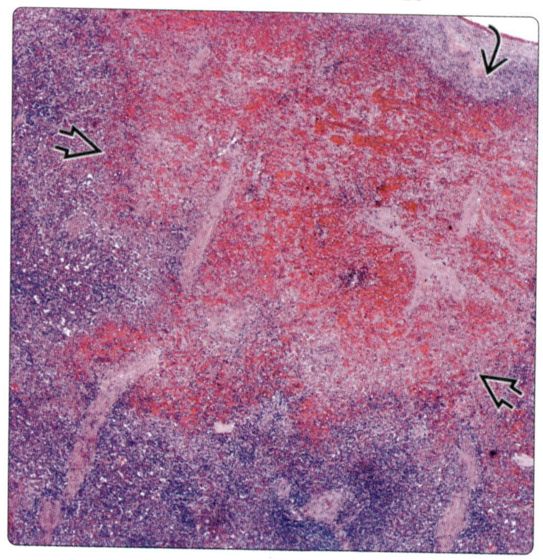

(Left) *The kidney is a common site of arterial emboli causing infarct. In this case, the area of infarction is somewhat less well demarcated, but it is characterized by a hemorrhage in a wedge shape .* **(Right)** *Microscopically, this kidney infarct had coagulative necrosis, and an organizing thromboembolus was noted in a vessel toward the base. Note the fibroblastic ingrowth and focal recanalization .*

Kidney Infarct

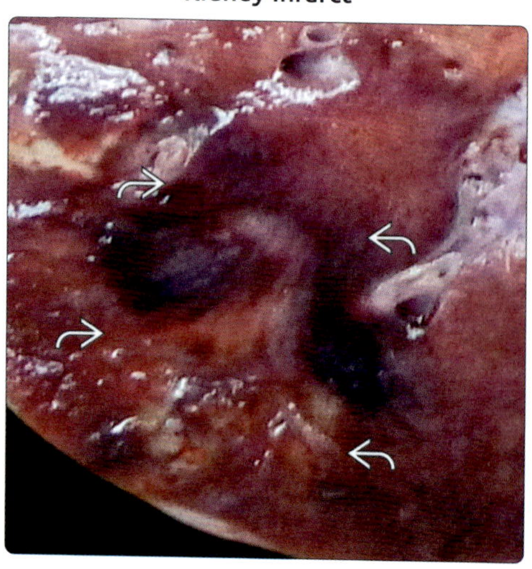

Kidney Infarct, Histology

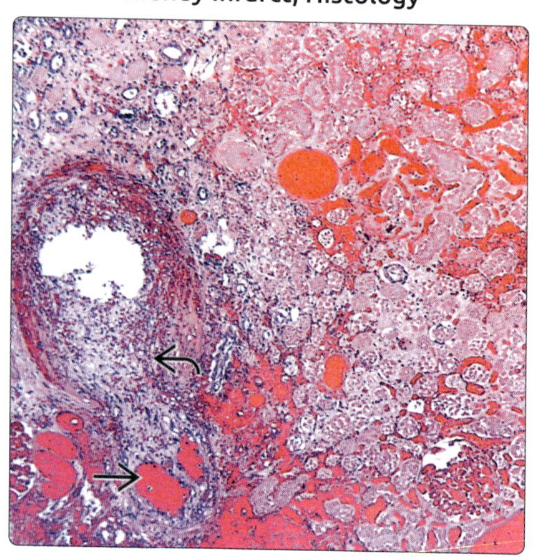

Patent Foramen Ovale

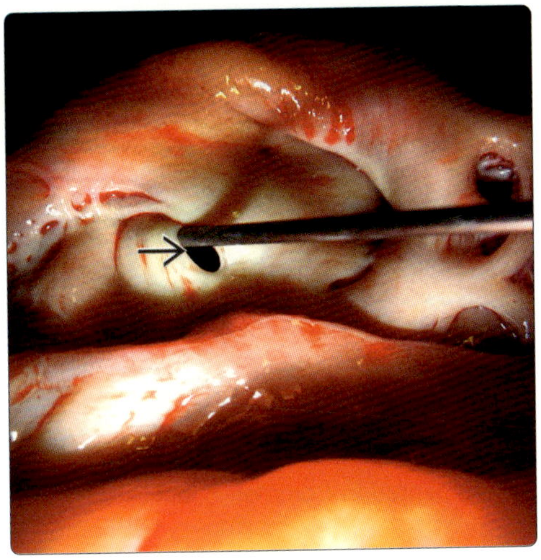

Right Atrial and Ventricular Thrombi

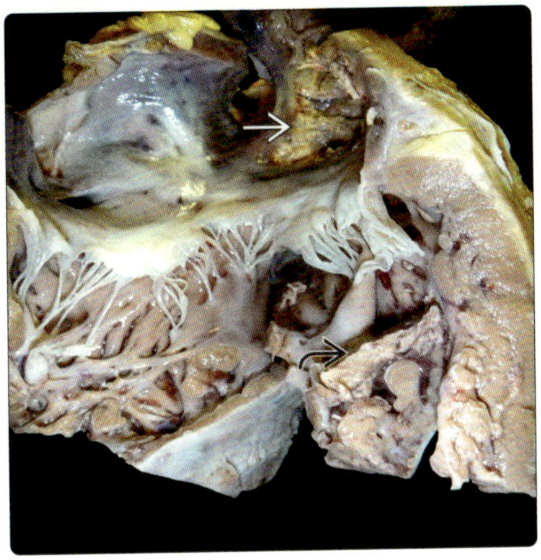

(Left) *Seen in ~ 27% of autopsies, patent foramen ovale is a flap-like opening between atrial septum primum and secundum. It is often present in paradoxical embolism where VTE cross to the arterial circulation.* **(Right)** *Rarely, pulmonary emboli ± infarcts arise from right heart thrombi. This cardiac transplant recipient had an extensive right ventricular thrombus and a right atrial thrombus overlying myocardial necrosis related to chronic rejection.*

Atrial Appendage Thrombus

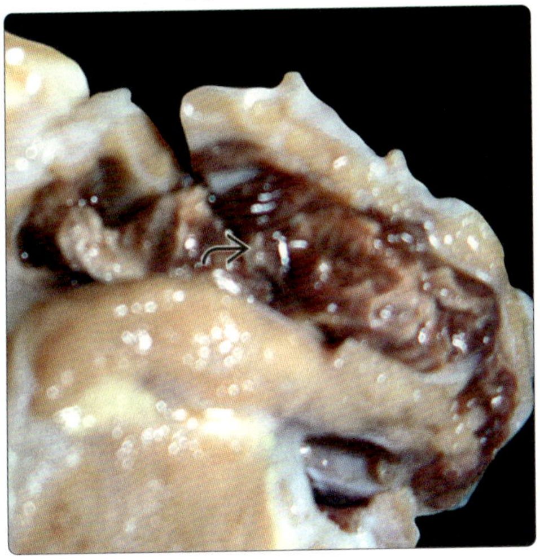

Cortical Infarct

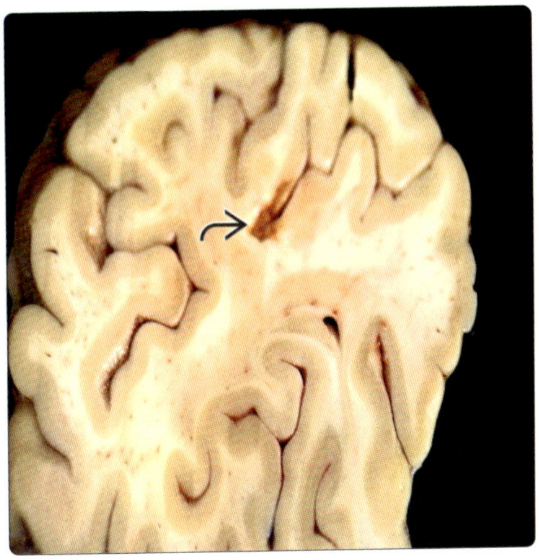

(Left) *Transected left atrial appendage demonstrates a large thrombus that was the source for systemic thromboemboli. This thrombus formed in a cardiac transplant patient with atrial fibrillation. Atrial thrombi are often seen in dilated atria associated with atrial fibrillation.* **(Right)** *Brain section shows small cortical infarct secondary to left atrial appendage thromboemboli. The CNS and lower extremities are 2 of the most common anatomic sites for systemic thromboemboli.*

Left Ventricle Mural Thrombus

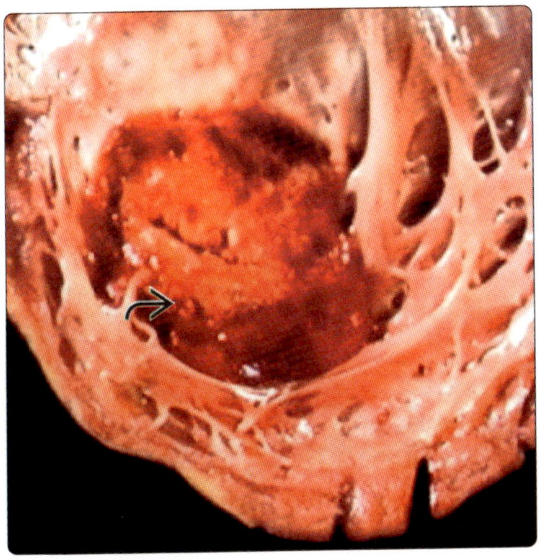

Mural Thrombus, Histology

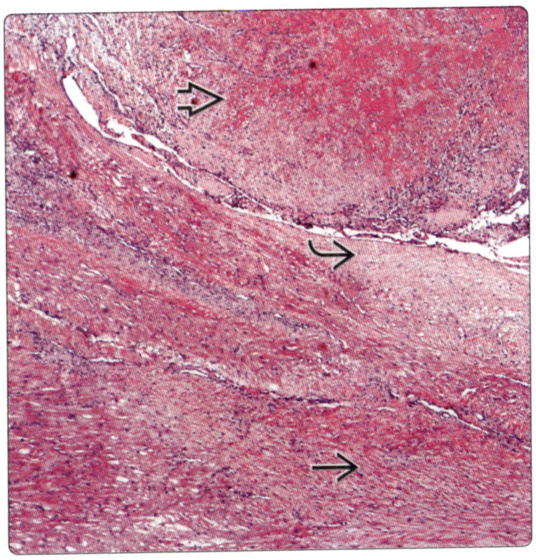

(Left) *Cardiac thrombi may form in the atria or ventricles. Ventricular thrombi most often form in the setting of myocardial infarction, as demonstrated here. These are often referred to as mural thrombi.* **(Right)** *H&E section of left ventricular wall demonstrates a mural thrombus attached to a thickened endocardium adjacent to an area myocardial fibrosis secondary to a prior infarct. This is the most common location for heart thrombus and the main source for systemic thromboemboli.*

Aortic Degenerative Diseases

KEY FACTS

TERMINOLOGY

- Degenerative changes of media of aorta and large elastic arteries, **nonspecific for etiology**, associated with aneurysms and dissections
- Medial degeneration components (2016 SCVP-AECVP nomenclature)
  - Mucoid extracellular matrix material accumulation (MEMA), elastic fiber fragmentation &/or loss, smooth muscle cell nuclei loss, and laminar medial collapse

ETIOLOGY/PATHOGENESIS

- Hypertension
- Bicuspid aortic valve syndrome
- Marfan syndrome, connective tissue diseases

CLINICAL ISSUES

- Usually presents with aneurysm, dissection, or rupture of aorta or large artery
- Surgery for large aneurysms, ascending aortic dissections
- Blood pressure control for small aneurysms, descending aortic dissections
- Steroids for aortitis or arteritis

MICROSCOPIC

- MEMA, elastic fiber alterations, loss of smooth muscle nuclei, collapse of elastic lamellar scaffold

ANCILLARY TESTS

- Always obtain elastic stain
- Submit for EM, if Ehlers-Danlos type IV is suspected

DIAGNOSTIC CHECKLIST

- Clinical correlation often helpful
  - MEMA-T: Common in Marfan and Turner syndromes
  - MEMA-I: Common in Loeys-Dietz syndrome
  - Elastic fiber fragmentation: Common in familial thoracic aneurysm syndrome and arterial tortuosity syndrome
- Autopsy performance should include examination for gross dysmorphology suggesting genetic disorder

Aortic Medial Degeneration

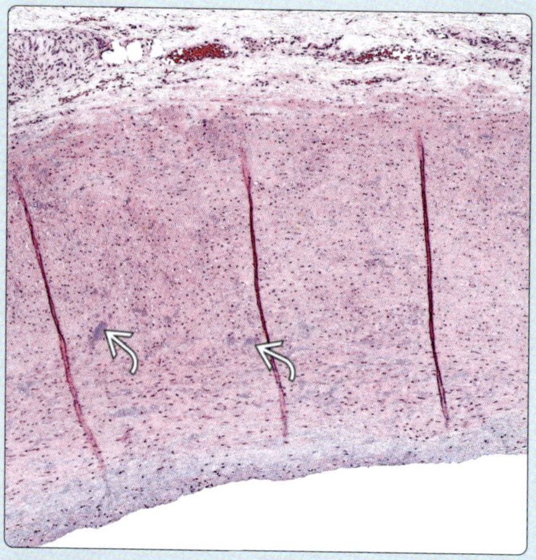

Aortic Medial Degeneration: Elastic Stain

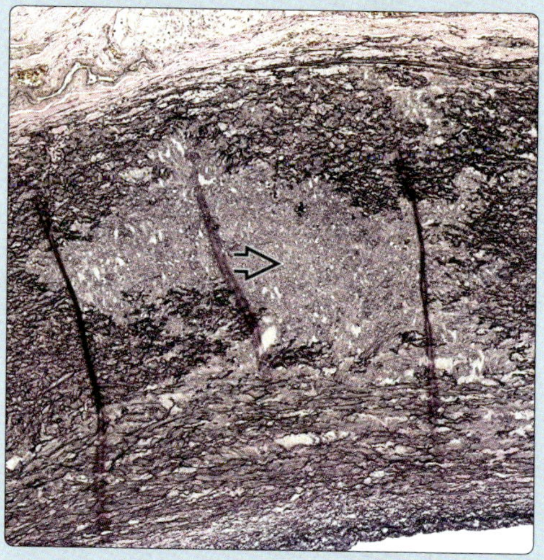

(Left) *H&E of the full-thickness aorta shows a patchy accumulation of mucoid extracellular matrix* →. **(Right)** *Elastic stain shows a large area of elastic fiber loss and translamellar accumulation of mucoid extracellular matrix material (MEMA-T)* ⇨.

Mucoid Extracellular Matrix Accumulation

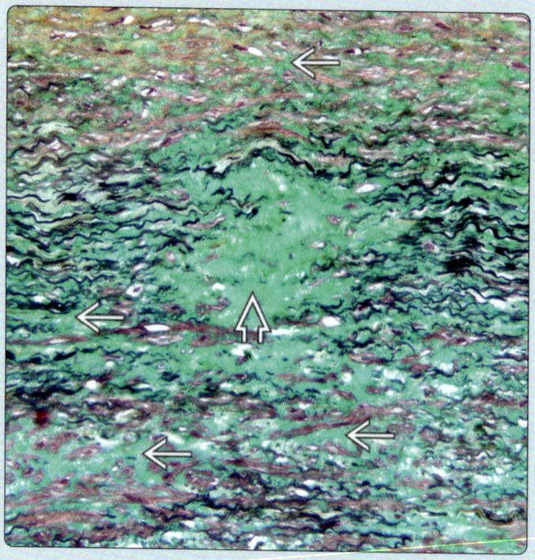

Aortic Wall Dissection

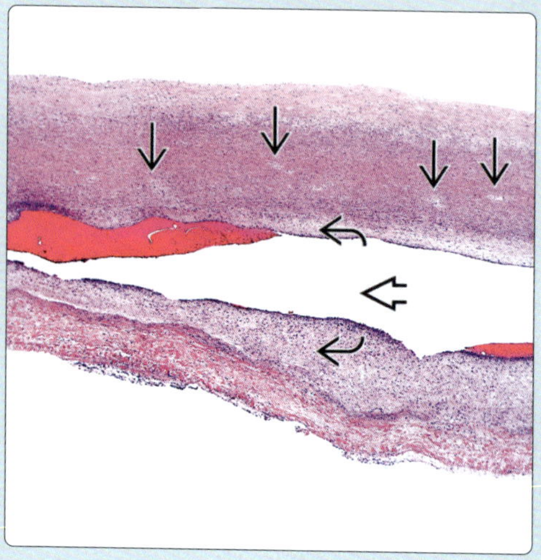

(Left) *Deposition of blue-staining proteoglycans* → *between smooth muscle cell layers is highlighted by Movat staining with cyst-like pooling* → *in an area devoid of black-staining elastic fibers.* **(Right)** *Medial degeneration may present with aortic dissection. Note the dissection tract* ⇨ *with neointima* ⇨. *Even by H&E staining, areas of degeneration are visible in the adjacent media* →.

TERMINOLOGY

Synonyms

- Cystic medial degeneration
- Cystic medial necrosis
- Myxoid medial degeneration

Definitions

- Medial degeneration components (2016 SCVP-AECVP nomenclature)
  - Mucoid extracellular matrix material accumulation (MEMA)
    - Intralamellar (MEMA-I): Increase in mucoid extracellular matrix that **does not** alter arrangement of lamellar units
    - Translamellar (MEMA-T): Increase in mucoid extracellular matrix that **does** alter arrangement of lamellar units to varying degrees
  - Elastic fiber fragmentation &/or loss
    - Elastic fibers fragmentation/loss with increasing translamellar spaces
  - Elastic fiber thinning &/or disorganization
  - Smooth muscle cell nuclei loss
    - Medial region with absent smooth muscle cell nuclei
  - Laminar medial collapse
    - Compaction of medial elastic fibers created by collapsed lamellar units showing band-like loss of smooth muscle cells
  - Medial fibrosis
    - Best appreciated on connective tissue stains (e.g., trichrome)
    - May be intralamellar or translamellar

ETIOLOGY/PATHOGENESIS

Hypertension

- Essential hypertension
- Weightlifting
- Cocaine abuse
- Pregnancy

Congenital Disorders

- Bicuspid aortic valve syndrome
- Turner syndrome
- Diverticulum of Kommerell

Inflammatory Disorders

- Takayasu arteritis
- Giant cell arteritis, others

Inherited Connective Tissue Diseases

- Marfan syndrome
- Loeys-Dietz syndrome
- Ehlers-Danlos syndrome, type IV
- Familial thoracic aortic aneurysms and dissections
- Arterial tortuosity syndrome, others

CLINICAL ISSUES

Presentation

- Aneurysm: Usually asymptomatic
- Dissection: Sudden severe chest pain, syncope, or shortness of breath
- Rupture: Severe chest pain; often sudden death

Treatment

- Surgical approaches
  - Large aneurysms or dissections involving ascending aorta (Stanford type A)
    - Replacement of diseased segment with synthetic graft
    - Endovascular stent graft placement
- Drugs
  - Antihypertensives for small aneurysms or dissections involving only descending aorta (Stanford type B)
  - Steroids, immunosuppressives for aortitis or arteritis

Prognosis

- Aneurysm
  - Larger lesions more likely to dissect or rupture
- Dissection
  - Stanford type A lesions do worse and are treated more aggressively
- Rupture
  - Grim prognosis

IMAGING

General Features

- Aneurysm, dissection, or rupture visible radiographically

MACROSCOPIC

General Features

- Aneurysms usually fusiform, nonatherosclerotic, noncalcified
- In cases of dissection, intimal tear often but not always identifiable

Sections to Be Submitted

- In all cases, submit minimum of 6 sections (fit into 2 cassettes), as histologic findings often patchy
- In cases of dissection, also submit intimal tear
- If Ehlers-Danlos type IV is suspected, submit for electron microscopy
- Always obtain elastic stain; trichrome also recommended

MICROSCOPIC

Histologic Features

- Histologic features nonspecific; identification of etiology usually not possible
- Fragmentation and loss of elastic fibers
- Accumulation and pooling of proteoglycans (mucoid extracellular matrix) between elastic lamellae
- Loss of intervening smooth muscle cell layers, absent nuclei and elastic lamellar collapse
- Clinical-pathologic associations
  - MEMA-T: Common in Marfan syndrome, Turner syndrome
  - MEMA-I: Common in Loeys-Dietz syndrome
  - Elastic fiber fragmentation: Common in familial thoracic aneurysm syndrome and arterial tortuosity syndrome

Inherited Causes of Aortic Medial Degeneration

	Gene Involved	Inheritance	Clinical Manifestations
Marfan syndrome	Fibrillin-1 (*FBN1*)	Autosomal dominant, variable penetrance	Aortic root aneurysm, ectopia lentis, tall stature, long slender limbs, decreased skeletal muscle mass, scoliosis, pectus excavatum carinatum, arachnodactyly
Loeys-Dietz syndrome	TGF-β type 1 and type 2 receptors (*TGFBR1*, *TGFBR2*) TGF-β2 and TGF-β3 SMAD2, SMAD3	Autosomal dominant	Pectus deformity, scoliosis, long fingers, dural ectasia, aortic root aneurysm, widely spaced eyes, bifid uvula, cleft palate, clubfoot deformity, translucent skin and easy bruising, dystrophic scars, cervical spine malformation
Ehlers-Danlos syndrome	Type 3 procollagen *COL3A1*, *FLNA*	Autosomal dominant	Thin skin, arterial or uterine rupture, bruising , small joint hyperflexibility
Familial aortic dissections	*TGFBR2*, *ACTA2*, *MYH11*, *MAT2A*	Autosomal dominant	Thoracic aortic aneurysm, aortic dissection, bicuspid aortic valve, patent ductus arteriosus
Arterial tortuosity syndrome	*SLC2A10*, *LOX*, *MFAP5*, *FOXE3*, MYLK, PRKG1, SLC2A10	Autosomal recessive	Extreme vascular tortuosity, dolichocephaly, malar hypoplasia, joint laxity

ANCILLARY TESTS

Histochemistry

- Verhoeff van Gieson (VVG) (elastic) stain
    - Stains elastic fibers black
    - Stains muscle and other tissues yellow
    - Stains collagen red
    - Does not differentially stain proteoglycans
- Movat elastic (pentachrome) stain
    - Stains proteoglycans blue
    - Stains elastic fibers black
    - Stains muscle red
    - Stains collagen yellow
    - Stains fibrin bright red

Electron Microscopy

- In Ehlers-Danlos type IV, unidentified fibrinogranular substance in extracellular matrix

DIFFERENTIAL DIAGNOSIS

Medial Degeneration of Specific Etiology

- Strong family history or characteristic clinical dysmorphology suggests inherited disorder
- Severe medial degeneration suggests inherited connective tissue disease
- Inflammation or giant cells in media indicates aortitis

DIAGNOSTIC CHECKLIST

Clinically Relevant Pathologic Features

- Clinical information often helpful (e.g., presence of bicuspid aortic valve)
- Active inflammation should always be noted if seen
- Autopsy performance should include examination for gross dysmorphology suggesting genetic disorder

Pathologic Interpretation Pearls

- Histologic features nonspecific for etiology
- Severe degeneration suggests connective tissue disease

SELECTED REFERENCES

1. Bhandari R et al: Diagnostic approach and management of genetic aortopathies. Vasc Med. 25(1):63-77, 2020
2. Faggion Vinholo T et al: Genes associated with thoracic aortic aneurysm and dissection: 2019 update and clinical implications. Aorta (Stamford). 7(4):99-107, 2019
3. Töpel I: Noninfectious aortitis: what the cardiologist needs to know. Curr Opin Cardiol. 32(6):692-8, 2017
4. Halushka MK et al: Consensus statement on surgical pathology of the aorta from the Society for Cardiovascular Pathology and the Association for European Cardiovascular Pathology: II. Noninflammatory degenerative diseases - nomenclature and diagnostic criteria. Cardiovasc Pathol. 25(3):247-57, 2016
5. Ladich E et al: Vascular diseases: aortitis, aortic aneurysms, and vascular calcification. Cardiovasc Pathol. 25(5):432-41, 2016
6. Ryan C et al: Non-infectious aortitis of the ascending aorta: a histological and clinical correlation of 71 cases including overlap with medial degeneration and atheroma--a challenge for the pathologist. J Clin Pathol. 68(11):898-904, 2015
7. Stone JR et al: Consensus statement on surgical pathology of the aorta from the Society for Cardiovascular Pathology and the Association for European Cardiovascular Pathology: I. Inflammatory diseases. Cardiovasc Pathol. 24(5):267-78, 2015
8. Romaniello F et al: Aortopathy in Marfan syndrome: an update. Cardiovasc Pathol. 23(5):261-6, 2014
9. Juraszek A et al: Evaluation of the intraoperative specimens of the thoracic and abdominal aorta. J Cardiothorac Surg. 8:110, 2013
10. Wu D et al: Molecular mechanisms of thoracic aortic dissection. J Surg Res. 184(2):907-24, 2013
11. Jain D et al: Causes and histopathology of ascending aortic disease in children and young adults. Cardiovasc Pathol. 20(1):15-25, 2011
12. Maleszewski JJ et al: Histopathologic findings in ascending aortas from individuals with Loeys-Dietz syndrome (LDS). Am J Surg Pathol. 33(2):194-201, 2009
13. Tadros TM et al: Ascending aortic dilatation associated with bicuspid aortic valve: pathophysiology, molecular biology, and clinical implications. Circulation. 119(6):880-90, 2009
14. Homme JL et al: Surgical pathology of the ascending aorta: a clinicopathologic study of 513 cases. Am J Surg Pathol. 30(9):1159-68, 2006

Normal Aortic Wall

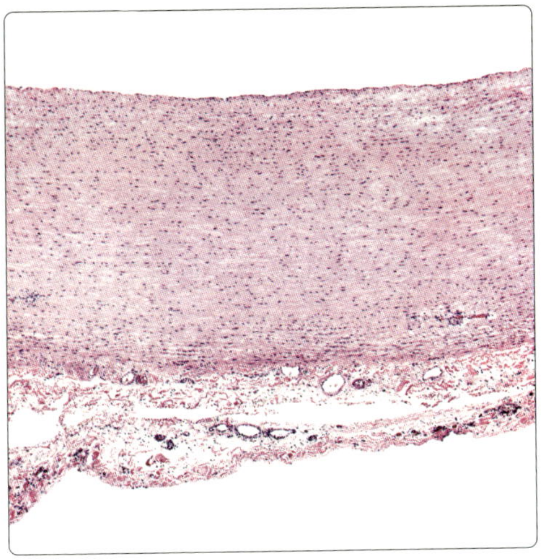

Normal Aortic Wall: Higher Power

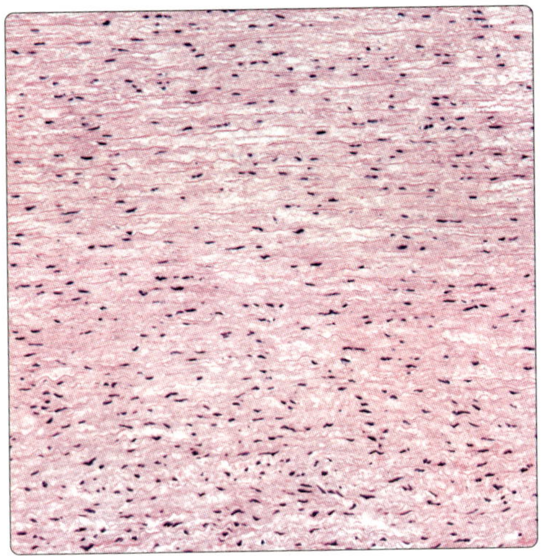

(Left) *On low power, the orderly, layered arrangement of medial smooth muscle and uniform thickness of the normal aortic wall is readily apparent, even on H&E staining.* **(Right)** *On higher power, the orderly arrangement of medial smooth muscle cells in the normal aorta is seen with evenly distributed scattered smooth muscle cell nuclei.*

Normal Aortic Wall: Elastic Stain

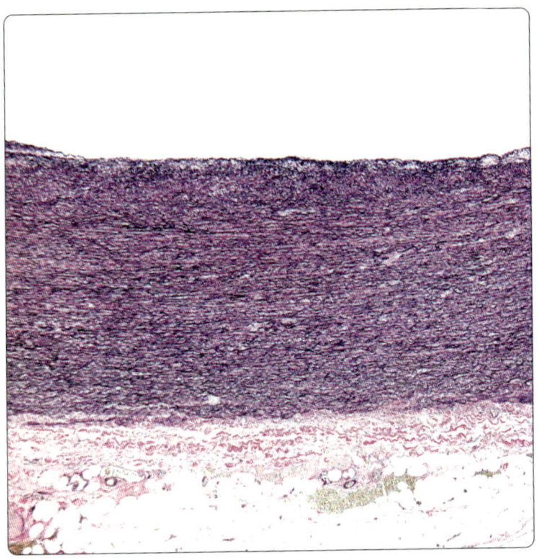

Normal Aortic Wall: Elastic Stain

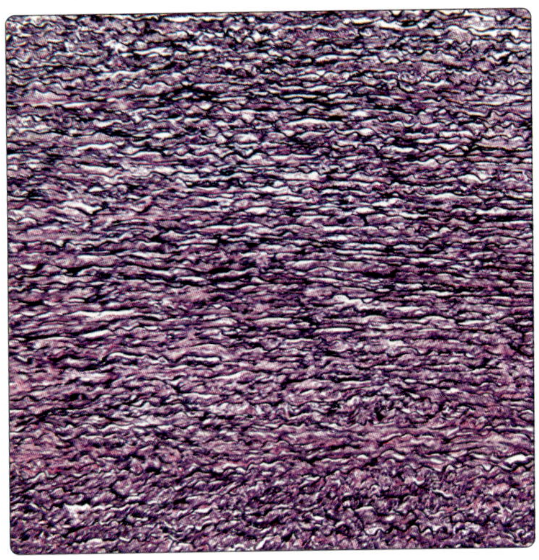

(Left) *Evaluation of elastic fibers is facilitated by Verhoeff van Gieson (VVG) elastic stain, which stains these fibers black. On low power, the orderly, layered arrangement and even distribution of elastic fibers throughout the entire medial thickness can be readily appreciated in the normal aorta.* **(Right)** *On higher power, the orderly, laminated arrangement of elastic fibers in the normal aortic media can be seen with uniform spacing of individual fibers by smooth muscle cells.*

Normal Aortic Wall: Movat Elastic Stain

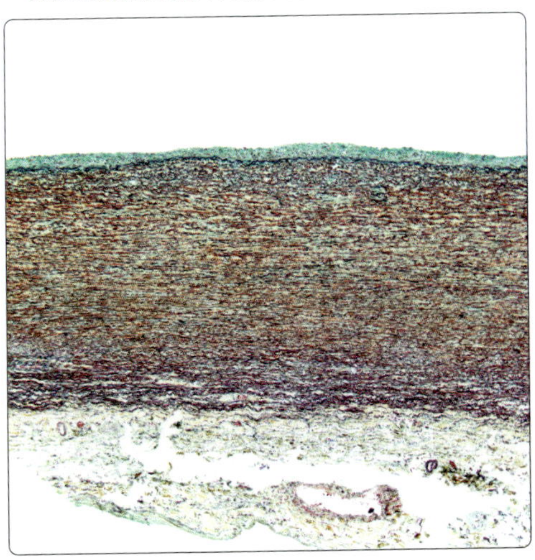

Normal Aortic Wall: Movat Elastic Stain

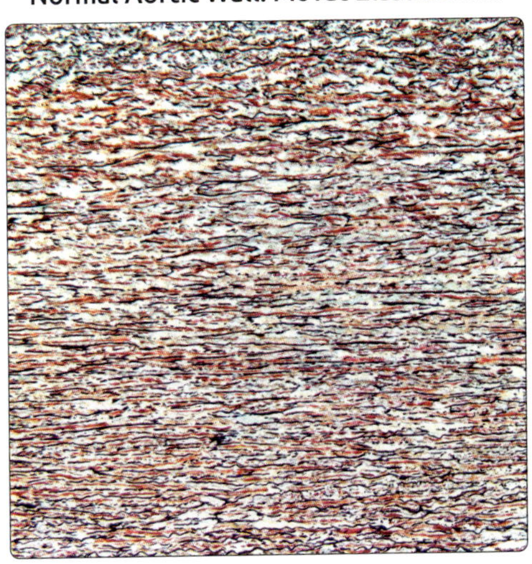

(Left) *Alternatively, elastic fibers can be evaluated by the Movat (pentachrome) stain by which these fibers also stain black. As with other elastic stains, the Movat stain highlights the orderly, laminated arrangement of elastic fibers in the normal aorta.* **(Right)** *On higher power, the uniform spacing of individual elastic fibers (black) by intervening smooth muscle cell layers (red) and collagen fibers (yellow) of Movat-stained aorta wall is apparent.*

(Left) *With medial degeneration, aortic wall thickness can be irregular, and cyst-like areas of medial proteoglycan accumulation* ⮕ *may be apparent on H&E staining, although the degree of medial degeneration may be significantly underestimated without elastic stain.* **(Right)** *In this example of severe medial degeneration, VVG elastic stain highlights broad areas of extensive elastic fiber fragmentation and loss* ⮕ *that were much less apparent by H&E staining.*

Mucoid Extracellular Matrix Accumulation

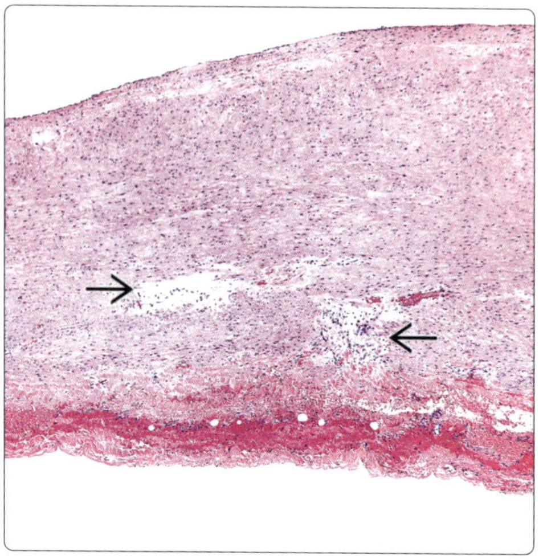

Aortic Medial Degeneration: Elastic Stain

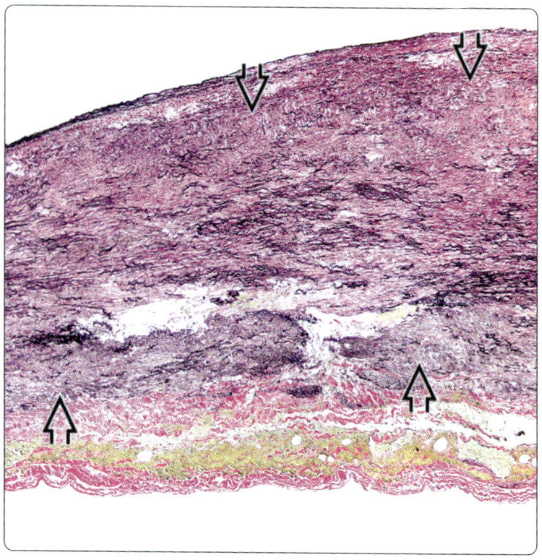

(Left) *When medial degeneration is extensive, areas of proteoglycan accumulation may appear myxoid* ⮕ *and are readily apparent by H&E staining, even at low power.* **(Right)** *On Movat-stained sections, proteoglycans appear blue. With medial degeneration, proteoglycans accumulate between smooth muscle layers and in areas of elastic fiber fragmentation, imparting a blue appearance to the aortic wall. Even at low power, cyst-like pools of accumulated proteoglycans are apparent* ⮕.

Mucoid Extracellular Matrix Accumulation

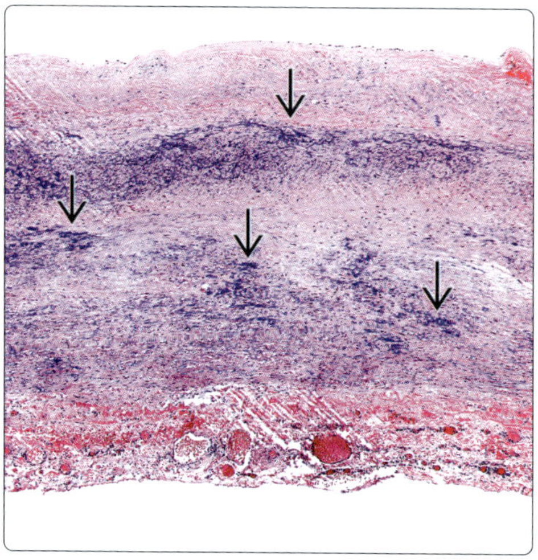

Medial Degeneration: Movat Elastic Stain

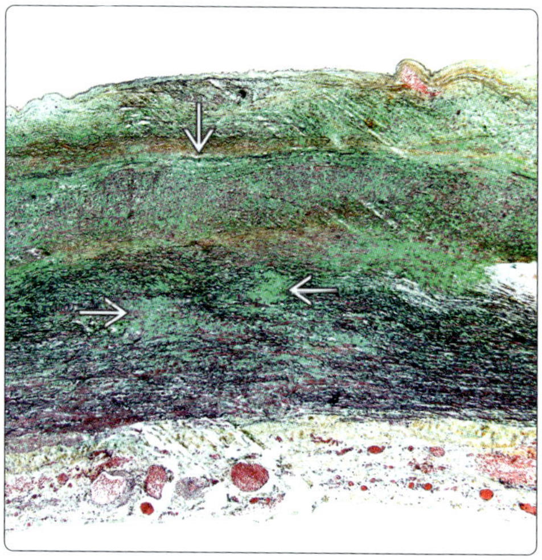

(Left) *On higher power, accumulated proteoglycans between smooth muscle cells often appear myxoid* ⮕ *by H&E staining.* **(Right)** *VVG elastic stain highlights areas of elastic fiber fragmentation and loss* ⮕ *in the aortic media with cyst-like areas of proteoglycan pooling between smooth muscle layers* ⮕*. Although not true cysts, in the past, these accumulations led some to refer to this change as cystic medial degeneration.*

Mucoid Extracellular Matrix Accumulation

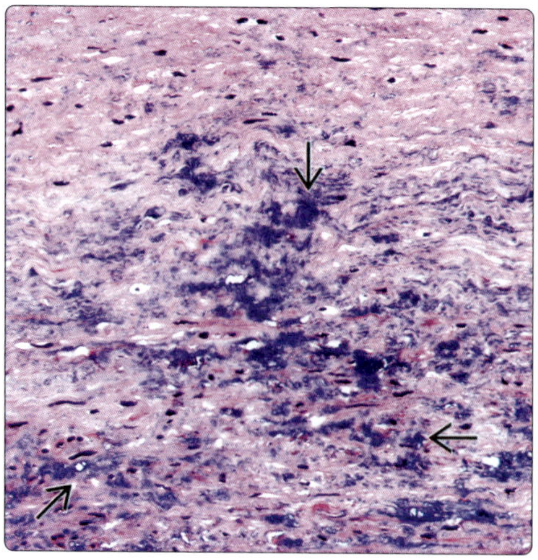

Mucoid Extracellular Matrix Accumulation: Elastic Stain

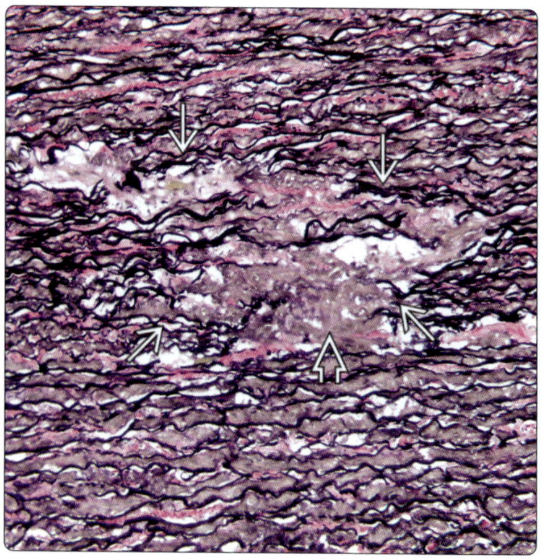

Marfan Syndrome Phenotype

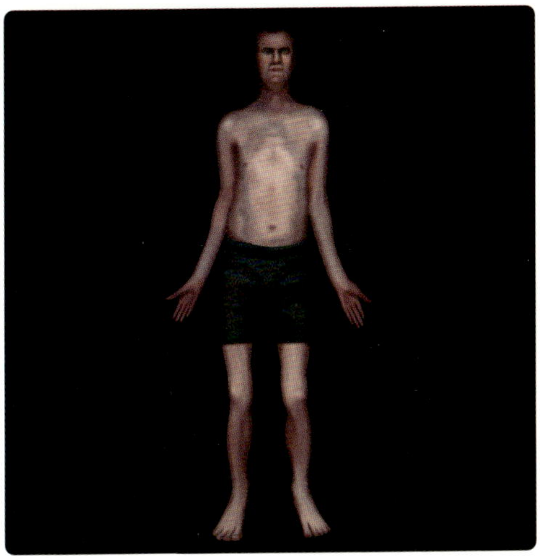

Loeys-Dietz Syndrome, Type 1

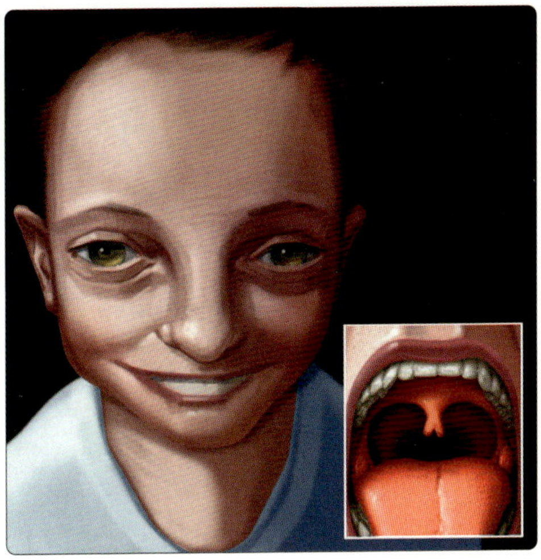

(Left) *Marfan syndrome is one of the inherited causes of aortic medial degeneration. The phenotype is characterized by a long, thin body habitus with long limbs compared to trunk, long fingers (arachnodactyly), pectus excavatum, and scoliosis.* **(Right)** *The Loeys-Dietz syndrome, type 1 phenotype includes hypertelorism (wide-set eyes), cleft palate/bifid uvula, and craniosynostosis. There is also overlap with Marfan phenotype.*

Media Degeneration

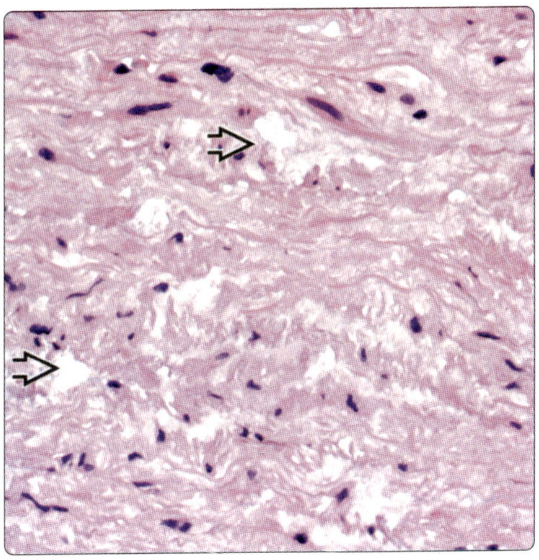

Aorta With Medial Degeneration: Elastic Stain

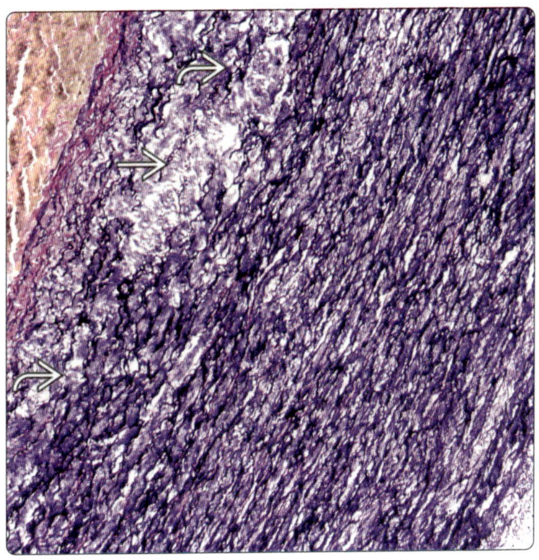

(Left) *Thoracic aortic wall shows cyst-like areas of medial proteoglycan accumulation → that appear basophilic on H&E stain. In cases of connective tissue disorders, this change is more prominent.* **(Right)** *The areas of media degeneration → are more evident on elastic stain, and it is possible to identify the areas of elastic fragmentation →.*

Takayasu Arteritis

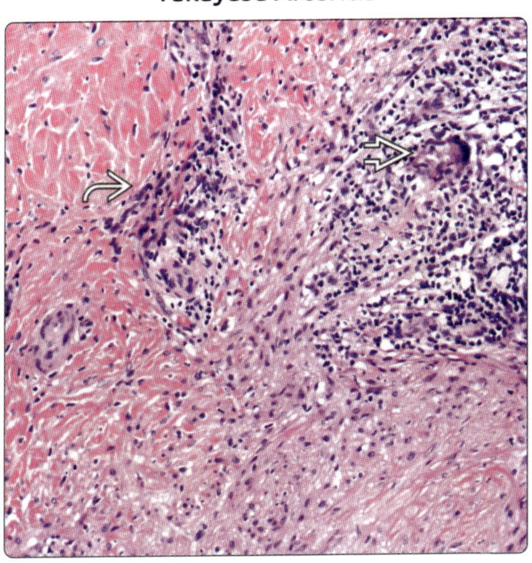

Takayasu Arteritis: Elastic Stain

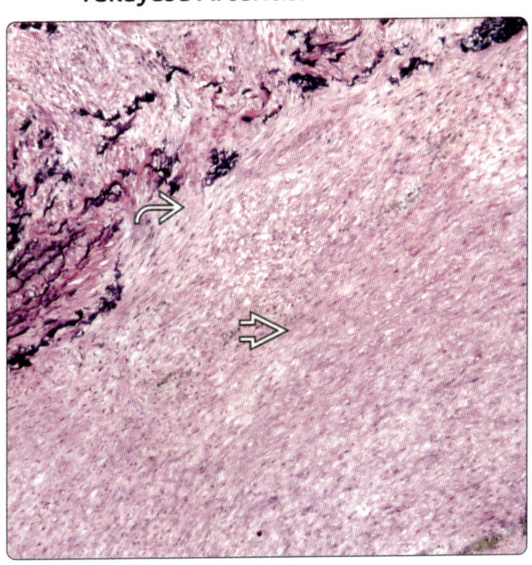

(Left) *Ascending aorta shows focal mononuclear inflammatory infiltrate → in the media admixed with scattered giant cells →. Inflammatory disorders can cause degenerative changes in the aortic wall.* **(Right)** *Aortic wall in a case of Takayasu arteritis shows marked disruption of the elastic lamina → as well as loss of elastic fibrils. There is also fibrous thickening of the media →. The presence of inflammation and giant cells is critical for the diagnosis of aortitis.*

(Left) *Dissection is often a consequence of medial degeneration →. Dissection tracts usually involve the outer 1/3 of the wall with formation of neointima over time →. Note the adventitia → and the thin portion of the media → on VVG elastic stain.* **(Right)** *In mild cases, the histologic changes can be much more subtle. An elastic stain should be obtained in all cases, as it facilitates recognition of focal areas of elastic fiber loss and proteoglycan accumulation →, as seen on VVG stain.*

Aortic Dissection: Elastic Stain

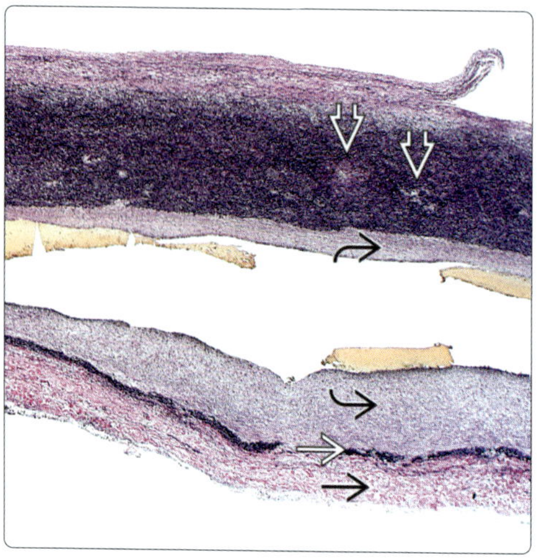

Aortic Dissection: Mild Changes

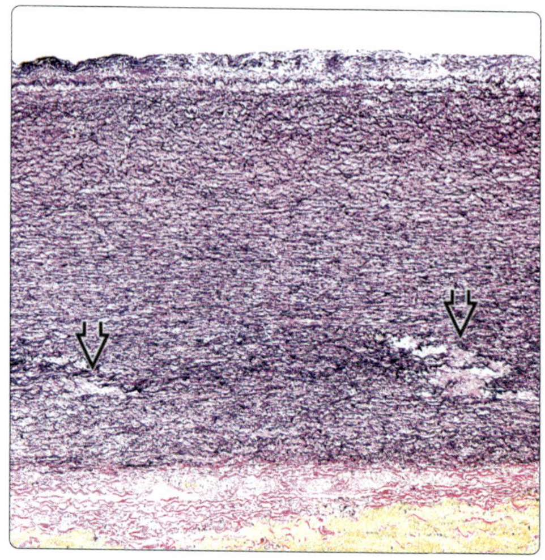

(Left) *Inflammation is an important cause of medial degeneration, and all such cases should be evaluated for aortitis, as these patients may benefit from steroids or immunomodulators. Note the lymphocytic infiltrate → and focal giant cells → in this case of giant cell aortitis.* **(Right)** *VVG elastic stain highlights extensive areas of medial degeneration → in this case of active giant cell aortitis.*

Giant Cell Aortitis

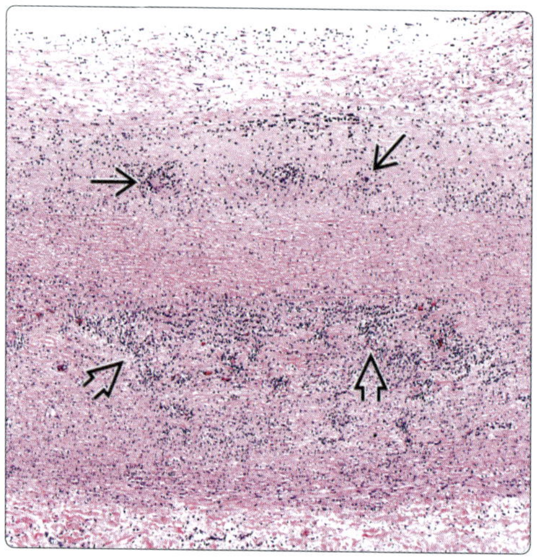

Giant Cell Aortitis: Elastic Stain

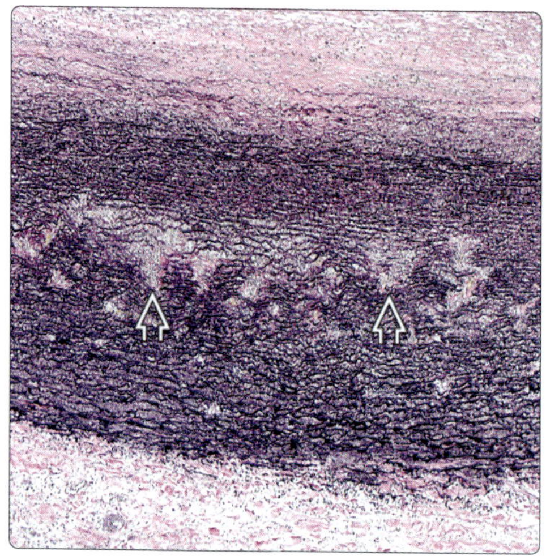

(Left) *Dissection may also occur as a consequence of aortitis with medial degeneration. Note the dissection tract with thrombus → with active aortitis involving the nearby media →. Necrosis of the dissected media → is extensive due to tearing of the vasa vasorum with medial infarction.* **(Right)** *VVG elastic stain highlights medial degeneration throughout the wall, including areas involved by dissection →. A nearly transmural tear is present in an area of active aortitis →.*

Aortitis Complicated by Dissection

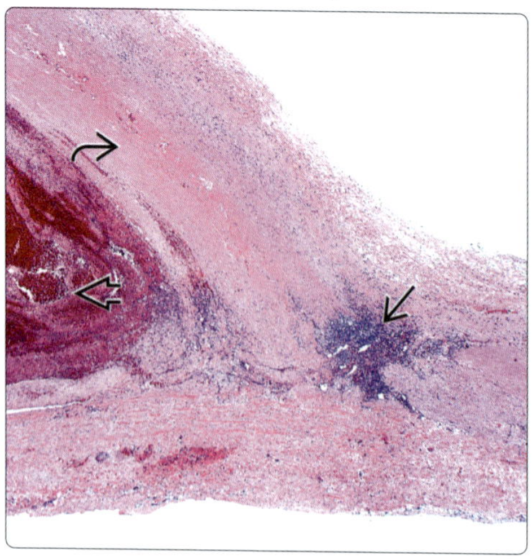

Aortitis Complicated by Dissection: Elastic Stain

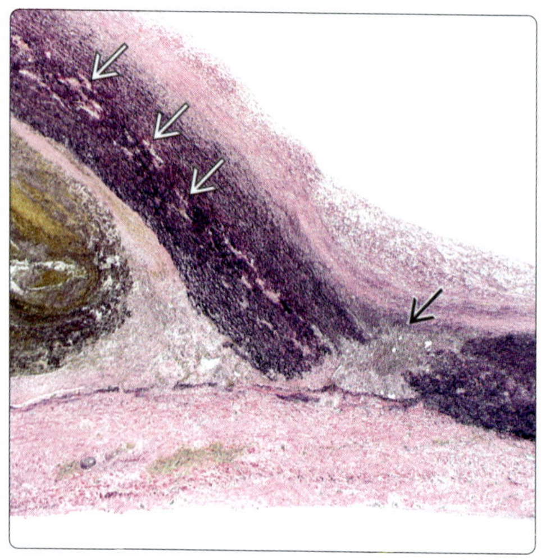

Laminar Medial Collapse

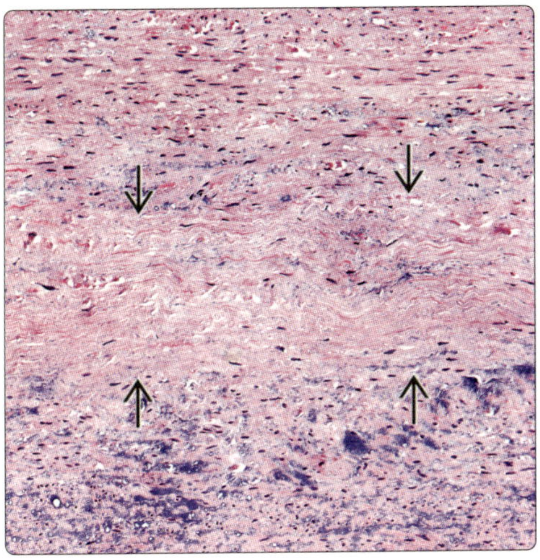

Laminar Medial Collapse: Movat Elastic Stain

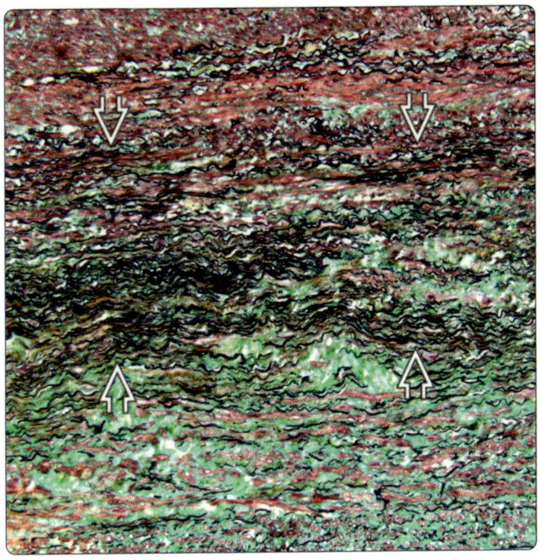

(Left) *On H&E staining, the hallmark of laminar medial collapse is a band-like area of smooth muscle necrosis with loss of smooth muscle cell nuclei* →*. Although it is considered to be a separate pathologic process from medial degeneration, it is often seen as a secondary feature in moderate to severe cases of medial degeneration.* **(Right)** *In laminar medial collapse, Movat stain highlights the collapse of elastic lamellae in layered areas of smooth muscle necrosis* ⇒*.*

Laminar Medial Collapse

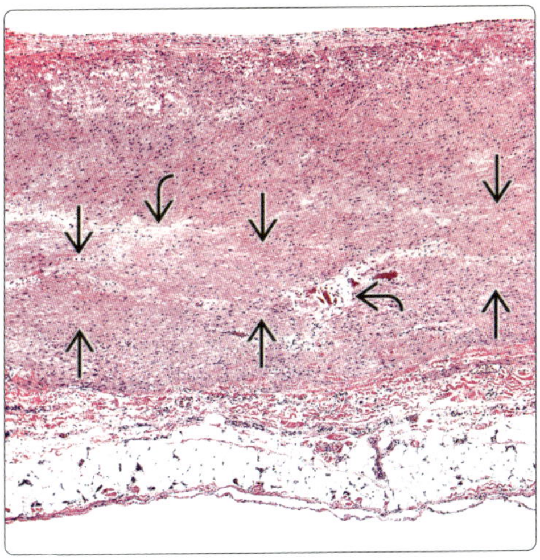

Laminar Medial Collapse: Elastic Stain

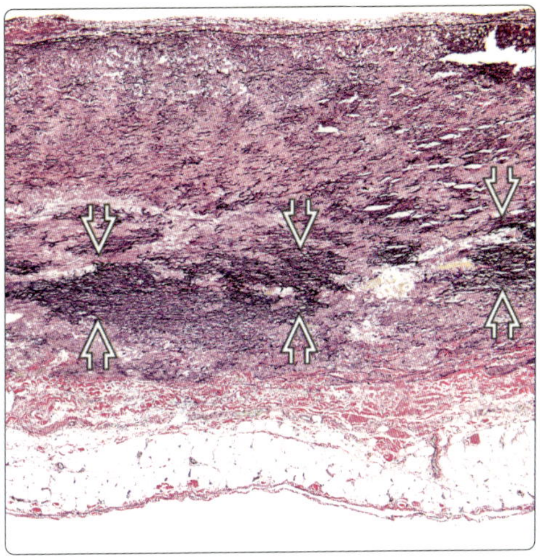

(Left) *Laminar medial collapse may be seen as a secondary feature in cases of medial degeneration. On H&E stain, this appears as a band-like area of smooth muscle nuclear loss* →*, although this process may be obscured by areas of coexisting medial degeneration* ↗*, as in this case.* **(Right)** *By staining elastic fibers black, VVG elastic stain facilitates detection of elastic lamellar collapse (decreased distance between individual fibers) in areas of laminar medial necrosis* ⇒*.*

Laminar Medial Collapse, Mild Changes

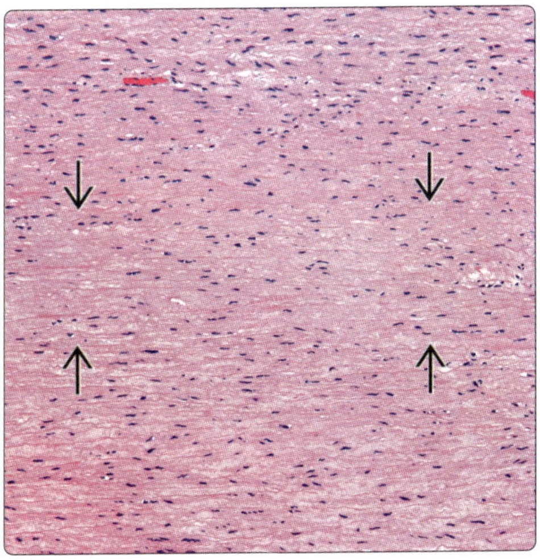

Laminar Medial Collapse, Mild Changes: Elastic Stain

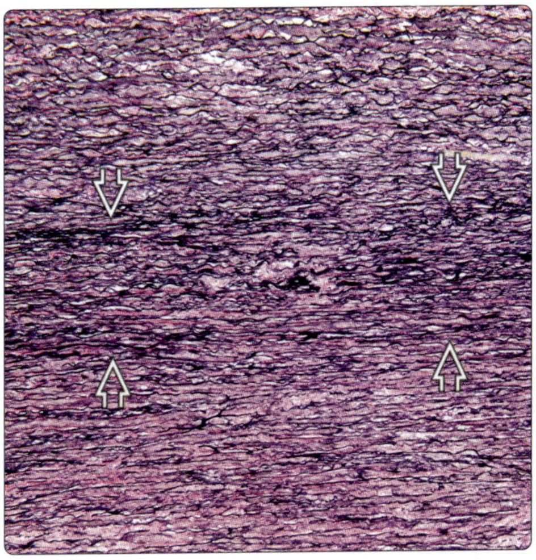

(Left) *In cases of early laminar medial collapse, histologic findings can be extremely subtle on H&E staining when areas of smooth muscle nuclear loss are small or incomplete* →*.* **(Right)** *In mild cases of laminar medial collapse, elastic stain is critical, as it facilitates detection of early elastic lamellar collapse. Subtle, darker bands* ⇒ *are seen due to loss of intervening smooth muscle cells and decreased distance between elastic fibers, which are spared on VVG stain.*

Genetic Diseases of the Aorta

KEY FACTS

TERMINOLOGY

- Genetic diseases affecting aorta (and sometimes other vessels), resulting in aneurysm, dissection, rupture, &/or obstruction

CLINICAL ISSUES

- MFS: Variable severity of disease with most surviving into mid to late adulthood
- LDS: Follows more aggressive course
- vEDS: Significantly shortened lifespan (50% mortality at 48 years); vessels may rupture without aneurysm
- TS: Adults at risk for cardiovascular morbidity and mortality (often related to rupture or dissection); 10% have aortic coarctation
- FTAAD: Typically without signs/symptoms apart from vascular complications; true prognostic information is unknown

MACROSCOPIC

- Typically manifests as fusiform aneurysm/dilatation
- May have medial dissection

MICROSCOPIC

- No specific aortic histopathologic features to distinguish genetic causes of aneurysm from nongenetic or between types of genetic causes
- Medial degeneration
  - Cystic or mucoid type
  - Dispersed type
- Laminar medial necrosis characterized by smooth muscle nuclear loss with concomitant collapse of lamellar units, usually in band-like pattern
- Medial disorganization characterized by nonparallel elastic fiber orientation
- Medial thinning
- Medial dissection characterized by medial separation with fibrin deposition &/or neointima formation

Aortic Aneurysm in Marfan Syndrome

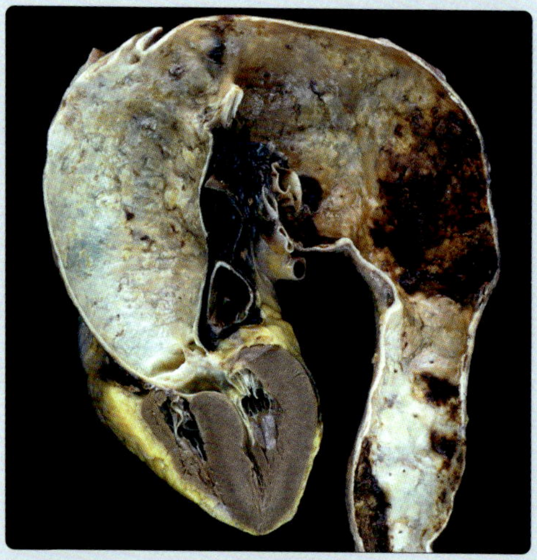

CT of Aortic Aneurysm in Marfan Syndrome

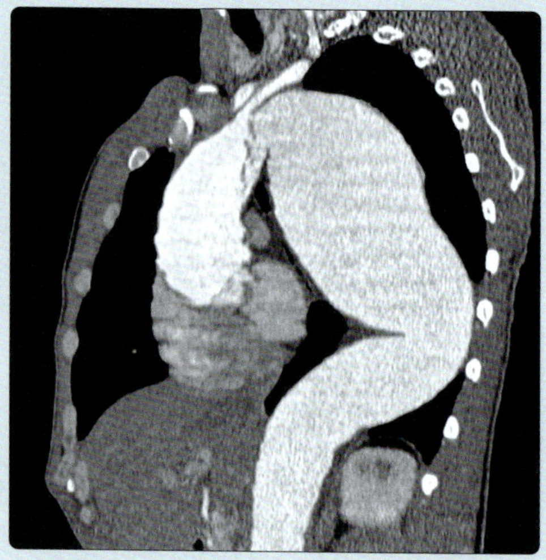

(Left) *This specimen from a patient with Marfan syndrome exhibits the massive (and occasionally multifocal) nature of aortic aneurysms in these individuals. Marked atherosclerosis is also present.* **(Right)** *CT exhibits massive multifocal aortic dilatation (aneurysms) characteristically seen in the setting of Marfan syndrome. Similar findings may be present in other genetic diseases involving the aorta.*

H&E Stain of Aortic Medial Degeneration

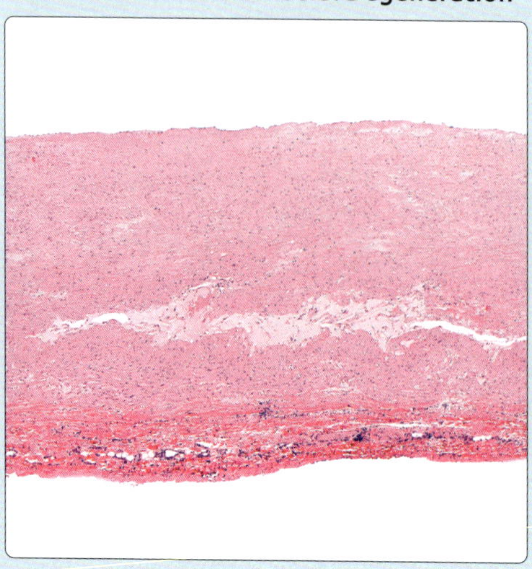

Elastic Stain of Aortic Medial Degeneration

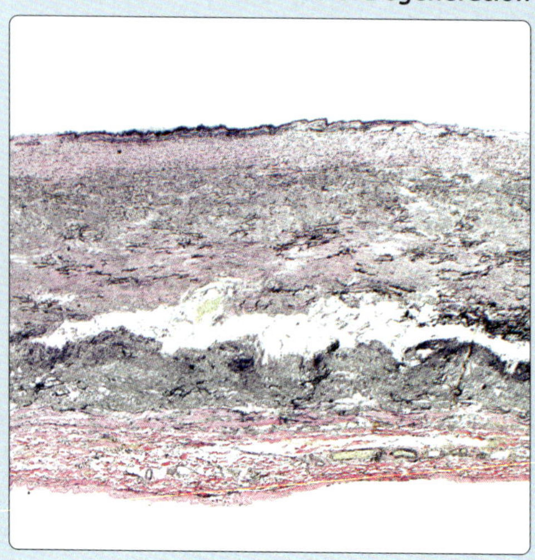

(Left) *Low-power view exhibits medial degeneration characterized by medial disruption with mucopolysaccharide/glycoprotein accumulation without medial inflammation. In this example, the process involves the media in a transmural fashion, but it is often more focal and patchy. The degree of elastic fiber disruption is not readily apparent on H&E.* **(Right)** *VVG elastic stain shows the prominent elastic fiber disruption throughout the media.*

Genetic Diseases of the Aorta

TERMINOLOGY

Definitions

- Genetic diseases affecting aorta (and sometimes other vessels), resulting in aneurysm, dissection, rupture, &/or obstruction

CLINICAL ISSUES

Epidemiology

- Incidence
  - Marfan syndrome (MFS): Between 1 in 3,000 and 1 in 5,000
  - Loeys-Dietz syndrome (LDS): Unknown
  - Vascular (type IV) Ehlers-Danlos syndrome (vEDS): Between 1 in 10,000 and 1 in 25,000 (for all EDS variants, vEDS represents 5-10% of these)
  - Turner syndrome (TS): 1 in 2,500 girls
  - Familial thoracic aortic aneurysm and dissection (FTAAD): Unknown

Presentation

- MFS
  - Tall and slender stature
  - Elongated fingers and toes (arachnodactyly)
  - Pectus deformity (excavatum or carinatum)
  - Spontaneous pneumothorax
  - Ectopia lentis, elongated globe, retinal detachment
- LDS
  - Widely spaced eyes (hypertelorism)
  - Bifid uvula and palate abnormalities
  - Craniosynostosis
- vEDS
  - Characteristic facial appearance
  - Thin, translucent skin and easy bruising
  - Joint hypermobility/laxity
- TS
  - Short stature
  - Absent/delayed puberty
  - Webbed neck
- FTAAD
  - Typically without signs/symptoms apart from vascular complications

Treatment

- Surgical approaches
  - Aortic root replacement (elective surgery prior to critical enlargement is preferred)
  - Thoracic or abdominal repair or replacement (endovascular or open)
- Drugs
  - β-blockers
  - Losartan (MFS and LDS)

Prognosis

- MFS: Variable severity of disease with most surviving into mid to late adulthood
- LDS: Follows more aggressive course
- vEDS: Significantly shortened lifespan (50% mortality at 48 years); vessels may rupture without aneurysm
- TS: Adults at risk for cardiovascular morbidity and mortality (often related to rupture or dissection); 10% have aortic coarctation
- FTAAD: True prognostic information is unknown

IMAGING

General Features

- Aneurysms, dissections, ruptures, and coarctations can all be visualized with various imaging modalities (CT, MR, US)

MACROSCOPIC

General Features

- Typically manifests as fusiform aneurysm/dilatation
- May have medial dissection

MICROSCOPIC

Histologic Features

- No specific aortic histopathologic features to distinguish genetic causes of aneurysm from nongenetic or between types of genetic causes
- Often exhibit 1 or more of following types of medial pathology
  - Medial degeneration (different morphologic patterns)
    - Cystic or mucoid type, characterized by elastic fiber loss with concomitant (often large) glycoprotein/mucopolysaccharide deposition
    - Dispersed type, characterized by lamellar widening (typically with elastic fiber loss) with small aggregates of glycoprotein/mucopolysaccharide
  - Laminar medial necrosis, characterized by smooth muscle nuclear loss with concomitant collapse of lamellar units, usually in band-like pattern
  - Medial disorganization, characterized by nonparallel elastic fiber orientation
  - Medial thinning
  - Medial dissection characterized by medial separation with fibrin deposition &/or neointima formation

ANCILLARY TESTS

Genetic Testing

- Identification of specific genetic mutation is mandatory for confirmation of diagnosis and clinical management

DIFFERENTIAL DIAGNOSIS

Inflammatory (Infectious or Noninfectious) Aneurysm

- Medial inflammation, ± giant cells

Atherosclerotic Aneurysm

- Prominent atherosclerosis, often with medial atrophy
- May be complicated by fact that genetic aneurysms may secondarily develop atherosclerosis

SELECTED REFERENCES

1. Luyckx I et al: Update on the molecular landscape of thoracic aortic aneurysmal disease. Curr Opin Cardiol. 37(3):201-11, 2022
2. Creamer TJ et al: Insights on the pathogenesis of aneurysm through the study of hereditary aortopathies. Genes (Basel). 12(2):183, 2021

(**Left**) *H&E-stained section of a normal aorta wall shows the orderly arrangement of smooth muscle cells. The early changes of media degeneration are subtle and may be missed in H&E stain. Elastic stain is always recommended when evaluating arterial wall diseases.* (**Right**) *VVG elastic stain of a normal aorta wall shows the orderly laminated arrangement of elastic fibers in the media. There is uniform spacing of individual fibers by smooth muscle cells.*

H&E Stain of Normal Aorta Wall

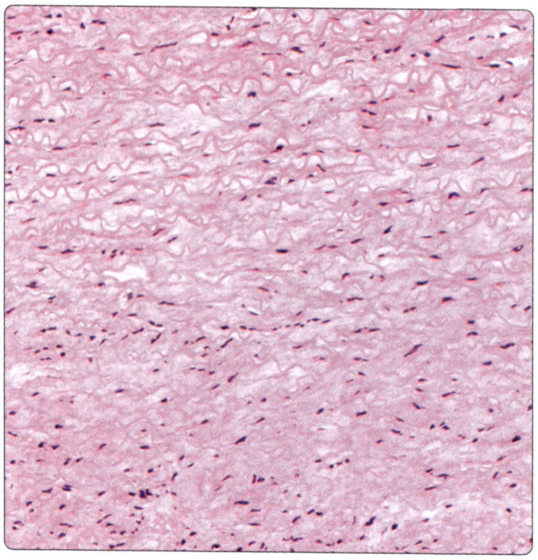

Elastic Stain of Normal Aorta Wall

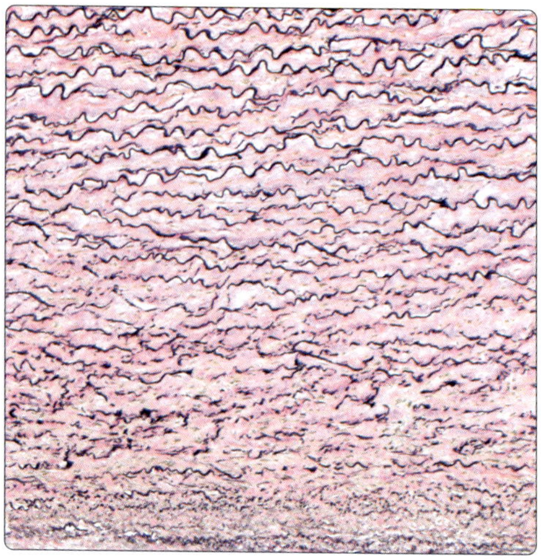

(**Left**) *H&E-stained section exhibits the mucoid type of medial degeneration. The term cystic medial necrosis has been used to describe this pattern, but, given that the lesion is neither cystic nor necrotic, the term medial degeneration is now preferred. The pools of basophilic material represent mucopolysaccharide/glycoprotein accumulation.* (**Right**) *VVG elastic stain shows the prominent elastic fiber fragmentation and loss within and around the glycoprotein pool.*

H&E Stain of Aortic Medial Degeneration

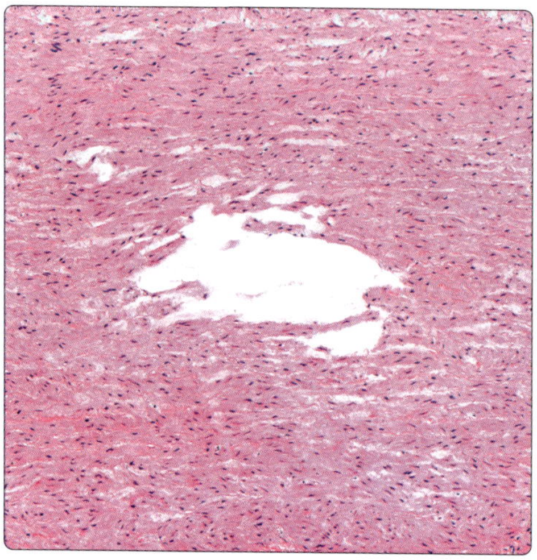

Elastic Stain of Aortic Medial Degeneration

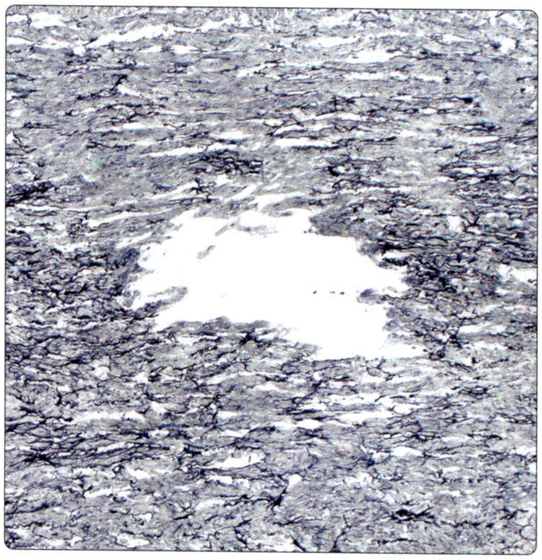

(**Left**) *H&E-stained section illustrates another pattern of medial degeneration, where the glycoprotein/ mucopolysaccharide accumulations are not as prominent. Given the subtlety of the findings on H&E, the importance of the VVG elastic stain becomes apparent.* (**Right**) *VVG elastic stain of an aorta wall in a case of medial degeneration shows marked transmural elastic fiber fragmentation that is not immediately apparent on H&E stain.*

H&E Stain of Aortic Medial Degeneration

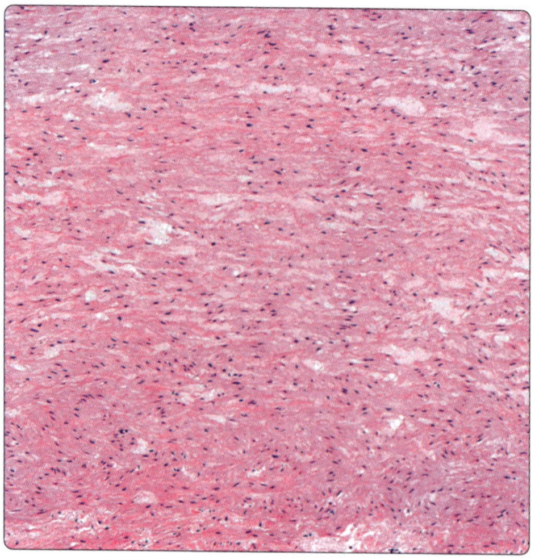

Elastic Stain of Aortic Medial Degeneration

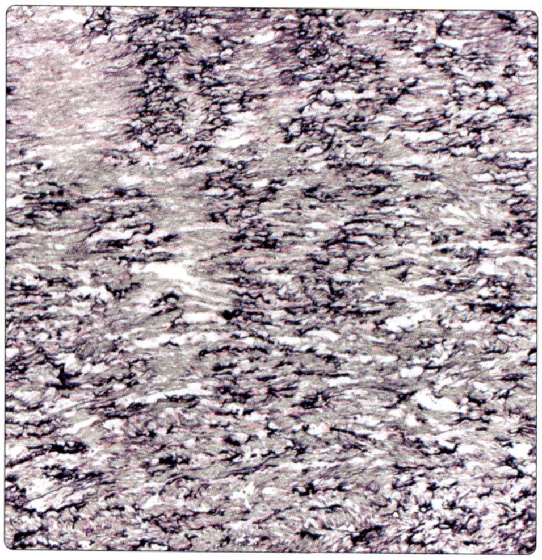

H&E Stain of Aortic Medial Dissection

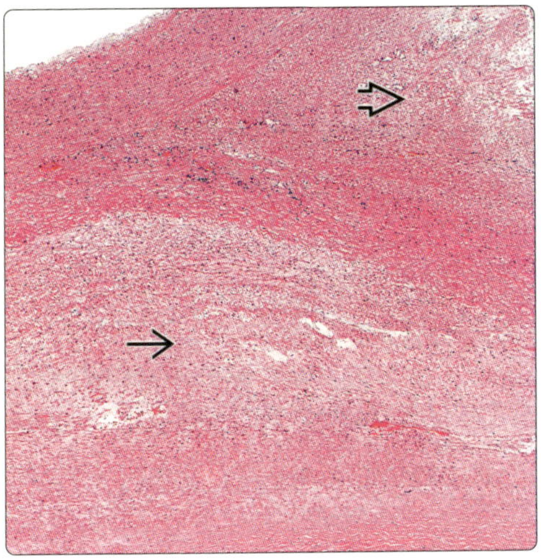

Elastic Stain of Aortic Medial Dissection

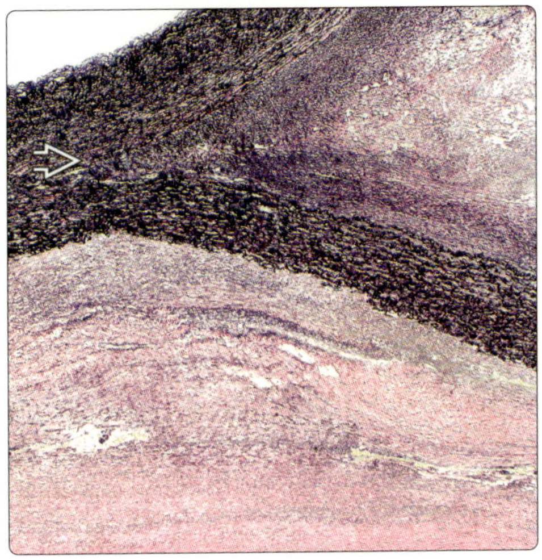

(Left) *H&E-stained section of an aorta resected from an individual with Marfan syndrome exhibits multiple dissection tracts. There is prominent neointima* ➡ *formation as well as a blind dissection tract* ⇨. **(Right)** *VVG elastic stain of an aorta resected from an individual with Marfan syndrome shows the splayed aortic media* ➡ *with the organized dissection tract contained therein.*

H&E Stain of Aortic Medial Dissection

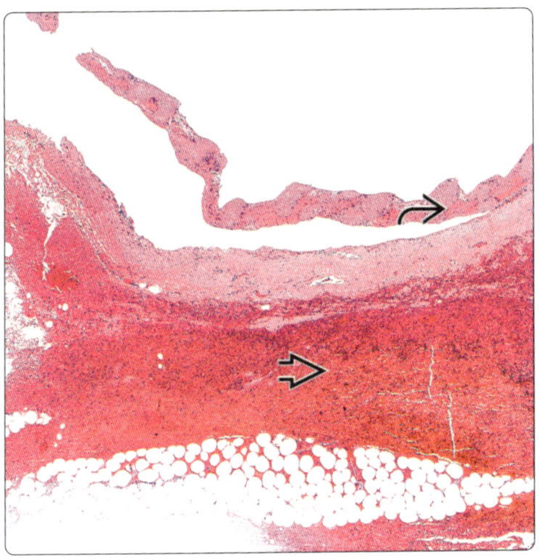

Elastic Stain of Aortic Medial Dissection

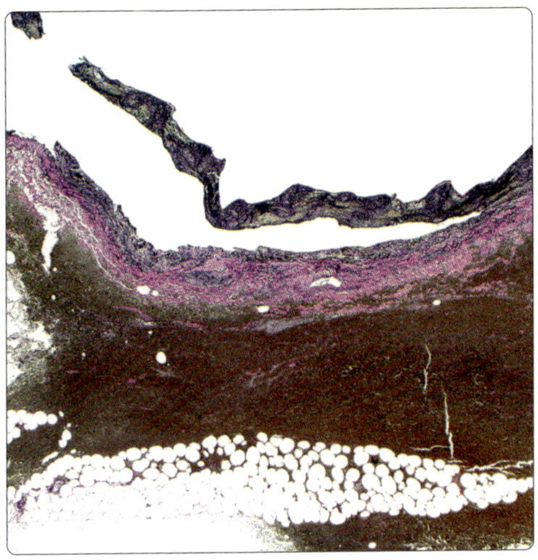

(Left) *Low-power view exhibits an acute aortic dissection with rupture from an individual with Loeys-Dietz syndrome. Fibrin deposition can be seen along the dissection tract* ↪. *The dissection involves the outer 1/3 of the media and, in this case, has ruptured through the media with prominent adventitial hemorrhage* ⇨ *present.* **(Right)** *VVG elastic stain highlights not only the medial dissection but also the underlying medial degeneration in a case of Loeys-Dietz syndrome.*

Aortic Coarctation in Turner Syndrome

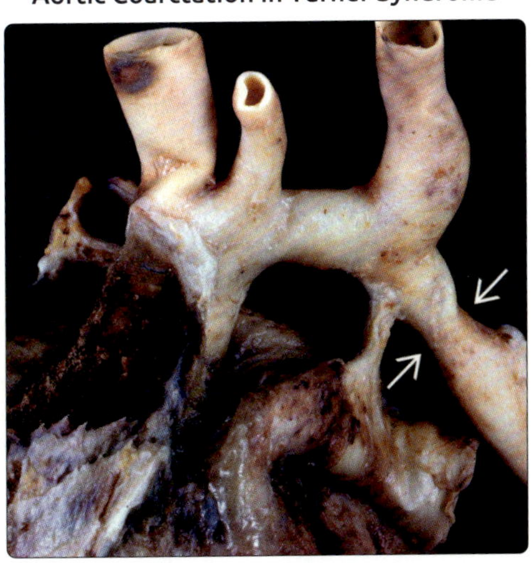

Elastic Stain in Turner Syndrome

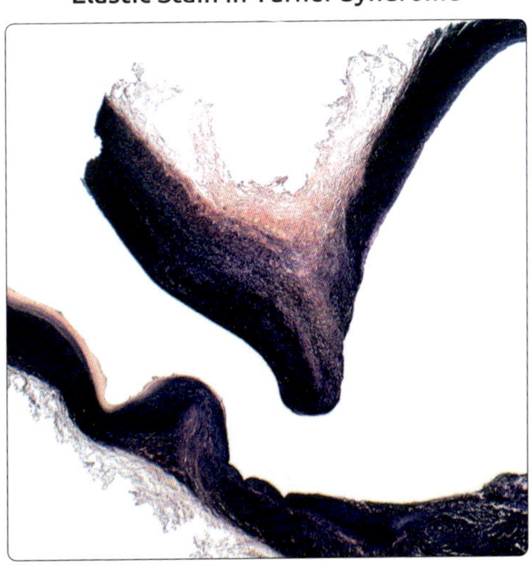

(Left) *Gross photograph of an autopsy specimen exhibits a juxtaductal aortic coarctation* ➡ *from an individual with Turner syndrome. Poststenotic dilatation is evident.* **(Right)** *Low-power view shows a surgically resected aortic coarctation. The coarctation ridge contains fibrotic and disorganized media. Ductal tissue is frequently identified extending into the aortic media, although the significance of this (beyond providing etiologic insights) is unknown.*

KEY FACTS

TERMINOLOGY

- Noninfectious aortitis
- Granulomatous aortitis
- Lymphoplasmacytic aortitis
- Not associated with infection or atherosclerosis

CLINICAL ISSUES

- Ascending aortic aneurysm
- ± systemic inflammatory symptoms
- ± vasculitis in other vessels

MICROSCOPIC

- Inflammation
  - Termed granulomatous due to prominence of histiocytes, but well-formed granulomas are not seen
- Laminar medial necrosis
- Medial degeneration
- Adventitial fibrosis

TOP DIFFERENTIAL DIAGNOSES

- Noninfectious aortitis is histologic pattern for cluster of clinical diseases that include
- Giant cell/temporal arteritis (with large vessel involvement)
  - Affects patients > 50 years of age with most cases presenting in 70s-80s
- Takayasu arteritis
  - Affects patients < 50 years of age with most cases presenting in teens and 20s
- Isolated aortitis
  - Idiopathic, occult active, or clinically isolated aortitis
  - Affects patients > 50 years of age, overlaps with giant cell/temporal arteritis
- IgG4-related aortitis
  - Often associated with marked adventitial and periadventitial fibrosis (periaortitis)
- Other rheumatologic disorders

(Left) *Aortic specimen from an asymptomatic 67-year-old man demonstrates giant cell aortitis characterized by transmural inflammation and numerous multinucleated giant cells (the intima faces downward).* **(Right)** *Multinucleated giant cells in giant cell aortitis are frequently seen "cuffing" broad areas of medial infarct-like dry necrosis. Medial lymphocytic infiltration is also seen in the background.*

Aortitis With Giant Cells

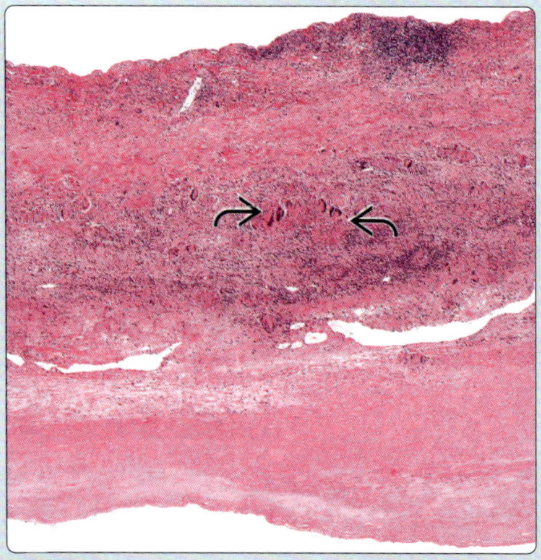

Multinucleated Giant Cells in Aortitis

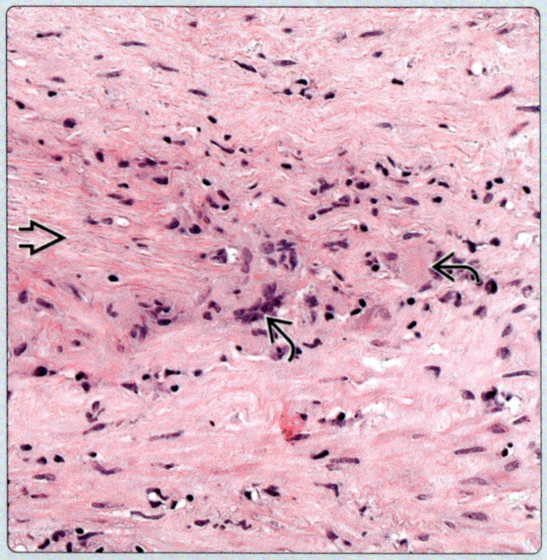

(Left) *Dense inflammatory infiltrate is shown within the aortic medial wall. Wide bands of media devoid of smooth muscle nuclei are also seen. These features are characteristic of aortitis.* **(Right)** *Elastic stain of aortitis shows areas of laminar medial collapse (elastic fibers without intervening smooth muscle). These areas correspond to absent medial smooth muscle nuclei in the H&E section.*

Noninfectious Aortitis

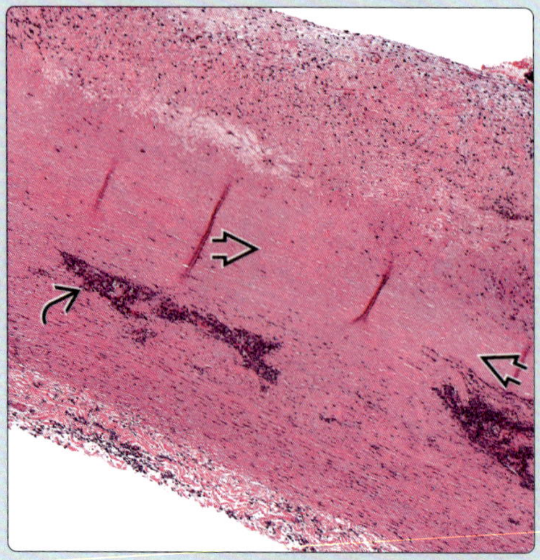

Noninfectious Aortitis (Elastic Stain)

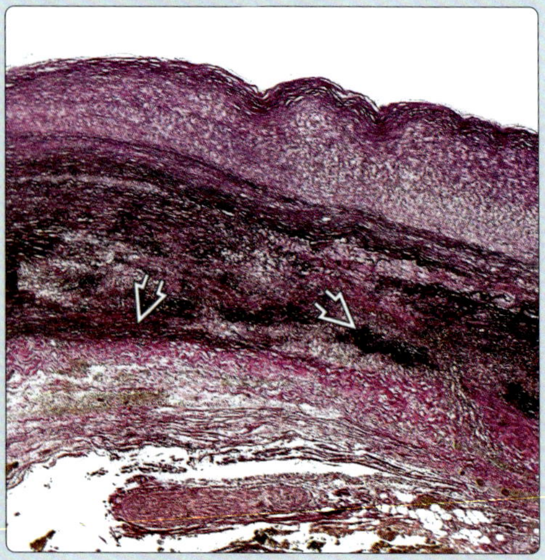

TERMINOLOGY

Synonyms

- Giant cell aortitis
- Granulomatous aortitis
- Lymphoplasmacytic aortitis

Definitions

- Inflammatory infiltrate primarily involving media and adventitia of aortic wall with associated destruction of smooth muscle cells and remnants of collapsed elastic lamina scaffolding (laminar medial necrosis)
  - By definition, not associated with infection or severe atherosclerosis
- Associated with different processes that are largely indistinguishable on histopathologic grounds; possibly representing final common pathway pattern of inflammation triggered by multiple inciting etiologies

ETIOLOGY/PATHOGENESIS

Autoimmune

- Often associated with systemic manifestations of vasculitis or other rheumatologic syndromes

Laminar Medial Necrosis Hypotheses

- Smooth muscle destruction due to direct cell-mediated immune injury with preservation of elastic lamina framework
- Smooth muscle loss due to midwall ischemia following damage to vasa vasorum with elastic lamina preservation
  - Neoangiogenesis and new vessel growth often seen adjacent to areas of laminar medial necrosis
  - Histiocyte-rich inflammatory infiltrate may represent secondary response to damage

CLINICAL ISSUES

Epidemiology

- Incidence
  - 2-16% of all ascending aortic aneurysm resections across several studies

Presentation

- Ascending aortic aneurysm
  - Incidental or at screening
  - Risk of dissection &/or rupture
- ± systemic inflammatory symptoms
- ± vasculitis in other vessels

Treatment

- Surgical approaches
  - Ascending aortic replacement (synthetic tube graft)
    - ± aortic root and valve replacement (Bentall procedure)
- Drugs
  - Antiinflammatory agents
    - Corticosteroids
    - Cytotoxic agents (azathioprine, cyclophosphamide)

MACROSCOPIC

General Features

- Aneurysmal dilatation
- Thickened aortic wall
- Irregular longitudinal intimal ridges (tree bark or cobblestone appearance)

MICROSCOPIC

Histologic Features

- Inflammation
  - Lymphocytes, histiocytes, and plasma cells primarily
  - Overall pattern is termed granulomatous due to prominence of histiocytes, although well-formed epithelioid granulomas are not seen
  - Giant cells are often seen if histiocytic inflammation is prominent but are not constant finding in giant cell aortitis (similar to giant cell arteritis)
  - Plasma cells and lymphocytes predominate in some cases; so-called lymphoplasmacytic aortitis pattern
    - IgG4 staining is recommended in such cases
  - Most prominent in adventitia and periadventitia but also in media layer (especially surrounding areas of laminar medial necrosis)
- Laminar medial necrosis
  - Loss of medial smooth muscle nuclei with persistence of elastic tissue strata, giving appearance of collapsed elastic scaffolding
  - Hypereosinophilic areas devoid of nuclei that appear black on elastic staining
- Medial degeneration
  - Loss of medial smooth muscle and elastic tissue with replacement by loose proteoglycan material
  - Typically, manifestation of noninflammatory connective tissue disorders but also occasionally seen in aortitis
- Adventitial fibrosis
  - Prominent in most cases, especially chronic Takayasu arteritis and IgG4-related aortitis
  - Storiform pattern should prompt careful evaluation for other features of hyper-IgG4 syndrome-associated aortitis

DIFFERENTIAL DIAGNOSIS

Giant Cell Temporal Arteritis (With Large Vessel Involvement)

- Horton disease or temporal arteritis
- Most common cause of aortitis overall (vs. isolated aortitis in some studies)
- Affects patients > 50 years of age with most cases presenting in 70s-80s
- Associated with symptoms of
  - Extracranial carotid branch ischemia and positive temporal artery biopsy
  - Polymyalgia rheumatica (proximal joint arthritis syndrome)
  - Systemic inflammation (malaise, fever, weight loss, night sweats)
- Elevated acute-phase reactants
  - Erythrocyte sedimentation rate
  - C-reactive protein

- Autopsy studies demonstrate frequent clinically occult cases, suggesting that signs and symptoms may be minor, and clinical course is indolent

Takayasu Arteritis

- "Pulseless" disease
- Besides aorta, primary aortic branches (arch vessels, celiac axis, renal arteries) and pulmonary artery (rarely) can be involved
- Proximal aortic aneurysmal dilatation but distal aortic narrowing and thrombosis
- Affects patients < 50 years of age with most cases presenting in teens and 20s
- Associated symptoms
  - Absent pulses in arms
  - Embolic or ischemic events (cerebrovascular, bowel, kidney)
  - Systemic inflammation

Isolated Aortitis

- Idiopathic, occult active, or clinically isolated aortitis
- Granulomatous aortitis encountered incidentally after resection of ascending aortic aneurysm
- Some cases of lymphoplasmacytic pattern have also been reported, including with increased IgG4
- Affects patients > 50 years of age, overlaps with giant cell/temporal arteritis
- No other systemic signs or symptoms of vasculitis or rheumatologic syndrome
- Treatment is controversial, but close observation is important
- Primary differential is with giant cell arteritis; difficult to distinguish in many cases since aortic involvement may precede temporal artery or other systemic involvement
- Increased risk of subsequent aneurysm development in aorta and systemically

IgG4-Related Aortitis

- Often associated with marked adventitial and periadventitial fibrosis ("periaortitis")
- Prominent plasma cells with IgG4: Total IgG ratio > 0.5 and > 50 IgG4 plasma cells per HPF
- Other histologic features include
  - Lymphoid follicle formation
  - Obliterative phlebitis
  - Storiform pattern of fibrosis (similar to IgG4-related disease of pancreas, orbit, and elsewhere)
- Represents 9-22% of thoracic aortitis cases in published series

Other Rheumatologic Disorders

- Rheumatoid arthritis
- Ankylosing spondylitis
- Behçet syndrome
- Systemic lupus erythematosus
- Granulomatosis with polyangiitis (Wegener)
- Relapsing polychondritis
- Tertiary syphilis
- Cogan syndrome

Pegfilgrastim (PEG-G-CSF)-Associated Aortitis

- Newly described entity; no histologic descriptions

DIAGNOSTIC CHECKLIST

Clinically Relevant Pathologic Features

- Giant cell aortitis is associated with several different disease processes that are largely indistinguishable on histopathologic grounds

Pathologic Interpretation Pearls

- Giant cell aortitis is not diagnosis but histologic pattern seen in several different conditions

SELECTED REFERENCES

1. de Boysson H et al: An updated review of cardiovascular events in giant cell arteritis. J Clin Med. 11(4):1005, 2022
2. Kadian-Dodov D et al: Inflammatory diseases of the aorta: JACC focus seminar, part 2. J Am Coll Cardiol. 80(8):832-44, 2022
3. Takahashi T et al: Granulocyte colony-stimulating factor-associated aortitis. Lancet Oncol. 23(3):e155, 2022
4. Amemiya K et al: Comparison of the damage to aorta wall in aortitis versus noninflammatory degenerative aortic diseases. Cardiovasc Pathol. 52:107329, 2021
5. Erdogan M: Aortitis: an update. Curr Opin Rheumatol. 33(1):34-40, 2021
6. Stone JR et al: Consensus statement on surgical pathology of the aorta from the Society for Cardiovascular Pathology and the Association for European Cardiovascular Pathology: I. Inflammatory diseases. Cardiovasc Pathol. 24(5):267-78, 2015
7. Siddiquee Z et al: Dense IgG4 plasma cell infiltrates associated with chronic infectious aortitis: implications for the diagnosis of IgG4-related disease. Cardiovasc Pathol. 21(6):470-5, 2012
8. Wang H et al: Comparison of clinical and pathological characteristics of isolated aortitis and Takayasu arteritis with ascending aorta involvement. J Clin Pathol. 65(4):362-6, 2012
9. Wang H et al: Giant cell aortitis of the ascending aorta without signs or symptoms of systemic vasculitis is associated with elevated risk of distal aortic events. Arthritis Rheum. 64(1):317-9, 2012
10. Laco J et al: Isolated thoracic aortitis: clinicopathological and immunohistochemical study of 11 cases. Cardiovasc Pathol. 20(6):352-60, 2011
11. Miller DV et al: The pathology of large-vessel vasculitides. Clin Exp Rheumatol. 29(1 Suppl 64):S92-8, 2011
12. Pipitone N et al: Idiopathic aortitis: an underrecognized vasculitis. Arthritis Res Ther. 13(4):119, 2011
13. Liang KP et al: Noninfectious ascending aortitis: a case series of 64 patients. J Rheumatol. 36(10):2290-7, 2009
14. Burke AP et al: Aortitis and ascending aortic aneurysm: description of 52 cases and proposal of a histologic classification. Hum Pathol. 39(4):514-26, 2008
15. Miller DV et al: Surgical pathology of noninfectious ascending aortitis: a study of 45 cases with emphasis on an isolated variant. Am J Surg Pathol. 30(9):1150-8, 2006
16. Tavora F et al: Review of isolated ascending aortitis: differential diagnosis, including syphilitic, Takayasu's and giant cell aortitis. Pathology. 38(4):302-8, 2006
17. Kerr LD et al: Occult active giant cell aortitis necessitating surgical repair. J Thorac Cardiovasc Surg. 120(4):813-5, 2000
18. Rojo-Leyva F et al: Study of 52 patients with idiopathic aortitis from a cohort of 1,204 surgical cases. Arthritis Rheum. 43(4):901-7, 2000

Giant Cell Aortitis

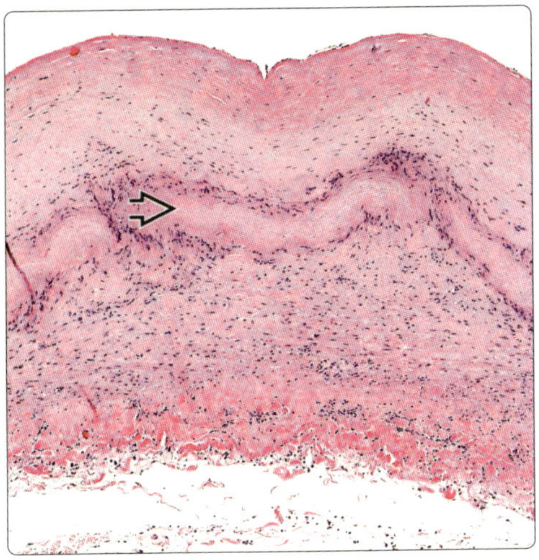

Elastic Laminar Collapse in Aortitis

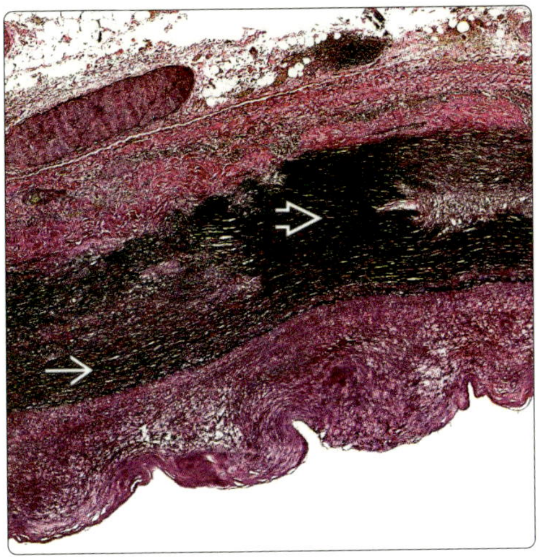

(Left) *Aortic specimen shows typical features of giant cell arteritis with a midwall band-like area of laminar medial necrosis surrounded by lymphohistiocytic inflammation with giant cells. Gaping, thin-walled vessels can also be seen adjacent to these areas.* **(Right)** *On elastic stain, the laminar medial necrosis appears solid black. There is loss of the intervening smooth muscle cell layers still seen in the preserved aortic wall.*

Mucoid Extracellular Matrix Accumulation in Aortitis

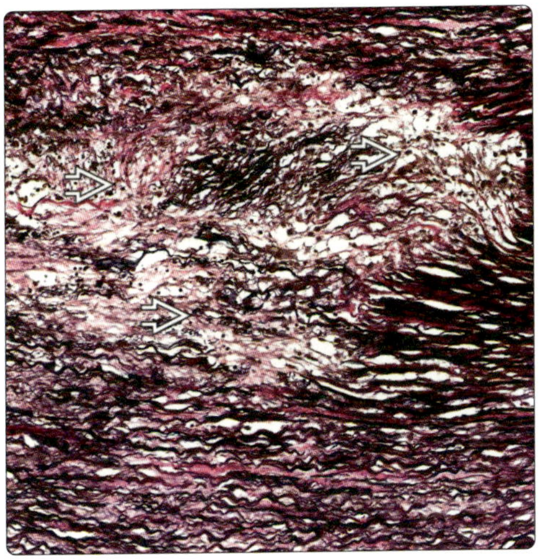

Medial Degenerative Changes in Aortitis

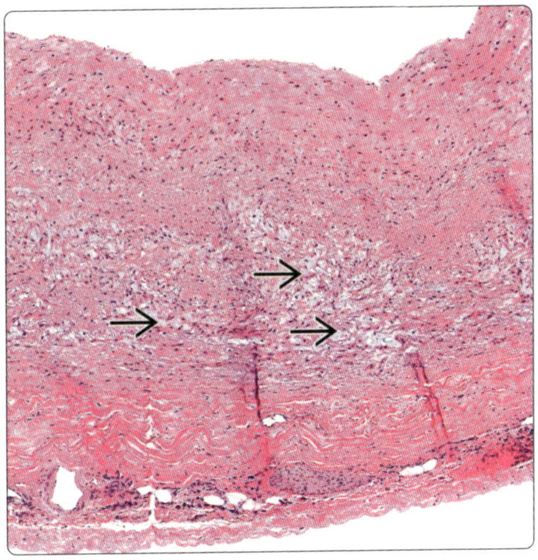

(Left) *Areas of active inflammation and loss of both medial smooth muscle and elastic tissue can often be seen focally as well as in giant cell aortitis.* **(Right)** *While medial degeneration (or cystic medial necrosis) is typically thought of in the context of connective tissue diseases, such as Marfan syndrome, areas of medial smooth muscle loss and replacement by proteoglycan material can also be seen in aortitis.*

Lymphoplasmacytic Aortitis

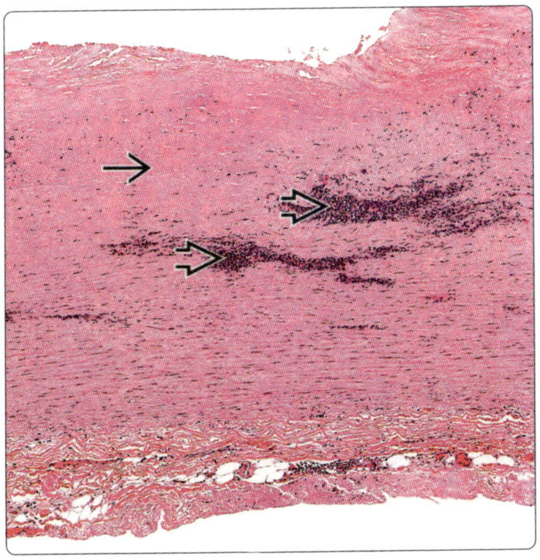

Lymphoplasmacytic Aortitis (High Power)

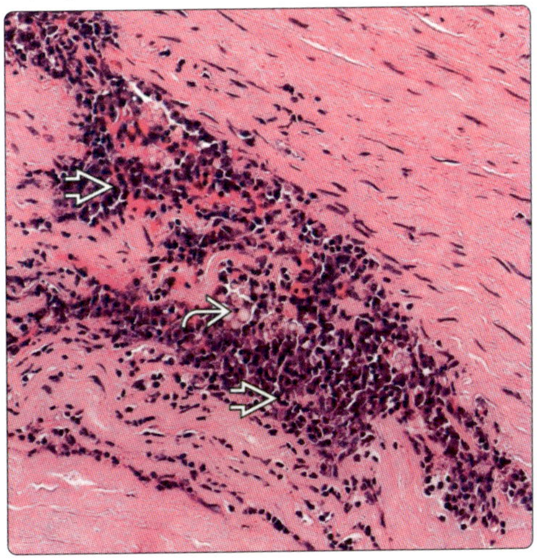

(Left) *A lymphoplasmacytic aortitis pattern can also predominate in some cases of aortitis. Areas of medial smooth muscle loss are seen, but the inflammation is much more dense and devoid of epithelioid histiocytes.* **(Right)** *On higher magnification, this example of lymphoplasmacytic aortitis shows a predominance of plasma cells. Extracellular, immunoglobulin-type crystals are also seen as part of this inflammatory infiltrate.*

Takayasu Arteritis

KEY FACTS

TERMINOLOGY

- Nonspecific chronic inflammatory arteriopathy of unknown cause affecting aorta, its primary branches, and (rarely) pulmonary artery

CLINICAL ISSUES

- Most common in southeast Asia, North Africa, and Mexico
- Uncommon in North America and Europe
- Median age of onset: < 25 years
- Almost exclusively in women
- Early preocclusive phase (systemic phase)
- Late occlusive phase (vascular phase)

IMAGING

- Angiography showing abrupt proximal (ostial) stenosis with poststenotic dilatation

MACROSCOPIC

- Aortic wall thickening (> 5 mm)
- Aortic intimal thickening and irregularity (tree bark change) in chronic phase

MICROSCOPIC

- Abundant transmural lymphohistiocytic inflammation, most prominent in adventitia
- Areas of microabscess-like necrosis (geographic) showing karyorrhectic "dirty" debris

TOP DIFFERENTIAL DIAGNOSES

- Infectious aortitis
- Rheumatologic disease
- Fibromuscular dysplasia

Aortic Arch Angiogram in Takayasu Arteritis

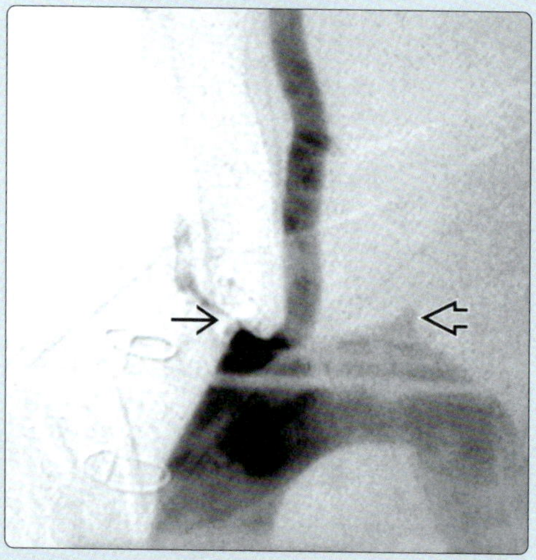

Thrombus in Takayasu Arteritis: Gross

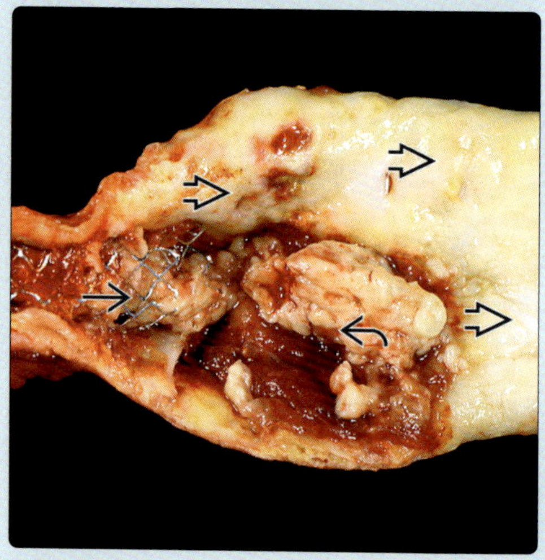

(Left) *Aortic arch angiogram shows near occlusion of the innominate → and left subclavian → arteries at their arch origin. This is typical of Takayasu arteritis, a.k.a. pulseless disease.* **(Right)** *Gross photograph shows prior stenting →, thrombosis →, and irregular intimal thickening →.*

Aortic Wall With Takayasu Arteritis

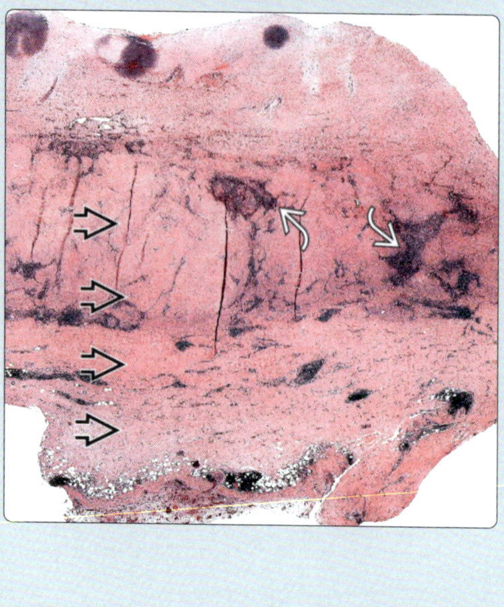

Granuloma in Takayasu Arteritis

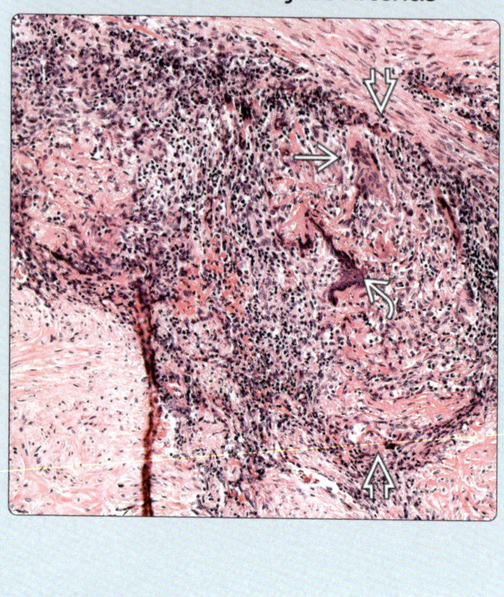

(Left) *Low-magnification view shows marked thickening of the aortic wall, mostly accounted for by the adventitial layer →. There are prominent inflammatory foci → visible, even at this power.* **(Right)** *High-magnification view shows well-formed granulomas → with multinucleated giant cells → and fragments of debris reminiscent of elastic fibers (Gamna-Gandy bodies →).*

TERMINOLOGY

Definitions

- Nonspecific chronic inflammatory arteriopathy of unknown cause affecting aorta, its primary branches, and (rarely) pulmonary artery

ETIOLOGY/PATHOGENESIS

Uncertain, Likely Multifactorial

- Genetic; ethnic predilection and positive monozygotic twin as well as HLA studies
- Infection (molecular mimicry); associations with mycobacteria, spirochetes, *Rickettsia*, and *Streptococcus*
- Autoimmune; antiendothelial antibodies found in many patients and weak association with disorders, such as Crohn, ankylosing spondylitis, systemic lupus erythematosus, and scleroderma

CLINICAL ISSUES

Epidemiology

- Incidence
  - Most common in southeast Asia, North Africa, and Mexico
  - Uncommon in North America and Europe
  - Estimated 100 new cases per year in Japan
- Age
  - Median age of onset: < 25 years
  - Per criteria, age of onset: < 50 years
- Sex
  - Almost exclusively in women
  - Takayasu arteritis and pregnancy
    - Common, given age distribution of this disease
    - Many pregnancies successfully carried to term
    - Chronic-phase disease and well-managed blood pressure help mediate risks

Presentation

- Early preocclusive phase (systemic phase)
  - Nonspecific systemic inflammatory symptoms
    - Fever
    - Malaise
    - Arthralgias
    - Myalgias
  - Typically lasts few weeks and often subclinical (not initially noticed or only felt to be significant in hindsight)
  - Thought to be when greatest vessel wall thickening is (or would have been) seen
- Late occlusive phase (vascular phase)
  - Arterial stenosis
    - Common carotid
    - Subclavian (post vertebral)
    - Renal
    - Celiac, superior mesenteric
    - Pulmonary
  - Episodic acute flare-ups (systemic inflammatory symptoms and elevated acute-phase reactants) lasting 1-2 weeks
  - Ocular manifestations
    - Hypertensive retinopathy
    - Ischemic retinopathy (rare)
  - Cardiac involvement
    - Aortic regurgitation (root and ascending aneurysmal dilatation)
    - Proximal coronary vasculitis
    - Pericarditis
    - Other valve involvement (valvulitis) (rare)
- Systemic signs and symptoms
  - Asymmetric or even absent pulses (a.k.a. pulseless disease)
  - Vascular bruits
  - Systemic hypertension
  - Heart failure
  - Acute renal failure
  - Intestinal angina
- Pulmonary artery involvement
  - Often asymptomatic but may progress to dyspnea, respiratory failure
  - 3 patterns of involvement
    - Proximal stenosis
    - Scattered distal stenoses ± proximal lesions
    - Arteriolitis without large vessel involvement (rare)
  - Arteriovenous malformations can result
  - Complex fistulous anastomotic connections between coronary, bronchial, and pulmonary arterial supplies
    - Catastrophic bleeding can result

Treatment

- Options, risks, complications
  - Goals are to improve systemic symptoms and prevent or halve further progress of vascular lesions
  - Medical
    - Corticosteroids (high dose initially, then long-term maintenance)
    - Methotrexate (for steroid-refractory cases)
    - Azathioprine and cyclophosphamide rarely used due to reproductive and other side effects in young women
    - Statin therapy effective in preventing accelerated atherosclerosis in late disease
    - Anticoagulation not demonstrated to help, except immediately post intervention
  - Surgical
    - Bypass strategies typically attempted to avoid active disease at anastomotic sites
    - Restenosis is common in active disease, especially if anastomotic site is involved
    - Postoperative steroids also given to prevent restenosis
  - Endovascular
    - Indicated only when there is imminent risk of hemodynamic compromise to downstream organ bed or significant risk of rupture
    - Often necessary in cervicocerebral, coronary, renal, and upper extremity arteries
    - Balloon angioplasty with stent placement is most common procedure
    - Restenosis is common (up to 30-40% at 1 year)

Prognosis

- 15- and 20-year survival 85% and 75%, respectively

- Common causes of death
  - Heart failure
  - Stroke
  - Renal failure
  - Postoperative complications
- Morbidity is high
  - 25-50% disability rates

Clinical Diagnostic Criteria

- Age < 40 years
- Limb claudication (especially arms)
- Brachial pulse diminution (≥ 1 arm)
- Humeral systolic pressure asymmetry (difference ≥ 10 mm)
- Subclavian or abdominal aortic bruit
- Abnormal arterial imaging
  - Aortic aneurysm
  - Narrowing or occlusion of aortic branches or distal aorta
  - Absent atherosclerosis and fibromuscular dysplasia features

IMAGING

Radiographic Findings

- Angiography showing abrupt proximal (ostial) stenosis with poststenotic dilatation
- MR, CT evidence of aortic mural thickening, aneurysm formation, distal aortic stenosis
- Stenosis of aortic arch vessels is pathognomonic

MACROSCOPIC

General Features

- Aortic wall thickening (> 5 mm)
- Aortic intimal thickening and irregularity (tree bark change) in chronic phase
- Thrombosis is rare
- Marked intimal thickening of smaller branch vessels

MICROSCOPIC

Histologic Features

- Active phase
  - Abundant transmural lymphohistiocytic inflammation, most prominent in adventitia
  - Giant cells, singly distributed and associated with histiocyte clusters
  - Areas of microabscess-like necrosis (geographic) showing karyorrhectic "dirty" debris
  - Adventitial fibroblast proliferation
  - Medial smooth muscle loss (laminar medial necrosis)
- Chronic phase
  - Little, if any, inflammation
  - Prominent adventitial fibrosis
  - Giant cells associated with areas of medial smooth muscle loss and elastic scaffold collapse
  - Plasma cells common
  - Otherwise indistinguishable from other forms of chronic aortitis

Pattern Variability

- Separation into active- and chronic-phase changes is somewhat arbitrary (and not supported by robust clinical correlative data)
- Most series report wide variation in histopathologic manifestations of this disease
- Separation from other forms of aortitis in particular is not possible on histologic grounds alone

ANCILLARY TESTS

Histochemistry

- van Gieson elastic to highlight areas of medial smooth muscle loss and collapsed elastic scaffolding

Immunohistochemistry

- IgG4 to exclude aortic involvement by hyper-IgG4 syndrome

DIFFERENTIAL DIAGNOSIS

Infectious Aortitis

- Tuberculosis
  - Acid-fast bacilli evident on staining
- Syphilis
  - Diagnosed on clinical grounds; organisms rarely identified
  - Predilection for sinotubular junction and sinuses of Valsalva (unlike Takayasu arteritis)
- Septic emboli (endocarditis)
  - Typically, valvular vegetations present

Rheumatologic Disease

- Acute articular rheumatism
- Sarcoidosis
- Adult Still disease
- Cogan syndrome
- Giant cell arteritis (in older patients)

Fibromuscular Dysplasia

- Stenoses and aneurysms but without inflammation

SELECTED REFERENCES

1. Kadian-Dodov D et al: Inflammatory diseases of the aorta: JACC focus seminar, part 2. J Am Coll Cardiol. 80(8):832-44, 2022
2. Pugh D et al: Large-vessel vasculitis. Nat Rev Dis Primers. 7(1):93, 2022
3. Stone JR et al: Consensus statement on surgical pathology of the aorta from the Society for Cardiovascular Pathology and the Association for European Cardiovascular Pathology: I. Inflammatory diseases. Cardiovasc Pathol. 24(5):267-78, 2015
4. Vaideeswar P et al: Pathology of Takayasu arteritis: a brief review. Ann Pediatr Cardiol. 6(1):52-8, 2013
5. Perrotta S et al: Aneurysmatic disease in patients with Takayasu disease: a case review. Herz. 37(3):347-53, 2012
6. Arnaud L et al: Pathogenesis of Takayasu's arteritis: a 2011 update. Autoimmun Rev. 11(1):61-7, 2011
7. Miller DV et al: The pathology of large-vessel vasculitides. Clin Exp Rheumatol. 29(1 Suppl 64):S92-8, 2011
8. Brunner J et al: Takayasu arteritis in children and adolescents. Rheumatology (Oxford). 49(10):1806-14, 2010
9. Mason JC: Takayasu arteritis–advances in diagnosis and management. Nat Rev Rheumatol. 6(7):406-15, 2010
10. Rav-Acha M et al: Coronary involvement in Takayasu's arteritis. Autoimmun Rev. 6(8):566-71, 2007

Takayasu Arteritis

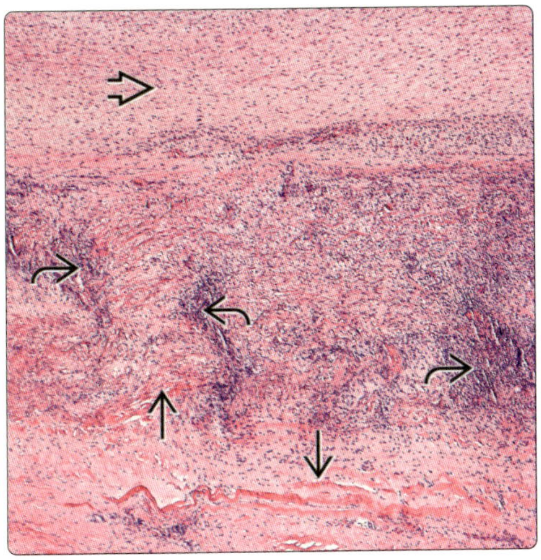

Takayasu Arteritis: Medial Changes

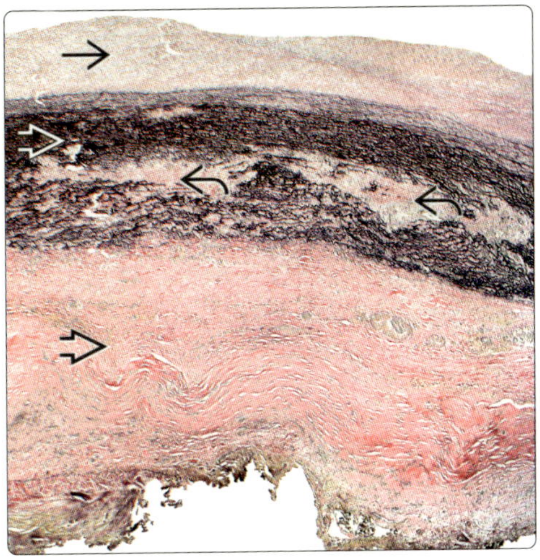

(Left) *Aortic wall involved by Takayasu arteritis shows relative preservation of the medial layer* → *with marked chronic adventitial inflammation* ↗ *and ropy adventitial dense collagen bands* →. **(Right)** *Elastic-stained aortic wall shows typical appearance of Takayasu arteritis with thickened intima* →, *inflammatory damage* ↪ *of the medial layer* →, *and marked adventitial fibrosis* →. *These changes are more consistent with chronic- (vascular) phase disease.*

Takayasu Arteritis: Abscess-Like Change

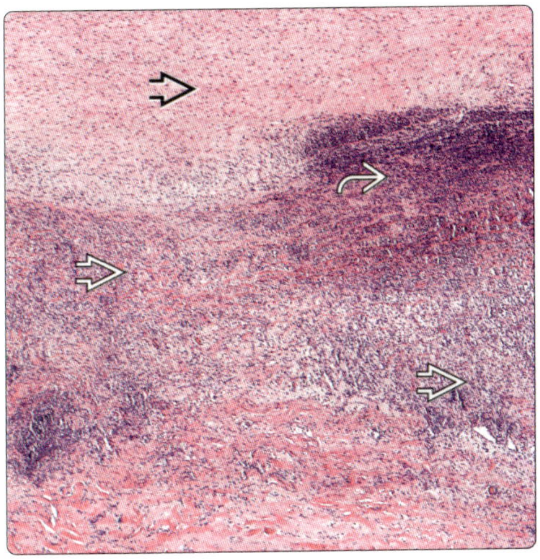

Takayasu Arteritis: Microabscess

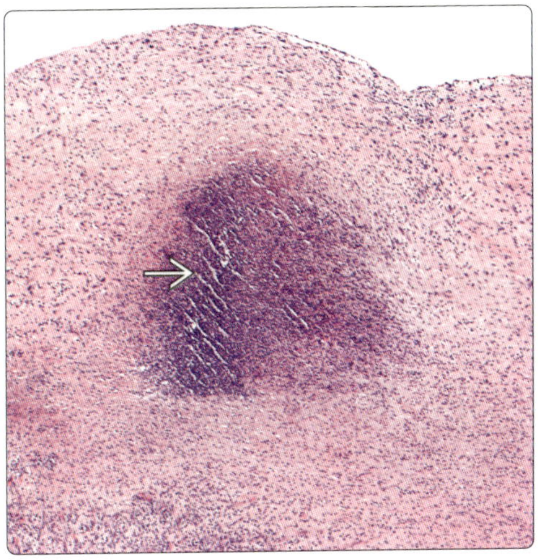

(Left) *Aortic wall shows more acute- (systemic) phase changes of Takayasu disease. The medial layer* → *is relatively preserved, but there is marked inflammation in the adventitia* →, *including a prominent acute necrotizing component* ↪. **(Right)** *Focal microabscess-like changes* → *are seen in this example of active-phase Takayasu arteritis. These changes resemble the type of geographic and "dirty" necrosis that is seen in granulomatosis with polyangiitis (Wegener).*

Takayasu Arteritis: Elastic Stain

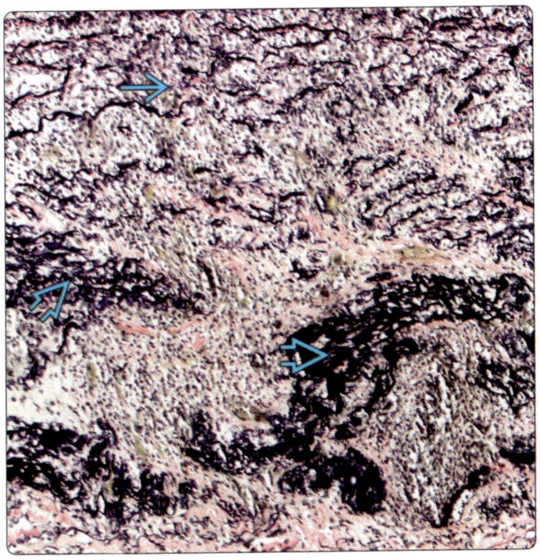

Takayasu Arteritis: Coronary Artery

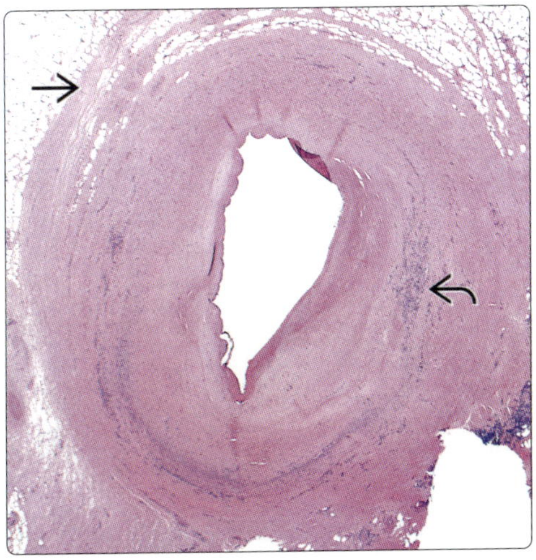

(Left) *Higher magnification view of an elastic-stained aorta involved by Takayasu arteritis shows active medial destruction* → *with fragmentation as well as loss of smooth muscle with resultant collapse of the elastic scaffold* →. **(Right)** *Takayasu arteritis may extend from the aorta to the proximal coronary arteries, as seen in this right coronary artery section from a patient with Takayasu arteritis. Transmural inflammation* ↪ *is seen as well as adventitial fibrosis* →.

Aortic Dissection

KEY FACTS

TERMINOLOGY

- Condition in which blood enters aortic wall, splaying elastic lamellae and creating hematoma
- Aortic dissection, dissecting aortic aneurysm, dissecting aneurysm, dissecting hematoma

CLINICAL ISSUES

- ~ 2,000 cases per year in United States
- Hypertension, especially in older men (comprises ~ 90% of aortic dissections)
- Hereditary syndromes and nonsyndromic hereditary disorders of connective tissue (especially in younger patients)
- Bicuspid aortic valve (BAV)
  - Affects up to 2% of population; more common in men
  - 5% of BAVs develop dissection
- Acquired connective tissue disorders (vitamin C deficiency, copper metabolism defects)
- Iatrogenic (complicating cardiac surgery or catheterization)
- Pregnancy or puerperium (rare)
- High mortality (1% per hour if left untreated), especially with dissection of thoracic aorta

MACROSCOPIC

- Intramural hematoma between inner 2/3 and outer 1/3 of aortic wall
- External rupture through adventitia, rare rupture back into true lumen (double-barrel aorta)

MICROSCOPIC

- Cystic medial degeneration is variably present and of variable severity
- Hematoma organizes with inflammation and pseudoneointima formation (chronic dissection) in survivors of acute event

ANCILLARY TESTS

- van Gieson elastic highlights disruption of elastic lamellae and areas of cystic degeneration

Type B Aortic Dissection

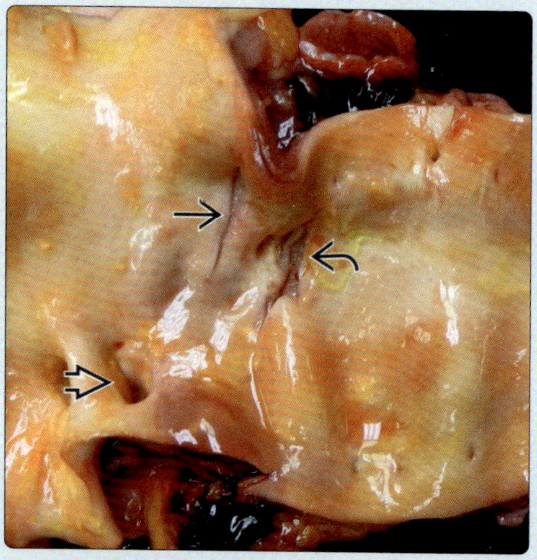

Cross Sections of Aortic Dissection and Bicuspid Aortic Valve Outflow Surface

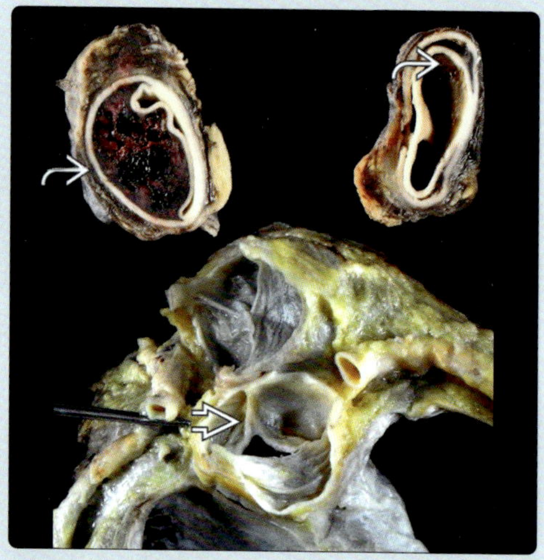

(Left) *In this aorta, there are 2 intimal tears distal to the subclavian ostium ⇨. One tear ⇨ extended proximally into an aortic dissection. The other tear ⇨ did not progress.* **(Right)** *This dissection highlights a bicuspid aortic valve that is viewed from the outflow (aortic) surface (abnormal cusp ⇨) and cross sections through the associated aortic dissection (false lumen ⇨). Of patients with bicuspid aortic valve, 5% will develop aortic dissection.*

Cross Section of Dissected Aortic Wall

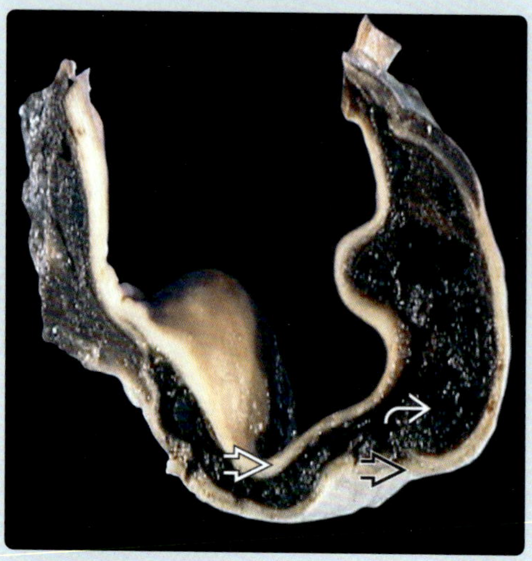

Aortic Dissection

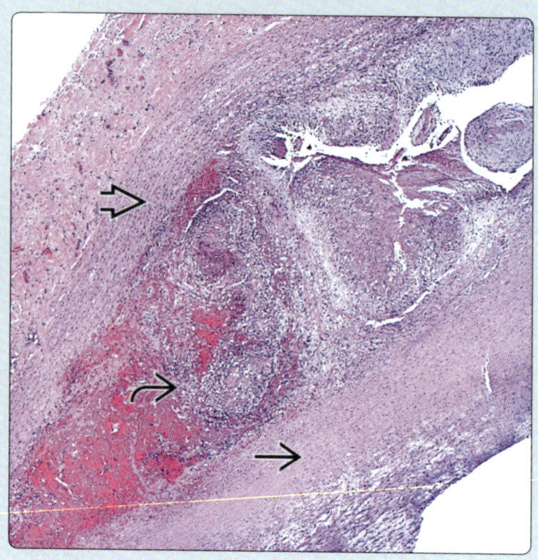

(Left) *This transmural section through an area of aortic dissection illustrates the intramural hematoma ⇨ between the inner 2/3 ⇨ and outer 1/3 ⇨ of the media.* **(Right)** *H&E-stained section through an aortic dissection reveals the false lumen ⇨ between the inner 2/3 ⇨ and outer 1/3 ⇨ of the media containing the intramural hematoma.*

TERMINOLOGY

Synonyms

- Aortic dissection, dissecting aortic aneurysm, dissecting aneurysm, dissecting hematoma
  - Since dissected aorta may or may not be dilatated, avoid synonyms containing "aneurysm"

Definitions

- Condition in which blood enters wall of aorta, splaying elastic lamellae and creating hematoma

ETIOLOGY/PATHOGENESIS

Hypertension

- Leads to medial degenerative change (pressure or ischemia-related injury)
- Ischemia in part through hyperplastic changes of media of vasa vasorum
- Extent of medial degeneration does not directly correlate with risk for dissection

Inherited or Acquired Connective Tissue Disorders

- Lead to variable amounts of aortic root dilatation and medial degeneration predisposing to dissection
- Many associated with upregulation of TGF-β activity in ascending aorta with medial remodeling and weakening "TGF-β-opathies" (e.g., Marfan syndrome, vascular Ehlers-Danlos syndrome, Loeys-Dietz syndrome)

CLINICAL ISSUES

Epidemiology

- Incidence
  - ~ 2,000 cases per year in United States
- Age
  - Most often in older patients (> 60 years of age)
  - In younger patients, think underlying heritable disorder of connective tissue, syndromic or nonsyndromic
- Sex: M > F (2-3:1)
- Risk factors
  - Hypertension, especially in older men (comprises ~ 90% of aortic dissections)
  - Hereditary syndromes and nonsyndromic hereditary disorders of connective tissue (especially in younger patients)
    - Marfan syndrome, vascular Ehlers-Danlos syndrome, Loeys-Dietz syndrome, autosomal dominant polycystic kidney disease, familial thoracic aortic aneurysm syndrome
    - Bicuspid aortic valve (affects up to 2% of population; more common in men; 5% develop dissection)
  - Acquired connective tissue disorders (e.g., vitamin C deficiency, copper metabolism defects)
  - Iatrogenic
    - Complicating cardiac surgery: Aortic cannulation and cross-clamp sites, aortotomy sites; complicating cardiac catheterization or intraaortic device implantation (intraaortic balloon pump)
  - Pregnancy or puerperium (rare)

Presentation

- Acute aortic syndrome
  - Pain and disruption of aortic media (e.g., aortic dissection, intramural hematoma, penetrating aortic ulcer, and other contained aortic ruptures)
- Related to obstruction of major branches
  - Stroke, myocardial infarction, mesenteric angina, pulse deficits, etc.
- Related to rupture
  - Death/shock, hemothorax/hemopericardium (tamponade), hemoperitoneum, retroperitoneal hematoma
- Related to valve dysfunction
  - Acute aortic regurgitation, acute congestive heart failure, shock

Prognosis

- Mortality is high (1% per hour if left untreated), especially with dissection of thoracic aorta

MACROSCOPIC

General Features

- Rupture (hemothorax, hemopericardium, etc.)
- ± aortic dilatation
- Classification based upon portion of aorta involved
  - Type A: Proximal aorta ± distal aortic involvement
  - Type B: Distal aorta, usually distal to subclavian artery
- Intimal tears noted in most aortic dissections
  - Transverse to oblique; within 10 cm of aortic valve; jagged edges; may be multiple
- Intramural hematoma between inner 2/3 and outer 1/3 of aortic wall
- External rupture through adventitia, rare rupture back into true lumen (double-barrel aorta)

MICROSCOPIC

Histologic Features

- Cystic medial degeneration is variably present and of variable severity
  - Loss of elastic fibers with pooling of excess ground substance (glycosaminoglycans) within aortic media
- Intramural hematoma within plane between inner 2/3 and outer 1/3 of media, splaying apart elastic lamellae
- Hematoma organizes with inflammation and pseudoneointima formation (chronic dissection) in survivors of acute event

ANCILLARY TESTS

Histochemistry

- van Gieson elastic highlights disruption of elastic lamellae and areas of cystic degeneration

SELECTED REFERENCES

1. Fujiyoshi T et al: Relationship between the aortic root Z-score and degree of translamellar mucoid extracellular matrix accumulation. Surg Today. 52(3):408-13, 2022
2. Cifani N et al: Stanford-A acute aortic dissection, inflammation, and metalloproteinases: a review. Ann Med. 47(6):441-6, 2015
3. Stone JR et al: Consensus statement on surgical pathology of the aorta from the Society for Cardiovascular Pathology and the Association for European Cardiovascular Pathology: I. Inflammatory diseases. Cardiovasc Pathol. 24(5):267-78, 2015

(Left) *Opening of the left chest cavity at autopsy shows a large hemothorax ➡ that was the consequence of a ruptured type A dissection. The lower lobe of the left lung is well visualized ⇨.* **(Right)** *Autopsy specimen demonstrates a distal aortic dissection ➡ occurring after replacement of the ascending aorta with a Dacron graft ➡. This dissection extended to the iliac arteries.*

Hemothorax Due to Ruptured Type A Dissection

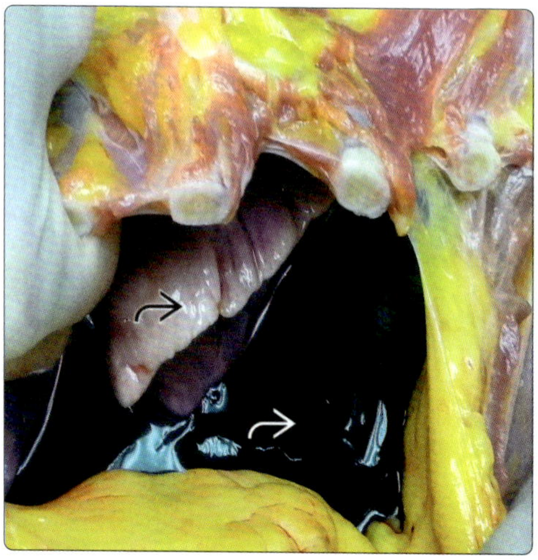

Dissection Post Graft Replacement

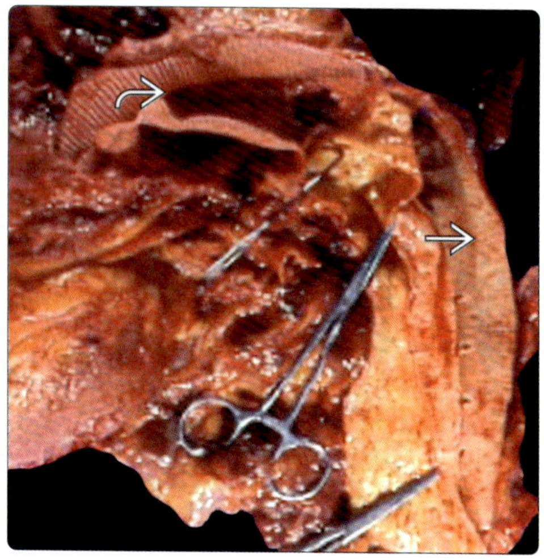

(Left) *Intimal tear ⇨ is still visible after surgical repair of the ascending aorta with a Dacron graft ⇨. It is in the most common location, close to the aortic valve ⇨, and transversely oriented. The commissures of the aortic valve have been supported by pledgeted sutures ➡ due to valve insufficiency.* **(Right)** *The other common site for intimal tear is just distal to the subclavian ostium. In dissections without intimal tears, blood is felt to enter the media via vasa vasorum.*

Ascending Aorta Repair and Intimal Tear

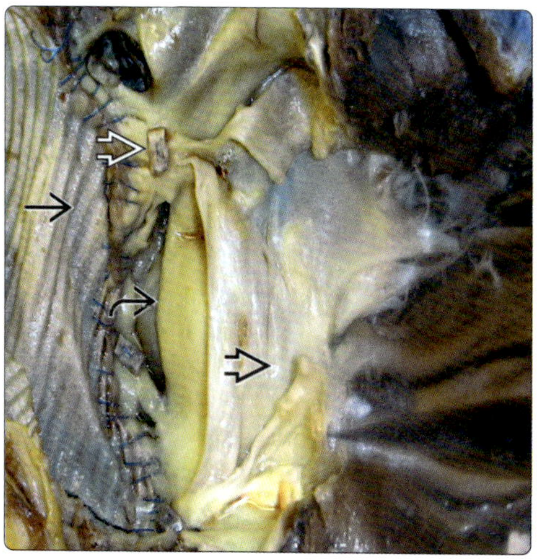

Type B Aortic Dissection

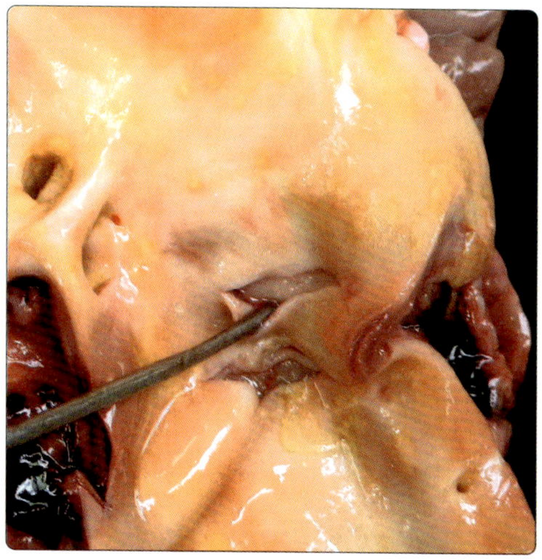

(Left) *The intimal surface of a surgically resected portion of an aortic dissection may appear deceptively normal with only mild atherosclerosis.* **(Right)** *Examination of the opposite surface of this specimen (i.e., the false lumen) reveals the hematoma ➡ and the rough granular surface of the dissected media ⇨.*

Intimal View of Dissected Aorta

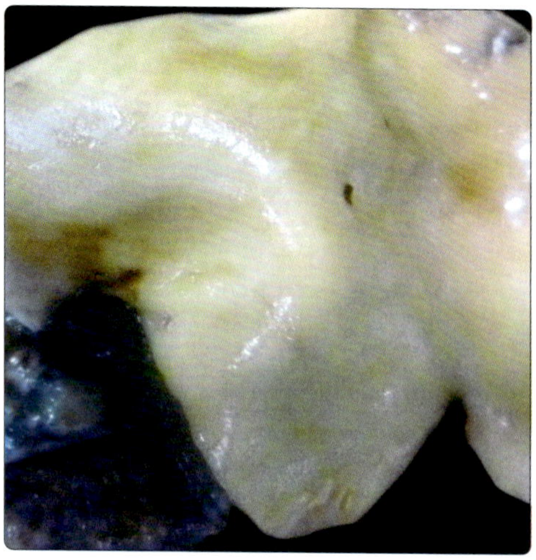

Posterior View of Dissected Aorta

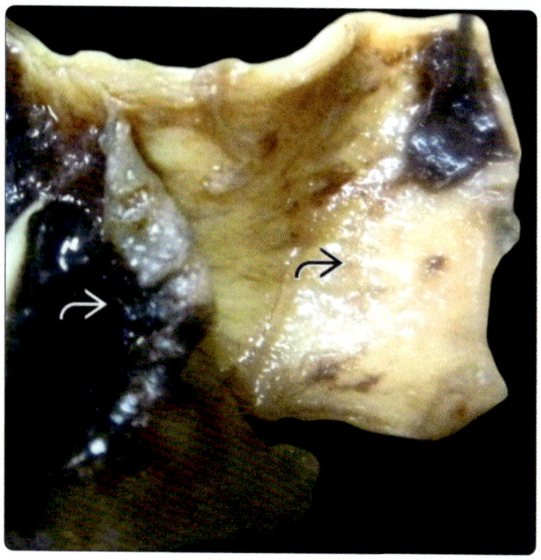

Elastic Stain of Dissected Aorta

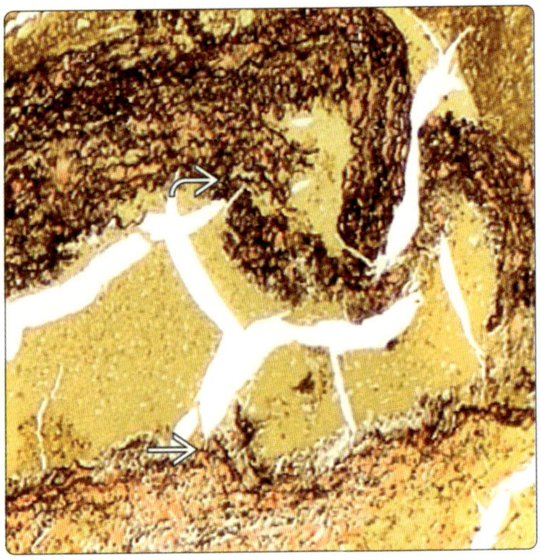

Elastic Stain of Dissected Aorta

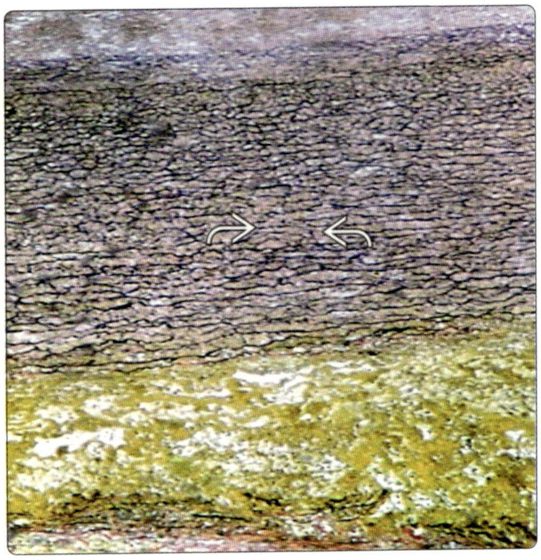

(Left) *Elastic stain of a recent dissection reveals the fragmented elastic lamellae lining the false lumen. The outer portion of this dissection is very thin.* **(Right)** *Elastic stain reveals only mild medial degenerative changes of thinning and loss of elastic lamellae in the aortic wall in an area of dissection. Medial degenerative changes are of varying severity in dissected aortas.*

Cystic Medial Degeneration

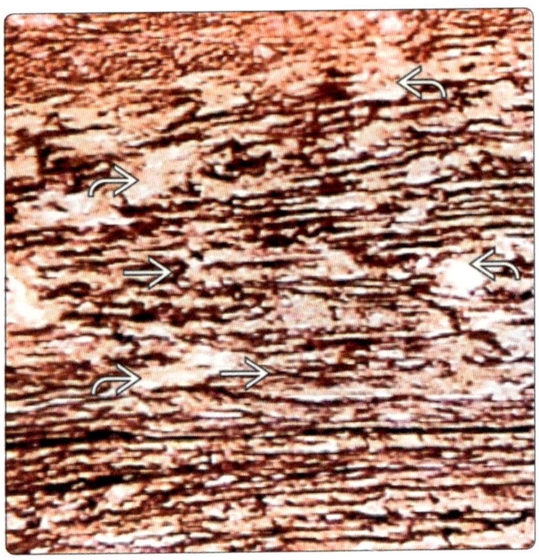

Healed Aortic Dissection

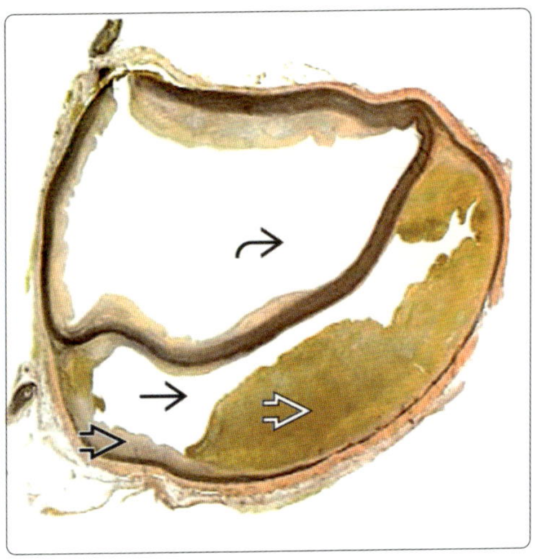

(Left) *More marked medial degenerative changes are noted in this aorta with areas of elastic fragmentation and pools of glycosaminoglycans accumulating in the media (cystic medial degeneration).* **(Right)** *This aorta has true and false lumina as a consequence of a healed aortic dissection. The true lumen shows mild intimal hyperplasia, whereas the false lumen within the media has healed with formation of a pseudoneointima. There is still hematoma present.*

Healed Aortic Dissection

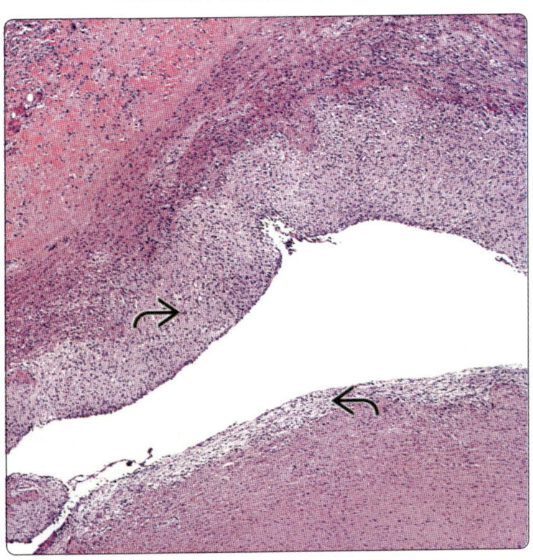

Healed Aortic Dissection

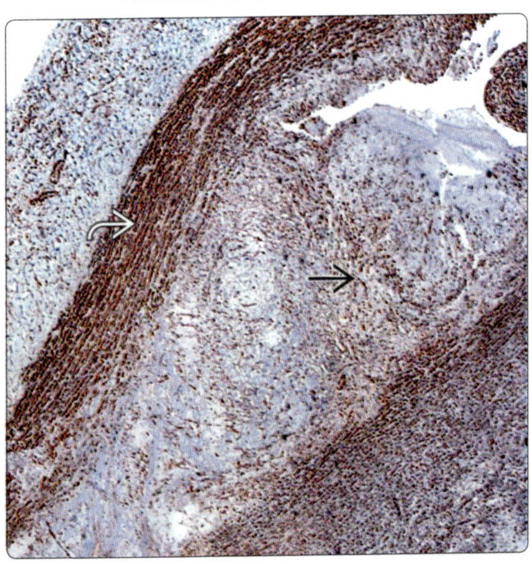

(Left) *H&E-stained section at higher magnification shows the healing false lumen of an aortic dissection, revealing the paler appearing pseudoneointima.* **(Right)** *SMA highlights the vascular smooth muscle cells of the aortic media and the smooth muscle cells that are forming the pseudoneointima. (Courtesy C. Minerowicz, MD.)*

Aortic Coarctation

KEY FACTS

TERMINOLOGY

- Common congenital cardiovascular defect characterized by discrete, ridge-like narrowing in descending aorta at site of aortic ductal attachment

CLINICAL ISSUES

- 1:3,000 live births
- Male predominance; estimated 2-4:1
- Present in 5-10% of cases with some form of congenital heart disease
- Dependent on site of stenosis to some extent
  - Proximal to ductus arteriosus: Earlier symptoms, more severe
  - Distal to ductus arteriosus: Later presentation, less severe

MACROSCOPIC

- Obstructing membrane or ridge of tissue at level of aortic isthmus
- Orienting specimen relative to insertion of ductus/ligamentum arteriosus is crucial
- Infantile type (preductal)
  - Long-segment narrowing proximal to ductus
  - Patent ductus arteriosus (PDA) supplies flow to distal aorta
  - Short segment of stenosis distal to ductus
- Adult type (post ductal)
  - Collateral vessels supply flow to distal aorta
  - Associated with bicuspid aortic valve and cerebral aneurysms

MICROSCOPIC

- Ductal tissue with variable penetration into adjacent aortic wall
- ± associated intimal hyperplasia overlying ductal insertion
- Increased collagen in medial and intimal layers overlying ductal insertion

Coronal View of Preductal Coarctation

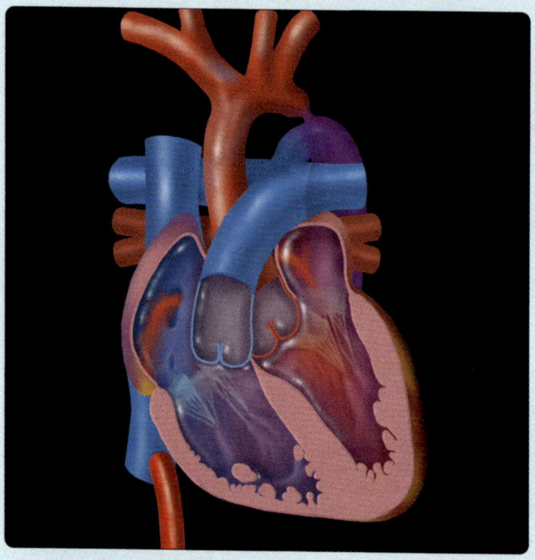

Sagittal View of Postductal Coarctation

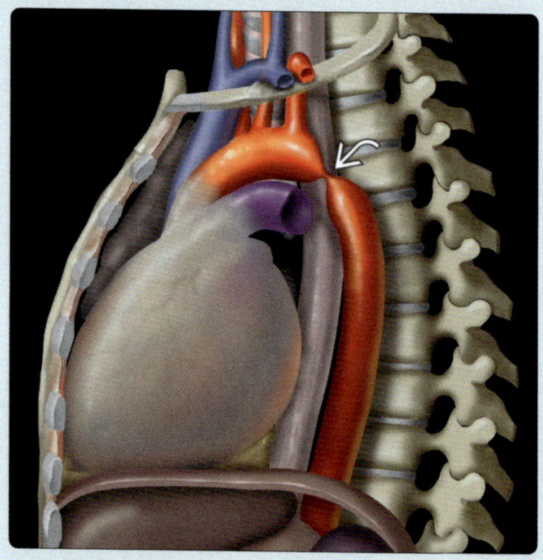

(Left) *Coronal graphic shows preductal coarctation with patent ductus arteriosus (PDA) and right-to-left shunt, resulting in decreased oxygenation in the descending aorta only.* **(Right)** *Sagittal graphic shows short-segment coarctation of the thoracic aorta distal to the ductus arteriosus ➔. Collateral vessels supply the distal aorta.*

CTA of Aortic Coarctation

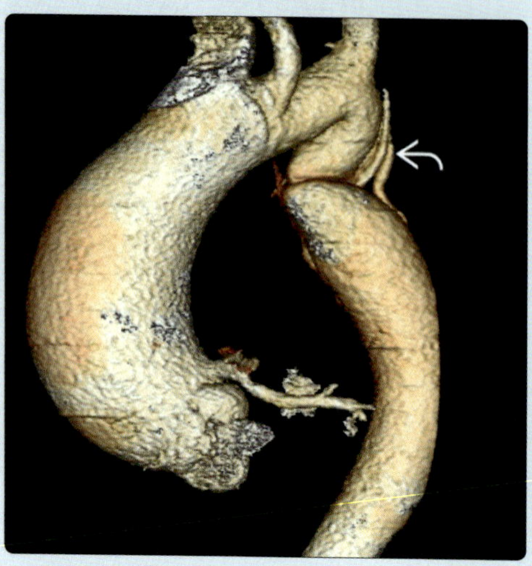

Gross Specimen From Aortic Coarctation

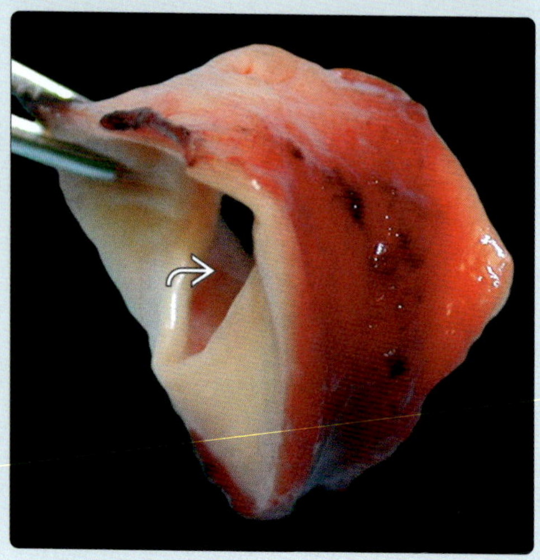

(Left) *Oblique CTA volume rendering shows aortic coarctation with hypoplastic arch and collaterals ➔. (Courtesy S. Abbara, MD.)* **(Right)** *This surgical "coarctectomy" specimen was removed at the time of aortic coarctation repair. The lumen shows marked stricturing ➔ relative to the overall diameter of the aorta at the resected ends.*

TERMINOLOGY

Definitions

- Common congenital cardiovascular defect characterized by discrete, ridge-like narrowing in descending aorta at site of aortic ductal attachment
  - May extend proximally to involve isthmus and aortic root (tubular hypoplasia)
- Literal translation means "drawing together," referring to encroachment on aortic lumen from all sides

ETIOLOGY/PATHOGENESIS

Developmental Anomaly

- Competing theories
  - Extension of ductal tissue into aorta wall proper, causing medial disruption/disorganization and resulting in constriction
    - Possibly also some downward mechanical traction (in direction of ductus)
    - Spatial transcriptomic studies show migration of extracellular matrix (ECM) and smooth muscle cells (SMCs) to subendothelial space
  - Hemodynamic hypothesis
    - Left-sided obstruction in utero due to aortic or mitral valve defects leads to decreased aortic flow and thus results in functional hypoplasia of ascending aorta (distal to isthmus)
- Both mechanisms may be involved simultaneously and to varying degrees from case to case

CLINICAL ISSUES

Epidemiology

- Incidence
  - 1:3,000 live births
  - 5-7% of all congenital heart disease
  - Present in 5-10% of cases with some form of congenital heart disease
- Sex
  - Male predominance; estimated 2-4:1
- Association with other congenital defects
  - Bicuspid aortic valve (50%)
    - Converse is not true (< 5% of bicuspid aortic valves are associated with coarctation)
  - Ventricular septal defect (33%)
  - Turner syndrome (4.4%)
  - Shone syndrome: Subaortic stenosis, parachute mitral valve, supravalvular mitral ring
  - Marfan syndrome
  - Atrial septal defect
  - Valvular stenosis (mitral/aortic)

Presentation

- Dependent on site of stenosis to some extent
  - Proximal to ductus arteriosus: Earlier symptoms, more severe
    - No collateral formation with aortic arch in utero
  - Distal to ductus arteriosus: Later presentation, less severe
    - Collateral circulation (e.g., intercostal arteries) forms to supply descending aorta
- Fetal
  - Disproportion of ventricular size to great vessel size on prenatal ultrasound
  - Association with other congenital heart defects
  - Chromosomal abnormalities (Turner syndrome)
- Neonate/infant
  - Peripartum collapse, acidosis
  - Heart failure
  - Heart murmur: Systolic, continuous, radiating to back
  - Weak/absent femoral pulses
  - Upper limb hypertension
  - Intracranial hemorrhage
- Child, adolescent, adult
  - Heart failure, including sudden cardiac arrest
  - Aortic dissection &/or rupture
  - Heart murmur: Systolic, continuous, radiating to back
  - Weak/absent femoral pulses
  - Upper limb hypertension
  - Exercise intolerance
  - Leg fatigue and claudication
  - Intracranial hemorrhage (cerebral aneurysms)
- Ductus arteriosus is patent in most cases of coarctation
- In patients with bicuspid aortic valve, coarctation associated (statistically) with left coronary dominance (44% vs. 14% for right dominance)

Treatment

- Surgical approaches
  - Resection of stenotic segment with extended end-to-end anastomosis
    - Most recommended and highest success rate (especially for infant and young child)
  - Repair with subclavian flap or synthetic graft
  - Endovascular stent placement
  - Intraluminal balloon angioplasty
    - Recommended for older patients
    - May result in restenosis and postdilatation aneurysm

Prognosis

- Dependent on age at presentation and degree of stenosis
  - Poor without surgical treatment
    - Uncontrolled hypertension
    - Congestive heart failure
    - Aortic rupture
    - Intracranial hemorrhage
  - Average age of death for patients diagnosed as adults: 42 years
  - Prognosis post surgery is generally good
    - Repaired before age 14: 90% 20-year survival
    - Repaired after age 14: 80% 20-year survival

IMAGING

Ultrasonographic Findings

- Narrowing of isthmus and posterior indentation shelf
- Color Doppler to highlight and quantitate gradient across coarctation

MR Findings

- T2 GRE: Length of systolic flow jet (dark) proportional to hemodynamic significance of coarctation

- MRA: Phase contrast to estimate pressure gradient
- T1: Cardiac-gated and 3D gadolinium sequences demonstrate morphology

CT Findings

- Aortic caliber change
- Collateral circulation anatomy
- Flow abnormalities in left subclavian artery
- Hypertrophy of intercostals with rib notching

Angiography

- Direct measurement of pressure gradient
  - If < 20 mm Hg, coarctation is mild
  - If > 20 mm Hg, intervention is required

MACROSCOPIC

General Features

- Obstructing membrane or ridge of tissue at level of aortic isthmus
- Infantile type (preductal)
  - Long-segment narrowing is proximal to ductus
  - Patent ductus arteriosus (PDA) supplies flow to distal aorta
  - Associated with heart defects
    - Ventricular septal defect
    - Atrial septal defect
    - Bicuspid aortic valve
    - Left ventricular outflow abnormalities (e.g., Shone syndrome)
    - Congenital mitral stenosis
- Adult type (post ductal)
  - Short segment of stenosis is distal to ductus
  - Collateral vessels supply flow to distal aorta
  - Associated with bicuspid aortic valve and cerebral aneurysms
- Poststenotic dilatation common
  - Intercostal artery orifices may be enlarged (relative to more distal ostia)

Sections to Be Submitted

- Orienting specimen relative to insertion of ductus/ligamentum arteriosus is crucial
- Transverse section in plane cutting through ductal tissue
  - Allows for evaluating extension of ductal tissue in aortic wall
  - Must include portion of wall opposite to ductal attachment
- Elastic staining useful in visualizing ductal tissue (vis-à-vis aortic wall)

MICROSCOPIC

Histologic Features

- Ductal tissue with variable penetration into adjacent aortic wall
  - ± associated intimal hyperplasia overlying ductal insertion
  - Increased collagen in medial and intimal layers overlying ductal insertion
  - If ductus closed surgically by previous operation, suture material embedded in dense collagen scar may be seen surrounding ductus
  - Consequent elastic fiber disarray caused by penetration of ductal wall into aorta
  - Medial degeneration can also be seen adjacent to coarctation site
    - Increasing long-term risk for subsequent dissection
- Adluminal (aortic wall opposite to ductal insertion side) "traction" hyperplasia
  - Hallmark histologic feature of coarctation
  - Mounded (fibromuscular dysplasia-like) intimal thickening contributing to stenotic narrowing
  - ± medial hypertrophy and degeneration
  - Thought to be due to hemodynamic shear stress from "kinking" at coarctation site
- Intimal and medial hyperplastic changes are dynamic and may be altered by interventions, such as duct closure

DIFFERENTIAL DIAGNOSIS

Takayasu Arteritis

- Acquired inflammatory narrowing of unknown etiology
- Not isolated to aortic isthmus

Interrupted/Atretic Aortic Arch

- More severe anomaly along same spectrum as tubular hypoplasia
- Complete occlusion and interruption of aorta
  - Fibrous cord remnant usually at isthmus or between left carotid and left subclavian arteries
  - Ductus arteriosus supplies aorta distal to interruption
- Often associated with malalignment-type ventricular septal defect with subaortic outflow tract obstruction

Vascular Rings

- May cause distortion of aortic contours that could be confused with coarctation
- Aberrant retroesophageal left subclavian artery is classic example, but many other variants are possible
- These anomalies result in arterial ring encircling trachea and esophagus
- Retroesophageal right subclavian (from otherwise normal innominate artery arising from aortic arch) is almost constant finding in coarctation (coarctation and vascular ring are not mutually exclusive)

SELECTED REFERENCES

1. Heider A et al: Histologic and morphologic character of pediatric abdominal aortic developmental coarctation and hypoplasia. J Vasc Surg. 76(2):556-63.e4, 2022
2. Zhou N et al: Coronary artery dominance and cardiovascular pathologies in patients with bicuspid aortic valve. Am J Med Sci. 363(2):147-50, 2022
3. Iwaki R et al: Evaluation of ductal tissue in coarctation of the aorta using x-ray phase-contrast tomography. Pediatr Cardiol. 42(3):654-61, 2021
4. Liu A et al: RNA sequencing analyses in infants patients with coarctation of the aorta. Hereditas. 158(1):32, 2021
5. Bigdelian H et al: Repair of aortic coarctation in infancy: a 10-year clinical experience. Asian Cardiovasc Thorac Ann. 24(5):417-21, 2016
6. Vonder Muhll IF et al: The adult with repaired coarctation: need for lifelong surveillance. Can J Cardiol. 32(8):1038.e11-5, 2016
7. Krieger EV et al: The adult with repaired coarctation of the aorta. Heart. 96(20):1676-81, 2010. Erratum in: Heart. 97(13):1112, 2011
8. Ho SY et al: Coarctation, tubular hypoplasia, and the ductus arteriosus. Histological study of 35 specimens. Br Heart J. 41(3):268-74, 1979

CECT of Aortic Coarctation

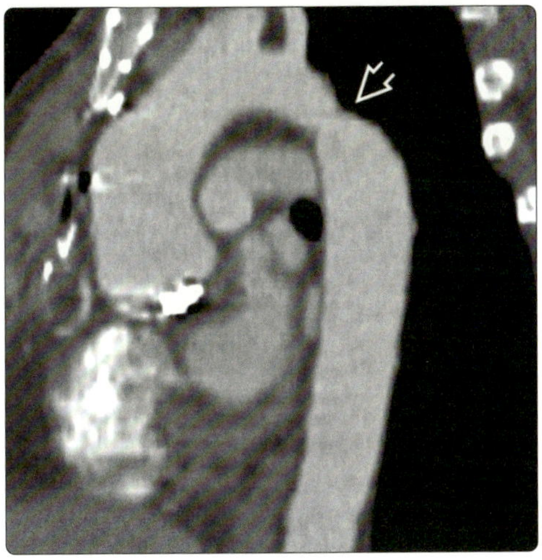

In Situ View of Aortic Coarctation at Autopsy

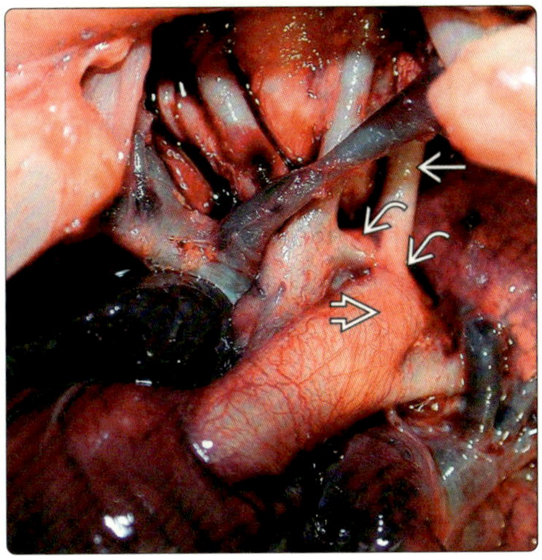

(Left) *Sagittal CECT shows a circumscribed, high-grade narrowing of the proximal descending thoracic aorta just distal to the ductus. (Courtesy T. Mohammed, MD.)* **(Right)** *In situ view of an aortic coarctation at autopsy shows a long, tubular-type coarctation with narrowing beginning after the left carotid origin and extending distally. The left subclavian artery and ductus are labeled for orientation.*

"Coarctectomy" Gross Specimen

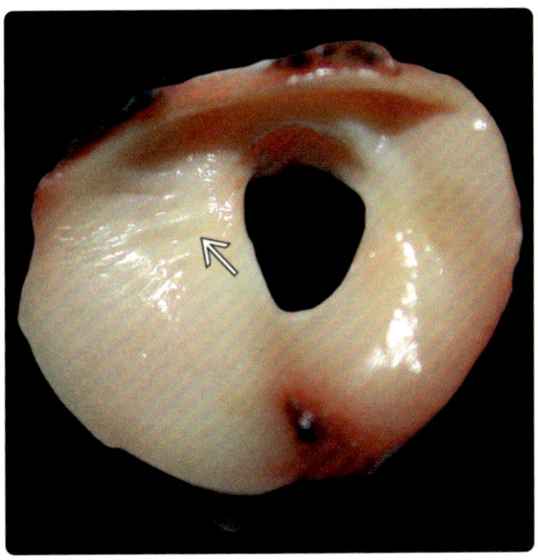

"Coarctectomy" Gross Specimen

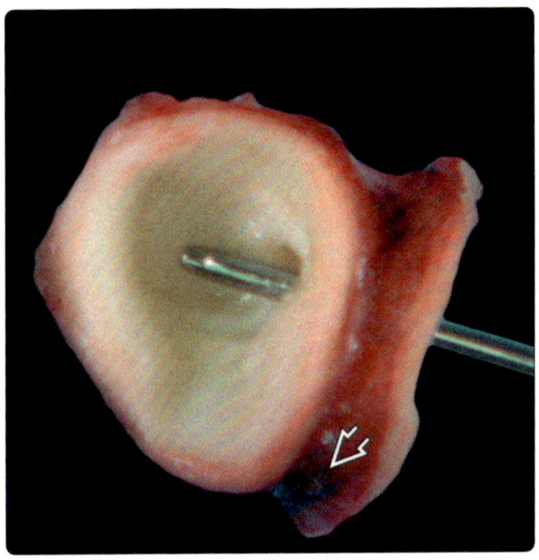

(Left) *En face view of a "coarctectomy" surgical specimen shows uniformity in the aortic wall lining the coarctation site. Focal radiating folds resemble a purse string cinching type of luminal narrowing.* **(Right)** *Surgical resection specimen shows a coarctation of the aorta that is only just probe patent (critical narrowing). A cauterized remnant of ligamentum arteriosus is seen.*

Histologic Features of "Coarctectomy" Specimen

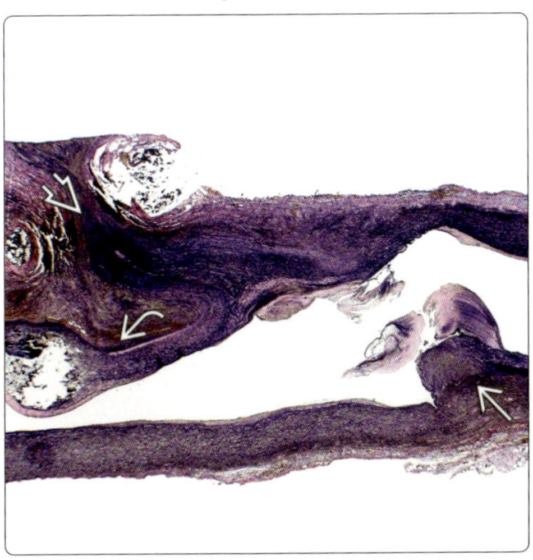

Histologic Features of "Coarctectomy" Specimen

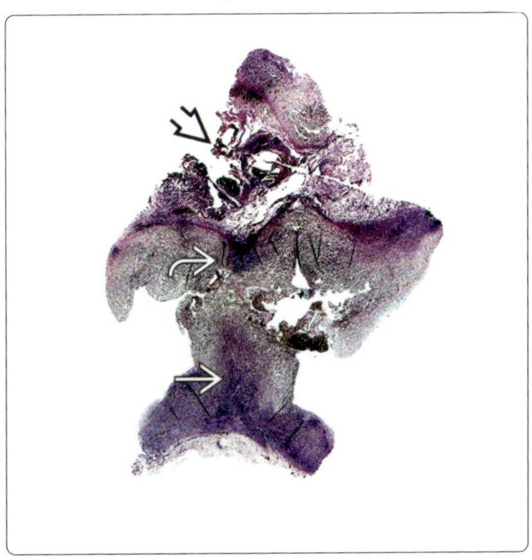

(Left) *Transverse section of a coarctation specimen shows the ductal remnant (surgically closed) and luminal narrowing due to intimal hyperplasia overlying the ductus connection as well as adluminal traction hyperplasia of the aortic wall. Sections submitted for microscopy should be oriented like this.* **(Right)** *Transverse section of a coarctation specimen shows the ductus with overlying intimal hyperplasia and adluminal traction hyperplasia.*

Aortic Atherosclerosis and Complications

KEY FACTS

TERMINOLOGY

- Atherosclerosis: Disease with chronic inflammation features and formation of atherosclerotic plaques
- Aneurysm: Localized permanent pathologic dilatation of vessel with diameter at least 50% > normal

CLINICAL ISSUES

- Major risk factors
  - Nonmodifiable: ↑ age, male sex, family history
  - Modifiable: Hypertension, ↑ lipid, smoking, diabetes mellitus
- Other: Systemic inflammation (↑ CRP), lipoprotein A, hyperhomocysteinemia, metabolic syndrome
- Abdominal aortic aneurysm (AAA)
  - Risk of rupture ↑ with ↑ diameter, high mortality rate: 4-5 cm 1%/year, 5-6 cm 11%/year, > 6 cm 25%/year

MACROSCOPIC

- AAA is usually fusiform and infrarenal
  - True aneurysm contains all layers of vessel wall
  - Very thick wall may be inflammatory aneurysm
  - ↑ diameter may have rupture; common site distal to renal arteries, left lateral

MICROSCOPIC

- Aortic atherosclerosis: Early lesions
  - Thickened intima with foam cells and scattered lymphocytes in fatty streak
- Aortic atherosclerosis: Atheromatous plaque progression
  - Intimal collection of extracellular lipid with inflammation, no significant fibrosis, and little change in media
  - Fibrosis around lipid, increasing thickening of intima, progressive degenerative changes of media
- Aortic atherosclerosis: Complicated lesions
  - AAA wall shows severe atherosclerosis, degeneration of media, mild adventitial inflammation, fibrosis of wall, dystrophic calcification, and nonorganized mural thrombus

Abdominal Aorta With Marked Atherosclerosis

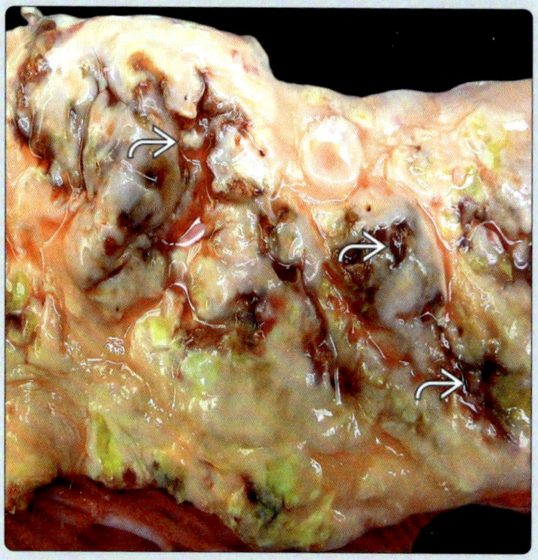

Infrarenal Aortic Aneurysm

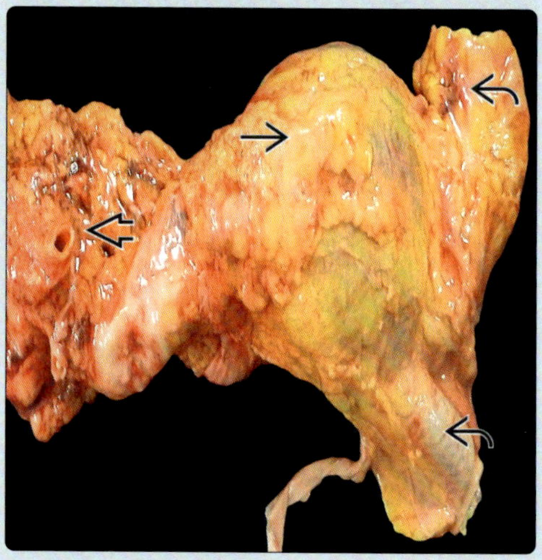

(Left) *This infrarenal aorta has a large atherosclerotic plaque burden and areas of plaque ulceration →. The aortic circumference is increased due to secondary degenerative changes of aortic media.* **(Right)** *This infrarenal, fusiform abdominal aortic aneurysm → is distal to the superior mesenteric artery → and renal arteries (not well visualized) and ends at the iliac vessels →. This is a common site for this complication.*

Histologic Features of Atherosclerotic Plaque

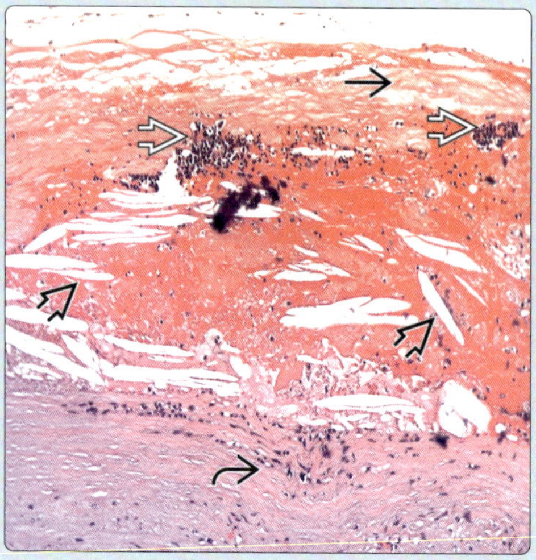

Histologic Features of Atherosclerotic Plaque

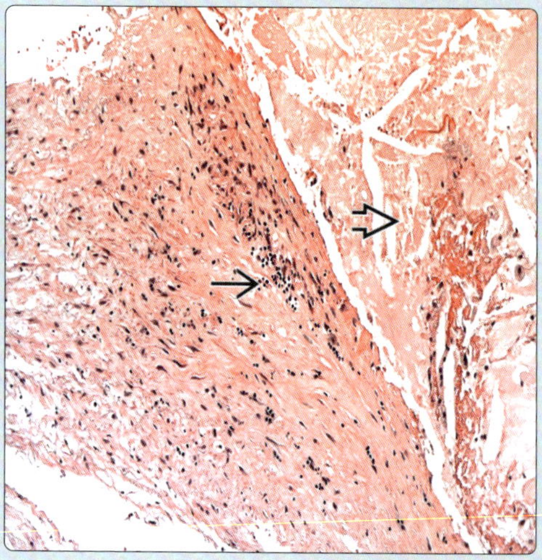

(Left) *This plaque hemorrhage expands the necrotic center (cholesterol crystals →) under a thin fibrous cap →. Dystrophic calcification and inflammation are noted →. The underlying media shows loss of staining of nuclei of smooth muscle cells and inflammation →.* **(Right)** *Inflammation is a component of atherosclerosis. Lymphocytes → are seen here in a fibrous cap adjacent to the necrotic core →.*

TERMINOLOGY

Definitions

- Atherosclerosis: Chronic, progressive inflammatory disease characterized by formation of atherosclerotic plaques in medium and large arteries
  - Intimal atherosclerotic plaques composed of intra- and extracellular lipid (often oxidized), inflammatory cells (T cells and macrophages), vascular smooth muscle cells (VSMCs), and extracellular matrix (collagen and proteoglycans)
    - Dystrophic calcification often present
  - Degenerative changes of media
- Aneurysm: Localized permanent pathologic dilatation of vessel with diameter at least 50% > normal
  - Normal diameter relates to age, location, body habitus, and daily workload
    - ↑ age, ↑ diameter ~ 1-2 mm/year; ↓ compliance
    - Ascending/descending < 2.1/< 1.6 cm/m²; abdominal < 3 cm
  - True aneurysm contains all layers of vessel wall
    - Shape: Fusiform-circumferential, symmetric; saccular-asymmetric bulging of portion of wall
    - Abdominal: Infrarenal (10 mm distal to ostia), juxtarenal (at ostia), suprarenal (extends proximal)
    - Thoracic: Ascending (annulus to innominate), arch, descending (distal to L subclavian)
  - False (pseudo) aneurysm
    - Contained rupture surrounded by adventitia, periadventitial connective tissue, or fibrous wall
- Penetrating aortic ulcer
  - Deeply ulcerated plaque extending into media

ETIOLOGY/PATHOGENESIS

Atherosclerosis: Response to Injury

- Endothelial injury [hemodynamic factors, toxins (smoke), ↑ lipid, hyperhomocysteinemia]
- Lipid accumulation
  - Oxidized low-density lipoprotein (LDL) and cholesterol crystals, foam cells, cytokines and growth factors, inflammation (monocytes), platelet adhesion,
  - Smooth muscle cell recruitment, proliferation, matrix production

Aneurysm Formation: Abdominal Aorta

- Progressive atrophy of media, inflammation, ↑ metalloproteinase activity (↓ metalloproteinase inhibitors activity), matrix destruction, wall weakening, dilatation/rupture
  - Atherosclerosis is most important initiating factor
  - May be genetic predisposition related to genes that regulate metalloproteinase or inflammation

Aneurysm Formation: Thoracic Aorta

- Hypertension is most important risk factor
  - Medial ischemia via vasa vasorum is one potential mechanism plus hemodynamic factors
- Genetic disorders affecting SMCs and connective tissue
  - TGF-β-related vascular disorders (Loeys-Dietz), fibrillin disorders (Marfan), type III collagen (Ehlers-Danlos)
- Tertiary syphilis rare cause of TAA
  - Immune reaction to infection → proliferative endarteritis of vasa vasorum → media ischemia

CLINICAL ISSUES

Epidemiology

- Major risk factors
  - Nonmodifiable: ↑ age, male sex, family history, ethnicity
  - Modifiable: Hypertension, ↑ lipid, smoking
- Other: Systemic inflammation (↑ CRP), lipoprotein A, hyperhomocysteinemia, metabolic syndrome

Presentation

- Aortic atherosclerosis
  - Long preclinical phase then complications
    - Atheroemboli and obstruction (kidney, extremity, CNS, intestine, coronary)
    - Systemic disease coronary/cerebrovascular ischemia
- Complications
  - Abdominal aortic aneurysm (AAA)
    - ~ 5-7% of population > 60 years of age, older men (> 50 years), smokers; M:F = 3.8-6:1
      - 10th leading cause of death in men > 55 years of age
    - Asymptomatic (~ 66-75%), pain, lack of pulses, claudication, emboli, pulsatile mass, branch obstruction, compression of adjacent structures (ureters, vertebral erosion), rupture
  - TAA
    - 3-4% of population > 65 years of age, ~ 95% asymptomatic (imaging Dx), usually hypertension history
      - Pain (impending rupture/dissection), aortic regurgitation, thromboemboli, mass effect (airway, superior vena cava, esophagus, vertebrae)
    - Rupture: Acute pain, shock, hemothorax, tamponade
    - Fistula formation: Hemoptysis, hematemesis, L → R shunt (airway, esophagus, pulmonary artery)
  - Inflammatory atherosclerotic aneurysm (IAA)
    - 2-15% of resected aortic aneurysms, usually in men, usually severe atherosclerosis
    - May have systemic signs of inflammation with elevated inflammatory markers (CRP)
    - Important to distinguish clinically from rheumatologic diseases, especially IgG4-related periaortitis
      - Check for autoimmune disease; may also be associated with retroperitoneal fibrosis/sclerosing mediastinitis
  - Penetrating aortic ulcer
    - Typically seen in men > 70 years of age; comorbidities (hypertension, smoking, coronary artery disease, COPD)
    - 2.3-11% of acute aortic syndromes
    - Contrast-enhanced CT: Outpouching ulcer crater, intimal calcification, localized intramural hemorrhage, severe atherosclerotic disease
  - Occlusive aortic thrombosis
    - Classic presentation Leriche syndrome in middle-aged men, usually smokers
      - Inability to maintain erection, leg fatigue on walking/standing, buttock/limb atrophy, foot pallor on standing

Treatment

- Modify risk factors with lifestyle and drug therapy
- Aneurysm repair: Surgical, endovascular (EVAR), and combination (EVAR + limited open surgery)

Prognosis

- AAA
  - Risk of rupture ↑ with ↑ diameter, F > M, high mortality rate
    - 4-5 cm: 1%/year; 5-6 cm: 11%/year; > 6 cm: 25%/year
  - Indications for repair
    - Diameter 5.5 cm or 2.5x normal or growth > 1 cm/year
- Thoracic aortic aneurysm (TAA)
  - Risk of rupture and dissection ↑ with ↑ diameter; F > M
    - < 6 cm: 5-6.5%; > 6 cm: 14%
- Penetrating aortic ulcer
  - When symptomatic risk of rupture > aortic dissection types A or B (40% vs. 7% and 3.6%)

MACROSCOPIC

General Features

- Aortic atherosclerosis: Early lesions
  - Intimal thickening around branch vessel ostia, posterior aspect of aortic wall
  - Progressive lipid deposition → fatty streaks
- Aortic atherosclerosis: Atheromatous plaque
  - Progressive extracellular lipid accumulation → soft necrotic core with overlying fibrous cap
  - Progressive fibrosis and calcification
- Aortic atherosclerosis: Complicated lesions
  - Ulceration of fibrous cap usually overlying thrombus
- Complications: Aneurysms
  - AAA
    - True, usually fusiform aneurysm, usually infrarenal, mural thrombus with lines of Zahn
    - ↑ diameter may have rupture; common site distal to renal arteries, left lateral
  - TAA
    - Atherosclerosis slightly less severe than AAA; thin wall due to degeneration of media
    - Fusiform true aneurysm, may have evidence of dissection
  - IAA
    - Markedly thick-walled aneurysm with extensive adhesions to adjacent structures
- Complications: Pseudoaneurysm
  - Localized periaortic hematoma, usually saccular shape
    - Often prior surgical/endovascular procedure with vascular disruption, penetrating aortic ulcer
    - Thin neck connecting vessel lumen to pseudoaneurysm
- Complications: Penetrating aortic ulcer
  - Deep ulceration of aortic atherosclerotic plaque into media, often descending thoracic
    - Intramural hematoma, pseudoaneurysm, rupture
- Complications: Occlusive aortic thrombosis
  - Distal aorta at bifurcation, severe atherosclerosis with thrombosis and markedly ↓ lumen

MICROSCOPIC

Histologic Features

- Aortic atherosclerosis: Early lesions
  - Thickened intima (VSMC migrating into intima)
  - Intimal foam cells (mostly macrophages) and scattered lymphocytes in fatty streak
- Aortic atherosclerosis: Atheromatous plaque progression
  - Intimal collection of extracellular lipid with inflammation, no significant fibrosis, and little change in media
  - Fibrosis around lipid, increasing thickening of intima, progressive degenerative changes of media with thinning, loss of SMCs, attenuation of elastic lamellae
- Aortic atherosclerosis: Complicated lesions
  - Rupture of fibrous cap overlying necrotic plaque center with thrombus, intraplaque hemorrhage
  - Increasing degeneration of aortic media
- AAA
  - Severe atherosclerosis, marked degeneration of media (loss of elastic tissue, SMCs), fibrosis, mild adventitial inflammation ± hemorrhage or hemosiderin-laden macrophages (evidence of rupture)
    - Media may no longer be visible
    - Overlying thrombus in aneurysm does not organize; newer thrombus abluminal with red blood cells, fibrin, leukocytes, and older thrombus peripheral with cellular degeneration
    - Recent hemorrhage in older thrombus material suggests aneurysm expansion
- TAA
  - Fragmentation of elastic fibers and cystic medial degeneration, variable intimal thickening, and variable atherosclerotic change (↑ with ↑ age at presentation)
- IAA
  - Aneurysm-type changes of aortic wall with marked fibrosis and inflammation in adventitia
    - Plasma cells, lymphocytes, lymphoid aggregates, arteritis and venulitis in adventitial vessels
    - Less frequent granulomatous inflammation with giant cells

ANCILLARY TESTS

Histochemistry

- Elastic stain

SELECTED REFERENCES

1. Hellawell HN et al: Abdominal aortic aneurysms part one: epidemiology, presentation and preoperative considerations. J Perioper Pract. 31(7-8):274-80, 2021
2. Kyriacou H et al: Abdominal aortic aneurysms part two: surgical management, postoperative complications and surveillance. J Perioper Pract. 31(9):319-25, 2021
3. Evangelista A et al: Penetrating atherosclerotic ulcer. Curr Opin Cardiol. 35(6):620-6, 2020
4. Ramos C et al: Perioperative outcomes for abdominal aortic aneurysm repair based on aneurysm diameter. Vasc Endovascular Surg. 54(4):341-7, 2020
5. Leone O et al: The complex interplay among atherosclerosis, inflammation, and degeneration in ascending thoracic aortic aneurysms. J Thorac Cardiovasc Surg. 160(6):1434-43.e6, 2020
6. Ullery BW et al: Epidemiology and contemporary management of abdominal aortic aneurysms. Abdom Radiol (NY). 43(5):1032-43, 2018
7. Maleszewski JJ: Inflammatory ascending aortic disease: perspectives from pathology. J Thorac Cardiovasc Surg. 149(2 Suppl):S176-83, 2015

Early Atherosclerotic Changes in Thoracic Aorta

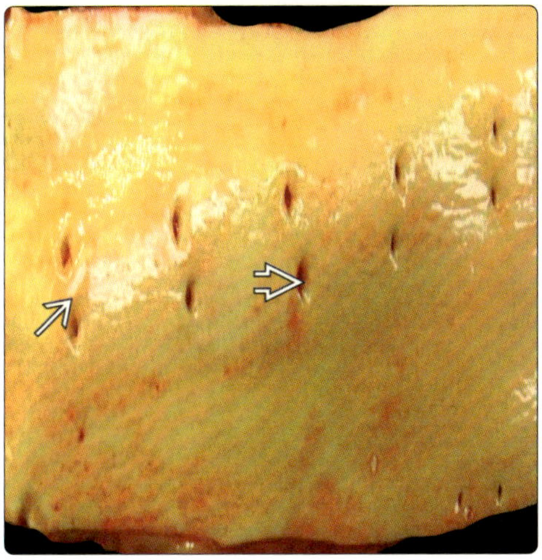

Complicated Atherosclerotic Plaque in Abdominal Aorta

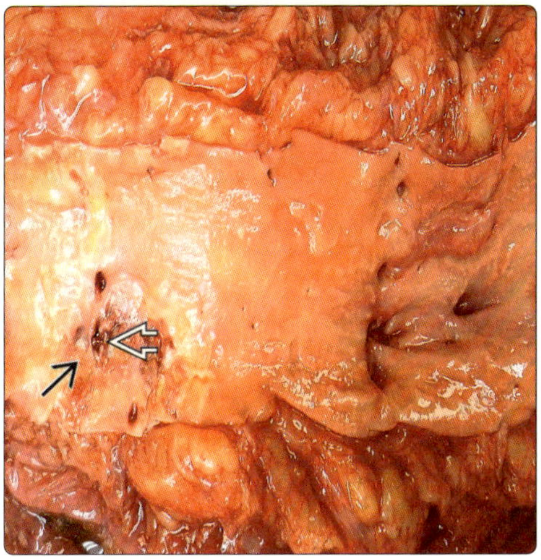

(Left) *Aortic intimal surface demonstrates early lesions of atherosclerosis with areas of intimal thickening ➡ predominantly around branch vessel ostia ➡. This preferential location is likely due to hemodynamics.* **(Right)** *This infrarenal aorta viewed from the intimal surface reveals complicated atherosclerotic plaque ⇨ with ulceration of the surface and overlying thrombus ➡. At this point in atherosclerotic disease, medial degenerative changes are not prominent.*

Histologic Features of Atherosclerotic Plaque

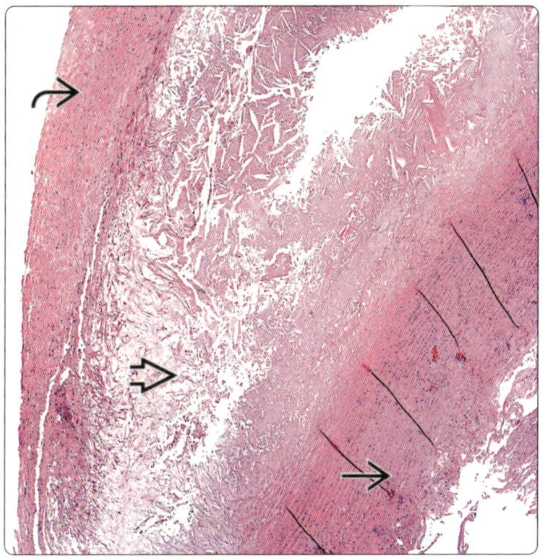

Cholesterol Embolization Involving Renal Artery

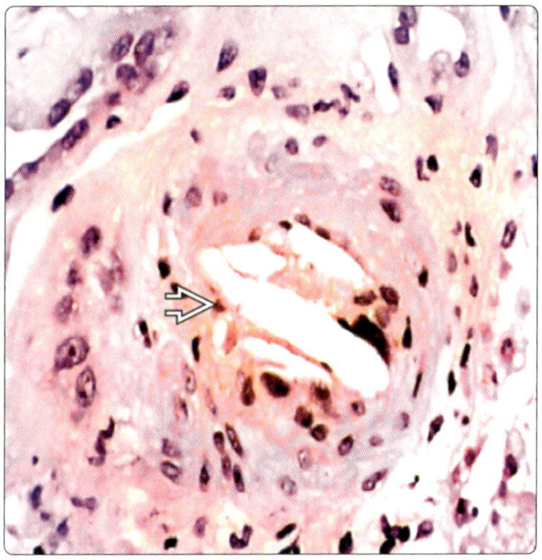

(Left) *This plaque has an intact fibrous cap ⇨, large necrotic center ⇨ with abundant cholesterol crystals, and a nondegenerated media ⇨, indicative of mild aortic atherosclerosis.* **(Right)** *Atheroembolic complications may be seen in atherosclerosis or aneurysmal disease. This renal artery is filled with cholesterol crystals ➡. The emboli arose from an abdominal aortic aneurysm.*

Advanced Atherosclerosis With Renal Artery Ostial Obstruction

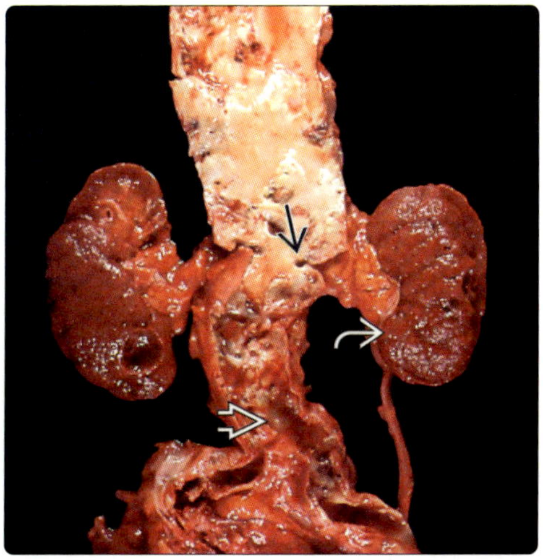

Aneurysm With Renal Artery Ostial Obstruction

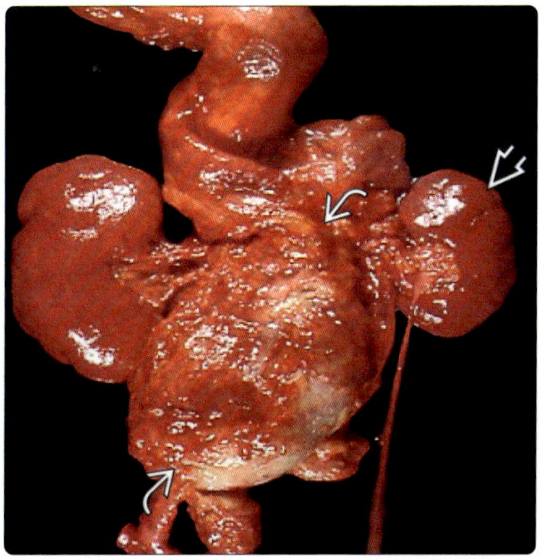

(Left) *Aorta with more advanced atherosclerosis becoming confluent in the infrarenal portion ➡ shows ostial obstruction, a complication of atherosclerosis. Right renal artery obstruction ⇨ is noted with associated renal atrophy ➡.* **(Right)** *Major branch obstruction is another complication of aneurysms. This juxtarenal abdominal aortic aneurysm ➡ is associated with obstruction of the left renal artery, as denoted by the atrophic left kidney ➡.*

Ruptured Infrarenal Aneurysm

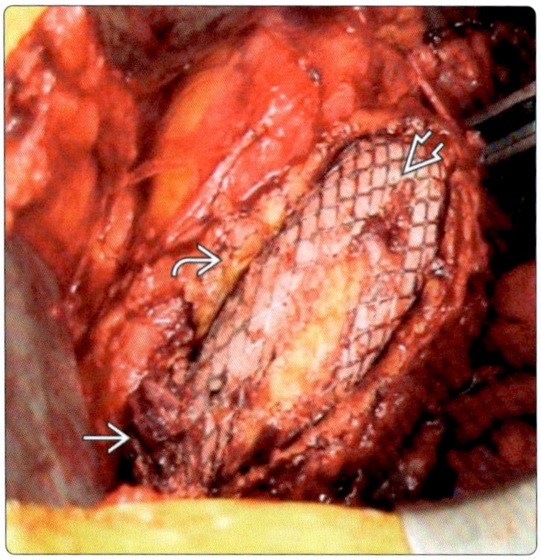

Histologic Features of Ruptured Aneurysm

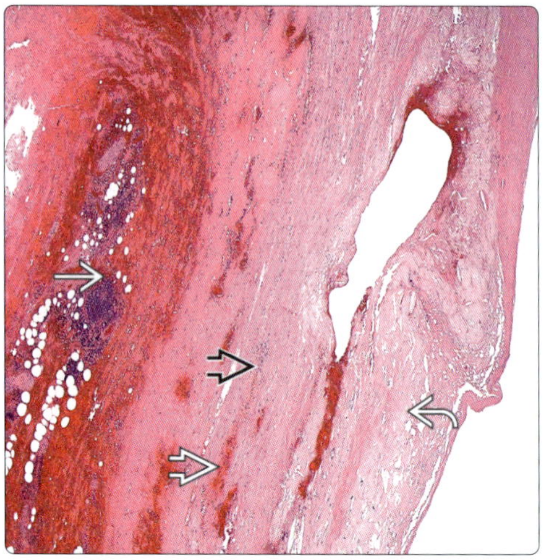

(Left) *This ruptured infrarenal aneurysm has an endovascular stent ➔. The aneurysm wall ↪ is thin, and there is hematoma → around the distal aneurysm due to rupture. (Courtesy S. A. Rahimi, MD.)* **(Right)** *Ruptured aneurysm shows plaque at the luminal surface ↩, hemorrhage through the wall ⇨, and recent adventitial hematoma as well as inflammation →. The media is quite thin ⇨. (Courtesy E. Sadimin, MD.)*

Elastic Stain of Aneurysm Wall

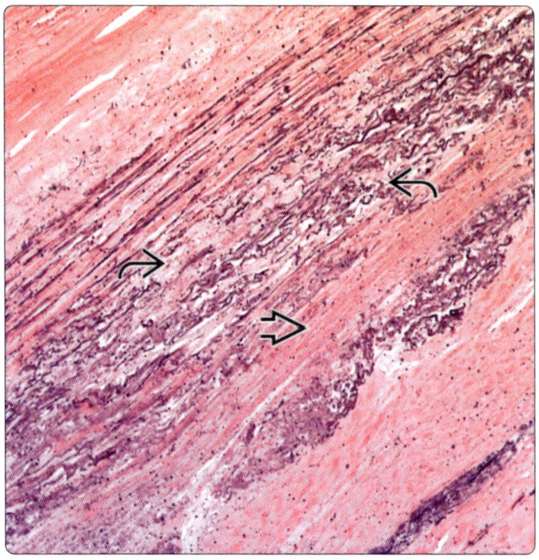

Adventitial Changes in Aneurysm Wall

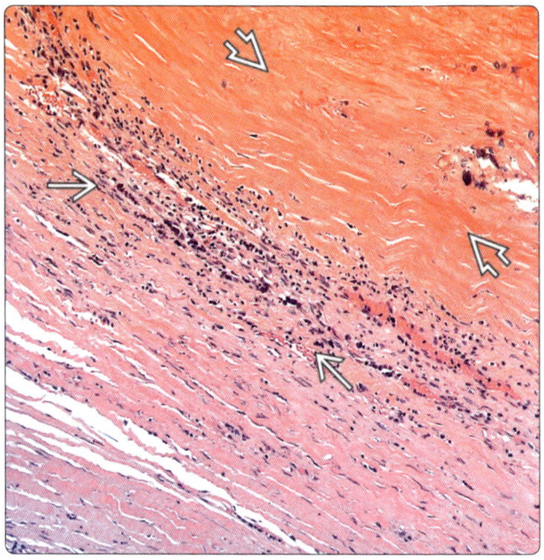

(Left) *Elastic stain of an aneurysm wall shows marked thinning and fragmentation of elastic lamellae ↪ and loss of elastic tissue ⇨.* **(Right)** *Inflammation, including lymphocytes and occasional plasma cells, is common in aneurysm walls. There is marked destruction of the media ⇨, and the inflammation is in the adventitial tissue →. Marked inflammation in a thick aneurysm wall with perianeurysmal adhesion would suggest inflammatory aortic aneurysm.*

CTA of Pseudoaneurysm

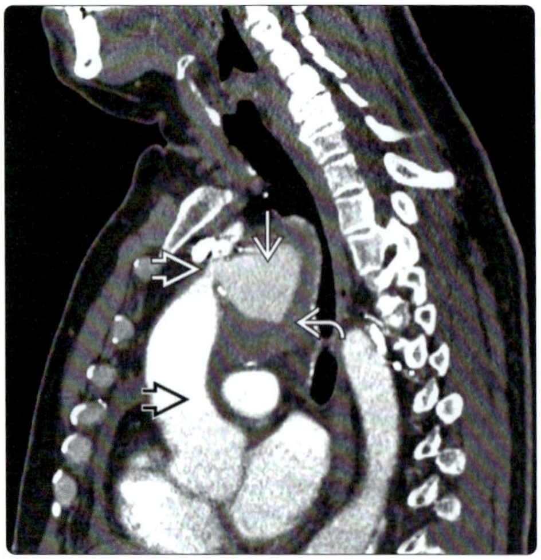

Aortic Pseudoaneurysm

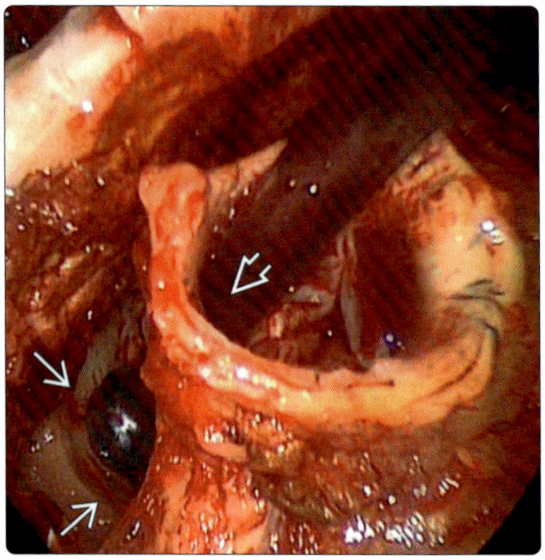

(Left) *CTA of an innominate artery pseudoaneurysm shows contrast in the aorta ⇨, the thin neck region ⇨ (perforation), and the pseudoaneurysm → with surrounding older hematoma that is less radiopaque ↩. (Courtesy G. Batsides, MD.)* **(Right)** *A cannula ⇨ is inserted through the ascending aorta into a pseudoaneurysm →. This pseudoaneurysm formed as a consequence of infection after ascending aortic repair. (Courtesy G. Batsides, MD.)*

Aneurysm Graft Thrombosis

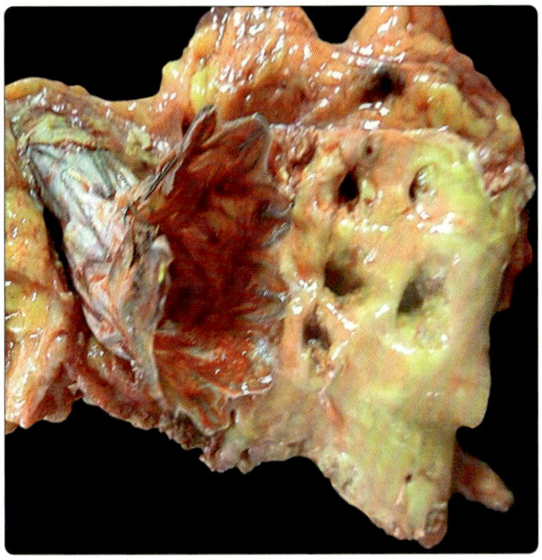

Proximal Portion of Endovascular Graft

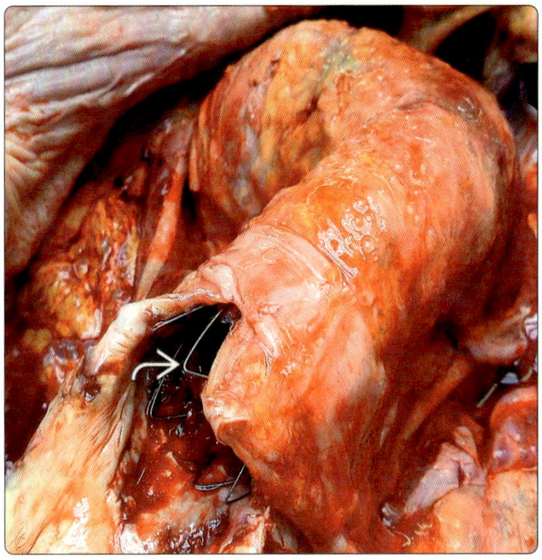

(Left) *Proximal graft inserted into this infrarenal aneurysm is covered with cloth and attached to the aorta beneath the renal artery ostia. In order to evaluate the aneurysm wall, it is necessary to peel away the tissue from around the graft. (Courtesy J. Chiaffarano, MD.)* **(Right)** *Some endovascular grafts have a bare metal proximal portion in order to allow perfusion to major vessels, such as renal arteries, if the aneurysm is juxta- or suprarenal.*

Ascending Aorta Aneurysm

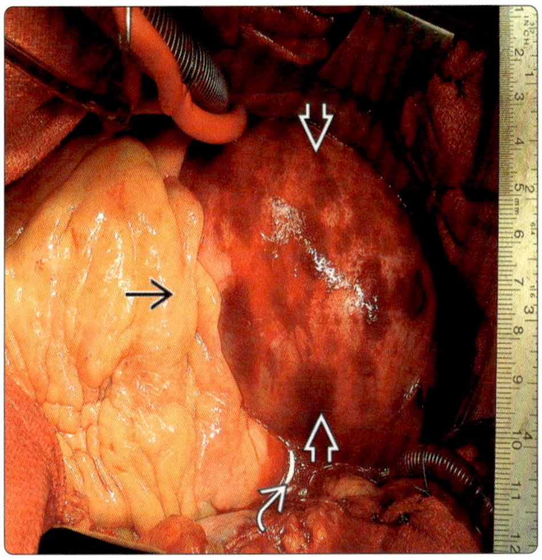

Thoracic Aorta Aneurysm Wall

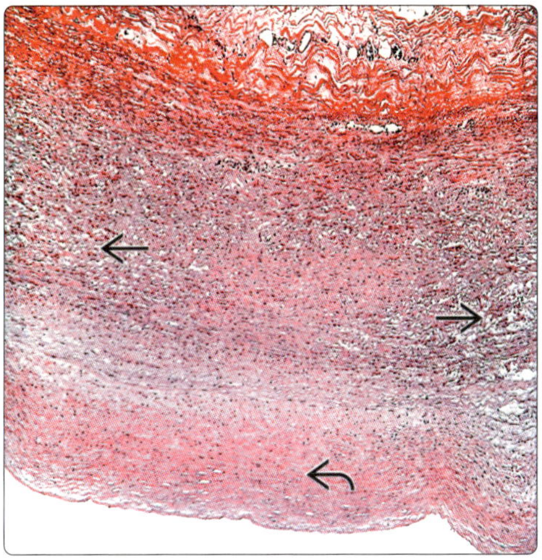

(Left) *This ascending aortic aneurysm (heart, pulmonary artery) required repair due to its large size. (Courtesy G. Batsides, MD.)* **(Right)** *Thoracic aneurysm wall shows degenerative changes in the media. There is intimal thickening without atherosclerotic plaque. The media demonstrates loss of staining of nuclei of smooth muscle cells and increase in proteoglycans.*

Thrombus Within Aneurysm

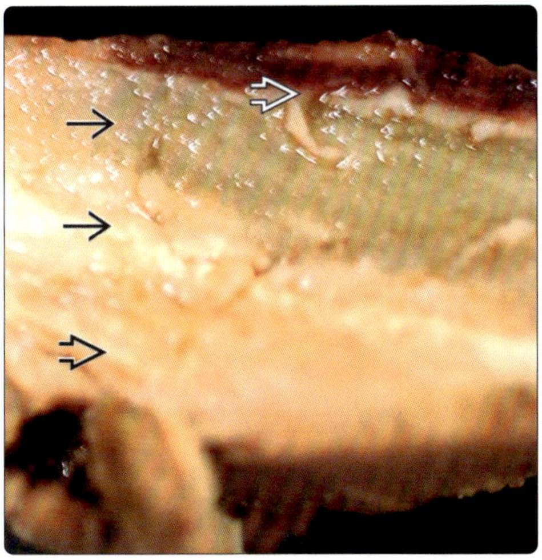

Thrombus Retrieved From Aortic Aneurysm

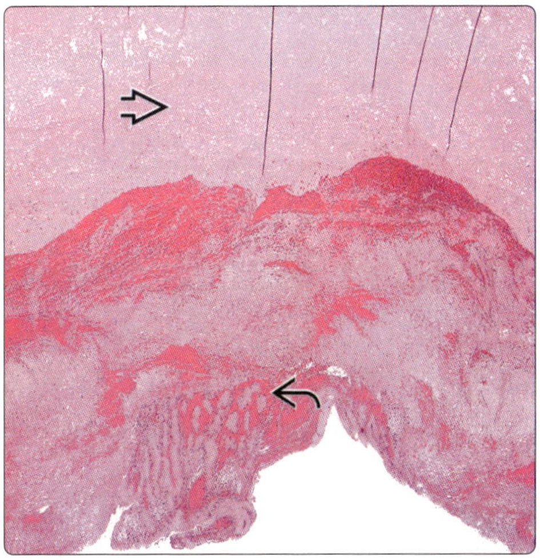

(Left) *Aneurysm thrombi do not organize, are laminated (lines of Zahn), and contain decolorized degenerated thrombus on the deep portion with more recent red-appearing thrombus along the lumen. Deep recent hemorrhage would indicate aneurysm growth.* **(Right)** *Histologically, these thrombi show more recent thrombus along the luminal surface (layered RBCs, fibrin) and homogeneous older thrombus without cellular detail. (Courtesy E. Sadimin, MD.)*

Chronic Periaortitis and IgG4-Related Disease

KEY FACTS

TERMINOLOGY

- Aortitis &/or periaortitis of thoracic &/or abdominal aorta, characterized by storiform fibrosis, plasma cell-rich inflammation, and increased proportion of IgG4-producing plasma cells

ETIOLOGY/PATHOGENESIS

- First recognized in autoimmune sclerosing pancreatitis but since reported in many organ systems

CLINICAL ISSUES

- Predominantly in older men
- Abdominal or back pain, malaise, fever
- Elevated acute-phase reactants
- Elevated levels of IgG4
- Ureteral obstruction and hydronephrosis
- Inflammatory abdominal aortic aneurysm
- Retroperitoneal fibrosis
- Ascending aortic aneurysm

MACROSCOPIC

- Marked mural thickening of aortic wall and fibrosis of periaortic tissue

MICROSCOPIC

- Adventitial scarring and lymphoplasmacytic inflammation
- Storiform pattern of dense adventitial sclerosis with entrapment of nerves, obliterative phlebitis, and thrombosed small arteries
- Adventitial lymphoid aggregates
- Exclusion criteria: Infection and granulomatous inflammation

ANCILLARY TESTS

- > 50 IgG4-positive plasma cells per standard 40x objective HPF
- IgG4:IgG ratio > 0.5 (counted in 3 HPFs with most IgG4 staining)

(Left) *Contrast-enhanced CT of the pelvis shows marked thickening of the aortic wall and fibrosis in the periaortic soft tissue. These findings are consistent with chronic periaortitis.* **(Right)** *High-magnification view of periaortic soft tissue in a case of chronic periaortitis shows abundant plasma cells, a substantial proportion of which stained positively for IgG4.*

CT Findings in Chronic Periaortitis

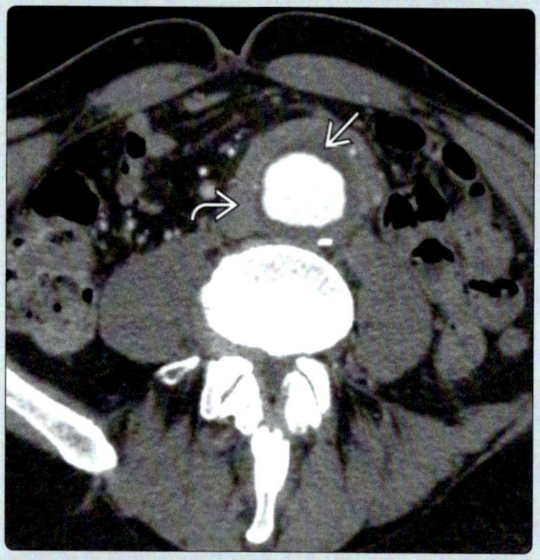

Periaortic Tissue

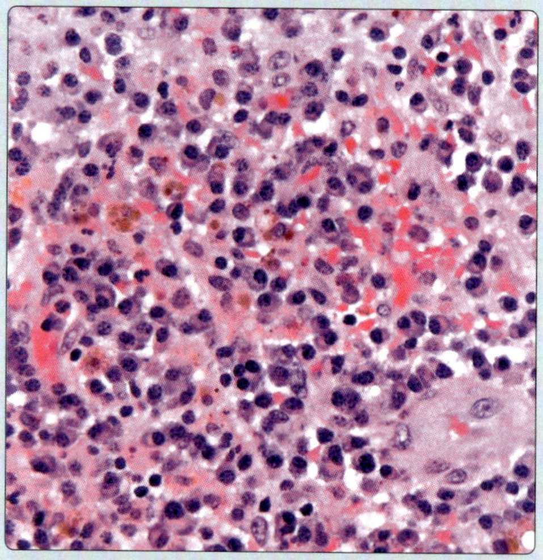

(Left) *Aortic wall shows a prominent lymphoplasmacytic infiltrate involving the media and adventitia. The plasma cells are aggregated in tight clusters.* **(Right)** *IgG4 shows abundant positive plasma cells. In IgG4-related disease, > 50 plasma cells are seen per HPF.*

Aorta Wall With Plasma Cell Infiltration of Media and Adventitia

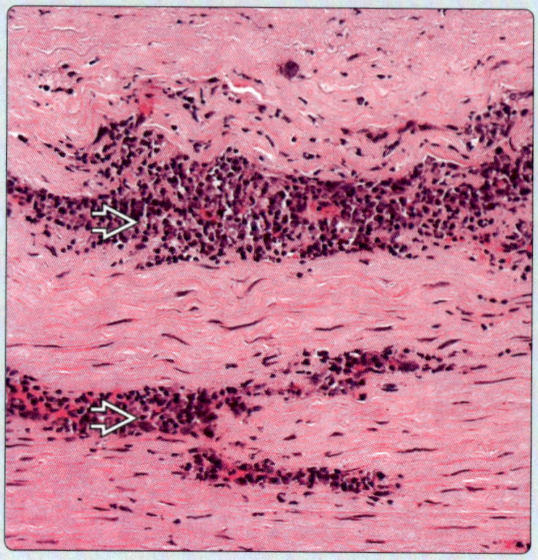

Immunohistochemical Stain for IgG4

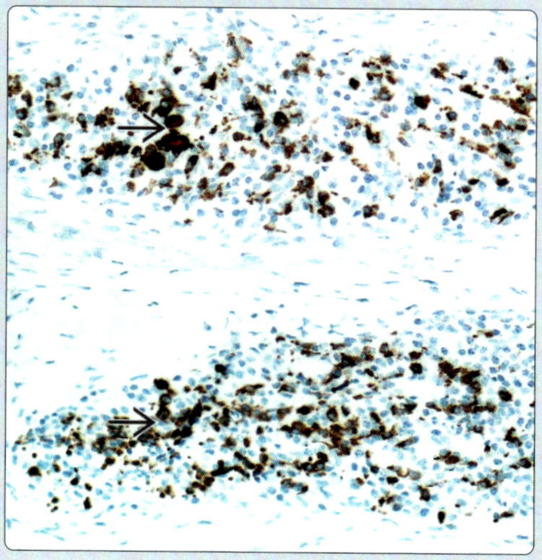

TERMINOLOGY

Synonyms

- Inflammatory abdominal aortic aneurysm
- Inflammatory periaortitis
- Hyper-IgG4 syndrome
- IgG4-related sclerosing disease

Definitions

- Aortitis &/or periaortitis of thoracic &/or abdominal aorta, characterized by storiform fibrosis, plasma cell-rich inflammation, and ↑ IgG4-producing plasma cells

ETIOLOGY/PATHOGENESIS

Idiopathic Sclerosing Disorder

- First recognized in autoimmune sclerosing pancreatitis but since reported as
  - Sialadenitis and lacrimal gland inflammation
  - Sclerosing cholangitis
  - Tubulointerstitial nephritis
  - Inflammatory pseudotumors (especially orbital)

IgG4 Characteristics

- In quiescent immune states, IgG4 is least abundant IgG subclass (< 5%)
- Noncomplement fixing
- Intermediate Fc portion affinity for antibody-dependent cell-mediated cytotoxicity
- Postulated role in development of tolerance to allergens

CLINICAL ISSUES

Presentation

- Predominantly in older men
- Abdominal or back pain, malaise, fever
- Elevated acute-phase reactants
- Ureteral obstruction and hydronephrosis

Laboratory Tests

- Elevated levels of IgG4 > 2x upper limits

Treatment

- Corticosteroids
- Surgical resection
- Endovascular stent grafting

Associated Manifestations

- Retroperitoneal fibrosis
- Sclerosing mesenteritis
- Sclerosing mediastinitis
- Ascending aortic aneurysm
- Multifocal fibrosclerosis (multiple organ systems involved)

IMAGING

Radiographic Findings

- Contrast-enhanced CT and MR best diagnostic modalities
  - Aortic wall thickening with relative posterior sparing
  - Periaortic soft tissue thickening with medial displacement of ureters

MACROSCOPIC

General Features

- Marked mural thickening of aortic wall and fibrosis of periaortic tissue
- ± atherosclerosis

MICROSCOPIC

Histologic Features

- Adventitial scarring and lymphoplasmacytic inflammation
  - Often with sheets of plasma cells
- Storiform pattern of dense adventitial sclerosis with
  - Entrapment of nerves
  - Obliterative phlebitis
  - Thrombosed small arteries
- Adventitial lymphoid aggregates

Exclusion Criteria

- Rule out infection
- Granulomatous inflammation should be absent

ANCILLARY TESTS

Immunohistochemistry

- IgG4
  - Consensus criteria
    - > 50 IgG4-positive plasma cells per standard 40x objective HPF
    - IgG4:IgG ratio > 0.5 (3 HPFs with most IgG4 staining)
- IgG or IgG1
  - To highlight all IgG-producing plasma cells (including IgG4), provide denominator for IgG4:IgG ratio
- CD138
  - To highlight all plasma cells present (useful if morphology is unusual)

DIFFERENTIAL DIAGNOSIS

Lymphoplasmacytic Aortitis

- No increase in IgG4 plasma cells

Atherosclerosis With Penetrating Ulcer

- Complicated atherosclerotic plaque associated with inflammation is present
- Occasionally aneurysmal dilatation, hematoma, or localized dissection are associated

Syphilitic Aortitis

- Involvement of proximal aorta is more frequent
- Aneurysm formation
- Lymphoplasmacytic inflammation involves vasa vasorum of adventitia with extension into media

SELECTED REFERENCES

1. Paratz ED et al: Intracoronary IgG4-related disease as an unusual cause of sudden cardiac arrest: a case series. Eur Heart J Case Rep. 6(2):ytac050, 2022
2. Takahashi K et al: IgG4-related periaortitis initially suspected of being an aortic intramural hematoma in the ascending aorta. Ann Vasc Dis. 14(4):380-3, 2021
3. Stone JR et al: Consensus statement on surgical pathology of the aorta from the Society for Cardiovascular Pathology and the Association for European Cardiovascular Pathology: I. Inflammatory diseases. Cardiovasc Pathol. 24(5):267-78, 2015

Mycotic Aneurysm

KEY FACTS

TERMINOLOGY

- Aneurysm that results from or is secondarily infected by organisms (usually bacteria) arising from distant site of infection

ETIOLOGY/PATHOGENESIS

- Primary: Infection of artery wall with secondary aneurysm development (uncommon)
- Secondary: Infection occurs in preexisting atherosclerotic aneurysm; usually arises from distant site (e.g., heart valve endocarditis, bacteremia)

CLINICAL ISSUES

- Incidence: Unknown, but estimated to be 0.65-2.00% of all aortic aneurysms
- Symptoms: Fever, localized pain, sepsis, pulsatile mass
- Formation of aneurysm may evolve rapidly, over course of days, or after initiation of aortitis
- Rupture is frequent (75%) without surgical and antibiotic treatment
- Mortality rate estimated at 67% without treatment

IMAGING

- Rapidly growing saccular aneurysm arising eccentrically from aortic wall
- Can involve any part of aorta wall or other vessels

MACROSCOPIC

- Saccular outpouchings are most common type
- Thin wall with periaortic inflammatory changes
- Marked edema of adventitia
- Calcification is uncommon

MICROSCOPIC

- Transmural acute inflammation with microabscesses, chronic inflammatory infiltrate, nonnecrotizing granulomatous inflammation; pseudoaneurysm, adventitia with chronic inflammation and dense fibrosis

Aorta Mycotic Aneurysm

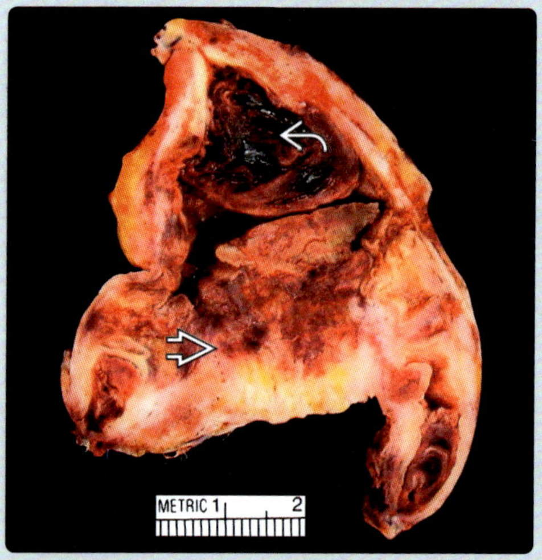

Histology of Mycotic Aneurysm

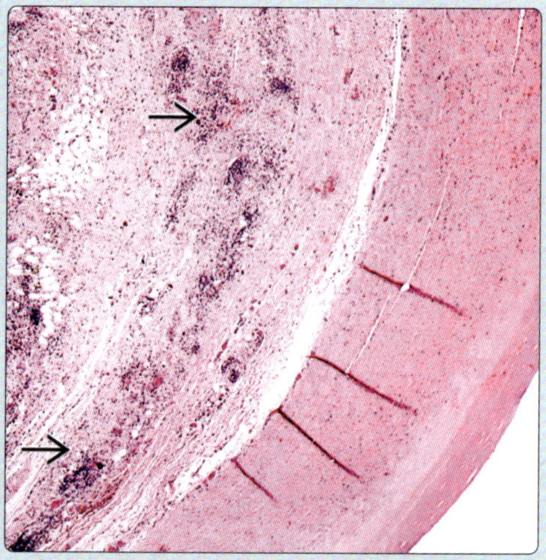

(Left) *Gross photograph of a mycotic aneurysm involving the aorta shows wall thickening as well as an organized thrombus in the lumen. The periaortic connective and adipose tissue show inflammatory changes.* **(Right)** *H&E-stained section of the aorta wall shows aggregates of inflammatory cells in the adventitia extending into the periaortic adipose and connective tissues in a case of mycotic aneurysm.*

Aorta Mycotic Aneurysm

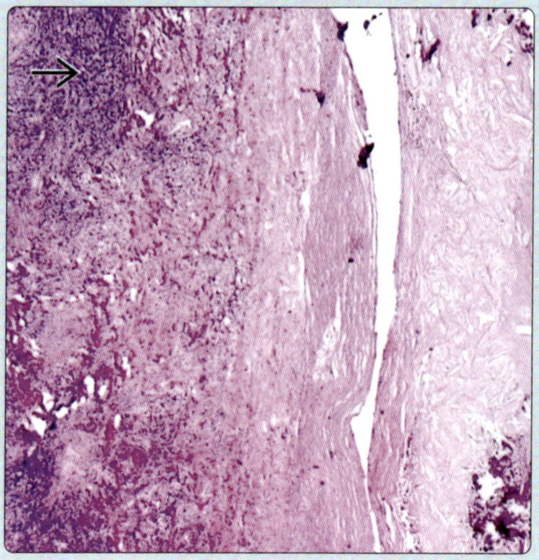

Gram Stain of Mycotic Aneurysm

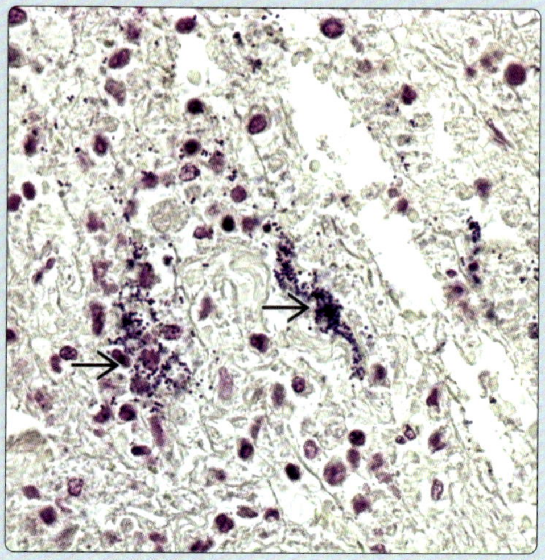

(Left) *H&E-stained section of the aorta wall shows atherosclerotic plaque, and in the media, there are aggregates of inflammatory cells. The inflammation extended into the adventitia and the periaortic adipose and connective tissues.* **(Right)** *Higher magnification Gram stain of the aorta wall mycotic aneurysm shows several aggregates of gram-positive cocci seen admixed with inflammatory cells.*

TERMINOLOGY

Synonyms

- Infectious aneurysm

Definitions

- Aneurysm that results from or is secondarily infected by microorganisms (usually bacteria) arising from distant site of infection

ETIOLOGY/PATHOGENESIS

Infectious Agents

- Most common organisms reported in preantibiotic era
  - *Treponema pallidum* (syphilis agent)
  - *Pneumococcus*
  - *Staphylococci*
  - *Gonococcus*
- Most common organisms reported in postantibiotic era
  - *Salmonella* species reported most frequently in Asia
  - *Staphylococcus aureus*
  - *Streptococcus species*
- Less common organisms: Gram positive (*Enteroccocci*, *Bacillus cereus*), gram negative (*Escherichia coli*, *Proteus*, *Bacteroides*, *Haemophilus*)
- Fungi (*Candida*, *Aspergillus*, *Cryptococcus*, *Paracoccidioides brasiliensis*)
- ~ 30% are culture negative

Pathogenesis

- Primary
  - Infection of artery wall with secondary aneurysm development
  - Uncommon type
- Secondary
  - Infection occurs in preexisting atherosclerotic aneurysm
  - Infection usually arises in distant site (e.g., heart valve endocarditis)
  - Seeding after bacteremia episode may also occur

Routes of Artery Wall Infection

- Implantation on intimal surface
  - Complication of recent or remote bacterial endocarditis
  - Most often seeding of existing lesion (atheroma or aneurysm)
- Embolization of bacteria into vasa vasorum
- Direct extension of infection from contiguous extravascular site
  - Complication of vertebral osteomyelitis
  - Pancreatitis
  - Psoas abscess
  - Mediastinal infection
- Traumatic inoculation of contaminated material into vessel wall
- Lymphatic spread

CLINICAL ISSUES

Epidemiology

- Incidence
  - Unknown but estimated to be 0.65-2.00% of all aortic aneurysms
    - In Taiwan, reported incidence is 13%
  - Increased risk in
    - IV drug users
    - Patients with prior bacterial endocarditis
    - Immunocompromised patients (e.g., diabetes mellitus, glucocorticoids use, chemotherapy, &/or malignancy)
    - Patients with vascular prostheses (valves, vascular grafts)
    - Intravascular procedures

Site

- Femoral artery (~ 56%)
- Abdominal aorta (~ 18%)
- Thoracic aorta (~ 15%)
- Mesenteric and peripheral arteries (~ 11%)

Presentation

- Fever
- Localized pain (e.g., back, abdomen)
- Rapidly enlarging pulsatile mass
- Sepsis

Laboratory Tests

- Blood and tissue cultures are necessary to identify microorganism and for diagnosis
  - Blood cultures reported positive in 74% in 1 series
  - Tissue cultures reported positive in 50% in 1 series
- Leukocytosis is frequent
- Elevated erythrocyte sedimentation rate and C-reactive protein

Natural History

- Formation of aneurysm may evolve rapidly, over course of days, after initiation of aortitis
- Rupture is frequent (75%) without surgical and antibiotic treatment

Treatment

- Surgical approaches
  - Open surgical repair
  - Endovascular repair is acceptable alternative
- Drugs
  - Intravenous broad-spectrum antibiotics

Prognosis

- Mortality rate estimated at 30-50% without treatment
  - Risk factors include older age, ruptured aneurysm, suprarenal location, extensive periaortic infection, psoas muscle abscess, aortoenteric fistula formation, and *S. aureus* infection

IMAGING

General Features

- Rapidly growing saccular aneurysm arising eccentrically from aortic wall
- Can involve any part of aorta wall or other vessels

MR Findings

- T1WI
  - Periaortic low signal intensity in absence of gadolinium
  - Aortic and periaortic enhancement post gadolinium

- T2WI
  - Periaortic high signal intensity on fat-suppressed images
- Contrast-enhanced MRA
  - 1 or more saccular aneurysms arising from aorta wall
  - Effacement of wall with possible leakage at rupture site

CT Findings

- NECT
  - Usually not calcified
  - Periaortic soft tissue stranding, edema, and fluid frequently present
  - Periaortic gas
  - Adjacent vertebral body abnormalities due to spread of infection
- CECT
  - 1 or more saccular aneurysms arising from artery wall
  - Lobular contours
  - Enhancement of periaortic soft tissue
  - Rim enhancement in cases with abscess

FDG PET/CT

- Increased uptake in infected aneurysm wall
- Gas bubbles and fat stranding

MACROSCOPIC

General Features

- Saccular outpouchings are most common type
- Thin wall with periaortic inflammatory changes
- Marked edema of adventitia
- Calcification is uncommon

Size

- Variable, ranging 2.2-17.5 cm in 1 study

MICROSCOPIC

Histologic Features

- 6 patterns of aorta wall changes have been described
  - Pattern 1
    - Transmural acute inflammation with microabscesses
    - Atherosclerotic changes and marked attenuation of media
  - Pattern 2
    - Marked atherosclerotic changes
    - Chronic inflammatory infiltrate (lymphocytes, plasma cells, histiocytes)
  - Pattern 3
    - Transmural acute inflammation with microabscesses
    - No atherosclerotic changes
  - Pattern 4
    - Nonnecrotizing granulomatous inflammation
    - Associated periadventitial fibrosis with chronic inflammation
  - Pattern 5
    - Pseudoaneurysm
    - No significant inflammation
  - Pattern 6
    - Adventitia with chronic inflammation and dense fibrosis

ANCILLARY TESTS

Histochemistry

- Gram, AFB, and Grocott stains may contribute to microorganism identification

DIFFERENTIAL DIAGNOSIS

Atherosclerotic Aneurysm

- Slow growing
- More often fusiform
- Severe atherosclerosis is present
- Calcification and bony metaplasia are common
- Laminated yellow-brown thrombus is frequently identified
- Absence of significant inflammation

Inflammatory Aneurysm

- Distal aorta and iliac involvement
- Fusiform
- Marked wall fibrosis and perianeurysmal chronic inflammation
- Retroperitoneal fibrosis
- Possible etiologies
  - Autoimmune
  - Localized manifestation of systemic vasculitis

Contained Rupture

- Focal disruption or gap in artery wall may be identified
- Hematoma instead of inflammatory process surrounding artery wall

SELECTED REFERENCES

1. Cox K et al: A review on the deeper understanding of inflammation and infection of the thoracic aorta. Vascular. 17085381211060928, 2022
2. Han M et al: Systematic review and meta-analysis of outcomes following endovascular and open repair for infective native aortic aneurysms. Ann Vasc Surg. 79:348-58, 2022
3. Liesker DJ et al: Patient-tailored approach for diagnostics and treatment of mycotic abdominal aortic aneurysm. Ann Vasc Surg. 84:225-38, 2022
4. Shirasu T et al: Meta-analysis finds recurrent infection is more common after endovascular than after open repair of infected abdominal aortic aneurysm. J Vasc Surg. 75(1):348-55.e10, 2022
5. Sörelius K et al: The microbiology of infective native aortic aneurysms in a population-based setting. Ann Vasc Surg. 78:112-22, 2022
6. Touma J et al: Mycotic/infective native aortic aneurysms: results after preferential use of open surgery and arterial allografts. Eur J Vasc Endovasc Surg. 63(3):475-83, 2022
7. Zhang N et al: Imaging features of mycotic aortic aneurysms. Quant Imaging Med Surg. 11(6):2861-78, 2021
8. Cinar I et al: Clinically isolated aortitis: pitfalls, progress, and possibilities. Cardiovasc Pathol. 29:23-32, 2017
9. Tsai CC et al: Infected aortic and iliac aneurysms: clinical manifestations in the emergency departments of two hospitals in southern Taiwan, China. World J Emerg Med. 8(2):121-5, 2017
10. Murphy DJ et al: Cross-sectional imaging of aortic infections. Insights Imaging. 7(6):801-18, 2016
11. Sörelius K et al: Nationwide study of the treatment of mycotic abdominal aortic aneurysms comparing open and endovascular repair. Circulation. 134(23):1822-32, 2016
12. Töpel I et al: Inflammatory diseases of the aorta: part 2: infectious aortitis. Gefasschirurgie. 21(Suppl 2):87-93, 2016
13. Molacek J et al: Acute conditions caused by infectious aortitis. Aorta (Stamford). 2(3):93-9, 2014
14. Johnstone JK et al: Endovascular repair of mycotic aneurysm of the descending thoracic aorta. Ann Vasc Surg. 27(1):23-8, 2013
15. Hsu RB et al: Surgical pathology of infected aortic aneurysm and its clinical correlation. Ann Vasc Surg. 21(6):742-8, 2007
16. Miller DV et al: Surgical pathology of infected aneurysms of the descending thoracic and abdominal aorta: clinicopathologic correlations in 29 cases (1976 to 1999). Hum Pathol. 35(9):1112-20, 2004

Axial CECT of Mycotic Aneurysm

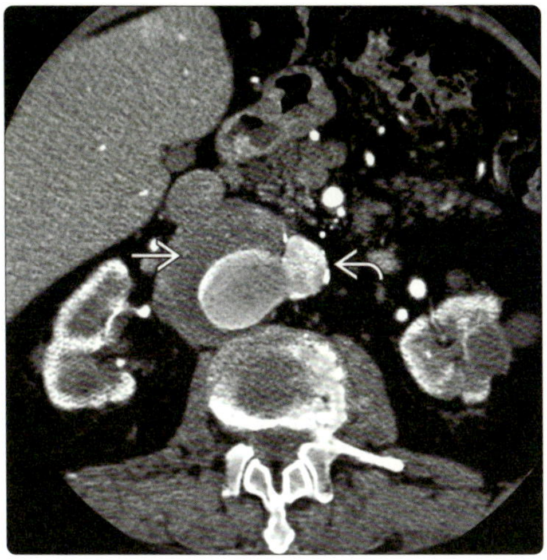

Mycotic Aneurysm, Pattern 2

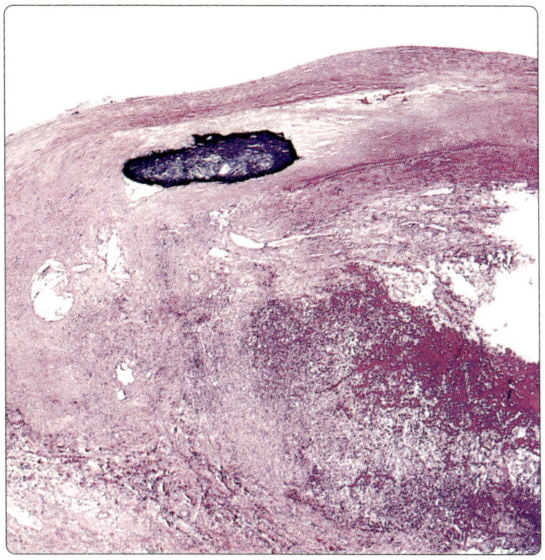

(Left) *Axial CECT shows a saccular outpouching from the abdominal aorta with mural thrombus corresponding to a mycotic aneurysm. Eccentric saccular appearance with involvement of a diseased segment of the arterial wall is characteristic. (Courtesy T. Grist, MD.)* **(Right)** *H&E-stained section of the aorta wall shows marked atherosclerotic changes with focal calcification. Scant inflammatory infiltrate involves the media, which also appears attenuated. These features correspond to pattern 2.*

Mycotic Aneurysm, Pattern 3

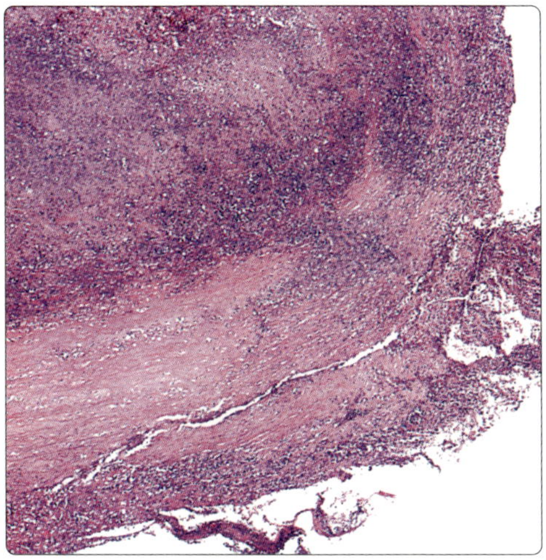

Mycotic Aneurysm, Pattern 3

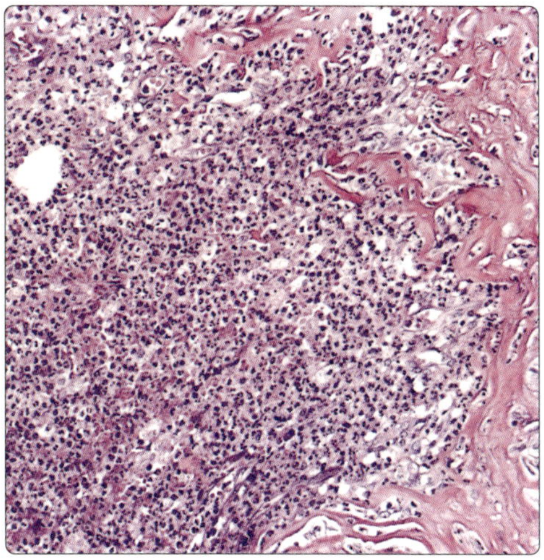

(Left) *H&E-stained section of a mycotic aneurysm shows marked inflammatory infiltrate involving all artery layers. There are no atherosclerotic changes or calcification. These features correspond to pattern 3. If atherosclerotic changes were present, these changes would correspond to pattern 1.* **(Right)** *At higher magnification, an H&E-stained section of a mycotic aneurysm shows marked neutrophilic infiltrate forming a microabscess. These features correspond to pattern 3.*

Elastic Stain of Mycotic Aneurysm, Pattern 6

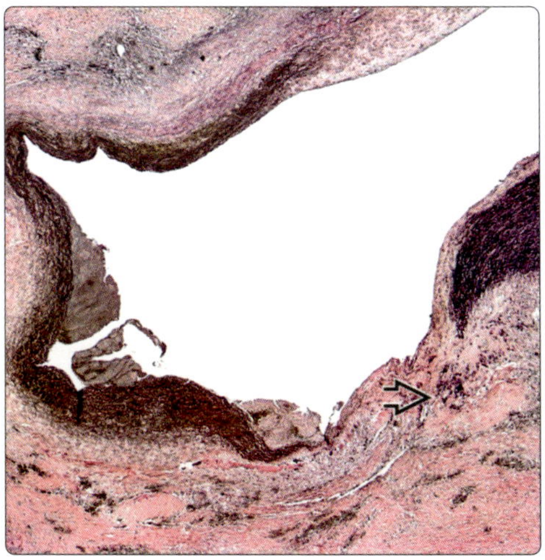

Elastic Stain of Mycotic Aneurysm, Pattern 6

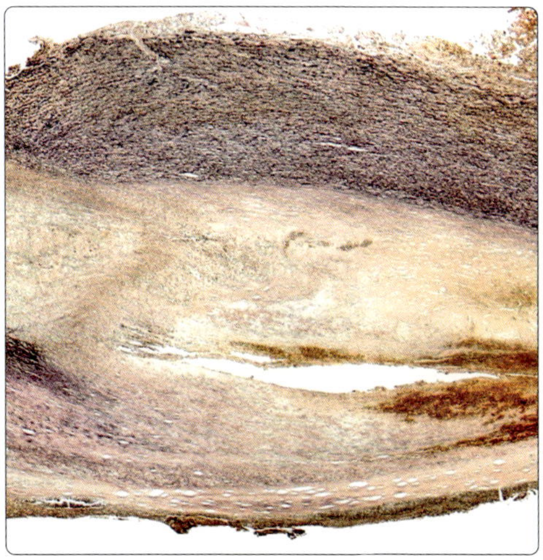

(Left) *Elastic stain of an aorta mycotic aneurysm shows segmental attenuation of the media layer, thickened adventitia with dense fibrosis, and scant chronic inflammatory infiltrate. These features correspond to pattern 6.* **(Right)** *Elastic stain of an aorta mycotic aneurysm shows thickened adventitia with dense fibrosis, but there is no significant inflammatory infiltrate. The media layer is not attenuated. These features correspond to pattern 6.*

KEY FACTS

TERMINOLOGY

- Progressive degenerative inflammatory disease characterized by accumulation of intra- and extracellular lipids, macrophages, T cells, proteoglycans, collagen, calcium in coronary artery intima

CLINICAL ISSUES

- Leading cause of acute coronary syndromes and death
- 1 in 3 males will suffer cardiac event before age 60
- Men more affected than premenopausal women
- Epicardial coronary arteries are most involved

MACROSCOPIC

- Gross evaluation of stenosis
  - Grade 1: < 25% cross-sectional luminal narrowing
  - Grade 2: 25-50% cross-sectional luminal narrowing
  - Grade 3: 50-75% cross-sectional luminal narrowing
  - Grade 4: > 75% cross-sectional luminal narrowing, considered critical stenosis

MICROSCOPIC

- American Heart Association classification
  - Grade 1: Isolated macrophages or foam cells
  - Grade 2: Intracellular lipid accumulation
  - Grade 3: Grade 2 lesions along with small, extracellular lipid pools
  - Grade 4: Grade 2 changes along with core of extracellular lipid
  - Grade 5: Lipid core and fibrous cap or multiple lipid cores and fibrous layers, calcific or fibrotic
  - Grade 6: More common grade 4 or 5 lesions with surface defect, &/or hematoma/hemorrhage, &/or thrombosis
- Plaque components
  - Cells: Smooth muscle, macrophages, T cells
  - Extracellular matrix, including collagen, elastic fibers, and proteoglycans
  - Lipids: Extra- and intracellular; mainly cholesterol and cholesterol esters

Atherosclerosis Pathogenesis

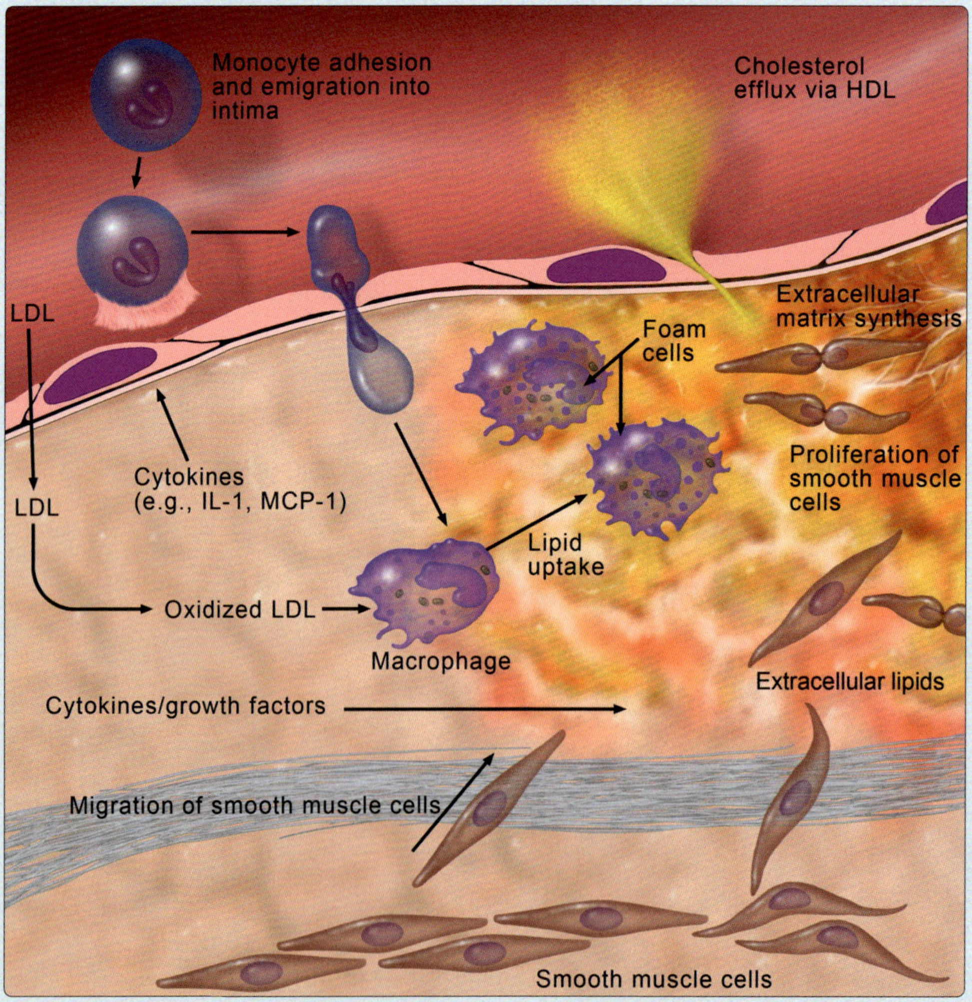

Graphic shows proposed cellular mechanisms of atherosclerosis pathogenesis. Hyperlipidemia and other factors cause endothelial injury, leading to adhesion of platelets and monocytes and the release of growth factors, inducing smooth muscle cell (SMC) migration and proliferation. SMCs produce extracellular matrix (collagen, proteoglycans). Foam cells result from macrophage differentiation through very low-density lipoprotein (VLDL) receptors and oxidized-LDL, recognized by scavenger receptors, and from SMCs by uncertain mechanisms. Extracellular lipid accumulation is 2nd to insudation from vessel lumen and degenerating foam cells.

TERMINOLOGY

Synonyms

- Coronary artery disease (CAD)

Definitions

- Progressive degenerative inflammatory disease characterized by accumulation of intra- and extracellular lipids, macrophages, T cells, proteoglycans, collagen, calcium in coronary artery intima
  - With obstruction of lumina and media weakening

CLINICAL ISSUES

Epidemiology

- Incidence
  - Leading cause of acute coronary syndromes and death
  - ~ 18.2 million Americans have CAD
  - 90% of cases are chronic obstructive CAD
- Age
  - 1 in 3 males will suffer cardiac event before age 60
- Sex
  - Men more affected than premenopausal women
- Ethnicity
  - White males more affected than Black males
  - Black females more affected than White females

Site

- Epicardial coronary arteries are most involved

Presentation

- Angina
  - Chronic stable
    - Chest pain on exertion
    - Released by rest or nitroglycerin use
  - Unstable
    - New-onset pain with minimal exertion
    - Chest pain at rest
  - Variant (Prinzmetal)
    - Chest pain exclusively at rest
    - ST segment elevation
- Acute myocardial infarction
  - Chest pain, persistent, crushing > 30-min duration
  - Retrosternal and radiating to left arm
  - Tingling sensation in hand and fingers
  - ST segment elevation and Q waves
  - CK and troponin elevation
- Sudden death
  - Death occurring within 24 hours of symptoms
- Chronic heart failure

Treatment

- Options, risks, complications
  - Primary prevention is critical to reduce risk factors to limit atherosclerosis progression and stabilize existing plaques
- Surgical approaches
  - Percutaneous transluminal coronary angioplasty
  - Coronary stenting
  - Coronary artery bypass graft
- Drugs
  - Lipid-lowering medications: HMG-CoA reductase inhibitors, PCKS9 inhibitors
  - Antihypertensive medication: β-blockers, angiotensin-converting enzyme inhibitors, angiotensin receptor blockers
  - Antiplatelet aggregate medications: Aspirin, P2Y12 inhibitors
- Complications: Restenosis, thrombosis

Risk Factors

- Elevated serum cholesterol
- Diabetes mellitus
- Hypertension
- Cigarette smoking
- Saturated fat diet
- Other factors: Homocystinuria, metabolic syndrome

IMAGING

MR Findings

- Coronary MR may characterize plaque components

CT Findings

- CTA differentiates calcified and noncalcified plaques but not lipid-rich and fibrous plaques
- Often underestimates plaque burden

Intravascular Ultrasound

- Can detect diseased segments in angiographic normal coronaries
- Lesion extent
  - Plaque area between lumen and internal elastic lamina
  - External elastic lamina, echolucent border
  - Can differentiate calcified from soft plaque
  - Detect plaque rupture and erosion
- Dissection also visualized

Angiography

- Conventional
  - Soft plaque may not be evident
  - Raised irregular lumen narrowing
  - Narrowing may be concentric or eccentric
  - May underestimate degree of atherosclerosis
- Angioscopy
  - Yellow plaques: Lipid-containing lesions with thin collagenous cap, more likely to rupture
  - White plaques: Thick fibrous caps and fibrous lesions

MACROSCOPIC

General Features

- Atherosclerosis is limited to epicardial arteries
  - Left anterior descending (LAD) artery most often involved, followed by circumflex
  - 70% of plaques are eccentric
  - Atherosclerotic plaques show variable gross appearance
    - White coloration (fibrous plaque)
    - Whitish yellow (fibrofatty plaque)
  - Artery lumen shows variable shapes
    - Elliptical
    - D-shaped
    - Polymorphic

  - Crescentic
  - Slit-like
- Gross evaluation of stenosis
  - Grade 1: < 25% cross-sectional luminal narrowing
  - Grade 2: 25-50% cross-sectional luminal narrowing
  - Grade 3: 50-75% cross-sectional luminal narrowing
  - Grade 4: > 75% cross-sectional luminal narrowing, considered critical stenosis
  - Comparing cross-sectional lumen stenosis to longitudinal angiographic "lumenogram" requires conversion factor
    - e.g., 90% longitudinal narrowing = 75% cross-sectional area reduction
- Thin cap fibroatheromas and ruptured plaques
  - Infrequent and focally distributed
  - Involve proximal aspects of LAD and left coronary artery
  - More uniformly distributed on right coronary artery
- Thick cap fibroatheromas
  - Less susceptible to rupture or erosion

MICROSCOPIC

Histologic Features

- American Heart Association classification
  - Grade 0: Normal histology or adaptive thickening without macrophages or foam cells
  - Grade 1: Isolated macrophages or foam cells
  - Grade 2: Intracellular lipid accumulation
  - Grade 3: Grade 2 lesions along with small, extracellular lipid pools
  - Grade 4: Grade 2 changes along with core of extracellular lipid
  - Grade 5: Lipid core and fibrous cap or multiple lipid cores and fibrous layers, calcific or fibrotic
  - Grade 6: More common grade 4 or 5 lesions with surface defect, &/or hematoma/hemorrhage, &/or thrombosis
- Plaque components
  - Different proportions of these components constitute plaques
    - Cells: Smooth muscle, macrophages (M1, M2, and Mhb), T cells (Th1, Th2, Treg)
    - Extracellular matrix, including collagen, elastic fibers, and proteoglycans
    - Lipids: Extra- and intracellular; mainly cholesterol and cholesterol esters
  - Plaques progressively enlarge and continuously change through cell death, degeneration, lipid accumulation, synthesis/degradation of extracellular matrix, and calcification
  - Plaque burden increases risk of acute cardiovascular events
- Plaque complications
  - Rupture-prone plaques
    - Large necrotic core (> 30% of plaque)
    - Thin fibrous cap (< 65 microns) with significant inflammation and few smooth muscle cells
    - Expansive remodeling preserving lumen
    - Neovascularization
    - Adventitial perivascular inflammation
    - Spotty calcification
  - Erosion-prone plaques
    - Scarce calcification
    - Sparse inflammation
    - Lipid poor
    - Proteoglycan and glycosaminoglycan rich
    - Internal and external laminae and media are nondisrupted
  - Hemorrhage
    - May contribute to necrotic core expansion, promote inflammation, and plaque vulnerability
  - Thrombosis
    - Plaque rupture exposes thrombogenic substances to clotting factors in luminal blood, leading to lumen thrombosis
    - Thought to be most common cause of acute coronary syndrome (> 70%)
    - Thought to cause quantized stepwise plaque progression
    - Occurs most often in 25-50% occlusive plaques with thin fibrous caps ("vulnerable plaques")
  - Calcification common process that increase with age
    - Spotty calcification more common in "vulnerable" plaques and associated with greater progression of plaque volume
    - Heavy calcification is seen in stable plaques
    - Total amount of calcification is marker of plaque burden

DIFFERENTIAL DIAGNOSIS

Ostial Stenosis

- Calcification of aorta sinotubular junction
- Takayasu arteritis
- Congenital malformations

SELECTED REFERENCES

1. Katta N et al: Obesity and coronary heart disease: epidemiology, pathology, and coronary artery imaging. Curr Probl Cardiol. 46(3):100655, 2021
2. Libby P: Inflammation during the life cycle of the atherosclerotic plaque. Cardiovasc Res. 117(13):2525-36, 2021
3. Mohindra R et al: Altered vascular extracellular matrix in the pathogenesis of atherosclerosis. J Cardiovasc Transl Res. 14(4):647-60, 2021
4. Udasimath S et al: Morphological changes of coronary arteries in cases of sudden death due to cardiac causes - an autopsy-based 10-year retrospective study. Heart Views. 22(3):189-95, 2021
5. Zheng J et al: Current progress of studies of coronary CT for risk prediction of major adverse cardiovascular event (MACE). J Cardiovasc Imaging. 29(4):301-15, 2021
6. Barrett TJ: Macrophages in atherosclerosis regression. Arterioscler Thromb Vasc Biol. 40(1):20-33, 2020
7. Fox KAA et al: The myth of 'stable' coronary artery disease. Nat Rev Cardiol. 17(1):9-21, 2020
8. Arbab-Zadeh A et al: From detecting the vulnerable plaque to managing the vulnerable patient: JACC state-of-the-art review. J Am Coll Cardiol. 74(12):1582-93, 2019
9. Mori H et al: Coronary artery calcification and its progression: what does it really mean? JACC Cardiovasc Imaging. 11(1):127-42, 2018
10. Parvand M et al: Recent developments in sex-related differences in presentation, prognosis, and management of coronary artery disease. Can J Cardiol. 34(4):390-9, 2018
11. Virmani R et al: The stress of plaque prognostication. JACC Cardiovasc Imaging. 1(3):472-5, 2018
12. Biessen EAL et al: Macrophage complexity in human atherosclerosis: opportunities for treatment? Curr Opin Lipidol. 28(5):419-26, 2017
13. Crea F et al: Acute coronary syndromes: the way forward from mechanisms to precision treatment. Circulation. 136(12):1155-66, 2017
14. Tesauro M et al: Arterial ageing: from endothelial dysfunction to vascular calcification. J Intern Med. 281(5):471-82, 2017

Grade 1 Atherosclerosis

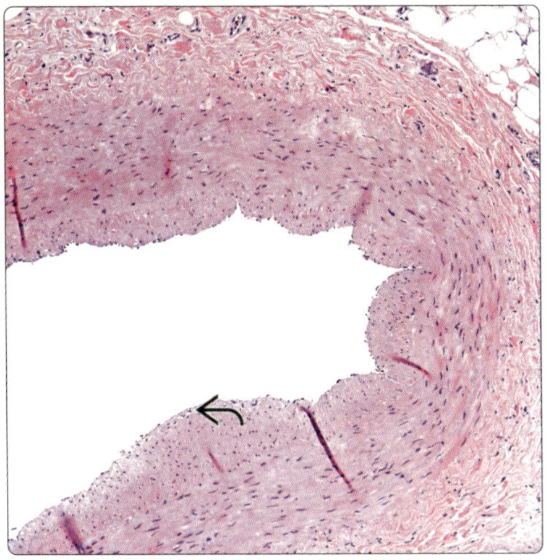

Grade 3 Atherosclerosis

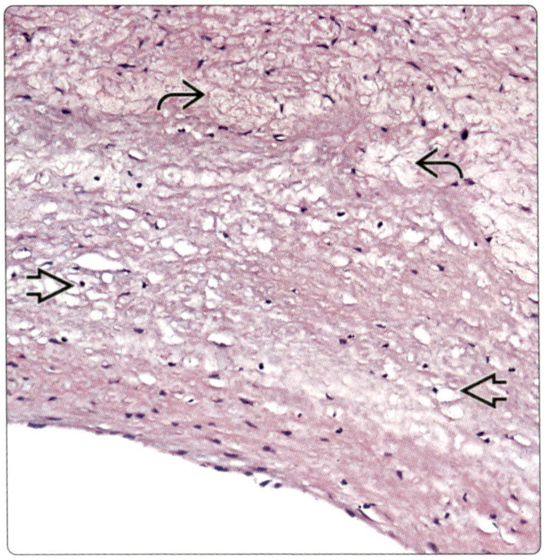

(Left) *H&E-stained section of a coronary artery shows rare foamy cells in the intima* ↪*; however, there is no thickening, and there are no deposits of extracellular lipids.* **(Right)** *H&E-stained section of a coronary artery shows numerous foamy cells in the intima* ⇨ *as well as deposits of extracellular lipids forming small pools* ↪*. There is mild fibrous thickening on the intima surface. Growth of plaque is secondary to the accumulation of cells, lipid, and extracellular matrix.*

Grade 5 Atherosclerosis

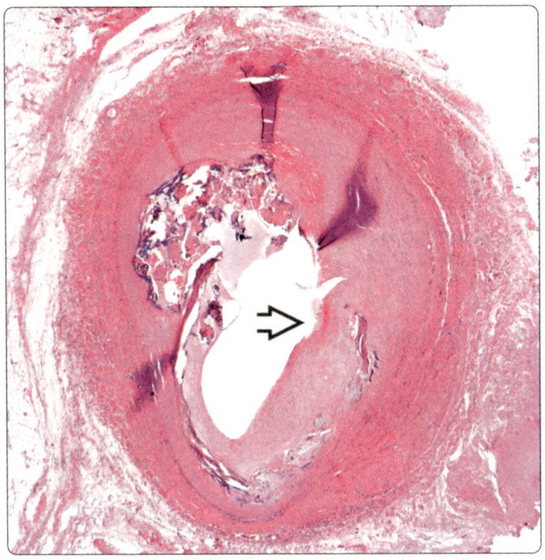

Grade 5 Atherosclerosis

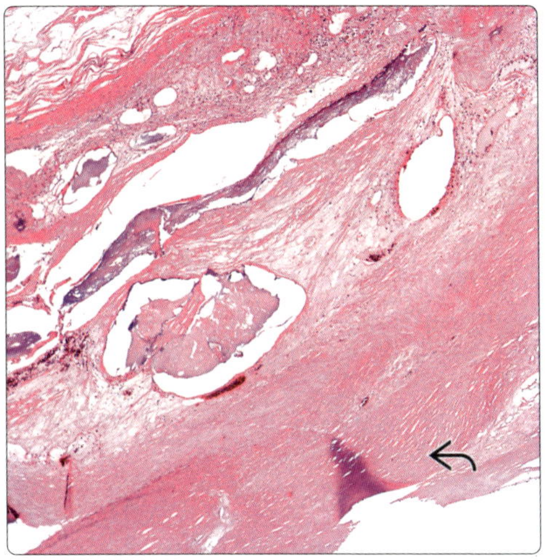

(Left) *H&E-stained section of a coronary artery shows a thick fibrous cap* ⇨ *with minimal accumulation of cells in the intima. There is focal calcification as well as surface ulceration. The lumen has an elliptical shape, and there is attenuation of the media.* **(Right)** *Higher magnification of an H&E-stained section of a coronary artery shows a thick fibrous cap atheroma* ↪*. There is focal calcification. This type of plaque is less susceptible to rupture or erosion.*

Grade 6 Atherosclerosis

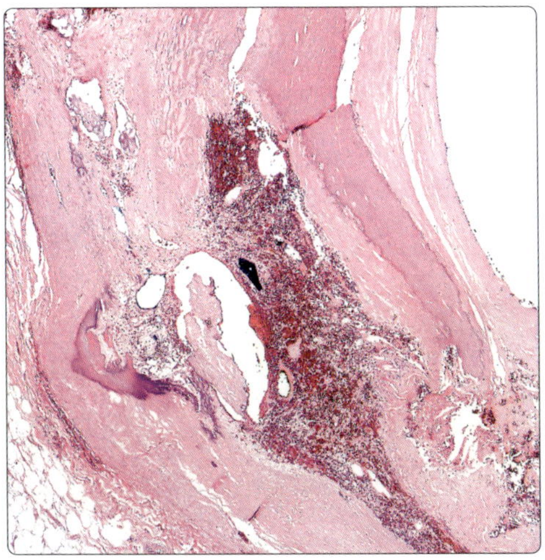

Coronary Plaque Thrombosis

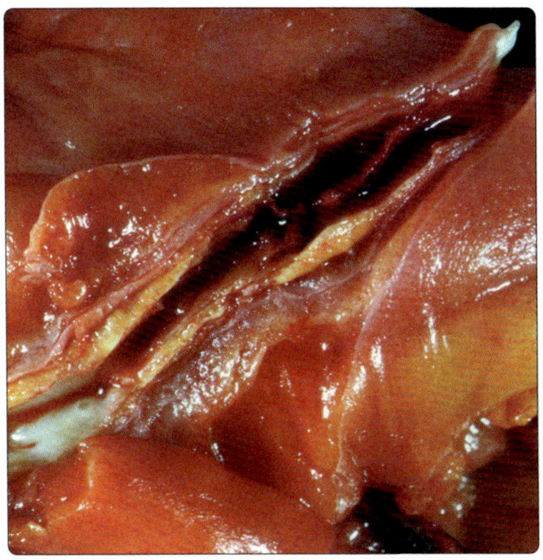

(Left) *H&E-stained section of a coronary artery shows hemorrhage into atherosclerotic plaque. This may occur after rupture of either the overlying fibrous cap or the thin-walled capillaries that vascularize the plaque. This will expand the plaque and reduce the lumen, leading to clinical manifestations.* **(Right)** *Anterior descending branch shows thrombus within the lumina. This was the final event, complicating coronary atherosclerosis and causing large myocardial infarct and the patient's death.*

Coronary Artery Dissection

KEY FACTS

TERMINOLOGY

- Coronary artery wall injury resulting from intimal tear with subsequent disruption of vessel wall or vasa vasorum rupture, which leads to intramural hematoma formation, obliteration of lumen, and secondary myocardial ischemia

ETIOLOGY/PATHOGENESIS

- Spontaneous
  - False lumen is formed either from intimal tear or through spontaneous hemorrhage arising from vasa vasorum
  - Pregnancy/post partum: Constitutional or acquired arterial wall weakness added to mechanical stress
- Iatrogenic
  - Postcoronary catheterization

CLINICAL ISSUES

- Young and middle-aged female patients without coronary disease have 3x higher occurrence than male patients
- Clinical presentation depends on extent of dissection flap and degree of luminal occlusion and varies from asymptomatic to sudden death
- Site involved
  - Most common involvement of left anterior descending branch (in females)
  - Right coronary (in males) and circumflex branch
  - Left main coronary rarely involved
- Conservative and surgical approaches vary based on localization, accessibility, and extent of dissection as well as patient stability and severity of ischemia

MICROSCOPIC

- Intimal tear may not be demonstrated
- Unremarkable media
- Adventitial eosinophils
- Angiomatous changes
- Myocardial ischemia may be present
- Vasculitis and cystic media necrosis are infrequent

Coronary Angiogram in Coronary Dissection

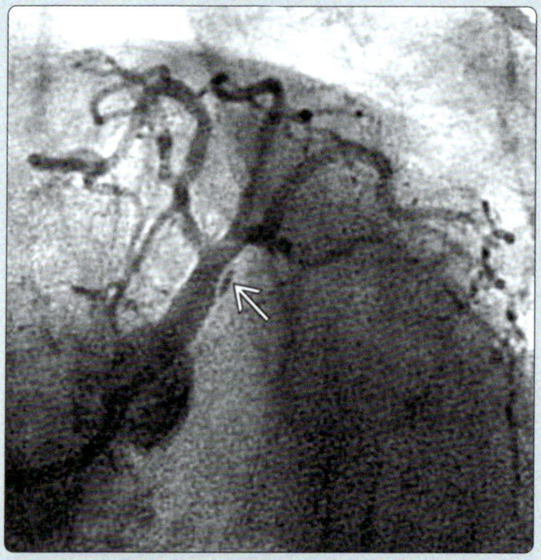

Acute Coronary Artery Dissection

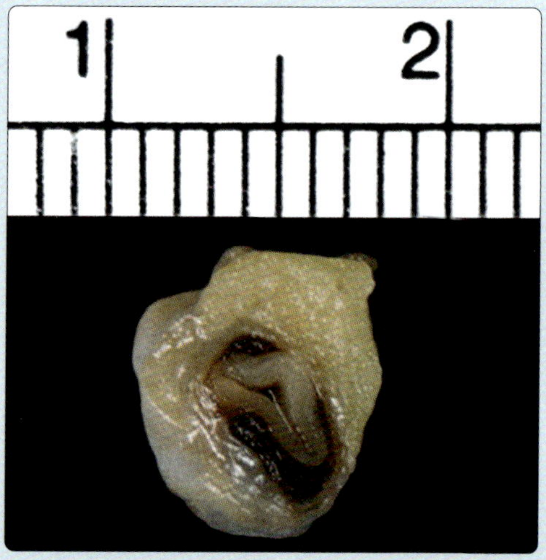

(Left) *Coronary angiogram demonstrates left main coronary artery dissection following stent wire manipulation. Contrast retention is seen in false lumina. (Courtesy J. Dodd, MD.)* **(Right)** *Gross photograph shows cross section of a coronary artery in a case of dissection with a hemorrhage surrounding the wall. The intima does not show atherosclerosis.*

Histology of Recent Coronary Artery Dissection

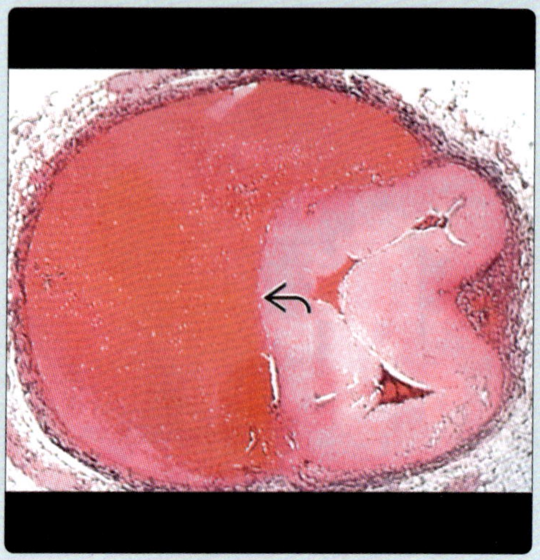

Healed Coronary Artery Dissection

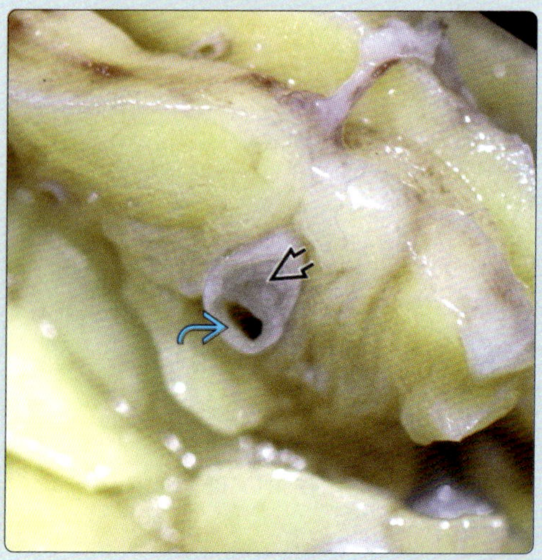

(Left) *Elastic-stained section of a coronary artery in a case of coronary artery dissection shows a hematoma localized in the outer aspect of the tunica media and contained by adventitia.* **(Right)** *Gross photograph shows the cross section of the left anterior descending coronary artery several years after dissection. There is fibrous tissue between the intima and media. The lumen is narrowed and eccentrically displaced. The intima does not show atherosclerosis.*

TERMINOLOGY

Abbreviations

- Spontaneous coronary artery dissection (SCAD)

Definitions

- Coronary artery wall injury resulting from intimal tear with subsequent disruption of vessel wall or vasa vasorum rupture, which leads to intramural hematoma formation, obliteration of lumen, and secondary myocardial ischemia

ETIOLOGY/PATHOGENESIS

SCAD

- False lumen is formed either from intimal tear or through spontaneous hemorrhage arising from vasa vasorum
- Pregnancy-associated SCAD: Constitutional or acquired arterial wall weakness added to mechanical stress
- Cocaine abuse: Vasospasm-induced coronary dissection

Iatrogenic

- Postcoronary catheterization

CLINICAL ISSUES

Epidemiology

- Incidence
  - Rare cause of coronary syndrome (1-4%) and sudden cardiac death (0.5%)
    - Spontaneous: Unknown, but annual incidence is estimated to be 2 per million
    - Iatrogenic: < 0.1% of patients undergoing coronary angiography or percutaneous intervention
- Age
  - In spontaneous dissection, young to middle-aged patients are most commonly involved
    - Median age at presentation: 45-53 years
    - Age range: 20-80 years
- Sex
  - Female patients without coronary disease have 3x higher occurrence than male patients
  - Up to 35% of women < 50 years of age presenting with myocardial infarct may be due to SCAD
  - SCAD is most common cause (43%) of pregnancy-associated myocardial infarct

Site

- Most common involvement of left anterior descending branch (in females)
- Right coronary (in males) and circumflex branch
- Left main coronary rarely involved in SCAD
- Multivessel SCAD occurs in 9-23% of cases

Presentation

- Depends on extent of dissection flap and degree of luminal occlusion
  - Asymptomatic
  - Chest pain most frequent presenting symptom
  - ST-segment elevation (26-87%) and non-ST-segment elevation (13-69%) myocardial infarct
  - Sudden death without myocardial infarction
  - Sudden death with acute myocardial ischemia
  - Ventricular arrhythmias

Laboratory Tests

- Elevation of troponin I has been reported

Treatment

- Options, risks, complications
  - Conservative and surgical approaches vary based on localization, accessibility, and extent of dissection as well as patient stability and severity of ischemia
- Surgical approaches
  - Percutaneous coronary intervention (PCI) with bailout stent implantation is associated with higher rates of complications and poor outcomes
  - Urgent coronary bypass grafting is indicated in cases of multiple vessel or left main coronary artery involvement or PCI failure
  - Heart transplantation
- Drugs
  - Antiplatelet therapy role is unclear and unsupported but should be used after PCI
  - Thrombolytic therapy is not indicated because it may exacerbate dissection
  - Antihypertensive medication and β-blockers are useful and can reduce risk of dissection recurrence
- Conservative approach
  - Favored in hemodynamically stable patients with maintained distal flow of dissected artery and without demonstrable ischemia
  - "Healing" of dissected area in SCAD has been reported in up to 73% of patients in clinical series
  - In-patient monitoring for 3-5 days after SCAD is recommended for early detection of dissection extension

Prognosis

- Mortality rate has decreased in SCAD to < 5% and is ~ 6% in iatrogenic dissection
- 10-year risk of recurrence, myocardial infarct, heart failure, or death is ~ 47%
- Recurrence risk is ~ 10-15% in recent series
- SCAD recurrence is higher in patients with hypertension and in some series with fibromuscular dysplasia and migraine headache
- Pregnancy-associated SCAD has worse outcomes with greater degree of heart muscle damage and higher likelihood of multivessel involvement

Risk Factors

- Spontaneous
  - Pregnancy (multiparity/older age at pregnancy)/post partum
  - Fibromuscular dysplasia (present in 68% of patients with SCAD)
    - Patients carrying rs9349379-A allele of PHACTR1 locus show increased risk to develop SCAD and fibromuscular dysplasia
  - Marfan, vascular Ehlers-Danlos, and Loeys-Dietz syndromes
  - Hormonal therapy
  - Immune or inflammatory diseases (systemic lupus erythematosus, Crohn disease, ulcerative colitis, rheumatoid arthritis, celiac disease)
- Iatrogenic

- Hypertension
- Coronary artery atherosclerosis with ostial involvement
- Use of guide catheters
- Possible triggers
  - Emotional stressors
  - Heavy physical exertion
  - Cocaine abuse

IMAGING

Coronary Angiography

- Intimal flap may appear as linear filling defect
- Flap may be fixed or mobile
- Dual lumen
- Contrast retention in false lumen
- Flow abnormalities
- Hematoma may simulate intracoronary thrombus
- Angiographic classification for SCAD
  - Type 1: Angiographic radiolucent flap and linear double lumen often associated with contrast hold-up
  - Type 2: Long diffuse and smooth stenosis predominantly located in mid to distal segments (most reported pattern)
    - 2a: Normal artery caliber proximal and distal to dissected area
    - 2b: Artery stenosis extends to distal segment of vessel without recovery of caliber
  - Type 3: Focal tubular stenosis similar to atherosclerotic disease
  - Type 4: Appears as total occlusion of distal vessel

Intravascular Ultrasound

- Helpful to confirm dissection and estimate extension
- Can demonstrate contrast or thrombus within false lumen
- Useful for stent sizing and implant

Optical Coherence Tomography

- Useful for characterization of true lumen and accurate measurement of intimal-medial membrane thickness and dimension of compressed lumen
- Can determine size, nature, and extent of false lumen
- Can demonstrate relationship of false lumen with side branches, fenestrations, and "entry tear"
- Helpful for locating position of guidewire in case of coronary revascularization

CT and MR Angiography

- Recommended for extracoronary screening of fibromuscular dysplasia in patients with SCAD

MACROSCOPIC

Sections to Be Submitted

- Middistal segments of epicardial coronary arteries should be evaluated

MICROSCOPIC

Histologic Features

- Intimal tear may not be demonstrated
- Hematoma seen in outer 1/3 of tunica media
- Media does not show abnormalities
- Adventitial eosinophils may be present
- Angiomatous adventitial changes may be present
- Vasculitis is unusual
- Cystic media necrosis only infrequently seen
- Acute myocardial ischemic changes seen in ~ 50% of reported cases

DIFFERENTIAL DIAGNOSIS

Embolic Coronary Disease

- Luminal obstruction caused by thromboemboli
- Atherosclerotic material, infected thrombi, &/or tumor emboli may be identified in artery lumina
- Absent intramural hematoma

Intraplaque Hemorrhage

- Occurs in complicated atherosclerotic plaques
- Intimal tear and false lumen not identified

SELECTED REFERENCES

1. Adlam D et al: Spontaneous coronary artery dissection: pitfalls of angiographic diagnosis and an approach to ambiguous cases. JACC Cardiovasc Interv. 14(16):1743-56, 2021
2. Bocchino PP et al: Invasive versus conservative management in spontaneous coronary artery dissection: a meta-analysis and meta-regression study. Hellenic J Cardiol. 62(4):297-303, 2021
3. Cerrato E et al: Antiplatelet therapy in patients with conservatively managed spontaneous coronary artery dissection from the multicentre DISCO registry. Eur Heart J. 42(33):3161-71, 2021
4. Díez-Villanueva P et al: Spontaneous coronary artery dissection in old patients: clinical features, angiographic findings, management and outcome. Eur Heart J Acute Cardiovasc Care. 10(8):926-32, 2021
5. Fukuta M et al: An autopsy case of spontaneous coronary artery dissection with eosinophilic coronary periarteritis and degeneration of medial smooth muscles. Am J Forensic Med Pathol. 42(4):387-91, 2021
6. Iismaa SE et al: Spontaneous coronary artery dissection and fibromuscular dysplasia: vasculopathies with a predilection for women. Heart Lung Circ. 30(1):27-35, 2021
7. Kermali M et al: Spontaneous coronary artery dissection: presentation and management options. Coron Artery Dis. 32(2):152-63, 2021
8. Kok SN et al: Recurrent spontaneous coronary artery dissection. Expert Rev Cardiovasc Ther. 19(3):201-10, 2021
9. Ramasamy A et al: Iatrogenic catheter-induced ostial coronary artery dissections: prevalence, management, and mortality from a cohort of 55,968 patients over 10years. Catheter Cardiovasc Interv. 98(4):649-55, 2021
10. Hayes SN et al: Spontaneous coronary artery dissection: JACC state-of-the-art review. J Am Coll Cardiol. 76(8):961-84, 2020
11. Krittanawong C et al: Recurrent spontaneous coronary artery dissection in the United States. Int J Cardiol. 301:34-7, 2020
12. Adlam D et al: Association of the PHACTR1/EDN1 genetic locus with spontaneous coronary artery dissection. J Am Coll Cardiol. 73(1):58-66, 2019
13. Clare R et al: Characteristics and clinical outcomes of patients with spontaneous coronary artery dissection. J Am Heart Assoc. 8(10):e012570, 2019
14. Main A et al: Percutaneous coronary intervention for the treatment of spontaneous coronary artery dissection. Interv Cardiol Clin. 8(2):199-208, 2019
15. Saw J et al: Canadian spontaneous coronary artery dissection cohort study: in-hospital and 30-day outcomes. Eur Heart J. 40(15):1188-97, 2019
16. Tan NY et al: Spontaneous coronary artery dissection: etiology and recurrence. Expert Rev Cardiovasc Ther. 17(7):497-510, 2019
17. Tanaka A: Shedding light on pathophysiology of spontaneous coronary artery dissection. JACC Cardiovasc Imaging. 12(12):2489-91, 2019
18. Adlam D et al: European Society of Cardiology, acute cardiovascular care association, SCAD study group: a position paper on spontaneous coronary artery dissection. Eur Heart J. 39(36):3353-68, 2018
19. Hayes SN et al: Spontaneous coronary artery dissection: current state of the science: a scientific statement from the American Heart Association. Circulation. 137(19):e523-57, 2018

Dissection of Left Main Coronary Artery

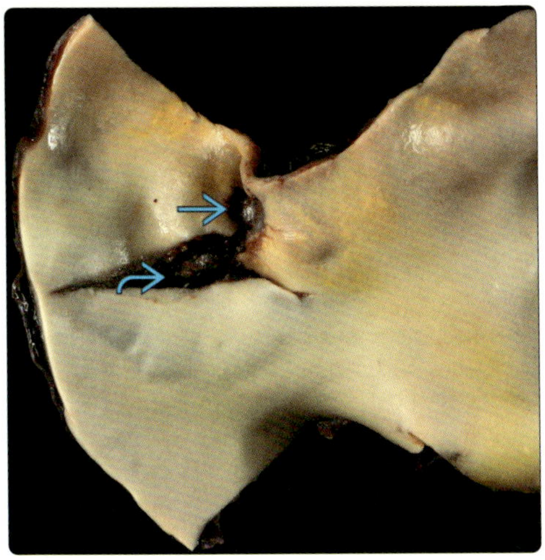

Gross Image of Spontaneous Coronary Artery Dissection

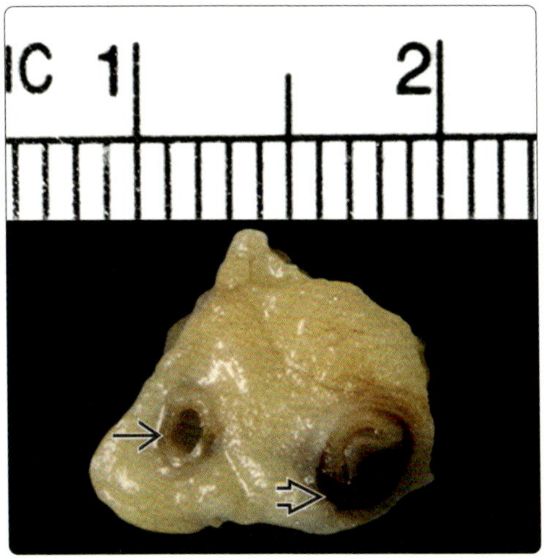

(Left) *The intimal surface of a portion of the aorta wall, including the left coronary ostium, demonstrates a hematoma surrounding the main left coronary artery in this case of sudden cardiac death due to coronary dissection. No significant atherosclerosis is present.* **(Right)** *Cross section of a coronary artery shows hemorrhage contained by adventitia in this case of coronary artery dissection. Significant atherosclerosis is not seen in the noninvolved coronary segment.*

Dissection of Left Anterior Descending Coronary Artery

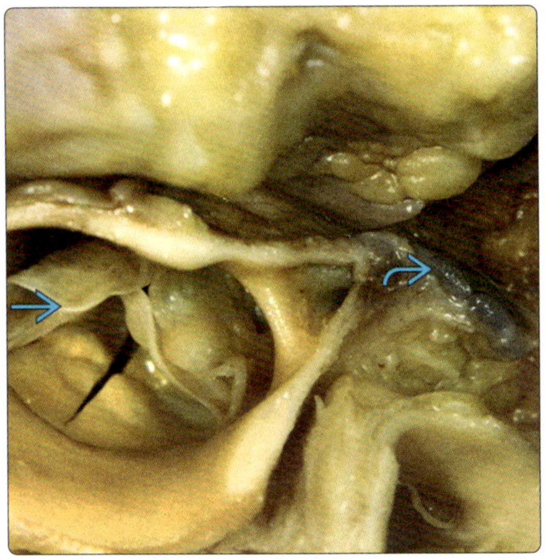

CTA in Coronary Dissection

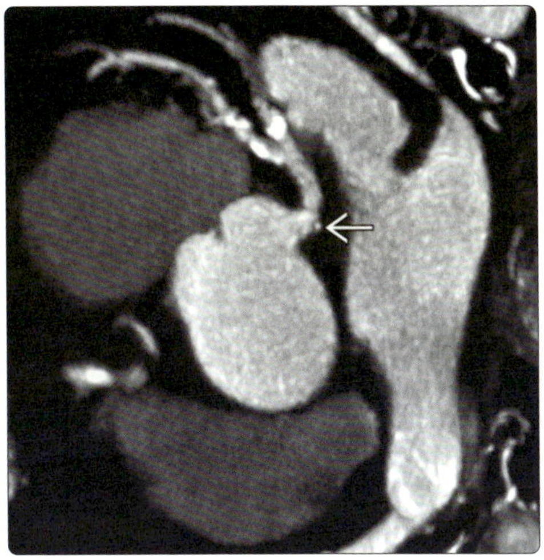

(Left) *The intimal surface of the aorta wall, including the aortic valve, demonstrates a hematoma surrounding the main left coronary artery with extension to the left anterior descending branch in this case of sudden cardiac death due to coronary dissection.* **(Right)** *CTA demonstrates a scant amount of contrast in the coronary artery wall corresponding to the area of dissection. (Courtesy J. Dodd, MD.)*

Histology of Healed Coronary Artery Dissection

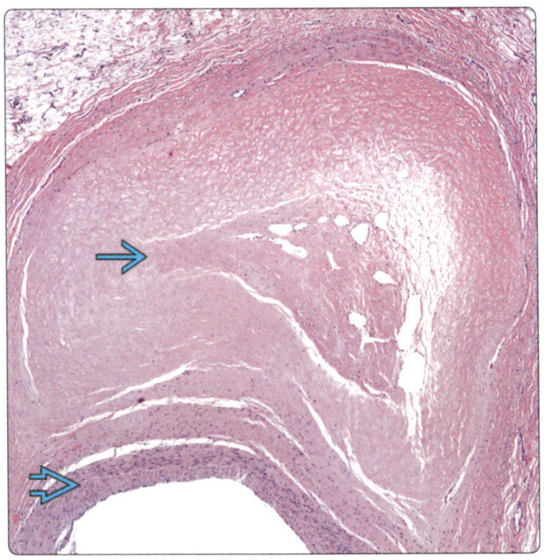

Myocardial Changes in Spontaneous Coronary Artery Dissection

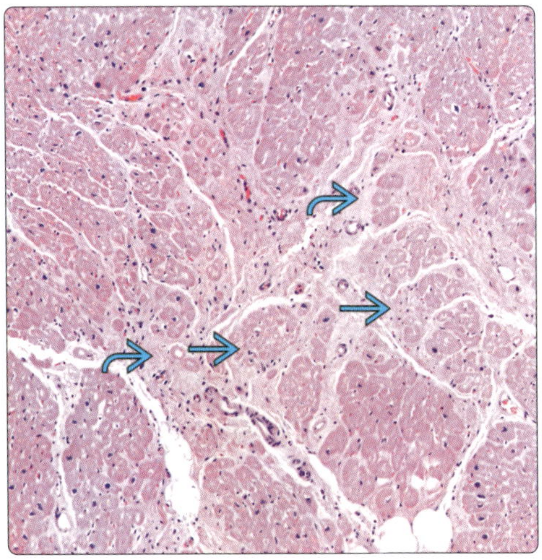

(Left) *Left anterior descending coronary artery shows fibrous tissue between adventitia and media layers replacing the prior intramural hematoma in this case of healed coronary dissection.* **(Right)** *Myocardium shows atrophic myocytes surrounded by areas of interstitial fibrosis. These changes are nonspecific, but, in this case of healed spontaneous coronary artery dissection, represent healed areas of prior ischemic injury.*

KEY FACTS

TERMINOLOGY

- Acute, self-limited vasculitis that primarily involves coronary arteries

CLINICAL ISSUES

- In USA, 76% of children < 5 years of age with median onset ~ 2 years of age
- Affects boys more than girls (1.5-1.7:1.0)
- More prevalent in Japan and in children of Japanese ancestry
- Fever for at least 5 days, usually 39 °C
- Nonpurulent conjunctivitis, polymorphous skin rashes, abnormalities of lip or oral mucosa
- Abnormalities of extremities and cervical lymphadenopathy
- Subacute phase: Coronary vasculitis in combination with elevated platelet count and hypercoagulable state
- Cardiac findings: Myocarditis, pericarditis, valvular and coronary artery abnormalities
- Noncardiac findings: Arthritis and arthralgias, vomiting and diarrhea

MACROSCOPIC

- Aneurysms occur as complication of Kawasaki disease in ~ 25% of cases without treatment
- Aneurysms are classified as small (internal diameter of vessel wall < 4 mm), medium (4-5 mm), and giant (> 8 mm)

MICROSCOPIC

- Coronary arteries with inflammatory cell infiltration of arterial wall, destruction of internal elastic lamina, necrosis of smooth muscle cells and myointimal proliferation, aneurysm formation, and wall thinning
- Other findings: Myocarditis and pericarditis, endocarditis with valvulitis, inflammation of atrioventricular node
- Healed phase: Aneurysmal dilatation and thinning of coronary arteries with calcification, myocardium with lymphoplasmacytic infiltrate and myocardial fibrosis, sequelae of valvulitis with valvular insufficiency

CT Angiography of Coronary Aneurysm in Kawasaki Disease | **Gross Image of Coronary Aneurysm in Kawasaki Disease**

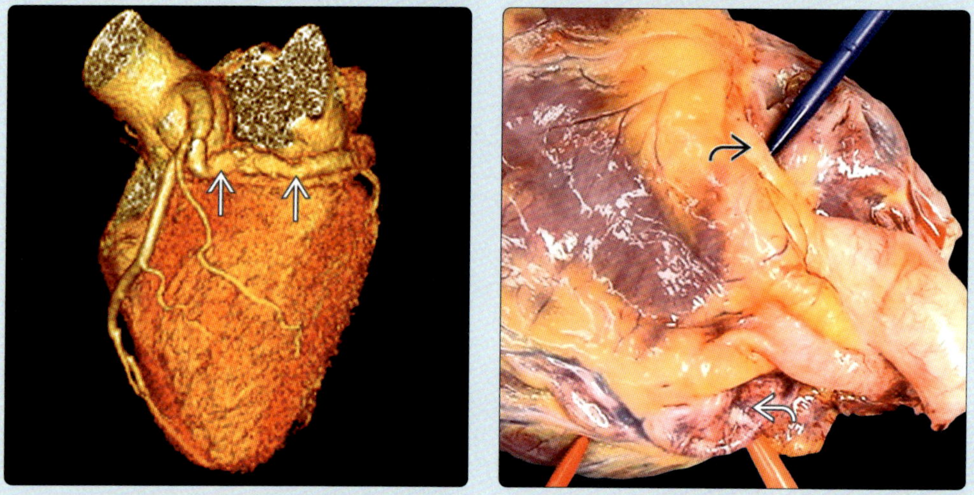

(Left) *Left anterior oblique volume-rendered cardiac CT shows left circumflex coronary aneurysm in a 37-year-old man with a childhood history of Kawasaki disease (KD). (Courtesy D. Green, MD and A. Soni, MD.)* **(Right)** *Gross photograph shows a giant aneurysm involving the proximal portion of the left anterior descending artery and an aneurysm involving the proximal portion of the right coronary artery.*

Histologic Changes in Coronary Artery | **Histologic Changes in Coronary Artery**

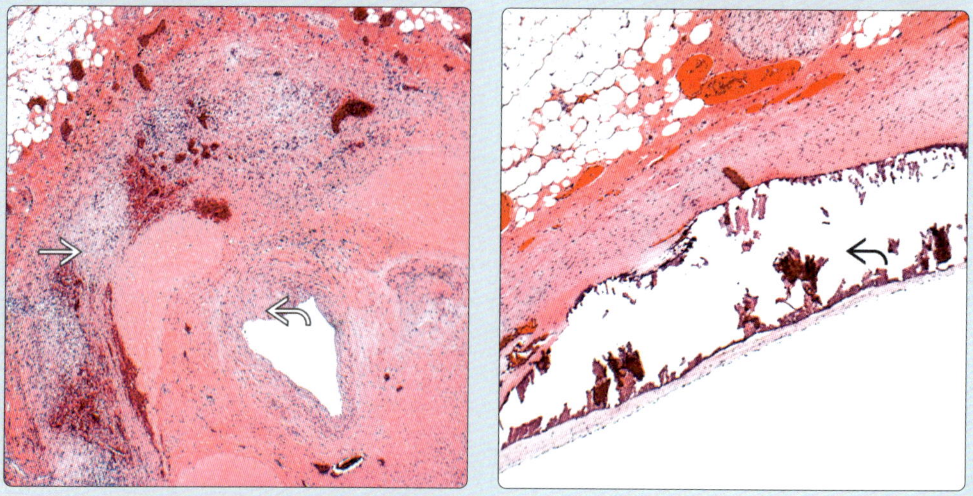

(Left) *Coronary artery section shows chronic inflammation and granulation tissue in the media. Intimal fibrosis and luminal stenosis are also present.* **(Right)** *At higher magnification, coronary artery shows aneurysm with marked thinning of the wall and intimal calcification in this case of KD.*

TERMINOLOGY

Abbreviations

- Kawasaki disease (KD)

Definitions

- Acute, multisystemic, febrile illness of unknown cause associated with self-limited vasculitis that primarily involves coronary arteries

ETIOLOGY/PATHOGENESIS

Infectious Agents

- Theory is that 1 or more widely distributed infectious agents evoke abnormal immunologic response in genetically susceptible individuals; however, no causative agent has been identified

T-Cell Activation

- Features seen in KD suggest T-cell involvement in pathogenesis
  - T-cell infiltration in artery walls
  - Elevation of soluble IL-2 receptor in serum
  - Imbalance of T-cell subsets (Th17 activation/lower T-reg response)
  - Functional variants in *ITPKC* gene (T-cell function regulator) in chromosome 19 have been identified

TGF-β

- Genetic variations in *TGF-β2* and *SMAD3* pathway genes influence susceptibility to develop KD and coronary artery aneurysms
- Promoting generation of myofibroblasts that mediate damage of arterial wall and recruitment of proinflammatory cells

CLINICAL ISSUES

Epidemiology

- Incidence
  - Annual incidence of 330.2 per 100,000 children of Japanese ancestry < 5 years of age
  - Annual incidence of 210 per 100,000 children of Japanese American ancestry < 5 years of age
  - 19.7 per 100,000 White children > 5 years of age in USA
- Age
  - In USA, 76% of children < 5 years of age with median onset ~ 2 years of age
- Sex
  - Affects boys more than girls (1.5-1.7:1.0)
- Ethnicity
  - More prevalent in Japan and in children of Japanese ancestry

Presentation

- Classic/complete: Fever (usually 39 °C) for at least 5 days with presence of at least 4 of following 5 principal clinical features
  - Nonpurulent conjunctiviti
  - Polymorphous skin rashes
  - Abnormalities of lip or oral mucosa: Erythema/cracking lips; "strawberry tongue"; erythema oral/pharyngeal mucosa
  - Abnormalities of extremities: Erythema/edema of hands and feet
  - Cervical lymphadenopathy: ≥ 1.5 cm in diameter, usually unilateral
- Atypical KD
  - Fever with 2 or 3 of classic KD clinical criteria
- Incomplete KD
  - With clinical features of KD but with additional clinical features not seen in KD
- Subacute phase: Coronary vasculitis in combination with elevated platelet count and hypercoagulable state
- Convalescent phase begins ~ 4-6 weeks when all signs of illness have disappeared; continues until acute-phase reactants have returned to normal
- Chronic phase: Long-term management of children with coronary artery abnormalities
  - Cardiac findings: Myocarditis, pericarditis, valvular abnormalities, coronary abnormalities
  - Noncardiac findings
    - Arthritis and arthralgias involving predominantly large joints
    - Gastrointestinal findings include abdominal pain, vomiting, diarrhea, and hepatic dysfunction
    - Encephalitis/encephalopathy, seizures, aseptic meningitis
    - Urinary system findings include urethritis, aseptic pyuria, microscopic/gross hematuria

Natural History

- Resolution without sequela
- Development of coronary artery abnormalities; ~ 6% regress in 1 year
- Cardiac involvement with myocarditis, aneurysm thrombosis, arrhythmia, myocardial infarction
- KD recurrence: ~ 3%

Treatment

- Surgical approaches
  - Coronary artery stenting
    - Indicated for localized severe stenotic lesions not involving ostia
    - When myocardial ischemia and fibrosis are present
    - Lower efficacy in comparison with coronary artery bypass grafting
  - Coronary artery bypass grafting
    - Recommended in younger children with ischemic myocardial changes and multivessel disease
  - Cardiac transplantation
    - For patients with end-stage cardiomyopathy, severe ventricular arrhythmias, inoperable multivessel coronary artery disease
- Drugs
  - Intravenous immunoglobulin; standard of care and reduces coronary artery complications (3-5% treated vs. 15-25% untreated)
  - Antiinflammatories
    - High doses of acetylsalicylic acid
    - Corticosteroid use is conditionally recommended when there is higher risk for aneurysm development or progression
  - TNF-α and IL-1 inhibitors in resistant cases

- Anticoagulants

Prognosis

- Regression of coronary artery aneurysm
  - Inversely related to severity of initial aneurysm and male sex
  - Positively related to early treatment
- Persistent aneurysms without stenosis
  - Rate of persistence is 72% at 1 year and 41% at 5 years
- Coronary artery aneurysm with stenosis
  - Most commonly seen in giant aneurysms (at inlet or outlet)
- Sudden cardiac death
  - May occur in older children and young adults years after episode of KD
- Risk factor for atherosclerosis
  - Controversial, but some reports indicate that acute vasculitis can result in coronary artery damage predisposing to thrombosis and progressive atherosclerotic changes
- Case-fatality rate < 0.2%
  - Principal cause of death is myocardial infarction from coronary artery occlusion

IMAGING

Radiographic Findings

- Coronary artery angiogram
  - Findings include
    - Fusiform and saccular dilatation of coronary arteries
    - If mural thrombus present, size of aneurysm can be underestimated
    - Degree of coronary artery stenosis can be estimated

MR Findings

- Lumen dark on double IR FSE
- Bright on GRE or b-SSFP unless thrombus present
- Myocardial fibrosis

CT Findings

- Cardiac-gated CT demonstrates
  - Aneurysmal dilatation
  - Calcification may be seen
  - Mural thrombus that may be occult in angiogram

MACROSCOPIC

Coronary Artery Aneurysms

- Aneurysms occur as complication of KD in ~ 25% of cases without treatment
- Aneurysms are classified as
  - Small (internal diameter of vessel wall < 4 mm)
  - Medium (4-5 mm)
  - Giant (> 8 mm)

MICROSCOPIC

Histologic Features

- Acute phase
  - Coronary arteritis with
    - Inflammatory cell infiltration of arterial wall (neutrophilic in initial phase)
    - Destruction of internal elastic lamina
    - Necrosis of smooth muscle cells and myointimal proliferation
  - Other findings: Myocarditis and pericarditis, endocarditis with valvulitis, inflammation of AV node
- Healed phase
  - Aneurysmal dilatation and thinning of coronary arteries with calcification
  - Myocardium with lymphoplasmacytic infiltrate and myocardial fibrosis
  - Sequelae of valvulitis with valvular insufficiency
- Other arteries involved with vasculitis and aneurysms, in approximate order of incidence: Axillary, common iliac, renal, subclavian, internal iliac, superior mesenteric, internal thoracic, femoral

DIFFERENTIAL DIAGNOSIS

Clinical Syndrome

- Infections
  - Viral: Measles, adenovirus, enterovirus, influenza, and SARS-CoV-2
  - Bacterial: Cervical adenitis, scarlet fever, staphylococcal scalded skin shock syndrome, leptospirosis
  - Rickettsial: Rocky Mountain spotted fever
- Immune mediated
  - Stevens-Johnson syndrome, serum sickness, rheumatic fever
  - Systemic vasculitis, connective tissue disorder (systemic lupus erythematosus)
  - Hereditary autoinflammatory syndromes
    - Tumor necrosis-associated periodic syndrome, hyper-IgD syndrome

Coronary Artery Aneurysm

- Congenital coronary artery aneurysm
  - Present from birth
  - No inflammatory infiltrate in artery wall
- Atherosclerotic aneurysm
  - Atherosclerotic intimal plaque
  - Only mild to moderate inflammation in artery wall
  - Older patients are more affected
- Polyarteritis nodosa
  - Presence of fibrinoid necrosis in media along with transmural wall inflammation
  - Epicardial and intramural arterial branches are affected

SELECTED REFERENCES

1. Gorelik M et al: 2021 American College of Rheumatology/Vasculitis Foundation guideline for the management of Kawasaki disease. Arthritis Rheumatol. 74(4):586-96, 2022
2. Hu J et al: Analysis of multiple organ involvement in Kawasaki disease. Eur J Pediatr. 181(3):951-7, 2022
3. Nabavizadeh SH et al: Assessing the association of Kawasaki disease symptoms and echocardiographic findings. Pediatr Cardiol. 43(4):816-20, 2022
4. Scherler L et al: Acute phase of Kawasaki disease: a review of national guideline recommendations. Eur J Pediatr. 181(7):2563-73, 2022
5. Chang L et al: Perspective of immunopathogenesis and immunotherapies for Kawasaki disease. Front Pediatr. 9:697632, 2021
6. Robinson C et al: Incidence and short-term outcomes of Kawasaki disease. Pediatr Res. 90(3):670-7, 2021
7. Zeng YY et al: An update on cardiovascular risk factors after Kawasaki disease. Front Cardiovasc Med. 8:671198, 2021
8. Rife E et al: Kawasaki disease: an update. Curr Rheumatol Rep. 22(10):75, 2020

Giant Aneurysm

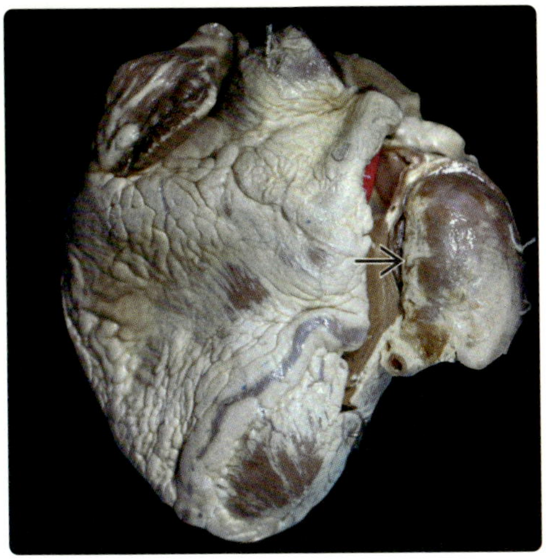

Thrombosed Aneurysm

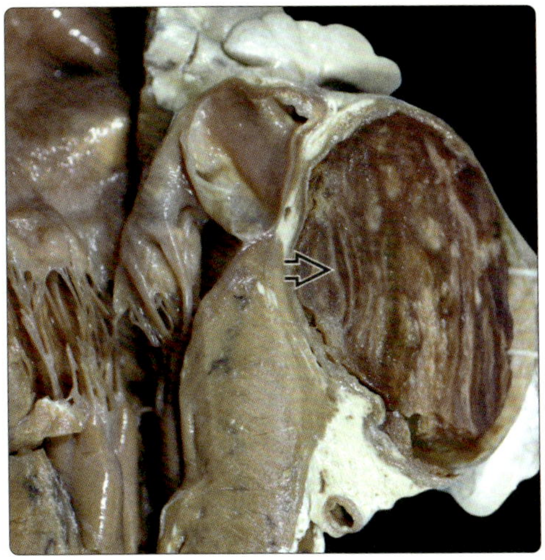

(Left) **(Left)** *Gross photograph of an explanted heart shows an anterior view of a giant aneurysm ➩ involving the left anterior descending coronary artery branch secondary to KD.* **(Right)** *Gross photograph of an explanted heart shows an anterior view of an open giant aneurysm involving the left anterior descending coronary artery branch secondary to KD. The aneurysm is occluded by an organized thrombus ➩.*

Histologic Changes in Coronary Artery

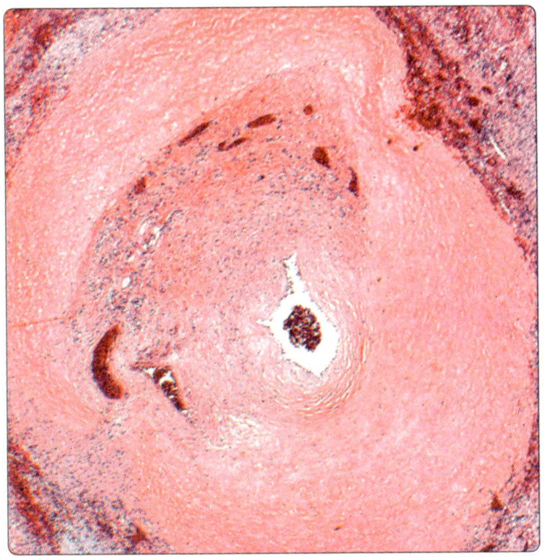

Histologic Changes in Coronary Artery

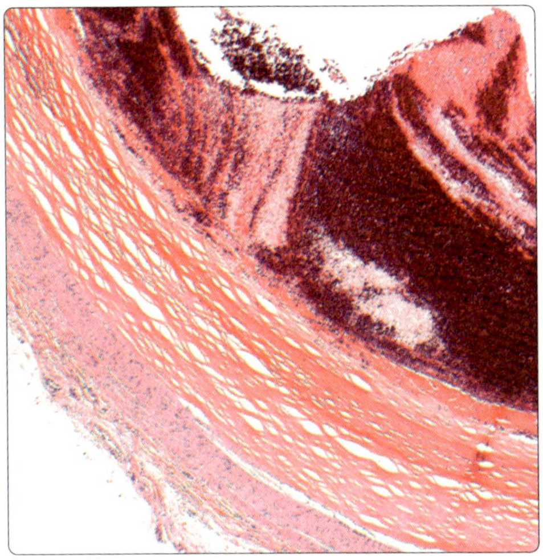

(Left) *H&E-stained section in a case of KD shows intimal fibrosis and organizing thrombus with near-complete obliteration of the lumen.* **(Right)** *H&E-stained section in a case of KD shows aneurysm with thinning of the coronary artery with recent fibrin platelet thrombus in the lumen. There are no significant inflammatory changes in this artery, consistent with a healing stage.*

Histologic Changes in Coronary Artery

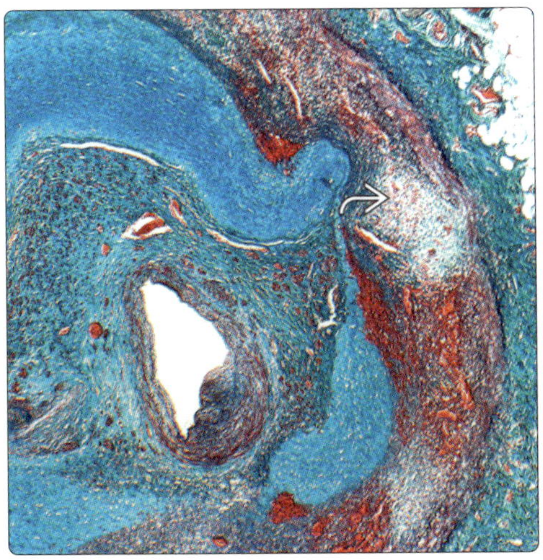

Trichrome Stain of Myocardium

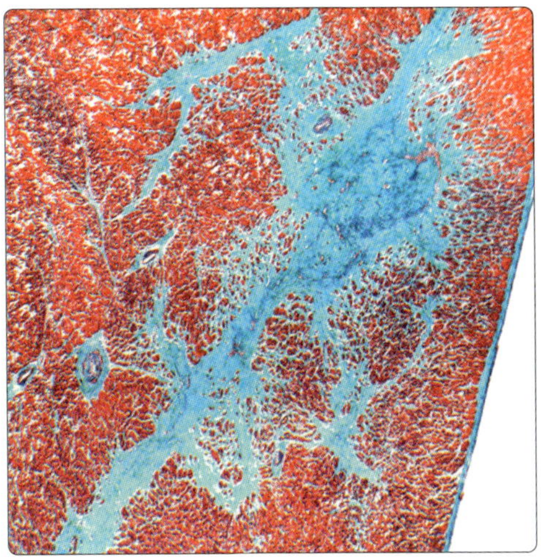

(Left) *Masson trichrome stain shows loss of elastic fibers in the media ➔ and replacement with granulation tissue and fibrosis. The healing phase of the arteritis is characterized by granulation tissue in the media.* **(Right)** *Masson trichrome stain in a case of KD shows an old healed microinfarct in the subendocardial region of the left ventricle. Infarcts may occur as a late complication.*

Coronary Artery Emboli

TERMINOLOGY

Definitions

- Coronary artery occlusion due to thrombus, tumor emboli, air, fat, calcified material, or foreign body, leading to myocardial ischemia

ETIOLOGY/PATHOGENESIS

Direct Coronary Embolization

- Endocarditis: Aortic or mitral valve
  - Nonbacterial
  - Infective: 1.5% in clinical series
- Heart mural thrombi
  - Atrial fibrillation [most frequent cardiac cause of coronary emboli (28.3%) in clinical series]
  - Myocardial infarct
  - Cardiomyopathy
- Mitral and aortic valve calcified deposits
- Myocardial infarction with rupture: Myocardial emboli
- Heart tumor: Myxoma (villiform variety)

Paradoxical Embolization

- Patent foramen ovale
- Atrial septal defect
- Pulmonary arteriovenous malformation from venous into systemic circulation

Iatrogenic Embolization

- Cardiac catheterization 0.1-0.3% of procedures
- Coronary CTA
- Endovascular devices coated with polymer material
- Cardiac surgery
  - Prosthetic valve replacement
  - Debridement of calcified valve or vessel
- Percutaneous balloon angioplasty (necrotic debris from native coronaries or bypass grafts)
- External cardiac massage

Other

- Tumor emboli from extracardiac malignancies
- Hypercoagulative state (antiphospholipid antibody syndrome)
- Trauma of large bones

Emboli Composition

- Platelet-fibrin emboli
- Calcium
- Talc
- Suture material
- Hydrophilic coating endovascular device polymer
- Cholesterol crystals
- Myocardium
- Air
- Fat
- Tumor fragments

CLINICAL IMPLICATIONS

Epidemiology

- Incidence
  - Rare cause of myocardial infarction (2.9% in clinical studies)
  - Prior to 1960, reported incidence ranged from 0.06-5.00% of cases of acute myocardial infarction
  - In autopsy reports, ~ 10-13% of myocardial infarcts are secondary to coronary artery emboli

Site

- Left coronary and branches are more commonly involved in noniatrogenic embolization

Presentation

- Clinical manifestations depend on type and size of emboli
- Acute cardiac event can occur in any type of emboli
  - Angina
  - Myocardial infarction
  - Arrhythmia
  - Sudden death
  - Cardiogenic shock
  - Pulmonary edema
  - Borderline elevated cardiac enzymes

Myocardial Infarct Secondary to Embolization

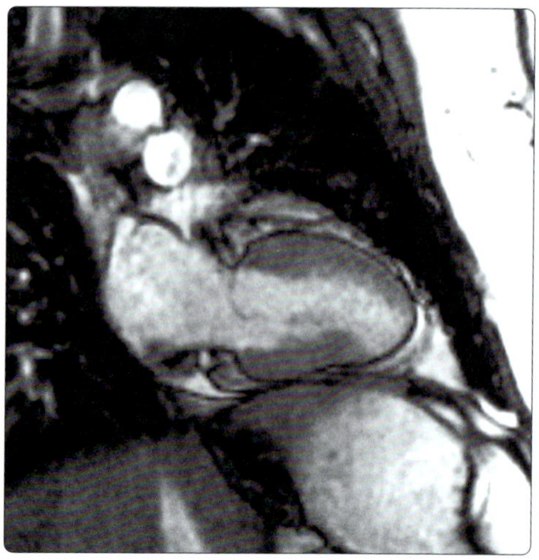

Coronary Artery Branch With Emboli From Coating Gel Device

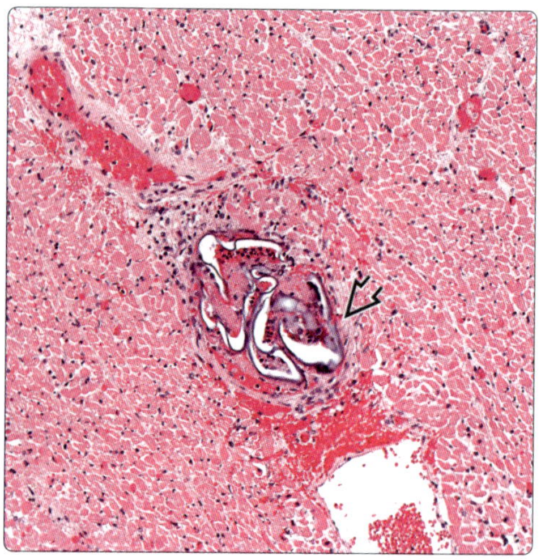

(Left) *Left ventricle long-axis SSPF MR shows transmural increased signal in the inferior apical wall, indicating small, acute infarct with corresponding edema. Coronaries were without atherosclerosis.* **(Right)** *H&E-stained section shows basophilic amorphous foreign material* ⇒ *within an intramyocardial vessel corresponding to polymer coating gel from a device used for coronary catheterization.*

- Septic emboli, in addition to acute cardiac event, may present with fever, heart murmur, splinter hemorrhages, splenomegaly

Treatment

- Options, risks, complications
  - Immediate treatment depends on type of emboli
- Surgical approaches
  - Aspiration thrombectomy should be considered in presence of high thrombus load
  - Stenting of occluded vessel is possible in select cases
  - Percutaneous transluminal coronary angioplasty
  - Air aspiration
  - Forceful injection of saline or contrast media to remove air emboli
  - Treatment of underlying cause (resection of myxoma or atrial thrombi)
- Drugs
  - Long-term anticoagulation is indicated to prevent thromboemboli in patients with valve prosthesis, mural thrombi, or cardiomyopathy
  - Antibiotics in cases of septic emboli are indicated
  - Thrombolytic therapy can be used depending upon etiology of embolization

Prognosis

- Long-term outcomes of ST-segment-elevation myocardial infarct patients secondary to coronary emboli are worse than atherosclerotic coronary disease due to acute onset and absent collateral circulation
- Recurrence is possible, especially if atrial fibrillation is present
- 50% mortality at 10 years has been reported

IMAGING FINDINGS

Echocardiography

- Can determine origin of thrombus in heart chambers
- Identify valve abnormalities: Vegetations, calcifications
- Presence of atrial septal defect or patent foramen ovale

CT Findings

- Cardiac-gated CTA may show
  - Subtle subendocardial perfusion defect
  - Regional akinesis
  - May identify underlying pathology (mural thrombus, tumor)

Coronary Angiogram

- Filling defects in multiple coronary territories
- Atherosclerotic disease is usually absent
- Abrupt occlusion of coronary branches
- No significant collateral vessels

MACROSCOPIC

General Features

- Gross findings depend on type of emboli

MICROSCOPIC

Histologic Features

- Types of emboli
  - Atheroemboli
    - Composed of fibrin, platelets, cholesterol clefts, and calcified material
    - Complication of coronary artery interventions in patients with atherosclerotic disease
  - Calcium emboli
    - Calcium material from aortic or mitral valves may be dislodged after surgical interventions
  - Septic emboli
    - Composed of fibrin and platelets; bacterial agents may be identified
    - Secondary to infectious endocarditis
  - Hydrophilic polymer gel-coated emboli
    - Nonpolarizable, nonrefractile granular material
    - Basophilic, eosinophilic, colorless, gray-black
    - Associated thrombosis and foreign body giant cell reaction
    - Negative stain for calcium
  - Tumor emboli
    - Most common from atrial myxoma or papillary fibroelastoma
    - Emboli may be composed of fibrin material overlying tumor
    - Fragments of myxoma or other malignant tumor may be identified within artery lumen
  - Myocardial emboli
    - Extremely rare
    - Sequela of ruptured myocardial infarct
    - Reported cases after septal myomectomy occur
  - Bone marrow emboli
    - Paradoxical emboli in extensive resuscitation
- Myocardial changes
  - Extent of myocardial injury depends on size of vessel involved and collateral circulation
  - Focal areas of ischemic necrosis

DIFFERENTIAL DIAGNOSIS

Atherosclerotic Coronary Disease

- Most common cause of coronary occlusion
- Atherosclerotic plaque

SELECTED REFERENCES

1. De Roeck F et al: Prosthetic aortic valve thrombosis complicated by left main coronary artery bifurcation embolism: case report and review of literature. Cardiovasc Revasc Med. 28S:72-4, 2021
2. Kariyanna PT et al: Coronary embolism and myocardial infarction: a scoping study. Am J Med Case Rep. 8(2):31-43, 2020
3. Xiang G et al: Clinical features and prognosis of acute myocardial infarction caused by non-tumor origin coronary artery embolism. Am J Emerg Med. 38(6):1185-91, 2020
4. Hickey TB et al: Iatrogenic embolization following cardiac intervention: postmortem analysis of 110 cases. Cardiovasc Pathol. 40:12-8, 2019
5. Vendittelli PS et al: Coronary artery embolism: two case reports and a review of the literature. Am J Med Sci. 357(4):333-7, 2019
6. Miyaoka M et al: Clinicopathological features of hydrophilic polymer emboli in Japanese autopsy cases. APMIS. 126(11):838-41, 2018
7. Popovic B et al: Coronary embolism among ST-segment-elevation myocardial infarction patients: mechanisms and management. Circ Cardiovasc Interv. 11(1):e005587, 2018
8. Raphael CE et al: Coronary embolus: an underappreciated cause of acute coronary syndromes. JACC Cardiovasc Interv. 11(2):172-80, 2018
9. Shibata T et al: Prevalence, clinical features, and prognosis of acute myocardial infarction attributable to coronary artery embolism. Circulation. 132(4):241-50, 2015

Giant Cell/Temporal Arteritis

KEY FACTS

TERMINOLOGY

- Vasculitis of large vessels with unique predilection for involvement of extracranial carotid artery branches (including temporal artery)
- Considered granulomatous arteritis in Chapel Hill classification due to abundance of histiocytes and absence of necrosis

CLINICAL ISSUES

- Older adults; Chapel Hill classification specifies that patients must be > 50 years old; most are typically in their 70s or 80s

MACROSCOPIC

- Because segmental involvement is common, evaluating multiple sections at multiple levels is recommended

MICROSCOPIC

- Transmural (intimal, medial, and adventitial) inflammatory infiltrate
- Giant cells are frequently absent and not required for diagnosis

TOP DIFFERENTIAL DIAGNOSES

- Prior traumatic injury
- Takayasu arteritis

DIAGNOSTIC CHECKLIST

- Temporal arteries are generally not affected by atherosclerosis
  - Intimal thickening should not be interpreted as atherosclerosis but should prompt thorough evaluation of media for healed arteritis features
- Mönckeberg medial calcific sclerosis and elastic laminar calcification are common in older patients and frequently seen
  - Giant cells seen in this context do not indicate giant cell arteritis (GCA) (if other features, such as transmural inflammation, are absent)

Intraoperative Photograph of Temporal Artery

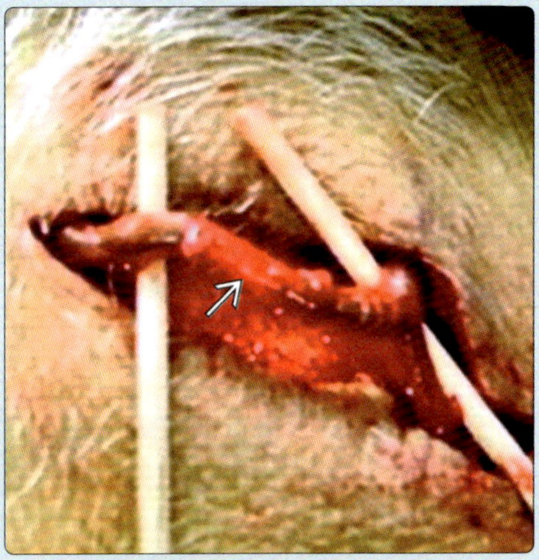

Cross Section of Giant Cell/Temporal Arteritis

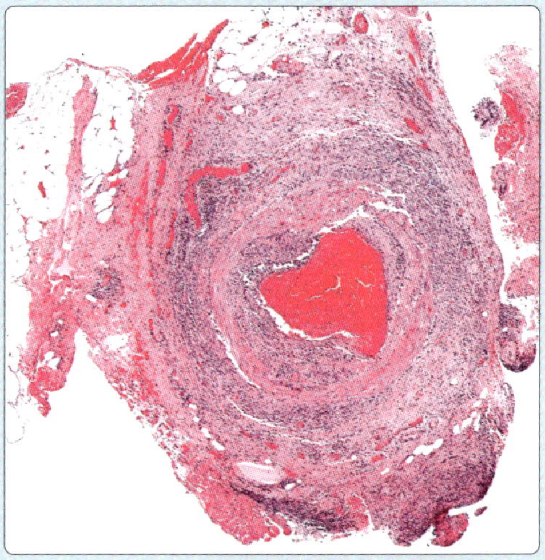

(Left) *This photograph taken just prior to a temporal artery biopsy shows the abnormal nodular and thickened appearance of a temporal artery ➡ involved by giant cell arteritis (GCA).* **(Right)** *This temporal artery involved by temporal arteritis shows transmural inflammation, the histologic hallmark of giant cell/temporal arteritis.*

Histologic Features of Giant Cell/Temporal Arteritis

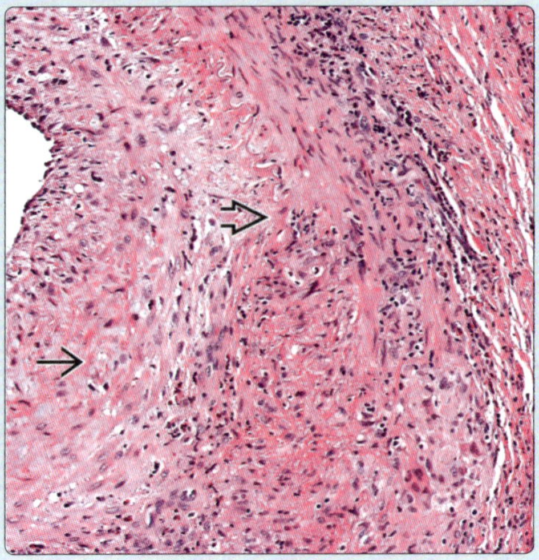

Histologic Features of Giant Cell/Temporal Arteritis

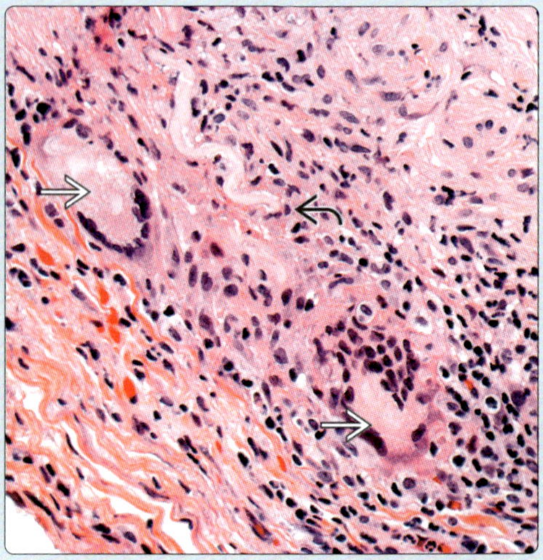

(Left) *Disruption of the internal elastic layer ⇨ is clearly seen on this H&E stain. The intimal layer ⇨ (inside the internal elastic layer) also shows pronounced thickening, typical of GCA. There is transmural inflammation, although no giant cells are seen in this case.* **(Right)** *Multinucleated giant cells ➡, GCA's namesake, are seen as part of a mixed transmural inflammation in this artery. There is also disruption of the internal elastic lamina ⇨.*

TERMINOLOGY

Abbreviations

- Giant cell arteritis (GCA)

Definitions

- Vasculitis of large vessels with unique predilection for involvement of extracranial carotid artery branches (including temporal artery)

CLINICAL ISSUES

Epidemiology

- Age
  - Older adults; most are typically in their 70s or 80s
- Sex
  - Female patients are affected 2-3x more often than male patients
- Ethnicity
  - Most common in people of northern European ancestry

Presentation

- Cranial ischemia
  - Headache (temporooccipital)
  - Scalp tenderness
  - Bulging nodular temporal artery
  - Jaw claudication (pain with chewing)
  - Partial or complete visual loss
- Polymyalgia rheumatica (proximal joint arthritis)
  - Present in 1/3 of GCA patients
- Other arterial involvement
  - Intracranial: Stroke, transient ischemic attack
  - Subclavian: Upper extremity claudication, asymmetric blood pressure
  - Ascending aorta: Aortic aneurysms ± rupture

Treatment

- Corticosteroids
  - Response is usually rapid
  - Eventual tapering is recommended; relapses common
  - Average duration of steroid treatment is 2 years

Prognosis

- Generally indolent, slowly progressing; responds to steroids
- Visual loss and aneurysm rupture are feared complications

IMAGING

Radiographic Findings

- Angiography (for small vessel involvement) shows smooth tapering and segmental distribution
- Tomographic angiography (for large vessel involvement) shows aneurysm formation and wall thickening
  - Sparing of proximal aortic arch branches is helpful in distinguishing from Takayasu arteritis

MACROSCOPIC

Sections to Be Submitted

- Because segmental involvement is common, evaluating multiple sections at multiple levels is recommended
- Because precise cross sections are difficult to obtain on wet specimens, processing whole vessel sampled and then scalpel sectioning and embedding is preferred

Temporal Artery Biopsy

- Wall thickening, luminal narrowing apparent grossly

MICROSCOPIC

Histologic Features

- Transmural (intimal, medial, and adventitial) inflammatory infiltrate
- Segmental destruction of internal elastic lamina
- Medial replacement fibrosis (and smooth muscle loss &/or disorganization)
- Lymphocytes and macrophages predominate
- Giant cells are occasionally seen without well-formed granulomas
  - Giant cells frequently absent, not required for diagnosis

Healed Arteritis

- Minimal to absent inflammation
- Evidence of elastic laminar disruption with associated medial fibrosis
- Controversial and difficult to diagnose definitively, but possibility should be raised in setting of these findings

ANCILLARY TESTS

Histochemistry

- Elastic stain to demonstrate elastic laminar disruption
- Connective tissue stains highlight fibrous replacement

DIFFERENTIAL DIAGNOSIS

Temporal Artery

- Prior traumatic injury
  - May show elastic laminar disruption and medial fibrosis (even pseudoaneurysm formation) in segmental pattern but usually without inflammation
  - May be difficult to differentiate on histopathology, but clinical correlation is usually helpful

Large Vessels

- Takayasu arteritis
  - More often has acute inflammatory component and "dirty" necrosis
  - Adventitial fibroinflammatory thickening common
  - Histopathology may be difficult to differentiate from GCA in many cases, but, clinically, patients are much younger and have different distribution of vessel involvement

SELECTED REFERENCES

1. Agostino A et al: Efficacy of bilateral temporal artery biopsies and sectioning of the entire block of tissue for the diagnosis of temporal arteritis. Cardiovasc Pathol. 59:107425, 2022
2. Shen A et al: Effect of temporal artery biopsy length and laterality on diagnostic yield. J Neuroophthalmol. 42(2):208-11, 2022
3. Frohman L et al: New developments in giant cell arteritis. Surv Ophthalmol. 61(4):400-21, 2016
4. Hussain O et al: Diagnosis of giant cell arteritis: when should we biopsy the temporal artery? Br J Oral Maxillofac Surg. 54(3):327-30, 2016
5. Cavazza A et al: Inflamed temporal artery: histologic findings in 354 biopsies, with clinical correlations. Am J Surg Pathol. 38(10):1360-70, 2014

(Left) *Normal temporal artery is characterized by minimal thickening of the intima → and a circumferentially intact elastic lamina →. A (normal) thick-walled branch vessel → is also seen.* **(Right)** *Section of temporal artery involved by GCA shows transmural inflammation with a mixed infiltrate involving the adventitial →, medial →, and intimal → layers. The elastic stain highlights elastic lamina disruption →.*

Normal Histology of Temporal Artery

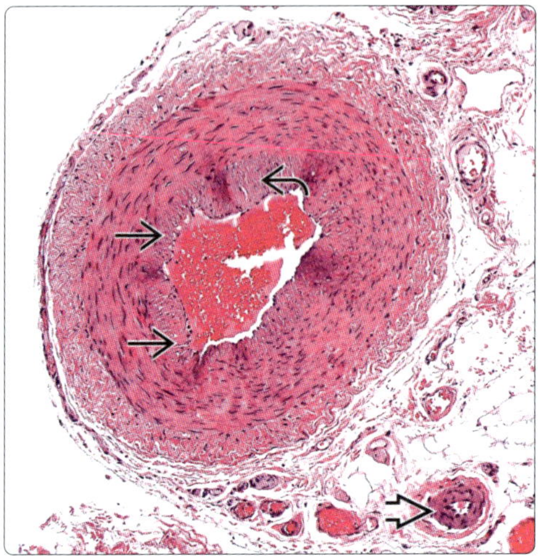

Elastic Stain of Temporal Arteritis

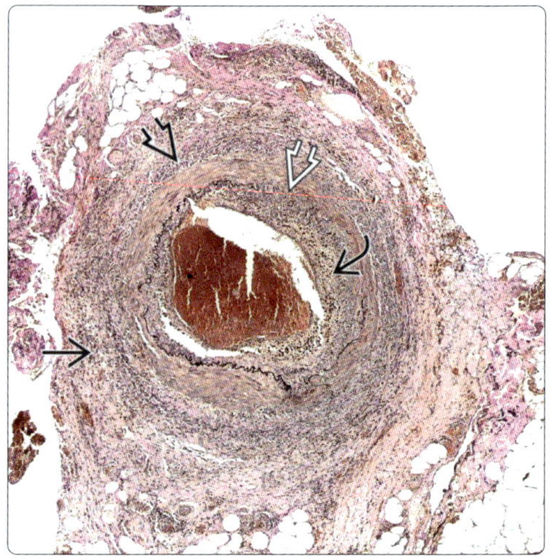

(Left) *This temporal artery is involved by GCA. There is transmural inflammation with a mixed infiltrate involving the adventitial →, medial →, and intimal → layers. The intima shows segmental loose fibrous thickening.* **(Right)** *This elastic-stained temporal artery segment in the same patient better delineates the vessel layers and shows discrete areas of internal elastic laminar disruption →.*

Histologic Features of Giant Cell/Temporal Arteritis

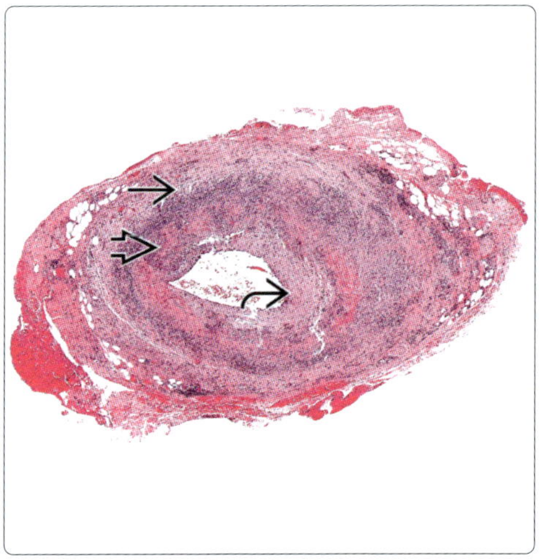

Elastic Stain of Giant Cell/Temporal Arteritis

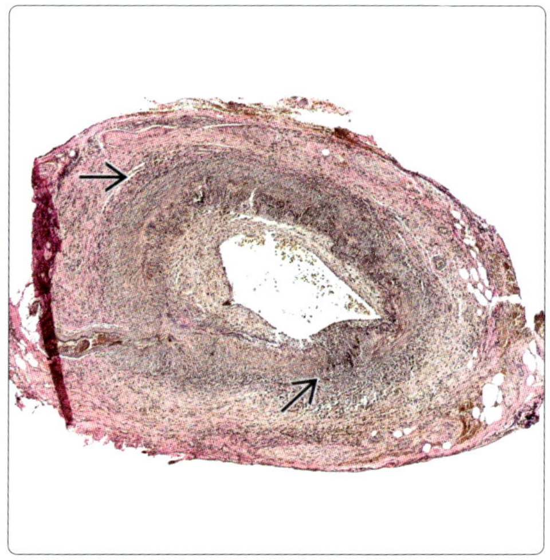

(Left) *This case of temporal arteritis shows mixed transmural inflammation that includes lymphocytes, eosinophils, neutrophils, plasma cells, and macrophages. In a few areas, the macrophages have coalesced into nascent giant cells →.* **(Right)** *Another multinucleated giant cell → is seen as part of the adventitial inflammatory component in this case of temporal arteritis. The presence of giant cells is not necessary for the diagnosis, and, frequently, no giant cells are seen.*

Histologic Features of Giant Cell/Temporal Arteritis

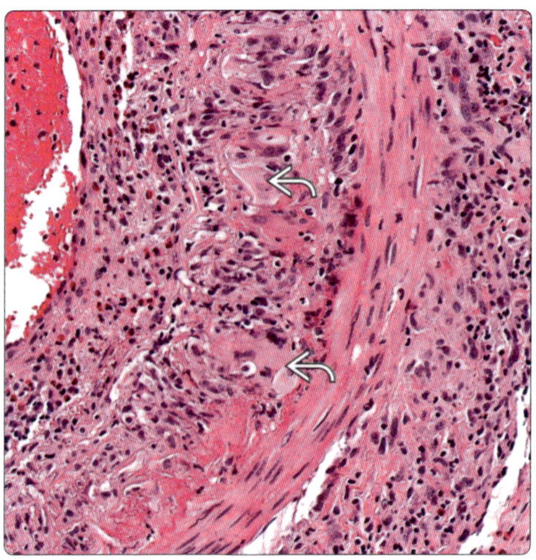

Histologic Features of Giant Cell/Temporal Arteritis

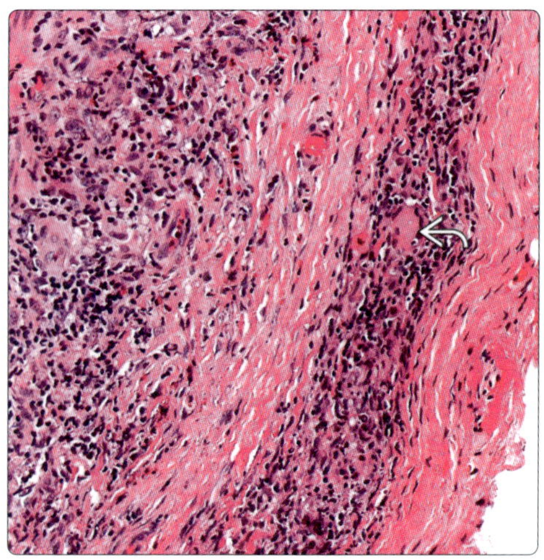

Histologic Features of Giant Cell/Temporal Arteritis

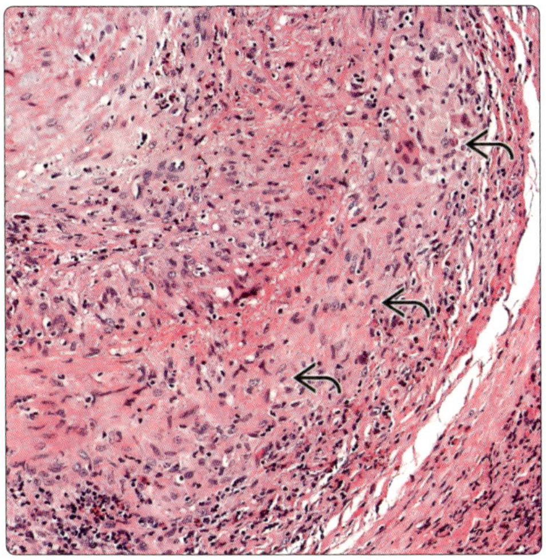

Elastic Stain of Giant Cell/Temporal Arteritis

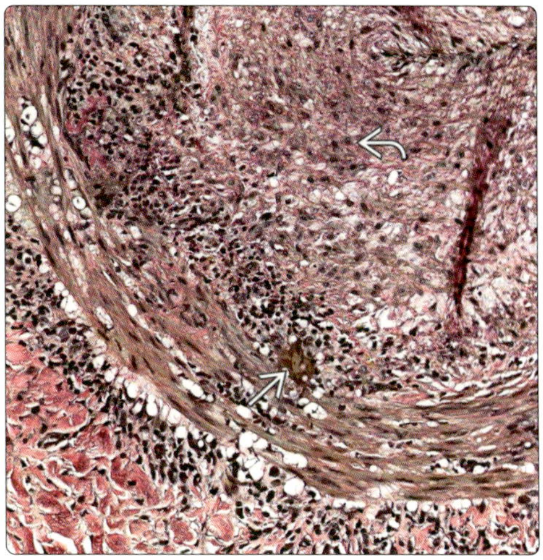

(Left) *This is an example of giant cell/temporal arteritis without giant cells. There is a very prominent histiocytic component ⇨ to the transmural inflammation, but no definitive multinucleated giant cells are seen.* **(Right)** *A multinucleated giant cell ➡ is seen in this level of an elastic-stained temporal artery. The intimal layer ➡ (inside the internal elastic layer) also shows pronounced thickening, which is typical of GCA.*

Histologic Features of Giant Cell/Temporal Arteritis in Healing Stage

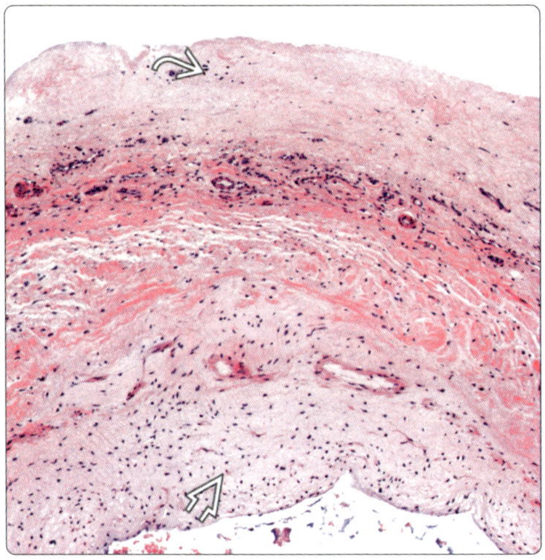

Histologic Features of Giant Cell/Temporal Arteritis in Healing Stage

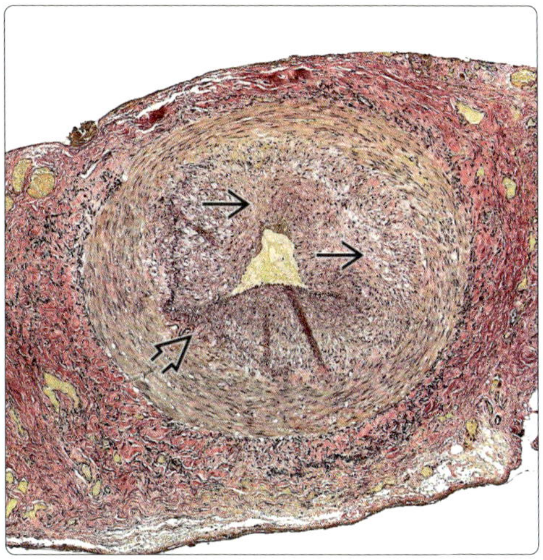

(Left) *This section of the temporal artery shows features of healed arteritis. There is no longer any significant inflammatory infiltrate but marked intimal thickening ➡ and periadventitial fibrosis ➡.* **(Right)** *This temporal artery shows features of healed arteritis. There is no longer any significant inflammatory infiltrate, but there is marked intimal thickening ⇨, and disruption of the internal elastic lamina ⇨ is seen.*

Traumatic Temporal Artery Injury

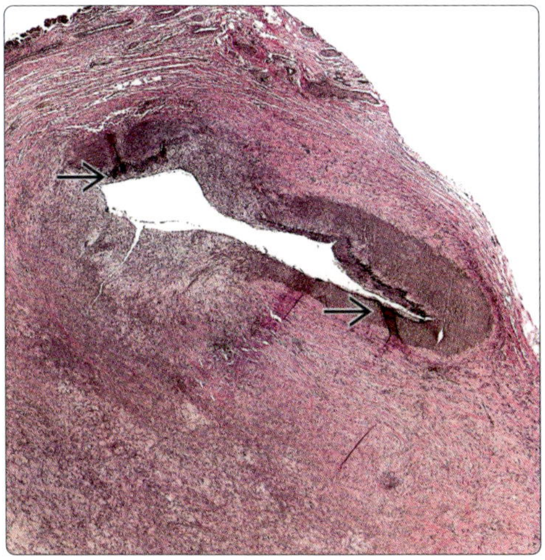

Traumatic Temporal Artery Injury

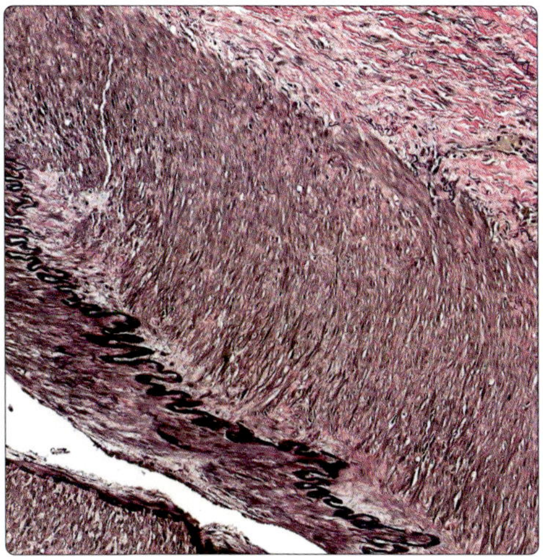

(Left) *This is an example of a traumatic temporal artery injury without arteritis. A contained rupture (pseudoaneurysm) has formed. There is a distinct break in the internal elastic layer ⇨. Trauma to this artery is not uncommon, given the superficial location.* **(Right)** *At higher magnification in the same patient, the artery involved by trauma shows no significant inflammation or replacement-type fibrosis in the medial layer. The internal elastic layer is intact, except at the area of trauma.*

Buerger Disease (Thromboangiitis Obliterans)

KEY FACTS

TERMINOLOGY

- Thromboangiitis obliterans: Progressive, nonatherosclerotic, segmental, inflammatory disease of small- and medium-sized vessels (arteries and veins) of lower and upper extremities

ETIOLOGY/PATHOGENESIS

- Exposure to any form of tobacco

CLINICAL ISSUES

- Disease of young smokers
  - Symptoms usually start before 45 years of age
- Originally thought to affect men only
  - Women also affected, especially smokers
- Ischemic symptoms
- Loss of sensation affects up to 70% of patients
- Raynaud phenomenon affects > 40% of patients and can be asymmetrical
- Complete cessation of all forms of tobacco to stop progression of clinical symptoms
- Patient's ability to discontinue tobacco most important factor affecting prognosis

IMAGING

- Multiple segmental, vascular occlusions of distal small- to medium-sized arteries
- Collateralization around obstructions ("corkscrew collaterals")

MICROSCOPIC

- Inflammatory thrombosis affecting arteries and veins
- Vessel wall inflammation
- Progressive thrombus organization
  - Associated with inflammatory cell infiltration (lymphohistiocytic, granulocytic, eosinophilic)
  - More prominent in thrombus compared to vessel wall
- Segmental distribution of disease

(Left) *The right lower limb shows dry gangrene of the toes in this 42-year-old man with history of smoking and no risk factors of atherosclerosis or other systemic vasculitic process. In this setting, these findings are compatible with Buerger disease.* **(Right)** *Artery of the lower limb shows lumen occluded by thrombus with associated inflammatory cell infiltration ↪. The internal elastic appears intact →, and no inflammation is seen. Early lesions are more useful for diagnosis.*

Dry Gangrene of Lower Extremity

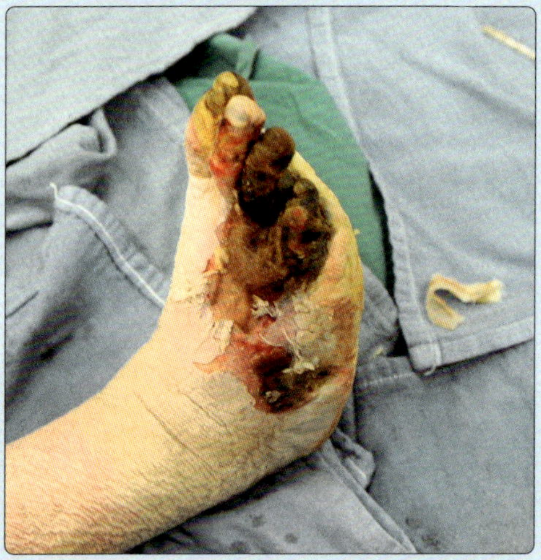

Acute Stage of Buerger Disease

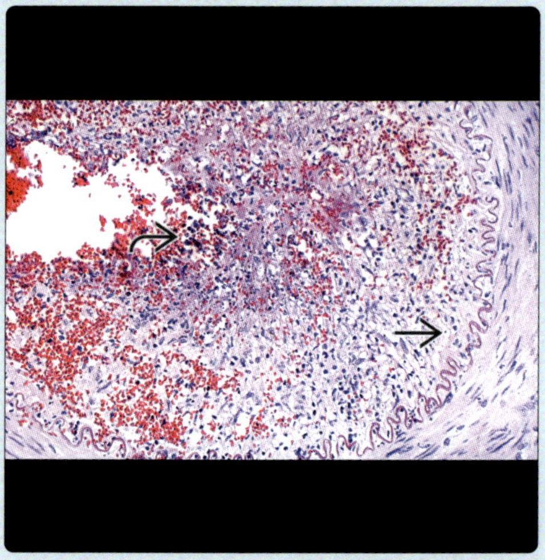

(Left) *Artery of the lower limb in a young man with a history of claudication and smoking shows chronic inflammatory cell infiltration in the wall → and an organized thrombus ↪.* **(Right)** *Artery wall shows lymphocyte infiltration, hemosiderin-laden macrophages, and intact internal elastic lamina →. These features are consistent with Buerger disease (subacute stage).*

Subacute Stage of Buerger Disease

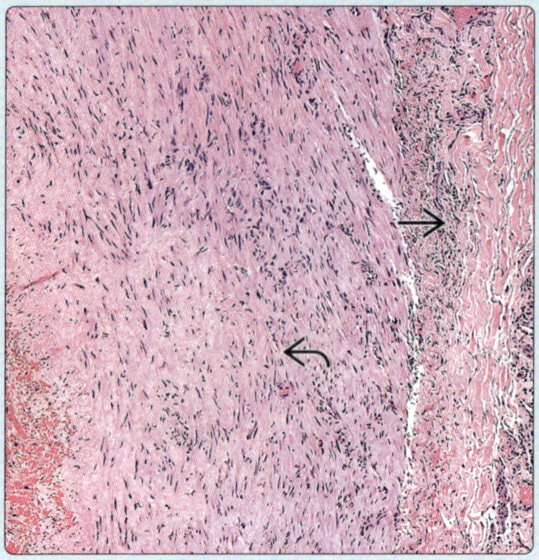

Subacute Stage of Buerger Disease

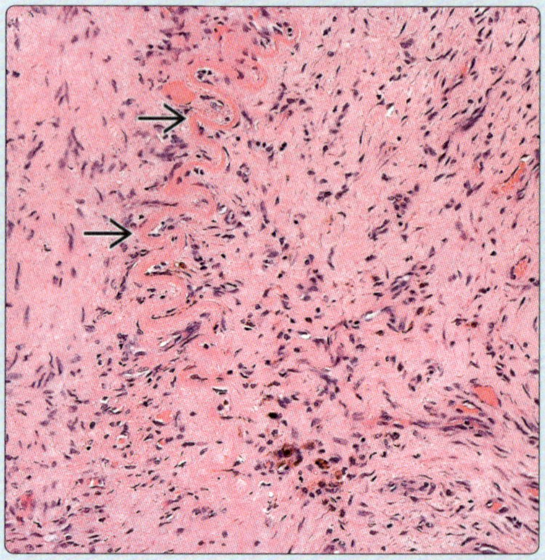

TERMINOLOGY

Synonyms

- Thromboangiitis obliterans (TAO)

Definitions

- Progressive, nonatherosclerotic, segmental, occlusive, inflammatory disease of small- and medium-sized vessels (arteries and veins) of lower and upper extremities

ETIOLOGY/PATHOGENESIS

Smoking

- Exposure to any form of tobacco; recent reports of cannabis as well
- Tobacco exposure plays key role in initiation and progression of disease

Autoimmune

- Anticardiolipin antibodies, antiendothelial antibodies
- ↑ cellular immunity to types I and III collagen
- ↑ linear deposits of immunoglobulins and complement along elastic lamina
- Autoimmune serologic testing (ANA, anti-dsDNA, anti-Smith, SCL-70, anticentromere, RNP, etc.)
- ↑ IL-17, IL-22, and IL-23 reported in TAO patients

Genetic

- Prothrombin gene mutation 202105
- Decrease in frequency of HLA-B12 antigen
- Disease-linked polymorphism in toll-like receptor *MYD88* ↑ susceptibility to TAO

Coagulation Abnormalities

- Hematocrit, RBC rigidity, and blood viscosity ↑ in TAO

Infection

- TAO associated with chronic anaerobic periodental infections in ~ 66% of patients
- "COVID toes" show some overlapping features

CLINICAL ISSUES

Epidemiology

- Incidence
  - Reported prevalence has declined in past decades, probably due to decline in tobacco use or due to ↑ in socioeconomic conditions
- Age
  - Disease of young smokers
  - Symptoms usually start before 45 years of age
- Sex
  - Originally thought to affect men only
  - Women also affected, likely due to ↑ cigarette smoking
  - Disease characteristics and prognosis do not seem to differ between men and women
- Ethnicity
  - More common in Middle Eastern and Asian nations (India 45-63%, Korea/Japan 16-66% prevalence in hospital-treated patients with occlusive peripheral vascular disease) but occurs in all populations

Presentation

- Ischemic symptoms
  - Pain and intermittent claudication of extremities; may radiate to central parts of body
  - Foot claudication occurs with infrapopliteal arterial occlusion
  - Calf claudication occurs if disease progresses to suprapopliteal segment
  - Pain may progress to persistent ischemic pain at rest
  - Ischemic ulcerations of toes, feet, or fingers may develop
  - Digital (dry) gangrene may occur, either with more advanced disease or, less commonly, spontaneously as ulceration
  - Gangrene does not always follow claudication and may even precede it
- Loss of sensation affects up to 70% of patients
- Raynaud phenomenon affects > 40% of patients and can be asymmetrical
- Superficial thrombophlebitis (venous involvement) distinguishes TAO from other vasculitides and atherosclerotic lesions
  - Patients may describe migratory pattern of tender nodules that follow venous distribution
- Vasculitis may involve mesenteric, cerebral, and coronary arteries and may even show multiorgan involvement

Treatment

- Adjuvant therapy
  - Complete cessation of all forms of tobacco to stop progression of clinical symptoms
  - Intermittent compression of arms and legs to ↑ blood flow to extremities
  - Spinal cord stimulation
- Surgical
  - Percutaneous transluminal angioplasty has been effective in some cases with critical limb ischemia
  - Amputation if gangrene affects limb
- Drugs
  - Iloprost (prostaglandin analogue): May cause pain relief and complete healing of trophic changes
  - Cilostazol (phosphodiesterase inhibitor): Indicated in ischemic ulcerations with no other possible revascularization strategies
  - Bosentan (endothelin receptor antagonists): Indicated in refractory cases, may ↑ distal flow with clinical improvement of trophic lesions
- Autologous bone marrow mononuclear cell transplantation
  - Effective treatment in some cases with critical limb ischemia with no other therapy options

Prognosis

- Patient's ability to discontinue tobacco most important factor affecting prognosis
- Death from TAO unusual but morbidity substantial

IMAGING

Angiography

- Typical angiographic findings
  - Multiple segmental, vascular occlusions of distal small- to medium-sized arteries
  - Collateralization ("corkscrew collaterals")
  - Proximal arteries should be normal with no evidence of atherosclerosis, aneurysm, or other source of emboli

- "Corkscrew collaterals" may be seen in other diseases
  - Connective tissue diseases: SLE, mixed connective tissue disease (MCTD), scleroderma, CREST syndrome

Echocardiography

- Excludes cardiac source of emboli

CECT With Contrast and MR

- Noninvasive vascular imaging
- Both useful in excluding arterial source of emboli
- Both define anatomy and extent of disease

MICROSCOPIC

Histologic Features

- Inflammatory thrombosis affecting arteries and veins
- Segmental distribution of disease
  - Normal areas interspersed with diseased segments
  - Variably intense inflammation in different segments
  - Acute phase of disease rare and most diagnostic
  - Chronic phase more common, less distinctive
- Acute stage: Inflammatory cell infiltration of thrombus more prominent compared to vessel wall
  - Polymorphonuclear leukocytes
  - Lymphohistiocytic inflammation
  - Occasionally, eosinophils
  - Microabscesses
    - Collection of polymorphs and multinucleated giant cells around thrombus
  - Vessel wall inflammation characterized by
    - Acute inflammatory cell infiltration involving all vessel layers and composed of
      - Polymorphonuclear leukocytes
      - Lymphohistiocytic inflammation
      - Eosinophils may also be found
- Subacute stage: Progressive thrombus organization
  - Associated with inflammatory cell infiltration (lymphohistiocytic, granulocytic, eosinophilic)
  - Variable vascularization of media
- Chronic stage: Complete organization of thrombus with extensive recanalization
  - Associated with lymphoid infiltration of organized thrombus
  - Variable wall and perivascular fibrosis
- Biopsy of early phlebitic lesions shows
  - Acute phlebitis without thrombus
  - Acute phlebitis with thrombus: Mixed inflammation of vessel wall with inflammatory thrombus
  - Granulomas
- Foci of residual inflammation in organized thrombi may suggest Buerger disease

ANCILLARY TESTS

Histochemistry

- Elastic stain should be performed to characterize internal elastic lamina

DIFFERENTIAL DIAGNOSIS

Systemic Lupus Erythematosus

- Immune complex deposition and autoimmune serologies (ANA, anti-dsDNA, anti-Smith) typically positive

Systemic Sclerosis (Scleroderma)

- Raynaud phenomenon with distal phalangeal ischemia part of spectrum of this autoimmune disease
- SCL-70 and anticentromere serologies
- CREST syndrome variant

Mixed Connective Tissue Disease

- RNP(+)

Hypothenar Hammer Syndrome (Repetitive Vascular Traumatic Injury)

- Usually, underlying intimal thickening and fibromuscular dysplasia-type changes present in vessel wall
- Superimposed thrombosis, usually with less prominent inflammation
- Veins typically not involved

Atherosclerosis Obliterans

- Stenotic atheromatous plaque causing luminal obstruction
- ± thrombosis

Distal Embolic Events

- Underlying vessel typically normal (or atherosclerotic)
- Echocardiogram, other imaging to assess source of embolism

SELECTED REFERENCES

1. Bergère G et al: Effect of cannabis consumption on characteristics and evolution of thromboangiitis obliterans. Vasa. 50(4):301-5, 2021
2. Sachdeva M et al: A review of COVID-19 chilblains-like lesions and their differential diagnosis. Adv Skin Wound Care. 34(7):348-54, 2021
3. Ehteshamfar SM et al: Humoral and cellular immune response to Buerger's disease. Vascular. 28(4):457-64, 2020
4. Mohamad Yusoff F et al: Long-term clinical outcomes of autologous bone marrow mononuclear cell implantation in patients with severe thromboangiitis obliterans. Circ J. 84(4):650-5, 2020
5. Li MD et al: Risk factors, mechanisms and treatments of thromboangiitis obliterans: an overview of recent research. Curr Med Chem. 27(35):6057-72, 2020
6. Kacmaz F et al: Clinical outcomes of extended endovascular recanalization of 16 consecutive Buerger's disease patients. Vascular. 27(3):233-41, 2019
7. Keramat S et al: Assessment of T helper 17-associated cytokines in thromboangiitis obliterans. J Inflamm Res. 12:251-8, 2019
8. Le Joncour A et al: Long-term outcome and prognostic factors of complications in thromboangiitis obliterans (Buerger's disease): a multicenter study of 224 patients. J Am Heart Assoc. 7(23):e010677, 2018
9. Sun XL et al: Pathogenesis of thromboangiitis obliterans: gene polymorphism and immunoregulation of human vascular endothelial cells. Atherosclerosis. 265:258-65, 2017
10. Rivera-Chavarría IJ et al: Thromboangiitis obliterans (Buerger's disease). Ann Med Surg (Lond). 7:79-82, 2016
11. Liew NC et al: Pathogenesis and management of Buerger's disease. Int J Low Extrem Wounds. 14(3):231-5, 2015
12. Klein-Weigel PF et al: Thromboangiitis obliterans (Buerger's disease). Vasa. 43(5):337-46, 2014
13. Kobayashi M et al: Endarteritis obliterans in the pathogenesis of Buerger's disease from the pathological and immunohistochemical points of view. Circ J. 78(12):2819-26, 2014

Plantar Aspect of Lower Extremity in Buerger Disease

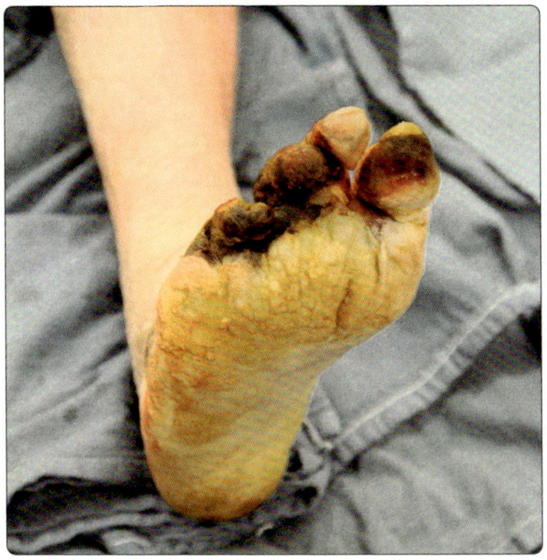

Elastic Stain of Arteries in Buerger Disease

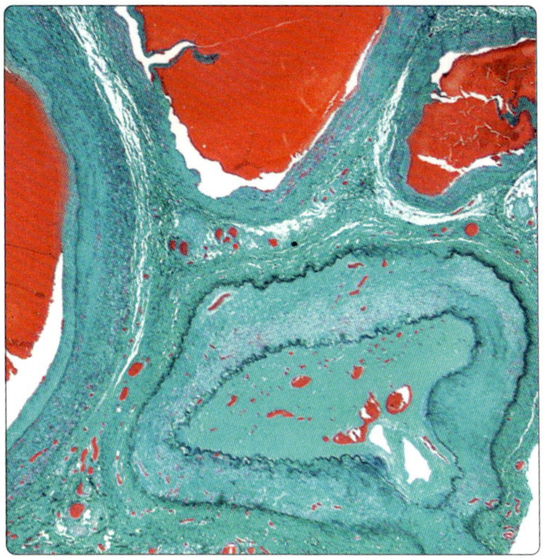

(Left) *The right lower limb shows dry gangrene of the toes in a 42-year-old man with a history of smoking and without other risk factors for atherosclerosis or vasculitic process.* **(Right)** *Lower limb vessels (posterior tibial) in the same patient show organized thrombotic occlusion, consistent with the vascular lesion of the chronic stage of Buerger disease.*

Artery Changes in Chronic Stage of Buerger Disease

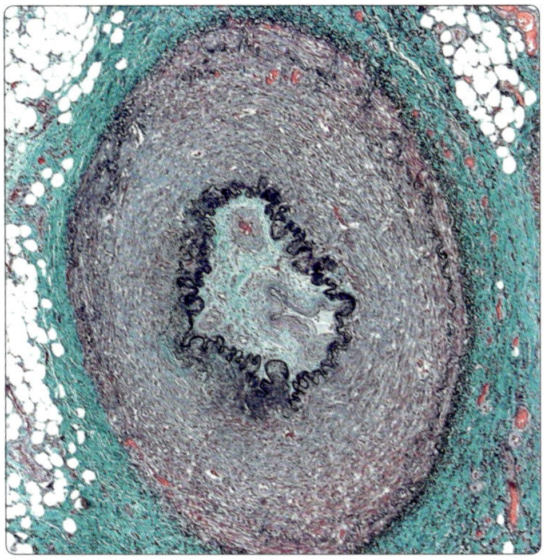

Chronic Stage of Buerger Disease

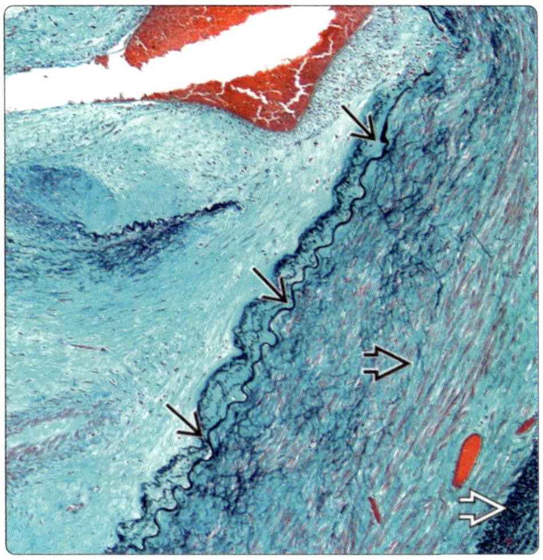

(Left) *Subcutaneous vessel of the lower limb in a smoker shows luminal occlusion by an organized thrombus. No inflammatory cells are seen in the vessel wall or thrombus. In an otherwise normal artery, this is consistent with the chronic stage of Buerger disease.* **(Right)** *Artery shows intact internal elastic lamina ⇨ with no evidence of atherosclerosis or wall inflammation in media ⇨ or adventitia ➡, but the lumen is occluded by an organized thrombus.*

Nonspecific Elastic Lamina Changes

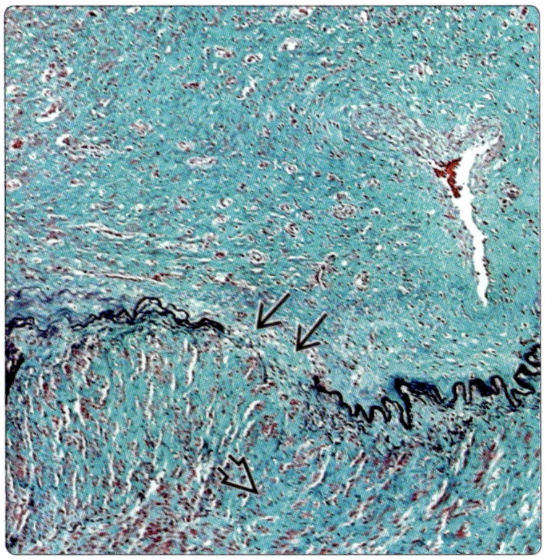

Nonspecific Elastic Lamina Changes

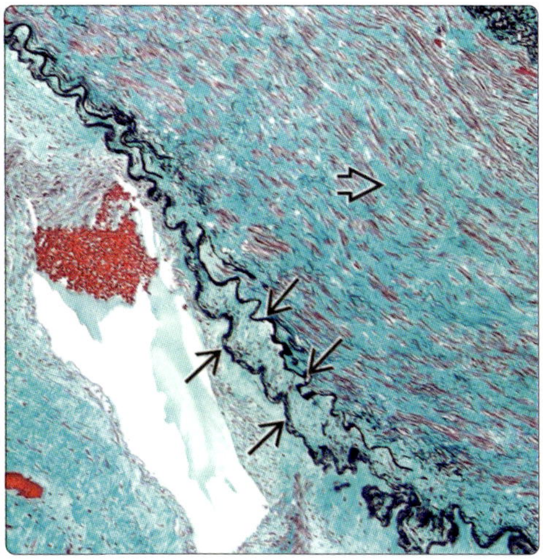

(Left) *Artery shows lumen occluded by an organized thrombus and foci of disruption of internal elastic lamina ⇨, indicating a nonspecific vascular injury. Media ⇨ is noted.* **(Right)** *Another area shows doubling of the internal elastic lamina ⇨, indicating a nonspecific finding of previous vascular injury. Media ⇨ is noted. In Buerger disease, the elastic lamina is usually well preserved.*

Fibromuscular Dysplasia

KEY FACTS

TERMINOLOGY

- Nonatherosclerotic, noninflammatory, fibrous, and fibromuscular proliferation of artery, typically stenosis &/or rupture

CLINICAL ISSUES

- Mostly young and female
- 60-90% involve renal artery, 50% bilateral
  - Commonly present with hypertension
  - May be asymptomatic
- Percutaneous transluminal renal angioplasty is treatment of choice

IMAGING

- String of beads pattern on angiography

MICROSCOPIC

- Intimal
  - Intimal hyperplasia resembles atherosclerosis but without lipid deposition
- Medial
  - Medial fibroplasia with abnormally oriented smooth muscle and aneurysms is most common
  - Perimedial fibroplasia with fibrous band in outer media
  - Medial hyperplasia with hyperplastic but otherwise normal media
- Periarterial (adventitial) fibroplasia
  - Circumferential adventitial fibrosis, normal media and intima

TOP DIFFERENTIAL DIAGNOSES

- Atherosclerosis
- Vasculitis
  - Typically has eccentric scarring, disruption of elastica, and no hyperplasia
- Dissecting aneurysm
  - Healed lesions may resemble perimedial fibroplasia
- Occasionally, normal arteries may appear to have disoriented smooth muscle

Fibromuscular Dysplasia: Elastic Stain

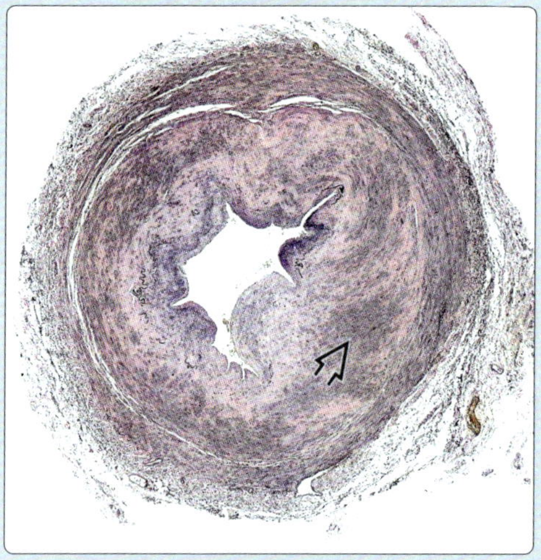

Renal Artery Angiogram in Fibromuscular Dysplasia

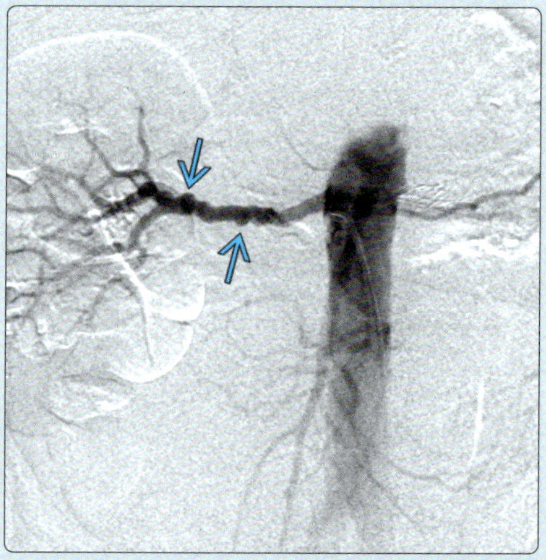

(Left) *Photomicrograph shows an artery in cross section with marked medial smooth muscle disorganization ⇨ and an irregular "festooned" luminal contour.* **(Right)** *Renal arteriogram shows a "string of beads" with multiple stenotic regions ⇨, consistent with fibromuscular dysplasia (FMD). (From DP: Kidney.)*

Pathologic Types of Fibromuscular Dysplasia

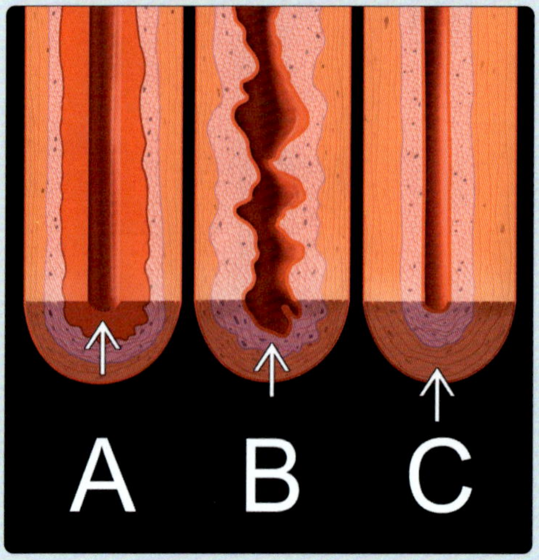

Medial-Type Fibromuscular Dysplasia: Trichrome Stain

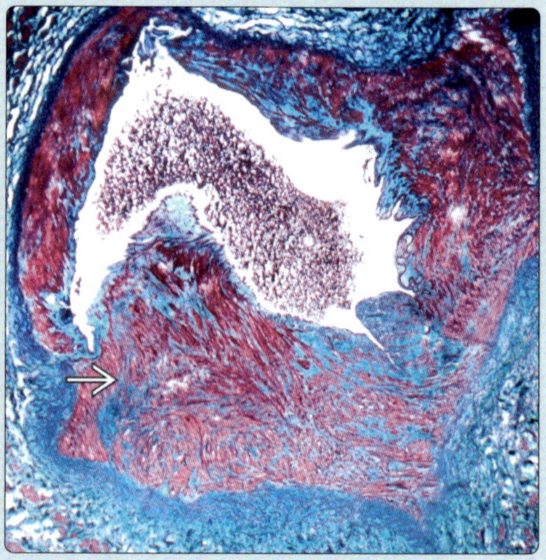

(Left) *FMD occurs in 3 main varieties: (A) Intimal fibroplasia, (B) medial FMD, and (C) periarterial (adventitial) fibroplasia.* **(Right)** *The medial fibroplasia form shows disoriented medial smooth muscle ➡ that protrudes into the lumen of the renal artery (trichrome stain).*

TERMINOLOGY

Abbreviations

- Fibromuscular dysplasia (FMD)

Synonyms

- Arterial fibrodysplasia
- Fibromuscular hyperplasia
- Intimal or periarterial (adventitial) fibroplasia

Definitions

- Idiopathic, segmental, noninflammatory, nonatherosclerotic small- and medium-sized artery diseases causing stenosis, occlusion, dissection, and aneurysms
- 2 major angiographic categories
  - Focal FMD: Single lesion involving any part of artery
  - Multifocal FMD: Alternating areas of stenosis and dilatation (string of beads) involving mid and distal portion of arteries
- 3 major histopathologic categories: Medial, intimal, and periarterial (adventitial)

ETIOLOGY/PATHOGENESIS

Genetic

- Sibling affected in 11% of patients
- Occasionally, associated Ehlers-Danlos syndrome type IV or Marfan syndrome
- Phosphatase and actin regulator 1 (*PHACTR1*) reported as susceptibility locus for FMD

Environment

- Smoking

Female Sex

- No link to estrogens or oral contraceptives proven

CLINICAL ISSUES

Epidemiology

- Incidence
  - ~ 4/1,000 for symptomatic renal FMD
    - Medial: 60-85%
    - Intimal: 1-5%
    - Periarterial: < 1%
  - 10-20% of patients with renal artery stenosis
- Age
  - Younger (15-50 years) for FMD
  - Older (> 50 years) for fibrotic forms
- Sex
  - Female predominance (medial form)
    - 90% affect women < 50 years old
  - Male predominance (intimal form)

Site

- 60-90% involve renal arteries
  - 50% bilateral
  - Distal 2/3 of renal artery
  - Extends into arcuates and interlobular arteries
    - May account for continued hypertension after correction of extrarenal stenosis
  - May have associated aneurysm
- May involve multiple vascular beds
  - Carotid arteries (26%)
  - Mesenteric/intestinal arteries (9%)
  - Iliac arteries (5%)
  - Popliteal, hepatic, coronary, and subclavian arteries (9%)
  - Less commonly, aorta and brachial, superficial femoral, tibial, and peroneal arteries

Presentation

- Hypertension, flank pain, abdominal bruit (renal artery)
- Headache, pulsatile tinnitus, dizziness, neck pain (carotid/vertebral arteries)
- Spontaneous coronary dissection may be associated to FMD
- Asymptomatic

Laboratory Tests

- Renin levels elevated

Treatment

- Surgical approaches
  - Surgical correction curative in ~ 70%
  - Percutaneous transluminal renal angioplasty is treatment of choice
  - Complex reconstruction, such as aortorenal bypass, is required in difficult cases
- Drugs
  - Hypertension may respond to ACE inhibitors but not most other antihypertensive agents
  - Antiplatelet therapy could prevent thrombotic and thromboembolic complications

Prognosis

- Good, if corrected
- If untreated, progressive narrowing may occur over course of 10 years (as judged by angiography)
  - Obstruction, dissecting aneurysms, and emboli may result
  - Sudden death, particularly in FMD of cardiac arteries (e.g., artery supplying sinus node) may occur
- Renal failure rare

IMAGING

General Features

- Catheter-based angiography considered gold standard for diagnosis but is invasive procedure
- CTA best noninvasive procedure to confirm/exclude diagnosis of FMD
- Contrast-enhanced MRA is option if CTA is contraindicated

MACROSCOPIC

General Features

- Beaded pattern of aneurysms and stenosis in renal artery branches

Size

- Kidney may show decreased cortical thickness

MICROSCOPIC

Histologic Features

- **Medial fibroplasia**

  - Aneurysms form as result of loss of smooth muscle and deficient elastic lamina
  - Fibrous and muscular ridges may be formed by alternating with areas of marked thinning and even aneurysm formation
  - Renal infarcts are more common with this type of lesion than other types of FMD
  - Thrombosis or rupture rarely occurs
  - Medial dissection may also occur in 5-10% of cases
    - Channel forms in outer 1/3 of vessel wall
    - Intimal fibroplasia may occur in area of dissection
- **Perimedial fibroplasia**
  - Dense, pale, fibrous tissue in outer media wall is well demarcated from hypertrophied circular muscle of inner media
    - Cellular fibrous tissue may extend transmurally
    - Adventitial fibrosis may extend into adjacent adipose and connective tissue, causing constriction (rare)
  - External elastic lamina outside fibrous zone may be replaced
    - Outer medial border may have circumferential aggregates of elastic tissue, which may appear as dense collagen on light microscopy, but electron microscopy shows them to be elastin
  - Thrombosis is more common in this form than in other types of renal artery dysplasia
  - Multifocal stenoses produce irregular beading with beads smaller than vessel diameter on radiographic examination
- **Medial hyperplasia**
  - Medial smooth muscle hyperplasia devoid of fibrosis showing normal orientation
  - Intima, elastica, and adventitia are normal
  - Angiographic appearance similar to intimal fibroplasia
- **Intimal fibroplasia**
  - Affects major branches of aorta, often bilateral
  - Irregular, long tubular stenosis in young adults; smooth, focal stenosis in older adults
  - Circumferential or eccentric intimal fibrosis
    - Intimal proliferation of loose, moderately cellular fibrous tissue inside internal elastic lamina without lipid or inflammatory cells
    - Internal elastic lamina is present
    - Media and adventitia are normal
- **Periarterial (adventitial) fibroplasia**
  - Collagenous fibroplasia encircles adventitia and extends into surrounding periarterial fibroadipose tissue
  - Few mononuclear cells may be present
  - Intima, internal elastic lamina, external elastic lamina, and media are usually normal
- **Parenchymal lesions, affected side**
  - Atrophy of tubules
    - Small, back-to-back tubules with simple epithelium and little interstitial fibrosis
  - Prominent juxtaglomerular apparatus
  - Small arteries spared changes of hypertension
- **Parenchymal lesions, contralateral side**
  - Compensatory hypertrophy of tubules and glomeruli
  - Vascular lesions related to hypertension
    - Intimal fibrosis of arcuate-sized arteries
    - Arteriolar hyalinosis

DIFFERENTIAL DIAGNOSIS

Atherosclerosis

- Resembles intimal form
- Lipid-laden cells, foam cells, and often, lymphocytes are present

Macroscopic Polyarteritis (Polyarteritis Nodosa)

- Can resemble perimedial fibroplasia or adventitial form
- Typically has eccentric scarring, disruption of elastica, and no hyperplasia

Dissecting Aneurysm

- Healed lesions may resemble perimedial fibroplasia
- Longer continuous involvement

Normal Artery

- Occasionally, normal arteries may appear to have disoriented smooth muscle
- Elastin stains reveal normal layers of elastic lamina

DIAGNOSTIC CHECKLIST

Pathologic Interpretation Pearls

- Elastin stains valuable for evaluation and classification

SELECTED REFERENCES

1. McNair PW et al: Spontaneous coronary artery dissection and its association with fibromuscular dysplasia and other vascular abnormalities. Am J Cardiol. 125(1):34-9, 2020
2. Gornik HL et al: First international consensus on the diagnosis and management of fibromuscular dysplasia. Vasc Med. 24(2):164-89, 2019
3. Krittanawong C et al: Prevalence, presentation, and associated conditions of patients with fibromuscular dysplasia. Am J Cardiol. 123(7):1169-72, 2019
4. Maas AHEM et al: Spontaneous coronary artery dissections and fibromuscular dysplasia: current insights on pathophysiology, sex and gender. Int J Cardiol. 286:220-5, 2019
5. Skeik N et al: Nonatherosclerotic abdominal vasculopathies. Ann Vasc Surg. 60:128-46, 2019
6. Hua X et al: Comparing coronary artery fibromuscular dysplasia with coronary atherosclerosis: from clinical to histopathological characteristics. Cardiovasc Pathol. 35:57-63, 2018
7. Ko M et al: Diagnosis and management of fibromuscular dysplasia and segmental arterial mediolysis in gastroenterology field: a mini-review. World J Gastroenterol. 24(32):3637-49, 2018
8. Narula N et al: Fibromuscular dysplasia: contemporary concepts and future directions. Prog Cardiovasc Dis. 60(6):580-5, 2018
9. Tasaki T et al: Aortic fibromuscular dysplasia complicated by dissection: a case report and review of literature. Cardiovasc Pathol. 31:41-6, 2017
10. Brinza EK et al: Fibromuscular dysplasia: advances in understanding and management. Cleve Clin J Med. 83(11 Suppl 2):S45-51, 2016
11. O'Connor SC et al: Recent developments in the understanding and management of fibromuscular dysplasia. J Am Heart Assoc. 3(6):e001259, 2014
12. Persu A et al: European consensus on the diagnosis and management of fibromuscular dysplasia. J Hypertens. 32(7):1367-78, 2014
13. Olin JW: Recognizing and managing fibromuscular dysplasia. Cleve Clin J Med. 74(4):273-4, 277-82, 2007
14. Plouin PF et al: Fibromuscular dysplasia. Orphanet J Rare Dis. 2:28, 2007
15. Alhadad A et al: Revascularisation of renal artery stenosis caused by fibromuscular dysplasia: effects on blood pressure during 7-year follow-up are influenced by duration of hypertension and branch artery stenosis. J Hum Hypertens. 19(10):761-7, 2005
16. Carmo M et al: Surgical management of renal fibromuscular dysplasia: challenges in the endovascular era. Ann Vasc Surg. 19(2):208-17, 2005
17. Pascual A et al: Renal fibromuscular dysplasia in elderly persons. Am J Kidney Dis. 45(4):e63-6, 2005
18. Boutouyrie P et al: Evidence for carotid and radial artery wall subclinical lesions in renal fibromuscular dysplasia. J Hypertens. 21(12):2287-95, 2003
19. Pannier-Moreau I et al: Possible familial origin of multifocal renal artery fibromuscular dysplasia. J Hypertens. 15(12 Pt 2):1797-801, 1997

Prominent Medial Fibrosis in Fibromuscular Dysplasia

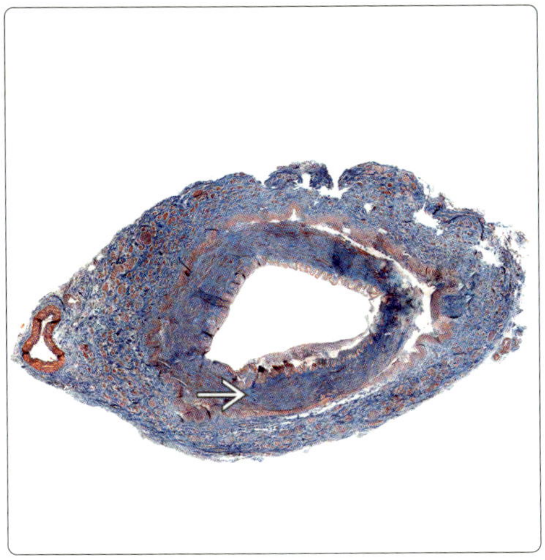

Perimedial Fibroplasia in Fibromuscular Dysplasia

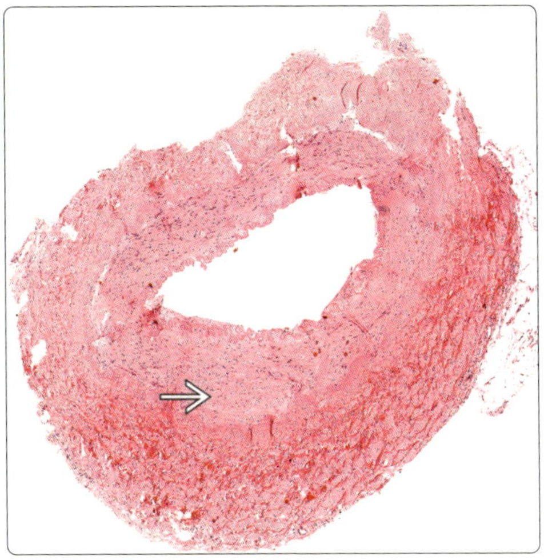

(Left) *Low-power view of the renal artery with perimedial fibroplasia shows that the outer media is occupied by a layer of blue-staining fibrous tissue ➡, as highlighted on this trichrome stain.* **(Right)** *Low-power view shows perimedial fibroplasia of the renal artery in which the outer media is occupied by a layer of fibrous tissue ➡ that is paler than the smooth muscle.*

Perimedial Fibroplasia: Trichrome Stain

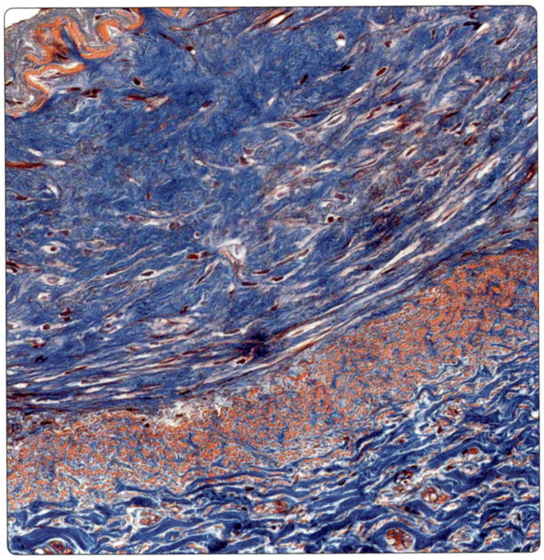

Dense Adventitial Collagen in Fibromuscular Dysplasia

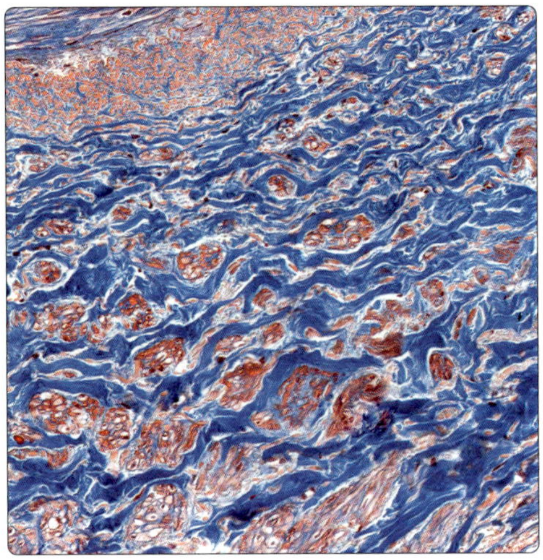

(Left) *Higher power trichrome stain of perimedial fibroplasia shows that the majority of the renal artery wall is composed of variably staining fibrous tissue.* **(Right)** *Higher power trichrome stain of perimedial fibroplasia of the renal artery shows that the arterial wall smooth muscle is infiltrated by dense fibrous tissue.*

Haphazard Arrangement of Medial Smooth Muscle Nuclei in Fibromuscular Dysplasia

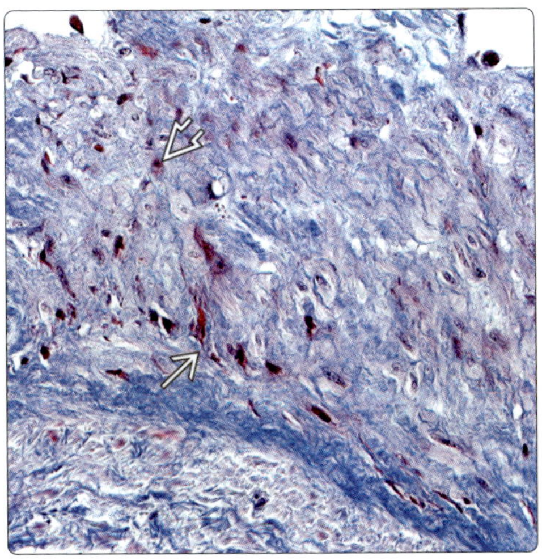

Fibrosis Between Medial Smooth Muscle Cells in Fibromuscular Dysplasia

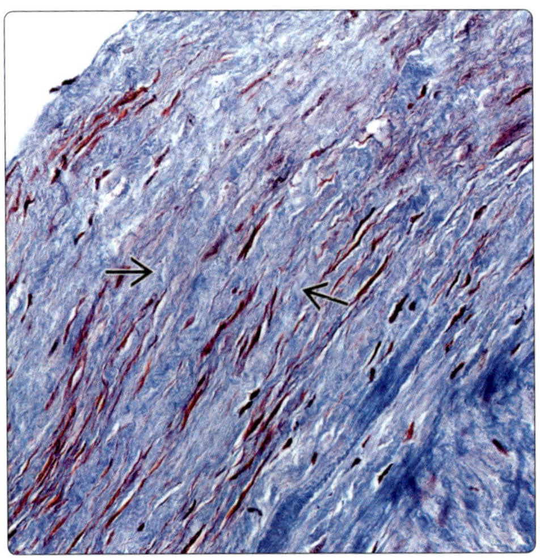

(Left) *Higher power trichrome stain of perimedial fibroplasia of the renal artery shows dense fibrous tissue between smooth muscle cells. Smooth muscle cells simulate both a spindled ➡ and epithelioid ➡ morphology.* **(Right)** *Higher power trichrome stain of perimedial fibroplasia of the renal artery shows dense fibrous tissue ➡ between smooth muscle cells. The smooth muscle cells have acquired a spindled morphology.*

(Left) *Disoriented medial smooth muscle cells protrude into the lumen of a renal artery alternating with abnormally thin regions, typical of the medial fibroplasia variant of FMD. This form is probably a congenital malformation.* **(Right)** *Alternating thick and thin segments of the renal artery wall are highlighted in this longitudinal section of an artery with FMD. Perimedial fibroplasia is also apparent.*

Bizarre Luminal Projections in Medial-Type Fibromuscular Dysplasia

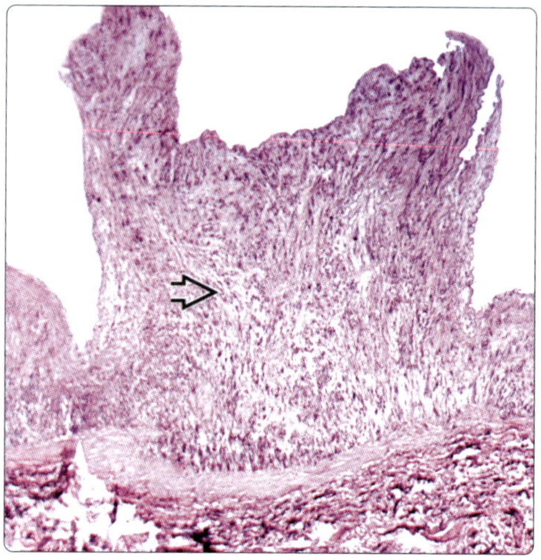

Alternating Thick-Thin Arterial Wall in Fibromuscular Dysplasia

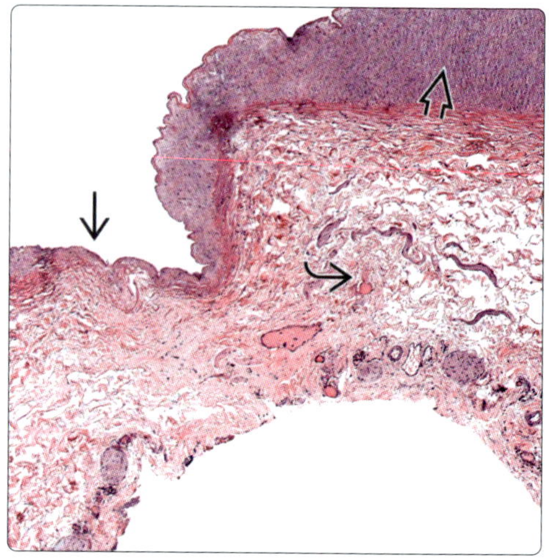

(Left) *PAS stain of the renal artery shows pale-staining loose fibrous tissue in the outer media, denser fibrous tissue admixed with smooth muscle in the inner media, and loose connective tissue in the adventitia in a case of perimedial fibroplasia of the renal artery.* **(Right)** *A higher power trichome stain of perimedial fibroplasia of the renal artery shows dense fibrous tissue between smooth muscle cells. Some smooth muscle cells are spindled and others simulate an epithelioid morphology.*

Segmental Medial Thinning in Fibromuscular Dysplasia

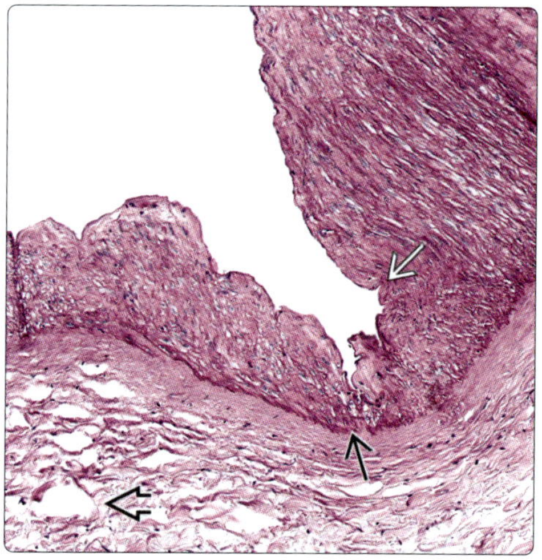

Segmental Medial Thinning in Fibromuscular Dysplasia: Trichrome Stain

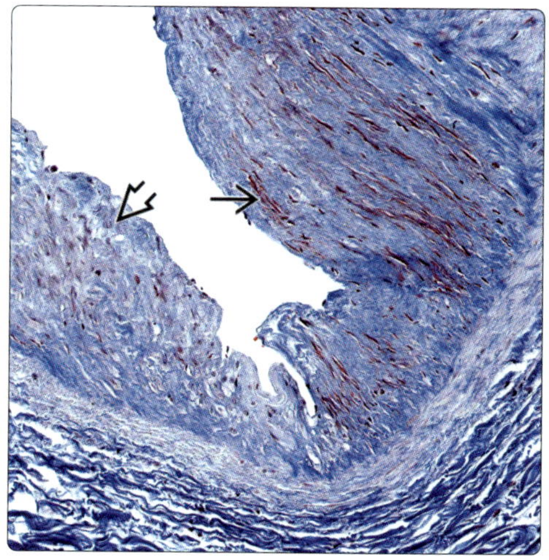

(Left) *Elastic stain of the renal artery involved by FMD shows pale-staining fibrous tissue filling the outer media with the inner media being filled by a darker layer, which alternates between being thick and thin, focally simulating aneurysm formation.* **(Right)** *Elastic stain of an artery with FMD shows an abnormally thin region of the media, which was probably dilated in vivo, forming an aneurysm. The outer media has dense bands of elastic fibers.*

Early Aneurysm Formation in Fibromuscular Dysplasia

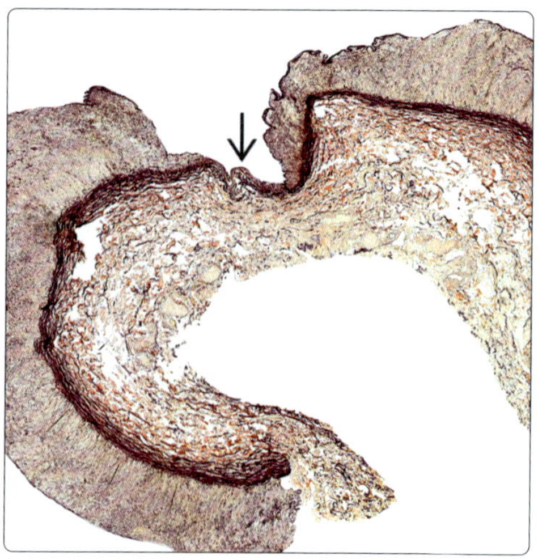

Early Aneurysm Formation in Fibromuscular Dysplasia: Higher Power

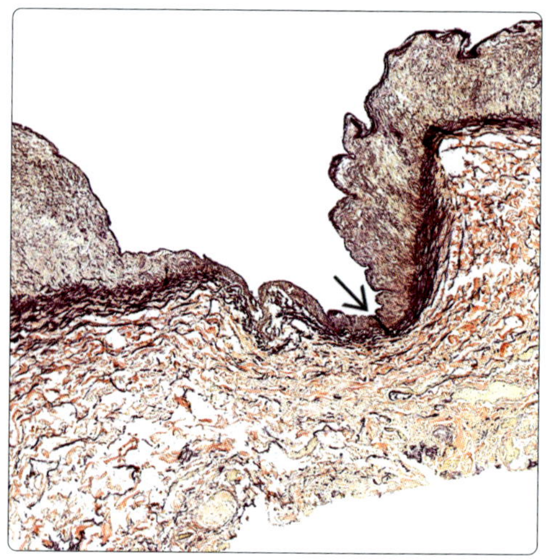

Disorganized Medial Smooth Muscle in Fibromuscular Dysplasia

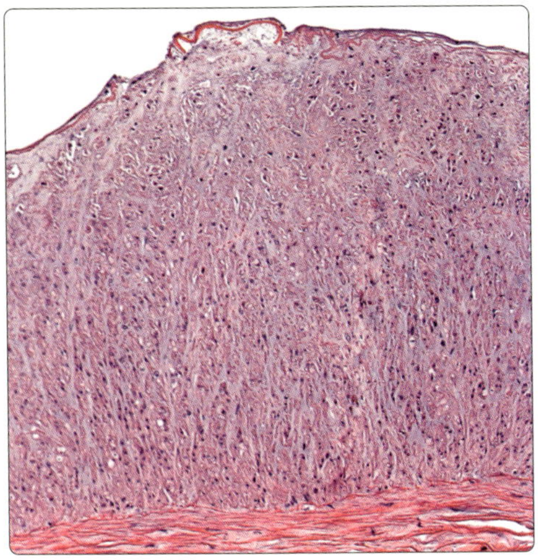

Intimal Fibroplasia in Fibromuscular Dysplasia

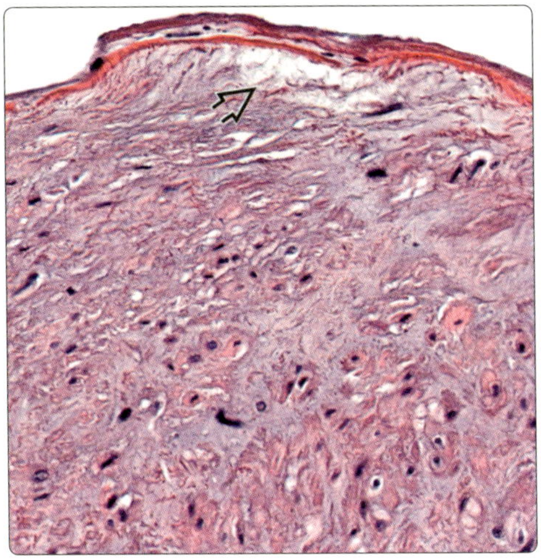

(Left) *Medium-power view shows FMD due primarily to perimedial fibroplasia in a proliferation in which loose, moderately cellular fibrous tissue leads to narrowing of the renal artery.* **(Right)** *H&E high-power view of perimedial fibroplasia with "secondary" intimal fibroplasia shows loose, cellular fibrous tissue ⇨ expanding the media and extending into the intima, leading to renal artery stenosis. This may simulate "endarteritis" seen in other contexts.*

Smooth Muscle Abnormalities in Fibromuscular Dysplasia: PAS

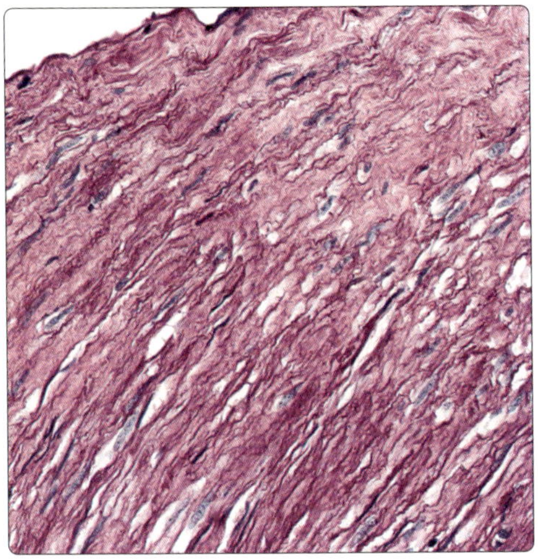

Smooth Muscle Vacuolation in Fibromuscular Dysplasia

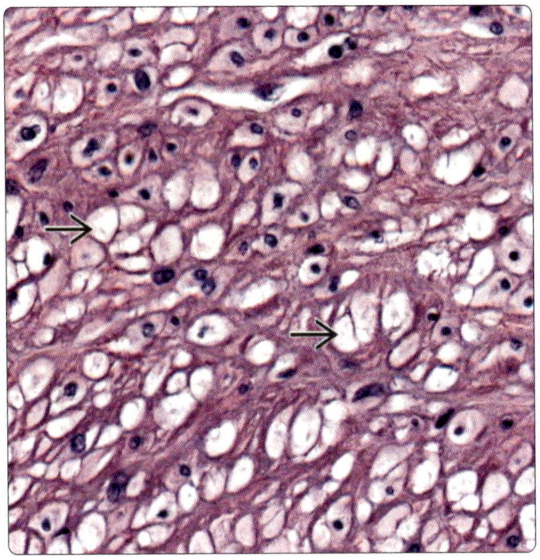

(Left) *Higher power view of a PAS stain of the renal artery in FMD shows dense fibrous tissue between smooth muscle cells.* **(Right)** *A higher power view of perimedial fibroplasia of the renal artery stained with PAS shows dense fibrous tissue between smooth muscle cells. The smooth muscle cells in this case acquire a clear cell appearance ⇨ due to glycogenation.*

Medial-Type Fibromuscular Dysplasia: PAS

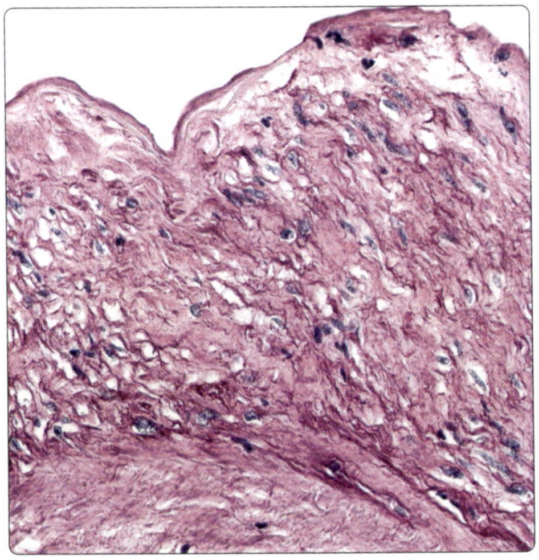

Fibromuscular Dysplasia Types in Carotid Model

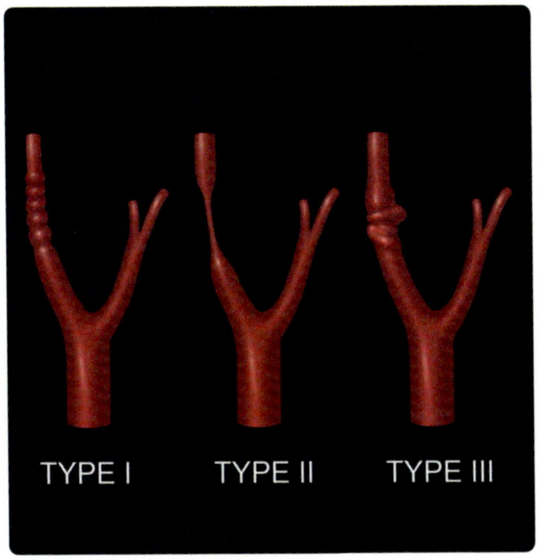

(Left) *A higher power view of FMD of the renal artery stained with PAS shows dense fibrous tissue between smooth muscle cells and disoriented smooth muscle cells.* **(Right)** *Graphic shows the 3 patterns of FMD as seen on angiography. Type I has a string of beads appearance, type II has tubular stenosis along a segment of the artery, and type III has unifocal abnormality/stenosis.*

KEY FACTS

TERMINOLOGY

- Synonym: Segmental mediolytic arteriopathy
- Rare arterial disease with characteristic pattern of medial smooth muscle loss in muscular arteries; leads to aneurysm and rupture

ETIOLOGY/PATHOGENESIS

- Possible precursor lesion to fibromuscular dysplasia
- Putative relationship to vasospasm

CLINICAL ISSUES

- Aneurysms and hemorrhages, most commonly involving specific arterial bed
- Middle-aged and older patients
- Aneurysms and hemorrhages, most commonly involving
  - Intraabdominal arteries
  - Retroperitoneal arteries
  - Intracranial arteries
  - Coronary arteries
  - Renal arteries

MICROSCOPIC

- Segmental medial smooth muscle loss
  - Elastic laminae are preserved
  - Smooth muscle vacuolation
  - Smooth muscle loss with replacement by loose matrix
  - Segmental involvement
- Pseudoaneurysm (contained rupture)
  - Abrupt break in normal arterial wall with outpouching "false" aneurysm bounded only by adventitial fibrous tissue

TOP DIFFERENTIAL DIAGNOSES

- Fibromuscular dysplasia
- Vasculitis (arteritis)

Multiple Discrete Aneurysms in Segmental Arterial Mediolysis

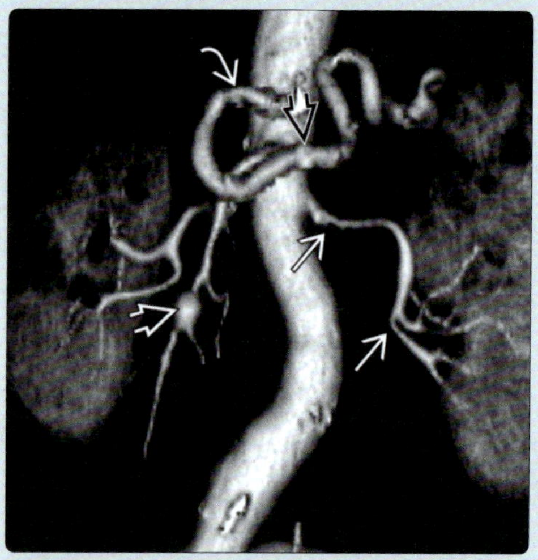

Chronic Reparative Phase of Segmental Arterial Mediolysis

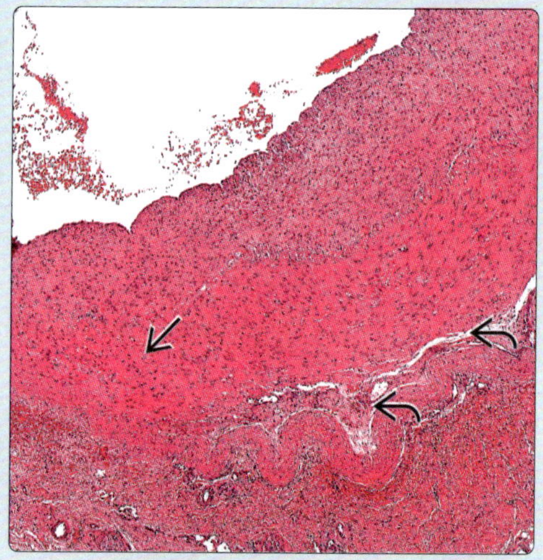

(Left) *Reconstructed 3D CTA highlights multiple aneurysms involving the proximal ➡ and more distal ⇨ superior mesenteric and left ➡ and right ➡ renal arteries.* **(Right)** *Artery shows features of segmental arterial mediolysis in chronic reparative phase. There is still separation at the external elastic lamina ⤻ and areas of mediolysis → in a segmental distribution pattern.*

Mediolysis in Segmental Arterial Mediolysis

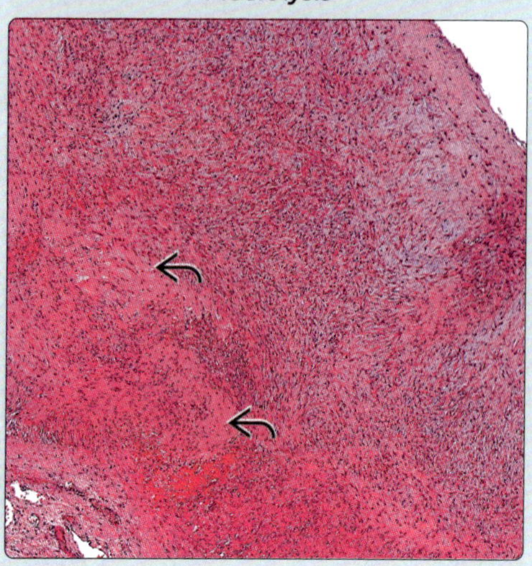

Segmental Medial Arteriolysis

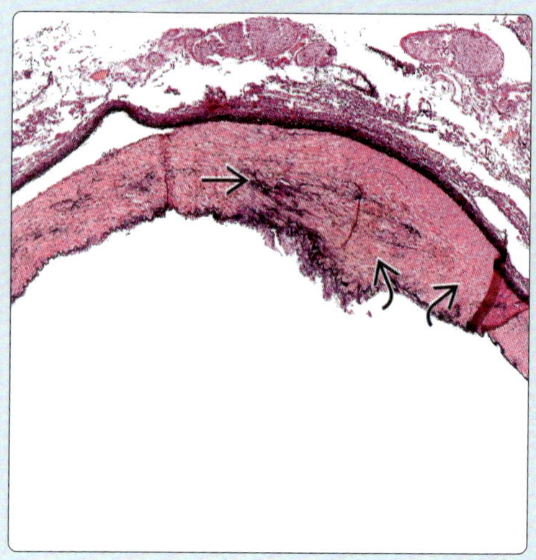

(Left) *Mediolysis ⤻ is apparent at higher magnification in this arterial wall.* **(Right)** *Elastic stain shows an obvious medial abnormality with disorganization of elastic fibers → and areas of mediolysis ⤻.*

TERMINOLOGY

Abbreviations

- Segmental arterial mediolysis (SAM)

Synonyms

- Segmental mediolytic arteriopathy

Definitions

- Rare arterial disease with characteristic pattern of medial smooth muscle loss in muscular arteries; leads to aneurysm and rupture
- Somewhat controversial entity given scarcity of this disease and majority of reports stemming from single pathologist

ETIOLOGY/PATHOGENESIS

Idiopathic

- Putative relationship to vasospasm
- Possible precursor lesion to fibromuscular dysplasia

Drug Related

- β-2 agonists
    - Animal models of ractopamine administration reproduce SAM lesions in renal, hepatic, and coronary arteries
        - Ractopamine is not for human use but is added to livestock feed to improve growth

Hypoxia

- Distinct form of SAM is described in neonatal coronary arteries following severe prolonged hypoxia

CLINICAL ISSUES

Presentation

- Aneurysms and hemorrhages, most commonly involving
    - Intraabdominal arteries
    - Retroperitoneal arteries
    - Intracranial arteries
    - Coronary arteries
    - Renal arteries
- Middle-aged and older patients
- No apparent sex predilection

Prognosis

- Natural history is unpredictable
- No established guidelines for when to intervene vs. when to observe

IMAGING

Angiographic Appearances

- Abrupt arterial dilatation
- Aneurysm(s)
- String of beads (successive aneurysms)
- Dissecting hematoma
- Stenosis and occlusion

MACROSCOPIC

General Features

- Aneurysm (true and false types)
    - Often with mural thrombus
- Intramural hematoma
- Arterial rupture site with hematoma
- Dissection

Anatomic Distribution

- Typically limited to specific locus, organ, or arterial bed
    - Celiac axis
    - Superior mesenteric artery
    - Inferior mesenteric artery
    - Renal artery
- Multiple discrete lesions along same vessel are common
- Involvement of multiple arterial beds is rare

MICROSCOPIC

Histologic Features

- Mediolysis
    - Disruption of smooth muscle cell membranes
    - Smooth muscle vacuolation
    - Smooth muscle loss with replacement by loose matrix
    - Elastic laminae are preserved
    - Progression of mediolysis has been proposed to occur in 2 phases
        - Injurious: Smooth muscle mediolysis and tearing along external elastic lamina
        - Reparative: Granulation tissue and eventual fibrous replacement
- Segmental involvement
    - Involving only portion or "arc" of arterial circumference in cross section
    - Predominantly in other media (with apparent inward progression)
- Pseudoaneurysm (contained rupture)
    - Abrupt break in normal arterial wall with outpouching "false" aneurysm bounded only by adventitial fibrous tissue

DIFFERENTIAL DIAGNOSIS

Fibromuscular Dysplasia

- Medial smooth muscle disorganization may be seen but not mediolysis (as in SAM)

Vasculitis (Arteritis)

- Internal elastic lamina is usually disrupted in vasculitis (but not in SAM)

SELECTED REFERENCES

1. Takeda A et al: A case of segmental arterial mediolysis of multiple visceral arteries following anti-COVID-19 vaccination: late complication or rare coincidence? Am J Case Rep. 23:e937505, 2022
2. Slavin RE: Segmental arterial mediolysis: a multiguised vasospastic arteriopathy with collateral mesangial cell hyperplasia and cardiac toxicity generated by norepinephrine and hyperdense adrenoceptors alone or by crosstalk with other pressor agents. Int J Vasc Med. 2021:2046566, 2021
3. Slavin RE: Segmental arterial mediolysis: course, sequelae, prognosis, and pathologic-radiologic correlation. Cardiovasc Pathol. 18(6):352-60, 2009
4. Slavin RE et al: Segmental arterial mediolysis with accompanying venous angiopathy: a clinical pathologic review, report of 3 new cases, and comments on the role of endothelin-1 in its pathogenesis. Int J Surg Pathol. 15(2):121-34, 2007
5. Slavin RE et al: Segmental arterial mediolysis: a precursor to fibromuscular dysplasia? Mod Pathol. 8(3):287-94, 1995

Mönckeberg Medial Calcific Sclerosis

KEY FACTS

TERMINOLOGY

- Calcification of internal elastic lamina and media of muscular arteries, usually without significant luminal encroachment

ETIOLOGY/PATHOGENESIS

- Associated with chronic renal failure, calciphylaxis, diabetes mellitus, osteoporosis

CLINICAL ISSUES

- Strongly age related (median: ~ 75 years)
- Extremities most commonly affected
  - Also head and neck, breast, uterus, thyroid
- Most cases are asymptomatic; usually no treatment is required
- Classically considered benign condition but not entirely without consequence
- Severe cases present with sequelae of distal ischemia
- Ischemia treated with bypass graft or amputation

IMAGING

- Calcification visible on x-ray imaging with ring-like (cross section) or tram-track (longitudinal section) appearance

MACROSCOPIC

- Markedly calcified, pipestem-like vessels

MICROSCOPIC

- Dystrophic medial calcification of small to medium-sized muscular arteries, typically centered on internal elastic lamina (IEL)
- Calcification may be focal, nodular, or extend circumferentially
- Mild to moderate intimal thickening may be present
- Disruption or reduplication of IEL sometimes seen
- Inflammation generally absent

DIAGNOSTIC CHECKLIST

- Unlike atherosclerosis, intima usually spared

Coronary Artery

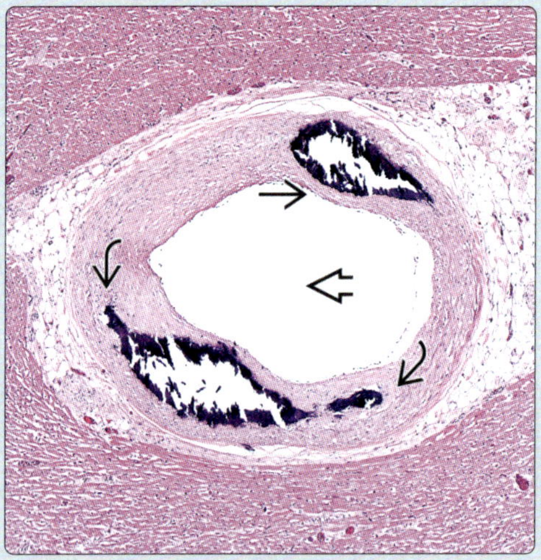

Subcutaneous Tissue

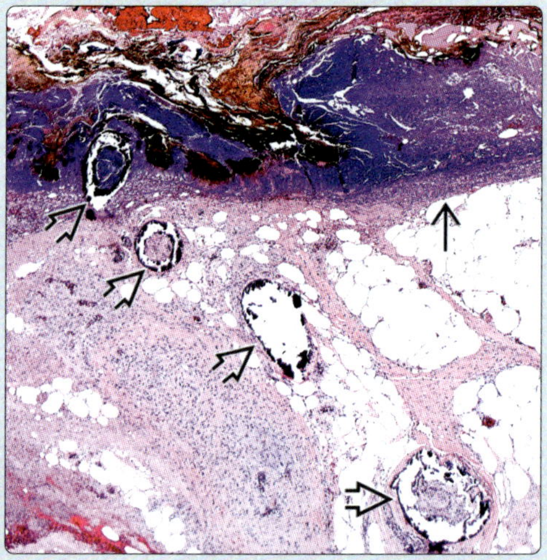

(Left) *Mönckeberg medial calcification of intramural coronary artery is shown. Calcification is centered on internal elastic lamina with circumferential extension ⮊ but preserves intima ⮊ and lumen ⮊.* **(Right)** *Although usually benign, severe cases of Mönckeberg calcification may be life threatening, especially in the setting of calciphylaxis. Subcutaneous arteries are occluded ⮊ with necrosis of overlying skin ⮊.*

Uterine Artery

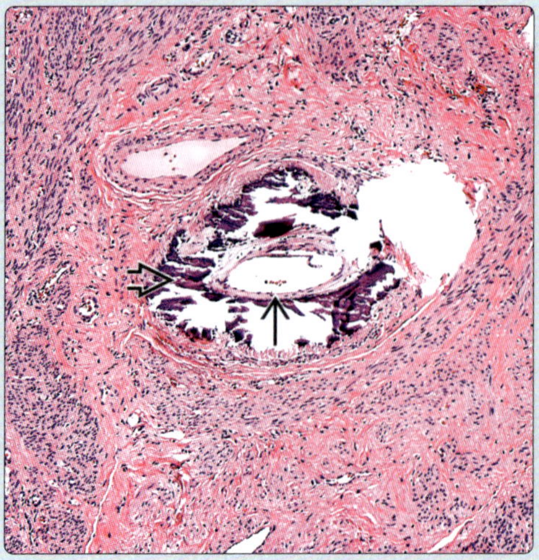

Punctate Calcification

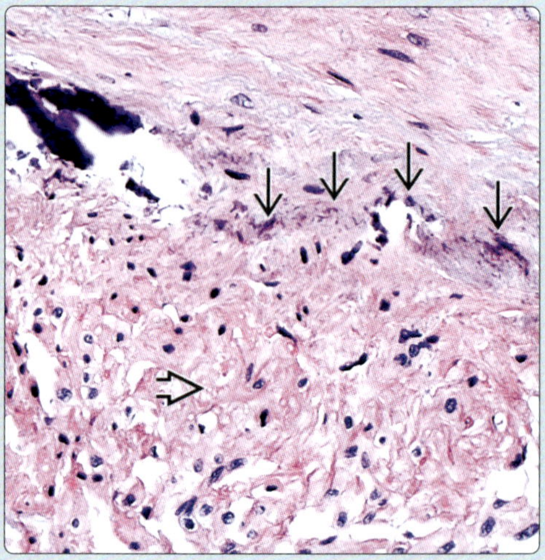

(Left) *Mönckeberg calcification in visceral organs is often incidental, as in this uterus. Note preservation of the intima ⮊ despite thick, circumferential calcification ⮊.* **(Right)** *Mönckeberg calcification begins as a punctate calcification ⮊ on the internal elastic lamina. In early lesions, media is uninvolved ⮊.*

TERMINOLOGY

Synonyms

- Medial calcific sclerosis
- Mönckeberg sclerosis

Definitions

- Calcification of internal elastic lamina (IEL) and media of muscular arteries, usually without significant luminal encroachment

ETIOLOGY/PATHOGENESIS

Etiology Unknown

- Likely related to dysregulated calcium handling
  - More common in chronic renal failure and hyperparathyroidism, especially in setting of calciphylaxis
  - More common in osteoporosis and diabetes mellitus
- Vascular smooth muscle cell damage and transdifferentiation to osteoblast-like cells

CLINICAL ISSUES

Epidemiology

- Incidence
  - Estimated prevalence ~ 13.3% for males and 6.9% for females
- Age
  - Strongly age related (median: ~ 75 years)
- Sex
  - M:F = 3:2

Site

- Small to medium-sized muscular arteries
  - Extremities most common: Dorsalis pedis artery, posterior tibial artery, radial artery, smaller arteries of extremities
  - Head and neck: Temporal artery, arteries in basal ganglia
  - Breast
  - Visceral arteries (particularly in diabetics): Pelvic arteries, thyroid

Presentation

- Most cases are asymptomatic
  - Discovered incidentally during imaging of extremities or at autopsy
  - Discovered incidentally in resected viscera, e.g., breast, uterus, or thyroid
- Severe cases present with sequelae of distal ischemia
  - Claudication, intractable pain
  - Chronic ulcers, gangrenous necrosis of extremity

Treatment

- Surgical approaches
  - Usually no treatment required
  - If symptomatic, arterio-arterial bypass may be performed with synthetic vascular graft if vessel sufficiently large
  - Amputation of extremity in severe cases

Prognosis

- Classically considered benign condition but not entirely without consequence
  - Decreased compliance, increased pulse pressure
  - May contribute to peripheral vascular disease
- In severe cases, stenosis causes significant morbidity

IMAGING

Radiographic Findings

- Calcification visible on x-ray imaging with ring-like (cross section) or tram-track (longitudinal section) appearance
- When present in breast, may mimic microcalcifications associated with breast malignancy

MACROSCOPIC

General Features

- Markedly calcified, pipestem-like vessels

MICROSCOPIC

Histologic Features

- Dystrophic medial calcification of small to medium-sized muscular arteries, typically centered on IEL
  - Calcification may be limited to IEL or extend into media
- Calcification may be focal, nodular, or extend circumferentially
- Mild to moderate intimal thickening may be present
  - Usually without luminal narrowing, but stenosis may be present, particularly in setting of calciphylaxis
- Disruption or reduplication of IEL sometimes seen
- Inflammation generally absent

DIFFERENTIAL DIAGNOSIS

Atherosclerosis

- Intimal thickening and atheromatous plaque formation, typically with luminal encroachment
- Calcification usually centered on intima
- Usually limited to aorta and its major branches

DIAGNOSTIC CHECKLIST

Clinically Relevant Pathologic Features

- May mimic breast carcinoma radiographically
- Generally benign process, but morbidity high with occlusion

Pathologic Interpretation Pearls

- Unlike atherosclerosis, intima usually spared

SELECTED REFERENCES

1. Fitzgerald J et al: Calcified facial and maxillary arteries: incidental radiographic findings indicative of Mönckeberg arteriosclerosis. J Am Dent Assoc. 152(11):943-6, 2021
2. Shichijo C et al: Intracranial Mönckeberg's atherosclerosis is frequently found in autopsy cases of advanced stage malignancy with cerebral infarction. Cancers (Basel). 13(20):5234, 2021
3. Tahmasbi-Arashlow M et al: Radiographic manifestations of Mönckeberg arteriosclerosis in the head and neck region. Imaging Sci Dent. 46(1):53-6, 2016
4. Lanzer P et al: Medial vascular calcification revisited: review and perspectives. Eur Heart J. 35(23):1515-25, 2014
5. Fishbein GA et al: Arteriosclerosis: rethinking the current classification. Arch Pathol Lab Med. 133(8):1309-16, 2009
6. Micheletti RG et al: Mönckeberg sclerosis revisited: a clarification of the histologic definition of Mönckeberg sclerosis. Arch Pathol Lab Med. 132(1):43-7, 2008

Behçet Disease

KEY FACTS

TERMINOLOGY

- Inflammatory vascular disease characterized by recurrent oral and genital aphthae, ocular abnormalities, skin lesions, and articular, neurologic, gastrointestinal, and pulmonary manifestations

ETIOLOGY/PATHOGENESIS

- Etiology unknown but characterized by vasculitis
- Vasculitis may affect both arteries and veins of all sizes

CLINICAL ISSUES

- Nearly all present with oral aphthous ulcers
- Genital aphthous ulcers in > 75%
- Cutaneous lesions in > 75%
- Ocular disease in 25-75%
- Neurologic disease in < 20%
- Systemic large vessel vasculitis may lead to aneurysms or thrombosis
- Arthritis
- Large vessel aneurysms may require surgical repair
- Prognosis poor with neurologic, ocular, or large vessel disease, which requires high-dose immunosuppression

MICROSCOPIC

- Wide spectrum of features, depending on site and clinical presentation
- Ulceration of epidermis or mucosa
- Small vessel arteritis &/or phlebitis, sometimes with intraluminal thrombi
- Inflammatory infiltrate mixed but neutrophils often prominent
- Leukocytoclastic vasculitis with fibrinoid necrosis

DIAGNOSTIC CHECKLIST

- Vasculitis may affect arteries &/or veins of any size
- Inflammatory infiltrates usually mixed but neutrophils often prominent
- Intraluminal thrombi often present

Vaginal Aphthous Ulcer

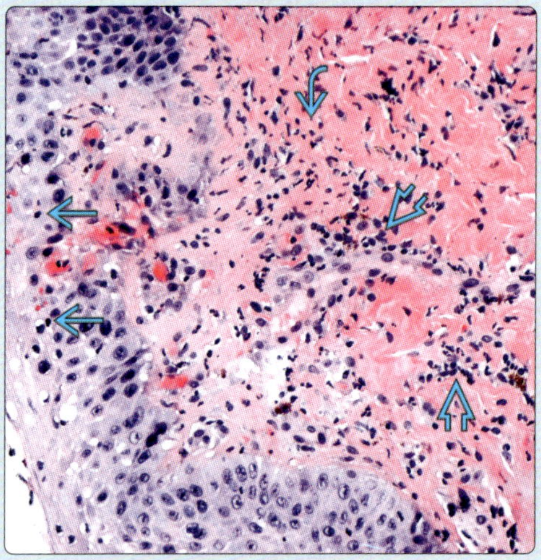

Vaginal Aphthous Ulcer

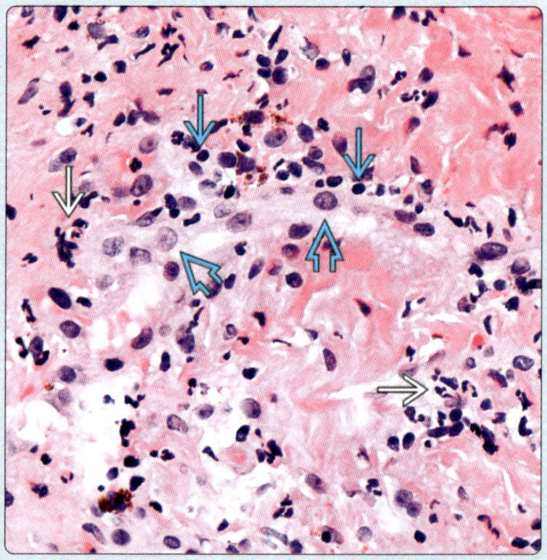

(Left) *Biopsy of a vaginal aphthous ulcer shows a submucosal mixed inflammatory infiltrate with perivascular accentuation and infiltration of the squamous mucosa at the ulcer margin.* **(Right)** *On high power, the mixed perivascular infiltrate in the vaginal submucosa is readily apparent with numerous neutrophils and lymphocytes associated with markedly reactive endothelial cells.*

Brain Involved by Behçet Disease

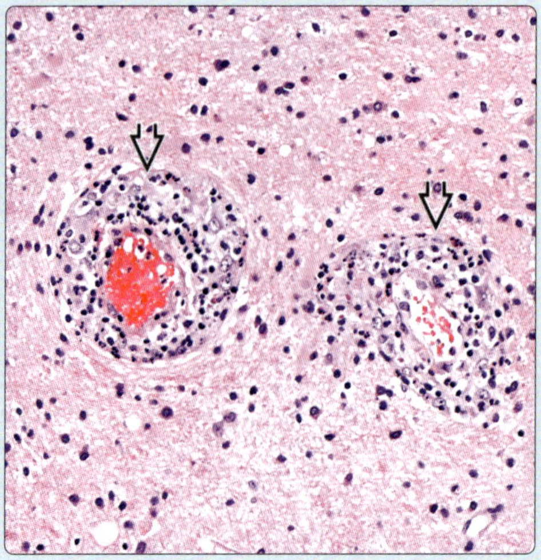

Brain Involved by Behçet Disease

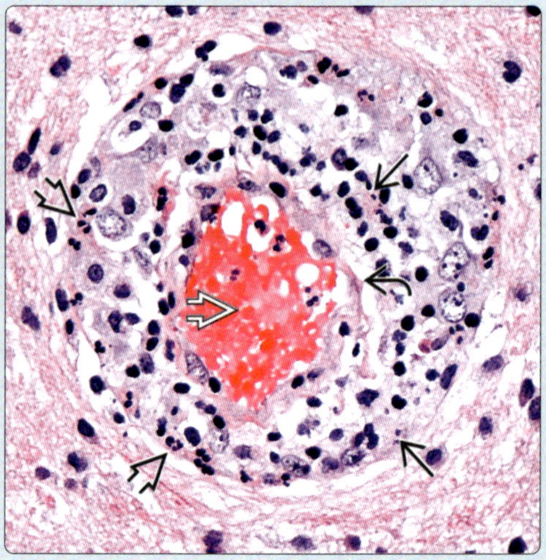

(Left) *True leukocytoclastic vasculitis with fibrinoid necrosis of small vessels may sometimes be seen, as in this case of Behçet disease with neurologic involvement.* **(Right)** *Vascular lesions may display frank leukocytoclasia with a marked neutrophilic infiltrate, "nuclear dust" from degenerating neutrophils, fibrinoid necrosis, and thrombosis.*

TERMINOLOGY

Definitions

- Inflammatory vascular disease characterized by recurrent oral and genital aphthae, ocular abnormalities, skin lesions, and articular, neurologic, gastrointestinal, and pulmonary manifestations

ETIOLOGY/PATHOGENESIS

Autoimmune Disorder

- Unknown endogenous target(s)
- Autoreactive T cells play critical role
- Humoral activation with autoantibodies &/or immune complexes
- Cross reactivity of human peptides with bacterial or viral proteins
- Associated with some human leukocyte antigen (HLA) subtypes, e.g., HLA-B51
- *IL10* gene mutations have been identified

Vasculitis

- Most, but not all, clinical manifestations secondary to vasculitis
- Vasculitis involving both arteries and veins
- Vasculitis may affect vessels of all sizes
- Endothelial dysfunction

CLINICAL ISSUES

Epidemiology

- Incidence
  - Most common in Turkey (80-370 cases/100,000)
  - Less common in North America and Europe (0.12-7.50 cases/100,000)
- Age
  - Young adults (20-40 years)
- Sex
  - Prevalence similar in men and women
  - Disease usually more severe in young men with severe pulmonary artery involvement

Presentation

- Nearly all present with painful oral aphthous ulcers
- Genital aphthous ulcers in > 75%
- Cutaneous lesions in > 75%
- Ocular disease in 25-75%, often progresses to blindness if not treated
  - Uveitis (anterior, posterior, or both; often bilateral)
  - Hypopyon (severe uveitis with pus in anterior chamber)
  - Retinal vasculitis
  - Vascular thrombosis
  - Optic neuritis
- Neurologic disease in < 20%, more common in men
  - Vasculitic lesions with associated parenchymal lesions and neurologic deficits
    - Thrombosis of small arteries or veins
    - Thrombosis of large arteries, veins, or sinuses
    - Arterial vasculitis
  - Aseptic meningitis or encephalitis
- Systemic vasculitis
  - Arterial involvement
    - Small artery involvement most common
    - Large artery involvement in 30%
    - Pulmonary artery aneurysms characteristic
    - Aorta, carotid, or iliac vessels may also be involved
    - Sequelae include hemorrhage, stenosis, aneurysms, thrombosis
  - Venous involvement
    - Superficial and deep venous thrombosis
    - Occlusion of dural sinuses, superior or inferior vena cava
    - Budd-Chiari syndrome (hepatic vein obstruction)
- Gastrointestinal aphthous ulcers in some cases
  - Especially terminal ileum, cecum, ascending colon
- Arthritis
- Renal, cardiac, or pulmonary disease in rare cases

Laboratory Tests

- No laboratory tests are pathognomonic
- C-reactive protein or erythrocyte sedimentation rate may be elevated (nonspecific)
- HLA typing may aid in diagnosis of some patients

Natural History

- Follows waxing and waning course with exacerbations and remissions

Treatment

- Surgical approaches
  - Large vessel aneurysms may require surgical &/or endovascular repairs
- Drugs
  - Minor manifestations (arthritis, mucocutaneous ulcers)
    - Colchicine/glucocorticoids
  - Major manifestations (neurologic, ocular, large vessel disease)
    - High-dose glucocorticoids
    - Other immunosuppressive agents (e.g., TNF antagonists-infliximab, cyclophosphamide, cyclosporine, azathioprine)
    - Anticoagulation for venous thrombotic events

Prognosis

- Variable, depending on manifestations
- Good with disease limited to mucocutaneous sites and joints
- Poor with neurologic, ocular, or large vessel disease but improving with immunosuppressive regimens

Clinical Diagnostic Criteria

- Recurrent oral aphthae (≥ 3x/year) plus at least 2 of following, in absence of other systemic disease
  - Genital aphthae
  - Synovitis
  - Posterior uveitis
  - Positive pathergy test (papule ≥ 2 mm developing 24-48 hours after insertion of needle into skin of forearm)

IMAGING

General Features

- Vascular aneurysms may be visible by radiography, CT, MR, &/or US

- Parenchymal lesions in central nervous system may be visible by MR

MACROSCOPIC

Aphthous Ulcers

- Round, punched-out appearance
- Usually 2-10 mm in diameter, occasionally up to 2 cm
- Oral, genital, and gastrointestinal lesions similar in gross appearance

Skin Lesions

- Acneiform lesions, vesicular/pustular eruptions, erythema nodosum-like nodules, erythema multiforme, superficial thrombophlebitis

MICROSCOPIC

Histologic Features

- Oral/genital aphthous ulcers
  - Mixed neutrophilic and mononuclear infiltrate at ulcer base with perivascular accentuation
  - Inflammatory infiltrate may extend into epithelium at ulcer margins
  - Diffuse immunofluorescence staining for IgM and C3 may be present in vessel walls
- Skin lesions
  - Wide spectrum of features, depending on clinical presentation
  - Erythema nodosum-like lesions show lymphocytic perivascular infiltrate in superficial and deep dermis
  - Septal panniculitis may be seen
  - Lymphocytic vasculitis may be present (lymphocytes invading vascular wall)
  - Neutrophils often prominent component of infiltrate
  - True leukocytoclastic vasculitis with fibrinoid change
  - Thrombi may be present in small vessels
  - Histiocytic granulomas generally not seen
- Gastrointestinal aphthous ulcers
  - Small vessel arteritis &/or phlebitis common in submucosa with associated mucosal ulceration
  - Thrombi often present in involved submucosal vessels
  - Inflammatory infiltrate may be predominantly neutrophilic, lymphocytic, or mixed
- Neurologic lesions
  - Small vessel arteritis &/or phlebitis, sometimes with intraluminal thrombi
  - Infarcts may be present with associated reactive parenchymal changes, including gliosis, gemistocytic astrocytes
  - Inflammatory infiltrate may be predominantly neutrophilic, lymphocytic, or mixed
  - Leukocytoclastic vasculitis with fibrinoid necrosis

DIFFERENTIAL DIAGNOSIS

Benign Aphthous Ulcers

- Often histologically indistinguishable from Behçet disease
- Diagnosed clinically by absence of other lesions
- Occur sporadically without frequent recurrence

Herpes Simplex Virus Infection

- May mimic aphthous ulcers of Behçet disease
- May also show vasculitis in dermis beneath ulcer
- Distinction made by identification of virus
  - Multinucleated keratinocytes with ground-glass nuclear viral inclusions at ulcer margin
  - Immunohistochemical stains or cultures for herpesvirus in difficult cases

Inflammatory Bowel Disease

- Aphthous ulcers often seen in Crohn disease
- Inflammatory infiltrate more diffuse
- Vasculitis not prominent
- Other Behçet disease-associated lesions not seen in IBD; clinical correlation often helpful
- Intestinal fissures, strictures, and granulomas usually not seen in Behçet disease

Stevens-Johnson Syndrome

- May mimic skin manifestations of Behçet disease
- Precipitated by exposure to various medications or by infections; clinical correlation essential
- True vasculitis generally not prominent

Pemphigus Vulgaris

- May also cause oral ulcers
- Suprabasal bullae with epidermal acantholysis
- Vasculitis generally not seen
- Immunofluorescence shows deposition of IgG in intracellular spaces of epidermis

Bullous Pemphigoid

- May also cause oral ulcers and subepidermal bullae
- Vasculitis generally not seen
- Immunofluorescence shows linear deposition of IgG along basement membrane

Other Systemic Diseases

- Cutaneous small vessel vasculitis, uveitis, arthritis, neurologic lesions, &/or large vessel disease seen in many autoimmune disorders and systemic illnesses
  - Systemic lupus erythematosus, ankylosing spondylitis, psoriatic arthritis, sarcoidosis, multiple sclerosis, syphilis, and other vasculitides
- Distinction often requires careful clinicopathologic correlation with associated clinical features and rheumatologic laboratory studies

DIAGNOSTIC CHECKLIST

Pathologic Interpretation Pearls

- Vasculitis may affect arteries &/or veins of any size
- Inflammatory infiltrates usually mixed but neutrophils often prominent
- Intraluminal thrombi often present

SELECTED REFERENCES

1. Hisamatsu T et al: Treatment and outcomes: medical and surgical treatment for intestinal Behçet's disease. Intest Res. 15(3):318-27, 2017
2. Lee HJ et al: Optimal diagnosis and disease activity monitoring of intestinal Behçet's disease. Intest Res. 15(3):311-7, 2017
3. Demirelli S et al: Cardiac manifestations in Behcet's disease. Intractable Rare Dis Res. 4(2):70-5, 2015
4. Stone JR et al: Consensus statement on surgical pathology of the aorta from the Society for Cardiovascular Pathology and the Association for European Cardiovascular Pathology: I. Inflammatory diseases. Cardiovasc Pathol. 24(5):267-78, 2015

Behçet Disease

Vaginal Aphthous Ulcer

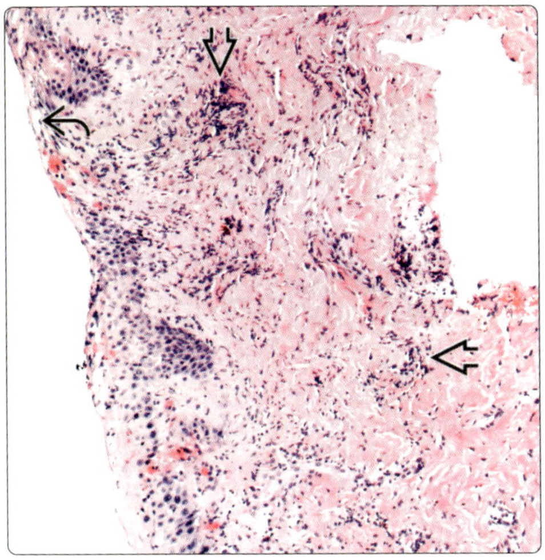

Lip Aphthous Ulcer

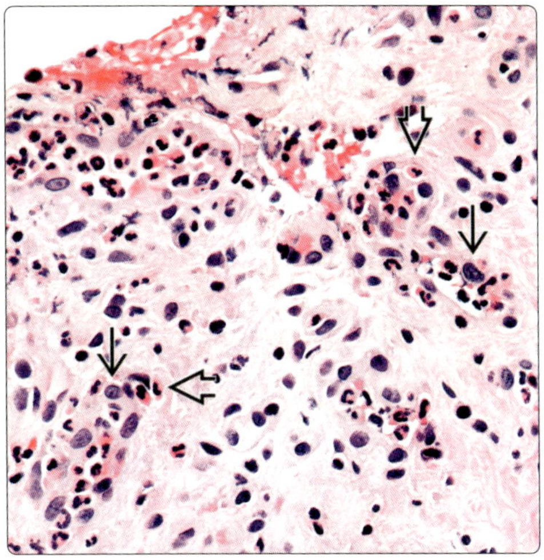

(Left) *Biopsy of a vaginal ulcer shows a perivascular inflammatory infiltrate ⇨ in the superficial submucosa with an overlying regenerating squamous mucosa ⇨.* **(Right)** *Neutrophils often predominate ⇨ as in this biopsy from an aphthous ulcer on the lip. Reactive endothelial changes include marked cell swelling and prominent nucleoli ⇨.*

Gastric Ulcer

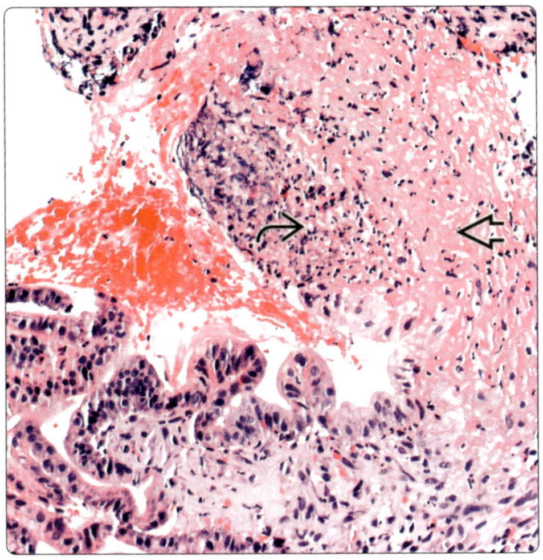

Brain Involved by Behçet Disease

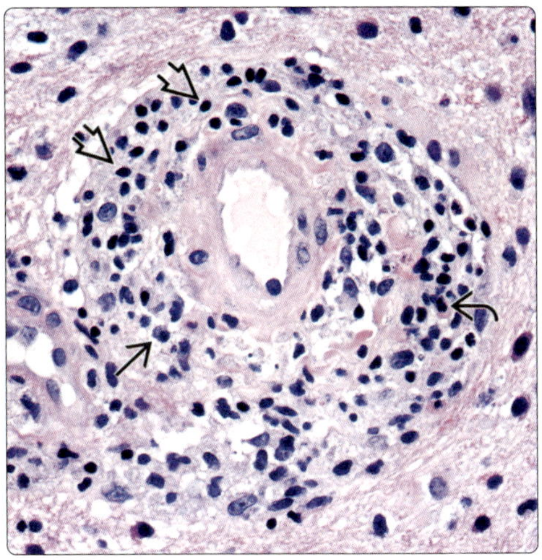

(Left) *Biopsy of a gastric ulcer shows mucosal erosion with abundant fibrinous material ⇨ and associated inflammation ⇨ that is consistent with Behçet disease in the right clinical setting.* **(Right)** *Inflammatory infiltrates are sometimes limited in a perivascular distribution without vascular wall involvement or fibrinoid necrosis. A mixture of lymphocytes ⇨, plasma cells ⇨, and occasional neutrophils ⇨ is seen in this case of neurologic involvement by Behçet disease.*

Colon With Small Vessel Vasculitis

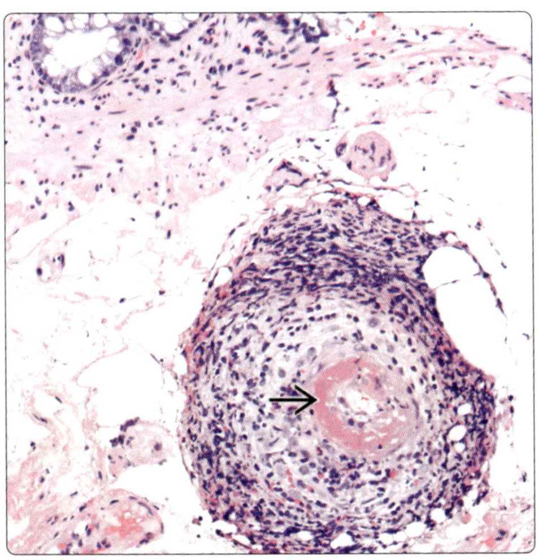

Small Vessel Vasculitis

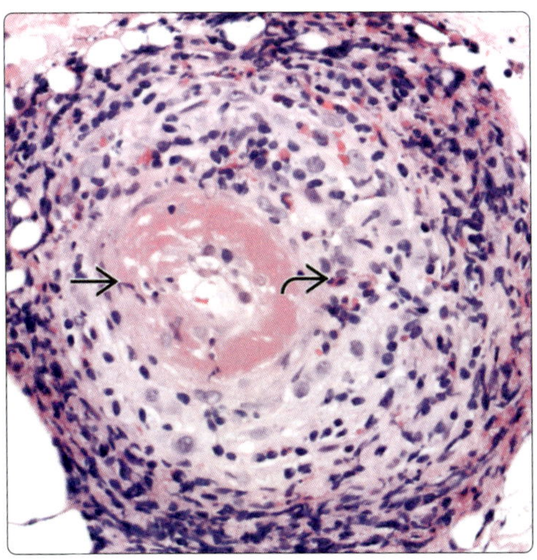

(Left) *ANCA-related small vessel vasculitis is in the differential diagnosis for Behcet disease; the presence of fibrinoid necrosis ⇨ is a feature more characteristic of ANCA-related small vessel vasculitis in correlation with a clinical history and serologic tests.* **(Right)** *Small artery shows fibrinoid necrosis ⇨ and mixed inflammatory infiltrate in the wall with prominent eosinophils ⇨ in this case of granulomatous with polyangiitis. Clinical history and serology studies are critical for correct diagnosis.*

Infectious Vasculitis

KEY FACTS

TERMINOLOGY

- Inflammation of blood vessels induced directly or indirectly by infectious organisms

ETIOLOGY/PATHOGENESIS

- May be primary, secondary by direct extension of nearby infection, or secondary to distant infection (immune complex mediated)
- Bacteria, often in setting of sepsis
- Fungi, especially *Aspergillus*, *Mucor*
- Viruses (often immune complex mediated)
- Parasites (rare)

CLINICAL ISSUES

- Immunocompromised status major risk factor
- Large vessel vasculitis: Aneurysms, hemorrhage, large infarcts
- Small vessel vasculitis: Hemoptysis, hematuria, neurologic deficits, multiple small infarcts
- Bacterial, fungal, and viral cultures essential
- Serologic tests useful to identify specific organisms
- Antibiotic therapy tailored to specific organism

MICROSCOPIC

- Acute, chronic, or mixed inflammation of vascular wall, often with endothelial swelling
- Fibrinoid necrosis with hemorrhage
- Microthrombi with infarction of surrounding tissue
- Fungal elements seen in fungal vasculitides
    - GMS, PAS stains often helpful
- Organisms usually not seen in bacterial vasculitis
    - Gram and silver stains occasionally helpful
    - Correlation with cultures usually required for identification

Cerebral Infectious Vasculitis

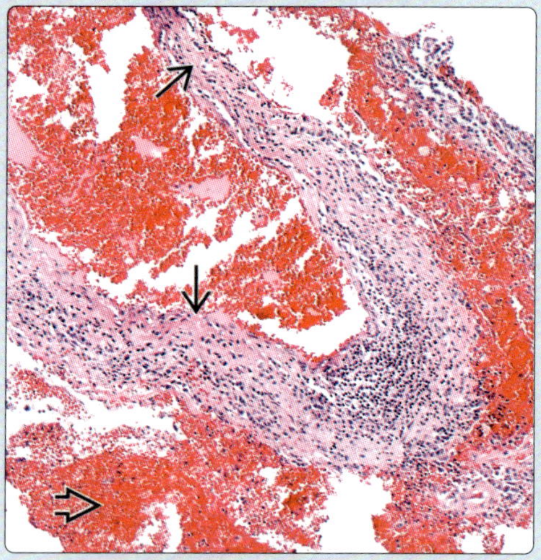

Invasive Aspergillosis

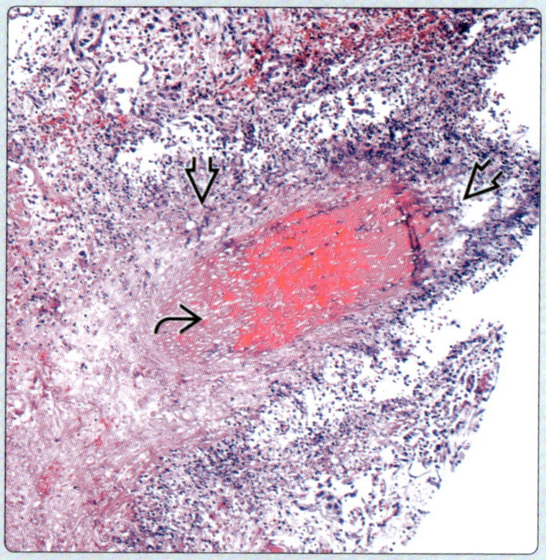

(Left) *H&E shows cerebral arteritis with fibrinoid necrosis of the vascular wall* ➙ *and fatal subdural hemorrhage* ➙ *in the setting of staphylococcal sepsis.* **(Right)** *H&E shows aspergillosis involving a small pulmonary artery with intraluminal hyphae* ➙ *and angioinvasive hyphae radiating through vascular media into the surrounding lung parenchyma* ➙*.*

Angioinvasive Mucormycosis

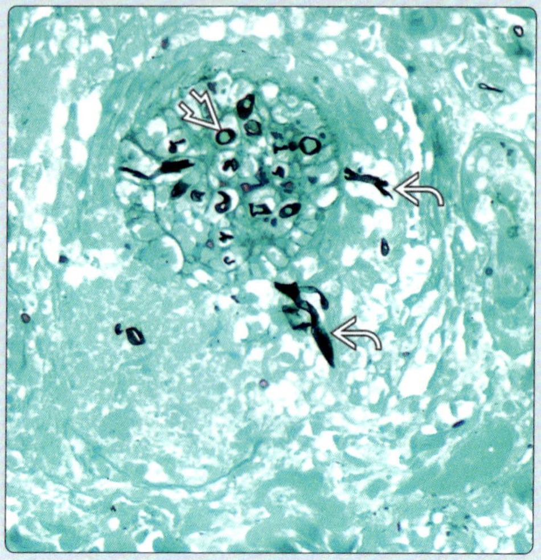

Vascular Granuloma With *Coccidioides*

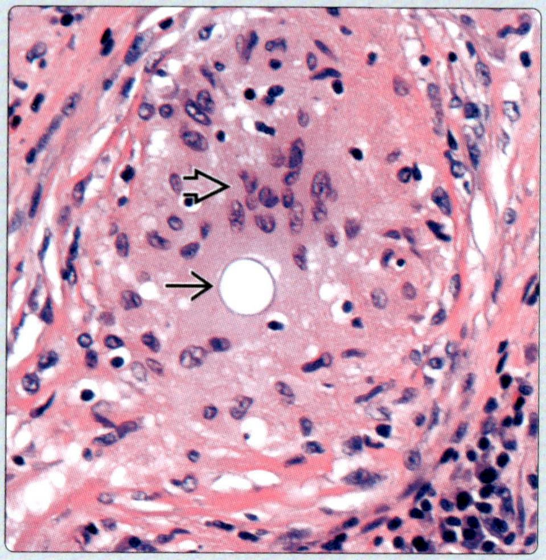

(Left) *GMS stain highlights intraluminal* ➙ *and angioinvasive* ➙ *fungal hyphae in a deep dermal arteriole in culture-confirmed mucormycosis.* **(Right)** *Although organisms may be scarce, a careful search in areas of granulomatous inflammation with giant cells* ➙ *may reveal engulfment of large empty spherules with refractile cell walls* ➙ *that are diagnostic for Coccidioides.*

TERMINOLOGY

Synonyms

- Mycotic vasculitis (primary), postinfectious vasculitis (secondary)

Definitions

- Inflammation of blood vessels induced directly or indirectly by infectious organisms

ETIOLOGY/PATHOGENESIS

Infectious Agents

- Bacteria
  - *Staphylococcus*, streptococci, *Neisseria*
  - *Salmonella*, *Escherichia*, other gram-negative rods
  - Rickettsiae, mycobacteria, others
- Fungi
  - *Aspergillus*, *Mucor*, other Zygomycetes
  - *Coccidioides*, others
- Viruses
  - Hepatitis B, hepatitis C
  - HIV
  - Cytomegalovirus, others
- Parasites
  - Amebae, *Schistosoma*, others

Pathogenesis

- Primary infection of vascular intima with centrifugal invasion through media into surrounding tissues
  - Most bacterial agents, in association with bacteremia
  - Most fungal agents, in association with fungemia
- Secondary vasculitis by centripetal erosion into vascular wall in setting of nearby infection
  - Mycobacteria, many fungi
- Secondary immune complex-mediated vasculitis
  - Streptococci, *Staphylococcus*
  - Most viruses, often with cryoglobulinemia

CLINICAL ISSUES

Presentation

- Variable; depends on vessel(s) and organ(s) involved
  - Large vessels
    - Secondary infection of preexisting aneurysm
    - Primary aneurysm formation (rare)
  - Small vessels
    - Hemoptysis with pulmonary involvement
    - Hematuria with renal involvement
    - Functional deficits with neurologic involvement

Laboratory Tests

- Bacterial, fungal, and viral cultures
- Serologic tests for specific organisms

Treatment

- Surgical approaches
  - Large aneurysms may require surgical repair
- Drugs
  - Antimicrobial therapy tailored to specific organism

Prognosis

- Depends on organism, location, speed of diagnosis
- Very poor for disseminated fungal infections

Risk Factors

- Immunocompromised status
  - Status post transplantation, corticosteroid therapy, acquired immunodeficiency syndrome, others

IMAGING

General Features

- Findings depend on vessel(s)/organ(s) involved
  - Pulmonary nodules, infiltrates, consolidation on thoracic imaging
  - Cerebral infarcts on CT or MR imaging of head
  - Large vessel aneurysms on thoracic/abdominal imaging

MACROSCOPIC

General Features

- Infarcts and aneurysms often grossly apparent

MICROSCOPIC

Histologic Features

- Acute, chronic, or mixed inflammation of vascular wall, often with endothelial swelling
- Fibrinoid necrosis may be present
- Fungal elements seen in fungal vasculitides
- Organisms usually not obvious in bacterial vasculitides
  - Pseudomonas is exception: Often shows marked vascular basophilia with abundant bacterial clusters obscuring vessel wall with tissue necrosis and conspicuously absent inflammation
  - Silver stains useful to detect *Treponema*

DIFFERENTIAL DIAGNOSIS

Noninfectious (Autoimmune) Vasculitides

- Large vessel vasculitides
  - Giant cell arteritis, Takayasu arteritis
- Medium vessel vasculitides
  - Polyarteritis nodosa, Kawasaki disease
- Small vessel vasculitides
  - Granulomatosis with polyangiitis (Wegener granulomatosis), Churg-Strauss syndrome, microscopic polyangiitis

SELECTED REFERENCES

1. Lötscher F et al: Spectrum of large- and medium-vessel vasculitis in adults: neoplastic, infectious, drug-induced, autoinflammatory, and primary immunodeficiency diseases. Curr Rheumatol Rep. 24(10):293-309, 2022
2. Pagnoux C et al: Vasculitides secondary to infections. Clin Exp Rheumatol. 24(2 Suppl 41):S71-81, 2006
3. Miller DV et al: Surgical pathology of infected aneurysms of the descending thoracic and abdominal aorta: clinicopathologic correlations in 29 cases (1976 to 1999). Hum Pathol. 35(9):1112-20, 2004

Diffuse Cerebral Arteritis in Sepsis

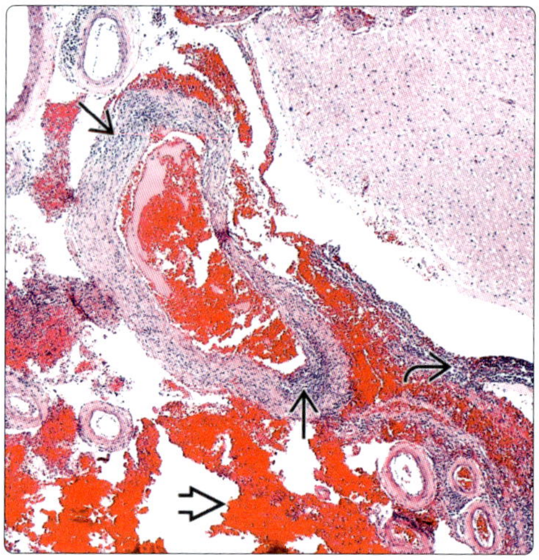

Lymphocytic Vasculitis in Cerebral Infection

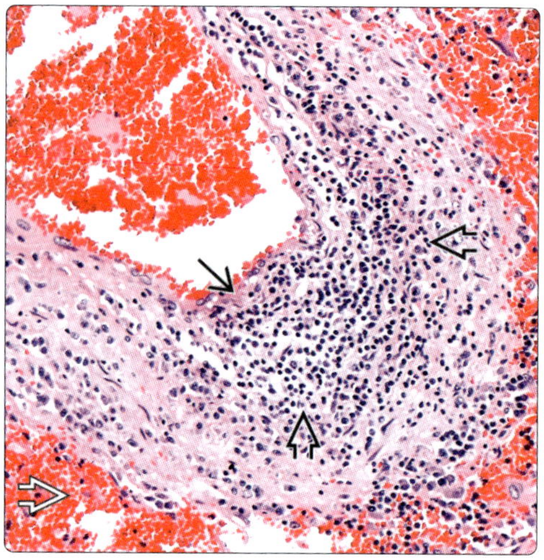

(Left) *Diffuse cerebral arteritis → is seen in a case of culture-confirmed Staphylococcus aureus sepsis with associated acute leptomeningitis → and massive fatal subdural hemorrhage →.* **(Right)** *H&E shows dense mixed inflammatory infiltrate → in the cerebral arterial wall with fibrinoid necrosis → and surrounding hemorrhage →.*

Transmural Necrosis in Infectious Cerebral Arteritis

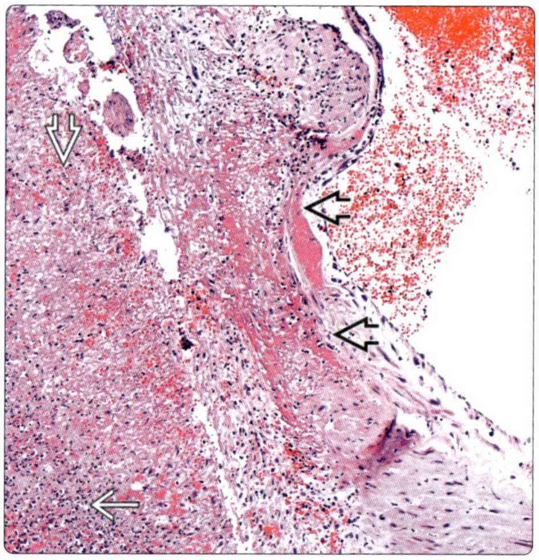

Diffuse Necrosis in Pulmonary *Pseudomonas* Infection

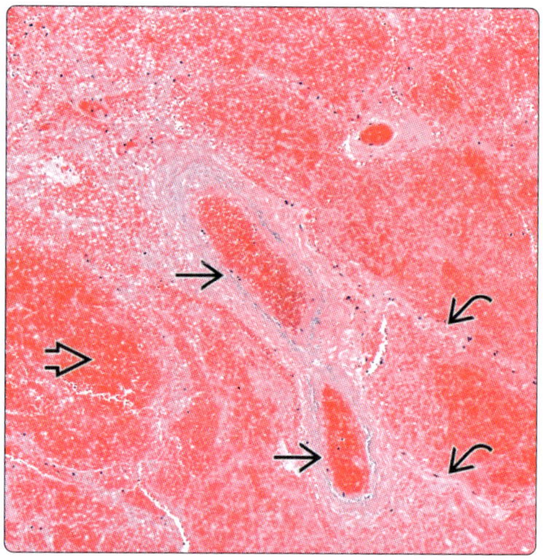

(Left) *Large cerebral artery in a case of staphylococcal sepsis with fatal subdural hemorrhage shows transmural fibrinoid necrosis →. Adjacent fibrin-rich thrombus → shows acute inflammation →, indicating extension of infection to leptomeningeal space.* **(Right)** *H&E shows pulmonary arteritis → with diffuse necrosis of pulmonary parenchyma → and massive fatal pulmonary hemorrhage → in a case of culture-confirmed Pseudomonas aeruginosa sepsis.*

Basophilic Necrosis of Artery Wall

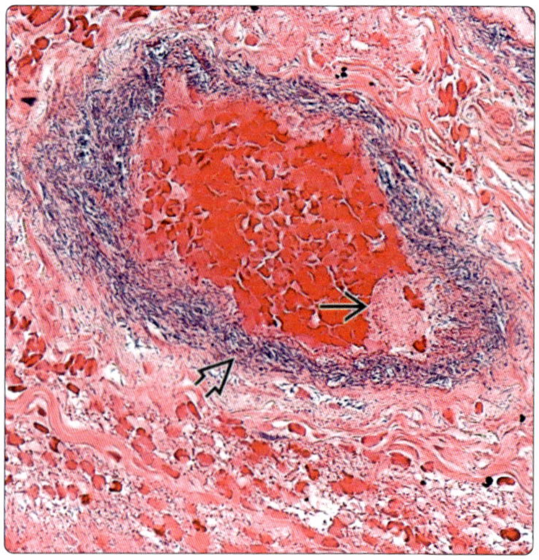

Bacterial Forms in Basophilic Necrosis

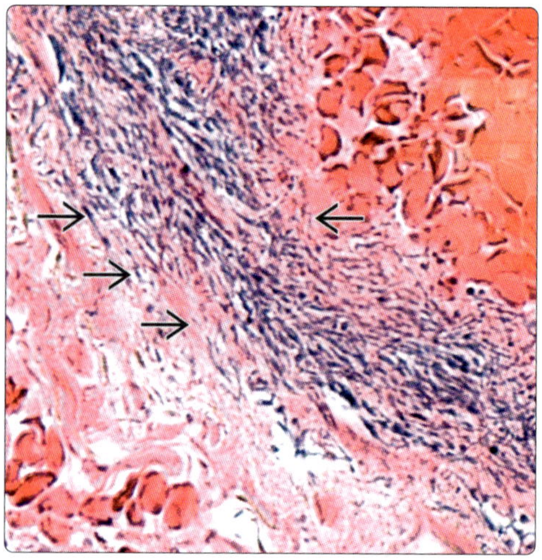

(Left) *H&E of the pulmonary artery in a case of Pseudomonas sepsis shows diffuse basophilia of the arterial wall → with partial thrombosis → without associated intramural inflammatory infiltrate.* **(Right)** *H&E of the pulmonary artery in a case of Pseudomonas sepsis shows closely clustered bacilli → densely infiltrating and obscuring vascular media with conspicuous absence of associated inflammatory infiltrates.*

Secondary Arteritis With Adventitial Infection

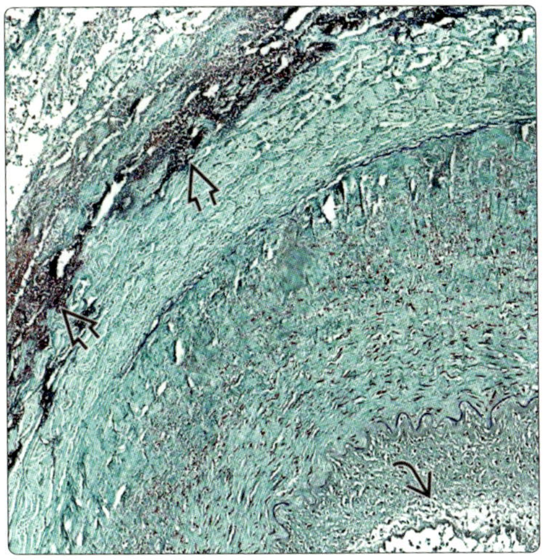

Gram-Positive Cocci in Infectious Vasculitis

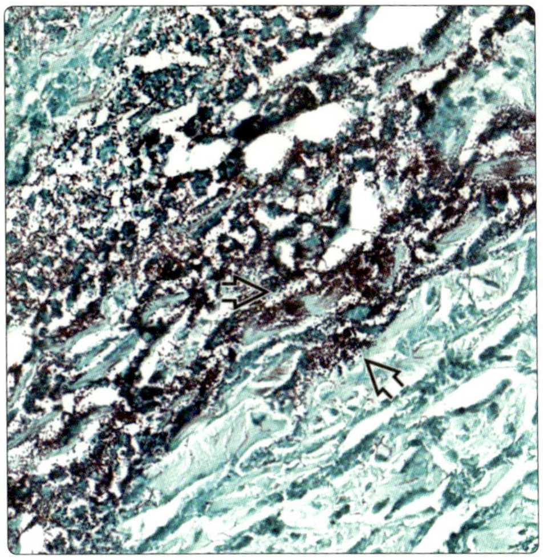

(Left) *Gram stain of the hepatic artery in a transplant patient with a porta hepatis abscess shows basophilic necrosis with gram-positive cocci invading the adventitia. Intimal inflammatory changes are also seen.* **(Right)** *Higher magnification of the basophilic necrosis in the same case shows gram-positive cocci (Gram stain).*

Granulomatous Infectious Vasculitis

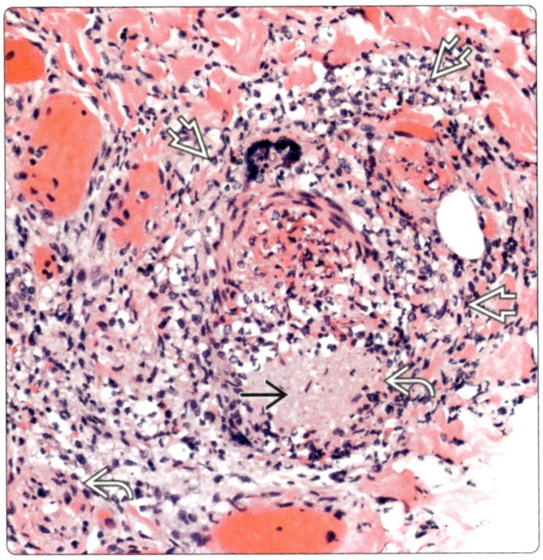

Granulomatous Infectious Vasculitis: Higher Magnification

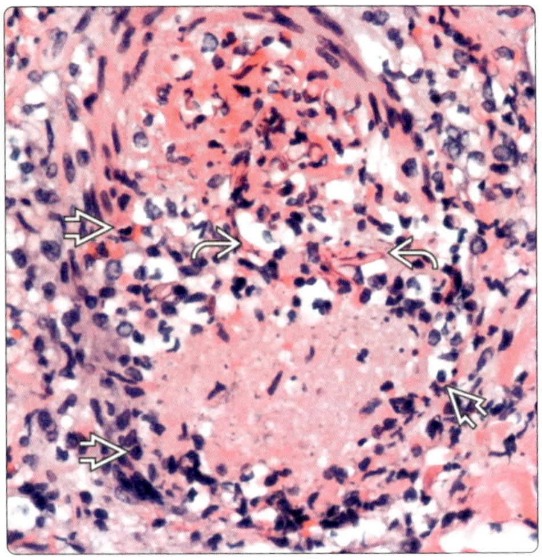

(Left) *On medium power, thrombosis and fibrinoid necrosis of small vessels are apparent in the deep dermis with associated dense perivascular mixed inflammatory infiltrate.* **(Right)** *On high power, intraluminal fungal hyphae are apparent with brisk mixed inflammatory infiltrate involving the vascular wall.*

Angioinvasive Fungal Hyphae

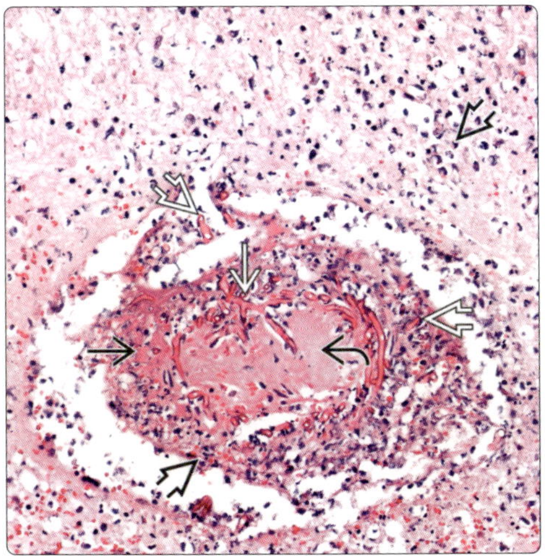

Angioinvasive Fungal Hyphae

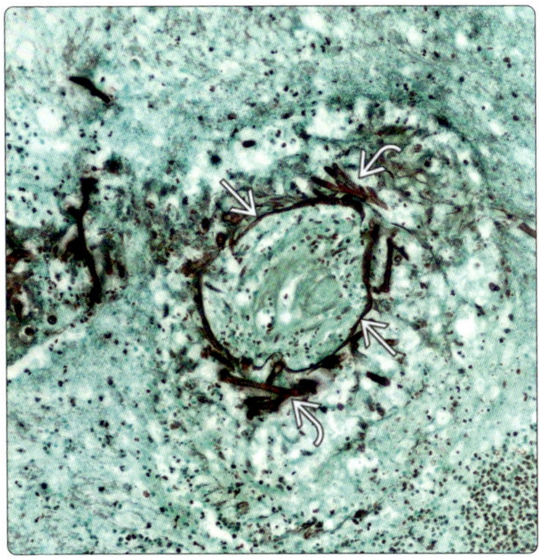

(Left) *H&E shows angioinvasive fungal hyphae with right-angle branching and associated vascular fibrinoid necrosis, thrombosis, and acute inflammation of the cerebral arterioles in this case of fatal disseminated mucormycosis.* **(Right)** *Fortuitous overstaining with GMS highlights internal elastic laminae of cerebral arterioles, aiding recognition of angioinvasive hyphae.*

Pulmonary Cavitary Coccidioidomycosis With Secondary Arteritis

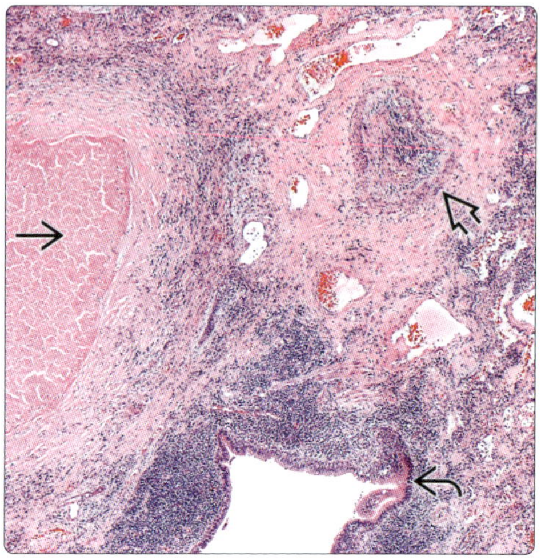

Secondary Vasculitic Lesion With Lymphoplasmacytic Inflammation

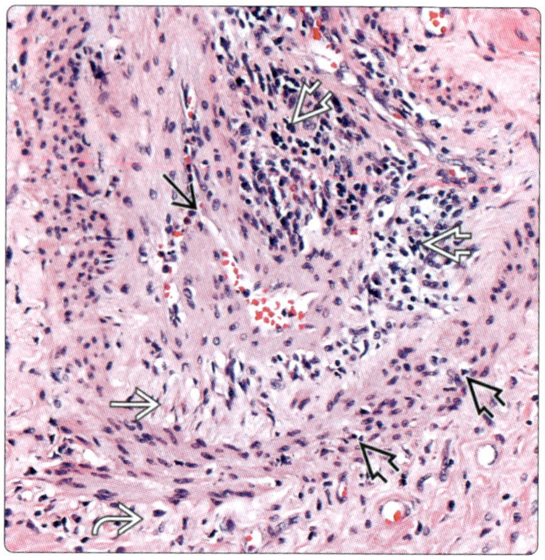

(Left) *Pulmonary cavitary coccidioidomycosis shows fibrocaseous granuloma with secondary vasculitis of nearby medium-sized pulmonary artery and secondary bronchiolitis.* **(Right)** *Higher magnification of secondary vasculitic lesion shows lymphoplasmacytic infiltration of vascular intima and media with luminal narrowing. At this magnification, internal and external elastic laminae aid recognition of this medium-sized pulmonary artery.*

Angiitis in Cutaneous Mucor Infection

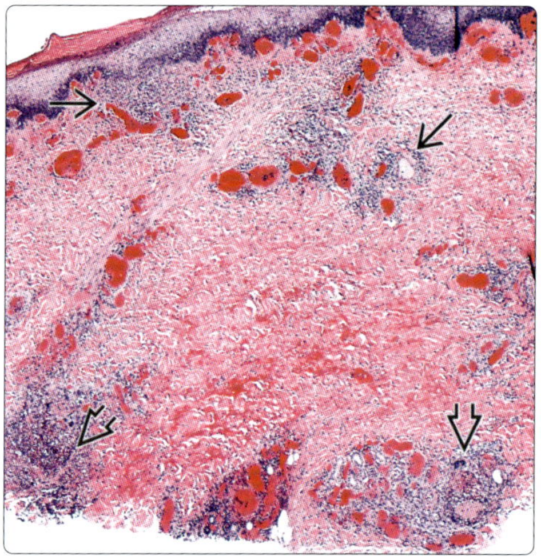

Mycelial Forms in Coccidioidomycosis

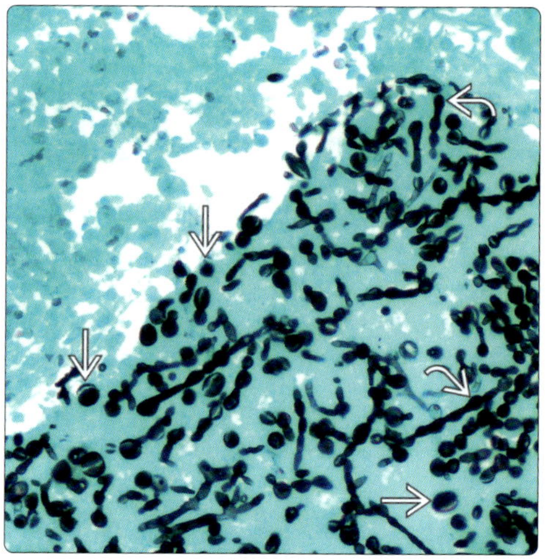

(Left) *Skin biopsy in systemic mucormycosis shows prominent perivascular inflammatory infiltrate in superficial and deep dermis.* **(Right)** *GMS staining in pulmonary cavitary coccidioidomycosis reveals mycelial forms with arthrospores and immature spherules of various sizes that may mimic hyphae and yeast of other fungal organisms.*

Vascular Involvement in Leptomeningeal Fungal Infection

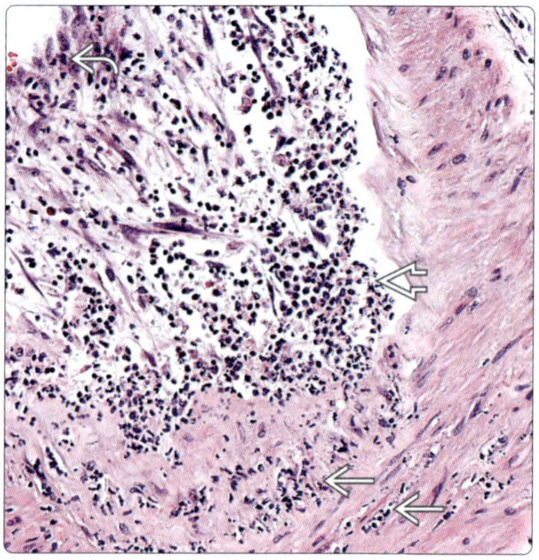

Coccidiomycosis Involving Leptomeningeal Vessels

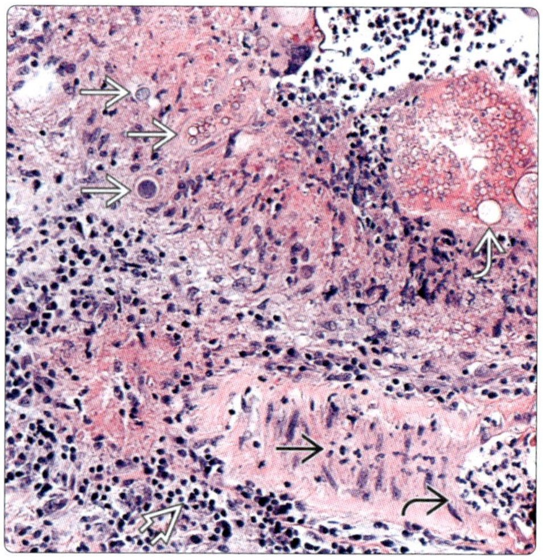

(Left) *Secondary involvement of large cerebral arteries in this case of fatal Coccidioides leptomeningitis shows a dense acute inflammatory infiltrate in vascular media and intima with subendothelial abscess formation.* **(Right)** *Spherules with and without endospores are seen in association with dense mixed perivascular inflammatory infiltrates that extend into vascular media and intima in a case of fatal leptomeningeal coccidioidomycosis.*

Angioinvasive *Aspergillus*: Lung

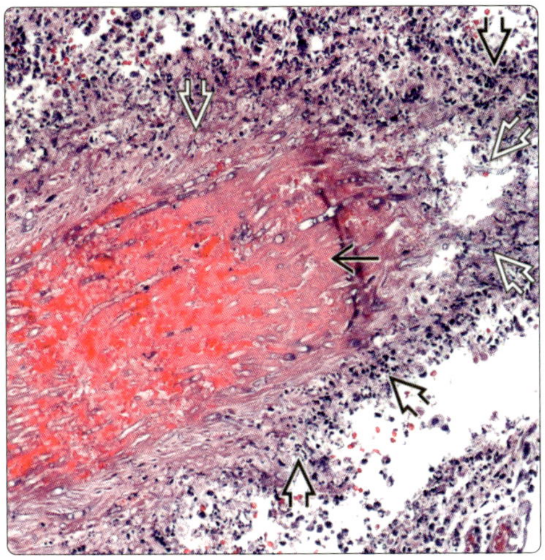

***Aspergillus* Immunoperoxidase**

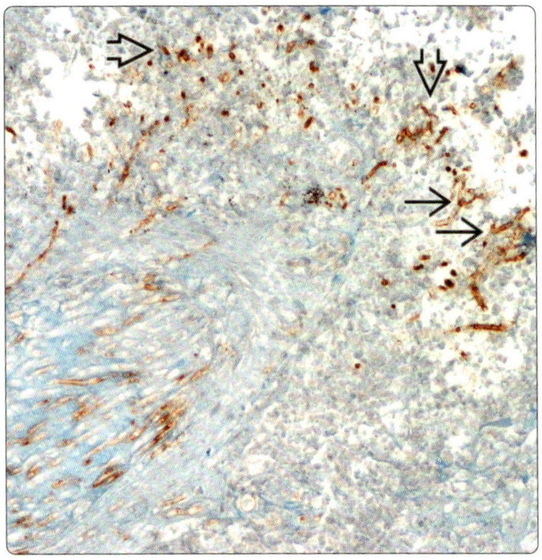

(Left) *Culture-confirmed angioinvasive pulmonary aspergillosis shows abundant fungal hyphae radiating into surrounding lung parenchyma ➡ with associated fibrinoid necrosis of a small pulmonary artery ⇨ and acute inflammation ⇨.* **(Right)** *Immunohistochemical staining for Aspergillus confirms invasion into surrounding lung parenchyma ⇨ and demonstrates acute-angle branching of fungal hyphae →.*

Cerebral Balamuthiasis

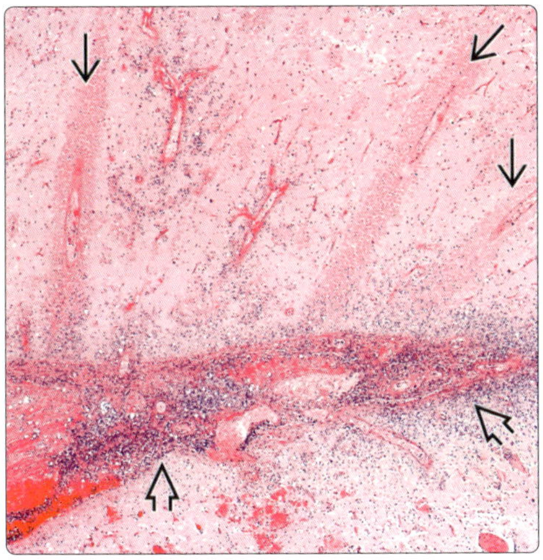

Cerebral Balamuthiasis: Higher Magnification

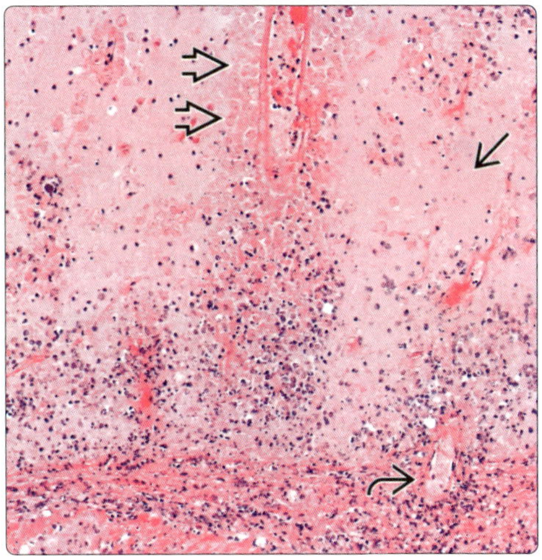

(Left) *A fatal case of solid organ transplant-transmitted cerebral balamuthiasis is shown. At low power, inflammatory infiltrate around cerebral vessels is apparent ⇨ with striking dense perivascular cuffing of nearby noninflamed vessels by parasites →.* **(Right)** *With increasing magnification, perivascular necrotic amebae become more apparent ⇨. Acute vasculitis with fibrinoid necrosis ↪ is seen with liquefactive necrosis of the brain parenchyma →.*

Cerebral Balamuthiasis in Transplant Patient

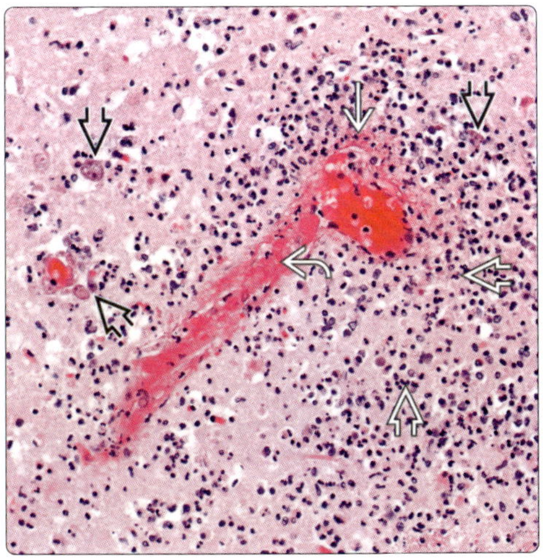

Ameba Forms in Cerebral Balamuthiasis

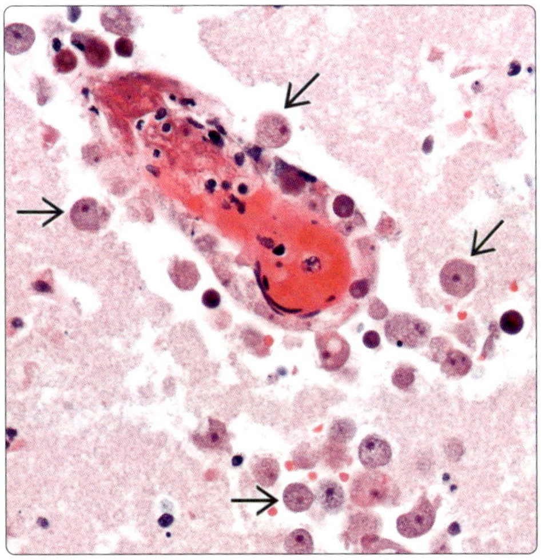

(Left) *H&E shows dense acute inflammation ➡ with fibrinoid necrosis ➡ and intraluminal thrombosis ➦ of the small cerebral arteriole in transplant-transmitted cerebral balamuthiasis. Scattered viable amebae are apparent near vessels ⇨.* **(Right)** *At high power, many viable amebae are seen cuffing small vessels →. Molecular testing confirmed their identity as Balamuthia mandrillaris.*

Lymphocytic Venulitis

KEY FACTS

TERMINOLOGY

- Slowly progressive chronic ischemic condition characterized by lymphocytic infiltration in veins and venules of intestinal wall and mesentery ± intimal hyperplasia

CLINICAL ISSUES

- Right colon is most frequently involved
- Middle-aged adults (range: 24-78 years)
- Vague abdominal symptoms mimicking inflammatory bowel disease
- Associations with microscopic colitis and diverticular disease have been rarely described
- Resection is indicated with clinical resolution in most cases and favorable prognosis

MACROSCOPIC

- Intestine segment may show wall thickening, strictures, and secondary changes due to ischemia
- Superficial mucosa lesions (ulceration, hemorrhage, edema)
- Transmural hemorrhagic infarction

MICROSCOPIC

- Lymphocytic inflammation of venules and veins in submucosa, subserosa, and pericolonic and mesenteric soft tissue with perivenular cuffing
- Arteries and arterioles free of inflammation
- Secondary thrombosis with associated intestinal ischemia
- Intimal hyperplasia with reduction of lumina seen in later stage

ANCILLARY TESTS

- Mixture of CD20 and CD3 lymphocytes with predominance of T cells
- Cytotoxic T cells positive for TIA-1

DIAGNOSTIC CHECKLIST

- Diagnosis is possible only after examination of resection specimen

(Left) *Colon section in a case of lymphocytic venulitis shows submucosal venules with marked wall thickening and chronic perivenular inflammation . (Courtesy K. Washington, MD.)* **(Right)** *Mesentery section in a case of lymphocytic venulitis shows an intact artery wall free of inflammation and a vein with sparse inflammation of the wall and perivenular cuffing of lymphocytes . (Courtesy K. Washington, MD.)*

Colon Submucosa

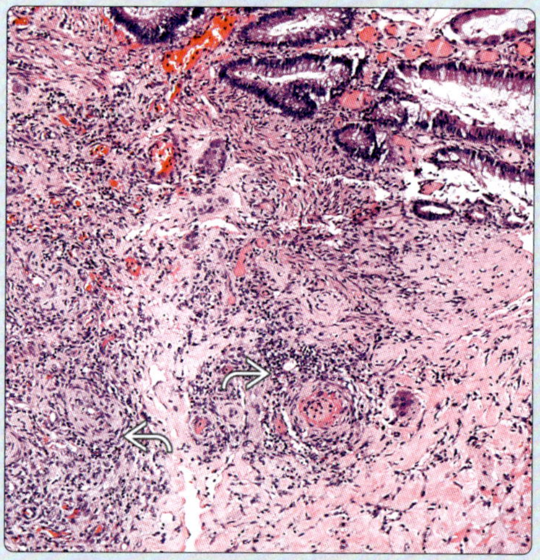

Mesentery

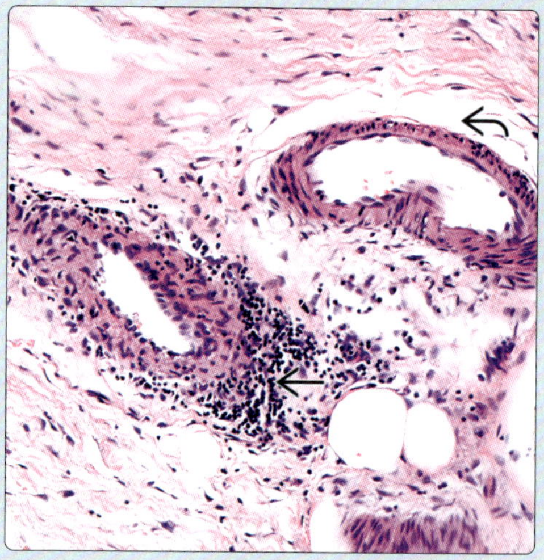

(Left) *Mesentery section in a case of lymphocytic venulitis shows intact artery wall and vein with intimal thickening and scant perivenular mononuclear inflammation . Myointimal thickening can be seen in cases with a long time from initial symptoms to surgery. (Courtesy K. Washington, MD.)* **(Right)** *At high magnification, this large mesenteric vein shows marked intimal hyperplasia and occlusion of the lumina . Scattered mononuclear inflammatory cells are seen in the wall. (Courtesy K. Washington, MD.)*

Intimal Hyperplasia

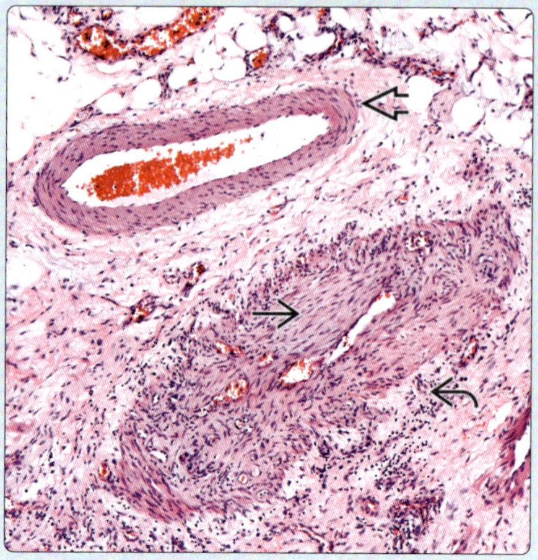

Occluded Vein

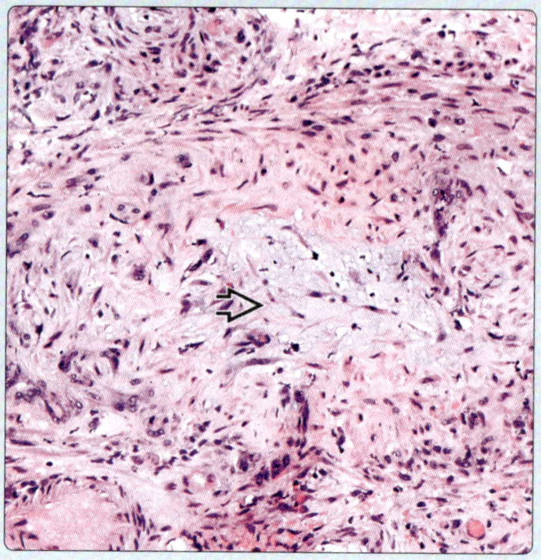

TERMINOLOGY

Synonyms

- Mesenteric inflammatory venoocclusive disease
- Enterocolic lymphocytic phlebitis
- Granulomatous phlebitis
- Intramural mesenteric venulitis

Definitions

- Slowly progressive chronic ischemic condition characterized by lymphocytic infiltration in veins and venules of intestinal wall and mesentery ± intimal hyperplasia

CLINICAL ISSUES

Epidemiology

- Incidence
  - Unknown
- Age
  - Middle-aged adults (range: 24-78 years)
- Sex
  - M:F = 2:1

Site

- Right colon is most frequently involved
- Small intestine
- Omentum
- Gallbladder

Presentation

- Vague abdominal symptoms mimicking inflammatory bowel disease
- Acute/chronic abdominal pain
- Mass
- Intussusception
- Acalculous cholecystitis
- Associations with microscopic colitis and diverticular disease have been rarely described

Treatment

- Surgical approaches
  - Resection is indicated with clinical resolution in most cases

Prognosis

- Favorable following surgical resection

IMAGING

General Features

- Imaging studies are not diagnostic of this process, and findings can overlap with other causes of venous mesenteric ischemia

MACROSCOPIC

General Features

- Intestine segment may show wall thickening, strictures, and secondary changes due to ischemia
  - Superficial mucosa lesions (ulceration, hemorrhage, edema)
  - Transmural hemorrhagic infarction

MICROSCOPIC

Histologic Features

- Lymphocytic inflammation of venules and veins in submucosa, subserosa, and pericolonic and mesenteric soft tissue
- Perivenular cuffing of lymphocytes can be seen
- Granulomatous inflammation occasionally present
- Arteries and arterioles free of inflammation
- Secondary thrombosis associated with intestinal ischemia
- Intimal hyperplasia with reduction of lumina in later stages

ANCILLARY TESTS

Immunohistochemistry

- Mixture of CD20 and CD3 lymphocytes with predominance of T cells
- Cytotoxic T cells positive for TIA-1

DIFFERENTIAL DIAGNOSIS

Systemic Vasculitis

- Arterial and vein involvement is present with prominent arterial changes
- Inflammatory infiltrate composed of neutrophils and eosinophils
- Fibrinoid necrosis of artery wall is commonly seen
- Extraintestinal manifestations are used to diagnose canonical systemic vasculitis syndromes
- Isolated intestinal involvement is unusual

Behçet Disease

- Systemic manifestations include inflammatory changes in oral, genital, and ocular distribution
- Ulceration of mucosa overlying Peyer plaque is common
- Lymphocytic inflammation involves arteries and venules
- Marked submucosal fibrosis seen in chronic lesions
- Granulomas are absent

Mesenteric Vein Thrombosis

- Relatively rare cause of intestinal ischemia mostly seen in adults in 6th-7th decades of life
- Associated with hypercoagulable states, inflammatory conditions, vascular injury, parasitic infections, neoplasia, cirrhosis
- No significant inflammation in vein walls

DIAGNOSTIC CHECKLIST

Pathologic Interpretation Pearls

- Diagnosis is possible only after examination of resection specimen

SELECTED REFERENCES

1. Okano S et al: Enterocolic lymphocytic phlebitis treated preoperatively with biologics and immunosuppressive agents. Case Rep Pathol. 2022:5120607, 2022
2. Farber ON et al: Not in the same vein: inflammatory bowel disease, malignancy, and enterocolic lymphocytic phlebitis. Dig Dis Sci. 66(2):413-18, 2021
3. Matsuda K et al: Successful surgical management of mesenteric inflammatory veno-occlusive disease. Surg Case Rep. 6(1):27, 2020
4. Nakaya M et al: Enterocolic lymphocytic phlebitis with marked myointimal hyperplasia and perivenous concentric fibrosis. Cardiovasc Pathol. 40:68-71, 2019

Varicosities

KEY FACTS

TERMINOLOGY

- Localized or diffuse dilatation of veins associated with lengthening and tortuosity

ETIOLOGY/PATHOGENESIS

- Saphenous vein varicosities (most common type) are secondary to valve incompetence with venous hypertension and primary changes in vein wall constituents leading to remodeling
    - Risk factors include heredity (strong), age, female sex, obesity, pregnancy, and prolonged standing
- Esophageal and gastric varicosities are due to hepatic portal hypertension (cirrhosis)

CLINICAL ISSUES

- In any location, may mimic neoplasm/cyst
- Peripheral: Dilated superficial varicose veins and soft tissue and skin changes, including edema, stasis dermatitis, lipodermatosclerosis, and venous ulceration with progressive disease
    - Stasis dermatitis changes of lower extremity skin in severe cases with venous ulcer
- Gastrointestinal and respiratory: Blood loss (hematemesis, hemoptysis)

MACROSCOPIC

- Varicose veins of lower extremity involve long and short saphenous veins and tributaries and are defined as palpably dilated veins > 4 mm in diameter
- Gut varicosities with dilated submucosal veins often with ulcer overlying area of rupture

MICROSCOPIC

- Variable patterns of vein wall remodeling: Intimal hyperplasia, subintimal and medial fibrosis, thrombus, increase or decrease vasa vasorum, and neovascularization of media
- Cardiac varix characteristically shows cystic structure lined by endothelium and often with associated thrombus and calcification

Esophageal Varices, Post Banding and Fulguration

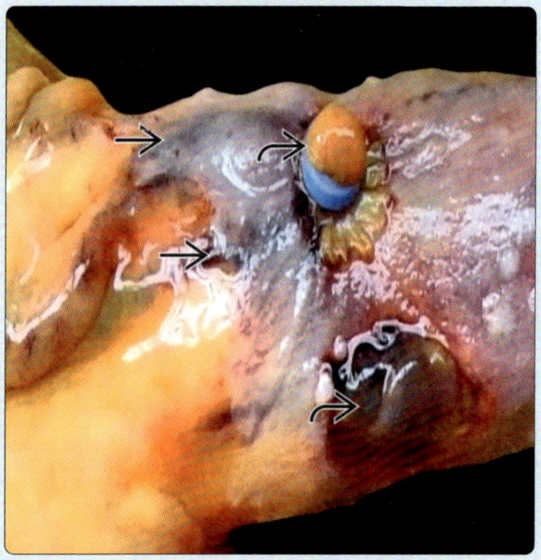

Vulvar Varicosities

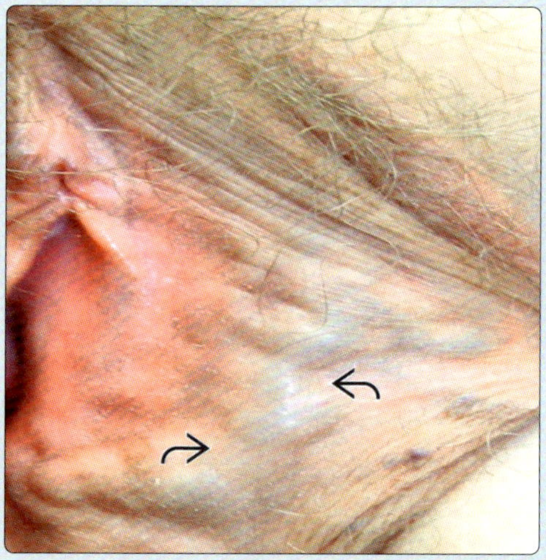

(Left) *This inverted esophagus from an autopsy of a cirrhotic patient shows fulgurated and banded areas that had clinically been bleeding. The esophageal varices can be seen as dilated submucosal veins. Banding of bleeding esophageal varices is recommended as 1st-choice treatment.* **(Right)** *Clinical photograph demonstrates a superficial blue serpiginous varicosity of the left vulva.*

Section From Cardiac Varix

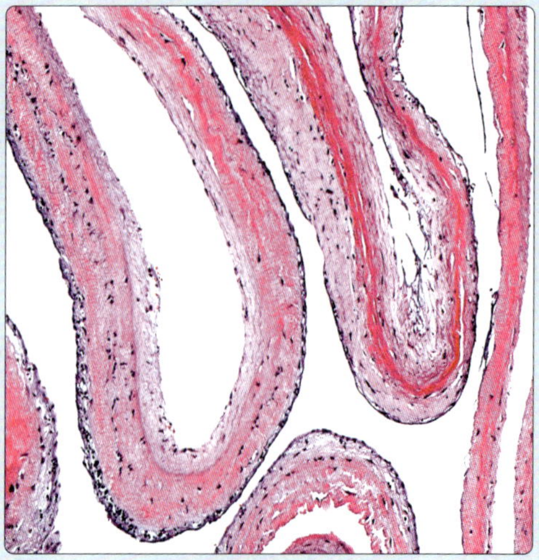

Saphenous Varicose Vein: Trichrome Stain

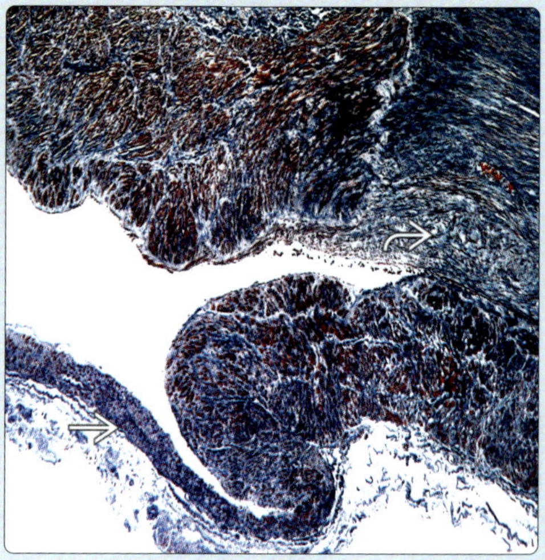

(Left) *Cardiac varix consists of a cystic structure lined by endothelium. It is usually located in the right atrium. Calcification and thrombus are not noted but are frequent in this entity.* **(Right)** *Saphenous vein wall segment from a vein stripping procedure demonstrates focal intimal hyperplasia and areas of wall thinning with loss of vascular smooth muscle cells.*

TERMINOLOGY

Synonyms

- Varix, varicose veins, varices

Definitions

- Localized or diffuse dilatation of veins associated with lengthening and tortuosity

ETIOLOGY/PATHOGENESIS

Congenital

- Venous malformation syndromes: Parkes Weber, Klippel-Trenaunay

Multifactorial

- Saphenous vein varicosities (most common type) are secondary to valve incompetence with venous hypertension and primary changes in vein wall constituents leading to remodeling
  - Risk factors include heredity (strong), age, female sex, obesity, pregnancy, prolonged standing, and history of deep vein thrombosis

Portal Hypertension

- Esophageal and gastric due to hepatic portal hypertension (cirrhosis)
  - Varices in atypical gut locations (e.g., small bowel) related to extrahepatic portal hypertension

Pregnancy

- Vulvar varicosities seen in 18-22% of pregnant women, rare outside of pregnancy
  - Usually resolves following pregnancy
  - Increased risk of recurrence and larger varicosities with subsequent pregnancy

CLINICAL ISSUES

Epidemiology

- Prevalence of peripheral varices estimated at 25-33% in women and 10-20% in men

Presentation

- Depends on anatomic location of varix
  - Peripheral: Dilated superficial varicose veins and soft tissue and skin changes, including edema, stasis dermatitis, lipodermatosclerosis, and venous ulceration with progressive disease
    - Stasis dermatitis changes of lower extremity skin in severe cases with venous ulcer
  - Gastrointestinal and respiratory: Blood loss (hematemesis, hemoptysis)
  - In any location, may mimic neoplasm/cyst
    - Cardiac varix most often mimics atrial myxoma

Treatment

- Adjuvant therapy
  - Compression stockings and phlebotonics for peripheral varicosities provide temporary relief but are not curative
- Interventional treatment for peripheral varicosities
  - Thermal ablation with external laser or endovenous catheter
  - Endovenous sclerotherapy
  - Mechanochemical ablation
  - Surgery: Ligation and stripping of great and small saphenous vein
- Interventional treatment for esophageal/gastric varicoses
  - Sclerotherapy, banding, balloon tamponade, esophageal stents, transjugular intrahepatic portosystemic shunts, endoscopic ultrasound glue injection
  - Surgical portosystemic shunts

IMAGING

Venous Duplex Ultrasonography

- Image flow in peripheral veins and measure waveforms and flow velocity

MACROSCOPIC

General Features

- Varicose veins of lower extremity involve long and short saphenous veins and tributaries and are defined as palpably dilated veins > 4 mm in diameter
  - May be associated with brown discoloration of lower extremity skin, thickening of epidermis, and venous ulcers
- Gut varicosities with dilated submucosal veins often with ulcer overlying area of rupture
- Other varicosities will present as cystic structures, hemorrhagic or containing thrombus, or recognized areas of dilated veins
  - Cardiac varix commonly in right atrium near limbus of fossa ovalis

MICROSCOPIC

Histologic Features

- Variable patterns of vein wall remodeling
  - Intimal hyperplasia
  - Subintimal and medial fibrosis
  - Thrombus
  - Increase or decrease vasa vasorum
  - Neovascularization of media
- Cardiac varix characteristically shows
  - Cystic structure lined by endothelium
  - Often with associated thrombus and calcification

ANCILLARY TESTS

Histochemistry

- Trichrome stain: Highlights intima hyperplasia and areas of loss of smooth muscle
- Elastic stain: Demonstrates disruption of elastic fibrils

DIFFERENTIAL DIAGNOSIS

Vascular Neoplasia

- Most important in nongastrointestinal visceral varices
- Gross and histologic examination will clarify diagnosis

SELECTED REFERENCES

1. Serra R et al: Clinical and pathological correlations in chronic venous disease. Ann Vasc Surg. 78:19-27, 2022
2. Whiteley MS: Current best practice in the management of varicose veins. Clin Cosmet Investig Dermatol. 15:567-83, 2022

Hypertensive Renovascular Diseases

KEY FACTS

TERMINOLOGY

- Renal vascular and glomerular disease secondary to hypertension (HTN) (blood pressure > 120/80 mm Hg)

ETIOLOGY/PATHOGENESIS

- Risk factors include obesity, lack of exercise, salt intake, Black race
- Arterial stiffening and increased pressure in afferent arterioles lead to hyalinosis

CLINICAL ISSUES

- ~ 30% of adults in United States have HTN
- ~ 95% due to essential HTN
- Effective drug therapy ameliorates sequelae

MACROSCOPIC

- Capsular surface usually granular with adherent capsule that strips with difficulty

MICROSCOPIC

- Granular surface of kidney due to alternating depressed scars, bulging spared, and hypertrophied nephrons
- Subcapsular sclerotic scars with sclerotic glomeruli, thickened arterioles, and atrophic tubules
- Arterial intimal fibrosis and arteriolar hyalinosis
- "Onion skinning," endothelial swelling, and fibrinoid necrosis of arterioles in malignant HTN

TOP DIFFERENTIAL DIAGNOSES

- Renal artery stenosis leading to renal atrophy
- Renal infarct
- Thrombotic microangiopathy, other causes
- Systemic sclerosis

(Left) *Nephrectomy specimen from a patient with hypertensive nephrosclerosis shows a characteristic coarsely granular surface with depressed scars.* **(Right)** *PAS stain shows arterioles with plump endothelial cells and muscular hypertrophy in a case of hypertensive renovascular disease.*

Kidney in Hypertension

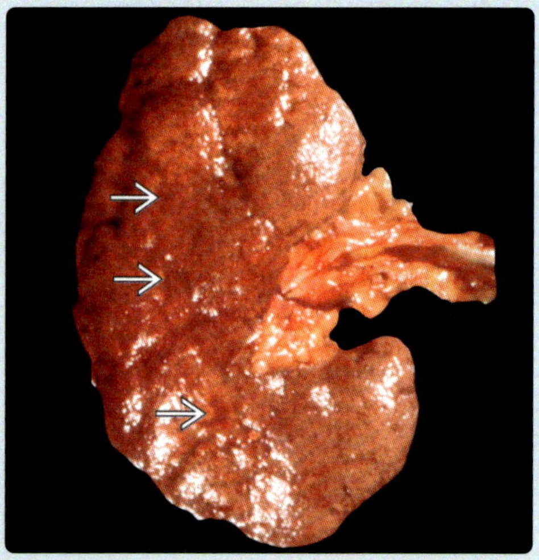

Arteriosclerosis: PAS Stain

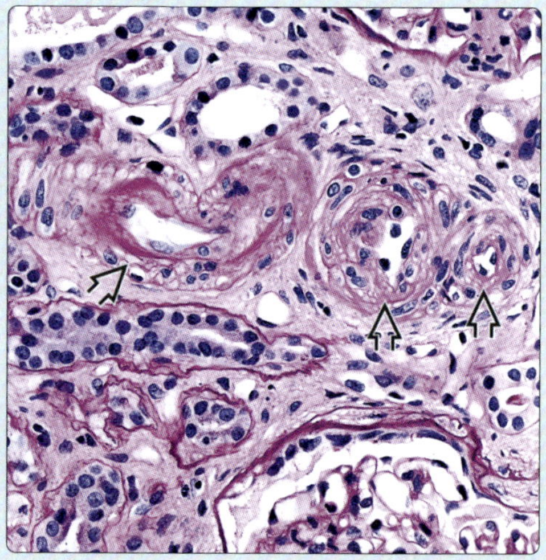

(Left) *Electron micrograph shows swollen endothelial cells, fragmented RBCs, and platelets in the glomerular capillary loops in a case of hypertensive renovascular disease. There is focal foot process effacement. There is also widening of the subendothelial zone.* **(Right)** *Elastic van Gieson stain highlights reduplication of the internal elastic lamina and fibrous intimal thickening in this interlobar-sized artery, changes that are commonly seen in hypertensive renovascular disease.*

Ultrastructural Changes in Malignant Hypertension: Electron Microscopy

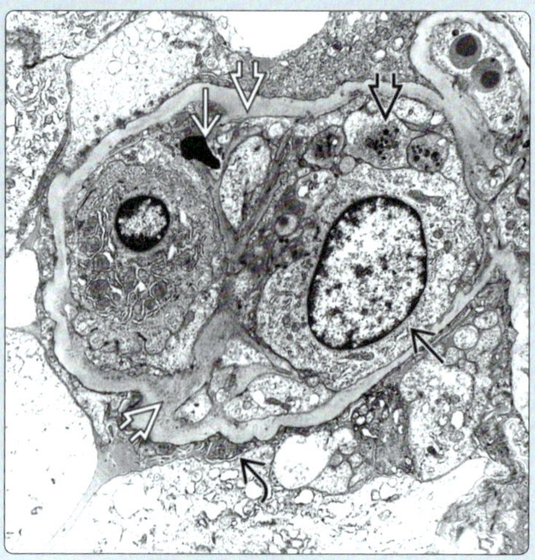

Arteriosclerosis: Elastic Stain

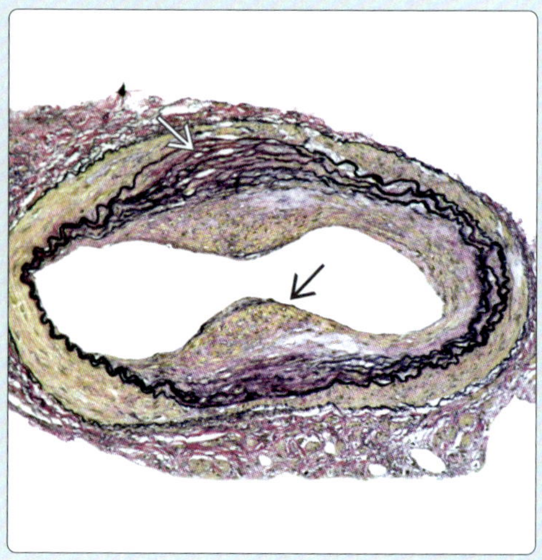

TERMINOLOGY

Abbreviations

- Hypertension (HTN)

Definitions

- Renal vascular and glomerular disease secondary to HTN (blood pressure > 120/80 mm Hg)

ETIOLOGY/PATHOGENESIS

Essential Hypertension

- ~ 95% of cases
- Risk factors include obesity, lack of exercise, salt intake, Black race
- Evidence for multigenic basis + environmental factors

Secondary Hypertension

- < 5% of cases
- Renal artery stenosis (Goldblatt HTN)
  - Increased production of renin by ischemic kidney
- Neoplasia
  - Pheochromocytoma, adrenal cortical tumors, renin-producing tumors
- Chronic renal disease

Malignant Hypertension

- Renin release causes cycle of vascular injury followed by more renin release
- Form of thrombotic microangiopathy

Effect of Hypertension on Arteries and Arterioles

- Direct injury to endothelium
- Arterial stiffening and increased pressure in afferent arterioles lead to hyalinosis

CLINICAL ISSUES

Epidemiology

- Incidence
  - ~ 30% of adults in United States have HTN
- Sex
  - Slightly more common in men
- Ethnicity
  - Black populations disproportionately affected

Presentation

- Papilledema, retinal hemorrhage, stroke, microangiopathic hemolysis when mean blood pressure > 160 mm Hg (malignant HTN)

Treatment

- Drugs
  - β-adrenergic antagonists, α-adrenergic antagonists
  - Smooth muscle dilators, endothelin antagonists
  - ACE inhibitors, vasopeptidase inhibitors, renin inhibitors
  - Diuretics, mineralocorticoid receptor antagonists

Prognosis

- Malignant HTN
  - If left untreated, survival is poor (20% 1-year survival)
  - Long-term survival is > 90% if blood pressure is controlled

MICROSCOPIC

Histologic Features

- Medium-sized arteries
  - Intimal fibrosis
  - Internal elastic lamina becomes multilayered (fibroelastosis); best seen on elastic stains
  - Smooth muscle hyperplasia
  - Diminished vascular lumen
- Arterioles
  - Hyaline arteriolosclerosis

Malignant Hypertension

- Small arteries
  - Mucoid (myxoid) intimal change and endothelial swelling in arterioles, a.k.a. "onion skinning"
  - Fibrinoid necrosis
- Arterioles
  - Arteriolar occlusion by endothelial swelling/edema-type change
  - Fibrin thrombi

DIFFERENTIAL DIAGNOSIS

Renal Artery Stenosis

- Renal tubular atrophy (endocrine type)
- Minimal renal interstitial fibrosis
- Intrarenal vessels often normal in renal artery fibromuscular dysplasia

Renal Infarct

- Usually larger, more focal than subcapsular scars of hypertensive disease, and wedge shaped

Thrombotic Microangiopathy, Other Causes

- Vascular and glomerular lesions similar to malignant HTN

Systemic Sclerosis

- Extrarenal and serologic features of systemic sclerosis are usually present

SELECTED REFERENCES

1. Freedman BI et al: Target organ damage in African American hypertension: role of APOL1. Curr Hypertens Rep. 14(1):21-8, 2012
2. Singh N et al: CKD in MYH9-related disorders. Am J Kidney Dis. 54(4):732-40, 2009
3. Hill GS: Hypertensive nephrosclerosis. Curr Opin Nephrol Hypertens. 17(3):266-70, 2008
4. Marcantoni C et al: A perspective on arterionephrosclerosis: from pathology to potential pathogenesis. J Nephrol. 20(5):518-24, 2007
5. Senitko M et al: An update on renovascular hypertension. Curr Cardiol Rep. 7(6):405-11, 2005
6. Fogo AB: Mechanisms in nephrosclerosis and hypertension-beyond hemodynamics. J Nephrol. 14 Suppl 4:S63-9, 2001
7. Perneger TV et al: Projections of hypertension-related renal disease in middle-aged residents of the United States. JAMA. 269:1272-7, 1993
8. Kasiske BL: Relationship between vascular disease and age-associated changes in the human kidney. Kidney Int. 31(5):1153-9, 1987
9. Kashgarian M: Pathology of small blood vessel disease in hypertension. Am J Kidney Dis. 5(4):A104-10, 1985
10. Ratliff NB: Renal vascular disease: pathology of large blood vessel disease. Am J Kidney Dis. 5(4):A93-103, 1985
11. Castleman B et al: The relation of vascular disease to the hypertensive state; the adequacy of the renal biopsy as determined from a study of 500 patients. N Engl J Med. 239(20):729-32, 1948

(Left) *In the kidney, intimal fibroplasia ➡ is often present in interlobar-sized arteries in hypertensive renovascular disease.* **(Right)** *In hypertension (HTN), the arterial media may also be markedly thickened ➡. This change represents an adaptive compensatory response in the setting of elevated pressure and increased vessel wall strain to protect the delicate glomerular capillary loops downstream.*

Intimal Fibrosis in Hypertension

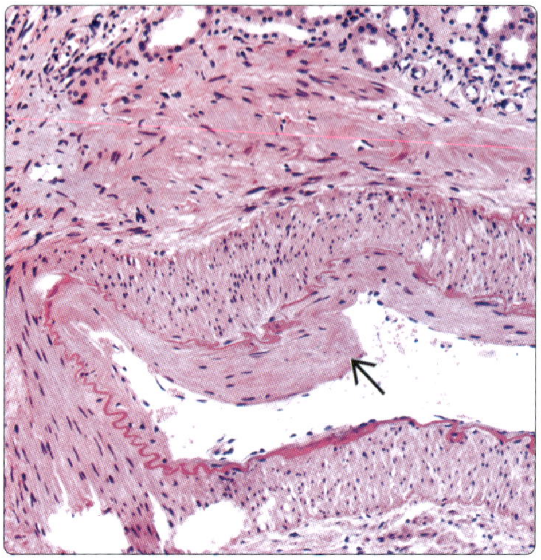

Medial Hypertrophy in Hypertension

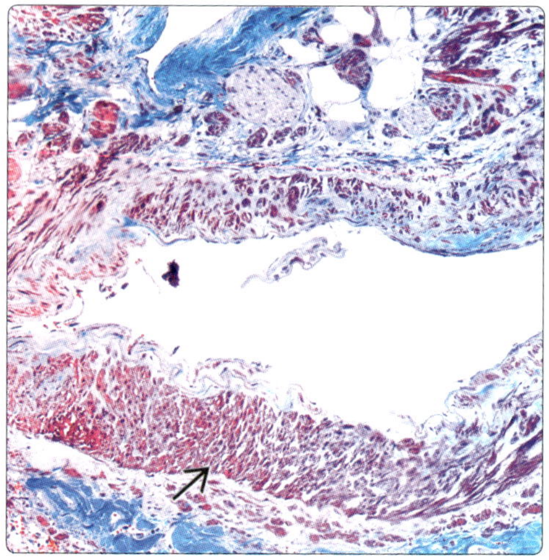

(Left) *Arterial intimal thickening ➡ and medial smooth muscle layer thinning ➡ may also be seen in hypertensive renovascular disease, as shown on this trichrome-stained section.* **(Right)** *In this interlobar-sized artery, trichrome stain shows medial thinning ➡ with thickening of the intima. There is also migration of fuchsinophilic medial muscle cells ➡ into the intima, a process called intimal fibroplasia.*

Arteriosclerosis in Kidney: Trichrome Stain

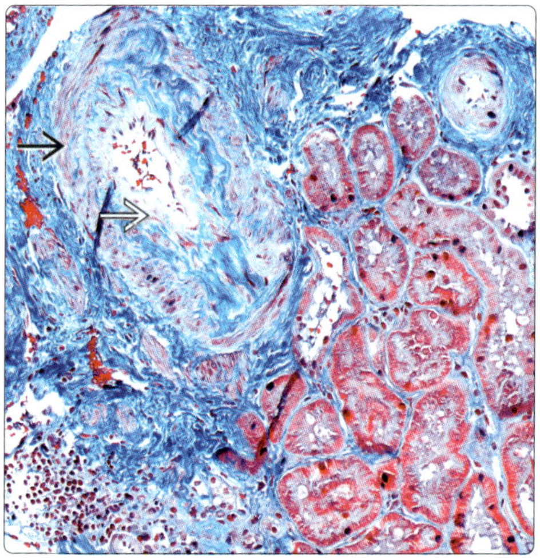

Intimal Fibrosis: Trichrome Stain

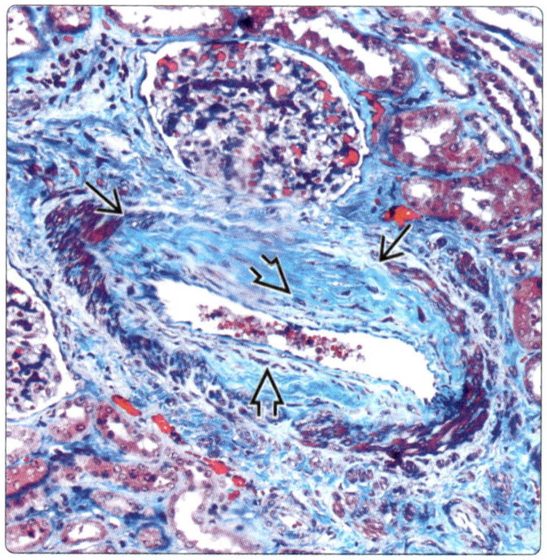

(Left) *In this PAS-stained renal biopsy from a patient with HTN, thickening and lamellation (reduplication) of the elastic lamellae ➡ is apparent in interlobar-sized arteries.* **(Right)** *Immunofluorescence for fibrin shows deposition in arterioles in hypertensive renovascular disease.*

Internal Elastic Lamina Changes in Hypertension

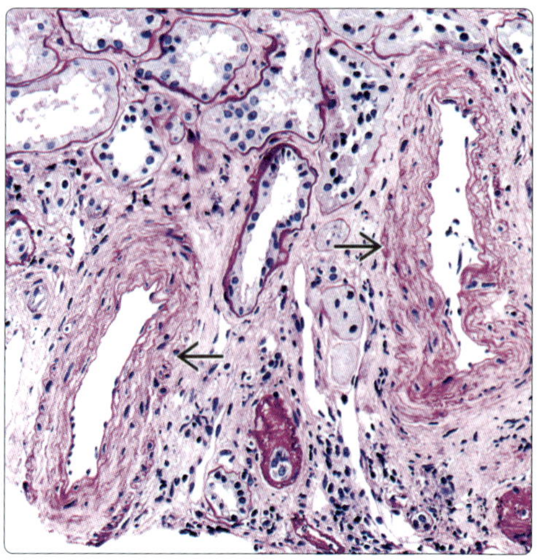

Fibrin Staining in Arterioles

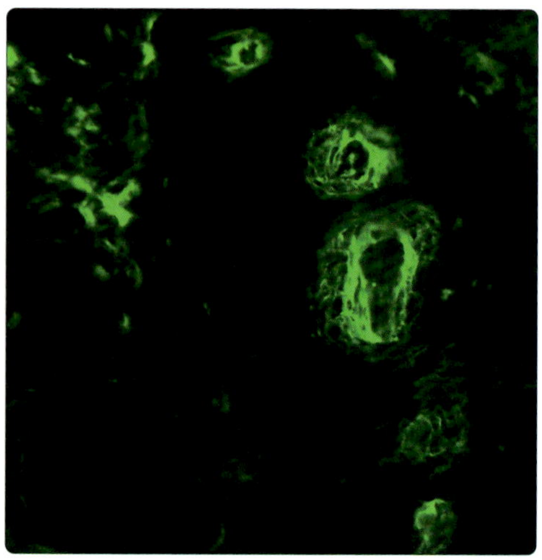

Marked Intimal Fibrosis

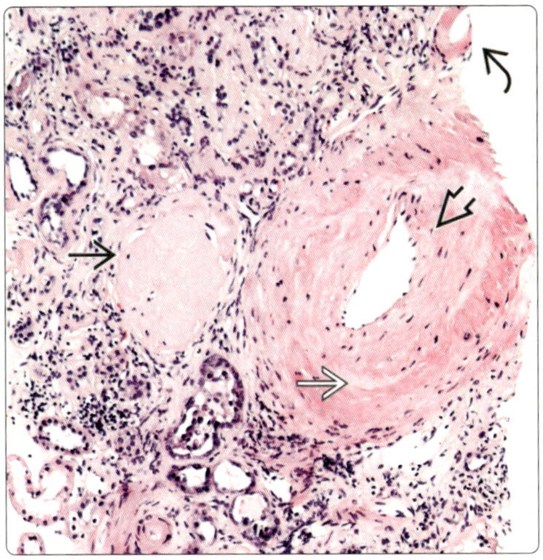

Arteriolar Hyalinosis in Hypertension

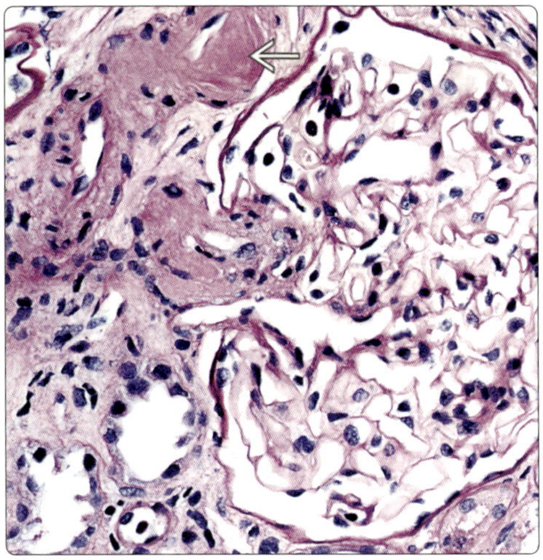

(Left) *Typical vascular changes of hypertensive nephrosclerosis include intimal fibrosis of an arcuate-sized artery and arteriolar hyalinosis. The internal elastica, the border between the intima and media, is indicated. Secondary features include interstitial fibrosis, tubular atrophy, and global glomerulosclerosis.* **(Right)** *Hyalinized arterioles are commonly found in a number of disorders, including HTN, diabetes, and calcineurin inhibitor toxicity.*

"Onion Skin" Change in Malignant Hypertension

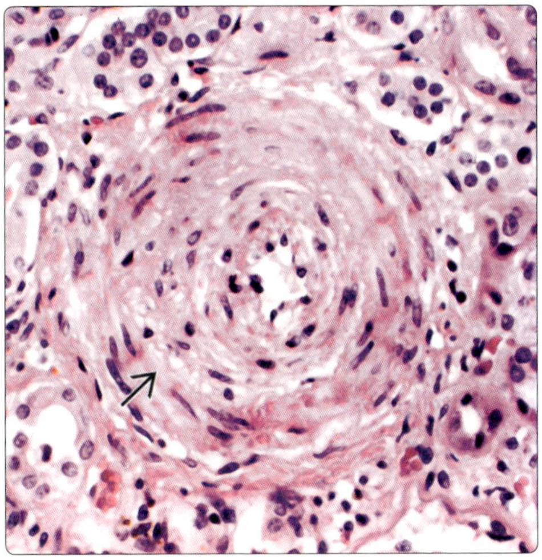

"Onion Skin" Change in Malignant Hypertension: Jones Stain

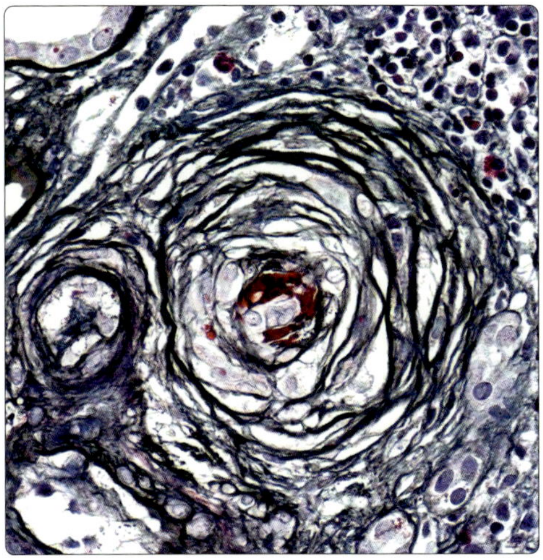

(Left) *Higher power view of this renal arteriole shows the "onion skin" change in the vessel wall due to concentric myointimal thickening in the setting of malignant HTN.* **(Right)** *Jones silver stain shows lamination ("onion skin" changes) of an arteriolar wall with near obliteration of the arteriolar lumen, a process that has been referred to as hyperplastic arteriolosclerosis in malignant HTN.*

Intimal Ultrastructural Changes in Hypertension: Electron Microscopy

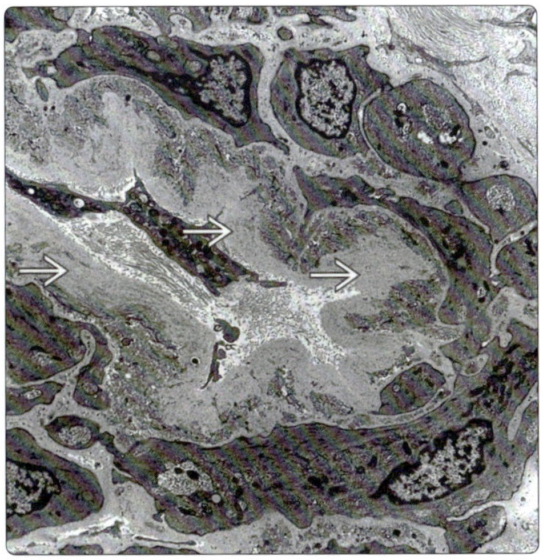

Arteriolar Hyaline: Electron Microscopy

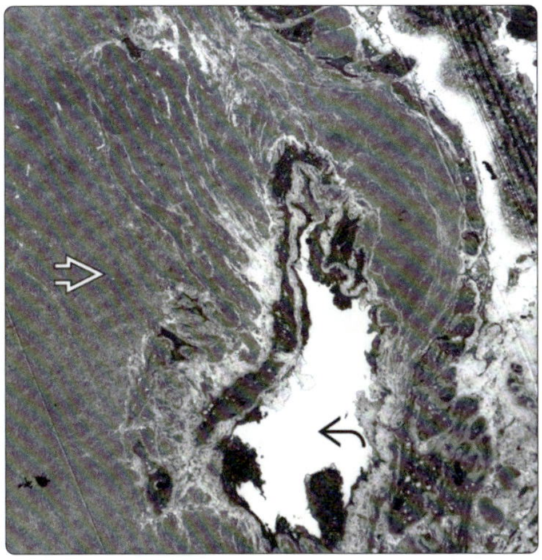

(Left) *Electron micrograph of a small renal artery shows accumulation of amorphous material between the endothelium and the media, probably the residua of "onion skin" thickening.* **(Right)** *Electron micrograph shows massive hyaline insudation in the intimal layer resulting in marked medial atrophy/replacement. The lumen is narrowed as a result.*

Vascular Graft Pseudoaneurysm

KEY FACTS

TERMINOLOGY

- Pseudoaneurysm: Hematoma formed by blood leaking from "break" in artery wall, not limited by all elements of vessel wall
- Develops outside vascular grafts (both native vessels and synthetic grafts), communicates with lumen, and is contained by surrounding soft tissues

ETIOLOGY/PATHOGENESIS

- Injury to graft due to iatrogenic trauma, infection, blunt injury, repeated puncture

CLINICAL ISSUES

- Commonly occurs at anastomotic sites
- Usually asymptomatic
- Patients may present with tender, pulsatile, gradually expanding mass at site of trauma
- Duplex ultrasonography is used as screening tool to assess peripheral vascular bypass graft surveillance
- Treatment: Small pseudoaneurysms can thrombose spontaneously, whereas others need definitive treatment
- Complications: Progressive enlargement of pseudoaneurysm; erosion of overlying skin, rupture, and hemorrhage
- Prophylaxis: Regular/planned rotation of needle puncture sites of graft to alternate sites

MACROSCOPIC

- Pseudoaneurysm in hemodialysis grafts may present as small orifice in graft material with stretching and thinning of overlying skin

MICROSCOPIC

- Pseudoaneurysm is formed outside arterial wall
- Contains thrombotic material
- Devoid of arterial wall layers
- Grafts used for hemodialysis access also show chronic changes in and around pseudoaneurysm area

Synthetic PTFE Graft With Pseudoaneurysm

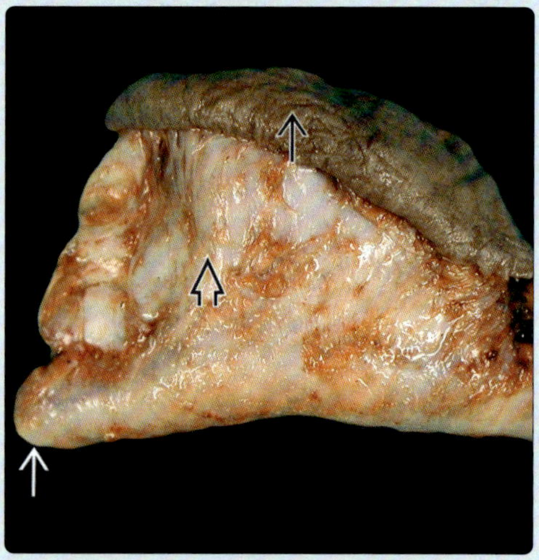

Thrombosed Dialysis Access Graft

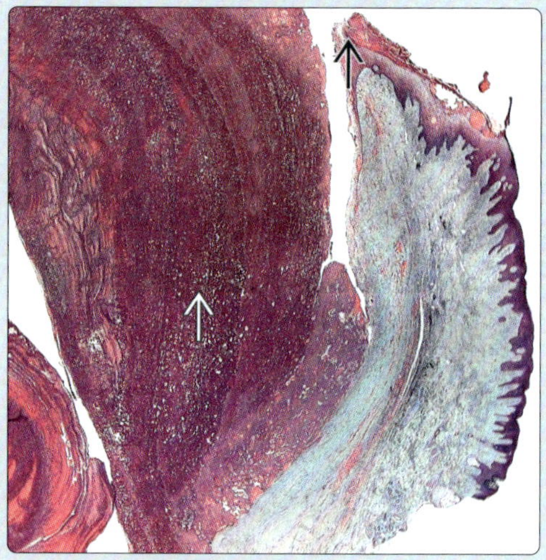

(Left) *Gross photograph of a synthetic polytetrafluoroethylene (PTFE) graft shows a large pseudoaneurysm localized under the skin with overlying ulceration.* **(Right)** *Low-power view of a Movat-stained section of dialysis access graft shows a large thrombus with ulceration of overlying skin. The skin changes occur because of scarring and loss of vascularization. Thrombosis within the graft leads to graft failure.*

Synthetic PTFE Graft

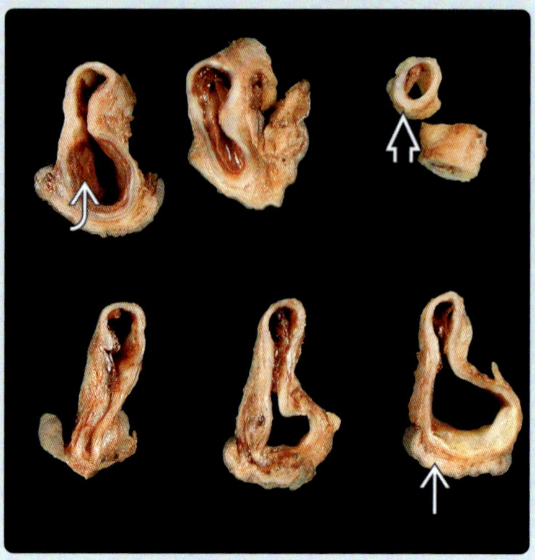

Histologic Features of Synthetic PTFE Graft

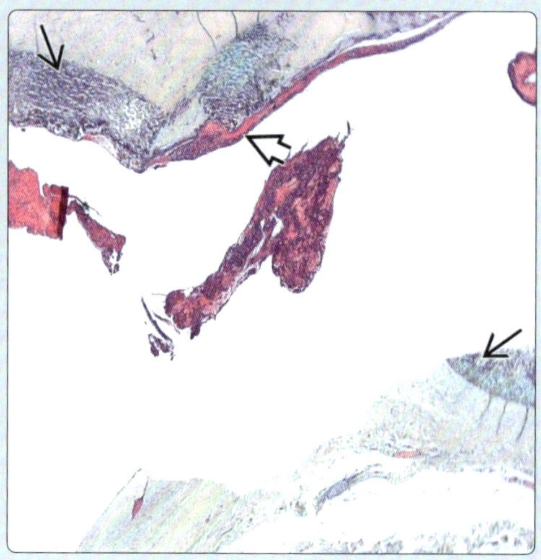

(Left) *Serial sections of synthetic PTFE graft show the normal-sized graft. The rest of the graft is aneurysmal with mural thrombus under the overlying skin.* **(Right)** *Low-power view of a Movat elastic-stained section of PTFE graft shows the pseudoaneurysmal graft wall with attached thrombus.*

TERMINOLOGY

Synonyms

- False aneurysm

Definitions

- Pseudoaneurysm: Hematoma formed by blood leaking from "break" in artery wall, not limited by all elements of vessel wall
- Develops outside vascular grafts (both native vessels and synthetic grafts), communicates with lumen, and is contained by surrounding soft tissues

ETIOLOGY/PATHOGENESIS

Mechanisms of Pseudoaneurysm Formation

- Trauma to vessel at time of harvest
- Presence of areas of weakness, such as valve sites in veins and branch points
- Hypertension and atherosclerotic degeneration of graft vessel wall
- Ischemia and necrosis of vessel wall
- Infection at site of insertion
- Dehiscence at anastomoses
- Iatrogenic trauma
  - Endovascular and surgical intervention, such as catheterization and stent placement
- Repeated puncture by dialysis needles at same location in graft
  - Causes damage to and breakdown of graft material
- Venous outflow stenosis with resultant increase in intragraft pressure
- Blunt or penetrating trauma leading to disruption of graft wall
- In arteriovenous shunt graft, pseudoaneurysm can also occur due to poor puncture technique before graft is fully mature

CLINICAL ISSUES

Epidemiology

- Incidence
  - Pseudoaneurysm of vascular graft is uncommon and occurs as late complication
  - Less frequent than true aneurysm
  - Pseudoaneurysm in aortobifemoral bypass grafts performed for abdominal aortic aneurysm (5%)
  - Dialysis access grafts (2-10%)
  - Pseudoaneurysm of saphenous vein graft (SVG) in coronary artery bypass grafting (CABG) is uncommon and occurs 12 ± 4.2 years after surgery
    - SVG to right coronary is most commonly involved

Site

- Pseudoaneurysms can occur in any vascular graft
  - Saphenous vein graft or internal mammary artery graft following CABG
  - Aortoiliac grafts performed for abdominal aortic aneurysm repair or peripheral vascular disease
  - Ascending thoracic aorta following aortic root or ascending grafting
  - Hemodialysis access graft (common) for treatment of renal failure
  - Vein grafts used for lower extremity arterial reconstruction following limb-threatening ischemia
- Pseudoaneurysms commonly occur at anastomotic sites, whereas true aneurysms involve graft midportion

Presentation

- Pseudoaneurysm of SVG in CABG
  - Suspected because of symptomatic manifestations (chest pain, dyspnea) soon after CABG
  - Can present as
    - Myocardial ischemia or infarction
    - Mediastinal mass
    - Fistula formation into cardiac chamber
    - Rupture
- Pseudoaneurysm of dialysis access grafts
  - May lead to mass effect
  - Distal ischemia
  - Embolization
  - Sepsis
  - Massive hemorrhage and death
  - Symptoms
    - Painful swelling at site of trauma or catheterization
- Pseudoaneurysm in other sites
  - Appear as tender, pulsatile, gradually expanding mass
  - May compress nerve leading to numbness

Treatment

- National Kidney Foundation Disease Outcomes Quality Initiative (KDOQI) has established guidelines for treatment of pseudoaneurysms
- Small pseudoaneurysms can thrombose spontaneously, whereas others need definitive treatment
  - Covered stent
    - Stent composed of metal and lined with polytetrafluoroethylene (PTFE) is placed endovascularly across "hole" through which pseudoaneurysm communicates with graft
    - This prevents pseudoaneurysm from receiving blood and allows thrombosis to occur
- Ultrasound probe compression of neck of pseudoaneurysm for ~ 20 min, during which blood within pseudoaneurysm clots
  - 1st line of treatment for femoral artery pseudoaneurysm < 4 cm in size
- Ultrasound-guided thrombin injection directly in pseudoaneurysm, causing blood clot
  - Suitable for pseudoaneurysms with neck as short as 5 mm and as wide as 4.3 mm
  - Complications
    - Distal embolization
    - Thrombosis of native artery
- Surgical ligation/graft removal (± distal bypass)
- Transcatheter intervention for SVG pseudoaneurysm in CABG

Complications

- Pseudoaneurysm can undergo
  - Calcification
  - Progressive enlargement

- Erosion of overlying skin
- Rupture
- Hemorrhage
- Turbulence in blood flow leading to graft thrombosis and graft failure
- Associated with cosmetic problems, infection, and difficulty in accessing graft
- Larger pseudoaneurysms are more prone to leakage and recurrences
- Pseudoaneurysm of SVG in CABG has in-hospital mortality rate of 15.7%
    - Increased risk of myocardial infarction, congestive heart failure, fistula formation, coronary artery embolization, and rupture

Prophylaxis for Dialysis Access Grafts Pseudoaneurysm

- Regular/planned rotation of needle puncture sites of graft to alternate sites
- Careful needle puncture techniques
- Aseptic precautions

IMAGING

Radiographic Findings

- Chest x-ray
    - Demonstrates enlarging heart silhouette, possibly related to heart failure

Ultrasonographic Findings

- Duplex ultrasound
    - Screening tool to assess peripheral vascular bypass graft surveillance
    - Sensitivity: > 90%
    - Confirms graft patency, anastomotic areas, stenosis, and thrombosis
- Color flow Doppler ultrasound
    - Shows aneurysmal swirl pattern of blood flow in graft

CT Findings

- CT shows pseudoaneurysm with mass effect
    - Thrombus can be identified showing laminated appearance
- CT angiogram identifies portion of graft involved by pseudoaneurysm

MACROSCOPIC

General Features

- Pseudoaneurysm in hemodialysis grafts may present as small orifice in graft material with stretching and thinning of overlying skin
- Skin overlying graft becomes scarred, avascular, and ulcerated

MICROSCOPIC

Histologic Features

- Pseudoaneurysm is formed outside arterial wall
- Contains thrombotic material
- Devoid of arterial wall layers
- Grafts used for hemodialysis access also show chronic changes in and around pseudoaneurysm area

DIFFERENTIAL DIAGNOSIS

True Aneurysm

- Localized dilatation of artery, whereas pseudoaneurysm forms outside arterial wall
- All layers of arterial wall are present in true aneurysm

Arterial Dissection

- Separation of arterial wall layers
- Blood accumulates between arterial layers
- Break/tear may be identified in intima

Penetrating Atherosclerotic Ulcer

- Crater-like defect in aorta media layer (usually descending thoracic portion) overlying atherosclerotic plaque
- Associated with intramural hematoma and wall dissection

DIAGNOSTIC CHECKLIST

Clinically Relevant Pathologic Features

- Pseudoaneurysm is formed outside arterial wall, devoid of artery wall layers, and contained by surrounding tissues

SELECTED REFERENCES

1. Li K et al: Graft infection after prosthetic bypass surgery for infectious femoral artery pseudoaneurysm in intravenous drug users: manifestation, management, and prognosis. Ann Vasc Surg. 70:449-58, 2021
2. Meola M et al: Ultrasound evaluation of access complications: thrombosis, aneurysms, pseudoaneurysms and infections. J Vasc Access. 22(1_suppl):71-83, 2021
3. Vinciguerra M et al: Management of patients with aortocoronary saphenous vein graft aneurysms: JACC state-of-the-art review. J Am Coll Cardiol. 77(17):2236-53, 2021
4. MacKenzie DJ et al: Early cannulation ePTFE arteriovenous access grafts are associated with a low incidence of pseudoaneurysm formation. Ann Vasc Surg. 64:270-5, 2020
5. Zucker DJS et al: Minimally invasive repair of ascending aortic pseudoaneurysms: an alternative to open surgical repair in high-risk patients. J Vasc Interv Radiol. 31(8):1342-7.e1, 2020
6. Kotelis D et al: Endovascular repair of pseudoaneurysms after open surgery for aortic coarctation. Interact Cardiovasc Thorac Surg. 22(1):26-31, 2016
7. Mudoni A et al: Aneurysms and pseudoaneurysms in dialysis access. Clin Kidney J. 8(4):363-7, 2015
8. Pan L et al: Application of stent-graft is the optimal therapy for traumatic internal carotid artery pseudoaneurysms. Int J Clin Exp Med. 8(6):9362-7, 2015
9. Hudzik B et al: Giant saphenous vein graft pseudoaneurysm compressing the right atrium and right ventricle and presenting as decompensated heart failure. Can J Cardiol. 27(3):390, 2011
10. Brewster DC: Mastery of Surgery. 5th ed. Lippincott Williams &Wilkins, 2007
11. Moszkowicz A et al: Occlusion of a rapidly expanding hemodialysis graft pseudoaneurysm with placement of a stent graft. Semin Intervent Radiol. 24(1):34-7, 2007
12. Yasim A et al: Complication of hemodialysis graft: anastomotic pseudoaneurysm: a case report. Transplant Proc. 38(9):2816-8, 2006
13. Zwiebel W et al: Introduction to Vascular Ultrasonography. WB Saunders, 2005
14. Memon AQ et al: Saphenous vein graft aneurysm: case report and review. Cardiol Rev. 11(1):26-34, 2003
15. Ryan JM et al: Technical innovation. Using a covered stent (wallgraft) to treat pseudoaneurysms of dialysis grafts and fistulas. AJR Am J Roentgenol. 180(4):1067-71, 2003
16. III: NKF-K/DOQI Clinical practice guidelines for vascular access: update 2000. Am J Kidney Dis. 37(1 Suppl 1):S137-81, 2001
17. Paulson EK et al: Treatment of iatrogenic femoral arterial pseudoaneurysms: comparison of US-guided thrombin injection with compression repair. Radiology. 215(2):403-8, 2000
18. Trop I et al: Anterior mediastinal mass in a patient with prior saphenous vein coronary artery bypass grafting. Chest. 115(2):572-6, 1999
19. Delorme JM et al: Vascular access for hemodialysis: pathologic features of surgically excised ePTFE grafts. Ann Vasc Surg. 6(6):517-24, 1992

Histologic Features of Synthetic PTFE Graft

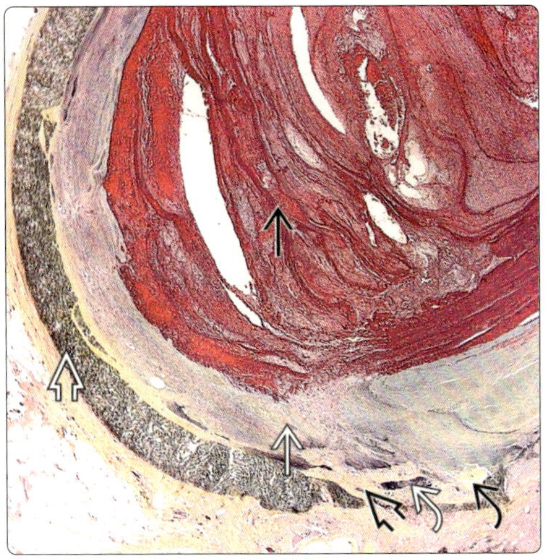

Histologic Changes in Synthetic PTFE Graft

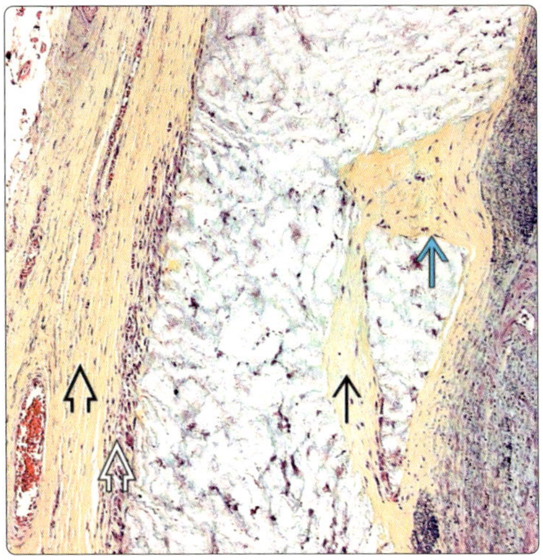

(Left) *Movat-stained section of a synthetic PTFE graft* ➡ *shows neointimal proliferation* ➡ *and large thrombus occluding the lumen* ➡*. The needle puncture tract is seen* ➡*, along with disrupted graft* ➡ *and pseudoaneurysm* ➡*.* **(Right)** *Movat-stained section of a synthetic PTFE graft at higher magnification shows perigraft fibrosis* ➡*, scant mononuclear cells* ➡*, puncture wounds* ➡*, and graft disruption* ➡ *secondary to puncture.*

Histologic Changes in Synthetic PTFE Graft

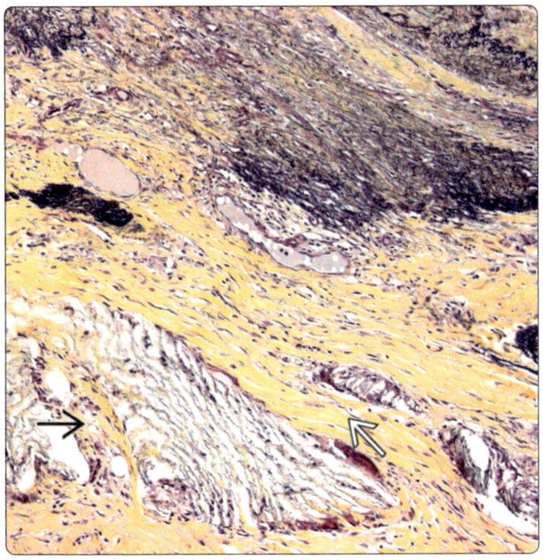

Histologic Changes in Synthetic PTFE Graft

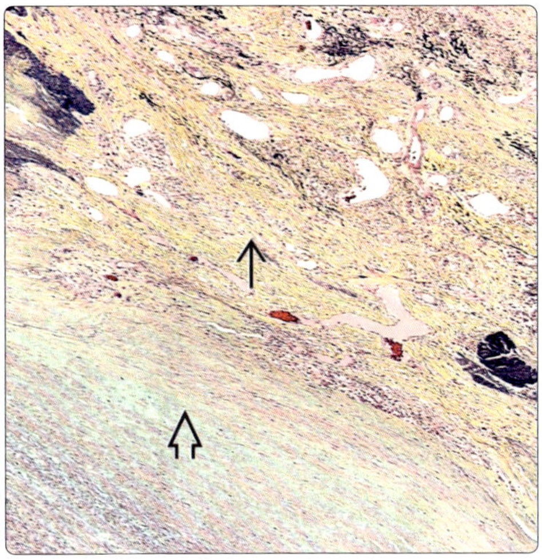

(Left) *Movat-stained section of a synthetic PTFE graft at low magnification shows puncture tracts* ➡ *leading to graft disruption* ➡*.* **(Right)** *Movat-stained section of a synthetic PTFE graft at higher magnification shows pseudoaneurysm* ➡*, which is contained by the surrounding tissue and devoid of arterial layers. Neointimal proliferation* ➡ *can also be appreciated.*

Histologic Changes in Synthetic PTFE Graft With Associated Infection

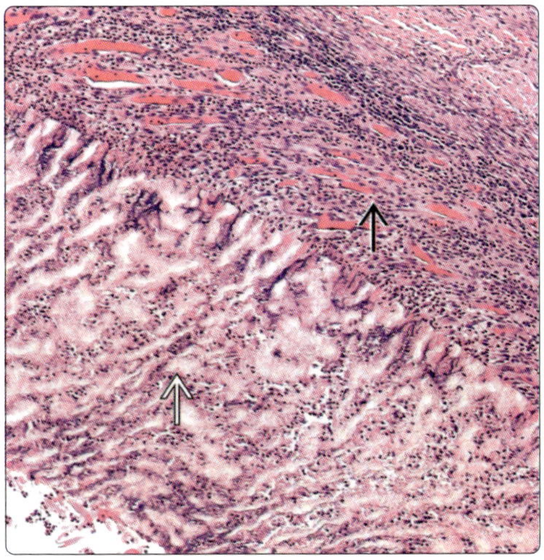

Degenerative Changes in Venous Graft

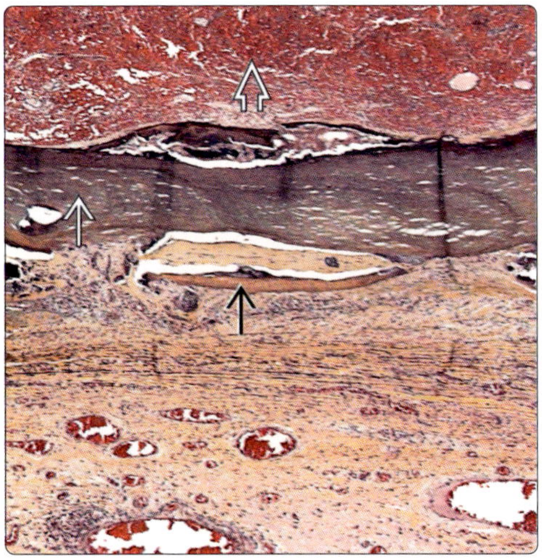

(Left) *H&E stain of a synthetic PTFE graft shows an infected graft* ➡ *with acute and chronic inflammatory cells surrounding* ➡ *and within the graft. Infection is one of the complications that can affect vascular grafts and may require removal.* **(Right)** *Movat-stained section of a venous graft shows calcification* ➡*, foci of bone formation* ➡*, and thrombus* ➡ *inside the vascular lumen.*

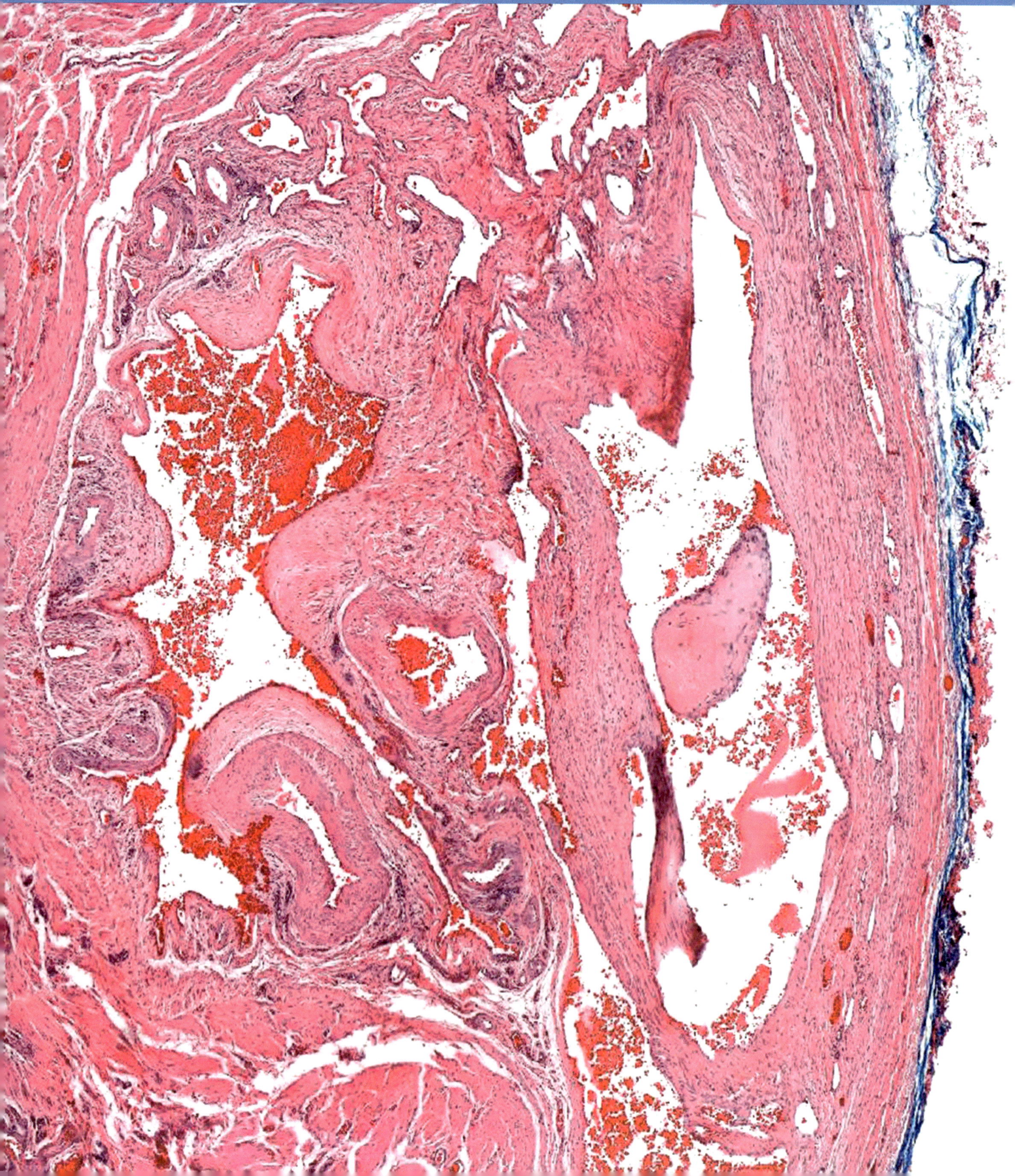

SECTION 8

Vascular Tumors

Benign

Malignant

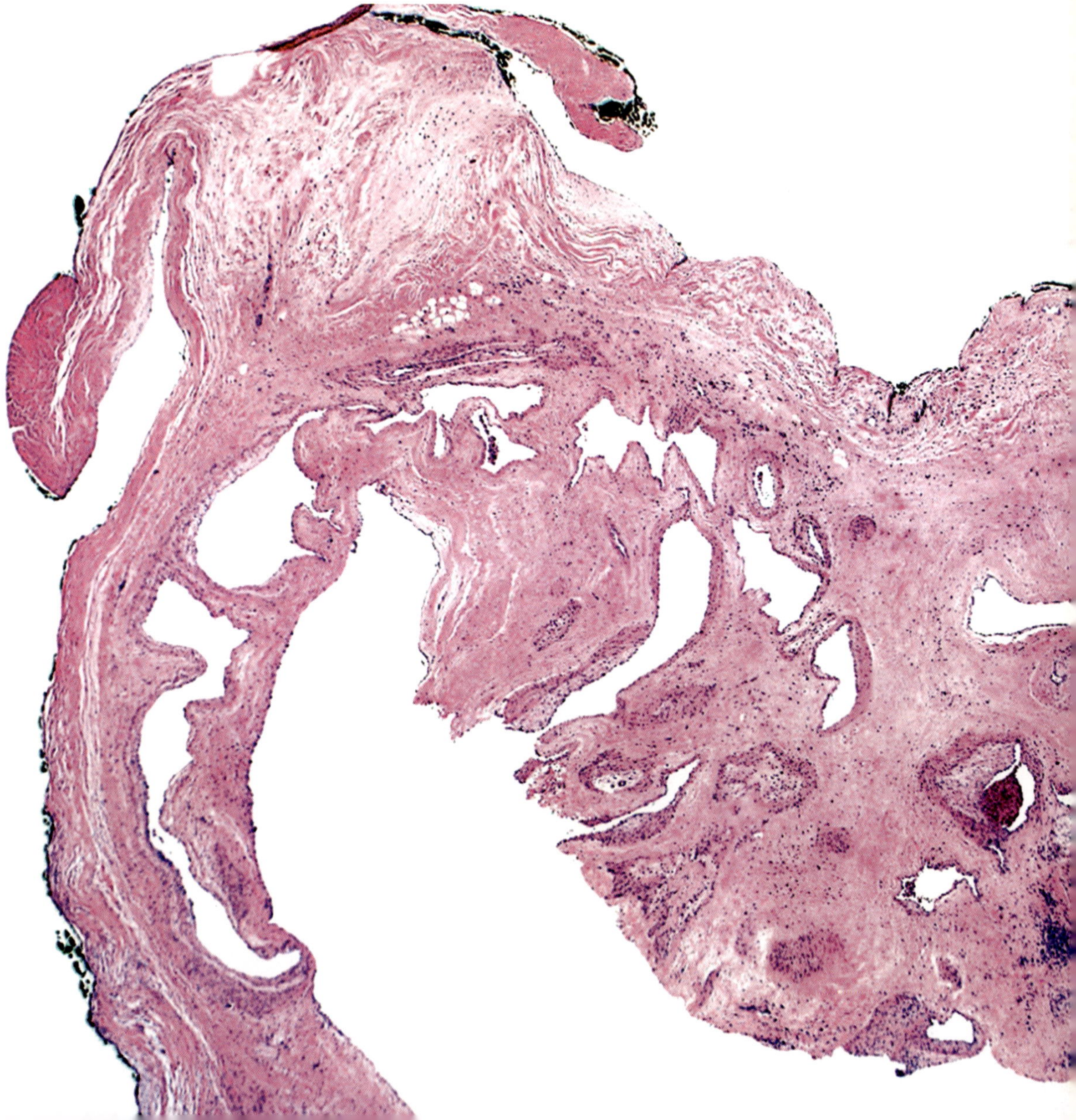

Hemangioma

KEY FACTS

TERMINOLOGY

- Benign, mass-like proliferation of blood vessels

ETIOLOGY/PATHOGENESIS

- Most are congenital; etiology is unknown

CLINICAL ISSUES

- Juvenile hemangiomas present in infancy
  - More common in female patients
  - Spontaneous regression occurs
- Other hemangiomas present at any age
  - Occur in skin, deep tissues, or viscera
  - Spontaneous regression does not occur
- Most are uncomplicated, requiring no treatment
- Essentially no malignant potential
- Surgery or medical therapy is reserved for clinically significant lesions involving vital structures
- High-output cardiac failure complicates large lesions

MACROSCOPIC

- Well-circumscribed, dark red nodule or mass
- Size widely variable

MICROSCOPIC

- Well-circumscribed proliferation of vessels
- Usually symmetric & multilobular
- No atypia or significant mitotic activity
- Pseudoinvasion is common in intramuscular hemangioma
- Surrounding chronic lymphocytic infiltrate may be prominent, often with abundant eosinophils in epithelioid hemangioma

ANCILLARY TESTS

- Elastic stains enable recognition of venous lesions
- GLUT1(+) in juvenile hemangiomas; expression indicates potential for regression
- CD31, CD34, FVIIIRAg, FLI1 (+)

(Left) *In this cavernous hemangioma, numerous thin-walled vascular spaces fill the superficial dermis. These vessels are lined by bland endothelial cells and are dilated and markedly congested.* **(Right)** *Capillary hemangiomas are composed of densely packed capillaries that may be only partially canalized. This example arose in the heart and shows mixed epithelioid and spindle cell features.*

Cutaneous Cavernous Hemangioma

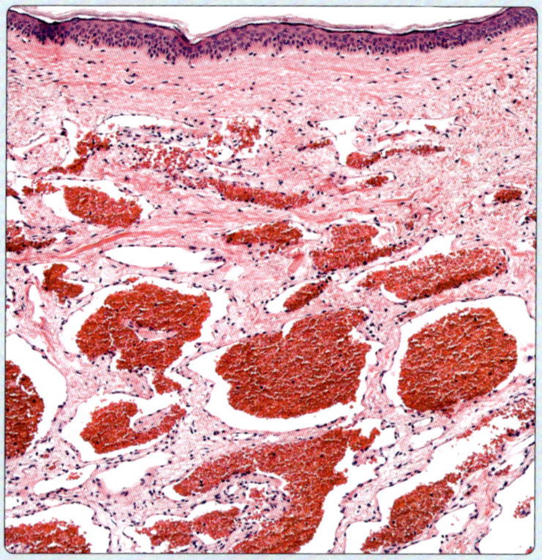

Capillary Hemangioma

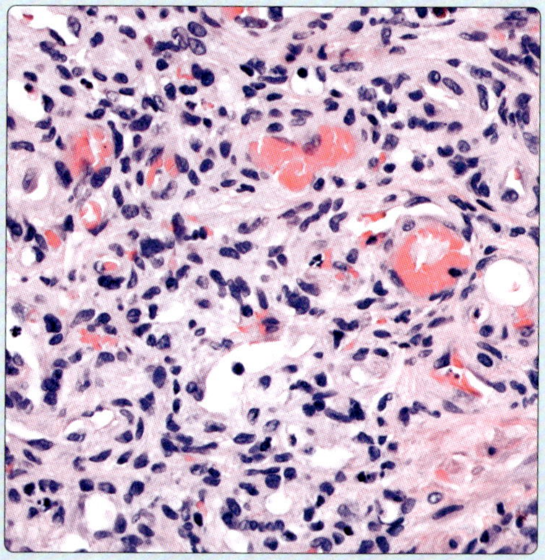

(Left) *This low-magnification photomicrograph shows a cavernous-type hemangioma of the heart with abnormally large and thick-walled irregular vascular spaces ➔.* **(Right)** *This higher magnification photomicrograph shows the irregular vascular channels ➔ permeating through the myocardium ⇨. Some of the channels appear thrombosed ⇨.*

Cardiac Hemangioma

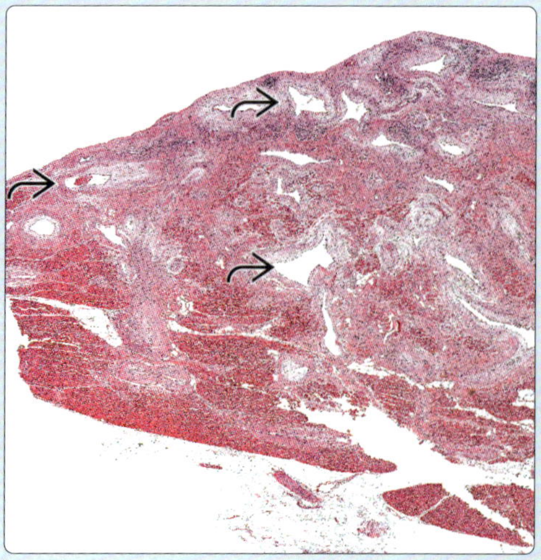

Cardiac Hemangioma

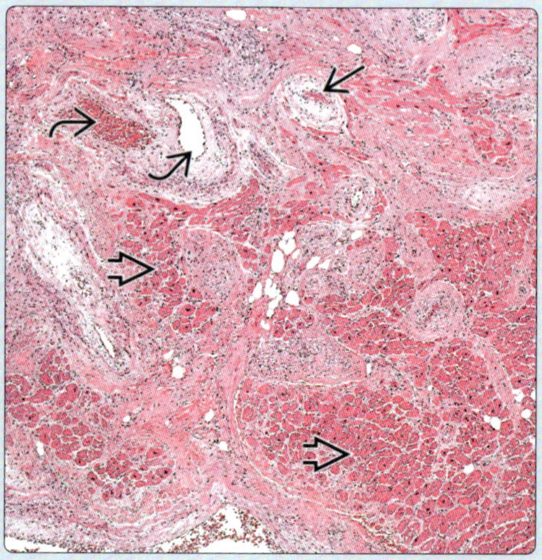

TERMINOLOGY

Synonyms

- Capillary hemangioma
  - Juvenile hemangioma: Infantile hemangioma, infantile hemangioendothelioma, strawberry nevus, cellular hemangioma of infancy
  - Lobular capillary hemangioma: Pyogenic granuloma, granuloma gravidarum (in pregnancy)
  - Other variants: Tufted hemangioma, verrucous hemangioma
- Cavernous hemangioma
  - Variants: Sinusoidal hemangioma, cherry angioma
- Intramuscular hemangioma: Skeletal muscle hemangioma
- Spindle cell hemangioma: Spindle cell hemangioendothelioma
- Epithelioid hemangioma: Angiolymphoid hyperplasia with eosinophilia, histiocytoid hemangioma, inflammatory angiomatous nodule

Definitions

- Benign, mass-like proliferation of blood vessels

ETIOLOGY/PATHOGENESIS

Developmental Anomaly

- Most are congenital
- Etiology is unknown: Some lesions may be hamartomatous; others are probably neoplastic

CLINICAL ISSUES

Presentation

- Capillary hemangioma
  - Juvenile hemangioma
    - Present at birth or arises in neonatal period
    - Slightly more common in female patients
    - Dark red macule, papule, plaque, or large tumor
    - Often involves head or neck
    - Size varies from small to very large & disfiguring
    - Enlarges quickly
    - Spontaneous regression over months to years
  - Lobular capillary hemangioma
    - Occurs at all ages; no sex predilection
    - Usually solitary, dark red nodule
    - Involves skin or mucosal membranes (especially of head, neck, or fingers)
    - Usually < 2 cm; grows rapidly
    - Spontaneous regression does not occur
    - Often ulcerates & bleeds
- Cavernous hemangioma
  - Occurs at all ages; no sex predilection
  - Less well circumscribed than capillary hemangiomas
  - Occurs in skin, deep tissue sites, or visceral organs
  - Spontaneous regression does not occur
- Intramuscular hemangioma
  - Usually in young adults; no sex predilection
  - Less well circumscribed than capillary hemangiomas
  - Most common in large leg muscles
  - Painful, especially after exercise
  - Spontaneous regression does not occur
  - Recurrence is common due to incomplete excision
- Spindle cell hemangioma
  - Occurs at all ages; more common in male patients
  - Usually in skin of distal extremities, especially hands
  - Spontaneous regression usually does not occur
- Epithelioid hemangioma
  - Usually middle-aged adults; no sex predilection
  - Usually in head & neck area, especially near ear
  - Spontaneous regression usually does not occur
  - Recurrence occurs in nearly 1/3 of cases
- Cardiac hemangioma
  - Usually cavernous morphology, often associated with Kasabach-Merritt syndrome

Treatment

- Nonintervention
  - Most are uncomplicated, requiring no treatment
- Surgical intervention
  - Reserved for clinically significant lesions involving vital structures
  - Options include laser surgery & excision
- Pharmacologic intervention
  - Reserved for clinically significant lesions involving vital structures

Prognosis

- Generally excellent, especially with small lesions
- Entirely benign; malignant transformation essentially never occurs
- Large lesions may be complicated by high-output cardiac failure

Syndromic Associations

- Maffucci syndrome
  - Multiple enchondromas, spindle cell hemangiomas, lymphangiomas
  - Usually evident in childhood
  - Pathologic fractures may occur, but lifespan is normal
- Kasabach-Merritt syndrome
  - Consumptive coagulopathy, thrombocytopenia, & hemorrhage; associated with hemangioma(s)
  - Typically presents in infancy or childhood
  - May lead to life-threatening hemorrhage
- Blue rubber bleb nevus syndrome
  - Multiple hemangiomas of skin & GI tract
  - Typically presents in childhood or early adulthood
  - May cause GI hemorrhage & anemia
- PHACE syndrome
  - **P**osterior fossa brain malformations (e.g., Dandy-Walker), **h**emangiomas (often large), **a**rterial lesions (especially involving large muscular arteries of head/neck), **c**ardiac anomalies, **e**ye abnormalities
- PELVIS syndrome
  - **P**erineal hemangioma, **e**xternal genital malformations (e.g., hypospadias), **l**ipomyelomeningocele, **v**esicorenal abnormalities, **i**mperforate anus, **s**kin tags

IMAGING

MR Findings

- T1: Intermediate intensity with flow voids
- T2: High intensity with flow voids

CT Findings

- Rapid enhancement following contrast infusion

MACROSCOPIC

General Features

- Well-circumscribed, dark red nodule or mass
- Size widely variable

MICROSCOPIC

Histologic Features

- Capillary hemangioma
  - Well-circumscribed proliferation of closely packed capillaries
  - Usually symmetric & multilobular
  - Capillaries may be only partially canalized
  - Atypia, multilayering, ↑ mitotic activity absent
- Cavernous hemangioma
  - Proliferation of dilated, thin-walled vascular spaces
  - Less circumscribed than capillary hemangiomas; invasive behavior absent
  - Atypia, multilayering, ↑ mitotic activity absent
  - Sinusoidal variant: Delicate, back-to-back, thin-walled, anastomosing vessels with minimal intervening stroma
- Intramuscular hemangioma
  - Well-formed vessels of variable thickness
  - Pseudoinvasion between individual myocytes
  - Stroma is often fibrous or myxoid
  - Adipocytic component is often present
  - Atypia & significant mitotic activity are absent
- Spindle cell hemangioma
  - Irregular, cavernous, thin-walled vessels surrounded by solid areas of spindled cells (noncanalized capillaries)
  - Vacuolated endothelial cells may be present
  - Atypia & significant mitotic activity are absent
- Epithelioid hemangioma
  - Relatively well-circumscribed, lobular proliferation of closely packed capillaries
  - Capillaries lined by plump, epithelioid endothelial cells
  - Surrounding chronic lymphocytic infiltrate may be prominent, often with abundant eosinophils
  - Atypia & significant mitotic activity are absent

ANCILLARY TESTS

Histochemistry

- van Gieson stain
  - Highlights single elastic lamina of venous lesions

Immunohistochemistry

- GLUT1
  - Expressed exclusively in juvenile hemangiomas
  - Aids in pediatric cases to distinguish from other vascular malformations
  - Expression indicates potential for regression
- CD34(+) in nearly all cases
  - Less specific; also expressed in other mesenchymal neoplasms
- CD31(+) in nearly all cases
  - Most specific endothelial marker
- FVIIIRAg(+) in nearly all cases
- FLI1(+) in nearly all cases

DIFFERENTIAL DIAGNOSIS

Arteriovenous Malformation

- Mixture of arterial & venous channels
- Elastic stains help to demonstrate arterial component (has internal & external elastic laminae)
- Often associated with significant shunt

Angiosarcoma

- Infiltrative pattern at low power
- Cytologic atypia is usually present
- Mitotic activity is greater, often with atypical mitoses

Kaposi Sarcoma

- Infiltrative pattern at low power; HHV8 IHC is positive

Angiolipoma

- Usually painful; prominent adipocytic component is present

Intravascular Papillary Endothelial Hyperplasia (Masson Lesion)

- Exuberant reactive proliferation in setting of organizing thrombus with recanalization
- Usually intravascular but may be seen in organizing hematomas
- Residual organizing thrombus is often present
- Abundant papillary formations of plump endothelial cells with hyalinized stalk

Hemangiomatosis

- Multifocal or diffuse hemangiomatous proliferations
- Usually mixture of capillaries, veins, cavernous spaces
- May involve skin, deep soft tissues, bones, &/or viscera
- Resection may be impossible; recurrence in most cases

Lymphangioma

- Distinction from cavernous hemangioma may be impossible
- Usually positive for D2-40 & CD31; CD34 often negative

DIAGNOSTIC CHECKLIST

Clinically Relevant Pathologic Features

- GLUT1 expression indicates potential for regression

Pathologic Interpretation Pearls

- Circumscription at low power favors benignity, particularly in spindled or epithelioid lesions

SELECTED REFERENCES

1. Kamata K et al: Exophytic cavernous hemangioma arising from the right ventricle: report of a rare case. Pathol Int. 71(4):267-71, 2021
2. Burke A et al: Tumors of the Heart and Great Vessels. American Registry of Pathology, 2015
3. Travis WD et al: WHO Classification of Tumours of the Lung, Pleura, Thymus and Heart. IARC, 2015
4. Bruder E et al: Vascular and perivascular lesions of skin and soft tissues in children and adolescents. Pediatr Dev Pathol. 15(1 Suppl):26-61, 2012
5. Ordóñez NG: Immunohistochemical endothelial markers: a review. Adv Anat Pathol. 19(5):281-95, 2012

Lobular Capillary Hemangioma

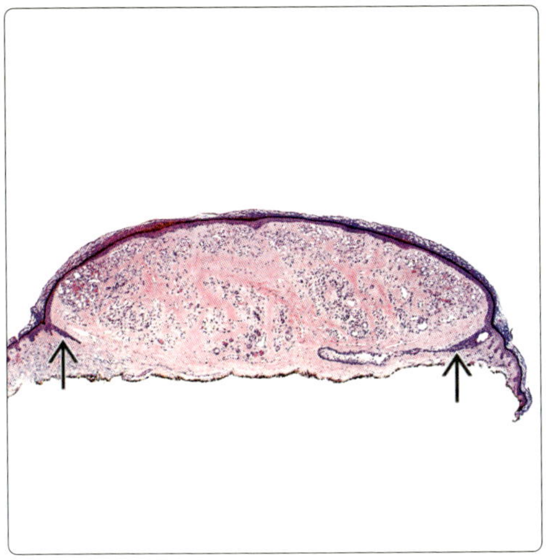

Capillaries in Lobular Capillary Hemangioma

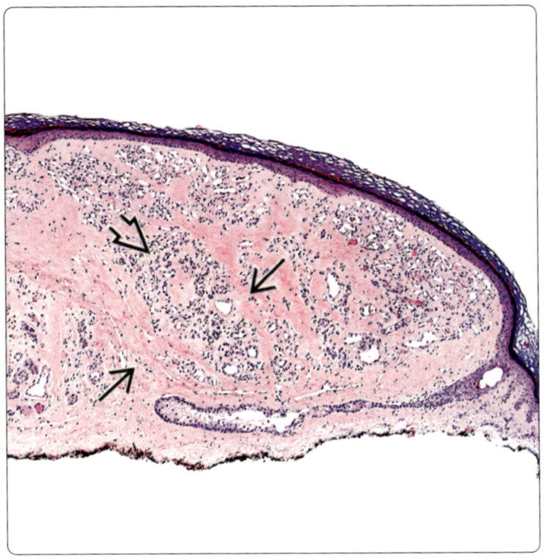

(Left) *At scanning magnification, a lobular capillary hemangioma is well circumscribed and is often relatively symmetric. Even at this magnification, the multilobular architecture is apparent. The lesion may sometimes be rimmed by an epithelial collarette →.* **(Right)** *At medium magnification, the lobular organization ➡ of the capillary channels is readily apparent. In this example, the lobules are surrounded by hypocellular and somewhat hyalinized collagenous stroma ⇨.*

Bland Endothelium in Hemangioma

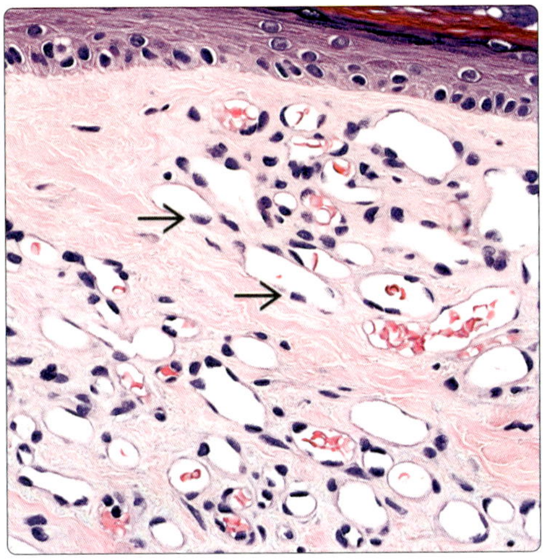

Capillary Hemangioma

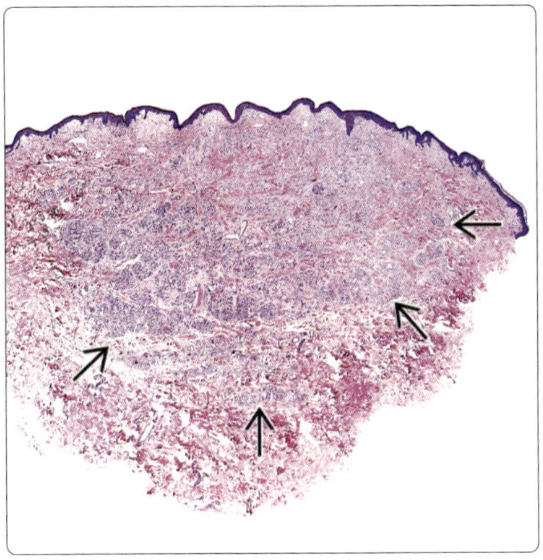

(Left) *At high power, the bland endothelial cell lining → of the densely packed capillary channels can be appreciated. Cellular atypia, multilayering, and mitotic activity are not seen in this lobular capillary hemangioma.* **(Right)** *In this capillary hemangioma, an epithelial collarette is not present, but the circumscription and symmetry of the lesion → are readily apparent at scanning magnification.*

Capillary Hemangioma

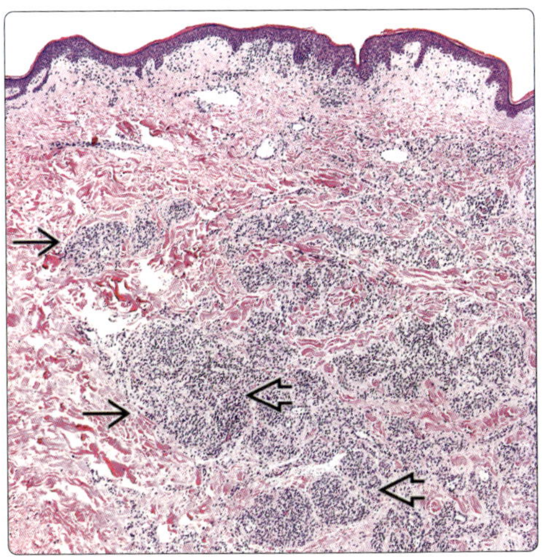

Feeder Vessel in Capillary Hemangioma

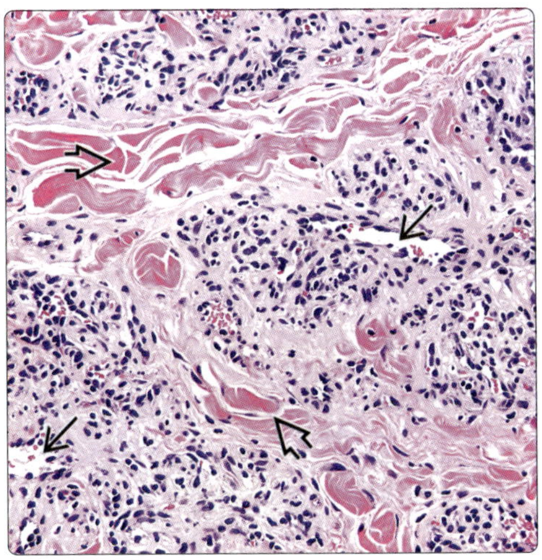

(Left) *At medium power, this capillary hemangioma shows lobules ⇨ of densely packed and largely uncanalized capillaries in the superficial dermis. The border → of the lesion is readily identifiable.* **(Right)** *At high power, this capillary hemangioma shows dense bands of fibrous tissue ⇨ that separate the lobules of slit-like and only partially canalized capillaries. Note the presence of a slightly larger "feeder vessel" → in the center of each well-organized lobule.*

(Left) *In this example of a cherry angioma from the trunk of an older adult patient, a well-circumscribed, symmetric proliferation of dilated and congested vascular channels is seen in the superficial dermis. The lobular architecture is easily identified. Note the surrounding epithelial collarette* ➙*, which is a typical feature of this lesion.* **(Right)** *At higher power, the bland, flat endothelial cell lining* ➙ *of the thin-walled vascular channels can be appreciated in this cherry angioma.*

Cherry Angioma

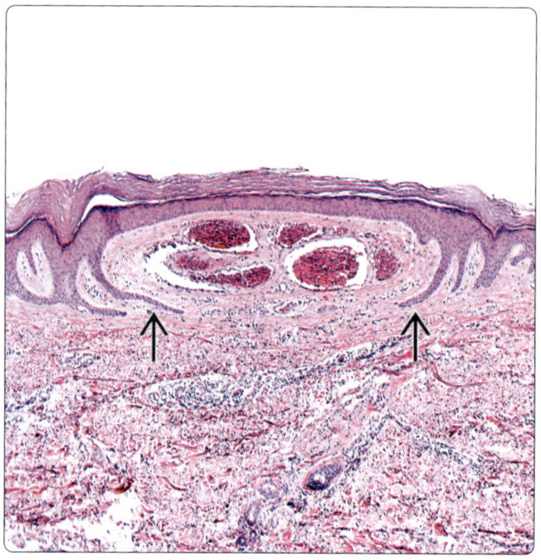

Cherry Angioma

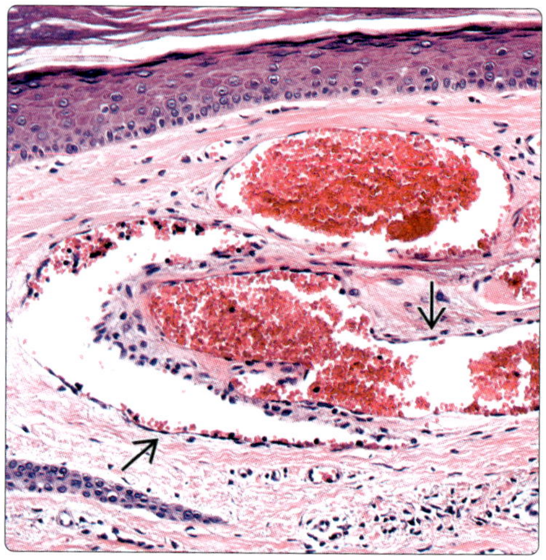

(Left) *Like other hemangiomas, the cavernous hemangioma displays a characteristic relatively well-circumscribed border* ➙ *that is easily appreciated at scanning magnification. Abundant congested vascular channels* ⇨ *fill the superficial dermis.* **(Right)** *At higher power, dilated and markedly congested, thin-walled vascular channels are readily appreciated in this cavernous hemangioma. These channels are lined by a single layer of flat, bland endothelial cells* ➙ *without atypia or significant mitotic activity.*

Cavernous Hemangioma

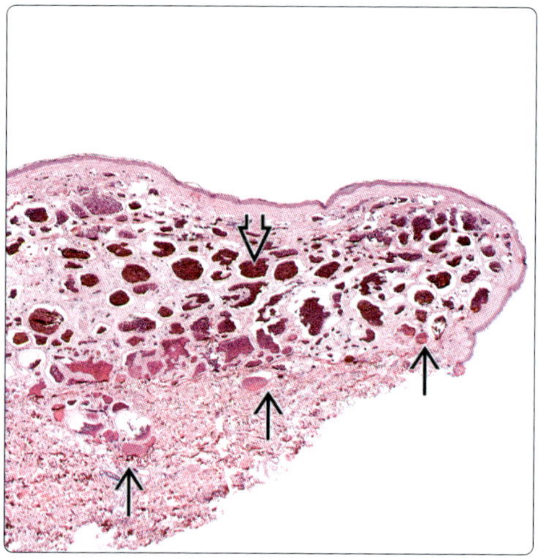

Bland Endothelium in Cavernous Hemangioma

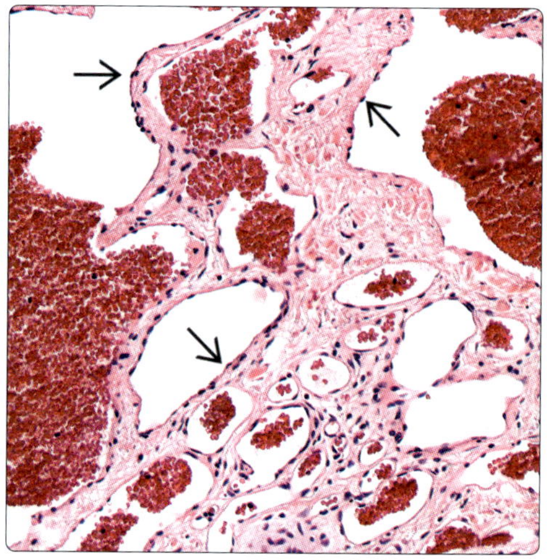

(Left) *In this example of a venous hemangioma, a well-circumscribed proliferation of vascular spaces is seen in the superficial dermis. The symmetry and lobular architecture of the lesion* ➙ *are readily appreciated at low power.* **(Right)** *At higher power, this venous hemangioma demonstrates a bland endothelial cell lining* ➙ *and surrounding vascular smooth muscle cells* ↪*. Atypia is not present.*

Venous Hemangioma

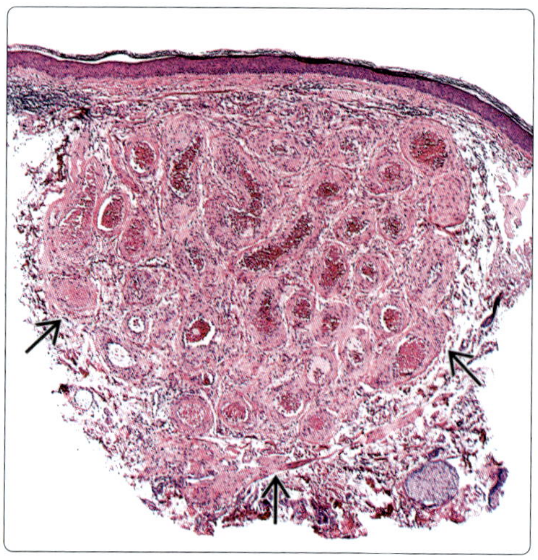

Bland Endothelium in Venous Hemangioma

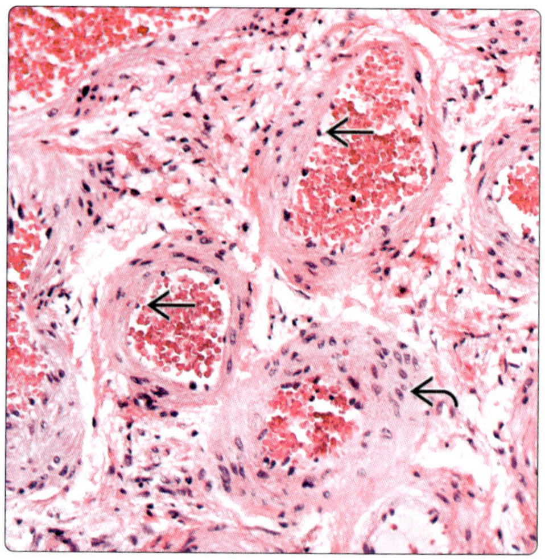

Intramuscular Hemangioma

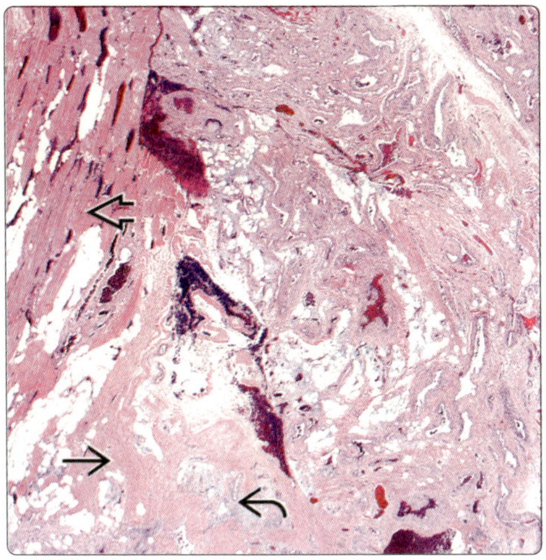

Intramuscular Hemangioma

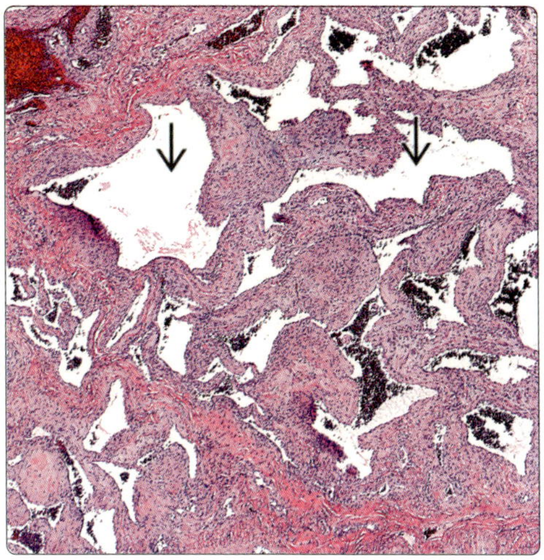

(Left) *At scanning magnification, abundant, variably sized vascular channels are present within the belly of a large skeletal muscle from the thigh. Even at this magnification, the heterogeneous nature of this proliferation is apparent with large, gaping vessels and smaller, slit-like vessels embedded in a fibrous and focally myxoid stroma.* **(Right)** *Large, thick-walled, anastomosing vascular channels are present in some areas of an intramuscular hemangioma.*

Angiolipoma of Muscle

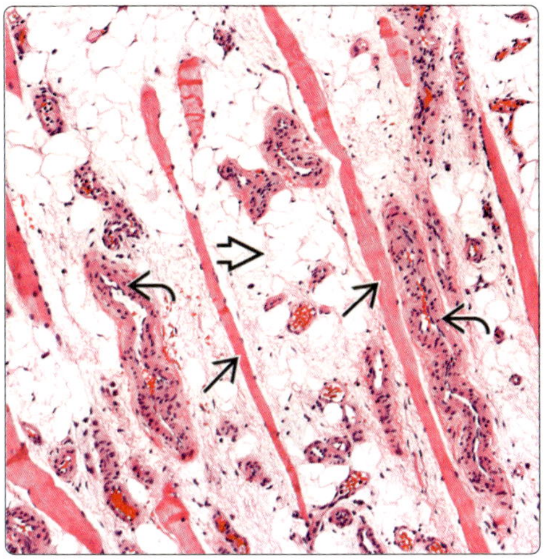

Intramuscular Angioma With Adipose Tissue

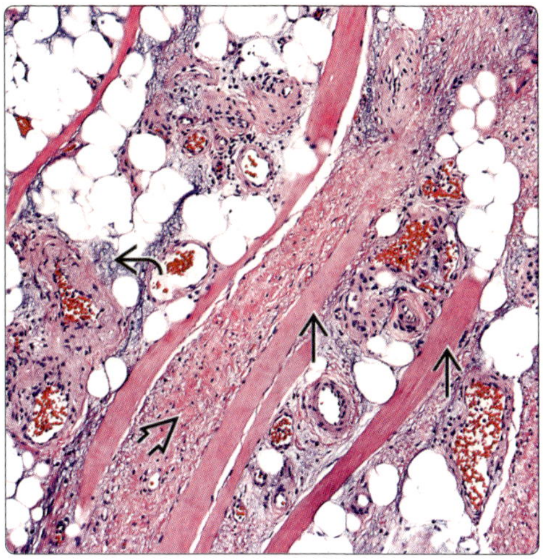

(Left) *In some areas, well-formed vessels dissect between individual myocytes. This should not be misinterpreted as invasive malignant behavior. Note the prominent adipocytic component, a feature often seen. In the past, these lesions were sometimes classified as angiolipomas of muscle.* **(Right)** *In other areas of an intramuscular hemangioma, a myxoid or fibrous stroma may be seen. Again, the presence of vessels between individual myocytes should not be misinterpreted as invasion.*

Organizing Thrombi in Hemangioma

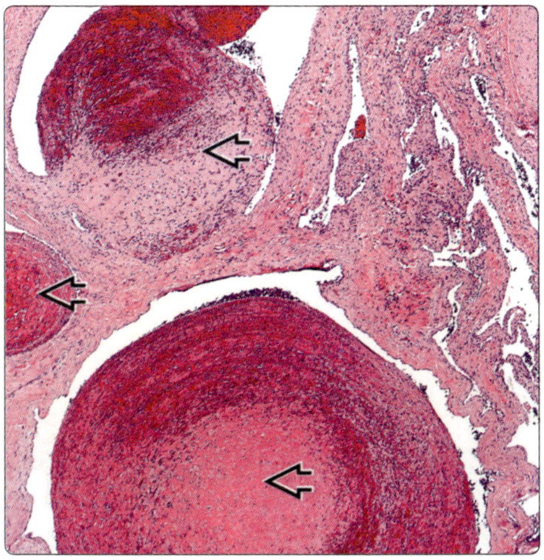

Old Organized Thrombi in Hemangioma

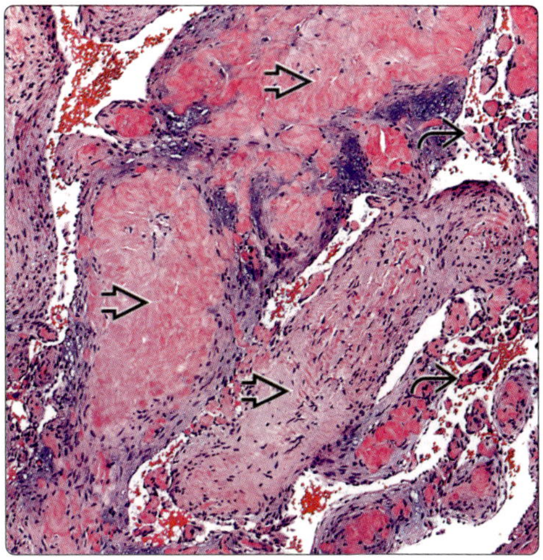

(Left) *Organizing thrombi are commonly present in the vascular spaces of hemangiomas, particularly in larger, cavernous channels.* **(Right)** *Older, organized, and hyalinized thrombi may also be seen in hemangiomas, including intramuscular hemangiomas, as in this case. Note the presence of focal intravascular papillary endothelial hyperplasia, a feature commonly seen in association with organizing or organized thrombi.*

(Left) *Although hemangiomas are relatively uncommon in the viscera, occasional cases may involve the heart. In this case, a cavernous hemangioma* ⇨ *involves the ventricular surface of a mitral valve leaflet.* (Right) *At low power, a Verhoeff-van Gieson elastic stain highlights the relative preservation of the underlying leaflet architecture* ⇨. *Although entirely benign, this lesion can have profound clinical consequences due to impaired valvular function.*

Mitral Valve Hemangioma

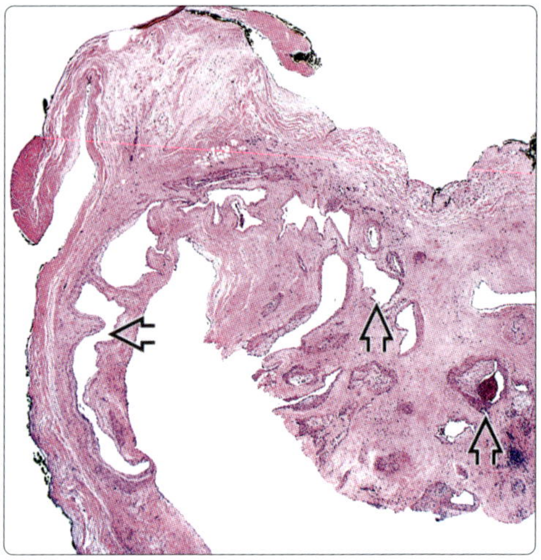

Mitral Valve Hemangioma (Elastic Stain)

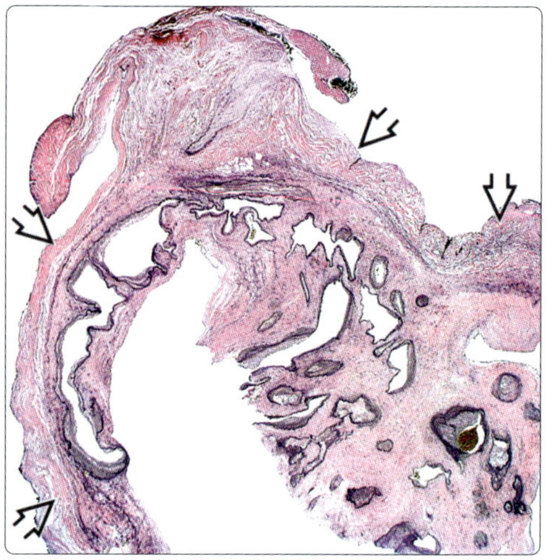

(Left) *On medium power, well-formed vascular channels can be seen. These channels are embedded within a fibrotic stroma* → *that probably represents native valve tissue.* (Right) *A Verhoeff-van Gieson elastic stain enhances recognition of vascular channels with a markedly irregular luminal profile* ↪ *and also accentuates the marked variation in wall thickness of other channels* →. *These irregularities would not be expected in typical postinflammatory valvular neovascularization.*

Mitral Valve Hemangioma

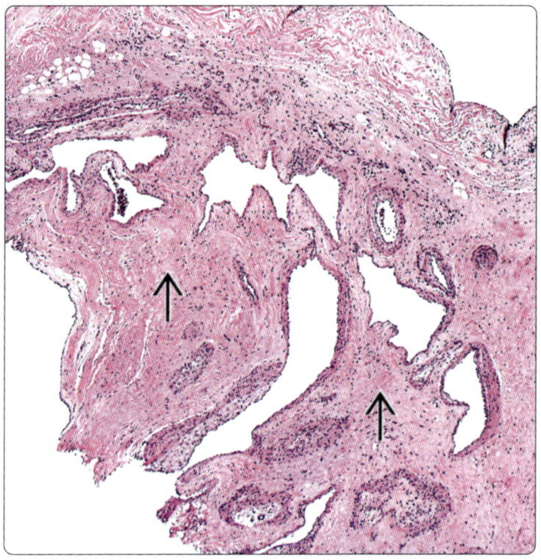

Mitral Valve Hemangioma (Elastic Stain)

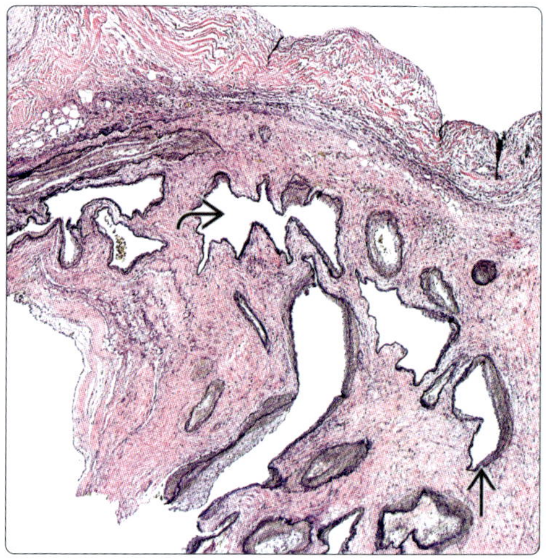

(Left) *At high power, the single layer of bland, flat endothelial cells* → *can be seen lining the vascular spaces. Atypia is not present. A variably thickened smooth muscle cell layer* ↪ *surrounds each channel.* (Right) *At high power, a Verhoeff-van Gieson stain highlights the single external elastic lamina (black)* → *and accentuates the variability of wall thickness. Based on these characteristics, these probably represent thickened venous channels.*

Bland Endothelium in Cardiac Hemangioma

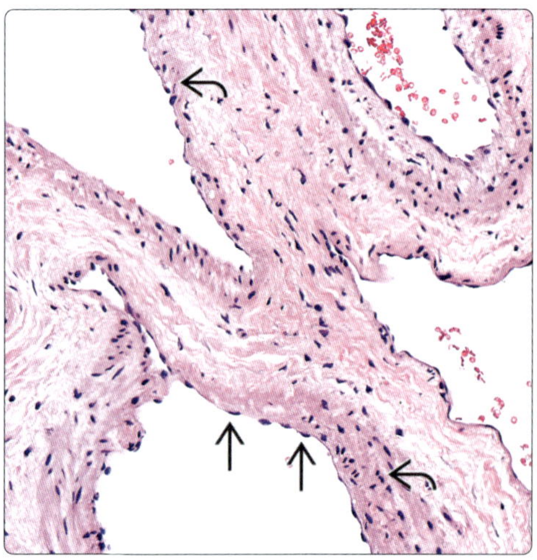

Endothelium in Cardiac Hemangioma (Elastic Stain)

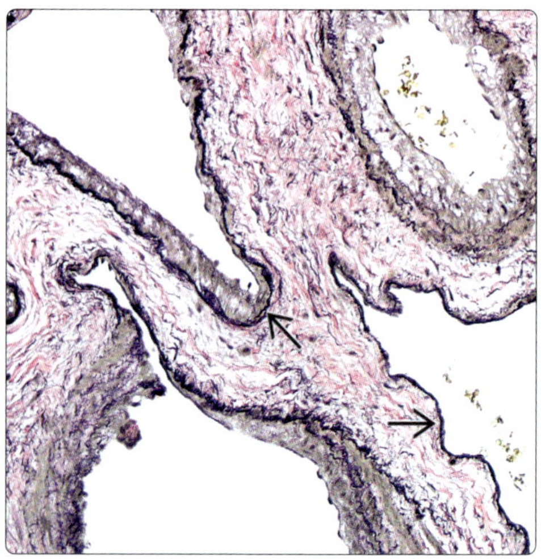

Cavernous Hemangioma

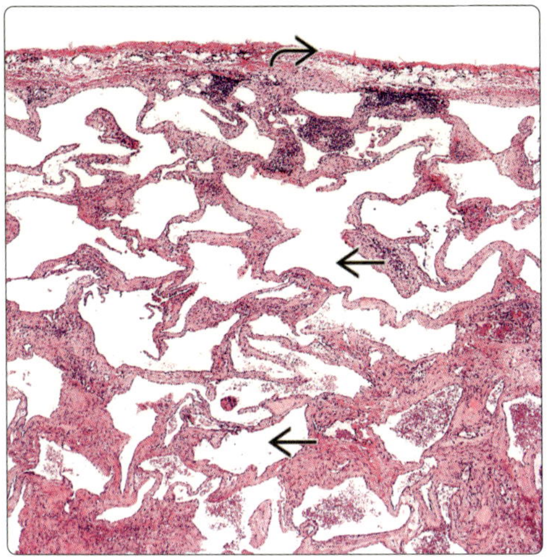

Bland Endothelium in Hemangioma

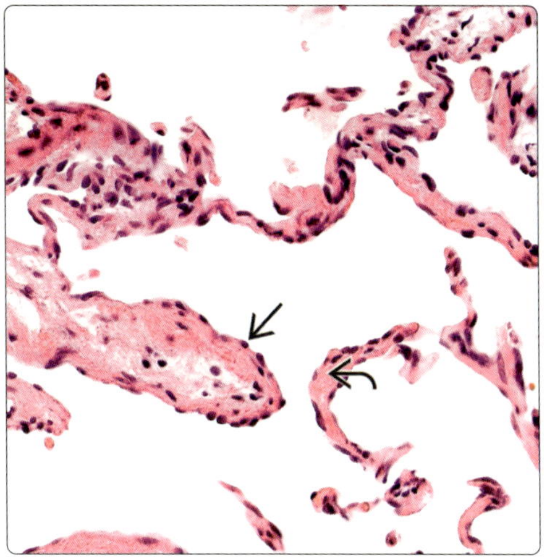

(Left) *The morphology of cardiac hemangiomas is variable. In this example of a large, cavernous cardiac hemangioma, a dense, lobular proliferation of back-to-back, thin-walled, irregular vascular channels* → *is seen. This lesion extends nearly to the epicardial surface* ↪. **(Right)** *On high power, sinusoidal architecture is focally present with back-to-back vascular spaces and little intervening stroma* ↪. *The blandness of the endothelial cell lining* → *is apparent.*

Cardiac Hemangioma

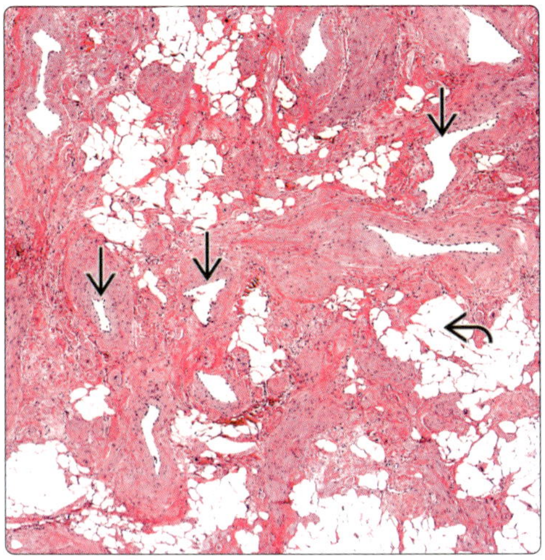

Myocyte Hypertrophy in Cardiac Hemangioma

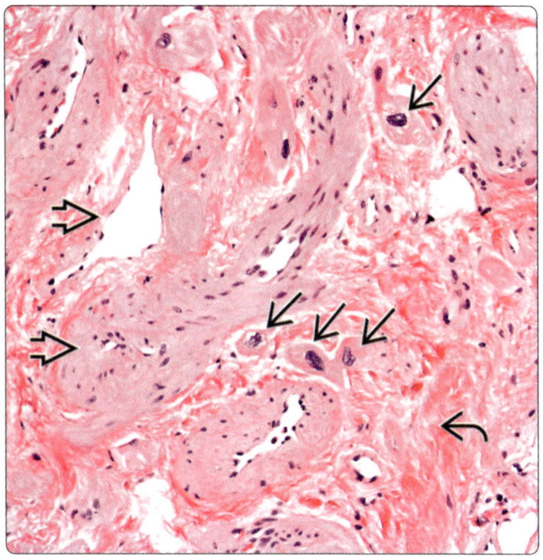

(Left) *In other cases of cardiac hemangioma, the lesion resembles hemangiomas involving skeletal muscle. Like intramuscular hemangiomas, an adipocytic component* ↪ *may be prominent between the proliferating vascular channels* →. **(Right)** *Markedly hypertrophied cardiomyocytes* → *with enlarged nuclei are entrapped among the well-formed, abnormal vascular channels within a densely fibrotic stroma* ↪. *Note the marked variation in vascular wall thickness* ⇨.

Cardiac Capillary Hemangioma

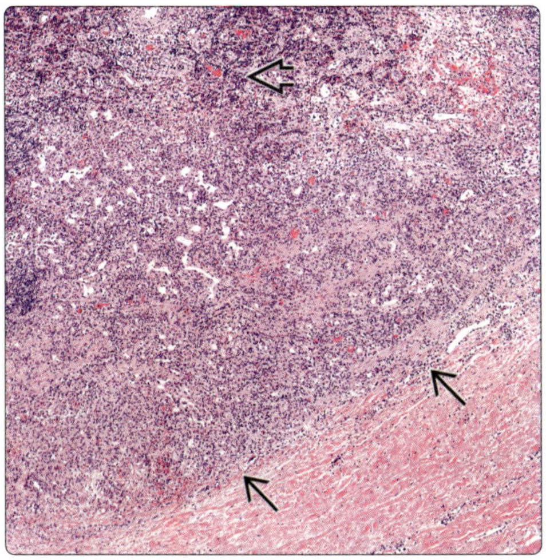

Lymphocytic Infiltrate in Epithelioid Hemangioma

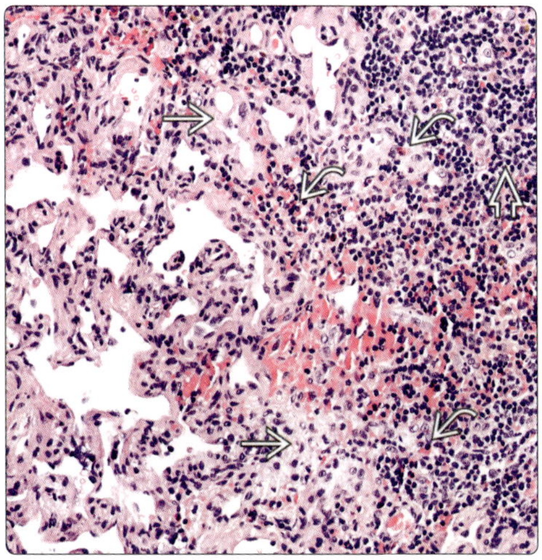

(Left) *Other cardiac hemangiomas are composed of dense capillaries. A chronic inflammatory infiltrate* ⇨ *masks this lesion's vascular nature. At low power, its circumscription* → *is readily apparent.* **(Right)** *A prominent lymphoid infiltrate is typical of epithelioid hemangiomas (a.k.a. angiolymphoid hyperplasia with eosinophilia). This cardiac hemangioma displays epithelioid features* ➡ *with a lymphocytic infiltrate* ⮕ *and scattered eosinophils* ↪.

(Left) *Although most hemangiomas involve the skin, occasionally, cases can involve deep tissues or visceral organs in virtually any location. This cavernous hemangioma involves the spleen. Note the distinct circumscription of this lesion ⇨, a feature typical of a benign vascular tumor.* **(Right)** *No atypia, multilayering, or significant mitotic activity is seen in this splenic hemangioma. On high power, bland endothelial cells → can be seen lining the thin-walled vascular channels.*

Cavernous Angioma of Spleen

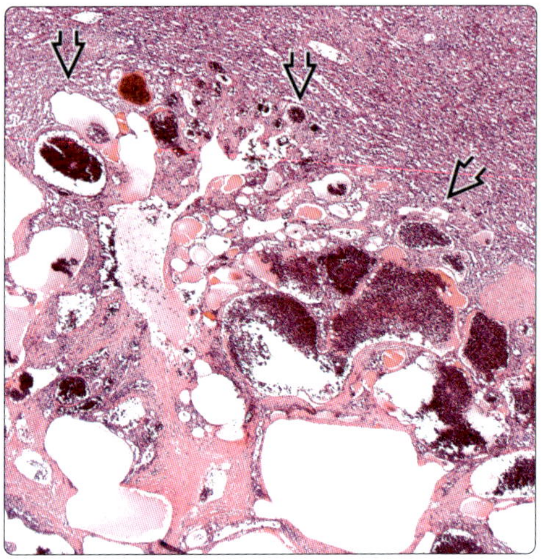

Bland Endothelium in Splenic Angioma

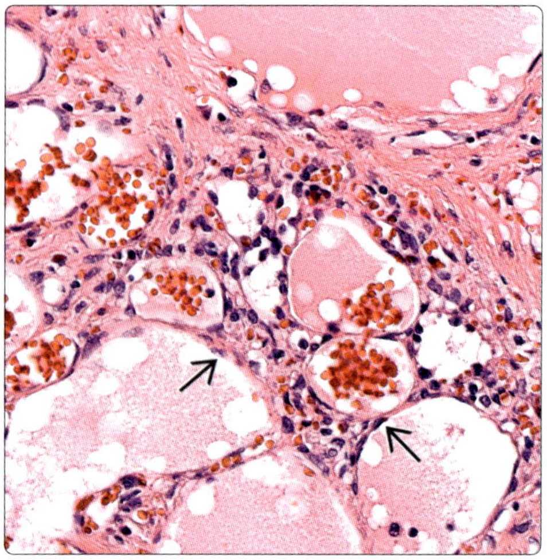

(Left) *Hemangiomas may arise within bones, most commonly in the axial skeleton, as in this cavernous hemangioma in the skull. Dilated, markedly congested vascular spaces → are present within the medullary cavity. This lesion completely replaces the marrow space but preserves the preexisting bony trabeculae ↶.* **(Right)** *Hemangiomas are occasionally found in the liver. In older adults, they may be sclerosed with few remaining vessels ↶ but remain well circumscribed ⇨.*

Hemangioma of Bone

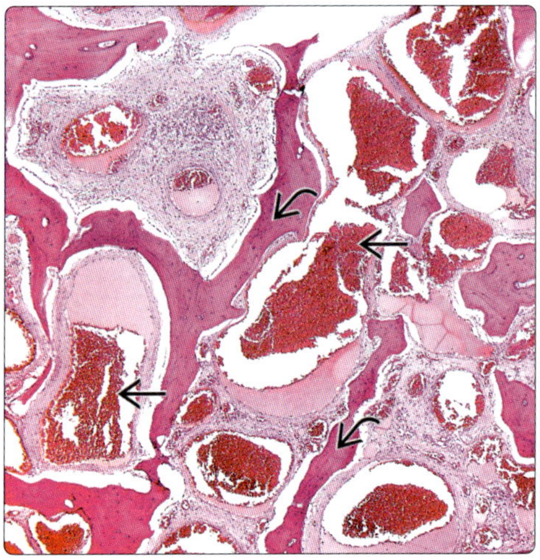

Hepatic Sclerosing Hemangioma

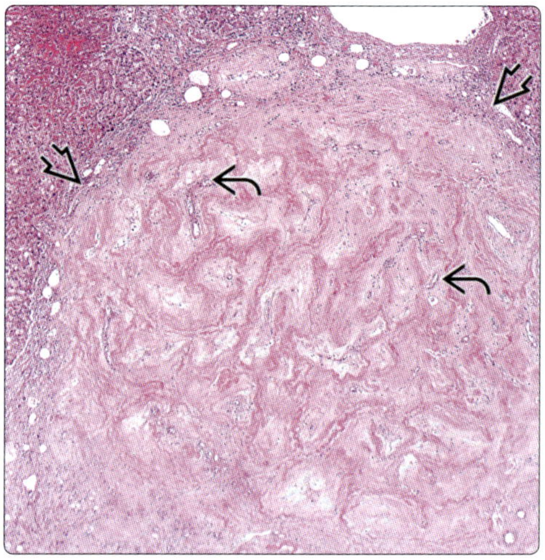

(Left) *In the liver, infantile hemangiomas are composed of dense, lobular proliferations of capillaries that are often not canalized. Bile ducts ↶ and other hepatic structures may be entrapped in these lesions, but the lesions are well circumscribed and entirely benign.* **(Right)** *At high power, extramedullary hematopoiesis ⇨ is often identified within the capillary channels of hepatic infantile hemangiomas. Note a lone megakaryocyte ↶ among numerous erythroid precursors.*

Hepatic Infantile Hemangioma

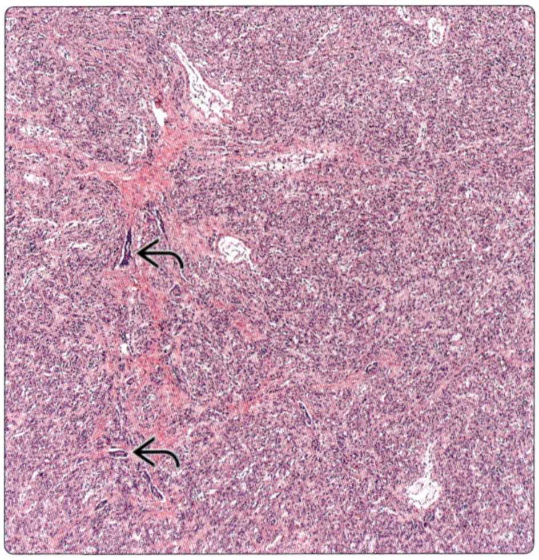

Extramedullary Hematopoiesis in Hepatic Infantile Hemangioma

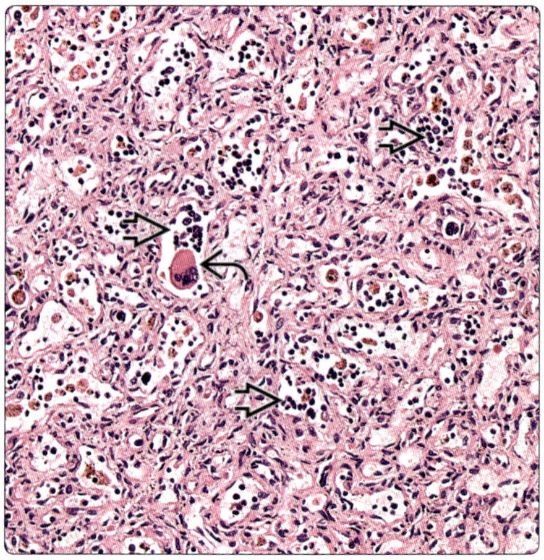

Angiolipoma

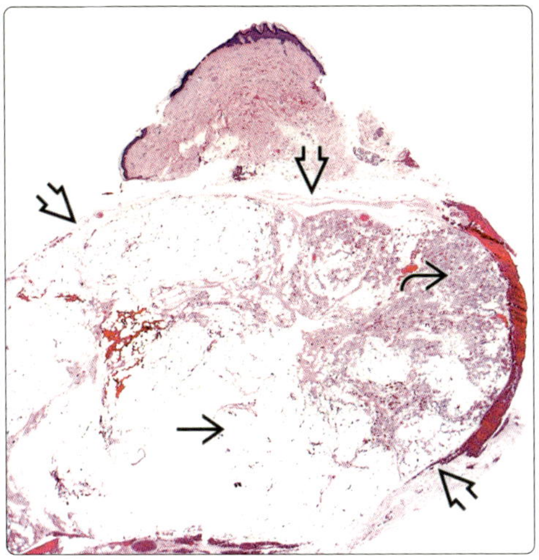

Angiolipoma

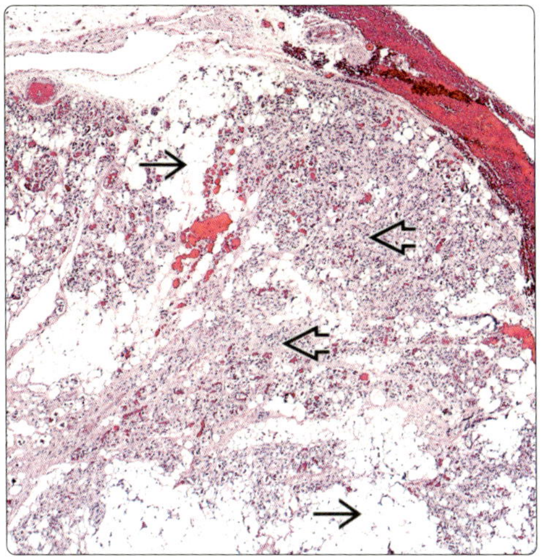

(Left) *The angiolipoma is a common lesion that may be related to hemangiomas. Typically presenting as a painful subcutaneous nodule, it is characteristically well circumscribed* → *at scanning magnification and displays a mixture of capillary* → *and adipocytic* → *components with the capillary component being more prominent at the periphery.* **(Right)** *At medium power, the capillary proliferation* → *is seen along with a prominent adipocytic component* →.

Thrombi in Angiolipoma

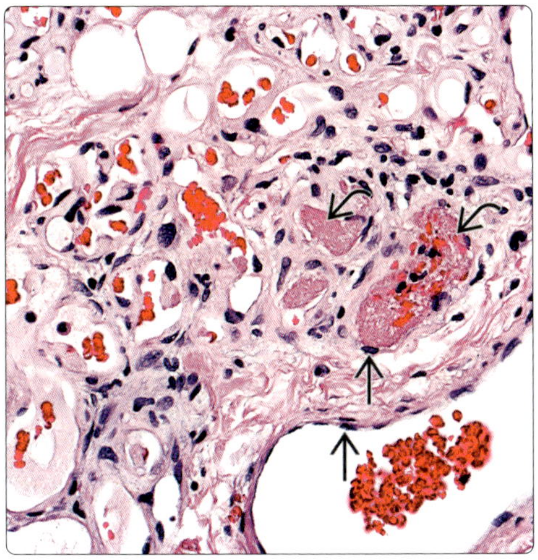

Intravascular Papillary Endothelial Hyperplasia

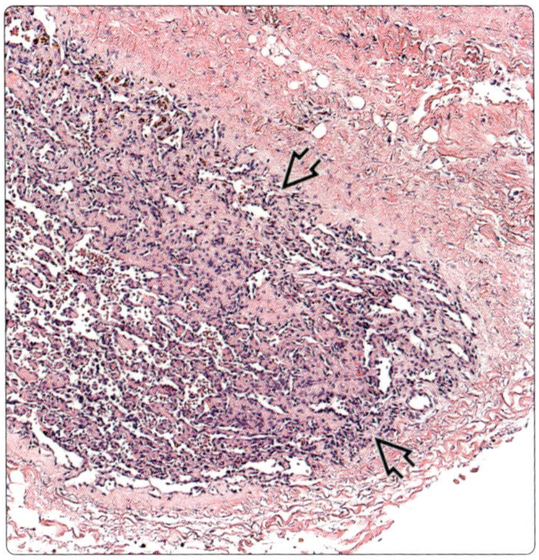

(Left) *At high power, angiolipomas often show fibrin microthrombi* → *within the lumina of capillary spaces, a supportive (but not specific) feature. The endothelial cells* → *are bland without atypia or significant mitotic activity.* **(Right)** *Intravascular papillary endothelial hyperplasia (formerly termed Masson lesion) is a reactive endothelial proliferation that is occasionally confused with hemangioma. At low power, its intravascular location is readily apparent* →.

Hemosiderin in Intravascular Papillary Endothelial Hyperplasia

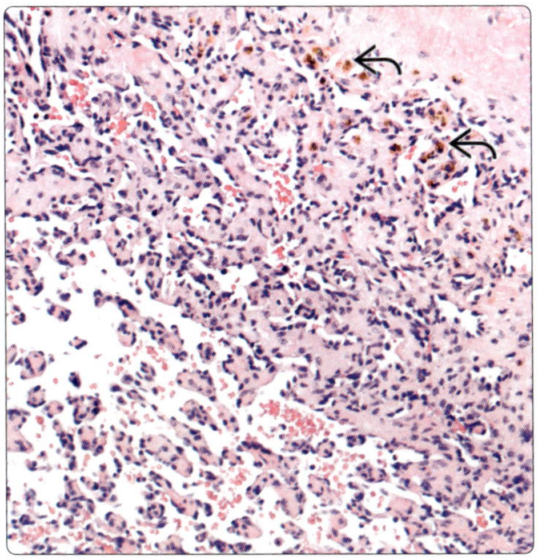

Hyalinization in Intravascular Papillary Endothelial Hyperplasia

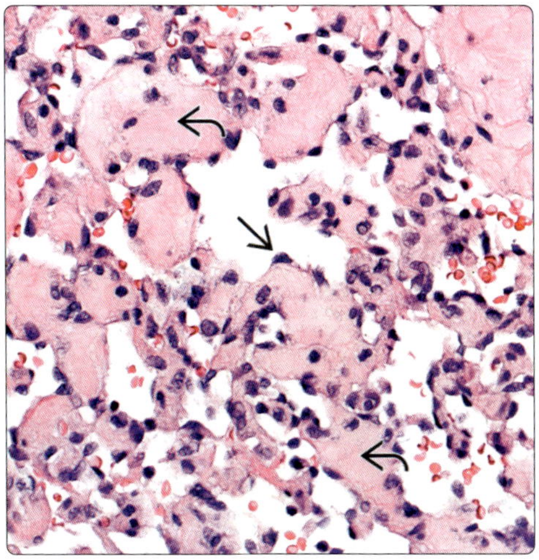

(Left) *Intravascular papillary endothelial hyperplasia represents exuberant endothelial proliferation in an organizing intravascular thrombus with vascular recanalization. Hemosiderin* → *is often found.* **(Right)** *In older lesions, the papillary cores become hyalinized* →. *Despite the architectural complexity, the endothelial cells* → *covering the papillary projections are bland, and atypia and multilayering are absent. These features distinguish this lesion from angiosarcoma.*

Angiomyolipoma

KEY FACTS

TERMINOLOGY

- Mesenchymal tumors believed to originate from perivascular epithelioid cell (PEC)
- Closely related to other PEC-type tumors (e.g., lymphangioleiomyomatosis, clear cell sugar tumors of lung, pancreas, and uterus, PEComas, and cardiac rhabdomyomas)

ETIOLOGY/PATHOGENESIS

- ~ 55-75% of patients with tuberous sclerosis develop renal angiomyolipoma (AML)
- < 50% of renal AML patients have tuberous sclerosis
- Associated with genetic alterations in tuberous sclerosis genes *TSC1* (9q34) and *TSC2* (16p13.3)

CLINICAL ISSUES

- Multifocality, bilaterality, larger size, faster growth, and younger age are more common characteristics in AML associated with tuberous sclerosis
- Overwhelming majority with benign clinical behavior

MACROSCOPIC

- Often well circumscribed but not encapsulated
- Cut surface is variable, reflecting relative proportion of fat, smooth muscle, or vessels in tumor

MICROSCOPIC

- Typically contains adipose tissue, smooth muscle, and dystrophic vessels in variable proportions
- Highly variable morphology
  - Predominantly lipomatous or leiomyomatous
  - Lymphangioleiomyomatous
  - Oncocytoma-like
  - Sclerosing type
  - AML with epithelial cysts
- Positive for melanocytic markers: HMB-45, Melan-A (MART-1), MITF

(Left) *Typical angiomyolipoma (AML) with fatty → and vascular ⇨ areas is shown. Leiomyoma-like areas may also be seen grossly. The tumor appears well circumscribed, but it is not encapsulated.* **(Right)** *Perivascular epithelioid cells (PECs) ⇨ surround a tumor vessel in this case of AML. The cells are the putative line of origin for these tumors.*

Gross Appearance

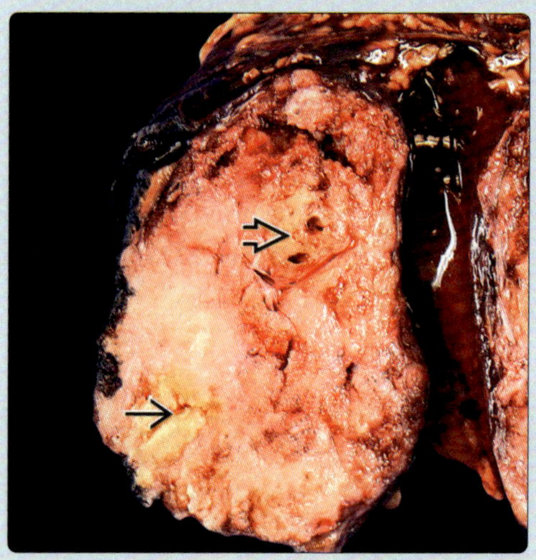

Perivascular Epithelioid Cells

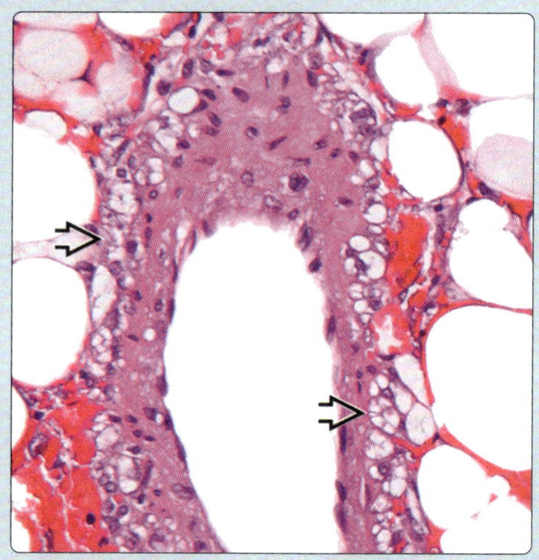

(Left) *Thin-walled vessel in a case of AML is shown. It is rimmed with a corona-like grouping of cells with clear cytoplasm →.* **(Right)** *The perivascular clear cells merging into this thin-walled vessel show strong cytoplasmic staining for HMB-45 →.*

Perivascular Clear Cells

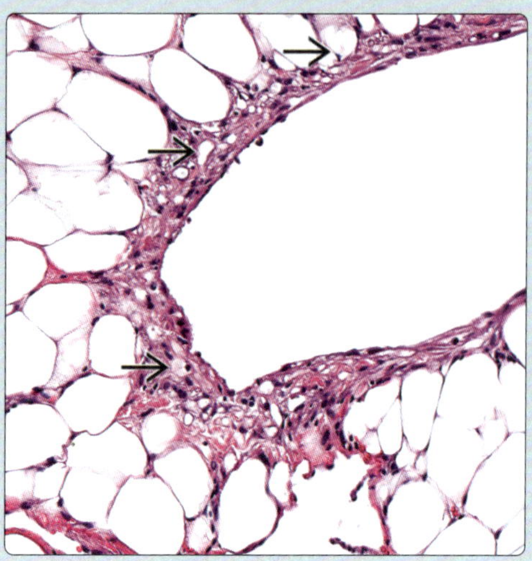

HMB-45 Staining

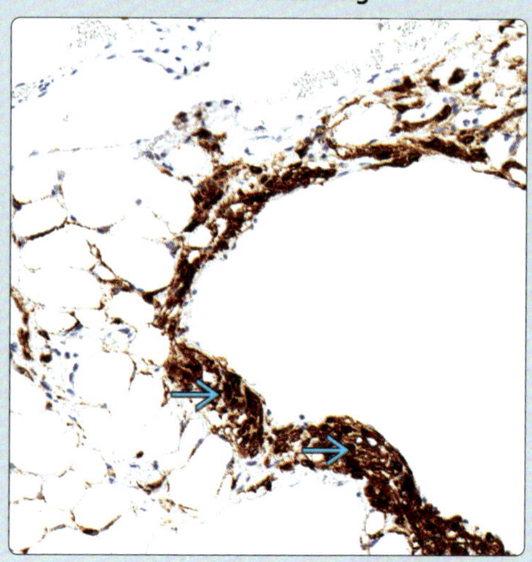

TERMINOLOGY

Abbreviations

- Angiomyolipoma (AML)

Definitions

- Mesenchymal tumor believed to originate from perivascular epithelioid cell (PEC)
- Closely related to other PEC-type tumors (e.g., lymphangioleiomyomatosis, clear cell sugar tumors of lung, pancreas, and uterus, PEComas, and cardiac rhabdomyomas

ETIOLOGY/PATHOGENESIS

Tuberous Sclerosis Complex

- Associated with genetic alterations in tuberous sclerosis genes, *TSC1* (9q34) and *TSC2* (16p13.3)
- 55-75% of patients with tuberous sclerosis develop renal AML
- < 50% of renal AML patients have tuberous sclerosis

Mammalian Target of Rapamycin Pathway

- Proteins encoded by *TSC1* (hamartin) and *TSC2* (tuberin) genes function as complex to negatively regulate mammalian target of rapamycin (mTOR) signaling
- Activated mTOR pathway markers are overexpressed in AML and related tumors

CLINICAL ISSUES

Presentation

- Multifocality, bilaterality, larger size, faster growth, and younger age are more common characteristics in AML associated with tuberous sclerosis
- Adipose-rich tumors are more easily diagnosed on imaging

Prognosis

- Typically benign clinical behavior
- Retroperitoneal hemorrhage is rare but often fatal complication
- Rare aggressive behavior, particularly in those with predominant epithelioid and other atypical features

MACROSCOPIC

Key Findings

- Often well circumscribed but not encapsulated
- Mean size: 6 cm (range: 0.5-25 cm) for resected tumors
- Cut surface is variable, reflecting relative proportion of fat, smooth muscle, or vessels in tumor

MICROSCOPIC

Histologic Features

- Typically contains adipose tissue, smooth muscle, and abnormal vessels in variable proportions
  - Smooth muscle component seen as fascicles of spindle cells or sheets of epithelioid cells with abundant eosinophilic granular cytoplasm
  - Thin-walled vessels showing hemangiopericytoma-like architecture and thickened, hyalinized vessels with eccentric lumina
- Uncommon types include predominantly lipomatous or leiomyomatous, lymphangioleiomyomatous, oncocytoma-like, and sclerosing type
- AML with epithelial cysts (AMLEC)
  - Epithelial cysts lined by cuboidal to hobnailed cells
  - Ovarian-like (CD10-positive) stroma

Lymph Nodes

- Regional lymph nodes occasionally contain AML
  - Considered tumor multicentricity
  - Disease progression has not been reported in cases with nodal involvement

ANCILLARY TESTS

Immunohistochemistry

- Expression of melanocytic markers: HMB-45, Melan-A (MART-1), MITF, tyrosinase, usually in epithelial cells
- Smooth muscle markers also positive
- Negative immunoreactivity for epithelial markers (cytokeratin, EMA/MUC1), except in AMLEC

DIFFERENTIAL DIAGNOSIS

Liposarcoma

- Mostly extrarenal, surrounding kidney
- Lack of dysmorphic vessels &/or smooth muscle component (unless part of dedifferentiation)
- Negative staining for melanocytic markers: HMB-45, Melan-A (MART-1), MITF
  - May be focal in AML
- Positive immunoreactivity for MDM2 and CDK4

Leiomyoma or Leiomyosarcoma

- Primary smooth muscle tumors are very rare in kidney
- No intratumoral fat or dysmorphic vessels are present, even after careful search
- Melanocytic markers are negative

Renal Oncocytoma

- Nested architecture, uniform nuclei
- Positive for epithelial markers and negative for melanocytic markers

DIAGNOSTIC CHECKLIST

Pathologic Interpretation Pearls

- Expression of melanocytic markers: HMB-45, Melan-A (MART-1), MITF, tyrosinase, usually in epithelial cells
- Adipose tissue, smooth muscle, and abnormal vessels in variable proportions
- Perivascular clear cells merging into walls of larger tumor vessels

SELECTED REFERENCES

1. Sanfilippo R et al: Role of chemotherapy, VEGFR inhibitors, and mTOR inhibitors in advanced perivascular epithelioid cell tumors (PEComas). Clin Cancer Res. 25(17):5295-300, 2019
2. Yan Z et al: Hepatic angiomyolipoma: mutation analysis and immunohistochemical pitfalls in diagnosis. Histopathology. 73(1):101-8, 2018
3. Aydin H et al: Renal angiomyolipoma: clinicopathologic study of 194 cases with emphasis on the epithelioid histology and tuberous sclerosis association. Am J Surg Pathol. 33(2):289-97, 2009

(Left) *Lipomatous AML grossly resembles liposarcoma. Generous sampling is essential, and recognition of abnormal blood vessels and perivascular epithelioid cells is necessary in such tumors.* (Right) *Typical triphasic AML is composed of fat, spindled smooth muscle fascicles ⇨, and a dysmorphic blood vessel. The smooth muscle cells have an epithelioid appearance and emanate from the vascular wall.*

Lipomatous Angiomyolipoma

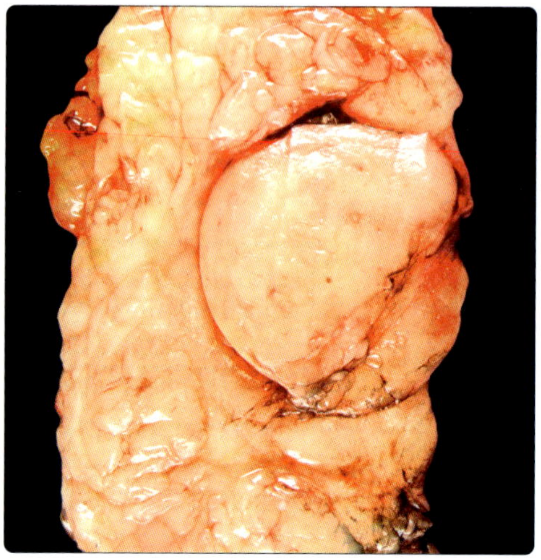

Smooth Muscle Fascicles

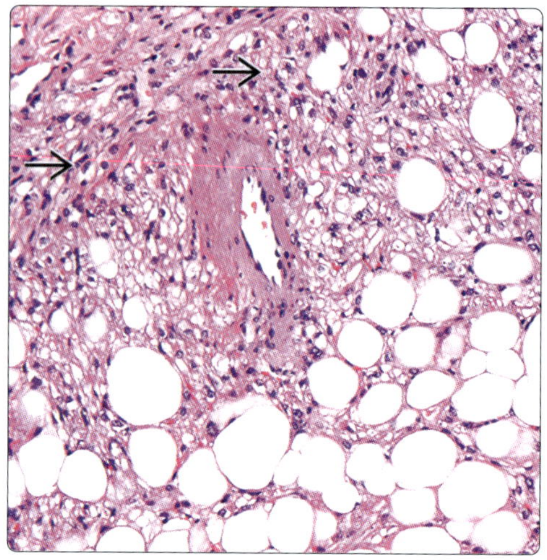

(Left) *AMLs are often well circumscribed, but most lack a capsule. At this low-power magnification, a distinct adipocytic component is recognized.* (Right) *Smooth muscle cells are often seen originating from a vessel wall ↪. This is a helpful diagnostic clue to the diagnosis in tumors with unusual histology (lipomatous or leiomyomatous AML).*

Border Interface

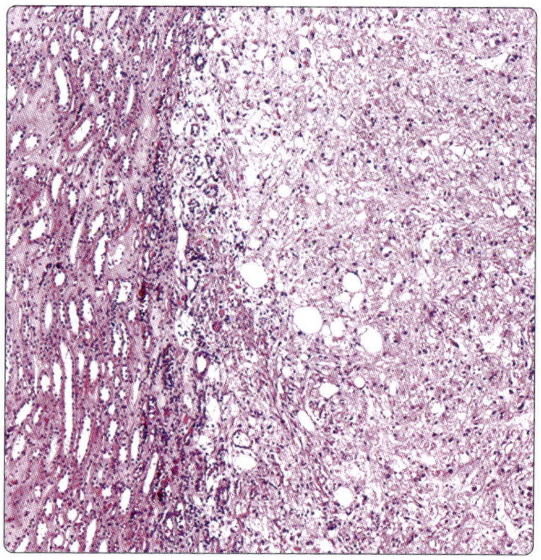

Perivascular Clear Cells

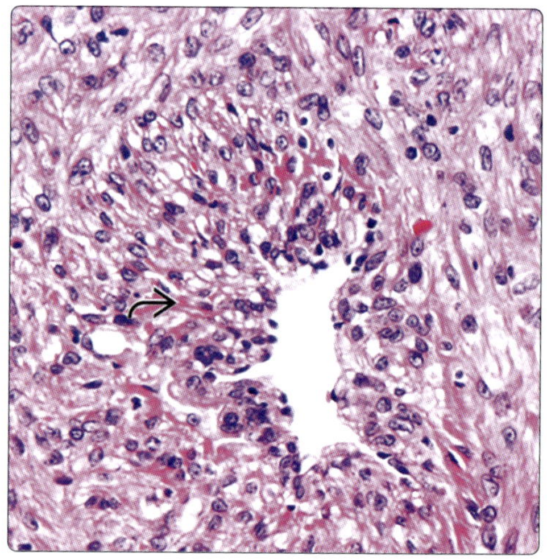

(Left) *HMB-45 [as well as Melan-A (MART-1)] is invariably positive in AML. The staining pattern may vary, but it is most prominent in epithelioid smooth muscle cells.* (Right) *SMA shows positivity in spindled and epithelioid smooth muscle cells. Note the positivity in a vessel wall ↪ that acts as an internal control. HMB-45 and Melan-A (MART-1) show stronger expression in epithelioid areas, whereas SMA is positive in spindled cells.*

HMB-45 Staining

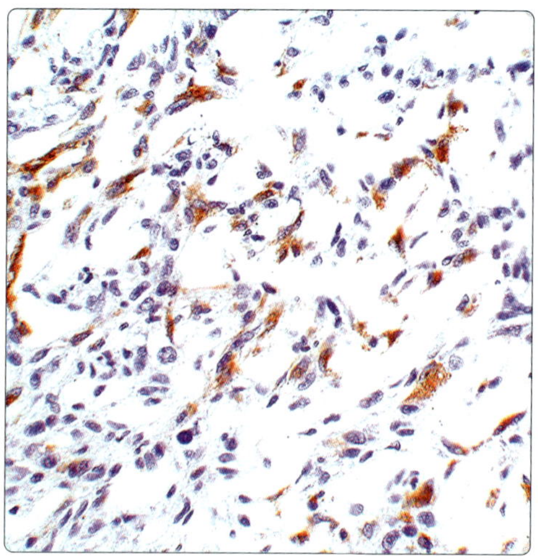

SMA Staining

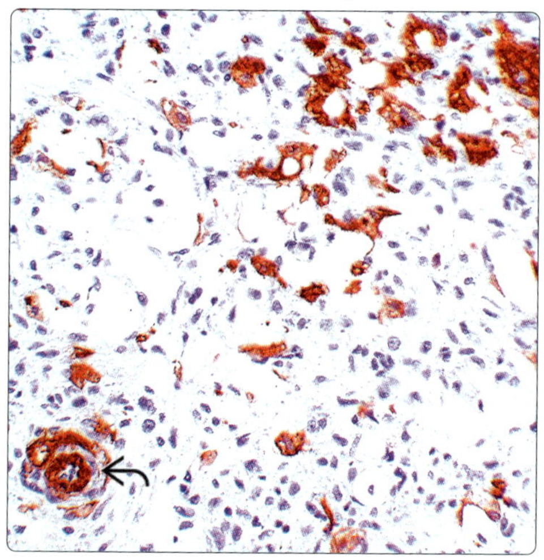

Entrapped Fat

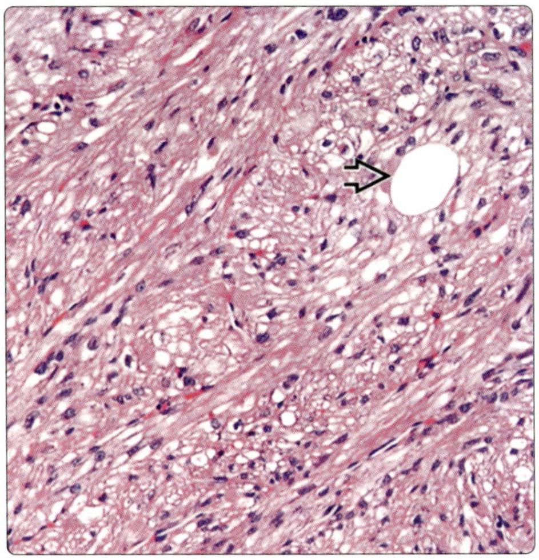

HMB-45 Staining in Smooth Muscle-Predominant Angiomyolipoma

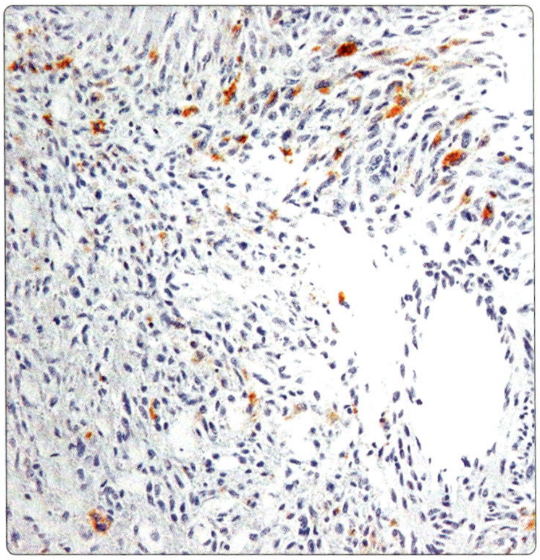

(Left) *Some cases of AML can resemble leiomyoma. Primary renal leiomyoma is very rare, and AML should always be considered in this setting. Even a single adipocyte ⇨ can be a helpful diagnostic clue. Immunostaining is also an important adjunct.* **(Right)** *HMB-45 shows smooth muscle-predominant AML. Often, only very focal positivity may be observed.*

Exophytic Renal Angiomyolipoma

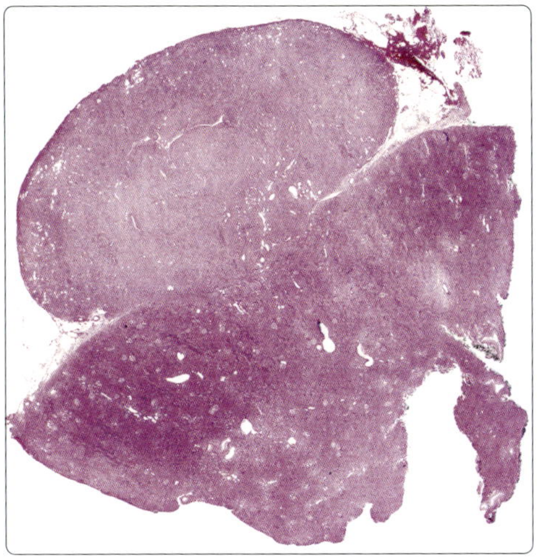

Core Needle Biopsy

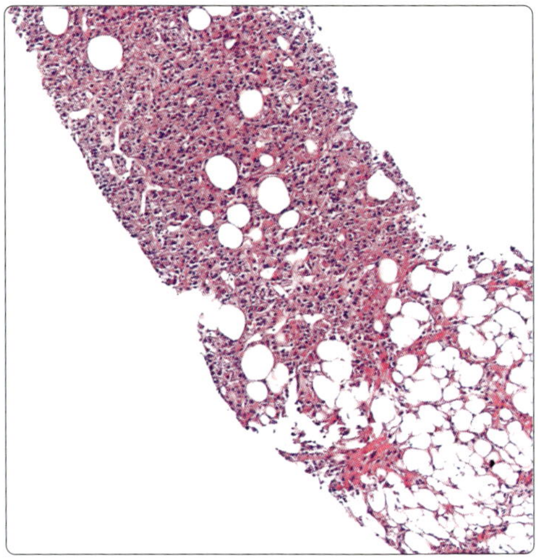

(Left) *Whole-mount of leiomyomatous AML arising from the renal capsule is shown. Such tumors are sometimes called renal capsuloma. Immunoexpression of melanocytic markers is confirmatory of AML.* **(Right)** *A definitive diagnosis of renal AML can be rendered on core needle biopsy, especially if the typical triphasic morphology is present.*

Epithelial Cysts

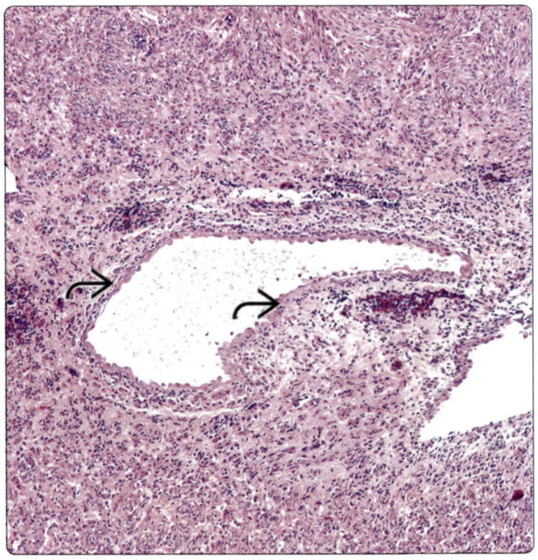

Oncocytoma-Like Angiomyolipoma

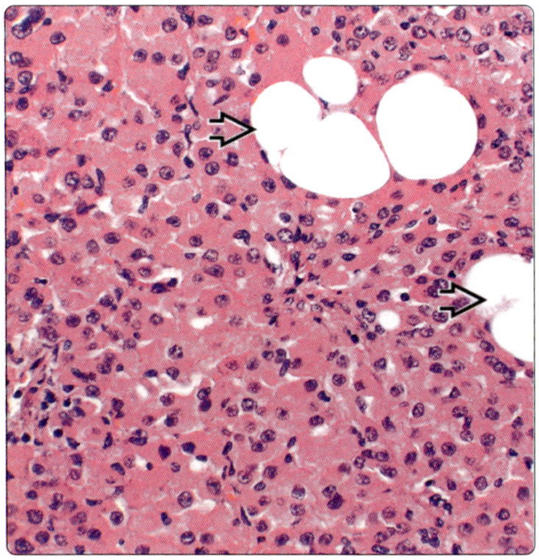

(Left) *AML with epithelial cysts (AMLEC) shows cysts lined by cuboidal epithelium with eosinophilic cytoplasm ↗. Occasionally, this cystic component may be conspicuous.* **(Right)** *Oncocytoma-like AML is a rare variant of AML. The presence of dysmorphic vessels, sclerosing areas, adipocytes ⇨, and nuclear variability should point toward the appropriate diagnosis. These are also diffusely positive for HMB-45/Melan-A (MART-1) and negative for epithelial markers.*

Glomus Tumor

KEY FACTS

TERMINOLOGY

- 3 major variants
  - Solid glomus tumor (glomus cell component only)
  - Glomangioma (glomus cell and vascular components)
  - Glomangiomyoma (glomus cell, vascular, and smooth muscle components)

CLINICAL ISSUES

- Most common in young adults
- Most commonly involves extremities, especially subungual area
- Usually arises in dermis or subcutis
- Rarely occurs in viscera
- Red-blue skin nodule, usually solitary
- Exquisitely painful, sensitive to cold
- Almost always benign
- Excision is usually curative; local recurrence is uncommon

MACROSCOPIC

- Unencapsulated dark red nodule
- Usually < 1 cm

MICROSCOPIC

- Composed of uniform, bland, round glomus cells with moderate amount of lightly eosinophilic cytoplasm
- Cell borders are usually well demarcated
- Sheets or nests of glomus cells surround thin, branching vascular channels
- Solid pattern most common
- Vascular component may be prominent and even cavernous (glomangioma)
- Rare cases also display smooth muscle component (glomangiomyoma)

ANCILLARY TESTS

- SMA and MSA strongly positive
- Cytokeratins virtually always negative

(Left) *Glomus tumors are characterized by proliferations of bland, round cells with distinct cytoplasmic borders → and eosinophilic cytoplasm surrounding vascular channels in a pericytic pattern ↶.* **(Right)** *Glomus cells may also form lacy nests and cords in a predominantly myxoid stroma, mimicking adenocarcinoma. Even in these cases, the perivascular distribution → is at least focally apparent.*

Glomus Tumor (High Magnification)

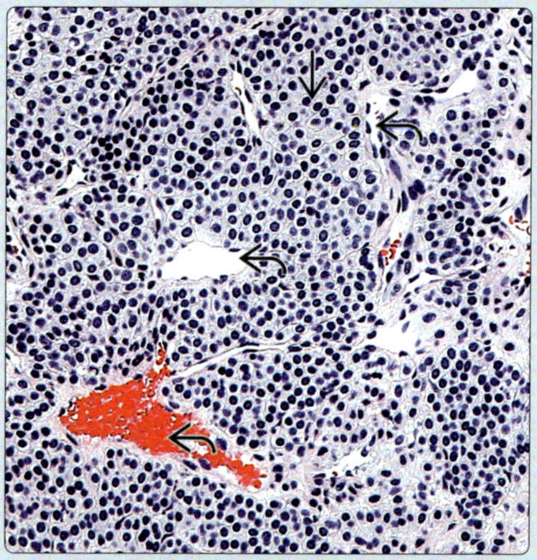

Glomus Tumor (High Magnification)

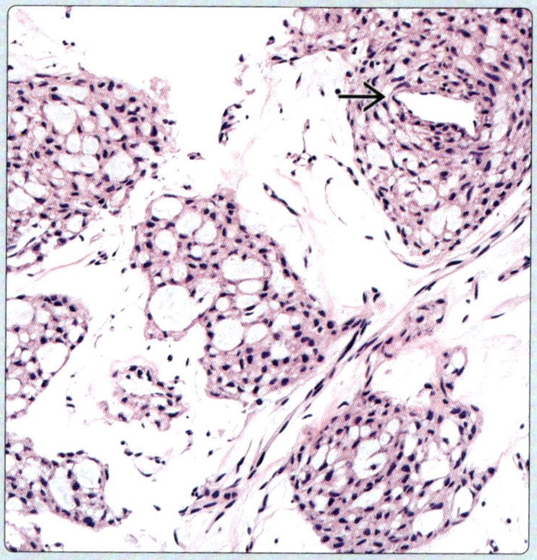

(Left) *H&E stain of a vagal glomus tumor demonstrates the classic zellballen pattern with rounded nests of cells →.* **(Right)** *Low-magnification H&E stain shows intravascular foreign material ⇨ introduced during an attempted endovascular embolization procedure. Ischemic tumor necrosis can be seen in such cases.*

Glomus Tumor (Low Magnification)

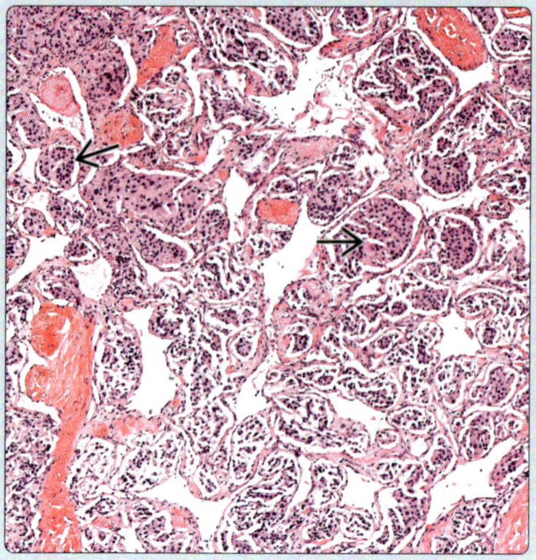

Glomus Tumor Following Embolization

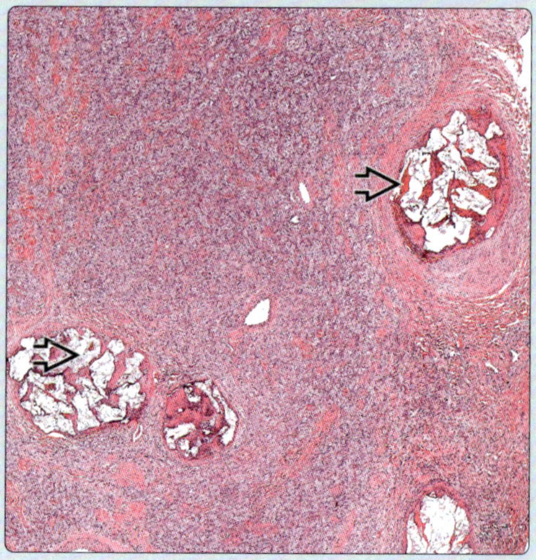

TERMINOLOGY

Definitions

- Family of neoplasms arising from modified perivascular smooth muscle cells of glomus body (Sucquet-Hoyer canal), which is involved in temperature regulation
- 3 major variants
  - Solid glomus tumor (glomus cell component only)
  - Glomangioma (glomus cell and vascular components)
  - Glomangiomyoma (glomus cell, vascular, and smooth muscle components)

ETIOLOGY/PATHOGENESIS

Sporadic Glomus Tumors

- Etiology unknown

Inherited Familial Glomangiomas

- Truncating mutations in glomulin gene on 1p21-22
- Usually autosomal dominant with incomplete penetrance

CLINICAL ISSUES

Epidemiology

- Age
  - Most common in young adults
- Sex
  - Subungual and digital lesions more common in female patients

Site

- Skin of extremities is most common location
  - Hands (digits and subungual)
  - Wrist, forearm
  - Foot
- Usually arises in dermis or subcutaneous tissues
- Rare cases reported in visceral organs and deep soft tissues

Presentation

- Red, purple, or blue skin nodule
  - Usually solitary; < 1 cm
- Pain (out of proportion to size), especially solid variant
  - Glomangiomas are not always painful
- May be sensitive to cold
- If multiple, suggests inherited disorder

Treatment

- Surgical approaches
  - Excision is usually curative

Prognosis

- Vast majority are benign
  - Local recurrence rare
- Rare cases of malignant glomus tumor (glomangiosarcoma) have been reported
  - Recurrence, metastasis, and death may occur

MACROSCOPIC

General Features

- Well-circumscribed, bulging, unencapsulated dark red nodule or mass

MICROSCOPIC

Histologic Features

- Solid glomus tumor
  - Most common pattern (~ 75% of cases)
  - Composed of uniform, round to ovoid cells with bland nuclear features, lightly eosinophilic cytoplasm, and well-demarcated cell borders (so-called glomus cells)
  - Sheets, nests, and trabeculae surround bland vessels
  - Hemangiopericytomatous pattern (staghorn-like, thin, branching vessels)
- Glomangioma
  - Prominent vascular component, cavernous vessels
  - Vessels surrounded by 2- to 3-cell layer of glomus cells
- Glomangiomyoma
  - Rare (~ 5% of cases)
  - Smooth muscle (myomatous) component is also present

ANCILLARY TESTS

Histochemistry

- Reticulin
  - Each glomus cell is surrounded by fine reticulin network

Immunohistochemistry

- SMA and SMA strongly positive
- Desmin occasionally focally positive
- CD34 occasionally positive
- Synaptophysin rarely positive but chromogranin negative
- Cytokeratins virtually always negative

DIFFERENTIAL DIAGNOSIS

Apocrine (Nodular) Hidradenoma

- Often displays ductal differentiation
- Stains for cytokeratins
- Frequently stains for CEA &/or EMA

Eccrine Spiradenoma

- Few duct-like structures are usually present
- Stains for cytokeratins

Intradermal Nevus

- Stains for melanocytic markers (e.g., S100, HMB-45)
- Displays maturation of melanocytes and smaller melanocyte nests with descent into dermis

Carcinoid Tumor

- Much more common than glomus tumor in viscera
- Positive for cytokeratins
- Stains for neuroendocrine markers (e.g., synaptophysin, chromogranin, CD56)
- Negative for muscle markers

SELECTED REFERENCES

1. Massey JNR et al: Excision of a rare cardiac tumor aided by endocardial electroanatomical mapping. J Card Surg. 36(12):4759-61, 2021
2. Castiglione V et al: What is hidden behind inferior negative T waves: multiple cardiac glomangiomas. JACC Case Rep. 1(4):657-62, 2019
3. Singh N et al: A large primary cardiac glomus tumour: a surgical dilemma. Eur J Cardiothorac Surg. 55(6):1237, 2019
4. Gombos Z et al: Glomus tumor. Arch Pathol Lab Med. 132(9):1448-52, 2008

(Left) *On scanning magnification, glomus tumors are typically well circumscribed → and usually < 1 cm in greatest dimension, as in this case of a solid glomus tumor arising in the subcutaneous tissue of the distal forearm.* **(Right)** *On low power, a thin capsule ↪ is seen. Numerous vascular channels → are apparent among the solid sheets of glomus cells. The channels are irregular, slit-like, branching, and staghorn-like, displaying the so-called hemangiopericytomatous pattern.*

Glomus Tumor (Low Magnification)

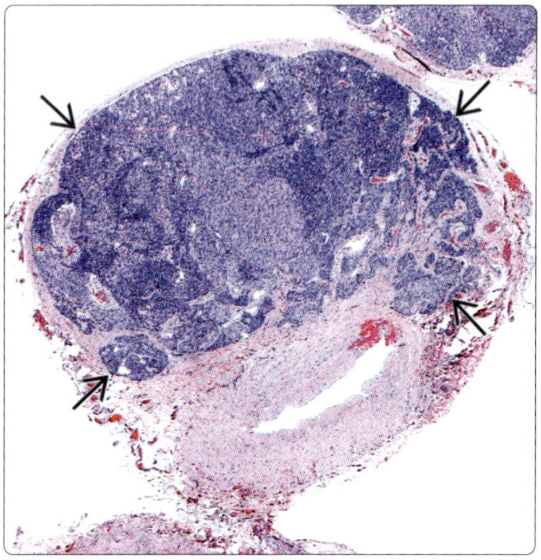

Glomus Tumor (Encapsulated)

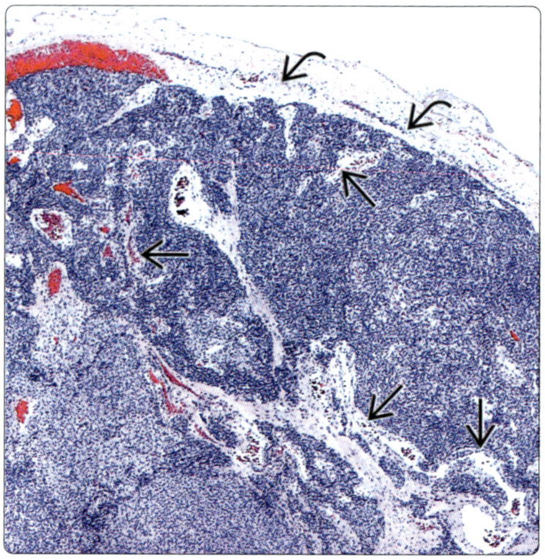

(Left) *Occasionally, glomus tumors are > 1 cm, although even these are well circumscribed and often encapsulated →. Note the areas of hemorrhage ↪, a feature seen when a superficial lesion is traumatized, as in this case from the lower leg.* **(Right)** *On medium power, solid sheets of glomus cells surround irregular, thin-walled vascular spaces that may be slit-like or, as in this case, ectatic →.*

Hemorrhage in Glomus Tumor

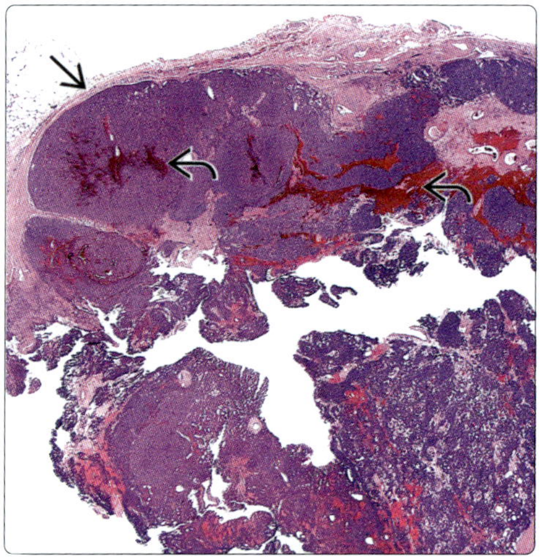

Glomus Tumor (Medium Magnification)

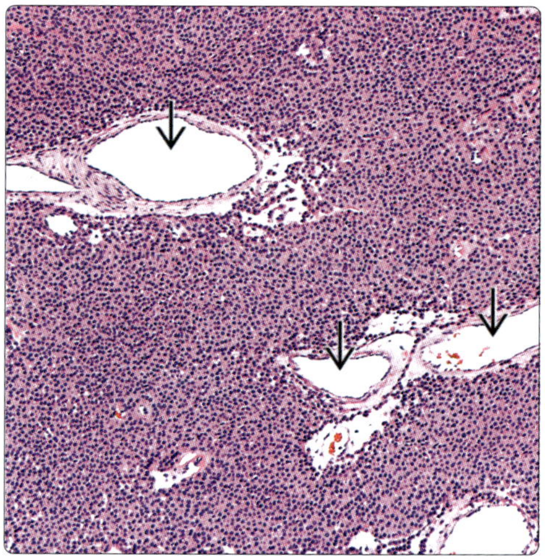

(Left) *On high power, glomus cells are small and round with lightly eosinophilic cytoplasm, prominent cell borders →, bland nuclear features, and very little mitotic activity. These cells surround irregular vessels in a so-called pericytic pattern. Vessels are lined by bland endothelial cells ↪.* **(Right)** *In some cases, glomus cells display oncocytic features with abundant, lightly eosinophilic granular cytoplasm and nucleoli. Note the compressed, slit-like vascular spaces →.*

Glomus Tumor (High Magnification)

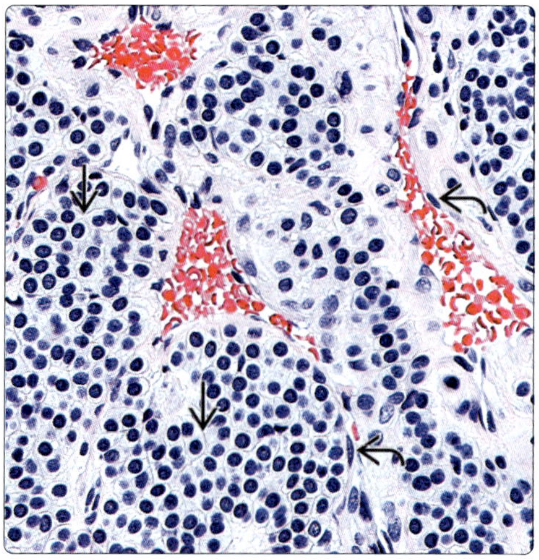

Glomus Tumor (High Magnification)

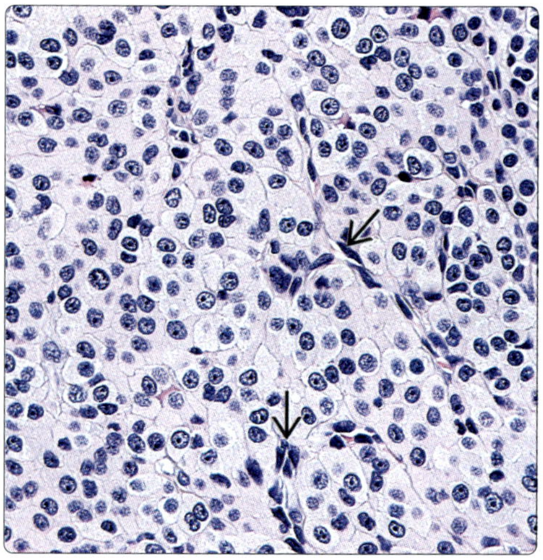

Glomus Tumor (High Magnification)

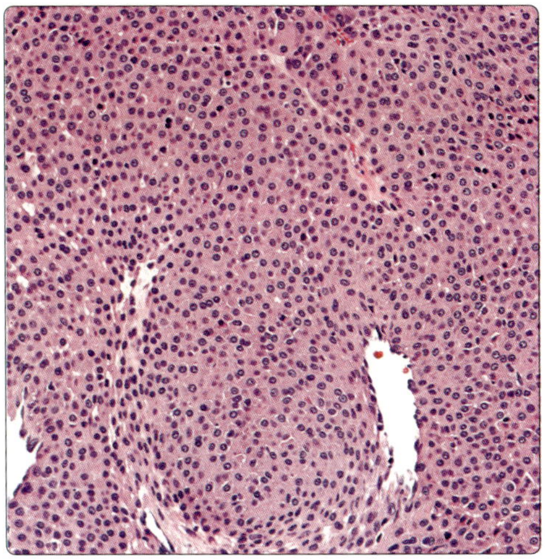

Hyaline Stroma in Glomus Tumor

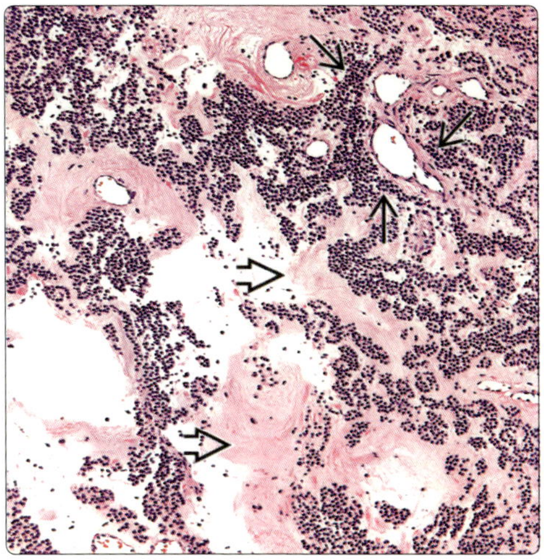

(Left) *In a typical case of a solid glomus tumor arising in the subcutaneous tissue of the shoulder, sheets of glomus cells surround vascular spaces with little, if any, intervening stroma.* **(Right)** *Other cases display nests of glomus cells within abundant myxohyaline stroma ⇨. In these cases, the abundant stroma may mask the pericytic relationship of glomus cells with associated vascular spaces. Careful searching will usually reveal pericytic morphology →, at least focally.*

Glomus Tumor (High Magnification)

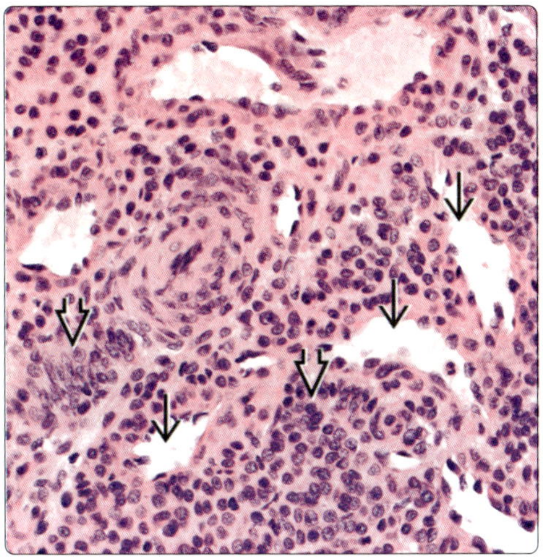

Glomus Tumor (Reticulin)

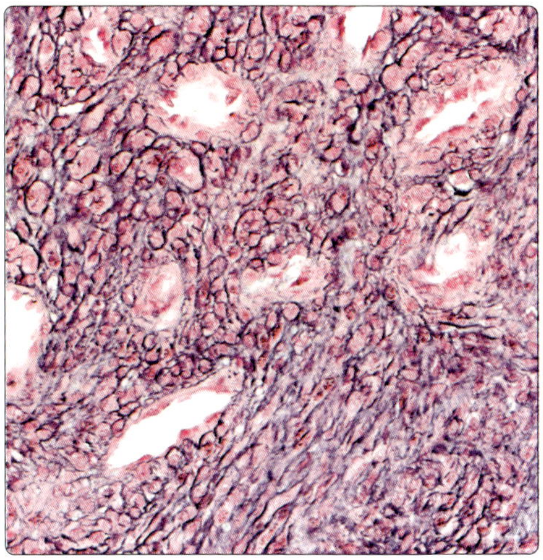

(Left) *In some cases, glomus cells may display crowding and become more oval ⇨, but even in these cases, the nuclear features are bland. Note the associated hemangiopericytomatous vascular channels →.* **(Right)** *A reticulin histochemical stain highlights a thin, lacy reticulin network that surrounds each individual glomus cell. This feature is characteristic of glomus tumors and may be used to differentiate them from other entities in difficult cases.*

Glomus Tumor (Low Magnification)

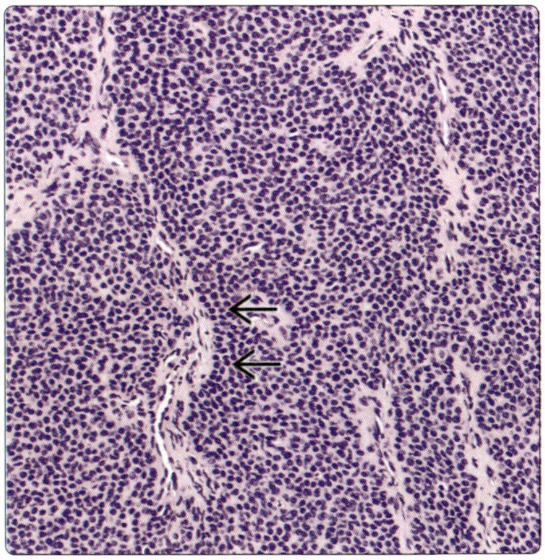

SMA in Glomus Tumor

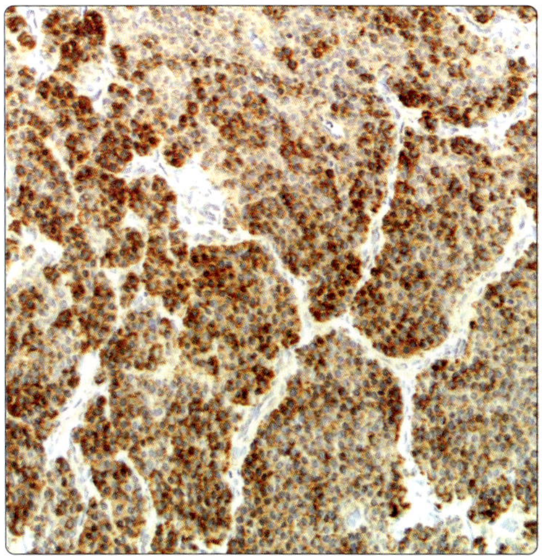

(Left) *In some cases, sheets of glomus cells with relatively little cytoplasm mimic small round blue cell tumors. Even here, the cells are very bland and can be seen surrounding irregular, slit-like vascular channels in a pericytic pattern →.* **(Right)** *In glomus cells, immunohistochemical staining for SMA is characteristically strong and diffuse. This staining pattern is very helpful for distinguishing glomus tumors from other entities in the differential diagnosis.*

(Left) *Some glomus tumors display extensive myxoid change, as in this unusual case from the 4th finger. At scanning magnification, irregular nests and cords are separated by hypocellular stroma ⇨.* **(Right)** *On medium power, the nests and cords of glomus cells display a lacy, somewhat cribriform appearance ⇨ and are separated from each other by abundant myxoid stroma. Vessels are present → but are masked throughout most of the lesion because of the lacy architecture.*

Myxoid Change in Glomus Tumor

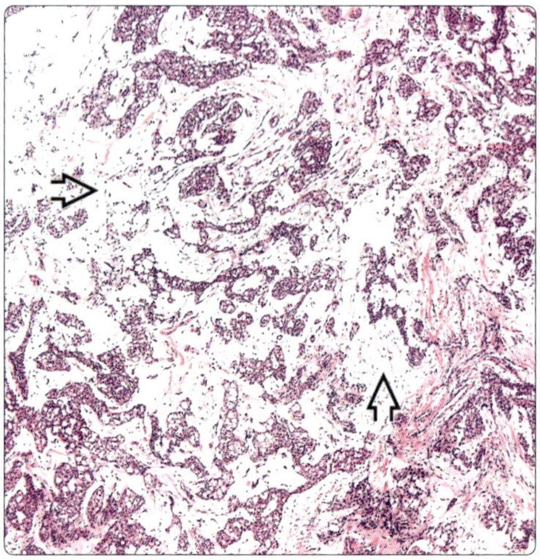

Glomus Tumor (Medium Magnification)

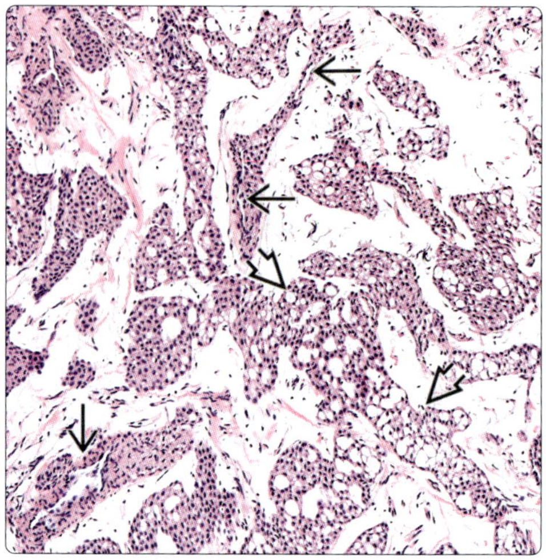

(Left) *On high power, lacy nests and cords of bland, round glomus cells seem to float in a loose myxoid stroma. This feature imparts a glandular or cribriform appearance to the nests and cords, mimicking adenocarcinoma.* **(Right)** *In cases displaying abundant myxoid stroma, areas of glomus cells surrounding hemangiopericytomatous vessels ⇨ are usually present, at least focally. A careful search for this feature can aid in the proper identification of the neoplasm.*

Glomus Tumor With Myxoid Stroma

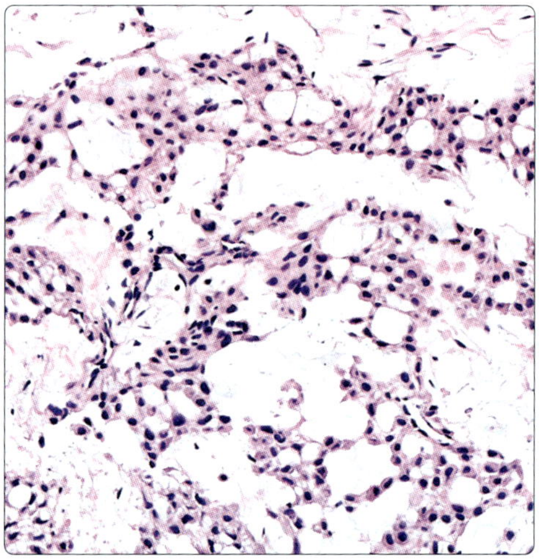

Glomus Tumor (High Magnification)

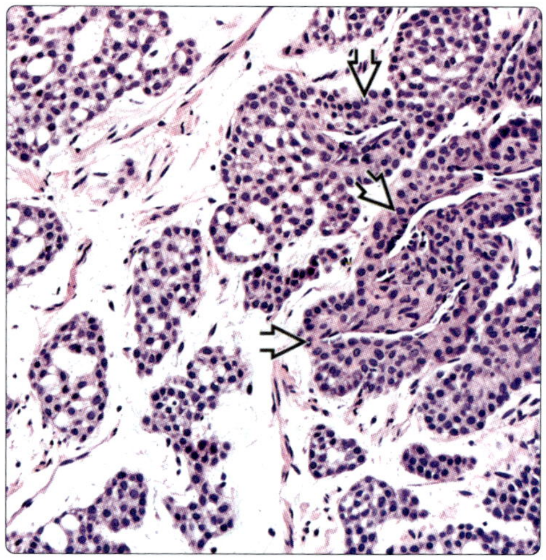

(Left) *Staining with mucicarmine highlights mucopolysaccharides, both within the stroma → and lacy nests ↪, indicating mucinous change. This change is occasionally seen in glomus tumors, and misdiagnosis of the lesion as an adenocarcinoma is a potentially disastrous pitfall.* **(Right)** *Immunostaining for SMA is diffusely positive in the lacy tumor nests →, and multiple immunostains for cytokeratins were negative (not shown), supporting a diagnosis of glomus tumor.*

Mucin in Glomus Tumor

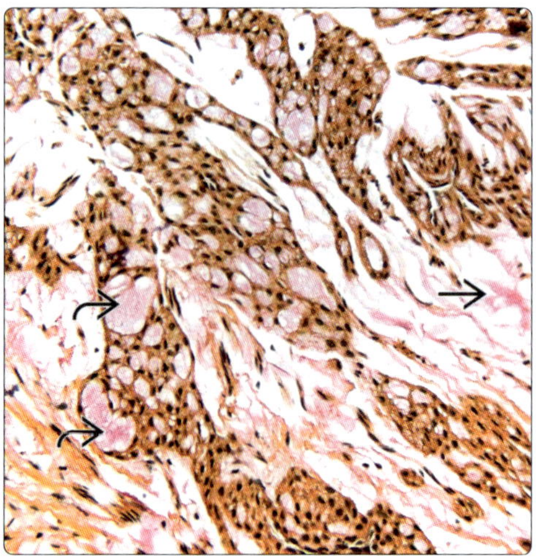

SMA in Glomus Tumor

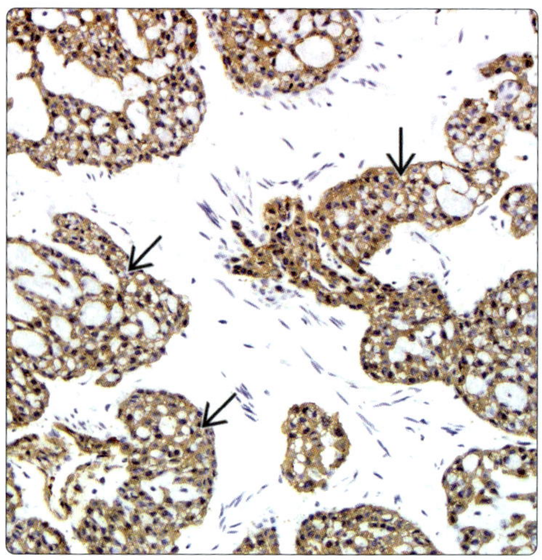

Glomangioma

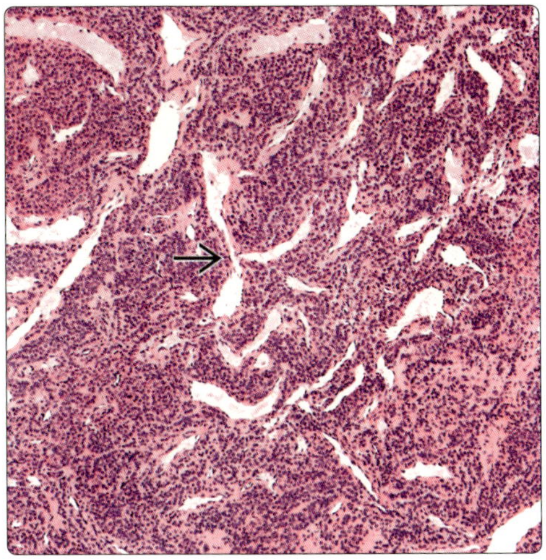

Glomangioma

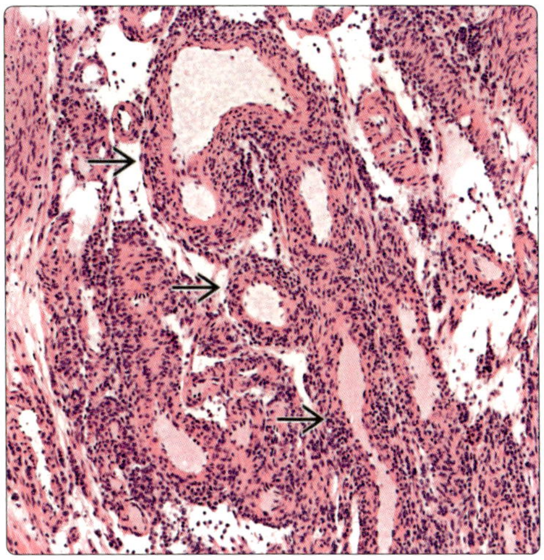

(Left) *Some glomus tumors display a prominent vascular component and are best classified as glomangiomas. In these cases, vessels display hemangiopericytomatous features* → *but are generally larger, thicker, and more abundant than in typical solid glomus tumors.* **(Right)** *In glomangiomas, the vascular component may be more obvious than the glomus cell component. Each thick-walled vascular space is surrounded by a thin cuff of glomus cells, usually 2-3 cells thick* →*.*

Perivascular Cuff in Glomangioma

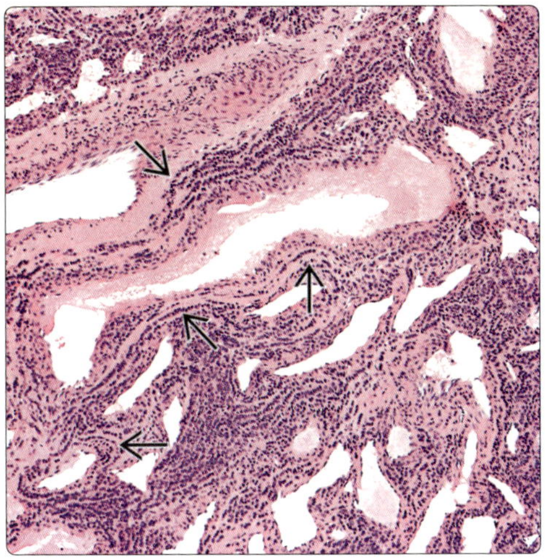

Triphasic Glomus Tumor

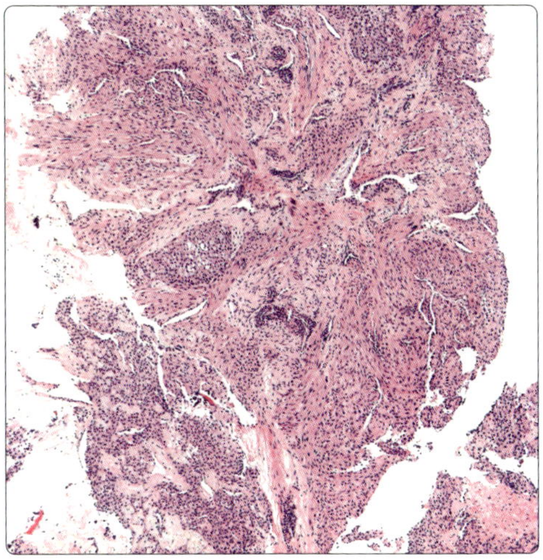

(Left) *In some glomangiomas, the perivascular cuff may form concentric "onion skin" layers* → *that appear to stream around each vessel. Even here, the perivascular cuffs are only a few glomus cells thick.* **(Right)** *In rare cases, glomus tumors display 3 components: Glomus cells, vessels, and smooth muscle cells. At low power, the haphazard admixture of these components is apparent. These tumors have been termed glomangiomyomas.*

Glomus Tumor Vessels

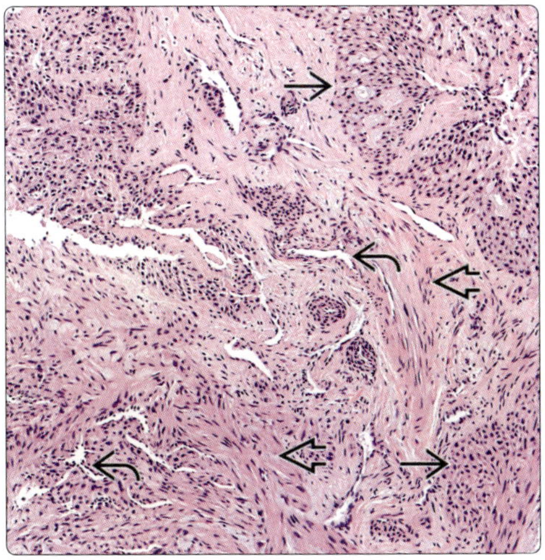

Glomus Tumor Vessels

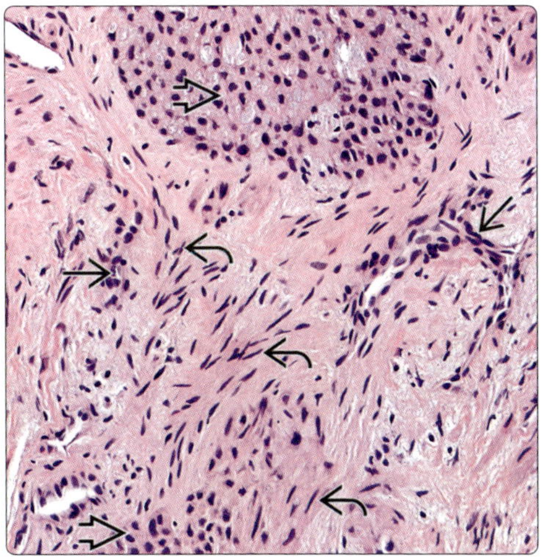

(Left) *At medium power, nests of glomus cells* →*, slit-like vascular channels* ↪*, and smooth muscle cell bundles* ⇨ *can all be seen in this lesion arising near the PIP joint of the 5th finger.* **(Right)** *At high power, solid nests of bland glomus cells* ⇨*, hemangiopericytomatous thin, branching vascular channels* →*, and irregular arrays of bland smooth muscle cells* ↪ *are all intimately admixed in this case of glomangiomyoma.*

Glomus Tumor

(Left) *Although glomus tumors usually occur in the skin, they occasionally arise in visceral sites and have been reported in virtually every organ. In this case, a large glomangioma* ⇨ *arose in the trachea with extension into the tracheal lumen. Note the tracheal cartilage* ↪ *and respiratory mucosa* →*.* **(Right)** *On medium power, the well-circumscribed lobules of vascular channels and glomus cells locally infiltrate and expand the superficial tracheal submucosa* →*.*

Glomus Tumor (Trachea)

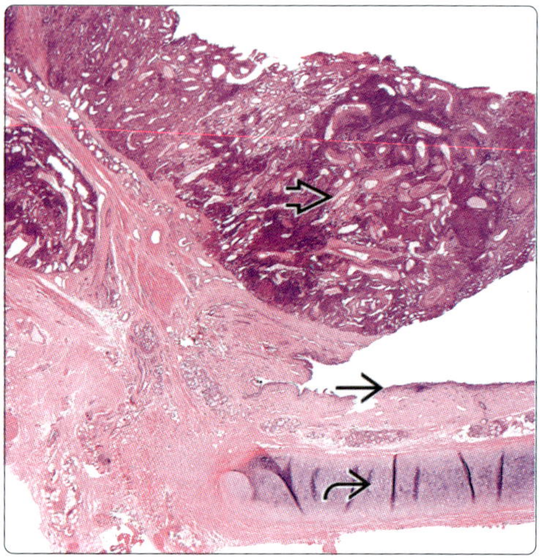

Glomus Tumor (Trachea)

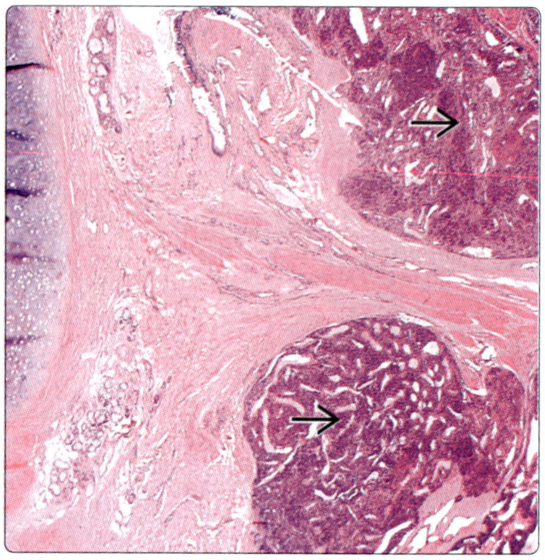

(Left) *Occasionally, glomus tumors arise in bones. Here, a primary intraosseous glomus tumor involves a phalanx of the great toe. As in other sites, cuffs of bland glomus cells surround numerous vascular channels in a pericytic pattern* →*.* **(Right)** *Glomus tumors occasionally arise in the gastrointestinal tract. In this case, a large glomus tumor involves the stomach wall. At scanning power, lobules of tumor locally invade the muscularis propria* → *without extragastric extension.*

Osseous Glomus Tumor

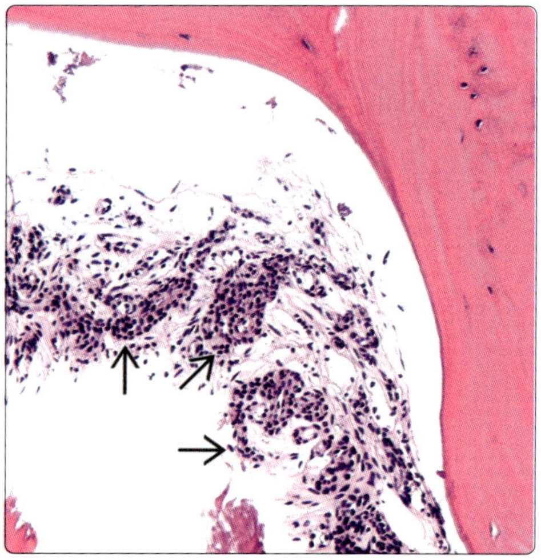

Glomus Tumor (Stomach)

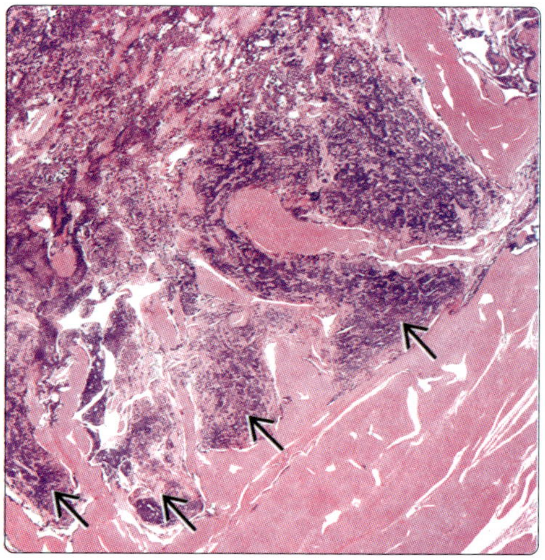

(Left) *Curiously, glomus tumors are sometimes rimmed by slit-like vessels* →*. Although a carcinoid tumor is an important diagnostic consideration, particularly in the gastrointestinal tract, these channels are an important clue that this may in fact represent a vascular neoplasm.* **(Right)** *On higher power, areas of classic glomus tumor morphology are seen in the stomach wall, including bland, round cells surrounding slit-like, hemangiopericytomatous vascular channels* →*.*

Glomus Tumor (Low Magnification)

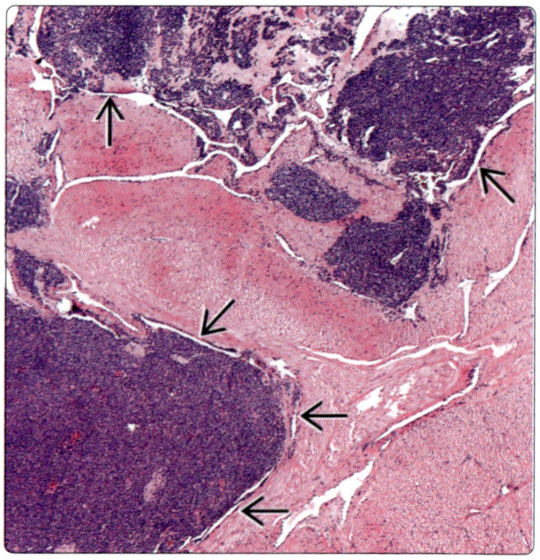

Glomus Tumor (Medium Magnification)

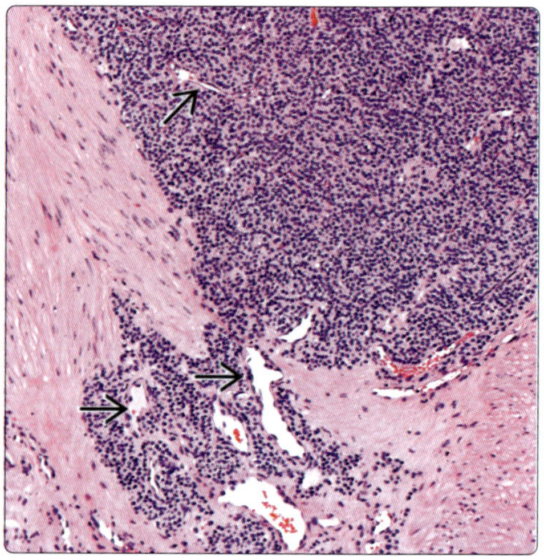

Glomus Tumor (High Magnification)

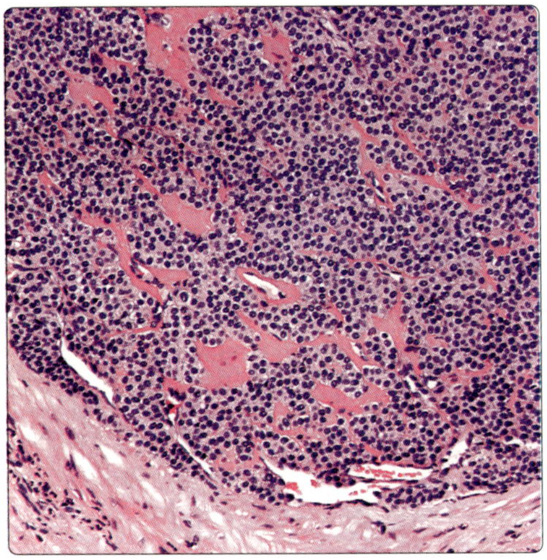

Negative Keratin Stain in Glomus Tumor

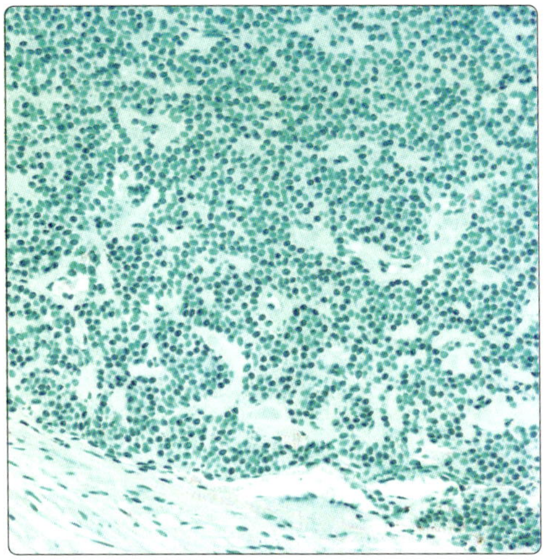

(Left) *In the gastrointestinal tract, glomus tumors can bear a striking resemblance to carcinoid tumors, as in this case of glomus tumor in the stomach.* **(Right)** *Immunohistochemistry can be an extremely useful tool to differentiate a glomus tumor from a carcinoid tumor. Unlike carcinoid tumors, glomus tumors do not express cytokeratins and will not stain with an antibody cocktail directed against low molecular weight CK8 and CK18 (CAM5.2), as seen here.*

SMA in Glomus Tumor

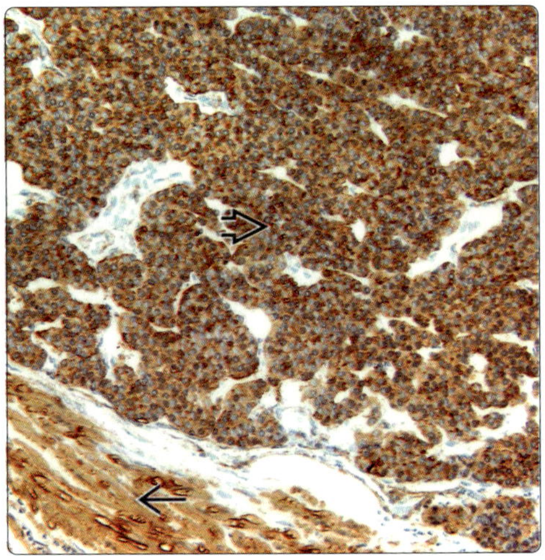

Low Ki-67 Index in Glomus Tumor

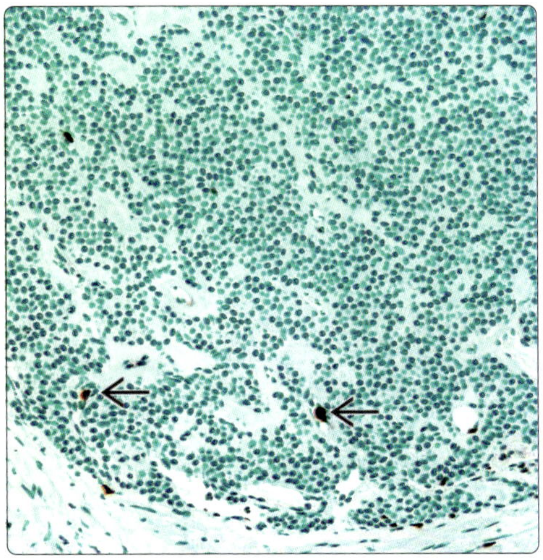

(Left) *Immunostaining for SMA is virtually always diffusely and strongly positive in glomus tumors ⇨, a feature not seen in carcinoid tumors. Note the positively staining muscularis propria →, a helpful internal control.* **(Right)** *Consistent with the benign behavior and extremely low proliferative rate of glomus tumors, immunostaining for Ki-67 reveals only rare, scattered individual glomus cells in the proliferative phase →.*

Synaptophysin in Glomus Tumor

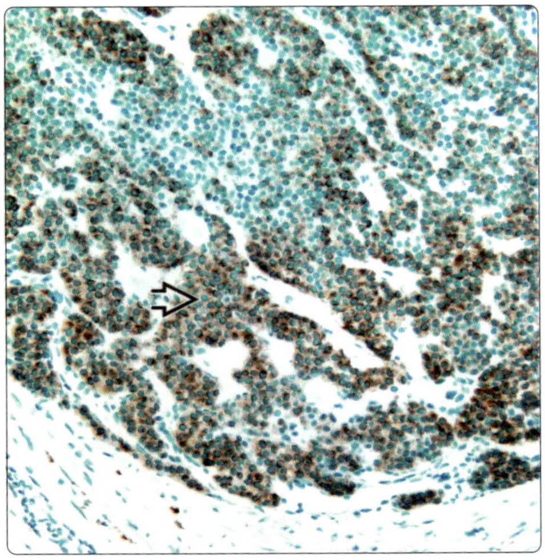

Negative Chromogranin in Glomus Tumor

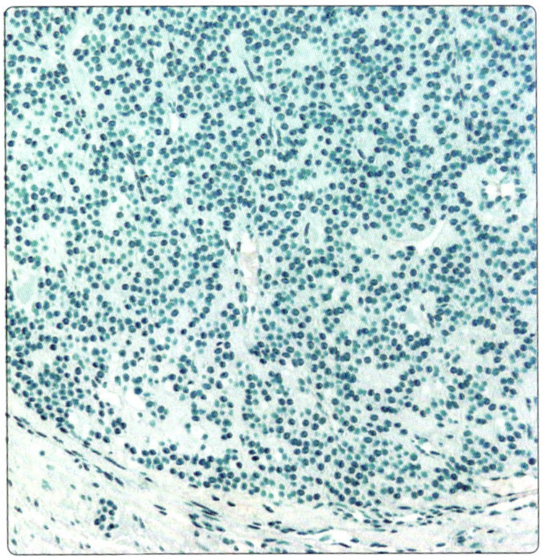

(Left) *Occasionally, glomus tumors show focal positive staining for synaptophysin. In rare cases, reactivity for synaptophysin is more extensive, as in this case ⇨, causing diagnostic confusion with carcinoid tumor. Immunostains with cytokeratin and SMA will ensure the correct diagnosis.* **(Right)** *Unlike synaptophysin, immunostains for chromogranin are virtually always negative in glomus tumors.*

Cystic Lymphangioma

KEY FACTS

TERMINOLOGY

- Benign tumor occurring mainly in pediatric patients and characterized by cystic dilatation of lymphatics

ETIOLOGY/PATHOGENESIS

- Malformations arising from sequestrations of lymphatic tissue that fail to communicate with lymphatic system
- 50-65% are present at birth

CLINICAL ISSUES

- In general, painless, soft, fluctuating mass that may enlarge; remains static or waxes and wanes
- Specific symptoms vary depending on location
- Complete surgical excision is standard treatment
- Although benign, may be associated with significant morbidity due to large size, critical location, or secondary infection

MACROSCOPIC

- Neck: Unicystic or multicystic bulging mass in superficial soft tissue
- Head (lips, cheek, tongue, and mouth): Cavernous-type lesion involving deep soft tissue
- Gastrointestinal: Solitary or multiple polypoid mass with spongy, cystic appearance on cut surface

MICROSCOPIC

- Cystic lymphangioma: Large, sharply demarcated, multiloculated, interconnected cystic spaces; significant fibrous connective tissue and smooth muscle stroma; aggregates of lymphocytes in cyst wall

ANCILLARY TESTS

- D2-40, CD31, and factor VIII are useful markers for identification of endothelium and diagnosis

(Left) *A large cystic lymphangioma (hygroma) of the neck is seen in this stillborn neonate. The size and location caused respiratory compromise leading to death. Although benign lesions, critical location, large size, and complications are associated with significant morbidity.* **(Right)** *Axial CECT shows a cystic lymphangioma as a thin-walled, water-density mesenteric mass with scattered calcifications in septa. (Courtesy M. Federle, MD and H. Dhatt, BA.)*

Autopsy Gross Specimen

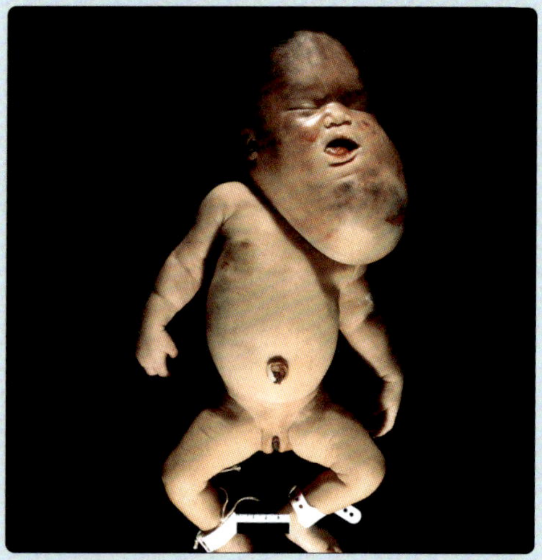

Axial CECT

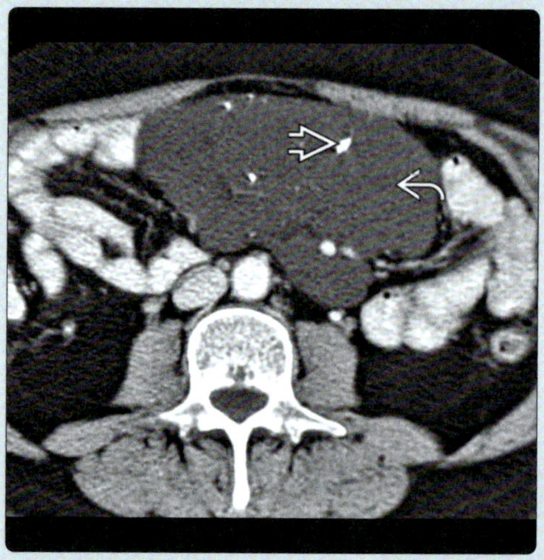

(Left) *Low-power view shows cystic spaces of varying sizes separated by delicate septa with scattered lymphoid aggregates in this intraabdominal lymphangioma.* **(Right)** *On higher magnification, neck lymphangioma shows honeycomb-like spaces lined by flattened endothelial cells. Benign lymphoid aggregates are also present. (Courtesy G. Ellis, MD.)*

Histologic Section

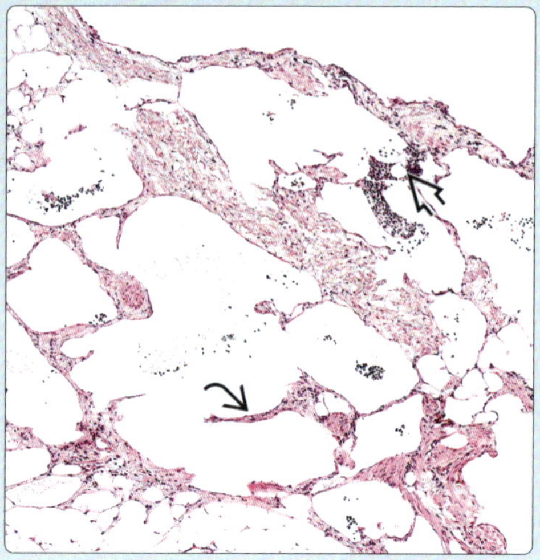

Histologic Section

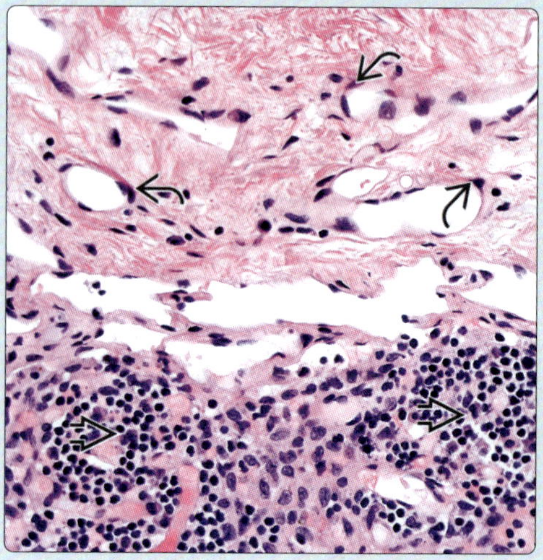

TERMINOLOGY

Synonyms

- Cystic hygroma

Definitions

- Benign tumor occurring mainly in pediatric patients and characterized by cystic dilatation of lymphatics

ETIOLOGY/PATHOGENESIS

Developmental Anomaly

- Malformations arising from sequestrations of lymphatic tissue that fail to communicate with lymphatic system
- Appear relatively early in life
- May occur as diffuse or multifocal disease (lymphangiomatosis)

Acquired

- Some lymphangiomas have developed following trauma, surgery, irradiation, or infection
- Likely represent lesions resulting from obstruction

CLINICAL ISSUES

Epidemiology

- Incidence
  - 1 in 6,000 births
  - 5% of benign tumors in infants and children
- Age
  - 50-65% present at birth
  - 80-90% diagnosed within 1-2 years of age
- Sex
  - Slight male predominance seen in some series

Site

- Head: Mouth, tongue
- Neck: Supraclavicular fossa of posterior cervical triangle, anterior cervical triangle; 10% extend into mediastinum
- Axillary region
- Mesentery of small intestine
- Sporadic involvement of solid organs: Lung, heart (more often involving visceral pericardium), spleen, liver, kidney, and bone

Presentation

- In general, painless, soft, fluctuating mass that may enlarge; remains static or waxes and wanes
- Specific symptoms vary depending on location
  - Head and neck lymphangiomas: Facial nerve paralysis, dysphagia or feeding problems, airway obstruction
  - Intraabdominal lymphangiomas: Gastrointestinal bleeding, acute abdomen secondary to obstruction
  - Cutaneous lymphangiomas: Asymptomatic or present with skin vesicles and lymphorrhea
  - Thoracic lymphangiomas: Cough, stridor, dyspnea, dysphagia, hemoptysis, superior vena cava syndrome
  - Intrauterine diagnosed lymphangiomas: Associated with nonimmune hydrops fetalis and Turner syndrome
    - Other associations include Noonan syndrome, familial pterygium colli, several chromosomal aneuploidies (trisomies 21, 18, and 13)

Treatment

- Complete surgical excision is standard treatment
- Recurrence after incomplete resection occurs in ≥ 10-15% of cases

Prognosis

- Benign but may be associated with significant morbidity due to large size, critical location, or secondary infection
- Rare cases of regression have been reported

IMAGING

Ultrasonographic Findings

- Primarily cystic lesion with internal septa of variable thickness, sometimes contains debris

MR and CT Findings

- Mass with low or intermediate signal intensity on T1WI and hyperintensity on T2WI
- Circumscribed cystic mass, nonenhancing content, and variable density

MACROSCOPIC

General Features

- Neck: Unicystic or multicystic bulging mass in superficial soft tissue
- Head (lips, cheek, tongue, and mouth): Cavernous-type lesion involving deep soft tissue
- Heart (visceral pericardium with most common location at right atrioventricular groove)

MICROSCOPIC

Histologic Features

- Cystic lymphangioma
  - Large, sharply demarcated, multiloculated, interconnected cystic spaces lined by endothelium
  - Fibrous connective tissue and smooth muscle stroma
  - Aggregates of lymphocytes, occasional germinal centers, and giant cells may be seen in cyst wall

ANCILLARY TESTS

Immunohistochemistry

- D2-40 (podoplanin), CD31, and factor VIII are useful markers for identification of endothelium and diagnosis

DIFFERENTIAL DIAGNOSIS

Cystic Mesothelioma

- Often affects large areas of peritoneum as multicystic mass composed of gland-like spaces
- Mesothelial cell lining is positive for cytokeratin and negative for vascular markers

Lymphangiomyoma

- Lymphatic spaces surrounded by smooth muscle cells positive for HMB-45

SELECTED REFERENCES

1. Pichler Sekulic S et al: Primary cardiac and pericardial lymphangiomas: clinical, radiologic, and pathologic characterization derived from an institutional series and review of the literature. Virchows Arch. 480(6):1211-21, 2022

Arteriovenous Malformations

KEY FACTS

TERMINOLOGY

- Arteriovenous malformation (AVM): Vascular malformation with abnormal connection between dysplastic arteries and arterialized veins (nidus) with blood flowing from arterial to venous system without intervening capillaries
  - Does not regress
  - Persists throughout life
  - May show commensurate growth during childhood
  - May worsen over time

ETIOLOGY/PATHOGENESIS

- Hereditary hemorrhagic telangiectasia (HHT), a.k.a. Osler-Weber-Rendu syndrome
  - Most common heritable AVM syndrome (1 in 5,000-10,000 patients)
  - *ENG*, *ACVRL1*, *SMAD4* mutations in HHT
- *PIK3CA* mutations associated with sporadic cerebral (cavernous) AVM

CLINICAL ISSUES

- Subarachnoid or CNS hemorrhage, GI hemorrhage, pulmonary hemorrhage

MACROSCOPIC

- Hemorrhagic, vascular-appearing lesion, regardless of location
  - May be associated with parenchymal (or cavity) hemorrhage
  - Larger vessels usually grossly apparent ± thrombus

MICROSCOPIC

- Abnormally large and irregular vessels (inappropriate size for tissue compartment)
  - Some recognizable as arteries with duplicated internal elastic lamina, others appearing to represent vein walls with thickened hyalinized walls
  - Large vascular spaces with intramural thick-walled vessels are helpful histologic finding

Cerebral AVM

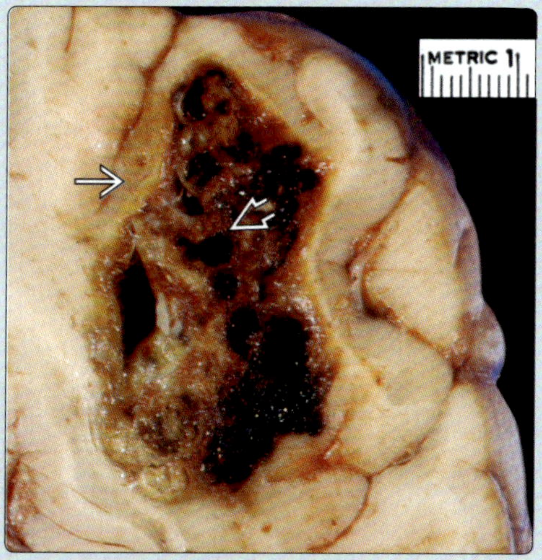

AVM With Onyx Polymer Embolization

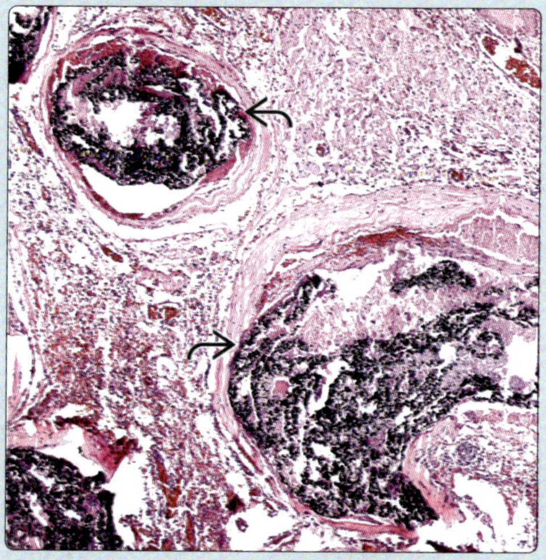

(Left) *Gross photograph of a cerebral arteriovenous malformation (AVM) ➡ in a patient with seizures shows variably sized vascular spaces and hemosiderin discoloration of the white matter ➡. (Courtesy R. Rhodes, MD.)* **(Right)** *AVM following Onyx polymer embolization shows black pigment ➡ within the vessel lumina. (Courtesy R. Rhodes, MD.)*

Intestinal AVM

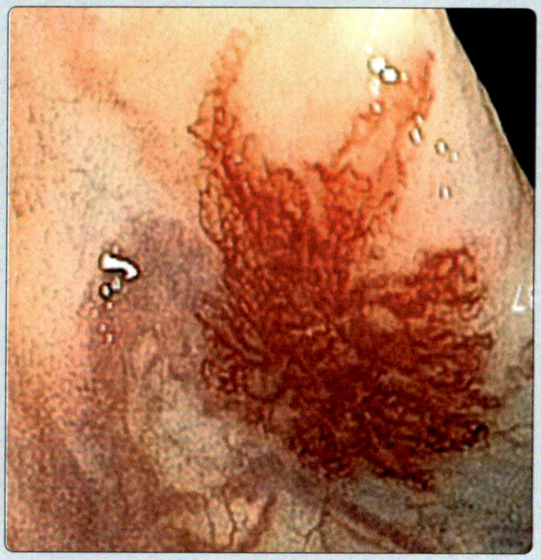

Intestinal AVM

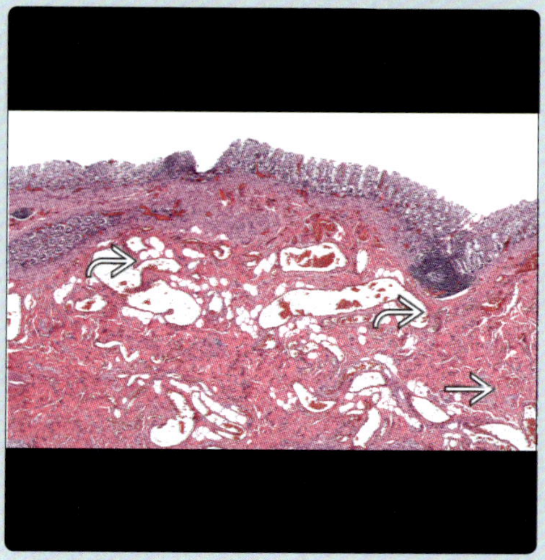

(Left) *Endoscopy in a 71-year-old man with aortic stenosis shows an intestinal AVM. There is thought to be an increased incidence of GI AVM in patients with aortic stenosis (Heyde syndrome). (Courtesy A. Manoukian, MD.)* **(Right)** *Submucosal AVM in the intestine shows gaping, thin-walled veins ➡ and other thicker walled vessels ➡ as well. The haphazard and variable nature of these vessels (compared to normal submucosal vasculature) is striking.*

TERMINOLOGY

Abbreviations

- Arteriovenous malformation (AVM)

Definitions

- Vascular malformation with abnormal connection between dysplastic arteries and arterialized veins (nidus) that enables blood to flow from arterial to venous system without intervening capillary system
  - Localized alteration of vascular morphogenesis does not regress, persists through life, may show commensurate growth during childhood, and may worsen over time

ETIOLOGY/PATHOGENESIS

Developmental Anomaly

- May be part of heritable syndrome
- Hereditary hemorrhagic telangiectasia (HHT), a.k.a. Osler-Weber-Rendu syndrome, is most common heritable AVM syndrome (1 in 5,000-10,000 patients)
  - Telangiectasias (skin, GI, mucous membranes) and AVMs (lungs, liver, brain, spinal cord)
  - 2 types of HHT, each distinguished by particular gene mutation
    - Endoglin (*ENG*) on chromosome 9q33-34 (HHT1)
    - Activin receptor-like kinase 1 (*ACVRL1*) on 12q (HHT2)
  - *SMAD4* gene mutation is seen in 10% of patients screening negative for HHT1 and HHT2
  - All 3 genes encode proteins involved in TGF-β signaling pathway, which is vital for normal vasculogenesis
  - No significant differences in phenotype are observed between HHT1 and HHT2
- *PIK3CA* mutations associated with sporadic cerebral (cavernous) AVM

CLINICAL ISSUES

Presentation

- Local effects
  - Pain, ulceration, bleeding; bruit often heard over lesion
  - Epistaxis is common early sign of HHT
  - CNS AVM: Most common vascular malformation
    - Subarachnoid or cerebral hemorrhage or seizures
    - M:F = 2:1
    - Spinal cord lesion: Foix-Alajouanine
- Systemic effects
  - CHF: Rare (< 2% of cases); usually infancy or puberty with rapidly enlarging limb AVM, embolic phenomena, and metastatic abscesses (pulmonary AVM)
- Schobinger clinical staging system for AVMs
  - I: Quiescence (mimics hemangioma; shunting noted on Doppler)
  - II: Expansion (with pulsation, palpable thrill, and tortuous veins)
  - III: Destruction (skin changes, ulceration, bleeding, tissue necrosis, lytic lesions)
  - IV: Decompensation (III + CHF)
- Puberty, pregnancy, and trauma are all risk factors for progression
- Curaçao criteria for diagnosis of HHT
  - Epistaxis (> 1 episode, especially nocturnal), multiple telangiectasias (lips, oral cavity, fingers, nose, GI tract), visceral AVMs (liver, pulmonary, cerebral, spinal), history of 1st-degree relative with HHT
- Heyde syndrome
  - Intestinal AVM in patients with aortic stenosis

Treatment

- Difficult due to recurrence, progression, and inability to completely remove
- Based on age of patient and location, size, and clinical stage

MACROSCOPIC

General Features

- Hemorrhagic, vascularized (regardless of location)
  - Subarachnoid or CNS hemorrhage, GI hemorrhage, or bleeding into body cavity (hemothorax is rarely reported with pulmonary AVM)
  - CNS AVM is typically in middle cerebral territory

MICROSCOPIC

Histologic Features

- Abnormally large vessels
  - Some recognizable as arteries with duplicated internal elastic lamina, others appear to represent vein walls with thickened hyalinized walls
- Endothelial lining is flat, not hobnailed or atypical
- IHC staining for WT1, thought to distinguish between vascular neoplasms (positive) and malformations (negative); may be positive in AVMs (only stage II AVMs were studied)
- Acute and organizing hemorrhage may be noted in surrounding tissue
- Intervening gliotic tissue can be seen in CNS AVMs

DIFFERENTIAL DIAGNOSIS

Arteriovenous Fistula

- Connection between artery and vein but without formation of nidus of vessels seen in AVM

SELECTED REFERENCES

1. Kohli P et al: Posterior mediastinal arteriovenous malformation: a rare catch. J Cardiovasc Thorac Res. 14(1):74-6, 2022
2. Wang K et al: Exome-wide analysis of de novo and rare genetic variants in patients with brain arteriovenous malformation. Neurology. 98(16):e1670-8, 2022
3. Peyre M et al: Somatic PIK3CA mutations in sporadic cerebral cavernous malformations. N Engl J Med. 385(11):996-1004, 2021
4. Schimmel K et al: Arteriovenous malformations-current understanding of the pathogenesis with implications for treatment. Int J Mol Sci. 22(16), 2021
5. Utami AM et al: A literature review of microvascular proliferation in arteriovenous malformations of skin and soft tissue. J Clin Transl Res. 7(4):540-57, 2021
6. Greene AK: Current concepts of vascular anomalies. J Craniofac Surg. 23(1):220-4, 2012
7. Kitajewski J: Arteriovenous malformations in five dimensions. Sci Transl Med. 4(117):117fs3, 2012
8. Lowe LH et al: Vascular malformations: classification and terminology the radiologist needs to know. Semin Roentgenol. 47(2):106-17, 2012
9. Meek ME et al: Management of pulmonary arteriovenous malformations. Semin Intervent Radiol. 28(1):24-31, 2011
10. Trindade F et al: Wilms tumor 1 expression in vascular neoplasms and vascular malformations. Am J Dermatopathol. 33(6):569-72, 2011
11. Batur P et al: Increased prevalence of aortic stenosis in patients with arteriovenous malformations of the gastrointestinal tract in Heyde syndrome. Arch Intern Med. 163(15):1821-4, 2003

(Left) *Angiogram shows a classic pulmonary AVM. The arterial communication is not seen clearly, but the draining vein is seen easily. Pulmonary AVMs are common in Osler-Weber-Rendu syndrome.* **(Right)** *3D reconstruction CTA shows a prominent AVM with its draining vein.*

Pulmonary AVM

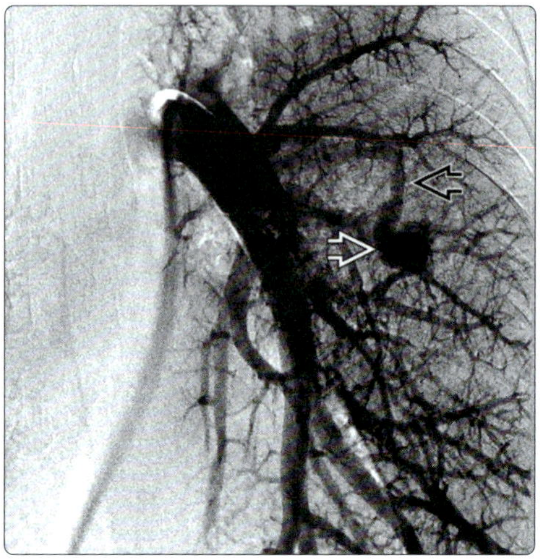

Pulmonary AVM

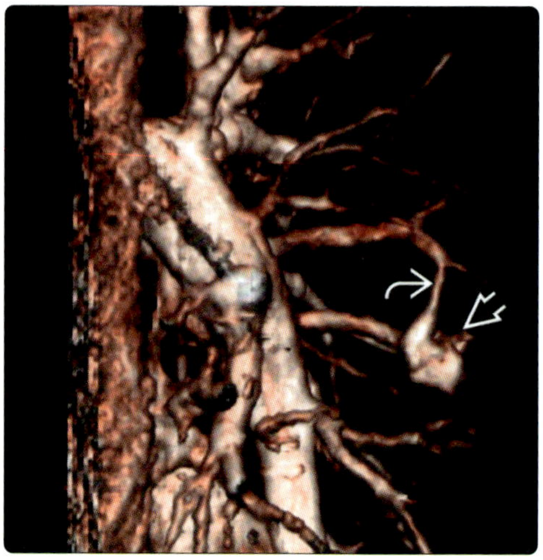

(Left) *Catheter angiography shows a complex AVM with multiple feeding arteries and draining veins. These are less common than simple AVMs (10%) and require embolization of all of the feeding arteries.* **(Right)** *Angiogram demonstrates a soft tissue AVM in the thumb. There is swelling surrounding the lesion, and myriad collateral small vessels are also seen. (From DI: Pediatrics.)*

Pulmonary AVM

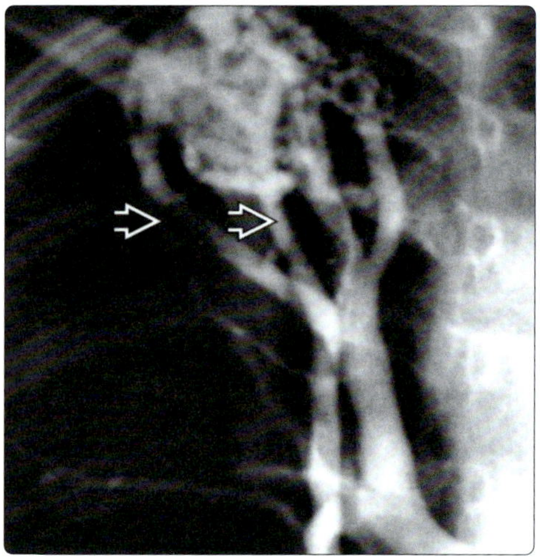

Soft Tissue AVM

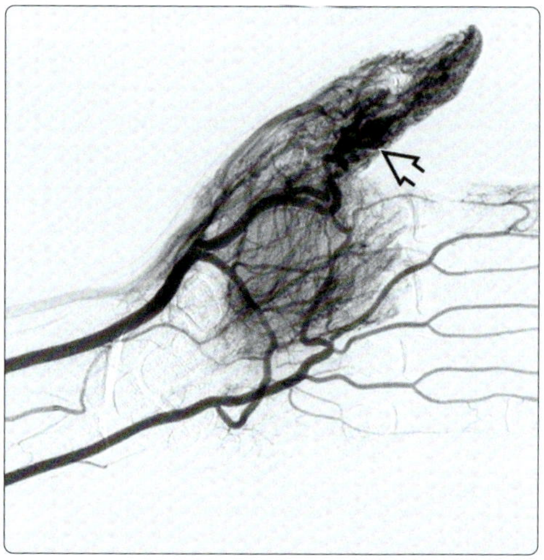

(Left) *Cross section of spinal cord with AVM shows enlarged vessels within the cord and in the surrounding leptomeninges, diagnostic for Foix-Alajouanine malformation. (Courtesy R. Rhodes, MD.)* **(Right)** *Pathognomonic features of AVM are shown. Within the wall of a vasculature structure with its lumen to the right, there are numerous thick-walled intramural vessels.*

Spinal Cord AVM

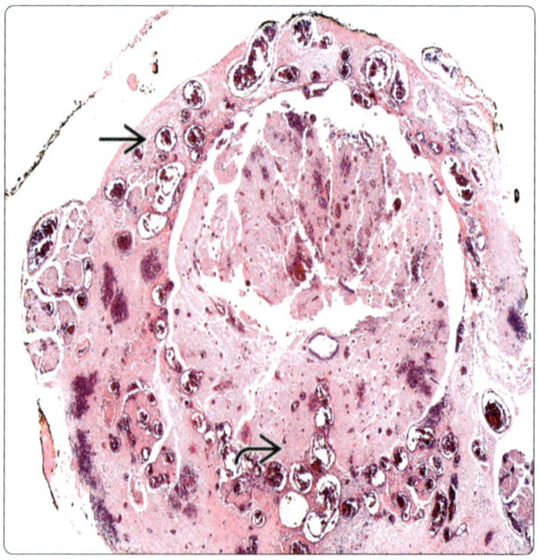

Intramural Vessels in AVM

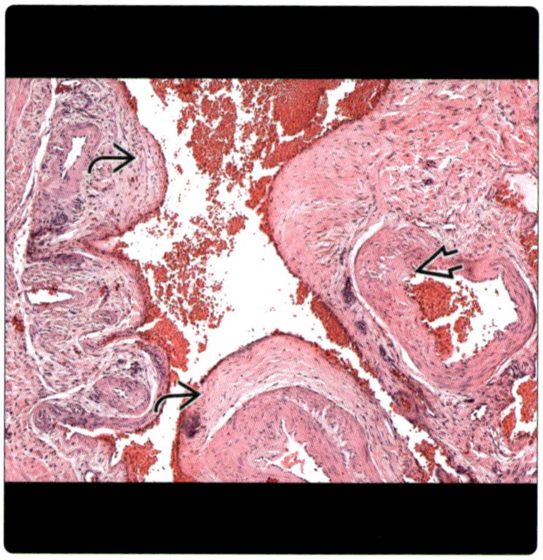

Cerebral AVM With Rupture

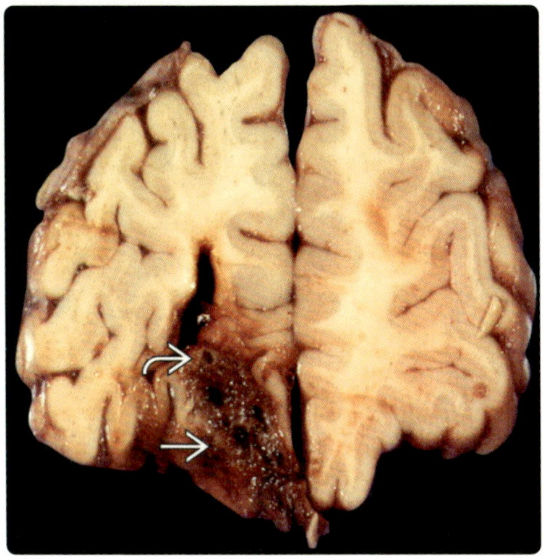

Cerebral AVM With Rupture

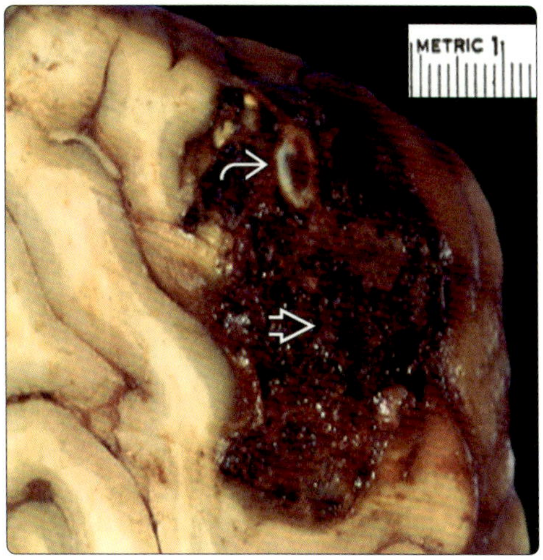

(Left) *Ruptured cerebral AVM of the frontal orbital lobe hemorrhaged into the subarachnoid space ➡. Large vascular spaces are seen ➡. (Courtesy R. Rhodes, MD.)* **(Right)** *Superficial AVM ➡ also ruptured, leading to subarachnoid hemorrhage. A large vessel with apparent thrombus can be seen ➡.*

Soft Tissue AVM

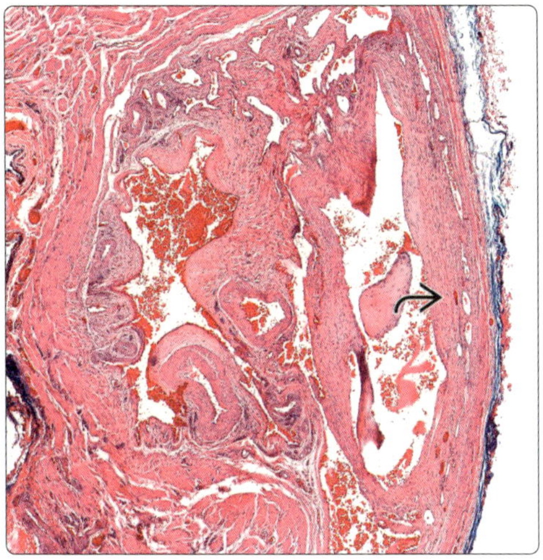

Intestinal AVM

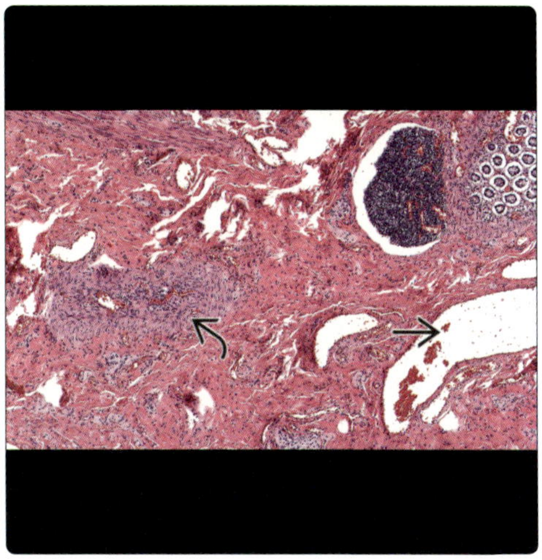

(Left) *Soft tissue AVM shows marked variability in luminal diameter, luminal contour, and vessel wall thickness. Fibrin is seen in the lumen focally ➡.* **(Right)** *Submucosal AVM in the intestine shows a disproportionately thick-walled vessel ➡ and multiple dilated, thin-walled vessels ➡.*

Intestinal AVM

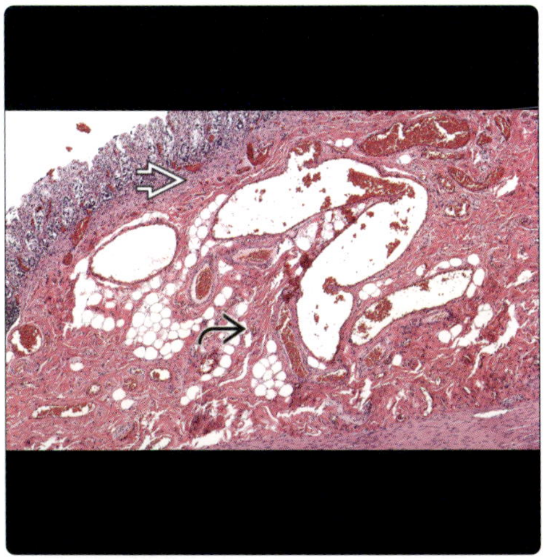

Intestinal AVM

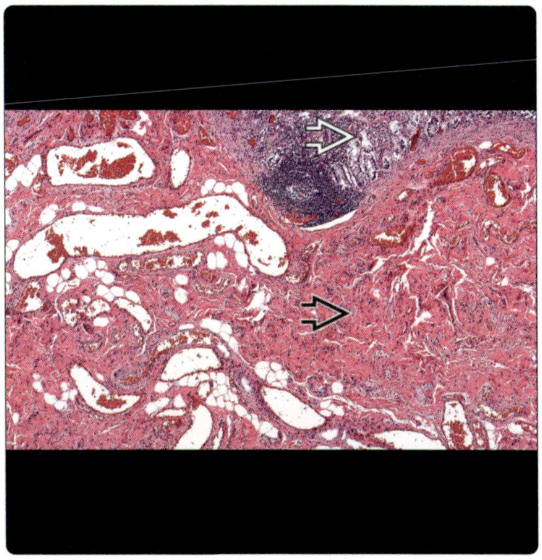

(Left) *Submucosal AVM in the intestine shows irregular and highly variable vessels of a size inappropriately large for the normal submucosal vasculature. Some residual fat is present ➡. The overlying mucosa shows ischemic changes ➡.* **(Right)** *The supporting stroma of this submucosal AVM in the intestine shows impressive dense collagenous fibrosis ➡. Ischemic mucosal changes are present ➡.*

Epithelioid Hemangioendothelioma

KEY FACTS

TERMINOLOGY

- Low-grade malignant vascular endothelial cell neoplasm with epithelioid cytomorphology

ETIOLOGY/PATHOGENESIS

- Translocation t(1;3)(p36;q25) almost always present

CLINICAL ISSUES

- Young to middle-aged adults
- More common in female patients
- Common sites include lung, liver, bone, soft tissue
- Treatment options include surgical resection, liver transplantation, or chemotherapy
- Course generally protracted but widely variable
- Prognosis better when lesions well defined
- Prognosis worse with infiltrative ill-defined lesions, extrapulmonary thoracic disease, pleural effusions

MACROSCOPIC

- Gray-white, very firm nodules; often multicentric
- May be focally calcified

MICROSCOPIC

- Epithelioid cells with eosinophilic cytoplasm
- Intracytoplasmic vacuoles with erythrocytes
- Abundant myxoid and variably hyalinized stroma
- Paucicellular in center, more cellular at periphery
- Mitotic activity low and necrosis minimal
- Vascular invasion common; mimics thrombi

ANCILLARY TESTS

- Vascular markers usually strongly positive, e.g., CD31, CD34, factor VIII-related antigen
- Keratins can be focally positive
- FISH assay for translocation helpful in difficult cases

Soft Tissue Epithelioid Hemangioendothelioma

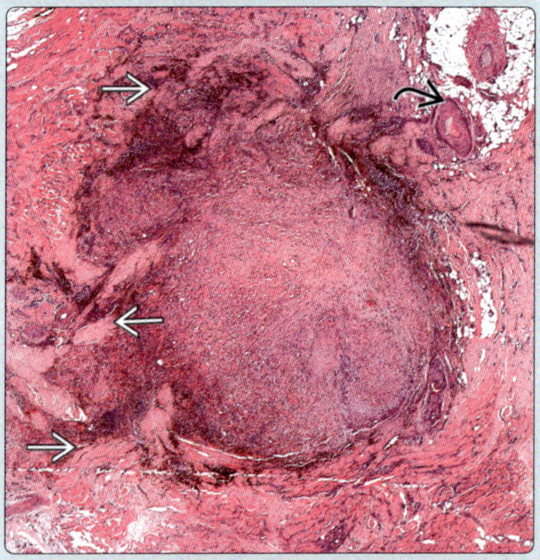

Epithelioid Hemangioendothelioma: Thrombus

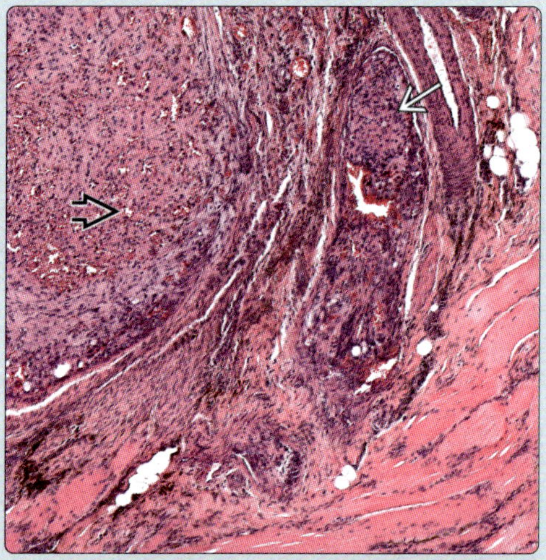

(Left) *Low-magnification view of an intramuscular epithelioid hemangioendothelioma (EHE) shows infiltrative borders. Prominent "feeder" vessels can also be seen.* **(Right)** *On higher magnification, the vascular nature of this EHE is apparent with irregular small vessel lumen contours. An apparent tumor thrombus is seen in a perilesional vessel.*

Epithelioid Hemangioendothelioma: Nodular Architecture

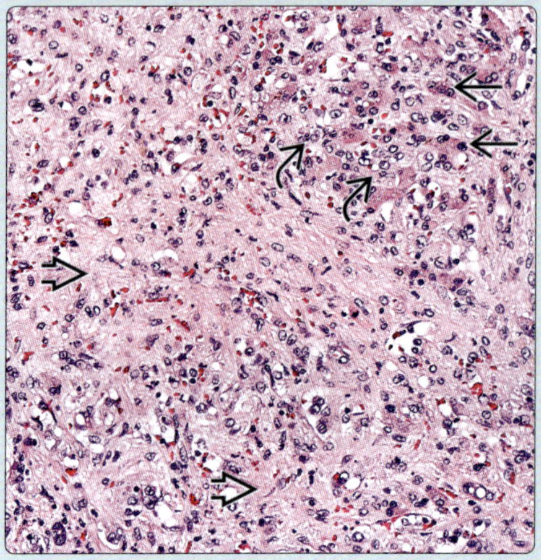

Epithelioid Hemangioendothelioma: Intracytoplasmic Lumina

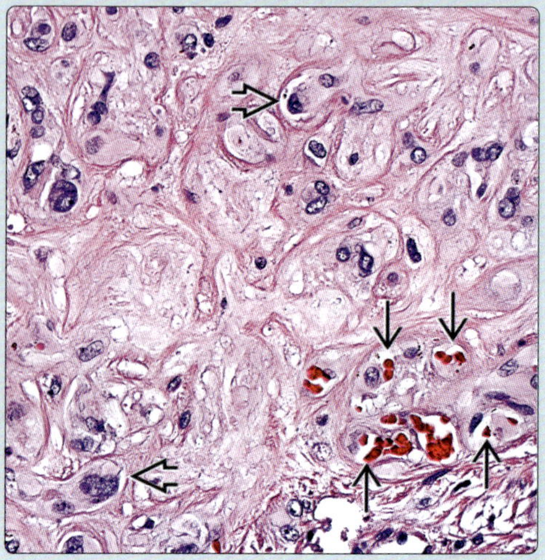

(Left) *EHE is characterized by solid nodules of epithelioid cells with myxohyaline stroma. In the liver, tumor cells infiltrate sinusoids between residual hepatocytes at the advancing edge.* **(Right)** *Large epithelioid cells are seen with abundant pink cytoplasm and mild atypia. Occasional intracytoplasmic vacuoles contain erythrocytes, a helpful feature that suggests a vascular neoplasm.*

TERMINOLOGY

Abbreviations

- Epithelioid hemangioendothelioma (EHE)

Definitions

- Low-grade malignant vascular endothelial cell neoplasm with epithelioid cytomorphology

ETIOLOGY/PATHOGENESIS

Chromosomal Translocation

- Fusion of *WWTR1* (WW domain-containing transcription regulator 1) with *CAMTA1* [calmodulin-binding transcription activator 1 t(1;3)(p36;q25)]
- Distinct (and rare) subset of *CAMTA1* translocation-negative cases with *YAP1*::*TFE3* fusion

CLINICAL ISSUES

Epidemiology

- Age
  - Young to middle-aged adults
- Sex
  - More common in female patients

Presentation

- Common sites: Lung, liver, skin, bone/soft tissue
- Clinical signs include pain, enlarging mass, pathologic fracture, cough/dyspnea, and hemorrhage

Treatment

- Surgical approaches
  - Resection of localized disease (often curative)
  - Liver transplantation for isolated hepatic disease
    - May be curative, but recurrence is common
- Chemotherapy
  - Conventional or antiangiogenic (e.g., bevacizumab)

Prognosis

- Better when lesions are discrete with well-defined borders
  - 1-, 5-, and 10-year survival rates: 96%, 84%, and 78%
- Worse with ill-defined lesions, extrapulmonary thoracic disease, pleural effusions, or extensive metastatic disease
  - 1-, 5-, and 10-year survival rates: 62%, 25%, and 10%

IMAGING

General Features

- Small, well-defined nodules; often multiple
- Lung: May involve parenchyma &/or pleura; often bilateral
- Liver: Often present in both lobes

MACROSCOPIC

General Features

- Often multicentric but occasionally solitary
- Gray-white, very firm nodules
- May be focally calcified

MICROSCOPIC

Histologic Features

- Epithelioid cells with eosinophilic cytoplasm
- Oval, vesicular nuclei with inconspicuous nucleoli
- Intracytoplasmic vacuoles, sometimes with erythrocytes
- Abundant myxoid and variably hyalinized stroma
- Calcification of dense, hyalinized stroma may occur
- Paucicellular in center, more cellular at periphery
- Mitotic activity and necrosis minimal to absent
- Vascular invasion common; mimics organizing thrombi

ANCILLARY TESTS

Immunohistochemistry

- CAMTA1 IHC highly specific
- Vascular markers usually strongly positive
  - CD31, CD34, factor VIII-related antigen
- Keratins often positive

In Situ Hybridization

- FISH for *WWTR1*::*CAMTA1* translocation

DIFFERENTIAL DIAGNOSIS

Carcinoma (Primary or Metastatic)

- Intracytoplasmic vacuoles may contain mucin but not erythrocytes
- Will stain for keratins but not vascular markers
- Greater nuclear pleomorphism

Epithelioid Angiosarcoma

- Mitotic activity and nuclear atypia more pronounced
- Necrosis more extensive

Epithelioid Sarcoma

- Stains for keratins, EMA, and CD34, but not CD31
- Displays more sheet-like growth

Myxoid Liposarcoma

- Displays characteristic fine, branching vessels
- Lipoblasts present
- Positive for S100 protein

DIAGNOSTIC CHECKLIST

Clinically Relevant Pathologic Features

- Infiltrative pattern portends worse prognosis

Pathologic Interpretation Pearls

- Significant atypia and mitotic activity indicate higher grade neoplasm, such as epithelioid angiosarcoma
- Potential pitfall: Keratins often positive; staining for vascular markers will prevent misdiagnosis

SELECTED REFERENCES

1. Deng Y et al: Primary cardiac epithelioid haemangioendothelioma. Eur Heart J. 42(15):1532, 2021
2. WHO Classification of Tumours Editorial Board: WHO Classification of Tumours: Thoracic Tumours. 5th ed. IARC Press, 2021
3. Agulnik M et al: An open-label, multicenter, phase II study of bevacizumab for the treatment of angiosarcoma and epithelioid hemangioendotheliomas. Ann Oncol. 24(1):257-63, 2013
4. Tanas MR et al: Identification of a disease-defining gene fusion in epithelioid hemangioendothelioma. Sci Transl Med. 3(98):98ra82, 2011
5. Deyrup AT et al: Epithelioid hemangioendothelioma of soft tissue: a proposal for risk stratification based on 49 cases. Am J Surg Pathol. 32(6):924-7, 2008

Epithelioid Hemangioendothelioma

(Left) *Formerly known as the intravascular bronchioloalveolar tumor, pulmonary EHE is characterized by lobulated nodules that expand and fill airspaces along a well-defined front* ➡ *without inducing a desmoplastic reaction.* **(Right)** *On higher power, the advancing edge of the tumor has a micronodular appearance due to its lepidic growth through the alveolar pores of Kohn, filling adjacent alveolar spaces and even airways* ↪ *while mostly preserving the alveolar walls* ➡*.*

Epithelioid Hemangioendothelioma in Lung

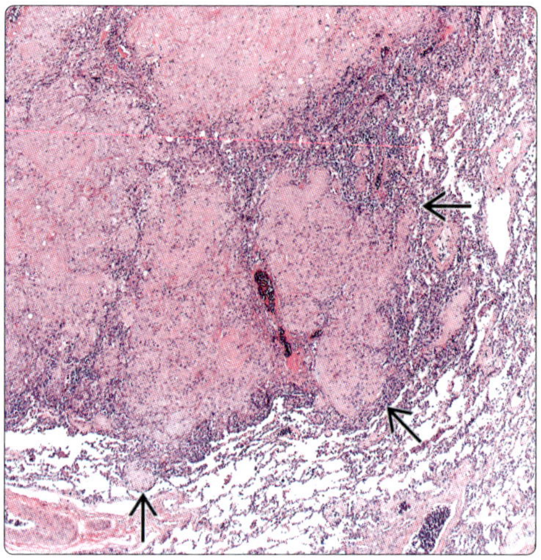

Epithelioid Hemangioendothelioma: Lepidic-Like Growth

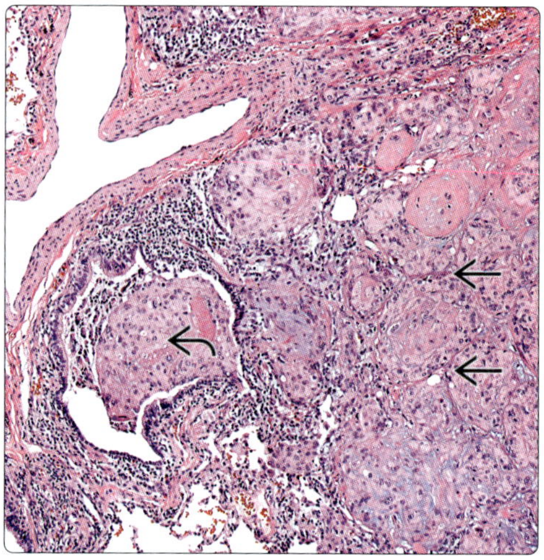

(Left) *The advancing edge of the tumor* ➡ *is often more hypercellular than are the central areas* ⇨*. In larger nodules, central areas can be hyalinized or necrotic with few remaining tumor cells (as in this case). Occasionally, central portions of tumor nodules may even undergo calcification.* **(Right)** *On higher power view, large epithelioid tumor cells with abundant eosinophilic cytoplasm and occasional intracytoplasmic vacuoles* ↪ *are embedded within a myxohyaline fibrous stroma.*

Epithelioid Hemangioendothelioma: Central Hyalinization

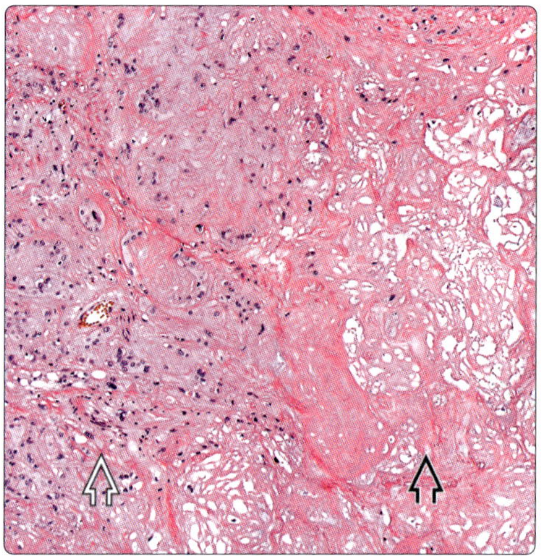

Epithelioid Hemangioendothelioma: High Magnification

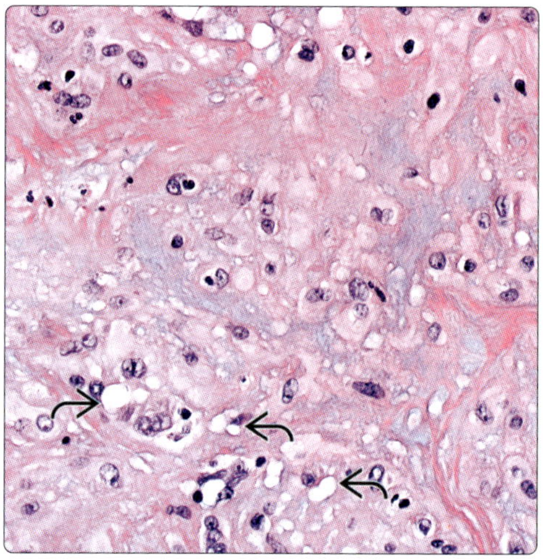

(Left) *At high power, cords and nests of tumor cells are seen in a background of dense, hyalinized fibrous stroma. In this case, the myxoid stromal element is much less apparent. Note the numerous intracytoplasmic vacuoles* ➡*, some of which contain erythrocytes* ↪*.* **(Right)** *CD31 immunohistochemistry highlights the large epithelioid tumor cells* ⇨ *of pulmonary EHE, confirming their endothelial differentiation, and also stains the native capillaries within alveolar walls* ➡*.*

Epithelioid Hemangioendothelioma With More Subtle Intracytoplasmic Lumina

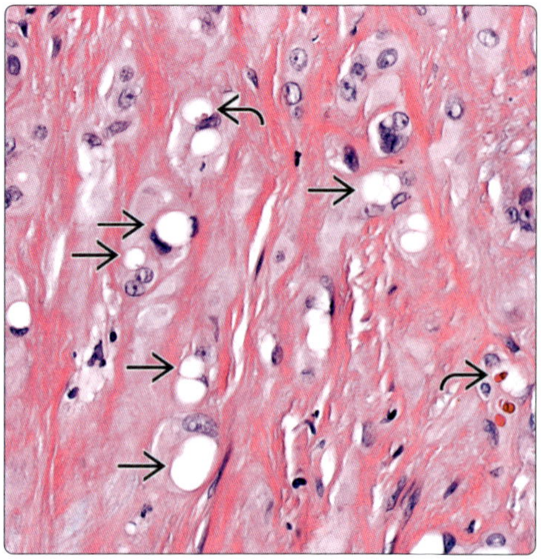

Epithelioid Hemangioendothelioma: CD31 Stain

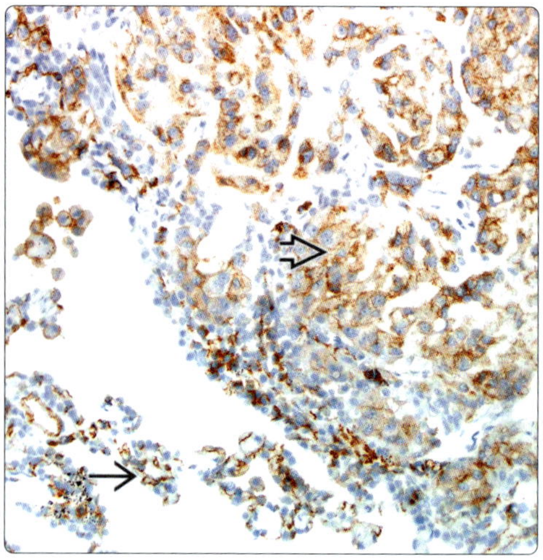

Epithelioid Hemangioendothelioma in Liver

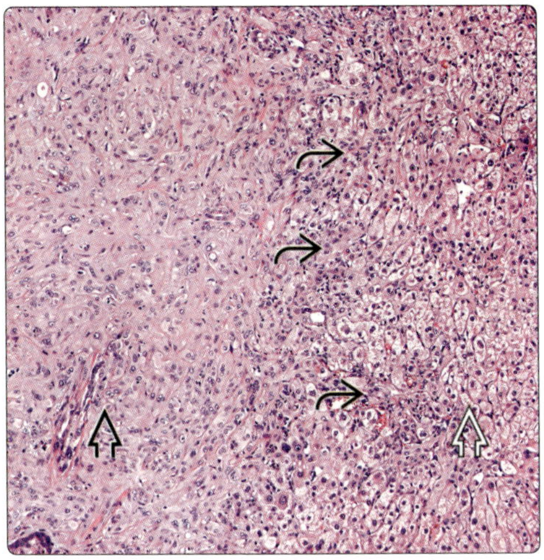

Epithelioid Hemangioendothelioma in Liver With Sclerotic Stroma

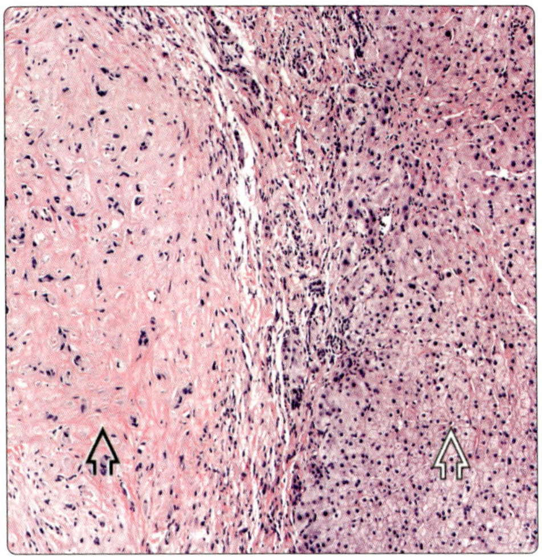

(Left) *Like its pulmonary counterpart, hepatic EHE is characterized by multiple nodules of epithelioid tumor cells in a myxohyaline stroma. At its advancing edge, infiltration of hepatic sinusoids ⇨ blurs the border between the tumor ⇨ and the adjacent hepatic parenchyma* ➡. **(Right)** *In more advanced lesions, the nodule ⇨ may become less cellular with stroma that is more sclerotic, and its border with the adjacent hepatic parenchyma* ➡ *may become more distinct.*

Epithelioid Hemangioendothelioma in Liver: Vascular Invasion

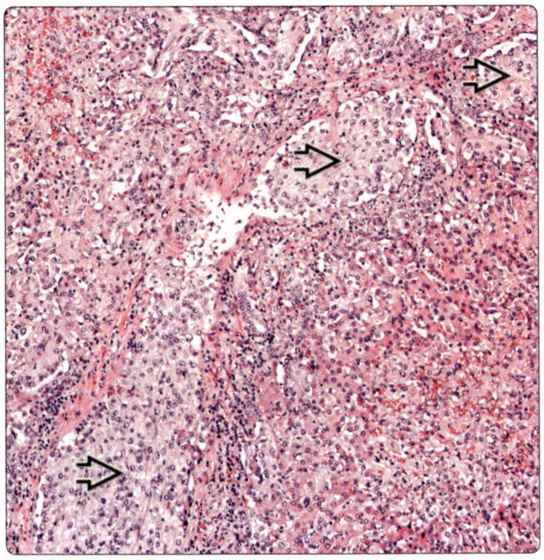

Myxohyaline Stroma in Epithelioid Hemangioendothelioma

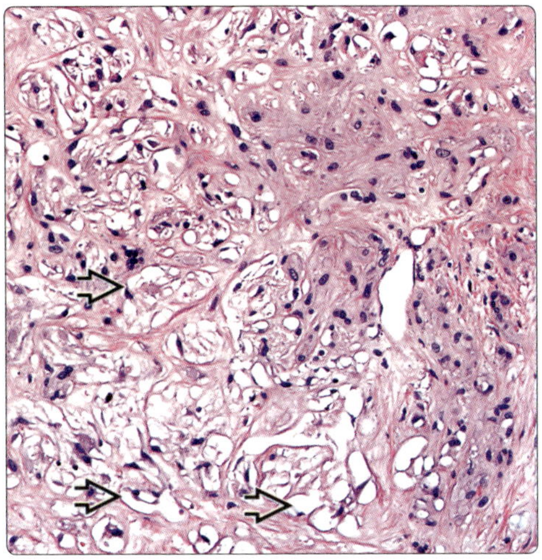

(Left) *EHE displays a penchant for vascular invasion. In this case, plugs of tumor cells ⇨ fill vessels, mimicking organizing thrombus. When observed near the main lesion, this phenomenon is readily recognized as vascular invasion. Farther away, particularly with inadequate sampling, this can be misdiagnosed as thrombus.* **(Right)** *Epithelioid tumor cells are embedded in a myxohyaline stroma. Intracytoplasmic vacuolization ⇨ is sometimes extensive.*

Epithelioid Hemangioendothelioma: High Magnification

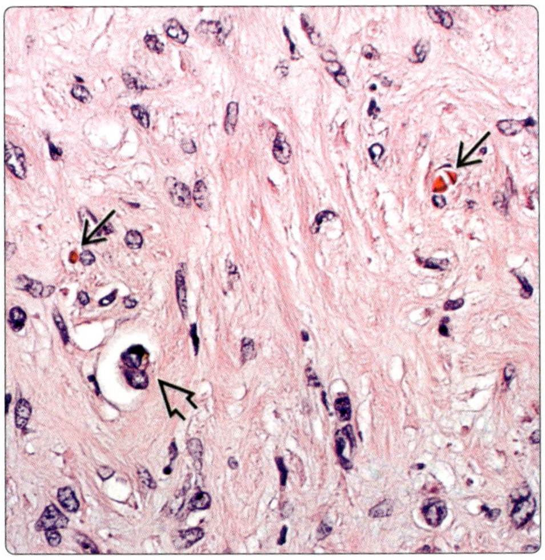

Metastatic Epithelioid Hemangioendothelioma in Lymph Node

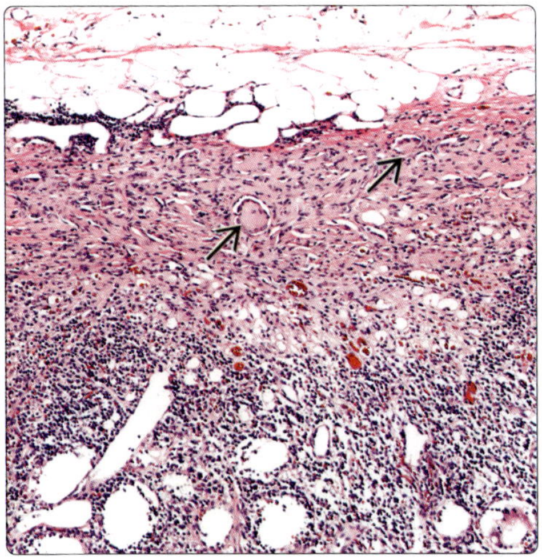

(Left) *On high power, papillary tufting of tumor cells is seen within a primitive vascular lumen ⇨, and occasional intracytoplasmic lumina contain erythrocytes ⇨. Both features are common in vascular neoplasms, including EHE.* **(Right)** *Metastasis to other sites may occur, including lungs, bones, and lymph nodes. In this case of hepatic EHE, metastatic tumor fills the subcapsular sinus of a lymph node. Note the prominent papillary tufting ⇨ within the metastatic deposit.*

Kaposi Sarcoma

KEY FACTS

TERMINOLOGY

- Low-grade malignant endothelial neoplasm associated with human herpesvirus 8 (HHV-8) infection
- 4 major types: Classic Kaposi sarcoma (KS), endemic KS, AIDS-associated KS, iatrogenic KS

CLINICAL ISSUES

- Skin lesions on feet &/or legs
  - 3 overlapping stages: Patch, plaque, nodular
- Classic KS usually indolent
- Endemic KS indolent in adults, aggressive in children
- AIDS-associated and iatrogenic KS often aggressive
- Local surgical excision, especially for single lesions
- Highly active retroviral therapy for AIDS-associated KS
- Systemic chemotherapy for widespread disease

MACROSCOPIC

- Reddish blue skin macules, plaques, or nodules

MICROSCOPIC

- Depends on stage
  - Patch: Irregular vascular channels in dermis
  - Plaque: Like patch stage but with spindle cell areas
  - Nodular: Predominantly spindle cell component
- Promontory sign: Vessel-around-vessel pattern
- Fascicles of spindle cells with sieve-like spaces
- Extravasated red cells and hyaline globules
- Scattered lymphocytes and plasma cells

ANCILLARY TESTS

- HHV8 positive in nearly all cases
- Other vascular markers often positive (e.g., CD31, CD34, FLI1; none are specific for KS)
- D2-40
  - Positive in > 1/2 of cases of KS

Kaposi Sarcoma: Low Magnification

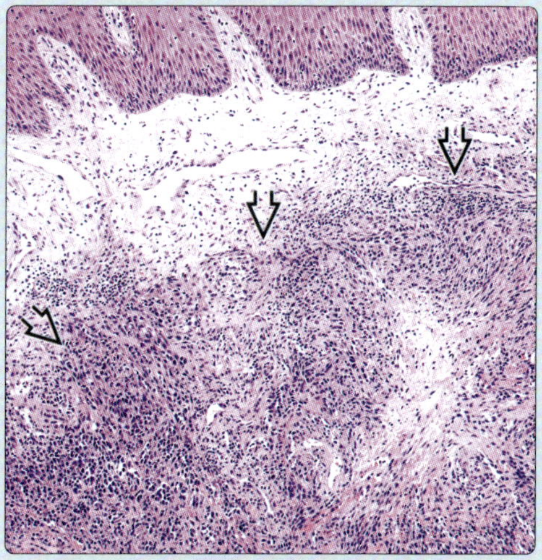

Kaposi Sarcoma: Higher Magnification

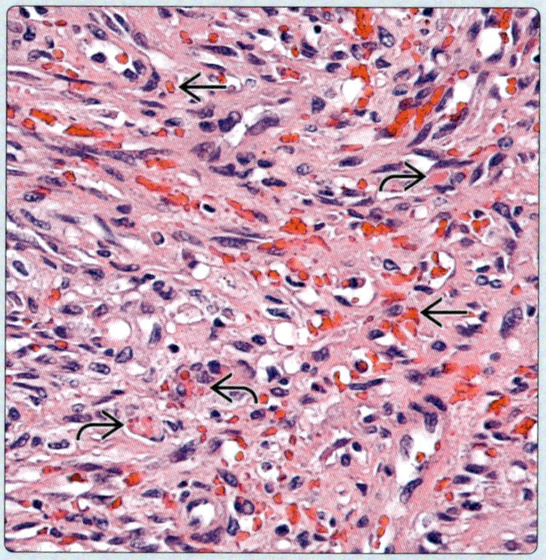

(Left) *Kaposi sarcoma (KS) usually presents on lower extremities as skin patches, plaques, or nodules (as in this case) and is characterized by neoplastic proliferations of vessels in the dermis due to human herpesvirus 8 (HHV-8) infection.* **(Right)** *Under high magnification, bland, spindled cells line sieve-like vascular spaces. Numerous extravasated erythrocytes and hyaline (eosinophilic) globules are present.*

Clinical Appearance of Kaposi Sarcoma: Thigh

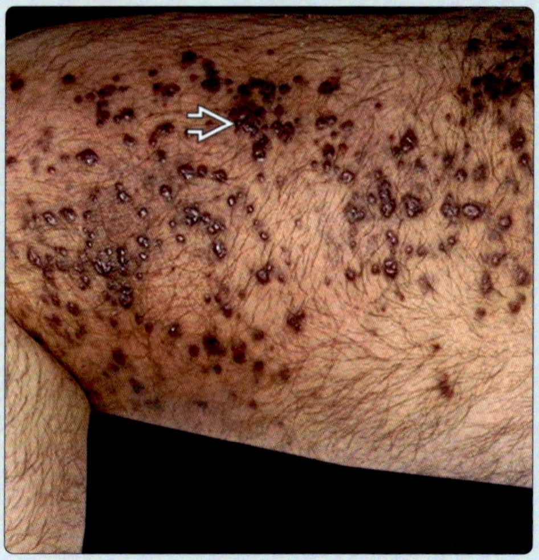

Clinical Appearance of Kaposi Sarcoma: Toes

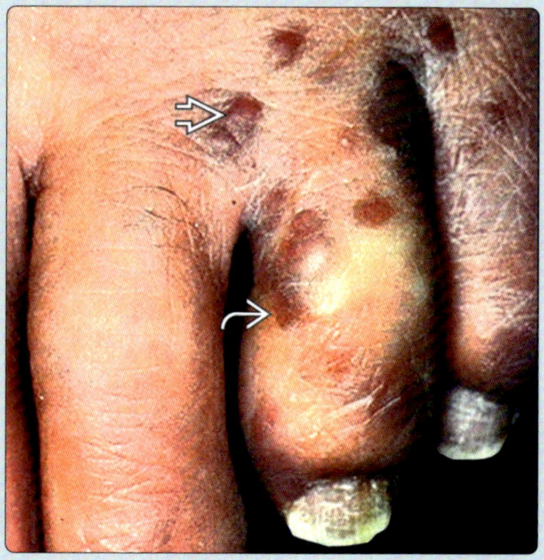

(Left) *In this patient, there are patches, plaques, and nodules. Lesions may remain unchanged for years or may grow rapidly and disseminate within weeks.* **(Right)** *KS typically involves the lower extremities, as in this example. Both flat, violaceous lesions and raised plaques are seen.*

TERMINOLOGY

Abbreviations

- Kaposi sarcoma (KS)

Definitions

- Borderline or low-grade malignant endothelial neoplasm associated with human herpesvirus 8 (HHV-8) infection
- 4 major types recognized
  - Classic (a.k.a. European, chronic)
  - Endemic (a.k.a. African, lymphadenopathic)
  - AIDS associated
  - Iatrogenic (a.k.a. immunosuppression or transplant associated)

ETIOLOGY/PATHOGENESIS

Infectious Agents

- HHV-8
  - a.k.a. KS-associated herpesvirus
  - Latent infection of endothelial cells

Predisposing Conditions

- Compromised immune status
  - Infectious (e.g., HIV infection or AIDS)
  - Iatrogenic (e.g., status post organ transplantation)

Classic Kaposi Sarcoma

- Older men, typically 50-70 years of age
  - M:F = 10-15:1
- Eastern European or Mediterranean descent
- Ashkenazi Jews

Endemic Kaposi Sarcoma

- Equatorial Africa (similar distribution as endemic Burkitt lymphoma)
- Children and younger adults
- More common in male patients

AIDS-Associated Kaposi Sarcoma

- May precede clinical recognition of AIDS
- Most cases (~ 95%) reported in homosexual or bisexual men
- Before highly active antiretroviral therapy (HAART), up to 1/3 of AIDS patients were affected
- Now KS is rare in AIDS patients treated with HAART (< 1%)

Iatrogenic Kaposi Sarcoma

- Especially after solid organ transplantation
  - Average time after transplant: 16 months
- Occasionally occurs after bone marrow transplantation

CLINICAL ISSUES

Presentation

- Skin lesions most common
  - Usually on feet &/or lower legs
  - 3 progressive and overlapping stages
    - Patches
    - Plaques
    - Nodules
  - May ulcerate and bleed easily, especially nodular lesions
  - May be accompanied by lymphedema of involved extremity
  - Growth rate is highly variable
    - Lesions may remain unchanged for years or may grow rapidly and disseminate within weeks
- Extracutaneous involvement is uncommon
  - Mucous membranes of GI tract
  - Lymph nodes (most common in endemic KS)
  - Visceral organ involvement (especially in AIDS-associated or iatrogenic KS)

Treatment

- Surgical approaches
  - Local excision, especially for single symptomatic lesions
- Drugs
  - HAART for AIDS-associated KS
  - Topical cis-retinoic acid, especially for AIDS-associated KS
- Radiation
  - KS is usually very sensitive to radiotherapy
  - Despite excellent initial responses, utility is limited by multifocal nature of disease and tendency to recur in nonirradiated areas
- Intralesional chemotherapy
  - Mostly for small or localized symptomatic lesions
- Systemic chemotherapy
  - For rapidly progressive, widespread, or bulky KS
  - Especially for AIDS-associated KS
- Observation
  - Especially for classic KS, when lesions are small and limited to lower extremities

Prognosis

- Depends on type of KS
  - Classic KS is usually indolent but rarely may be aggressive and disseminated
  - Endemic KS is usually indolent in adults but aggressive in children
  - AIDS-associated KS may be aggressive or indolent and may regress with HAART
  - Iatrogenic KS may be aggressive or indolent and may regress with modification of immunosuppressive regimen

MACROSCOPIC

General Features

- Skin lesions range from small macules/patches to larger plaques, and eventually to bulky nodules or masses
- Color of lesions may be purplish, reddish blue, dark brown, or black

Size

- Lesions range from few millimeters to many centimeters in greatest dimension

MICROSCOPIC

Histologic Features

- Similar in all types of KS
- Patch stage
  - Subtle proliferation of irregular, jagged vascular channels in superficial dermis

- Channels surround adnexal structures and normal vessels
  - Promontory sign: Vessel-around-vessel growth pattern with proliferating channels rimming normal vessels
- Channels lined by single layer of minimally to mildly atypical endothelial cells
- Extravasated red cells, intracellular and extracellular hyaline (eosinophilic) globules, and hemosiderin often present
- Scattered lymphocytes and plasma cells often seen

- Plaque stage
  - Similar to patch stage but also shows progressively increasing spindle cell component
  - Short fascicles of spindle cells with sieve-like vascular spaces; occasional mitotic figure
- Nodular stage
  - Large, well-circumscribed nodular proliferation in dermis &/or subcutis
  - Nodules consist almost entirely of spindle cell component with sieve-like vascular spaces
  - Mitotic figures may be frequent

ANCILLARY TESTS

Histochemistry

- PAS-D
  - Staining pattern: Hyaline globules stain strongly and are diastase resistant

Immunohistochemistry

- HHV8
  - Positive in nearly all cases and all variants
  - Stains nuclei
  - Number of positive-staining cells may vary
  - Highly specific for KS
    - Other vascular neoplasms virtually always negative
- Other vascular endothelial markers (none specific for KS)
  - CD34
    - Positive in > 90% of cases of KS; especially stains spindle cell component
    - Also stains variety of other vascular, mesenchymal, and hematologic neoplasms
  - CD31
    - Positive in up to 75% of cases of KS
    - Also stains variety of other vascular neoplasms
  - FLI1
    - Positive in up to 75% of cases of KS
    - Also stains angiosarcoma and Ewing/peripheral neuroectodermal tumor family of tumors
  - D2-40
    - Positive in > 1/2 of cases of KS
    - Also stains lymphatic channels

In Situ Hybridization

- Alternatively, HHV-8 may be detected by this method

PCR

- Rarely performed now that antibodies directed against HHV-8 are widely available for immunohistochemistry

DIFFERENTIAL DIAGNOSIS

Benign Vascular Proliferations

- Acroangiodermatitis
  - Vascular channels generally not irregular
  - Does not involve adnexal structures or show promontory sign
  - Does not stain for HHV-8
- Bacillary angiomatosis
  - Endothelial cells usually more epithelioid
  - Mixed inflammatory infiltrate usually more pronounced, including numerous neutrophils
  - *Bartonella* organisms present (may be identified by Warthin-Starry or Giemsa stain, immunohistochemistry, or PCR)
  - Does not stain for HHV-8
- Aneurysmal fibrous histiocytoma
  - Giant cells and foam cells often present
  - Does not stain for HHV-8
- Vascular transformation of lymph node sinuses
  - Vascular channels more distinct, without hyaline globules
  - Does not stain for HHV-8

Benign Spindle Cell Proliferations

- Spindle cell hemangioma
  - Typically displays some cavernous foci
  - Lacks hyaline globules; does not stain for HHV-8
- Angioleiomyoma
  - Lacks dense, sieve-like vessels
  - Lacks hyaline globules
  - Does not stain for HHV-8
  - Smooth muscle bundles stain positive for desmin

Malignant Neoplasms

- Kaposiform hemangioendothelioma
  - Usually in infants or young children, usually < 2 years old
  - Usually forms lobules separated by fibrous septa
  - Does not stain for HHV-8
- Angiosarcoma
  - Usually shows marked cytologic atypia
  - Mitotic activity usually prominent
  - May show endothelial multilayering
  - Does not stain for HHV-8

DIAGNOSTIC CHECKLIST

Pathologic Interpretation Pearls

- HHV-8 is positive in virtually all cases and is highly specific, but extent of HHV-8 positivity varies

SELECTED REFERENCES

1. WHO Classification of Tumours Editorial Board: WHO Classification of Tumours: Thoracic Tumours. 5th ed. IARC Press, 2021
2. Grabar S et al: Differential impact of combination antiretroviral therapy in preventing Kaposi's sarcoma with and without visceral involvement. J Clin Oncol. 24(21):3408-14, 2006
3. Cheuk W et al: Immunostaining for human herpesvirus 8 latent nuclear antigen-1 helps distinguish Kaposi sarcoma from its mimickers. Am J Clin Pathol. 121(3):335-42, 2004
4. Patel RM et al: Immunohistochemical detection of human herpes virus-8 latent nuclear antigen-1 is useful in the diagnosis of Kaposi sarcoma. Mod Pathol. 17(4):456-60, 2004

Kaposi Sarcoma: Subtle Patch Stage at Low Magnification

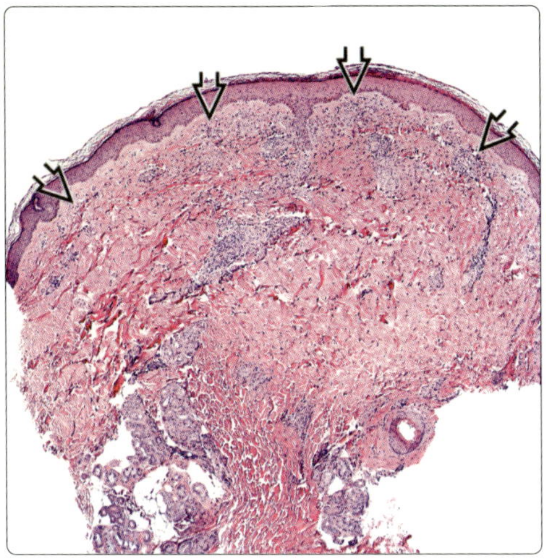

Kaposi Sarcoma: Subtle Patch Stage at Medium Magnification

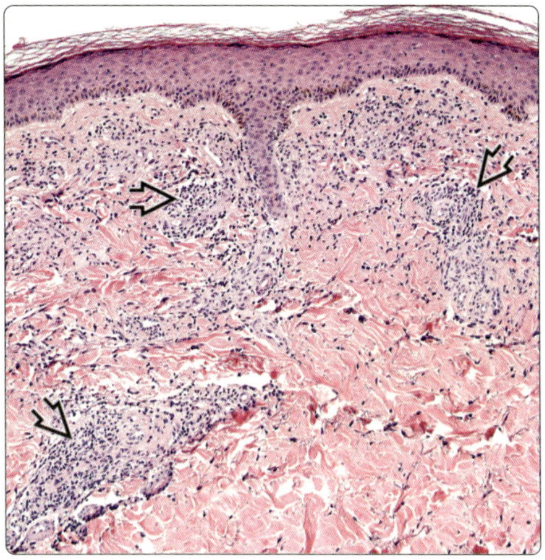

(Left) *At scanning magnification, the patch stage of KS can be extremely subtle with vague hypercellular areas ⇨ in the superficial dermis. At this magnification, the proliferating vascular channels are inapparent.* **(Right)** *At medium magnification, histologic findings in the patch stage remain subtle. Scattered lymphocytes ⇨ surround dermal vessels, a finding that may be misinterpreted as a mild inflammatory dermatosis.*

Kaposi Sarcoma: Subtle Patch Stage at High Magnification

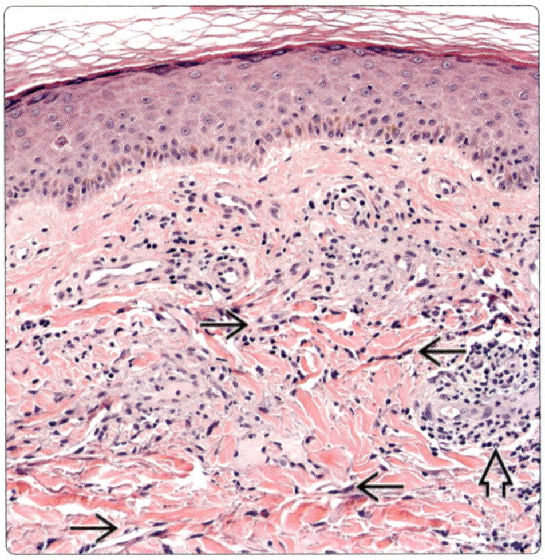

Kaposi Sarcoma: High Magnification With Slit-Like Channels

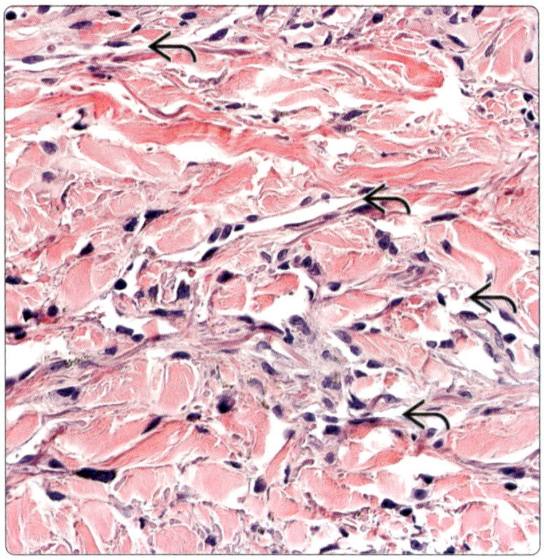

(Left) *At higher magnification, the distinction of the patch stage of KS from an inflammatory dermatosis is more apparent. Irregular, slit-like vascular channels → are present in the superficial dermis and are generally arranged parallel to the epidermis. A chronic mixed inflammatory infiltrate ⇨ is commonly seen in KS.* **(Right)** *At high power, irregular, slit-like vascular channels ↶ dissect between dermal collagen bundles. These channels are lined by bland endothelial cells.*

Kaposi Sarcoma: CD31 Stain

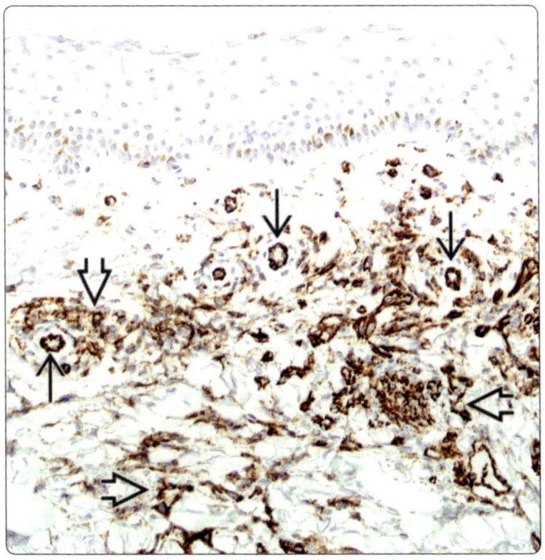

Kaposi Sarcoma: HHV8 Stain

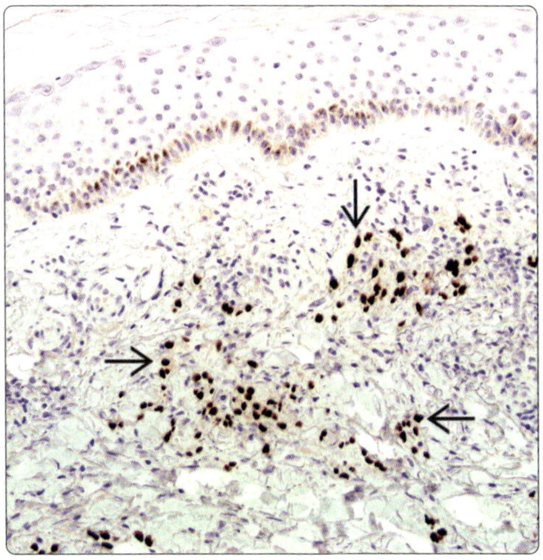

(Left) *Immunohistochemical staining for CD31 is often strongly positive in KS, highlighting neoplastic vascular channels ⇨ in the superficial dermis. This stain may enable recognition of the extent of tumor growth, which may be underestimated on H&E stains alone. Note the positive staining of nonneoplastic vessels in the superficial dermis →.* **(Right)** *In the patch stage of KS, immunohistochemical staining for HHV8 highlights nuclei of scattered neoplastic endothelial cells →.*

(Left) *At scanning magnification, the plaque stage of KS shows neoplastic vascular channels* → *in the superficial and middermis with relative preservation of deeper tissues* ⇨*. In other areas, a solid spindle cell component* ↪ *is readily identified.* **(Right)** *On medium power, irregular vascular channels* → *invade the dermis. Many are oriented parallel to the epidermis. A spindle cell component* ⇨ *is also present with abundant hyaline globules* ↪ *seen even at this power.*

Kaposi Sarcoma: Plaque Stage, Low Magnification

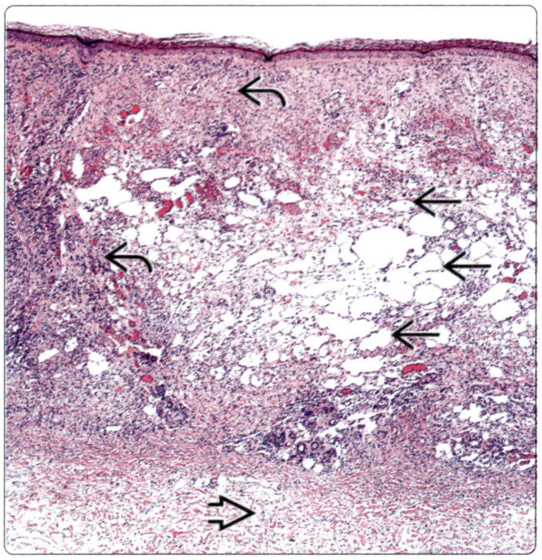

Kaposi Sarcoma With Spindled Cells

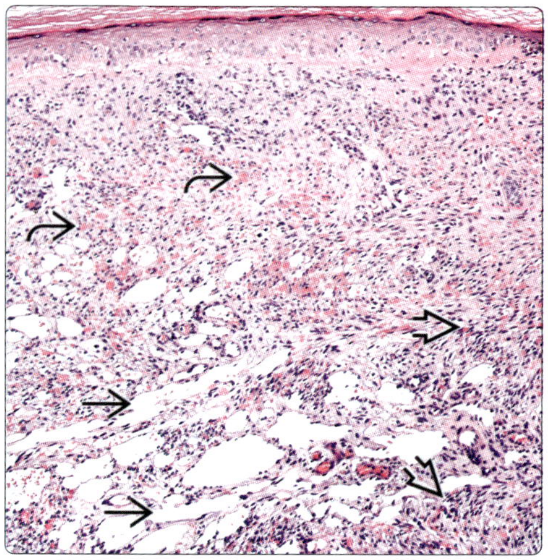

(Left) *At higher power, irregular, slit-like vascular channels* → *dissect not only between collagen bundles but also between deeper dermal adnexal structures, as in this case involving eccrine glands* ⇨*.* **(Right)** *Although not specific for KS, the promontory sign is often seen in the patch or plaque stages. Nonneoplastic vessels* ↪ *protrude into dilated neoplastic vascular spaces, like a high promontory of a rock jutting into the sea, to form a vessel-around-vessel pattern.*

Kaposi Sarcoma With Eccrine Involvement

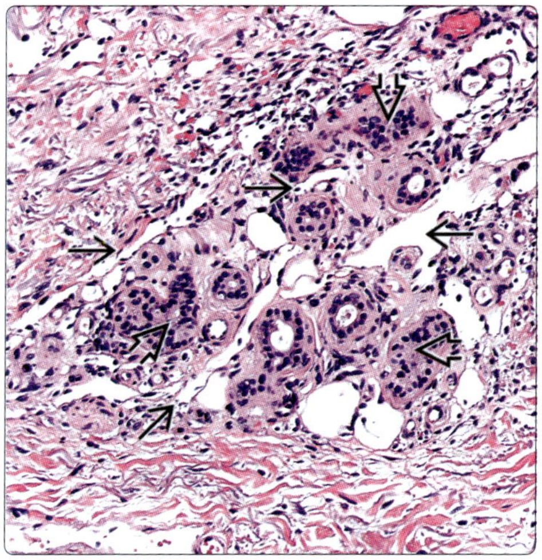

Promontory Sign in Kaposi Sarcoma

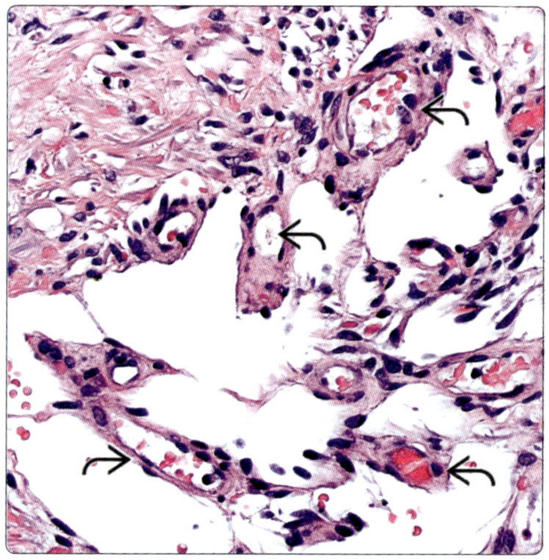

(Left) *The promontory sign may be formed not only by nonneoplastic vessels but also by adnexal structures. Note the single layer of bland endothelial cells* → *that surrounds an adnexal duct* ➥*. This phenomenon is produced by dilated neoplastic vascular channels as they completely envelop native structures.* **(Right)** *As in the patch stage, HHV-8 infection can be detected in the plaque stage by immunohistochemistry. The relative density of HHV-8-infected cells is greater in the plaque stage.*

Promontory Sign in Kaposi Sarcoma: Adnexal Structures

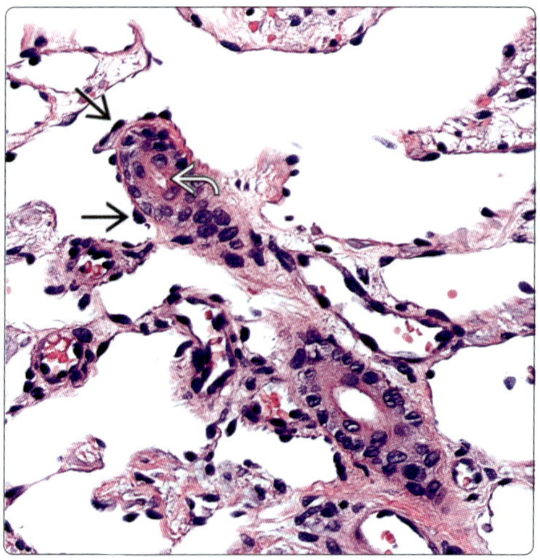

Kaposi Sarcoma: HHV8 Stain (Diffusely Positive)

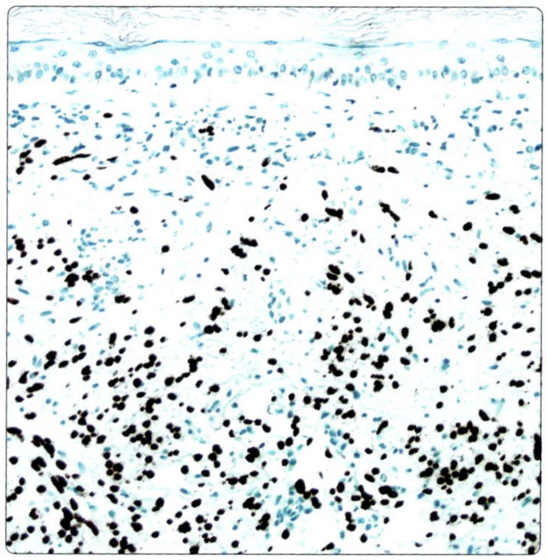

Kaposi Sarcoma: Nodular Stage (Low Magnification)

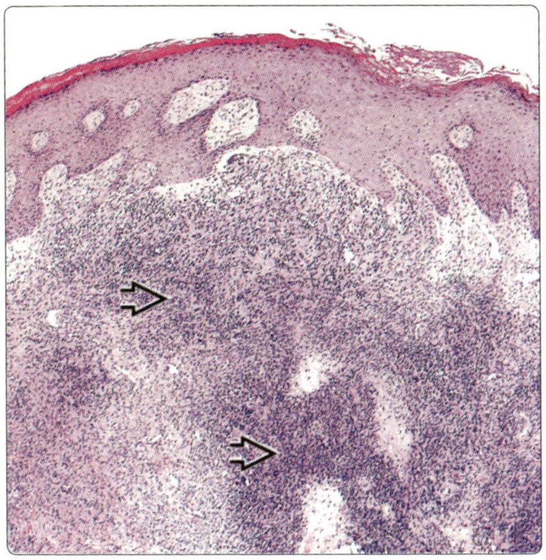

Kaposi Sarcoma: Nodular Stage

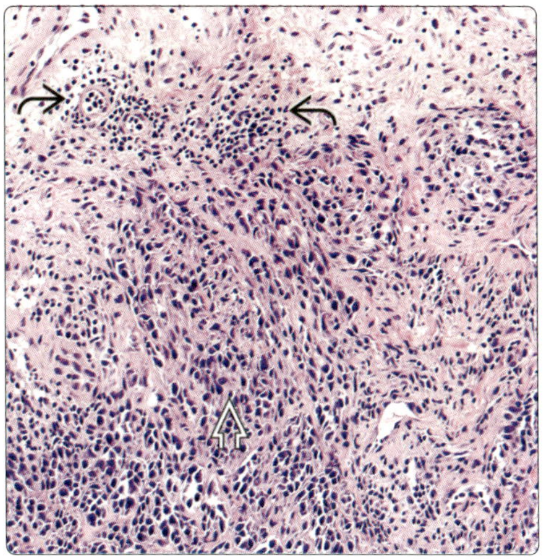

(Left) *At scanning magnification, the nodular stage of KS shows solid areas of spindled cells that efface the underlying dermal architecture. At this power, its vascular nature may not be immediately apparent.* **(Right)** *On higher power, the dense, sieve-like vascular channels are lined by endothelial cells that are plump but lack significant pleomorphism. At the edge of KS lesions, chronic inflammatory cells are often seen, even in the nodular stage.*

Kaposi Sarcoma: Epithelioid Morphology

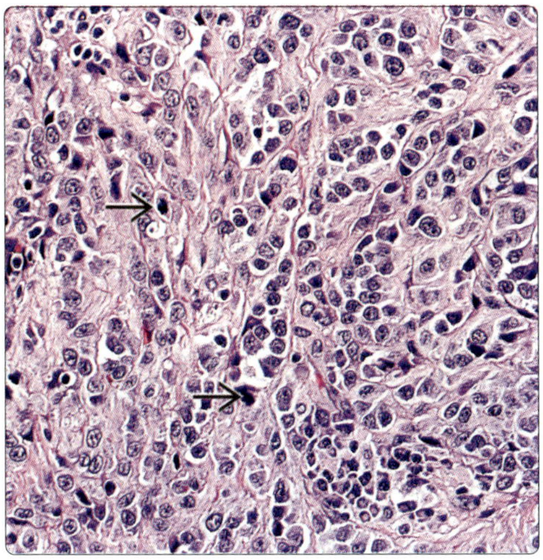

Kaposi Sarcoma: CD34 Stain

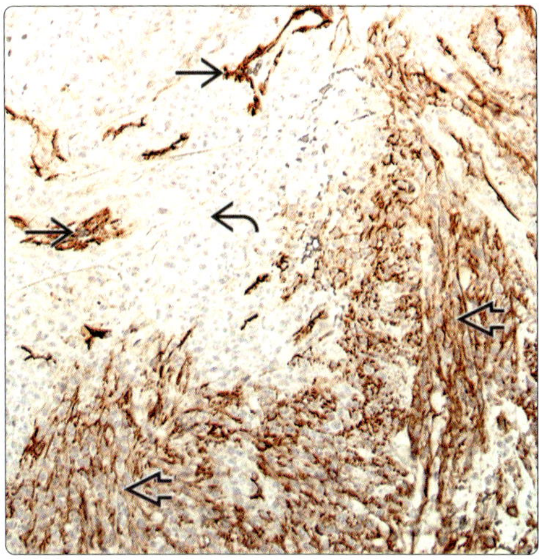

(Left) *In some cases, KS may acquire an epithelioid morphology, a feature that may make diagnosis difficult without adequate sampling or appropriate immunostains. Note the focally increased mitotic activity.* **(Right)** *CD34 immunohistochemistry is often positive in the spindle cell component, although CD34 may be absent in other areas. In this case, areas with epithelioid morphology lack CD34 expression. Note the entrapped CD34-positive nonneoplastic vessels.*

Kaposi Sarcoma: HHV8 Staining in Nodular Stage

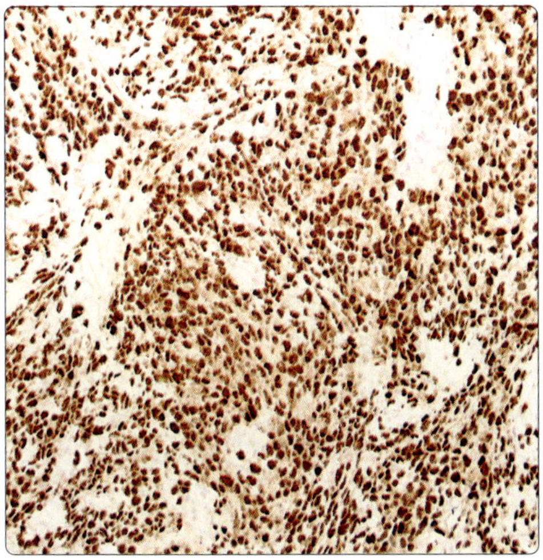

Kaposi Sarcoma: Lymph Node Metastasis

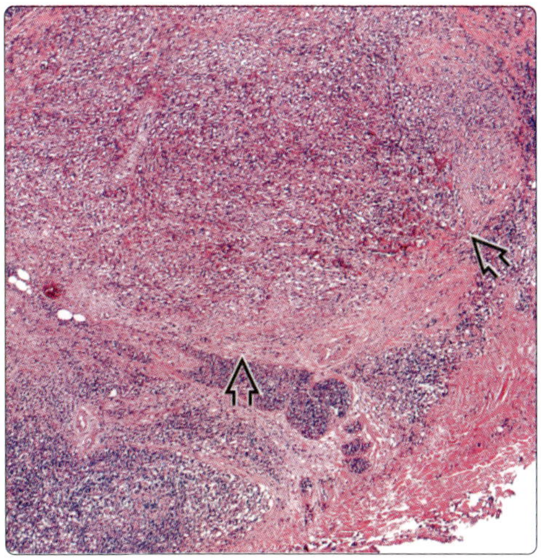

(Left) *Compared with the patch and plaque stages of KS, the density of HHV8 immunohistochemical staining is greatest in the nodular stage with virtually every spindle cell staining positive.* **(Right)** *Although lymph node involvement is unusual (except in children with endemic KS), bulky lymphadenopathy occasionally occurs in other types, particularly in cases of disseminated disease, as in this case of AIDS-associated nodular-stage KS with lymph node metastasis.*

Angiosarcoma

KEY FACTS

TERMINOLOGY

- Aggressive malignant vascular neoplasm

CLINICAL ISSUES

- Violaceous skin patches, nodules, and soft tissue masses
- Treated with wide excision, amputation, radiation, and chemotherapy
- Poor prognosis (5-year survival ~ 20%)
- Most common sites
  - Skin of head and neck in older patients
  - Skin of extremities
  - Skin irradiated during treatment for other malignancy
  - Rarely occurs in deep soft tissues, visceral organs
- Widespread metastasis common, especially to lungs

MACROSCOPIC

- Hemorrhagic friable nodules or masses
- Generally with infiltrative borders

MICROSCOPIC

- Anastomosing vascular channels lined by markedly atypical endothelial cells
  - Nuclear hyperchromasia, abundant mitoses
  - Invasion between collagen fibers of stroma
  - Perineural, perivascular, periadnexal invasion
- Many cases exhibit necrosis
- Some cases may exhibit epithelioid features
  - Epithelioid variant particularly aggressive
- Solid, undifferentiated component may be present

ANCILLARY TESTS

- Vascular markers (CD31, FLI1, ERG, CD34, FVIIIRAg) usually positive
- May express low molecular weight keratins
  - Especially epithelioid variant, which mimics carcinoma
  - Stains usually weak or patchy but may be strong

Cutaneous Angiosarcoma

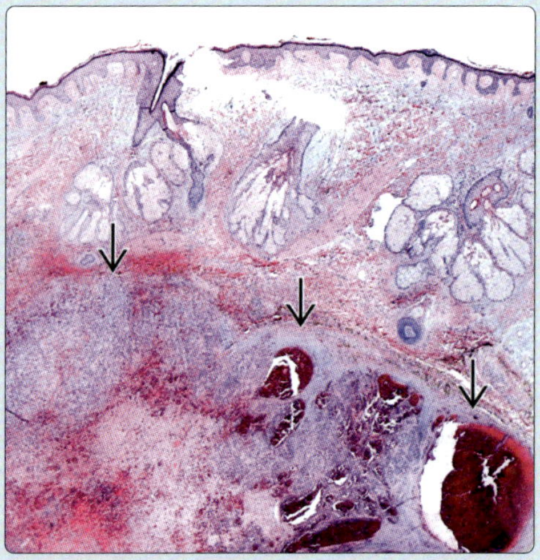

Atypia in Angiosarcoma

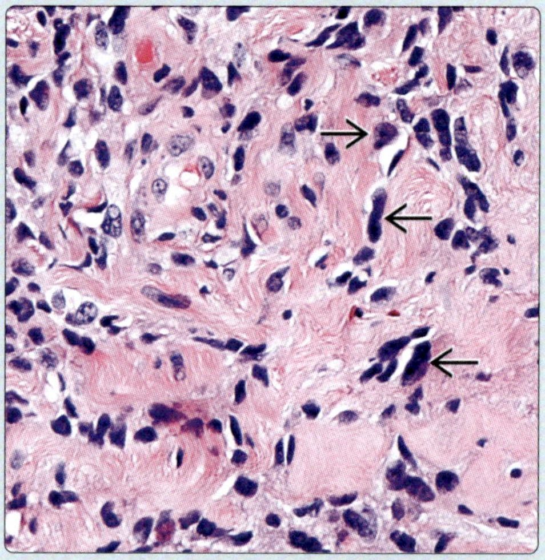

(Left) *Angiosarcoma most commonly involves the skin of the head and neck of older patients, where neoplastic vascular channels* → *of various sizes deeply invade the dermis and subcutaneous tissue.* **(Right)** *On high power, highly atypical endothelial cells with hyperchromatic nuclei* → *line slit-like rudimentary vascular channels that dissect between dermal collagen fibers.*

Interanastomosing Channels in Angiosarcoma

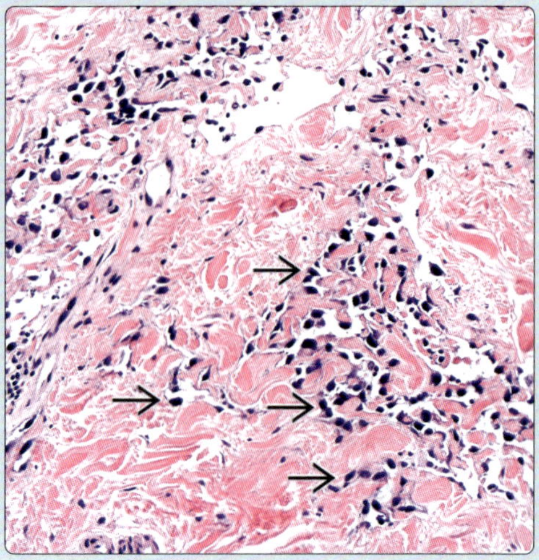

CD31 in Angiosarcoma

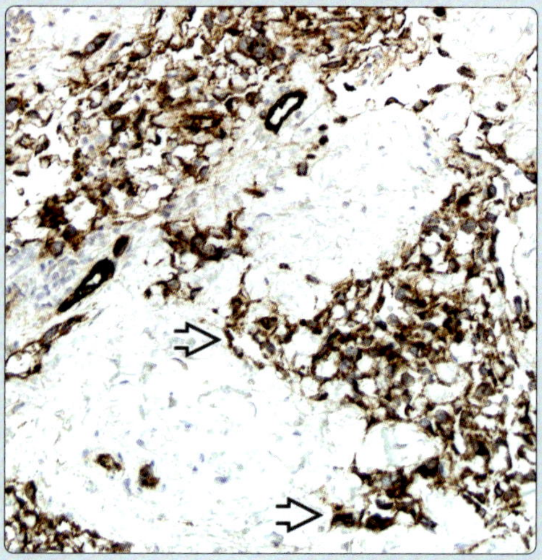

(Left) *Freely anastomosing irregular vascular channels* → *appear to dissect between dermal collagen fibers. These channels are lined by markedly hyperchromatic and atypical endothelial cells, cytologic features that help to differentiate a true angiosarcoma from benign and low-grade vascular neoplasms.* **(Right)** *CD31 shows malignant cells with strong cytoplasmic staining* ⇨*, a marker highly specific for endothelial differentiation.*

TERMINOLOGY

Abbreviations

- Angiosarcoma (AS)

Definitions

- Aggressive malignant neoplasm exhibiting vascular or lymphatic endothelial differentiation

ETIOLOGY/PATHOGENESIS

Environmental Exposure

- Radiotherapy for other malignancy
  - Breast and gynecologic malignancies, Hodgkin lymphoma
- Vinyl chloride, arsenic, other industrial chemicals
  - Associated with angiosarcoma of liver
- Indwelling foreign materials
  - Shrapnel, steel, plastic, synthetic grafts, others

Longstanding Lymphedema

- Usually after axillary lymphadenectomy
- Congenital
- Infectious
- Traumatic
- Pathogenesis unknown

CLINICAL ISSUES

Epidemiology

- Incidence
  - < 2% of all soft tissue sarcomas
  - In heart, AS represents ~ 40% of all cardiac sarcomas
- Sex
  - Distribution varies by site

Site

- Most common: Skin of scalp, face, and neck
  - Usually in older men
- Skin with chronic lymphedema (Stewart-Treves syndrome)
  - Arms
    - Seen after mastectomy with lymphadenectomy
    - May present decades after original surgery
  - Legs
    - Less common than cases involving arms
    - Etiology
      - Congenital
      - Traumatic
      - Filarial infections
      - Post surgery
- Skin irradiated during treatment for other malignancy
  - Breast most common location
    - Usually presents years after irradiation
- Deep soft tissues and bone
  - Usually in older patients, especially men
- Visceral organs
  - Liver, spleen, lung, heart, others
    - Rare location
    - In recent series, right atrium was most common location in heart

Presentation

- Violaceous skin patches, blue-black nodules
  - Often ulcerated, painful, nonhealing, bleeding
  - May be confused with bruising, edema, or infection
  - Breast radiation-associated AS may present
    - Skin rash, ecchymosis, or skin thickening on or near previous cancer and surgical site
- Deep soft tissue masses
  - May bleed, causing anemia
    - Hematoma, hemothorax, hemoperitoneum

Treatment

- Surgical approaches
  - Wide excision, amputation
  - May improve overall survival
- Radiation
  - Usually following surgery
  - Improves local control
- Chemotherapy
  - Less effective but used with unresectable tumors

Prognosis

- Poor, regardless of location, with 5-year survival ~ 20%
- Widespread metastasis common, especially to lungs

MACROSCOPIC

General Features

- Hemorrhagic, friable nodules or masses; often multiple
- Generally with infiltrative borders

MICROSCOPIC

Histologic Features

- Anastomosing vascular channels lined by markedly atypical endothelial cells, dissecting between stromal collagen
  - Nuclear hyperchromasia and abundant mitoses
  - Invasion around nerves, vessels, adnexal structures
- Many cases exhibit necrosis
- Solid, undifferentiated component may be seen
  - Intracytoplasmic lumina containing erythrocytes helpful, if present
- Some cases exhibit epithelioid features
  - Epithelioid variant particularly aggressive
- Biphasic pattern with spindle and epithelioid morphology can be seen

ANCILLARY TESTS

Immunohistochemistry

- Vascular markers usually positive
  - CD31
    - Most specific for endothelial differentiation
  - ERG
    - Highly sensitive endothelial marker
  - FLI1
    - Also expressed in Ewing sarcoma/peripheral neuroectodermal tumor (PNET) family
  - CD34
    - Less specific, expressed in variety of other mesenchymal and hematopoietic neoplasms
  - FVIIIRAg

 – Highly specific but least sensitive
- May express low molecular weight keratins &/or EMA
  - Especially epithelioid variant, which mimics carcinoma
  - Stains usually weak or patchy but may be strong

Genetic Testing

- Overall, *CIC* abnormalities occurred in 9% (9/98) of cases, affecting younger patients with primary AS with inferior disease-free survival
  - In contrast, *PLCG1* and *KDR* mutations occurred in both primary and secondary AS cases, accounting for 9.5% and 7%, respectively, with predilection for breast and bone/viscera location, regardless of *MYC* status
  - *MYC* amplification was present in most secondary AS related to breast cancer (91%) compared with other causes (25%) or primary AS (7%)
  - *FLT4*-amplified AS lacked *PLCG1/KDR* mutations, occurring predominantly in *MYC*-amplified population, and showed poor prognosis
- *CIC* rearrangements
  - Younger age, more solid morphology, shorter survival
- *PLCG1/KDR* mutations
  - Primary and secondary AS (especially breast and bone)
- *MYC* amplification
  - Secondary AS (especially breast)
  - Some primary AS (especially high grade)
- *FLT4* amplification
  - Often accompanies *MYC* amplification, portending even worse prognosis

DIFFERENTIAL DIAGNOSIS

Pseudoangiomatous Squamous Cell Carcinoma of Skin

- Dysplasia of overlying epithelium suggests squamous cell carcinoma
- Stains for p63 and high molecular weight keratins (HMWK) but not CD31 or CD34
- Potential pitfall: AS sometimes stains for low molecular weight keratins (LMWK) &/or EMA, especially epithelioid variant

Pseudoangiomatous Stromal Hyperplasia of Breast

- Lacks atypia, hyperchromasia, brisk mitotic activity
- Pitfall: Stains for CD34 but not CD31 or FVIIIRAg

Atypical Vascular Lesions

- Single/multiple pink papules in skin
- Usually develop 2-5 years post radiotherapy
- Focal proliferation of dilated vascular channels with single endothelial lining in papillary/reticular dermis
- Hyperchromatic nuclei but without atypia or mitosis
- Negative for *MYC* overexpression or amplification

Pseudoangiomatous Mesothelioma

- Stains for mesothelial markers (HMWK, calretinin, WT-1, others)
- Lacks vascular markers [occasionally CD34(+)]
- Pitfalls: AS usually stains for WT-1 and sometimes for LMWK &/or EMA, especially epithelioid variant

Epithelioid Hemangioendothelioma

- Lacks cytologic atypia and significant mitotic activity

Kaposi Sarcoma

- Lacks cytologic atypia
- Positive immunostaining for HHV8 in nearly all cases

DIAGNOSTIC CHECKLIST

Clinically Relevant Pathologic Features

- Epithelioid variant particularly aggressive

Pathologic Interpretation Pearls

- Atypia &/or mitoses help to exclude benign or low-grade neoplasm
- Immunohistochemical stains for vascular markers critical for diagnosis

SELECTED REFERENCES

1. Yin K et al: Survival outcomes in patients with primary cardiac sarcoma in the United States. J Thorac Cardiovasc Surg. 162(1):107-15.e2, 2021
2. Tyebally S et al: Cardiac tumors: JACC CardioOncology state-of-the-art review. JACC CardioOncol. 2(2):293-311, 2020
3. Chen TW et al: Primary cardiac sarcomas: a multi-national retrospective review. Cancer Med. 8(1):104-10, 2019
4. Linfeng Q et al: Cardiac angiosarcoma: a case report and review of current treatment. Medicine (Baltimore). 98(49):e18193, 2019
5. Zhang C et al: Clinical characteristics associated with primary cardiac angiosarcoma outcomes: a surveillance, epidemiology and end result analysis. Eur J Med Res. 24(1):29, 2019
6. Leduc C et al: Cardiac angiosarcoma: histopathologic, immunohistochemical, and cytogenetic analysis of 10 cases. Hum Pathol. 60:199-207, 2017
7. Agaimy A et al: Angiosarcoma arising in association with vascular Dacron grafts and orthopedic joint prostheses: clinicopathologic, immunohistochemical, and molecular study. Ann Diagn Pathol. 21:21-8, 2016
8. Huang SC et al: Recurrent CIC gene abnormalities in angiosarcomas: a molecular study of 120 cases with concurrent investigation of PLCG1, KDR, MYC, and FLT4 gene alterations. Am J Surg Pathol. 40(5):645-55, 2016
9. Shah S et al: Radiation-associated angiosarcoma of the breast: clinical and pathologic features. Arch Pathol Lab Med. 140(5):477-81, 2016
10. Udager AM et al: MYC immunohistochemistry in angiosarcoma and atypical vascular lesions: practical considerations based on a single institutional experience. Pathology. 48(7):697-704, 2016
11. Amitabha C et al: Primary pericardial angiosarcoma: a case report and review of literature. J Cardiothorac Surg. 10 Suppl 1:A36, 2015
12. Burke A et al: Tumors of the Heart and Great Vessels. American Registry of Pathology, 2015
13. Patel SH et al: Angiosarcoma of the scalp and face: the Mayo Clinic experience. JAMA Otolaryngol Head Neck Surg. 141(4):335-40 2015
14. Look Hong NJ et al: Cardiac angiosarcoma management and outcomes: 20-year single-institution experience. Ann Surg Oncol. 19(8):2707-15, 2012
15. Young RJ et al: Angiosarcoma. Lancet Oncol. 11(10):983-91, 2010
16. Lucas DR: Angiosarcoma, radiation-associated angiosarcoma, and atypical vascular lesion. Arch Pathol Lab Med. 133(11):1804-9, 2009
17. Weaver J et al: Postradiation cutaneous vascular tumors of the breast: a review. Semin Diagn Pathol. 26(3):141-9, 2009
18. Lydiatt WM et al: Angiosarcoma of the head and neck. Am J Surg. 168(5):451-4, 1994
19. Cooper PH: Angiosarcomas of the skin. Semin Diagn Pathol. 4(1):2-17, 1987

Subtle Example of Angiosarcoma

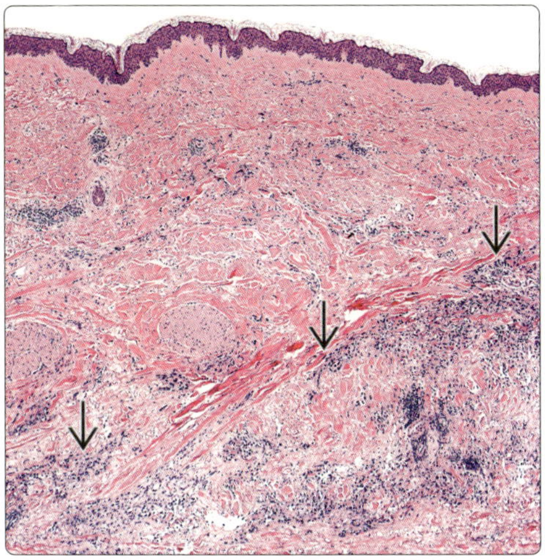

Angiosarcoma in Subcutis

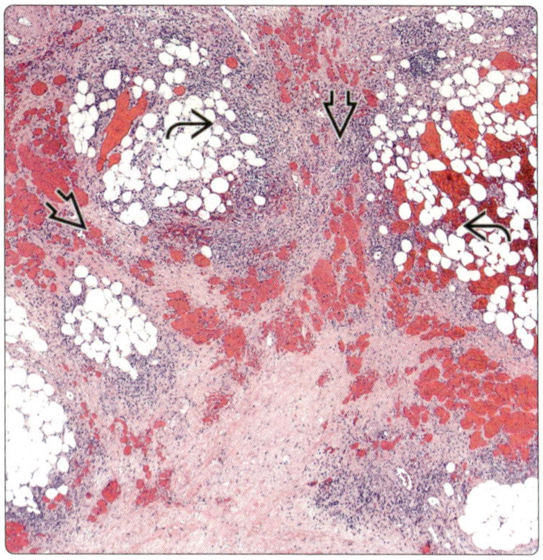

(Left) *The dermis displays patchy increased cellularity that may be subtle, mimicking perivascular inflammation. However, unlike inflammatory infiltrates, the malignant cells of angiosarcoma are markedly hyperchromatic and often enlarged ⇒, features that are appreciable even at low power.* **(Right)** *In the skin, congested vascular channels deeply invade the subcutis, tracking along interlobular septa ⇒ and invading into lobules between individual adipocytes ⇒.*

CD31 in Angiosarcoma

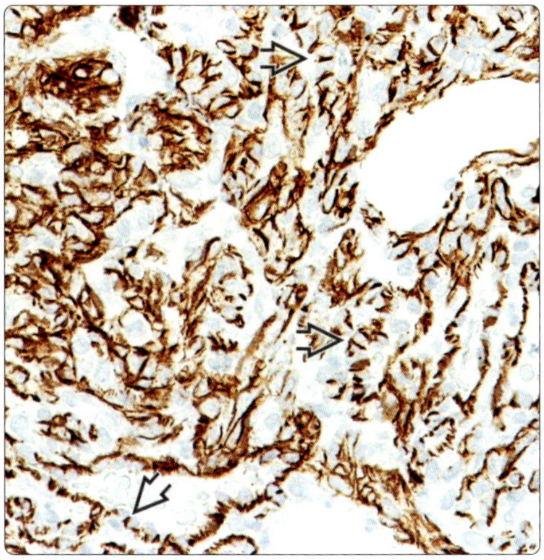

CD34 in Angiosarcoma

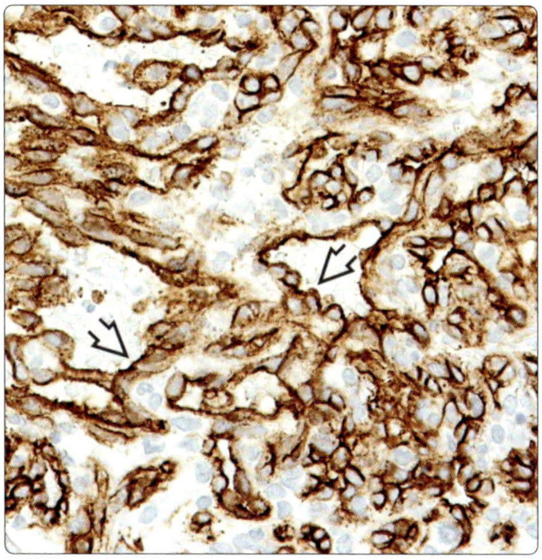

(Left) *Alternatively, CD31 may highlight interendothelial membranes ⇒, resembling rows of dominoes seen from above. This pattern is usually seen in benign vessels but may also be seen in angiosarcoma, as in this case.* **(Right)** *CD34 strongly stains neoplastic endothelial channels of angiosarcoma, typically with a membranous pattern ⇒. Although not entirely specific, in the appropriate morphologic setting, this marker is supportive of vascular differentiation.*

Endothelial Atypia in Angiosarcoma

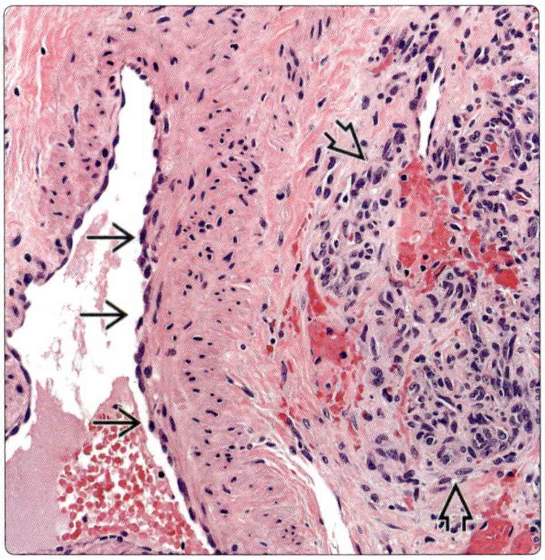

Hemorrhage in Angiosarcoma

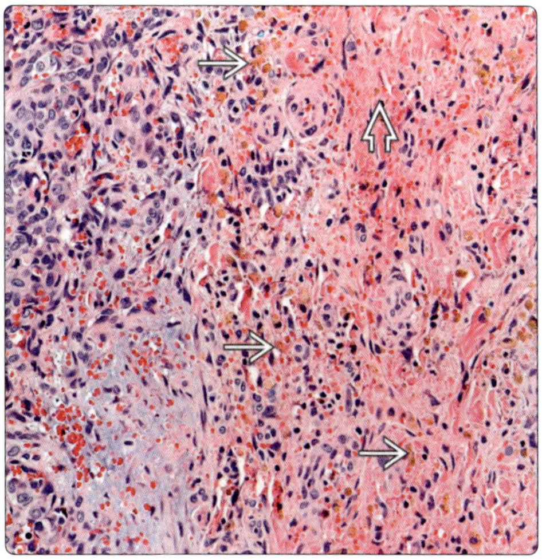

(Left) *In comparison with benign endothelial cells of a nearby small artery ⇒, the malignant endothelial cells of angiosarcoma ⇒ are larger, darker, more crowded, and pleomorphic.* **(Right)** *Erythrocyte extravasation and frank hemorrhage are often seen in angiosarcoma and may lead to hemosiderin deposition ⇒, particularly in areas adjacent to tumor necrosis ⇒.*

(Left) *Postirradiation angiosarcoma of the breast shows irregular, congested, necrotic vascular channels infiltrating a densely sclerotic stroma. The hypocellular background may make identification of malignant cells challenging, but the low-power appearance should raise strong suspicion of a malignant vascular neoplasm.* **(Right)** *Scattered, hyperchromatic, large, malignant cells* → *are present in areas of degenerating channels. Note the residual benign atrophic breast duct* →.

Postirradiation Angiosarcoma of Breast

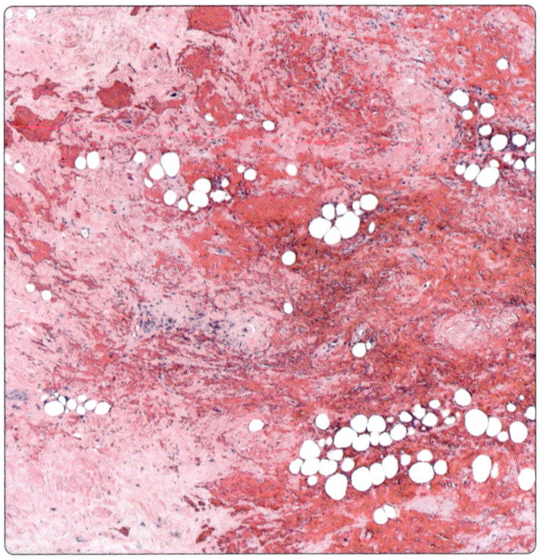

Postirradiation Angiosarcoma of Breast

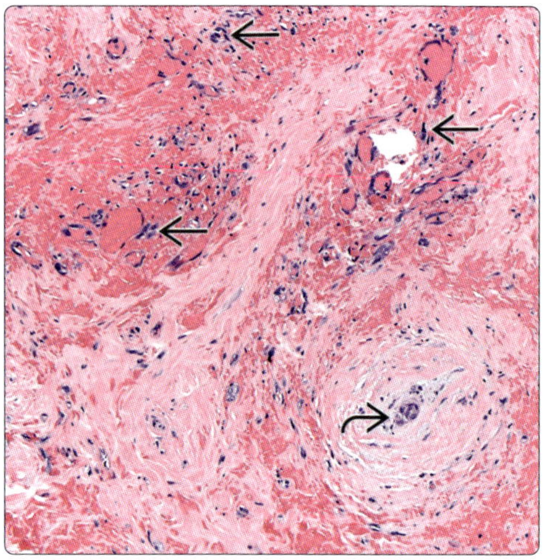

(Left) *Postirradiation angiosarcoma may be hypocellular with sclerotic stroma, mimicking pseudoangiomatous stromal hyperplasia (PASH). Atypical hyperchromatic cells display intracytoplasmic lumina* →, *some even containing erythrocytes* →, *a feature specific for vascular differentiation that is not seen in PASH.* **(Right)** *Although distinctly uncommon, primary angiosarcoma occurs in visceral organs, including the liver, spleen, lung, heart, and even the bladder, as shown.*

Sclerotic Postirradiation Angiosarcoma

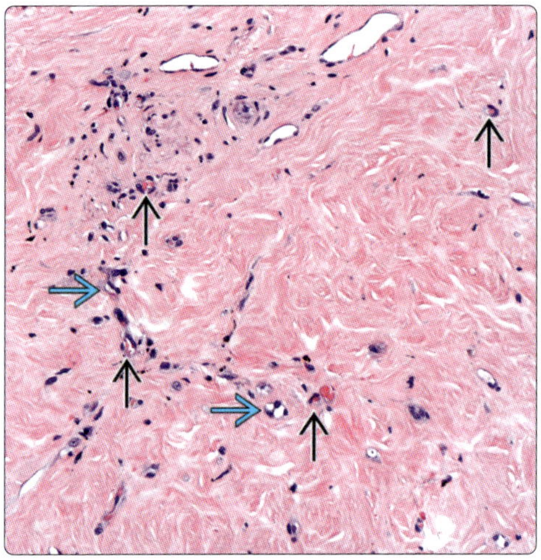

Bladder Angiosarcoma

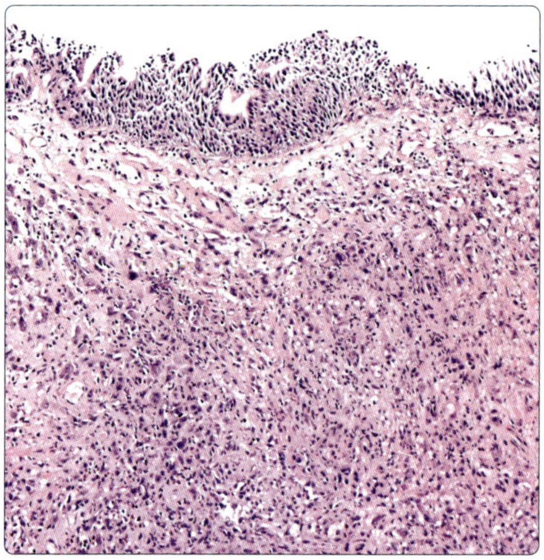

(Left) *In this high-grade epithelioid angiosarcoma involving the skin, plump malignant cells with abundant cytoplasm* → *invade the dermis, entrapping benign vessels* →. **(Right)** *Despite its vascular nature, epithelioid angiosarcoma may outgrow its own vascular supply, causing ischemic necrosis* → *of its core. Necrosis, when present, can help distinguish a true angiosarcoma from benign angiomas or vascular neoplasms of low-grade malignant potential (hemangioendotheliomas).*

Benign Vessel Entrapment by Angiosarcoma

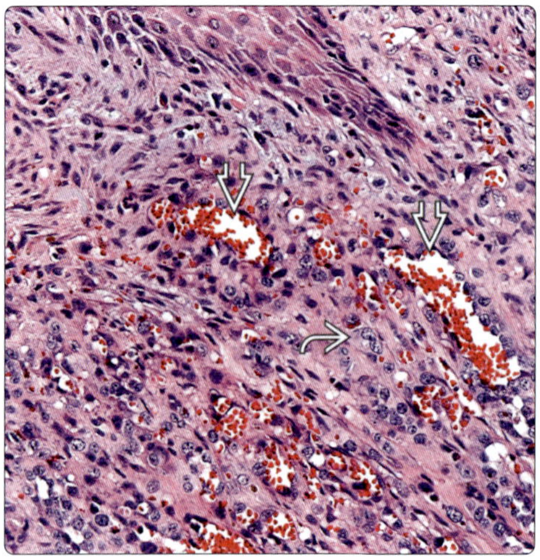

Necrosis in Angiosarcoma

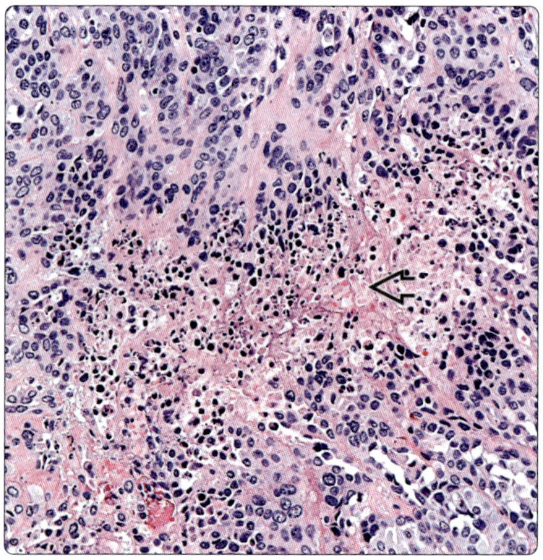

Epithelioid Change in Angiosarcoma

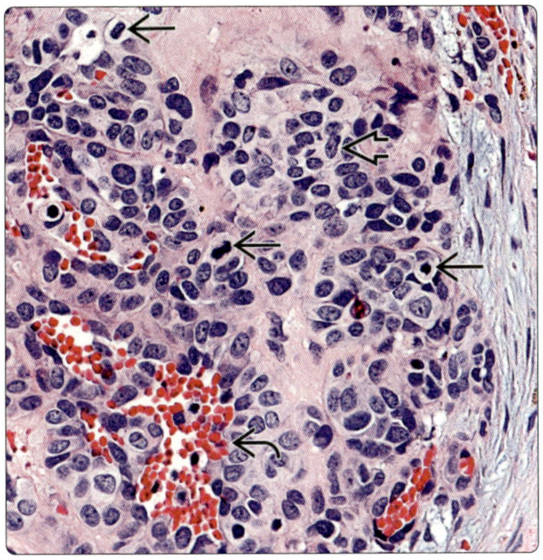

Atypical Mitosis in Angiosarcoma

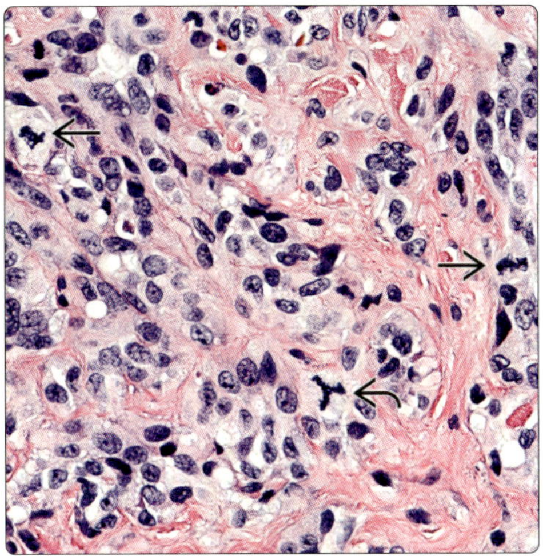

(Left) *Epithelioid angiosarcoma is a highly aggressive malignancy. Note the plump endothelial cells with abundant cytoplasm and well-defined cell borders, forming invasive vascular channels* ↪ *and solid clusters* ⇨*. Mitoses are numerous* →*.* **(Right)** *Mitotic activity is characteristically brisk* → *in epithelioid angiosarcoma, consistent with its aggressive behavior, and may include atypical or tripolar mitotic figures* ↪*.*

Epithelioid Angiosarcoma

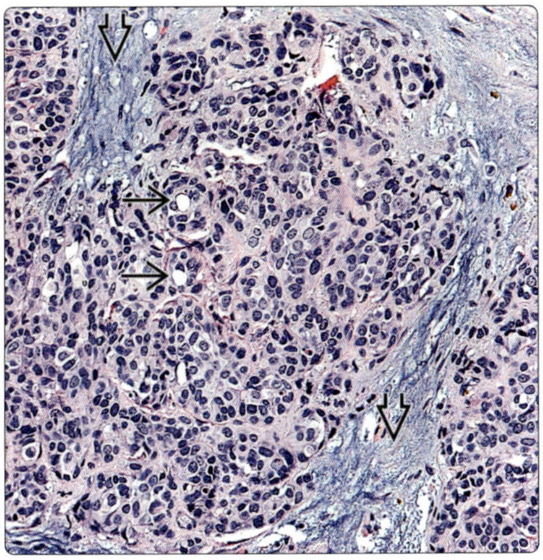

Perineural and Perivascular Invasion in Angiosarcoma

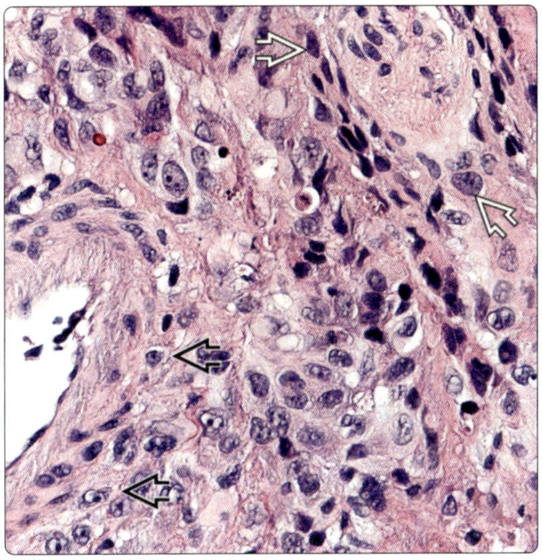

(Left) *Epithelioid angiosarcoma may display solid or nested growth and prominent myxoid stroma* ⇨*. Note the intracytoplasmic lumina* →*. Differential diagnosis includes poorly differentiated adenocarcinoma and squamous cell carcinoma (among others), but remember that epithelioid angiosarcoma often expresses cytokeratins &/or EMA.* **(Right)** *Perineural* ⇨ *and perivascular* ⇨ *invasion are common features of epithelioid angiosarcoma.*

Metastatic Epithelioid Angiosarcoma to Lung

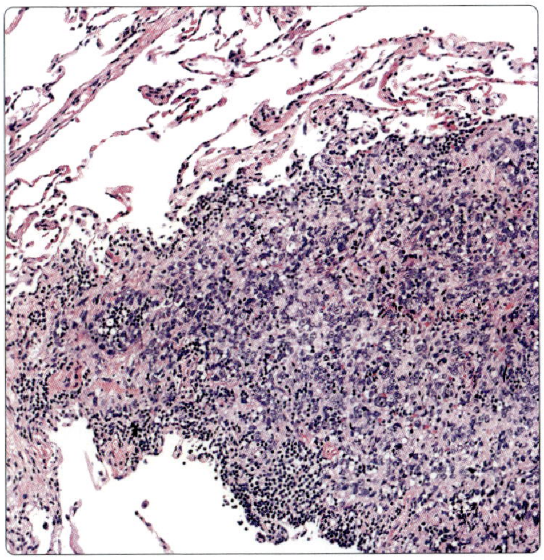

FLI1 in Angiosarcoma

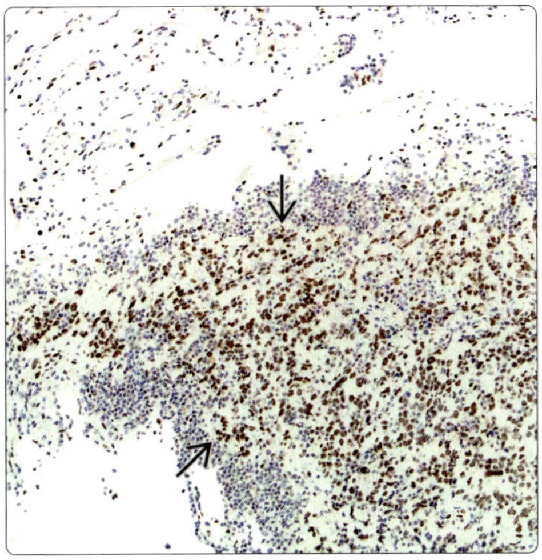

(Left) *Vascular differentiation is not always apparent. In the lung, metastatic epithelioid angiosarcoma may display solid growth and be mistaken for primary pulmonary carcinomas, melanoma, or other metastatic poorly differentiated neoplasms.* **(Right)** *FLI1 is highly sensitive and relatively specific for vascular differentiation (although it also stains the Ewing/PNET family of tumors). The malignant epithelioid cells display strong nuclear staining for FLI1* →*, consistent with metastatic epithelioid angiosarcoma.*

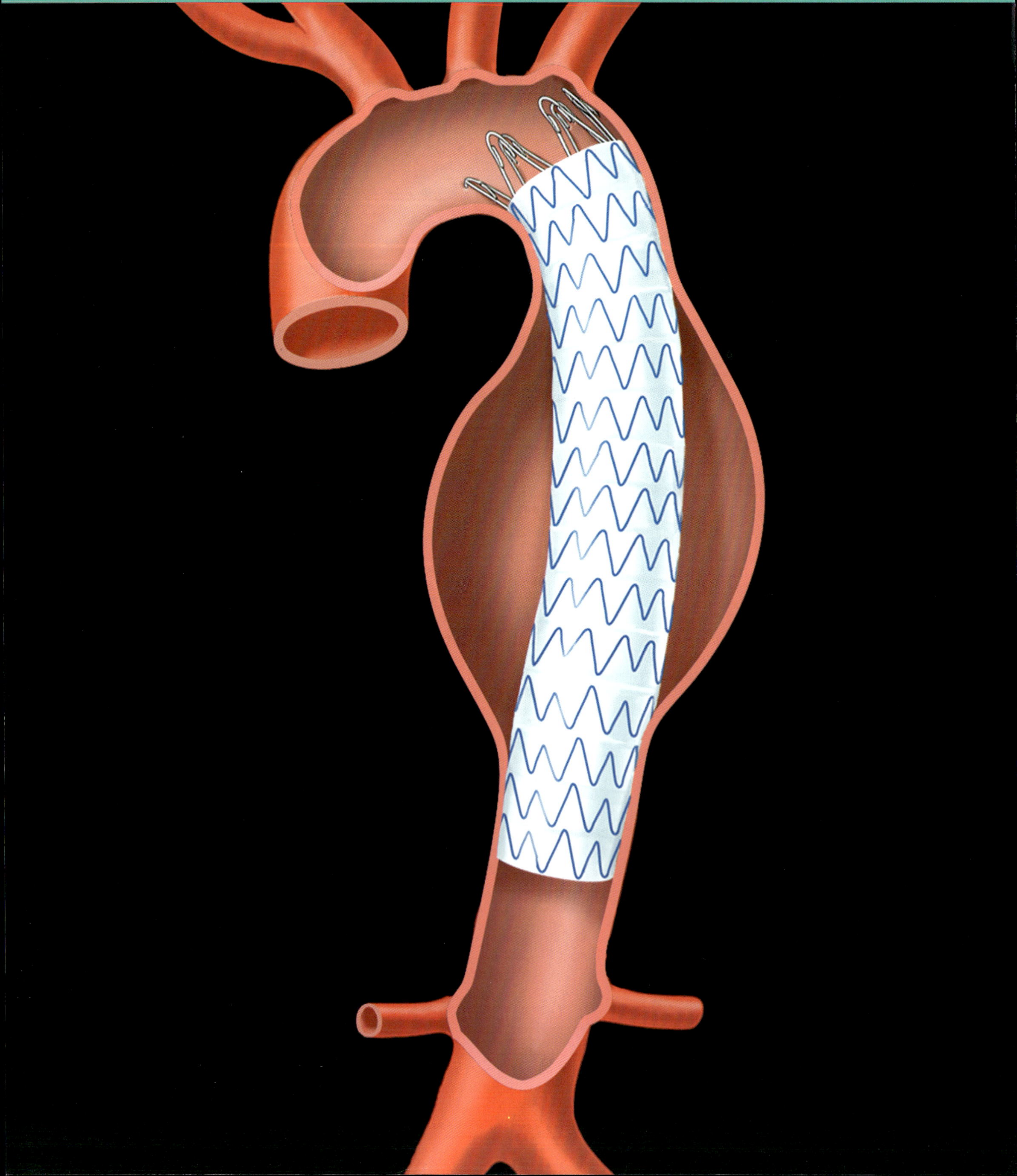

SECTION 9

Autopsy

Cardiac

Vascular

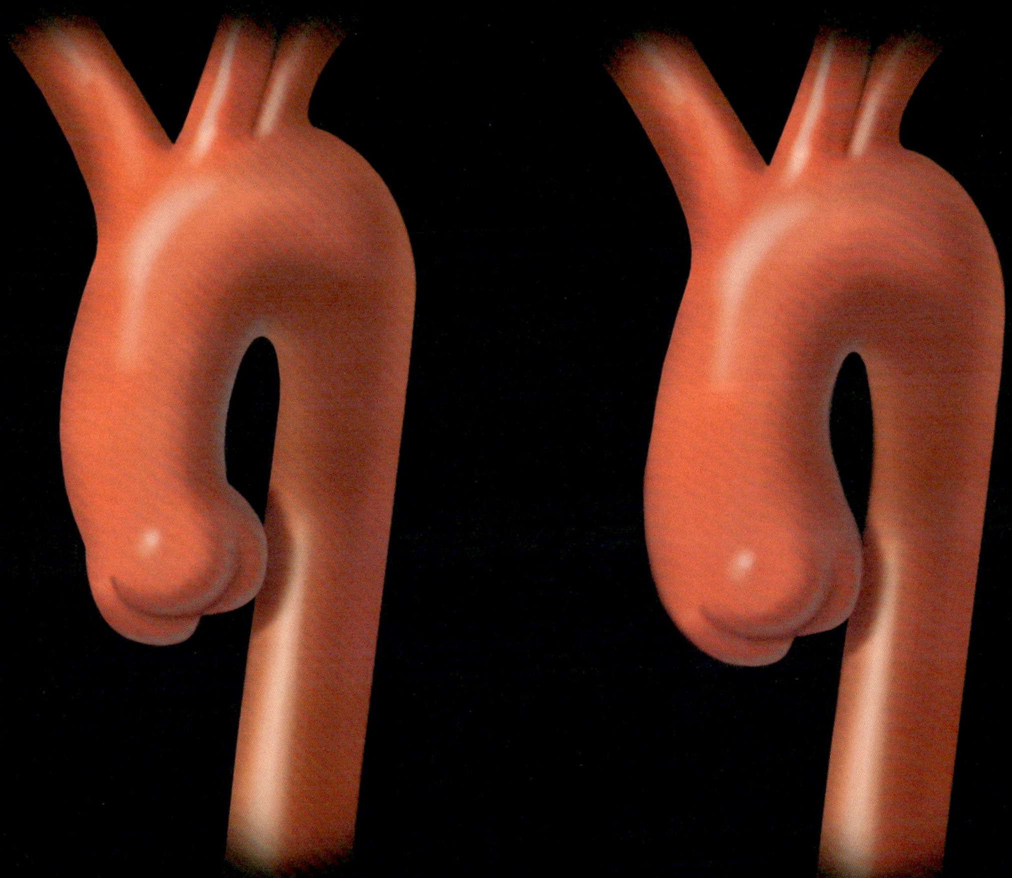

Coronary Artery Bypass Grafting

KEY FACTS

CLINICAL ISSUES

- Operative reports or coronary angiograms relevant to grafting targets and conduits are key to success in post coronary artery bypass grafting (CABG) heart evaluation
- Internal mammary artery graft: 90% patency at 10 years
- Saphenous vein graft (SVG): 20-30% patency at 10 years
- Once primary intervention for coronary artery disease, CABG has largely been replaced by percutaneous endovascular procedures (angioplasty and stenting)
- Patient outcomes post stenting are not better than post CABG, but stenting is obviously less invasive
- Dense pericardial adhesions may make it difficult to identify some grafts
- Left internal mammary artery (LIMA) grafts are easily obliterated upon removal of sternal chest plate

MACROSCOPIC

- For each bypass target vessel, document
  - Graft body: Serially sectioned with areas of plaque, thrombus, or other stenosis selected for microscopy
  - Distal anastomosis: Serial cross sectioning along axis of either native vessel or graft body
  - Distal native vessel runoff: Serial cross sectioning to evaluate potential for flow beyond target site
- Common sources of graft conduits
  - Veins: Saphenous, gastroepiploic/inferior epigastric
  - Arteries: Internal mammary, radial
- For each bypass target vessel, document
  - Graft body: Serially sectioned with areas of plaque, thrombus, or other stenosis selected for microscopy
  - Distal anastomosis: Serial cross sectioning along axis of either native vessel or graft body; submitted entirely
  - Distal native vessel runoff: Serial cross sectioning to evaluate potential for flow beyond target site
- Labeling and nomenclature
  - Convention: Label graft according to target vessel and graft body type

Autopsy Heart Specimen With Bypass Grafting

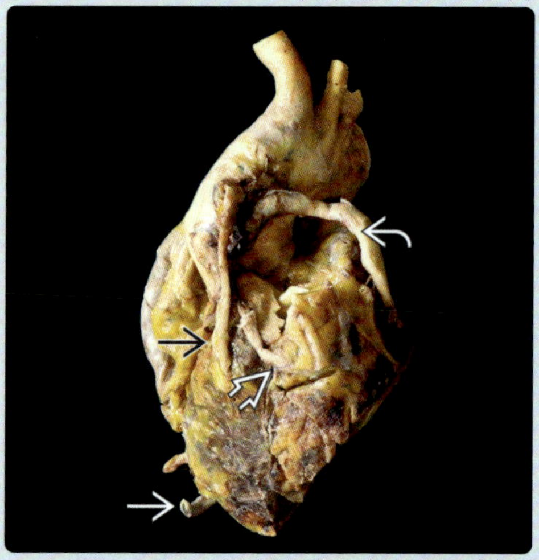

3D Reconstruction CT of Bypass Grafts

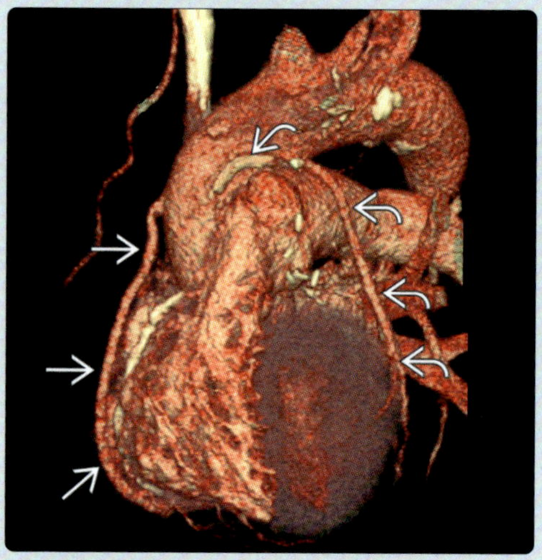

(Left) *Anterior gross photograph of an autopsied heart shows aortocoronary saphenous vein grafts (SVGs) to the right coronary, left anterior descending (LAD), and obtuse marginal targets. An additional posterior descending graft has been cut.* **(Right)** *3D reconstruction CT angiogram shows bypass grafts to the posterior descending and obtuse marginal coronary branches.*

Specimen Radiograph of Removed Bypass Graft Segments

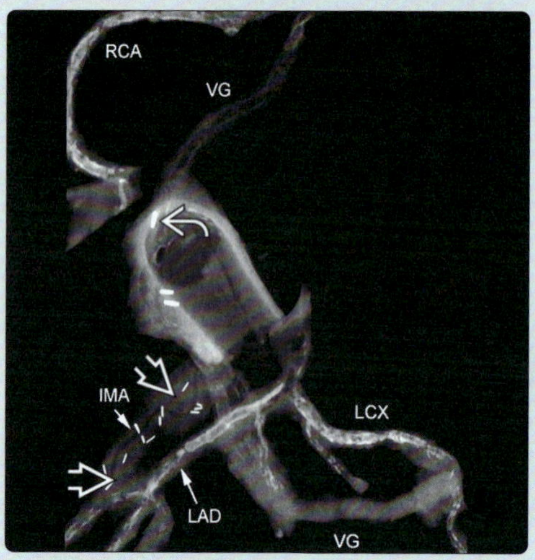

Bypass Graft Anastomosis, Elastic Stain

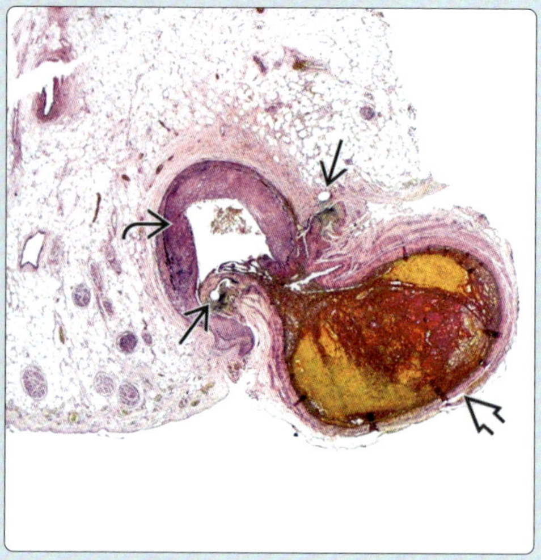

(Left) *Specimen radiograph of the coronary tree after dissecting free from the heart shows calcification in native vessels as well as bypass grafts. The left internal mammary artery (LIMA) graft is surrounded by numerous surgical clips. Larger clips are seen in association with the right vein graft.* **(Right)** *This section shows the typical figure-8 configuration of a bypass anastomotic site. Suture holes are helpful in identifying this. Both the native artery and vein graft are seen in cross section.*

TERMINOLOGY

Abbreviations

- Coronary artery bypass grafting (CABG)

CLINICAL ISSUES

Clinical Overview

- Once primary intervention for coronary artery disease, CABG has largely been replaced by percutaneous endovascular procedures (angioplasty and stenting)
- CABG is still performed in setting of
  - Patients with coronary disease and valve disease or other need for open-heart surgery
  - Certain patients with severe multifocal disease
- Patient outcomes post stenting are not better than post CABG, but stenting is obviously less invasive

Patient History Review

- Operative reports or coronary angiograms relevant to grafting targets and conduits are key to success in post-CABG heart evaluation
  - Left internal mammary artery (LIMA) grafts are easily obliterated upon removal of sternal chest plate
  - Old thrombosed graft conduits may become thread-like and difficult to identify
- Mention of triple, quadruple, etc., bypass refers to number of target vessel anastomoses, rather than number of graft conduits

Expected Graft Conduit Longevity

- Internal mammary artery graft: 90% patency at 10 years
- Saphenous vein graft (SVG): 20-30% patency at 10 years

Complications

- Early
  - "Kinking" or obstruction of graft body
  - Acute thrombosis (often due to hypercoagulability)
- Late
  - Fibrointimal proliferation and atheromatous plaques

IMAGING

Specimen Radiographic Findings

- Identify course of graft (clips along LIMA and SVG from graft harvesting): "Connect the dots"
- Calcific plaque in native vessels and grafts
- Reveal any metallic stents

MACROSCOPIC

General Features

- Common sources of graft conduits
  - Veins: Saphenous, gastroepiploic/inferior epigastric
  - Arteries: Internal mammary, radial
  - Scar patterns on external (skin) exam provide clues
    - Endoscopic vein harvesting may leave only subtle scars
- Common target vessels
  - Left anterior descending (LAD)
    - Ramus intermedius branch: Small branch arising at bifurcation of LAD and left circumflex (LCX) (trifurcation instead of bifurcation)
    - Diagonal branches: Primary branches of LAD serving anterior left ventricle (LV)
    - LIMA grafts almost exclusively to LAD due to anatomic constraints and adjacency
  - LCX
    - Obtuse marginal branches: Primary branches (or sometimes terminal course of LCX) serving lateral LV
  - Right coronary artery (RCA)
    - Posterior descending: Terminal course of RCA serving posterior/inferior LV
    - Posterior descending may be terminal course of LCX in ~ 10% of patients (left dominant circulation)
    - Posterolateral branch: Branch extending beyond posterior descending artery serving posterolateral LV

Sections to Be Submitted

- Proximal native coronary arteries
  - All vessels should be examined per routine to document need for CABG and apparent collateral (retrograde) flow
- For each bypass target vessel, document
  - Graft body: Serially sectioned with areas of plaque, thrombus, or other stenosis selected for microscopy
  - Distal anastomosis: Serial cross sectioning along axis of either native vessel or graft body; submitted entirely
  - Distal native vessel runoff: Serial cross sectioning to evaluate potential for flow beyond target site
- Proximal anastomosis for SVG can often be inspected grossly for patency and does not routinely need to be submitted

MICROSCOPIC

Histologic Features

- Evaluate for plaque and thrombosis, ± recanalization
  - Percentage of stenosis, recent/organized, shallow/occlusive
- SVG: Single elastic layer, adventitial smooth muscle bundles
  - Arterialization
    - Distinct internal elastic lamina, intimal fibroplasia, and plaque
- Anastomosis
  - Usually elongated, "figure 8," or otherwise distorted lumen contour with part of vessel circumference made of native artery and part from graft body
  - Paired suture holes serve as useful landmarks for anastomosis ("snake eyes")

REPORTING

Key Elements to Report

- Report percentage of stenosis of native target vessel, graft body, anastomosis, and distal vessel

Labeling and Nomenclature

- Convention: Label graft according to target vessel and graft body type
- Examples
  - LAD-D1-LIMA: Left internal mammary graft to 1st diagonal branch of LAD
  - LCX-OM2-SVG: SVG to 2nd obtuse marginal branch of LCX
  - RCA-PL-SVG: SVG to posterolateral branch of RCA

Autopsy Heart (Posterior) With Bypass Grafts

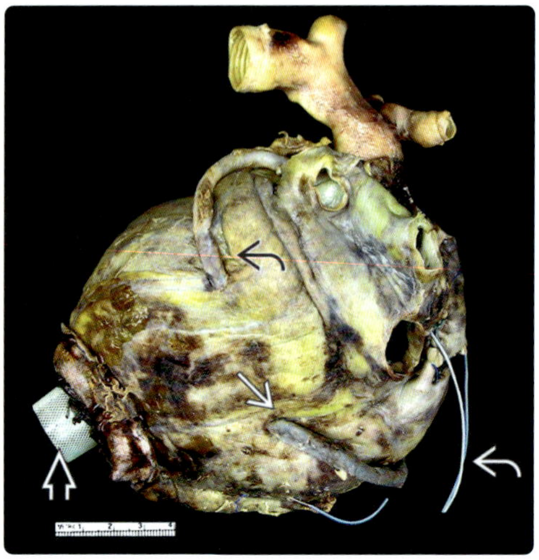

Autopsy Heart (Anterior) With Bypass Grafts

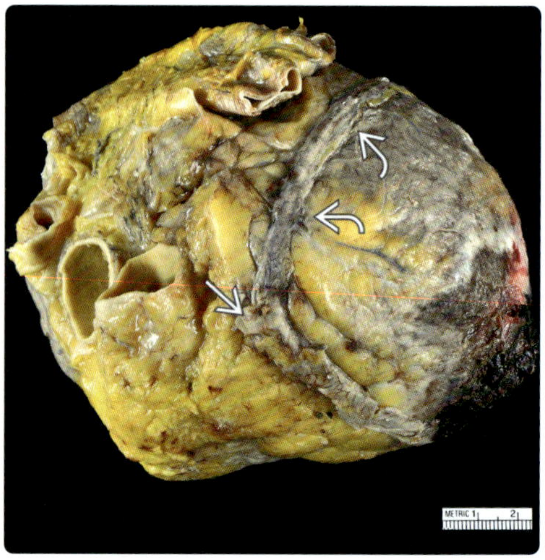

(Left) *Gross photograph of a heart that has had multiple cardiac procedures shows external pacing wires and a left ventricular assist device inflow cannula. There are also bypass grafts to the posterior descending and posterolateral coronary branches.* **(Right)** *This obviously dilated heart shows a sequential T graft with side-to-side anastomosis to the LAD (graft body mostly removed) and then continuing around to the posterolateral branch (end-to-side).*

Coronary Bypass Graft (Removed From Heart)

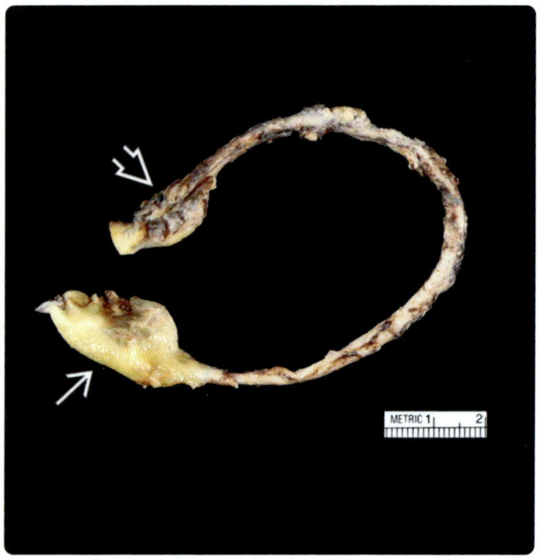

Coronary Bypass Graft, Distal End

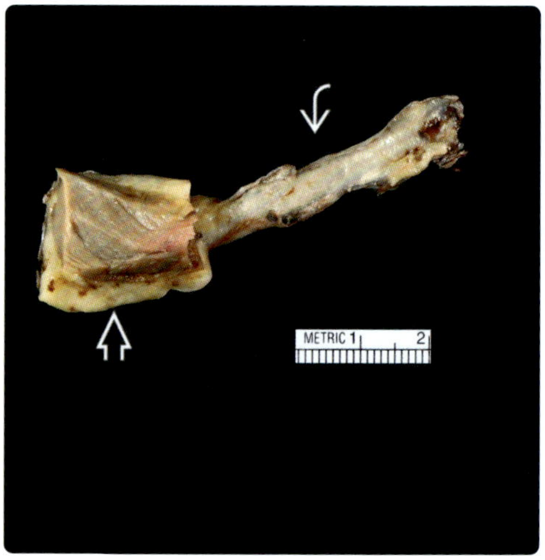

(Left) *Gross photograph shows a bypass graft that has been dissected free from the heart. The proximal portion contains the ostium and a portion of the aorta. The distal portion includes ventricular muscle surrounding the anastomotic site.* **(Right)** *Gross photograph shows a distal portion of the SVG that includes a portion of the graft body. A generous tissue block is taken around the anastomotic site to avoid disrupting delicate structures. The entire anastomosis area should be sectioned and submitted.*

Bypass Anastomoses in Cross Section

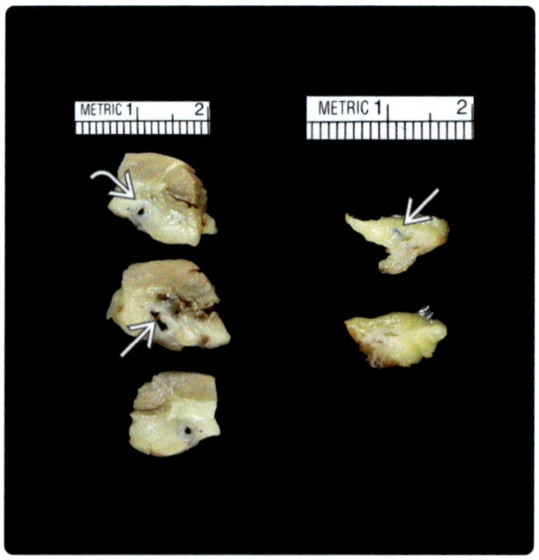

Autopsy Heart With Bypass Grafts

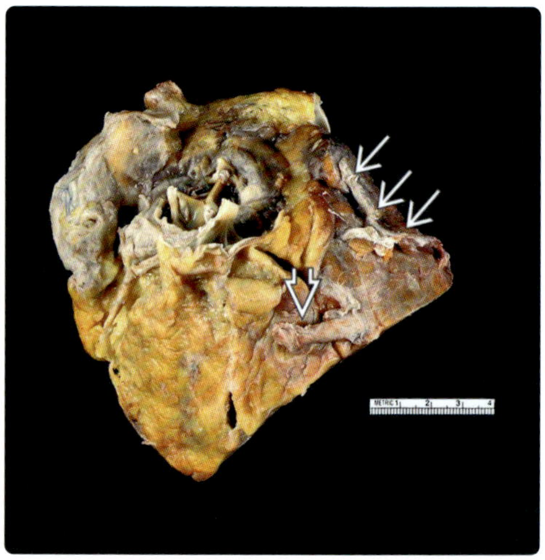

(Left) *Gross photograph shows 2 separate graft anastomoses. The site can be identified by a figure-8-shaped contour. The native vessel is also seen in cross section.* **(Right)** *This autopsy heart specimen (shown after short-axis sectioning of the ventricles) shows 2 coronary artery bypass grafts. There is a left internal mammary artery (LIMA) graft to the proximal circumflex as well as an SVG to the mid LAD.*

Bypass Anastomosis, Elastic Stain

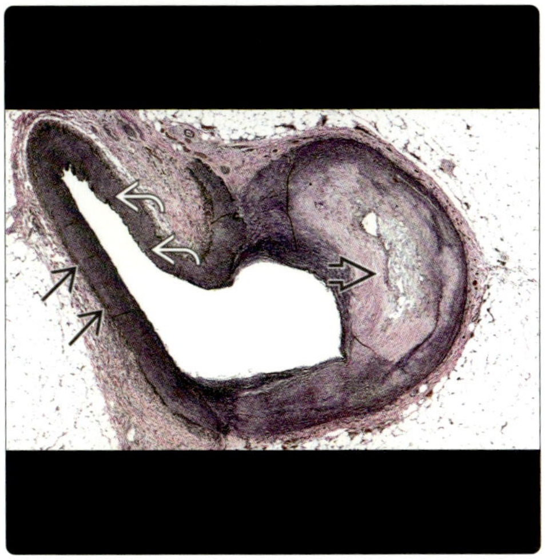

LIMA Graft Anastomosis, Elastic Stain

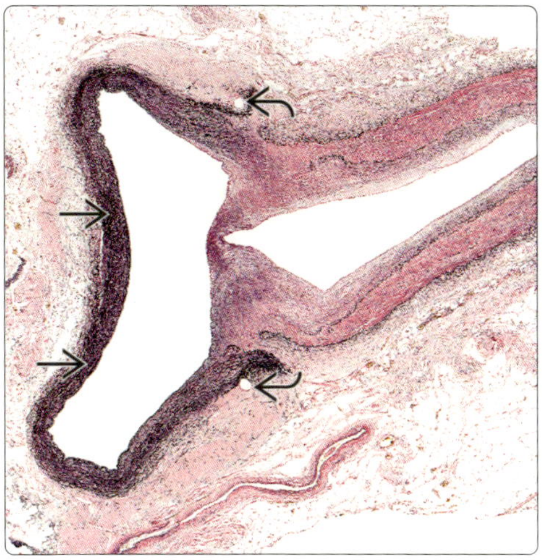

(Left) *Elastic stain section shows a muscular (radial) artery graft body characterized by distinct external and internal elastic layers. The target native vessel shows significant plaque with old plaque hemorrhage. The site is patent without fibrous intimal ingrowth.* **(Right)** *Paraffin section shows a LIMA to LAD anastomosis. The LIMA can be identified by its characteristic multilaminar elastic wall. Paired suture holes are present at the union site.*

Anastomotic Thrombosis (Acute)

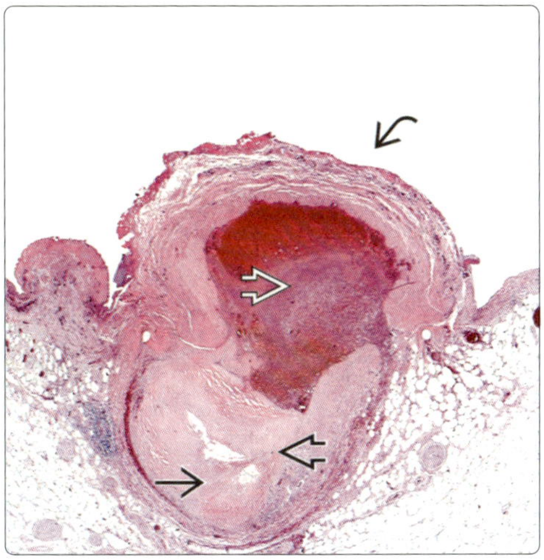

Anastomotic Thrombosis (Acute), Elastic Stain

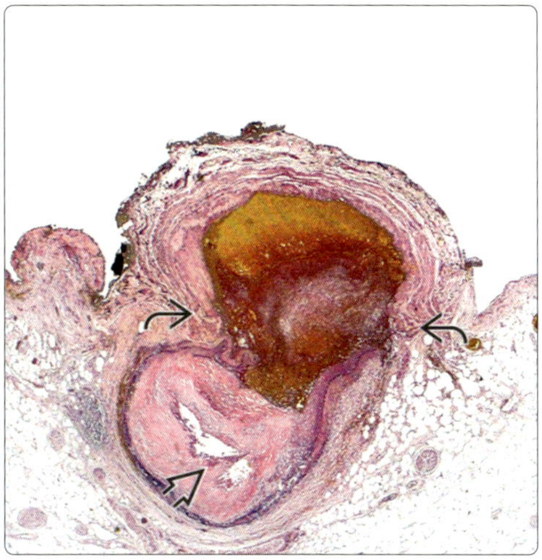

(Left) *Photomicrograph of a bypass anastomosis shows the native coronary artery with obstructive plaque forming the bottom 1/2 of the wall and the vein graft forming the top 1/2. This graft is acutely thrombosed.* **(Right)** *Elastic stain of the same anastomotic site illustrates how the native coronary artery can be differentiated from the vein graft by its internal elastic lamina. Suture holes are also a landmark for the anastomosis.*

Chronic Graft Body Occlusion, Elastic Stain

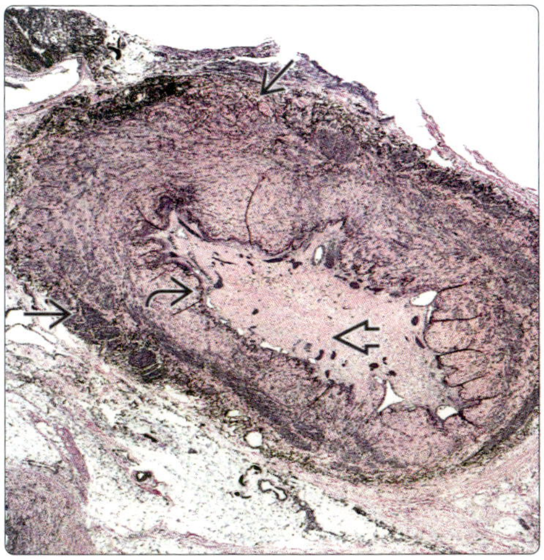

Bypass Graft Anastomosis With Calcific Plaque

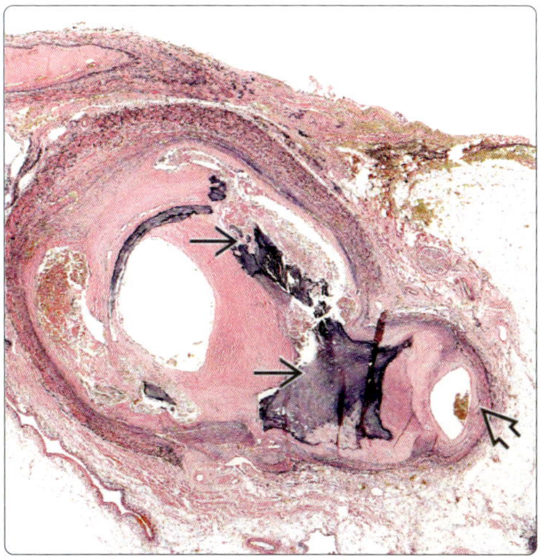

(Left) *Section of the SVG body shows old thrombotic occlusion. The vein graft has undergone "arterialization" with formation of a distinct internal elastic layer. Adventitial smooth muscle bundles confirm the venous nature of the vessel.* **(Right)** *Graft anastomosis site shows minor native vessel disease but severe calcific plaque involving the body and anastomotic site.*

Valve Replacement (Including Transcatheter)

KEY FACTS

CLINICAL ISSUES

- Type of prosthesis will determine which complications may be seen at autopsy
  - Mechanical: Very durable but requires anticoagulation
  - Bioprosthetic: No anticoagulation but structural deterioration common
  - Catheter deployed: Less invasive but numerous unique complications
  - Failure may cause stenosis &/or regurgitation
  - Failure may affect heart, lungs, and other organs

MACROSCOPIC

- Causes of prosthetic valve failure
  - Thrombosis (especially mechanical valves)
  - Structural deterioration (especially bioprosthetic valves)
  - Paravalvular leak, pannus formation, and infective endocarditis affect all valves
  - Incomplete expansion (catheter deployed only)
  - Suboptimal seating (catheter deployed only)
- Other complications: Hemorrhage, embolism, infarcts, hemolytic anemia, etc.
- Autopsy performance considerations
  - Examine prosthetic valves from both sides
  - Examine for perivalvular leaks, annular abscesses
  - Obtain radiographs to evaluate cusp calcification, integrity of metallic components (e.g., struts)
  - Photograph abnormalities
  - Evaluate for secondary cardiac/pulmonary disease
  - Submit vegetations for microbiologic cultures
  - Submit vegetations, perforations, abscesses, thrombi, and adherent tissues for microscopy

MICROSCOPIC

- Infective endocarditis: Thrombotic material with destruction of prosthetic valve tissue, necrosis, and dense inflammation; microorganisms may or may not be present
- Thrombi: Laminated appearance with alternating layers of RBCs/WBCs and platelets/fibrin seen in recent thrombi

(Left) *Cusp degeneration is a common cause of failure in bioprosthetic valves. Note the nodular calcified deposits* → *on the cusps of this bovine pericardial bioprosthesis, which resulted in valve stenosis.* **(Right)** *Infective endocarditis may involve prosthetic valves of any type. Here, vegetations* → *have formed on a bileaflet mechanical valve, restricting leaflet mobility and causing severe stenosis.*

Bioprosthetic Valve With Cusp Degeneration

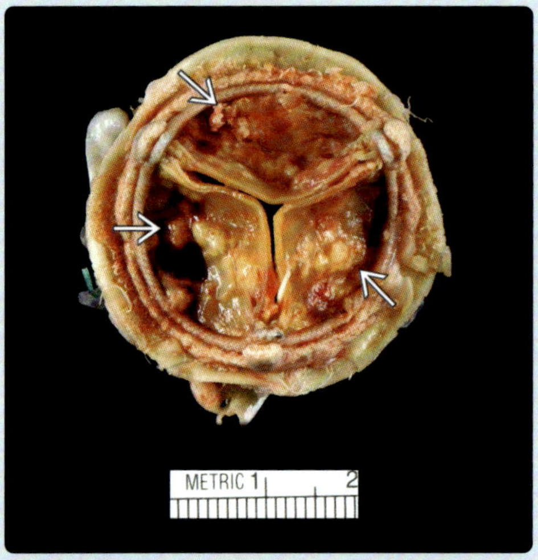

Prosthetic Valve Endocarditis

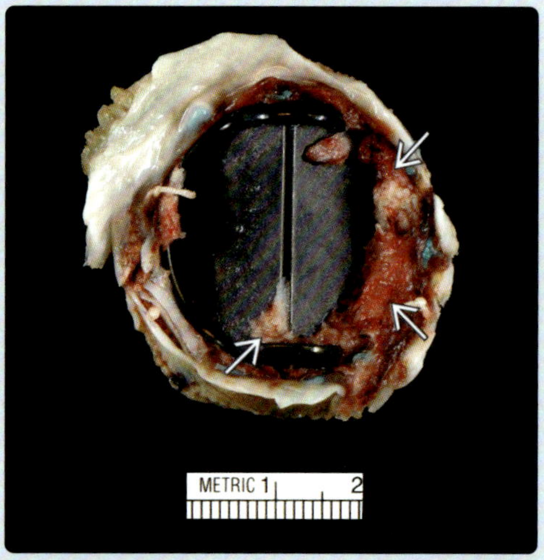

(Left) *Autopsy specimen demonstrates a surgically implanted bioprosthetic valve in mitral location* → *with early thrombosis* →*. Thrombosis in bioprosthetic valves occurs less often than in mechanical valves. It is usually due to inadequate anticoagulation.* **(Right)** *Marked calcification* → *of the cusps in this bioprosthetic valve is present on the ventricular surface. Degenerative changes are common complications in prosthetic valves, leading to stenosis and valve dysfunction.*

Atrioventricular Prosthetic Valve Thrombosis

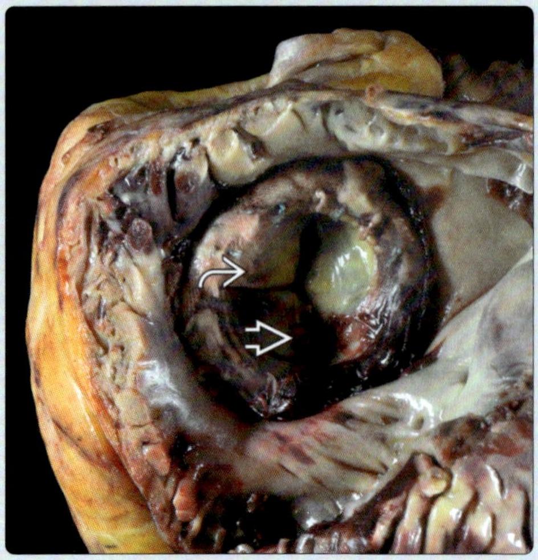

Degenerative Changes in Bioprosthetic Valve

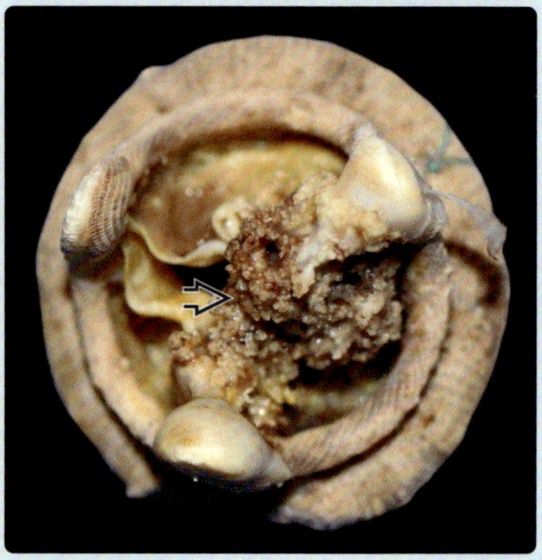

TERMINOLOGY

Abbreviations

- Prosthetic valve (infective) endocarditis (PVE)
- Transcatheter aortic valve replacement (TAVR)

Major Types of Prosthetic Valves

- Mechanical: Ball-in-cage, tilting disc, bileaflet
- Bioprosthetic: Porcine, bovine pericardial, cadaveric homograft
- Catheter-deployed bioprosthetic: Edwards SAPIEN, Medtronic CoreValve, Medtronic Melody, others
- MitraClip for percutaneous mitral valve repair
- Other devices

Hemodynamic Categories of Failure

- Prosthetic valve stenosis
- Prosthetic valve regurgitation

CLINICAL ISSUES

Clinical Overview

- Selection of type of valve prosthesis driven by combination of patient factors and inherent advantages and disadvantages of each prosthesis
- Type of prosthesis will determine which complications might be seen during autopsy
- Mechanical prosthetic valves
  - Advantages: Excellent durability (most remain functional for 20-30 years)
  - Disadvantages: Require lifelong anticoagulation (risk of hemorrhage, teratogenicity in women of child-bearing age), hemolytic anemia from mechanical trauma to RBCs
- Bioprosthetic valves
  - Advantage: No anticoagulation required
  - Disadvantage: Structural deterioration common (30-35% fail within 10-15 years)
- Catheter-deployed bioprosthetic valves
  - Advantages: Less invasive (for patients with high surgical risk); option when surgery is technically challenging or impossible; valve-in-valve procedures possible
  - Disadvantages: ↑ risk of stroke, long-term durability unknown, unique complications as outlined below

Patient History Review

- Clinical, operative, and echocardiography help plan and avoid complications and hemodynamic effects
  - Review can guide postmortem evaluation of prosthetic valve

Etiology of Prosthetic Valve Failure

- Thrombosis
  - More common with mechanical valves (inadequate anticoagulation)
  - May cause stenosis &/or regurgitation
  - May be embolize; downstream infarcts
- Structural deterioration
  - Primarily involves bioprosthetic valves
  - Cusp calcification usually causes stenosis
  - Cusp tear causes regurgitation
    - Usually tear occurs at commissure
    - Results in cusp prolapse
- Paravalvular leak: Central, commissural, paravalvular, or supraskirtal
  - May occur with any type of prosthetic valve
  - Results in regurgitation
- Pannus formation
  - May occur with any type of prosthetic valve
  - Annular fibrous ingrowth causes stenosis
- Infective endocarditis
  - May occur with any type of prosthetic valve
  - Causes regurgitation if valve structures are destroyed (e.g., perforations, cusp tears) or if surrounding native tissue is involved (with valve dehiscence)
  - Causes stenosis if vegetations are large
  - Infectious agents: *Staphylococcus epidermidis*, *Staphylococcus aureus*, streptococci, Gram-negative bacilli, fungi
  - Bioprosthetic infective endocarditis
    - May involve cusps &/or sewing ring
    - Sometimes complicated by annular abscess
  - Mechanical prosthetic infective endocarditis
    - Vegetations involve sewing ring
    - Usually complicated by annular abscess
  - Annular abscess
    - May burrow, perforate, &/or cause valve dehiscence
    - May extend to involve other valves
    - High operative mortality rate
  - Septic embolism

Complications Specific to Catheter-Deployed Valves

- Incomplete expansion
  - Proper leaflet coaptation requires full expansion to predesigned functional circumference
  - Incomplete expansion may cause "tenting" of cusps and fixed regurgitation
  - Overexpansion is rarely seen due to usual calcification and sclerosis of aortic anulus in aortic stenosis
- Suboptimal seating and attachment failure
  - Success requires alignment at level of anatomic annulus
  - Improper seating; becomes loose and embolizes
- Embolization of calcified debris from native cusps
  - Dislodged during balloon expansion prior to valve deployment
  - May cause strokes or infarcts in downstream organs
- Inverted orientation
  - Valve deployed via transfemoral or transapical approach; must be properly oriented in catheter sheath to prevent inverted (backward) deployment
  - Rare but may be fatal
- Annular rupture
  - Rare but may be fatal; due to aggressive balloon predilatation
- Coronary ostial obstruction with myocardial infarction
  - Rare; due to device itself or calcified debris from native aortic valve
- Complications specific to transapical approach
  - Hemopericardium with cardiac tamponade
  - Damage to mitral valve
  - Left ventricular (LV) pseudoaneurysm formation
  - LV arrhythmias
- Complications specific to transfemoral approach

- Access site infection or hematoma
- Aortofemoral injury: Rupture, pseudoaneurysm, dissection, stenosis/thrombosis/occlusion
- Distal embolization of dislodged femoral, iliac, or aortic atherosclerotic plaque

Other Complications

- Hemorrhage: Primarily with mechanical valves (due to anticoagulation)
- Embolism and infarcts due to thrombosis or infective endocarditis
- Hemolytic anemia: Primarily with mechanical valves (due to mechanical trauma to RBCs)

MACROSCOPIC

External Examination

- If recent surgical intervention, inspect incision site for signs of infection (purulence, necrosis, dehiscence)
- If recent transcatheter intervention, inspect percutaneous cannulation site (groin, small left thoracotomy) for hematoma or vascular complication
- Other scars indicating previous cardiac interventions
  - Median sternotomy
  - Other thoracotomy
  - Saphenous vein or radial artery harvesting

Internal Examination

- Brain and other viscera
  - Evaluate for infarcts due to embolization of valve thrombus or vegetations
- Lungs
  - Evaluate for edema or other evidence of congestive heart failure due to failed valve prosthesis
- Body cavities
  - Evaluate for evidence of procedure complications (e.g., hemopericardium, hemothorax)

Organ Examination

- Heart
  - Evaluate for disease of prosthetic valve
    - Carefully remove great vessels &/or atria to expose valves ("base of heart" dissection method)
    - If vegetations or annular abscesses are present, obtain material in sterile fashion for microbiologic cultures
    - Examine prosthetic valves from both sides (inflow and outflow)
    - Examine perivalvular tissues for abnormalities (e.g., perivalvular leaks, annular abscesses)
  - Evaluate for evidence of valvular heart disease
    - Record heart weight and standard measurements: LV, right ventricular (RV), septal wall thicknesses; LV internal short-axis chamber diameter, RV internal short-axis chamber dimensions, annular circumferences of native valves
    - Cardiac disease may be caused by native valve disease, prosthetic valve abnormalities, or both
  - Examples of secondary cardiac effects of common valve diseases
    - Aortic stenosis: LV pressure hypertrophy **without** LV dilatation; left atrial (LA) dilatation; RV/right atrial (RA) dilatation
    - Aortic regurgitation: LV pressure and volume hypertrophy with massive 4-chamber dilatation
    - Mitral stenosis: Normal LV, massive LA dilatation, RV/RA dilatation
    - Mitral regurgitation: LV pressure and volume hypertrophy with 4-chamber dilatation
  - Evaluate for other coexisting cardiovascular abnormalities
- Specimen radiography
  - Useful to determine extent of cusp calcification
  - Useful to evaluate for strut fractures and incomplete expansion of catheter-deployed valves
- Photograph abnormalities whenever possible
  - Valuable for medicolegal and educational purposes
- At minimum, submit following abnormalities for microscopy
  - Vegetations, cusp perforations, other features suggestive of infection
  - Annular abscesses
  - Thrombi (to evaluate for infection)
  - Any other tissue adherent to device
  - Conduction system should be examined in cases that developed conduction block &/or arrhythmia

MICROSCOPIC

Histologic Features

- Infective endocarditis
  - Abundant thrombotic material with destruction of prosthetic valve tissue, necrosis
  - Dense neutrophilic, lymphoplasmacytic, or granulomatous inflammation
  - Microorganisms may or may not be visualized
  - Stains for microorganisms (e.g., Gram, GMS) can help, but negative result does not rule out infection
- Thrombi
  - Recent thrombi show laminated appearance with alternating layers of RBCs/WBCs and platelets/fibrin
  - Older thrombi organization with capillary proliferation
  - Absence of microorganisms and dense neutrophilic inflammation

SELECTED REFERENCES

1. Sellers SL et al: Transcatheter aortic heart valves: histological analysis providing insight to leaflet thickening and structural valve degeneration. JACC Cardiovasc Imaging. 12(1):35-145, 2019
2. Yahagi K et al: Pathology of self-expanding transcatheter aortic valves: findings from the CoreValve US pivotal trials. Catheter Cardiovasc Interv. 91(5):947-55, 2018
3. Chamandi C et al: Latest-generation transcatheter aortic valve replacement devices and procedures. Can J Cardiol. 33(9):1082-90, 2017
4. Dasi LP et al: On the mechanics of transcatheter aortic valve replacement. Ann Biomed Eng. 45(2):310-31, 2017
5. Lim WY et al: Mechanical and surgical bioprosthetic valve thrombosis. Heart. 103(24):1934-41, 2017
6. van Kesteren F et al: Autopsy after transcatheter aortic valve implantation. Virchows Arch. 470(3):331-9, 2017
7. Yahagi K et al: Pathology of balloon-expandable transcatheter aortic valves. Catheter Cardiovasc Interv. 90(6):1048-57, 2017
8. Dangas GD et al: Prosthetic heart valve thrombosis. J Am Coll Cardiol. 68(24):2670-89, 2016
9. Amat-Santos IJ et al: Prosthetic valve endocarditis after transcatheter valve replacement: a systematic review. JACC Cardiovasc Interv. 8(2):334-46, 2015

Base of Heart View of Valves

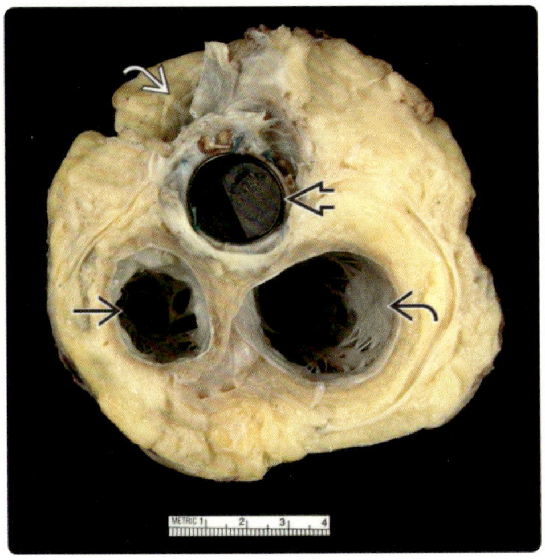

Valve Calcification in Bioprosthetic Valve

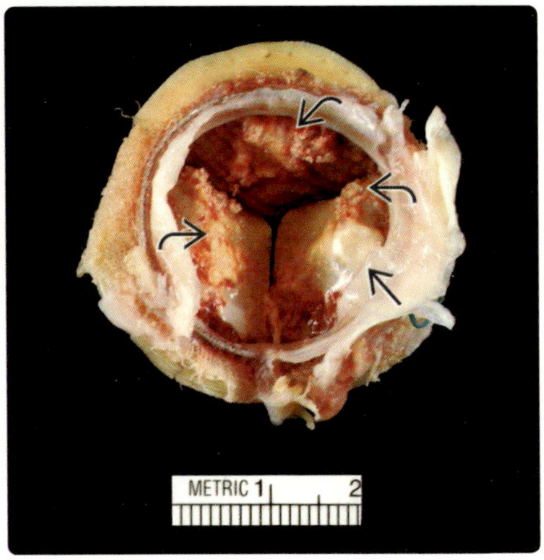

(Left) *Visualization of prosthetic valves is facilitated by the "base of heart" dissection method, whereby the atria are removed, revealing all 4 valves. Note the bileaflet mechanical prosthetic valve in the aortic position as well as native tricuspid, mitral, and pulmonary valves.* **(Right)** *Fibrocalcific degeneration of all 3 prosthetic cusps and formation of pannus on the surface of 1 cusp resulted in stenosis of this bioprosthetic aortic valve.*

Bioprosthetic Valve Thrombosis

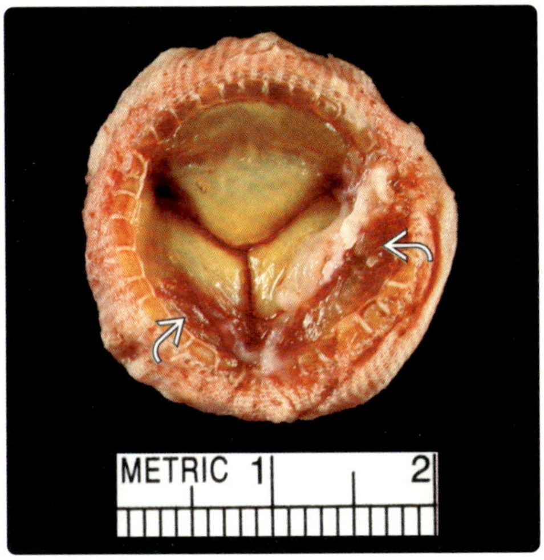

Valve Structural Degeneration

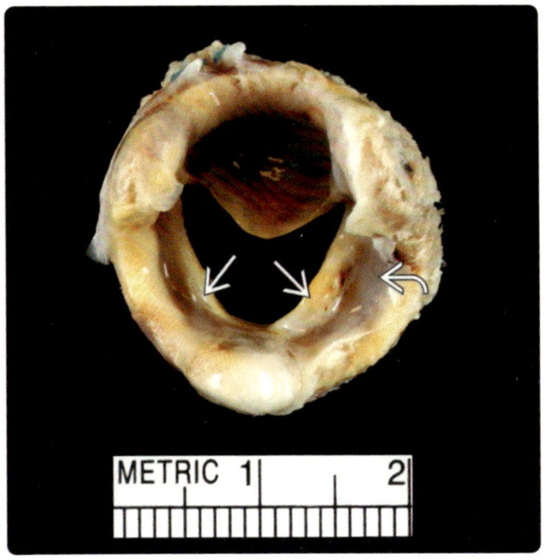

(Left) *Although more common on mechanical valves, thrombus may also form on the cusps of bioprosthetic valves, causing significant stenosis and potentially resulting in embolism and infarcts downstream.* **(Right)** *Structural degeneration is an important cause of failure of bioprosthetic valves. Here, significant fibrotic retraction of 2 cusps has resulted in torrential regurgitation of this porcine bioprosthetic valve. Also note focal pannus formation adjacent to 1 cusp.*

Valve Structural Degeneration

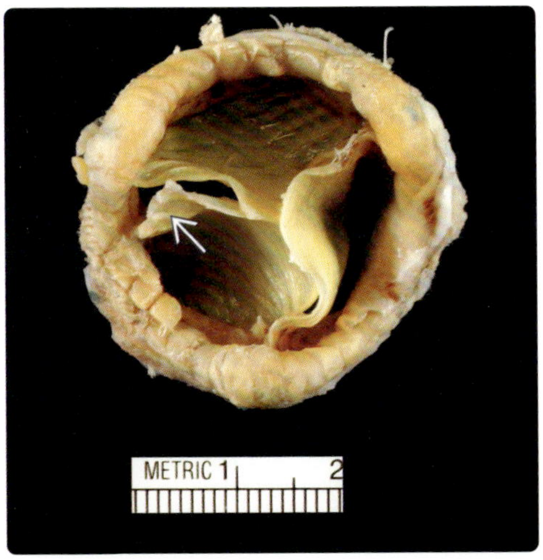

Bioprosthetic Valve With Cusp Tear

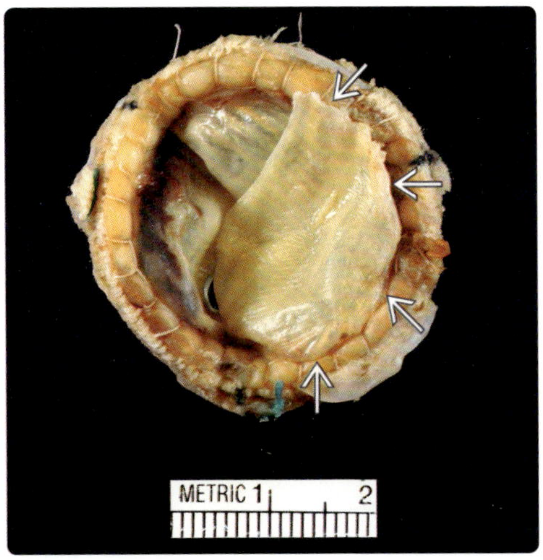

(Left) *Structural degeneration of bioprosthetic valves may also result in cusp tears, which usually form at commissures where mechanical strain and wear on the prosthetic cusp are greatest. Here, a large cusp tear has formed on this porcine bioprosthetic valve, resulting in severe regurgitation.* **(Right)** *On the reverse (inflow) side of this same valve, the extent of cusp tearing is more evident. The tear involves nearly the entire annular attachment of the involved cusp.*

(Left) *Dehiscence is an important cause of prosthetic valve failure. Here, dehiscence of a cadaveric-valved aortic homograft has resulted in formation of a perivalvular fibrotic cavity.* **(Right)** *Infective endocarditis can involve valve prostheses of all types. Hemodynamic consequences include both regurgitation and stenosis, depending on the size of vegetation and status of the cusps. Here, vegetations have resulted in perforation of 1 cusp, causing regurgitation.*

Prosthetic Valve Dehiscence

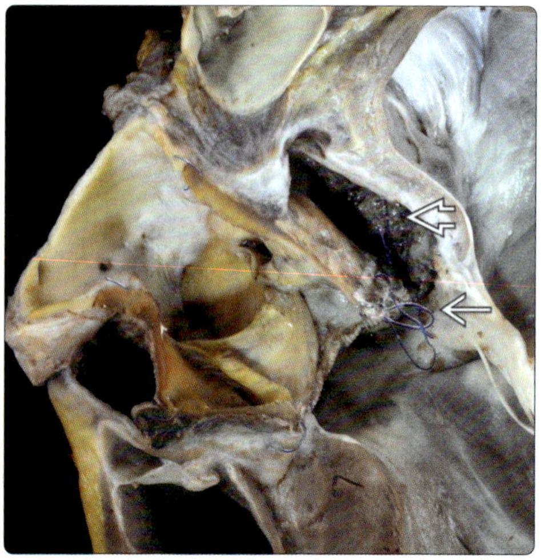

Bioprosthetic Valve Endocarditis

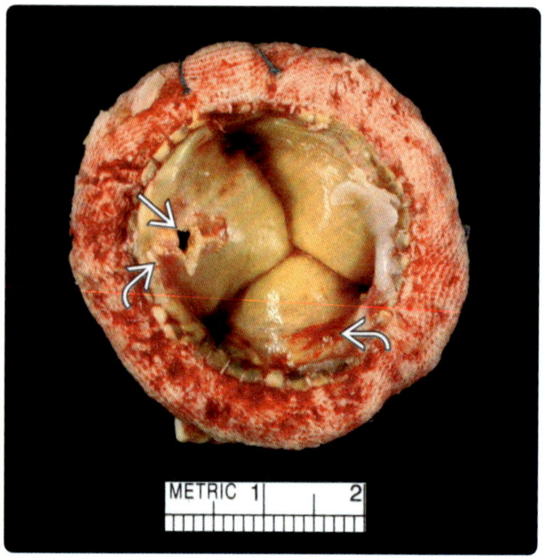

(Left) *In contrast, large infective vegetations may obstruct the valve orifice and result in significant prosthetic valve stenosis.* **(Right)** *Infective endocarditis may also involve mechanical valves, as in this case where bulky vegetations restrict mobility of the prosthetic leaflets, resulting in severe stenosis. Cultures and histologic sections should be obtained to confirm the infectious nature of the process and to identify the culprit microorganism.*

Bioprosthetic Valve Endocarditis

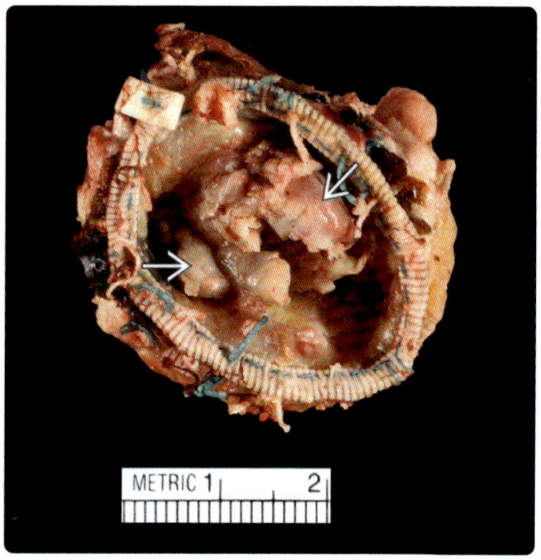

Mechanical Valve Endocarditis

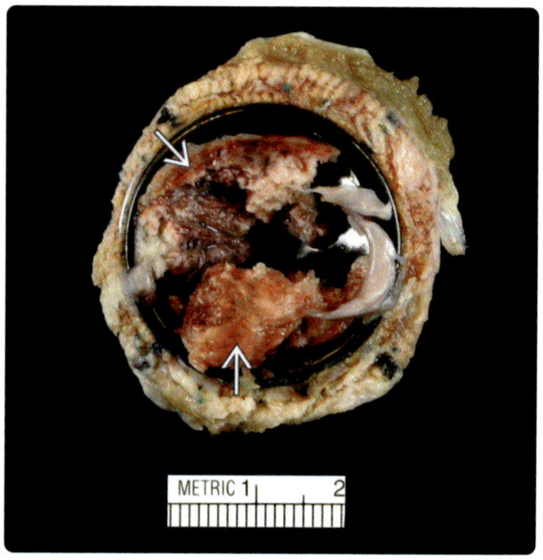

(Left) *Histologically, infective endocarditis involving a bovine pericardial bioprosthetic valve shows destruction of the cusp with adherent, fibrin-rich thrombotic vegetation material containing numerous irregular, "fuzzy" bacterial colonies.* **(Right)** *Gram stain highlights gram-positive bacterial colonies within the thrombotic vegetation and also within the partially destroyed cusp. Cultures confirmed the presence of Propionibacterium acnes.*

Infective Endocarditis: Histology

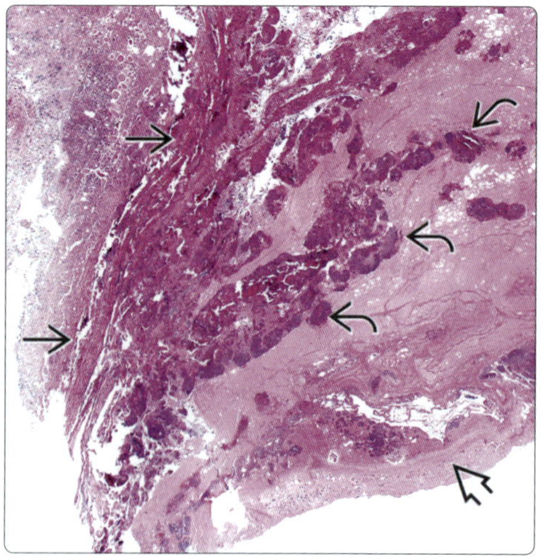

Gram Stain in Thrombotic Endocarditis

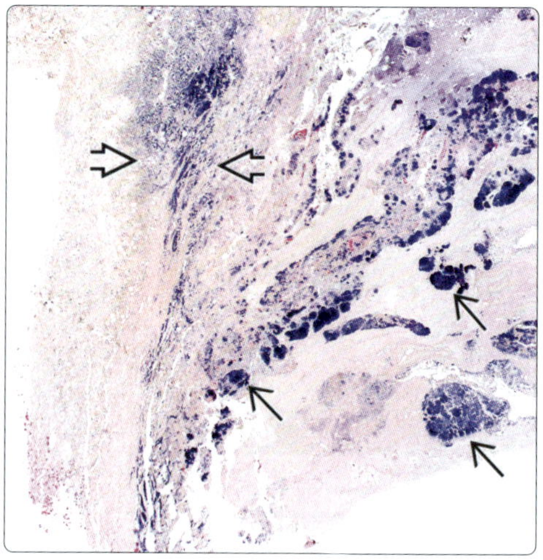

Transcatheter Aortic Valve Replacement With Bioprosthetic Valve

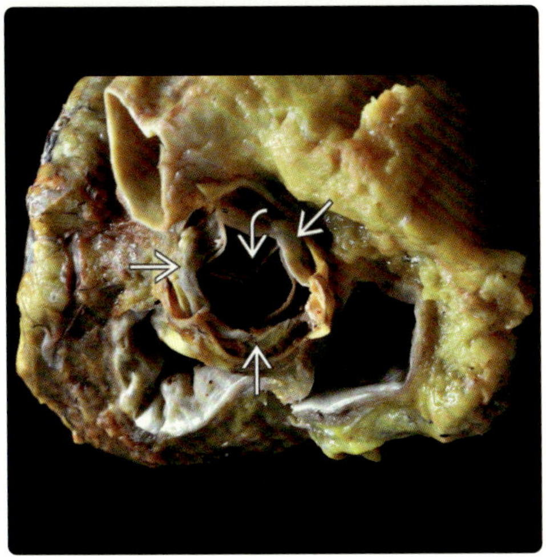

Catheter-Deployed Bioprosthetic Valve

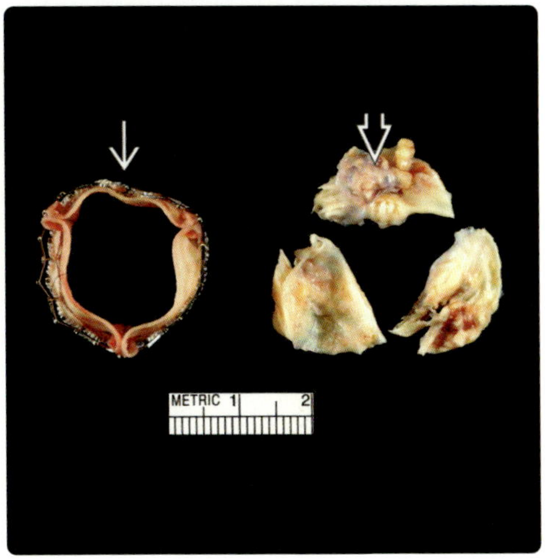

(Left) *Catheter-deployed bioprosthetic valves are positioned within a diseased valve without surgical removal thereof. Here, the atria have been removed, revealing a catheter-deployed bioprosthesis within a diseased aortic valve. Native cusps have been pushed aside by balloon dilatation prior to deployment of the device.* **(Right)** *Here, a catheter-deployed SAPIEN bioprosthetic valve is displayed alongside the excised calcified aortic valve cusps that surrounded it.*

Catheter-Deployed Bioprosthetic Melody Valve

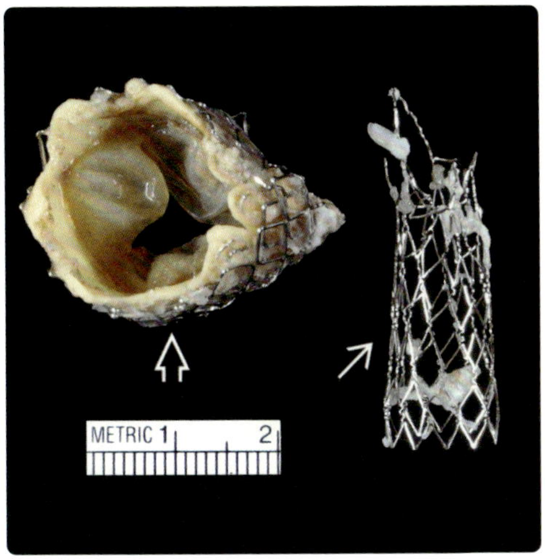

Catheter-Deployed Aortic Bioprosthetic Valve

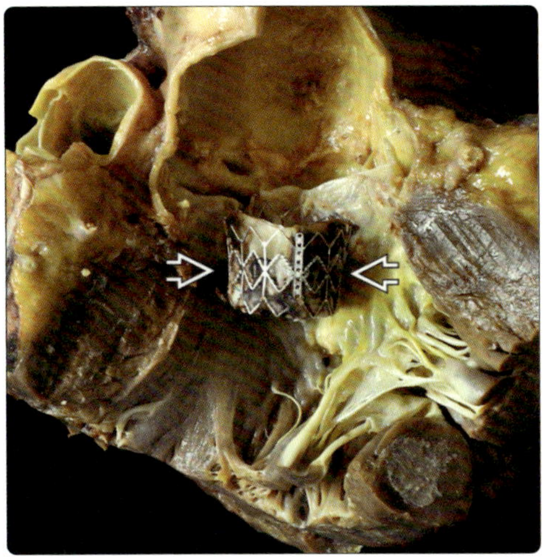

(Left) *This patient with tetralogy of Fallot underwent stenting of the right ventricular outflow tract and deployment of a Melody valve . Devices should be assessed for deformation and strut fractures, which in this case were due to surgical removal.* **(Right)** *This catheter-deployed bioprosthesis was properly seated within the aortic valve annulus. Autopsy evaluation should include assessment of device position, expansion, cusp coaptation, and the potential for perivalvular leaks.*

Inverted Prosthetic Valve Deployment

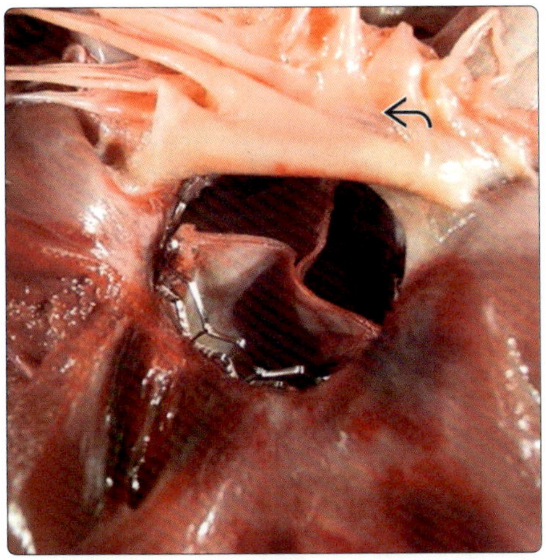

MitraClip Devices in Mitral Valve

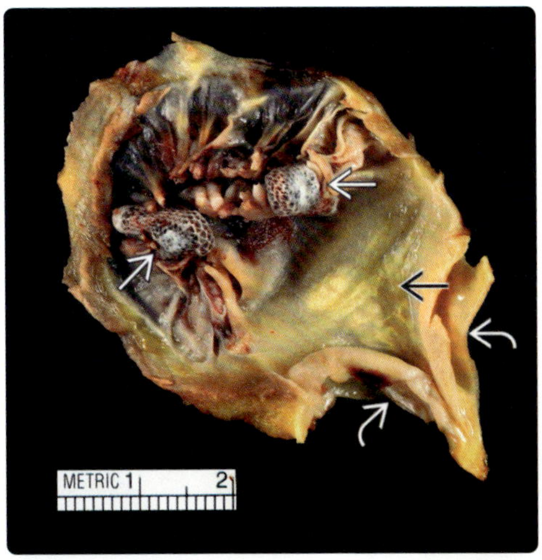

(Left) *Catheter-deployed valves may be placed transfemorally or transapically and must be properly oriented in the catheter sheath to prevent inverted (backward) deployment, as occurred in this unfortunate fatal case. Note the anterior mitral leaflet .* **(Right)** *This mitral valve is shown from the ventricular side. Two MitraClip devices were used to fix the anterior leaflet to segments of the posterior leaflet. Note the portion of the aortic valve and the aortomitral continuity .*

Infective Endocarditis

KEY FACTS

TERMINOLOGY

- Inflammation of endocardium (typically refers to infections on valve surfaces)

ETIOLOGY/PATHOGENESIS

- *Staphylococcus aureus* (31%)
- Viridans streptococci (17%)
- Microbe portal of entry
  - IV drug abuse, dental procedure
- Valve surface damage
  - Degenerative, rheumatic, congenital

CLINICAL ISSUES

- 3-10 episodes per 100,000 person-years
- Mean age: 51-65 years
- M > F (1.2-2.5:1.0)
- Hospital mortality rate: 9.6-26%

MACROSCOPIC

- Vegetations
  - Fleshy, soft, clot-like, friable
  - Septic emboli and infarcts (brain, spleen, kidneys, liver)

MICROSCOPIC

- Vegetations
  - Acute
    - Fibrin, platelets, neutrophils, microorganisms
  - Subacute
    - Granulation tissue, fibroblasts, collagen, plasma cells, absent microbes
- Valve annulus abscess
- Myocardial abscess

TOP DIFFERENTIAL DIAGNOSES

- Nonbacterial thrombotic endocarditis

Mitral Valve Endocarditis: Long-Axis View

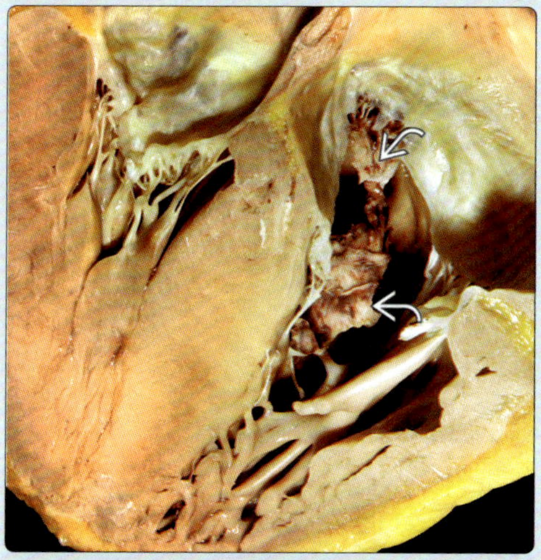

Endocarditis: Gram Stain

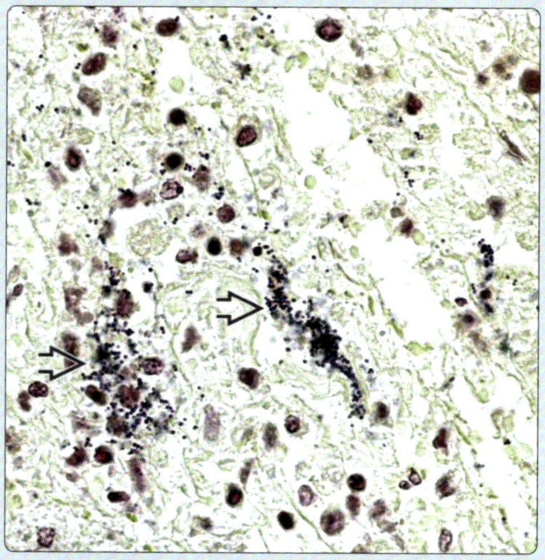

(Left) *Gross photograph of an autopsied heart shows a large, pedunculated vegetation involving the tricuspid valve. The vegetation appears to arise at a septal leaflet commissure.* **(Right)** *Tissue Gram stain from vegetation in the same patient shows gram-positive cocci, the most common type of bacteria seen in endocarditis. Necrotic debris, fibrin, and inflammation are also seen.*

Healing Endocarditis: Aortic Valve

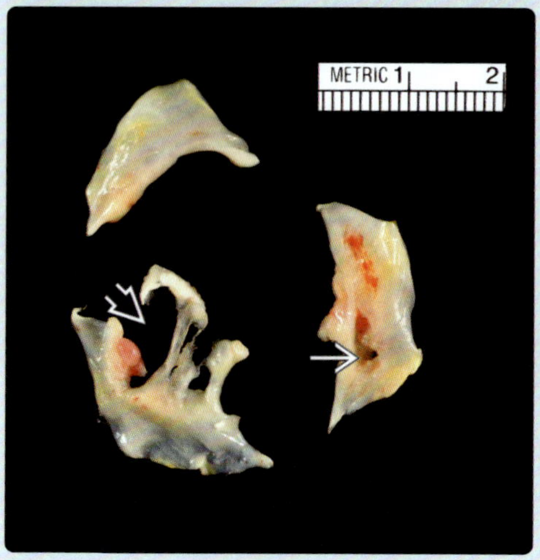

Mitral Valve Endocarditis

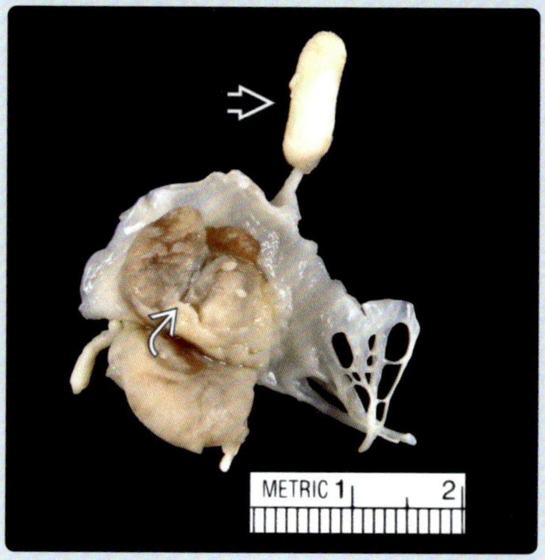

(Left) *Gross photograph of a surgically excised (3-leaflet) aortic valve shows evidence of endocarditis affecting 2 cusps. There are perforations and significant destruction of leaflet tissue. Bulky vegetations are not seen, as is often the case in the later phases of endocarditis.* **(Right)** *Gross photograph shows a large vegetation is present on this surgical mitral valve. One of the cords has ruptured and has vegetative growth as well.*

TERMINOLOGY

Definitions

- Inflammation of endocardium (typically refers to infections on valve surfaces)

ETIOLOGY/PATHOGENESIS

Infectious Agents

- *Staphylococcus aureus* (31%)
- Viridans streptococci (17%)
- Coagulase-negative staphylococci (11%)
- Enterococci (11%)
- Other streptococci (12%)
- Gram-negative *Haemophilus*, *Aggregatibacter*, *Cardiobacterium*, *Eikenella*, and *Kingella* species (HACEK) (2%)
- Gram-negative non-HACEK (2%)

Risk Factors

- Microbe portal of entry
  - IV drug abuse
  - Indwelling catheter
  - Hemodialysis
  - Dental procedure
- Valve surface damage
  - Degenerative
  - Congenital
  - Rheumatic

CLINICAL ISSUES

Presentation

- 3-10 episodes per 100,000 person-years
- Mean age: 51-65 years
- M:F = 1.2-2.5:1.0
- Hospital mortality rate: 9.6-26%
- Acute
  - Rapid onset and progression
  - Acute valvular insufficiency
  - Septic emboli
- Subacute
  - Protracted, insidious/smoldering course
  - Duke criteria
    - Positive blood culture (2 separate draws)
    - Positive imaging study (vegetation by echocardiogram, abscess by CT, etc.)
    - Minor criteria: Predisposition, fever, emboli, glomerulonephritis

Treatment

- Antibiotic therapy (intravenous) often followed by surgery several weeks later

Prosthetic Valve Endocarditis

- More common in people whose native valves had infective endocarditis
  - Often with same organism

IMAGING

Echocardiography

- Vegetations
- Regurgitant jets (Doppler), paravalvular leak
- Abscesses

MACROSCOPIC

Heart Findings

- Vegetations
  - Typically atrial aspect of atrioventricular valves and ventricular aspect of semilunar valves
  - Fleshy, soft, clot-like, friable
- Ruptured cordae
- Leaflet perforation
- Cusp aneurysm (old healed endocarditis)
- Infraction (septic emboli to coronary arteries)
- Perivalvular (ring) abscess

Extracardiac Findings

- Septic emboli and infarcts (brain, spleen, kidneys, liver)
- Mycotic (pseudo) aneurysms
- Postinfectious glomerulonephritis
- Secondary infection of abdominal aortic aneurysm

MICROSCOPIC

Histologic Features

- Vegetations
  - Active: Fibrin, platelets, neutrophils, microorganisms
  - Healing: Granulation tissue, fibroblasts, collagen, plasma cells, absent microbes
- Tendinous cord and leaflet destruction, erosion

ANCILLARY TESTS

PCR

- Next-generation bacterial DNA detection (paraffin tissue)
  - Especially when cultures and special stains are negative

DIFFERENTIAL DIAGNOSIS

Nonbacterial Thrombotic Endocarditis

- Fibrin, platelets without bacteria or purulent inflammation
- Typically small, dotting closing surfaces of leaflets
- Specific types
  - Marantic: Associated with malignancy
  - Libman-Sacks: Associated with lupus, other autoimmune disease

SELECTED REFERENCES

1. Rodríguez-García R et al: Evaluation of 16S rDNA heart tissue PCR as a complement to blood cultures for the routine etiological diagnosis of infective endocarditis. Diagnostics (Basel). 11(8):1372, 2021
2. Lieberman JA et al: Case report: comparison of plasma metagenomics to bacterial PCR in a case of prosthetic valve endocarditis. Front Pediatr. 8:575674, 2020
3. Castonguay MC et al: Surgical pathology of native valve endocarditis in 310 specimens from 287 patients (1985-2004). Cardiovasc Pathol. 22(1):19-27, 2013
4. Boland JM et al: Fungal prosthetic valve endocarditis: Mayo Clinic experience with a clinicopathological analysis. Mycoses. 54(4):354-60, 2011
5. Thiene G et al: Pathology and pathogenesis of infective endocarditis in native heart valves. Cardiovasc Pathol. 15(5):256-63, 2006

(Left) *Gross photograph of an autopsied heart shows a friable vegetation associated with the mitral valve. Significant left ventricular hypertrophy and mitral annular calcification are also present (unrelated to endocarditis).* **(Right)** *Endocarditis can involve other nonvalvular endocardial surfaces, such as this right atrial vegetation associated with an infected catheter tip. The metal probe passes under the Thebesian valve of the coronary sinus ostium.*

Healing Mitral Valve Endocarditis

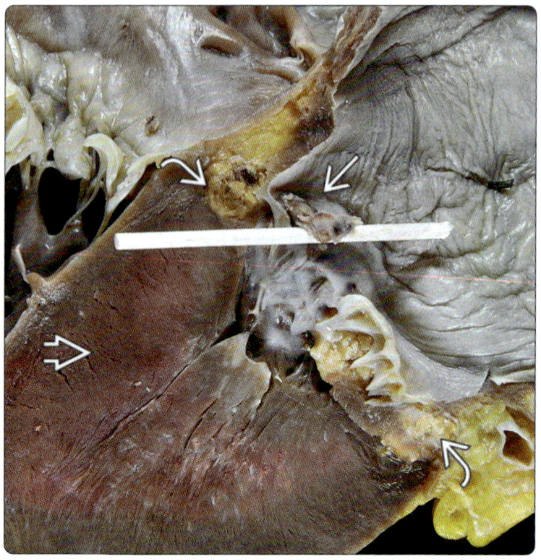

Nonvalvular Endocarditis: Right Atrium

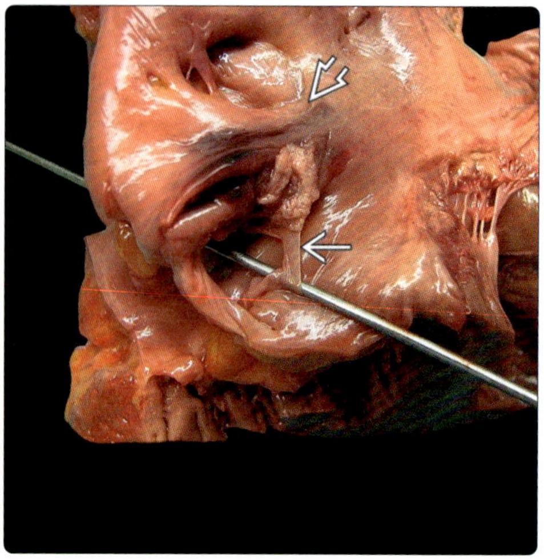

(Left) *Endocarditis can also involve prostheses, such as this valved conduit specimen. The texture of the vegetation is similar to thrombus and is often crumbly and friable. The embolic potential of masses like this is obvious.* **(Right)** *Gross photograph shows the leaflets of this Melody valve prosthesis have been perforated and eroded by active endocarditis. The cusp edges show fleshy, friable, pink vegetative material.*

Prosthetic Valve Endocarditis: Valved Conduit

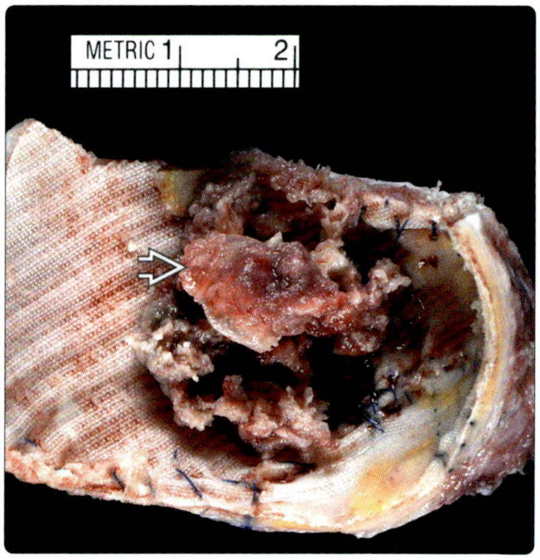

Prosthetic Endocarditis: Transcatheter Aortic Valve Replacement

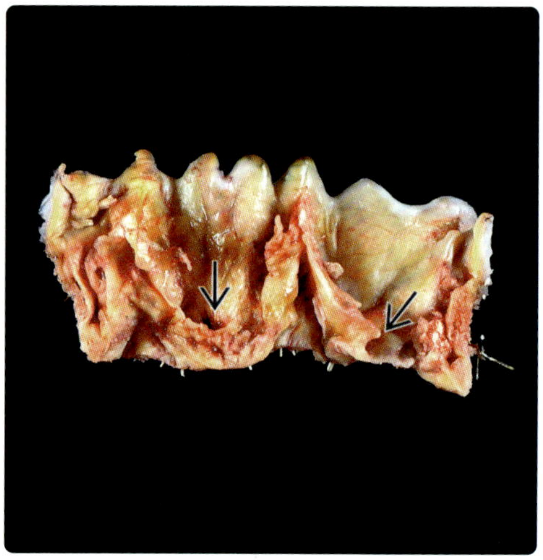

(Left) *Gross photograph of this congenitally malformed aortic valve was secondarily infected. Old healed endocarditis has resulted in a persistent leaflet perforation that would have resulted in significant valvular incompetence. The leaflet shows significant thickening due to fibroelastosis, consistent with postinflammatory disease.* **(Right)** *Lambl excrescences, as seen on this gross photograph of the aortic valve cusp, are normal anatomic variants and should not be mistaken for endocarditis.*

Healed Endocarditis: Unicommissural Aortic Valve

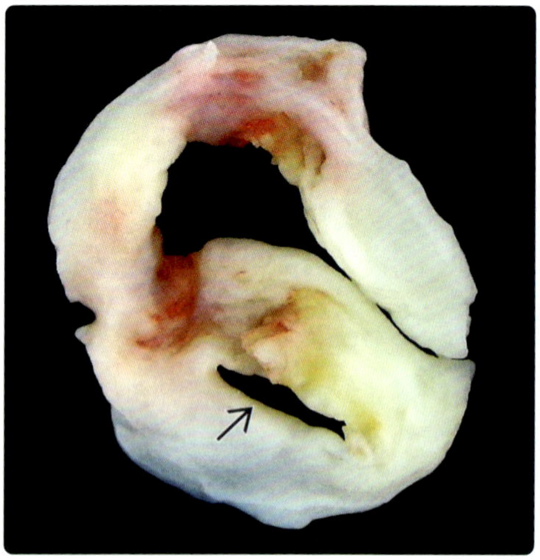

Lambl Excrescence

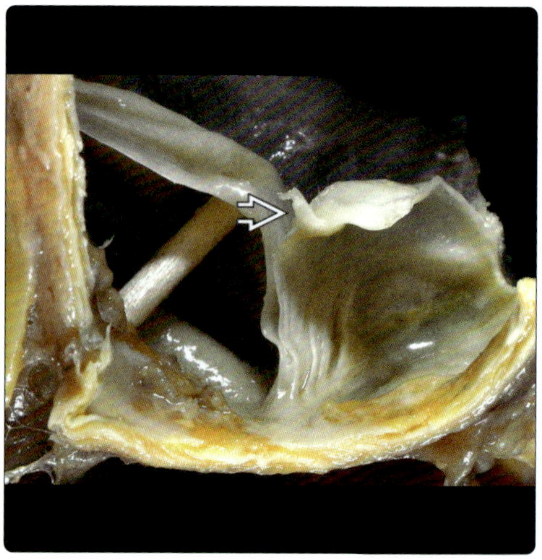

Bicuspid Aortic Valve With Vegetation (Superior)

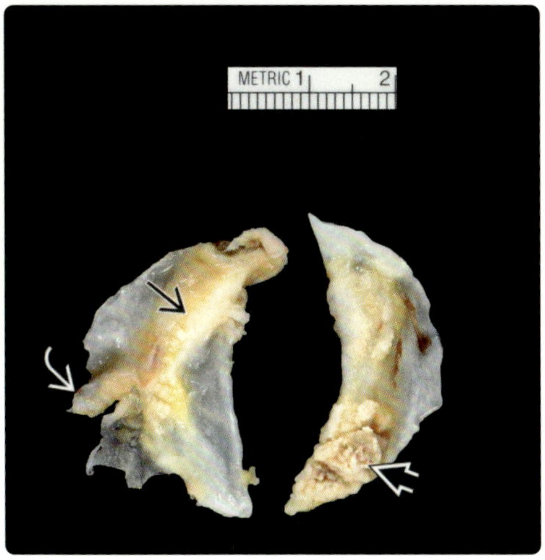

Bicuspid Aortic Valve With Vegetation (Inferior)

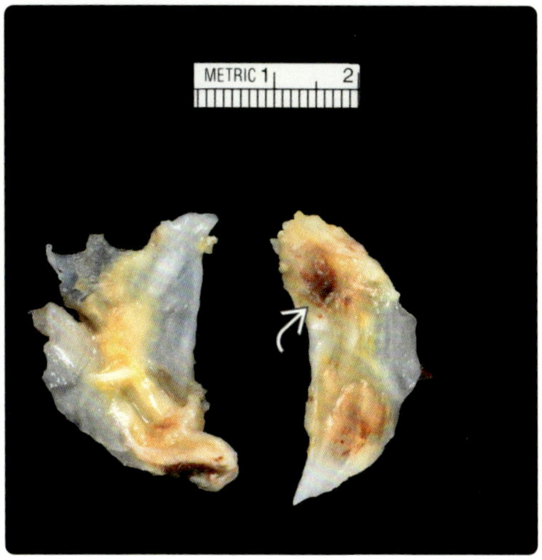

(Left) *Gross photograph of this congenitally malformed aortic valve shows a raphe* ➡ *on the conjoined leaflet. Bulky vegetation* ➡ *is seen on the other leaflet. Typical calcific deposits* ⇨ *from sclerosis associated with bicuspid valve are also seen. Bicuspid valves are a risk factor for endocarditis.* **(Right)** *Gross photograph of the undersurface of this bicuspid valve with endocarditis shows a perforation* ➡ *of the nonconjoined leaflet leading to aortic regurgitation.*

Bulky Vegetation of Bicuspid Aortic Valve

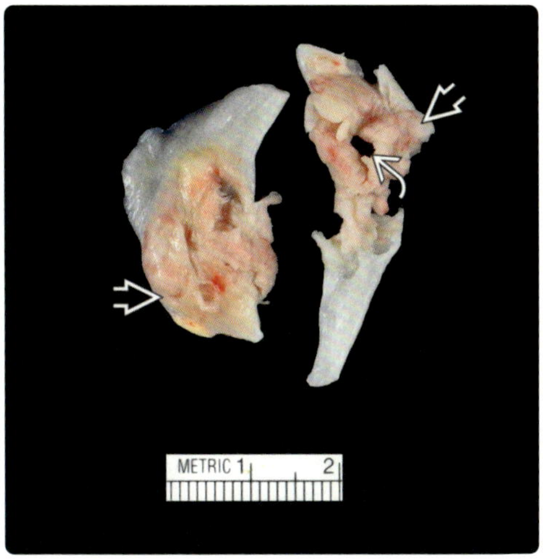

Old Healed Endocarditis

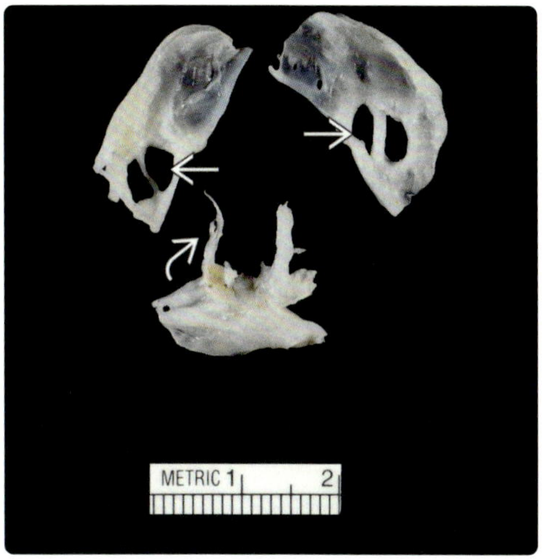

(Left) *Gross photograph of this congenitally bicuspid valve shows prominent bulky vegetations* ➡ *of both leaflets with destruction and perforation* ➡ *of the leaflet to the right. A bicuspid aortic valve is a predisposing risk factor for endocarditis.* **(Right)** *Gross photograph of this 3-leaflet aortic valve shows perforations* ➡ *involving 2 cusps. No active vegetations are seen. This is diagnostic of old healed endocarditis. An incidental Lambl excrescence is seen on the uninvolved cusp* ➡.

Active Endocarditis: Mitral Valve

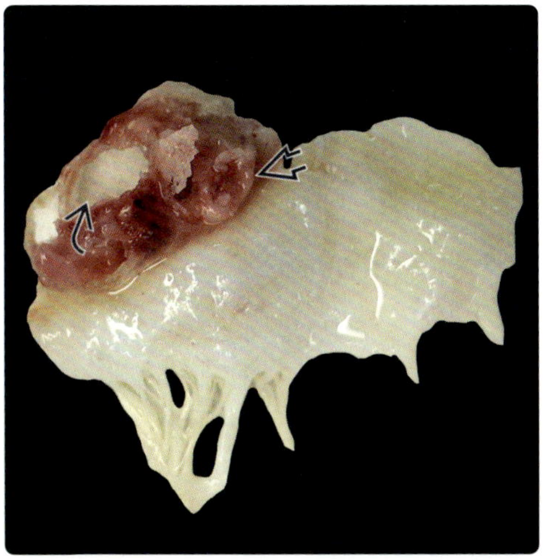

Mitral Valve Vegetation: Perforation

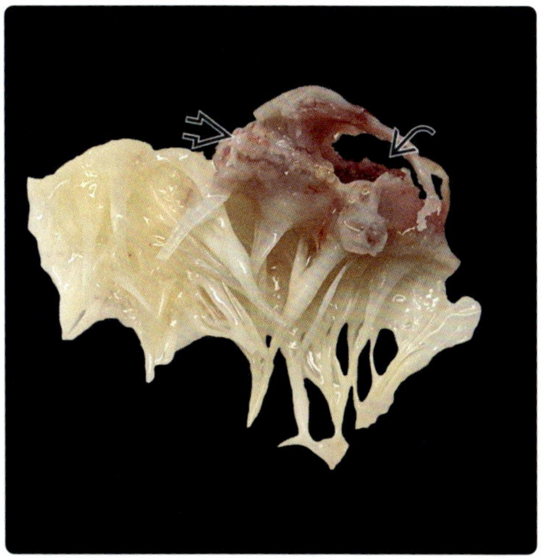

(Left) *Gross photograph of the atrial surface of this anterior mitral leaflet shows a fleshy vegetation* ⇨ *with perforation* ⇨ *leading to acute mitral insufficiency.* **(Right)** *Gross photograph of the ventricular surface of this anterior mitral leaflet shows a destructive, infective vegetation* ⇨ *with perforation* ⇨ *leading to acute mitral insufficiency.*

(Left) *Gross photograph shows both the anterior (left) and a segment of the posterior (right) mitral leaflets are involved by endocarditis. Prominent vegetations* → *are seen but no perforation is evident.* **(Right)** *Gross photograph shows multiple fragments of delicate (normal) leaflet tissue are involved by vegetations* → *of infective endocarditis. Some fragments consist entirely of vegetation* →.

Mitral Valve Endocarditis

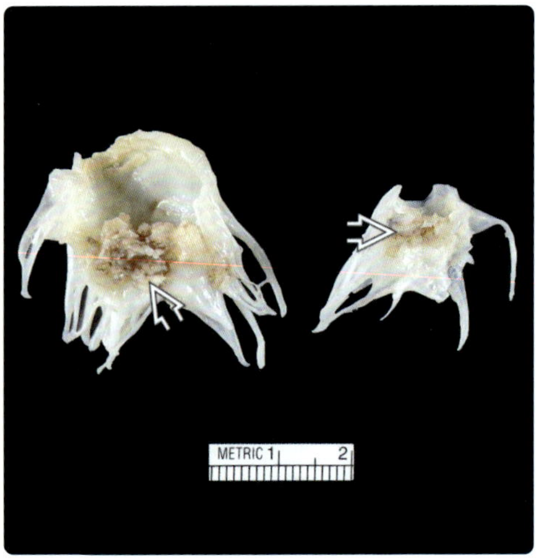

Tricuspid Valve Endocarditis

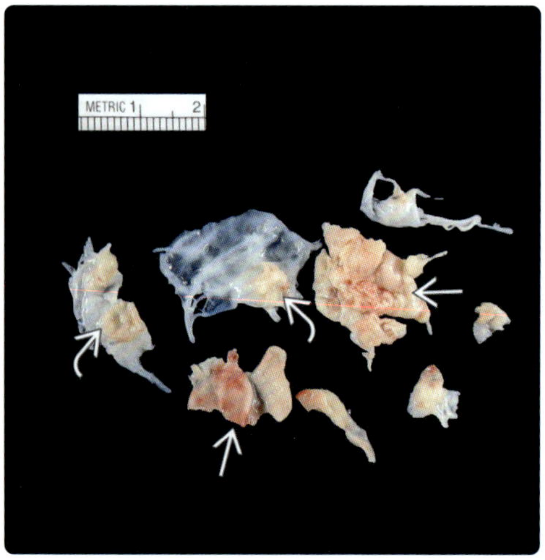

(Left) *Gross photograph of this specimen includes both a bicuspid aortic valve (left) with nodular calcific deposits* → *and a perforation* → *due to endocarditis and a mitral valve (right) with vegetations* →. **(Right)** *The mitral leaflet (left) shows moderate, rubbery thickening. This valve previously underwent repair using a synthetic annuloplasty ring (right). This subsequently became infected, leading to vegetation* → *formation.*

Aortic and Mitral Valve Endocarditis

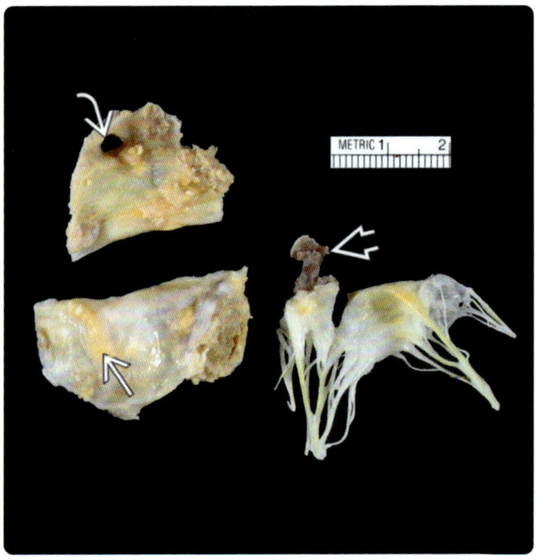

Mitral Annuloplasty Ring Vegetation

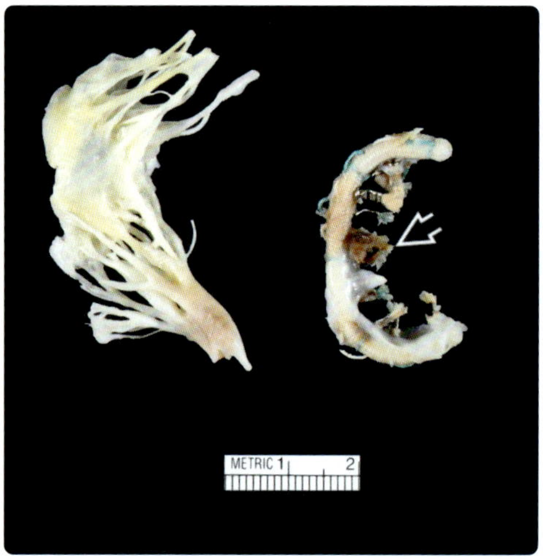

(Left) *Gross photograph of a 3-leaflet aortic valve shows dramatic nodular white vegetations* → *growing on 2 leaflets.* **(Right)** *This photomicrograph shows a destructive inflammatory process* → *damaging the valve tissue. Preexisting calcification* → *is seen at the edge of this valve. There is Gram-positive bacterial growth* → *along the bottom surface.*

Aortic Valve Endocarditis: Massive Vegetation

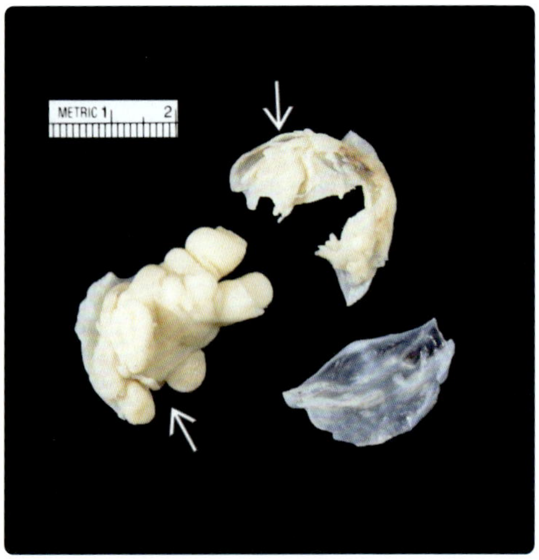

Mitral Valve Endocarditis (Gram Stain)

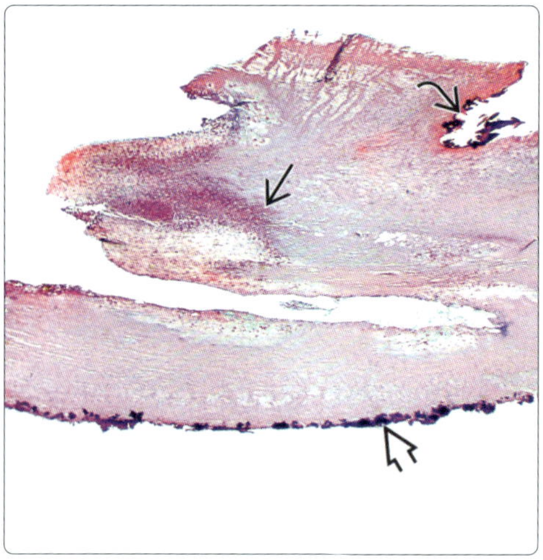

Endocarditis: Low Magnification

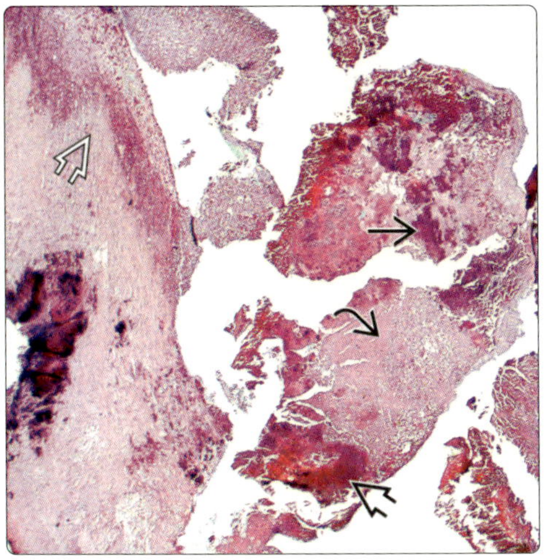

Bacterial Forms: H&E Stain

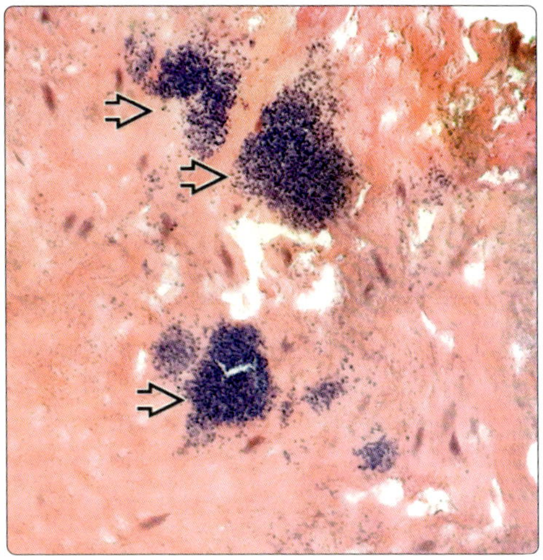

(Left) *Low-power view shows a destructive inflammatory process affecting the underlying valve. The vegetation is composed of bacteria, fibrin, and blood elements.* **(Right)** *"Colonies" or clusters of bacterial organisms can often be seen well on the H&E stain alone in active endocarditis. Gram staining is needed to assess the Gram reaction. After prolonged antibiotic treatment, they may be harder to appreciate.*

Microscopic Features of Fungal Endocarditis

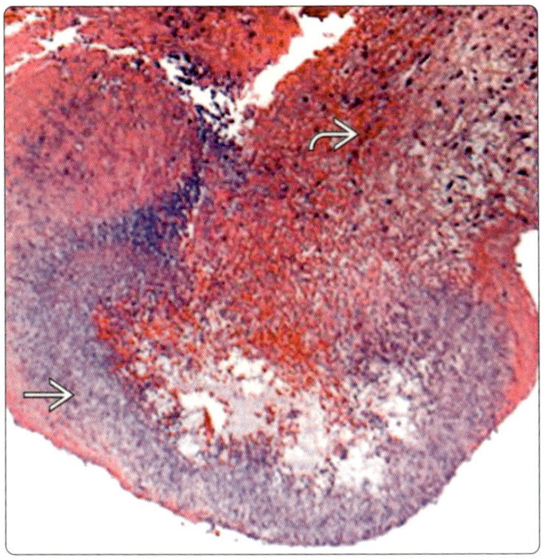

Microscopic Features of Fungal Endocarditis

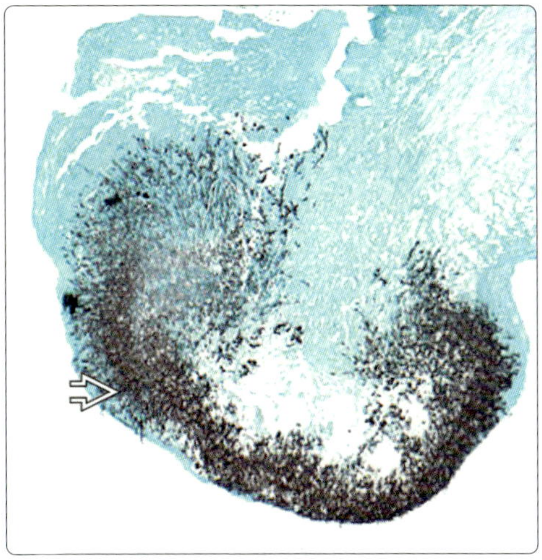

(Left) *H&E-stained section shows thrombotic debris admixed with numerous fungal elements.* **(Right)** *Gomori methenamine silver-stained section shows numerous fungal elements in this case of fungal endocarditis. Fungi are uncommon microorganisms causing endocarditis.*

Warthin-Starry Stain: Endocarditis

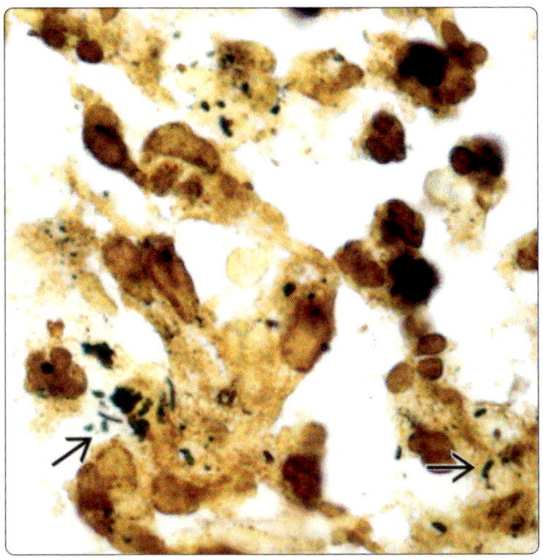

Gram-Positive Bacilli: Endocarditis

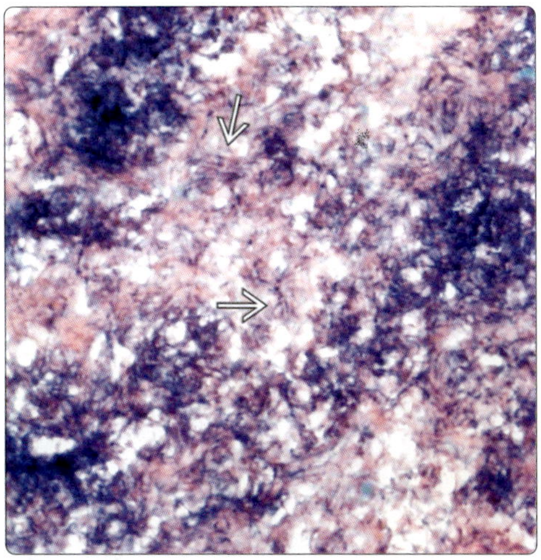

(Left) *In some cases, a silver-based stain (such as Warthin-Starry or Steiner methods) may reveal the presence of microbes when other techniques (Gram and GMS) are negative. This is especially true for syphilis and HACEK organisms.* **(Right)** *Gram-stained section of an endocarditis vegetation is shown. The microscopic field is replete with elongated Gram-positive bacilli (Lactobacillus in this case).*

Ventricular Assist Device Insertion

KEY FACTS

CLINICAL ISSUES

- 4 main clinical settings: Bridge to recovery, bridge to transplant, destination therapy, bridge to decision
- Pros/cons of extracorporal ventricular assist devices (VADs): Easier to inspect and replace components but more invasive, carry higher infection risk, less portable
- Pros/cons of intracorporal VADs: Harder to replace components (only driveline exits body) but carry lower infection risk, very portable
- Total artificial heart reserved for severe biventricular failure

MACROSCOPIC

- Photographic documentation of
  - All extracorporeal and intracorporeal components in situ
  - Device components after disassembly
  - Thrombi and any other abnormalities
- Examine skin at site(s) of device entry for infection; obtain samples for cultures
- Inside body, evaluate device in situ for infection, malorientation of outflow conduit, etc.
- Evaluate sheath at left ventricular apex for thrombus, pannus formation
- Open all conduits, examine blood contact surfaces for thrombus
- Confirm cannula patency
- Examine pump chamber for surface abrasions, wear
- Document serial numbers and findings

MICROSCOPIC

- Thrombus: Alternating layers of RBCs/WBCs and fibrin/platelets
- Sample skin at device entry site(s)
  - Dense neutrophilic inflammation/abscesses indicate infection
  - Perform GMS and Gram stains to identify microorganisms

(Left) *Gross photograph demonstrates all components of a HeartMate II left ventricular assist device (LVAD) in situ at autopsy, including the sewing ring, inflow cannula, pump, outflow conduit, and driveline.* **(Right)** *The CardioWest total artificial heart (TAH) consists of artificial right and left ventricles connected to the atria (behind device), main pulmonary artery, ascending aorta, and pneumatic drivelines.*

In Situ View of HeartMate II LVAD

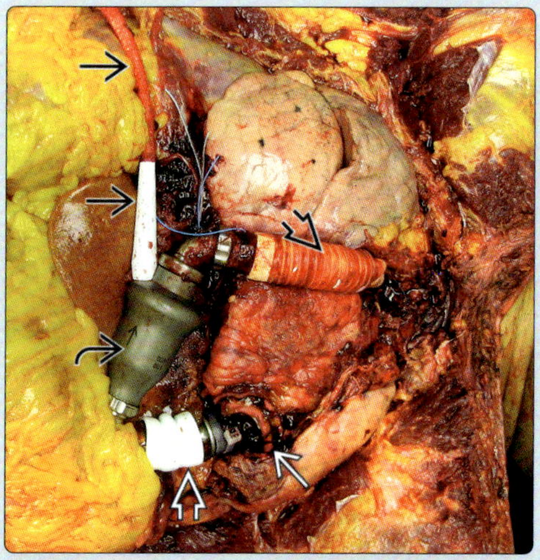

Autopsy Specimen Block With CardioWest Total Artificial Heart

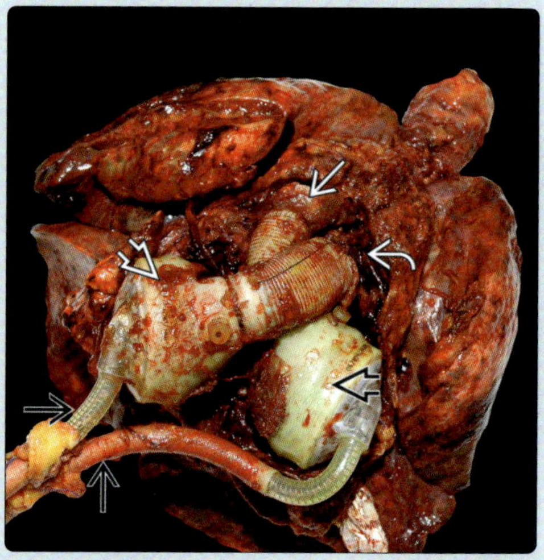

(Left) *The HeartWare HVAD is implantable within the pericardium with the pump attached directly to the left ventricular apex and the outflow conduit attached to the ascending aorta. The driveline is partially hidden under the specimen in this view.* **(Right)** *The CardioWest TAH is attached directly to the atria after surgical removal of the rest of the heart. Note artificial ventricles, drivelines, and Velcro connecting the ventricles.*

HeartWare HVAD Explant

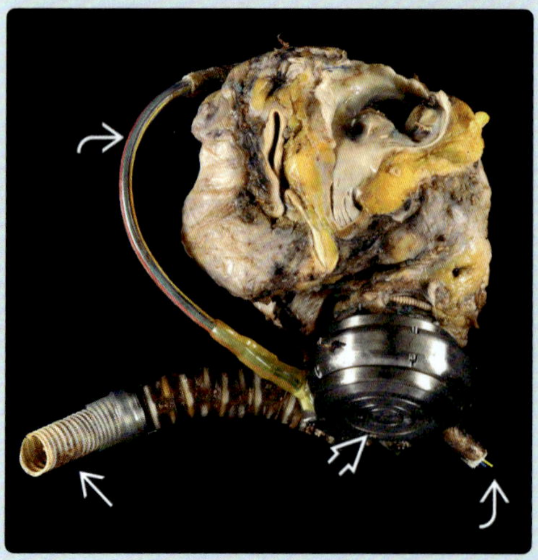

CardioWest Total Artificial Heart

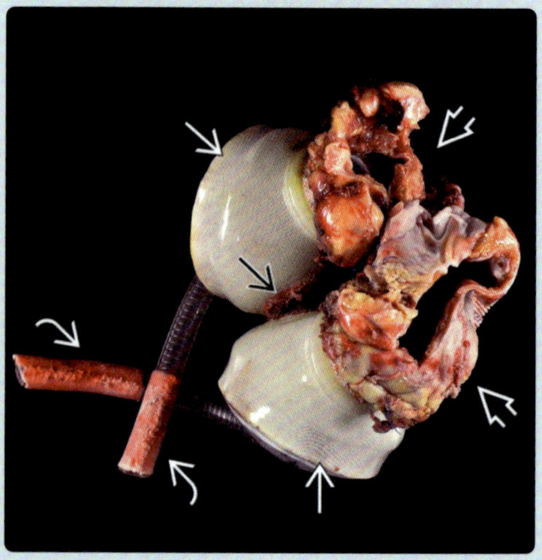

TERMINOLOGY

Abbreviations

- Ventricular assist device (VAD)
- Left VAD (LVAD)
- Right VAD (RVAD)
- Bi-VAD (BiVAD)

CLINICAL ISSUES

Ventricular Assist Devices in Clinical Practice

- Use of VADs has increased exponentially since FDA approval of HeartMate II in USA in 2008
- Support circulation during profound heart failure
  - Bridge to recovery: Temporary support until ventricular function is regained
    - Useful for potentially reversible cardiac conditions, such as myocarditis, postpartum cardiomyopathy
  - Bridge to transplant: Until donor heart available
  - Destination therapy: Provides support indefinitely (for patients who are not candidates for transplantation)
    - Increasingly becoming viable alternative
    - Survival with VAD is expected to approach that of transplantation (10-15 years average) in future
    - Avoids expense and complications of immunosuppression and rejection monitoring
  - Bridge to decision: Support while determining candidacy for transplantation
    - Later transitioned to either destination therapy or transplantation

Ventricular Assist Device Applications

- LVAD most commonly used
  - Right-sided (pulmonary) circulation generally improves with "unloading" of left ventricle
- In profound right heart failure, RVAD may be used
- In biventricular failure, Bi-VAD or total artificial heart (TAH) may be used

Interagency Registry for Mechanically Assisted Circulatory Support

- Monitors VAD use and outcomes
- > 10,000 patients followed
- For continuous flow pumps, current actuarial survival is 80% at 1 year and 70% at 2 years

Research Opportunities

- Myocardial recovery
  - Ongoing investigations into mechanisms during myocardial rest/unloading afforded by VAD support
  - Tissues commonly obtained at time of VAD implantation and at time of VAD removal (including not only at time of recovery or transplantation but also at autopsy)

Types of Ventricular Assist Devices

- Extracorporeal
  - Pump and controller external to body (e.g., Berlin EXCOR Pediatric, BVS 5000)
  - Clinically easier to inspect circuit and replace components in event of thrombus formation
  - More invasive
  - Higher infection risk
  - Less portable
- Intracorporeal
  - Intracardiac (e.g., HeartMate II, HeartMate III, HeartWare HVAD)
    - Direct cannulation of left ventricular apex for inflow, ascending aorta for outflow
    - Only driveline exits body
    - Lower infection risk
    - Very portable (small battery and consoles)
  - Extracardiac (Tohuku EHAM)
    - Pneumatically driven sheath placed around apex
    - Sheath device compresses and relaxes, mimicking cardiac massage
    - Still in developmental testing phase
  - TAH (SynCardia CardioWest)
    - Ventricles and all valves surgically removed, device sewn to atrial cuffs, and outflow cannulae anastomosed to proximal ascending aorta and main pulmonary artery
    - Only pneumatic drivelines exit body
    - FDA approved Freedom portable driver in 2014, enabling discharge from hospital
    - Reserved for patients with severe biventricular failure

Ventricular Assist Device Complications

- Thrombosis
  - Local: Pump thrombosis reported incidence 12.2%, increases rate of morbidity and mortality
    - Risk factors include recent implantation, young age, declining renal function, large stature, less severe ventricular dysfunction, inadequate antiplatelet, or anticoagulation therapy
  - Systemic
    - Thromboembolic events causing ischemic strokes (13-29% annualized rate)
    - Stroke risk during LVAD support is related to pump rather than to patient-related factors
- Bleeding
  - Local: Soft tissues surrounding pump
  - Systemic
    - Cerebral bleeding: Probably secondary to changes in cerebrovascular endothelial function and structure
    - Gastrointestinal bleeding (25-40% annualized rate)
      - Higher rate with continuous flow pumps
      - Probably secondary to acquired von Willebrand syndrome, anticoagulation, activation of fibrinolytic systems, presence of angiodysplasia
- Infection: Risk increases with duration of device implantation
  - Local: Pocket/drive-line infection, prevalence varies from 14-28%; pump endocarditis has 50% mortality rate (bacteria and fungi have been found in vegetations); device infection is risk factor for worse survival
  - Systemic: Sepsis most common fatal complication
- Life-threatening ventricular arrhythmia
  - Occurs in early postimplantation period with high mortality rate; incidence: 22-59%
- Mechanical failure
- Others: Right ventricular failure

Summary of Pulsatile Flow Pump Ventricular Assist Devices

Device	Manufacturer	Notes
Berlin EXCOR Pediatric	Berlin Heart	Extracorporeal, pediatric applications
CardioWest	SynCardia Systems, Inc.	Total artificial heart
Thoratec pVAD II	Thoratec	Short to midterm support, left ventricular assist device, right ventricular assist device, or biventricular assist device
Novacor LVAD	Novacor	1st generation, now discontinued
BVS 5000	Abiomed	1st generation, now discontinued
HeartMate XVE	Thoratec	1st generation, now discontinued

Summary of Continuous Flow Pump Devices

Device	Manufacturer	Notes
HeartMate III	Abbott	Intrapericardial implantation, larger profile than HVAD
HeartMate II	Thoratec	1st FDA approval
HeartWare HVAD	HeartWare, Inc.	Small size allows intrapericardial implantation
Heart Assist 5	MicroMed Cardiovascular, Inc.	Direct flow sensing and management
DuraHeart	Terumo Heart, Inc.	Centrifugal flow magnetic levitation pump
2000 FlowMaker	Jarvik Heart, Inc.	Axial flow magnetically driven pump
Impella	Abiomed	Augments rather than replaces ventricle function
DeBakey Child	MicroMed Cardiovascular, Inc.	Small, intracorporeal, pediatric applications
Evaheart	Sun Medical	Centrifugal flow magnetic levitation pump
Synergy Pocket Micro-Pump	HeartWare, Inc. (formerly CircuLite, Inc.)	Size of AA battery, partial-assist of less sick patients

MACROSCOPIC

Photographic Documentation

- Essential for medical, legal, and educational purposes
- Photograph all extracorporeal and intracorporeal components in situ
- Photograph device components after disassembly
- Photograph thrombi, any other abnormalities

External Examination

- Examine skin at site(s) of driveline or cannula entry and exit for purulence, necrosis, erythema, signs of infection
- If signs of infection present, obtain samples for microbiologic culture

Internal Examination

- Evaluate device in situ for signs of infection, disconnection of components, scarring with change in orientation of outflow conduit, other abnormalities
    - Sewing ring and sheath at left ventricular apex
        - Evaluate for thrombus and pannus formation
    - Device components: Inflow cannula, pump, outflow conduit and anastomosis to ascending aorta, driveline
- Disassemble device and examine components
    - Open all conduits and examine blood contact surfaces for thrombus and confirm cannula patency
    - Examine pump chamber for surface abrasions, wear, etc. (using beam lighting and magnification or, if possible, pump disassembly)
    - Examine housings and diaphragms
- Document serial numbers and any abnormalities

MICROSCOPIC

Histologic Features

- Thrombus
    - Alternating layers of RBCs/WBCs and platelets/fibrin
    - Must be distinguished from postmortem clot; shows heavier blood components (WBCs) settling to one side of clot, in gravity-dependent fashion
- Skin at device entry and exit sites
    - Dense neutrophilic inflammation and abscess formation indicate infection
    - Special stains (e.g., GMS and Gram) to identify and characterize microorganisms

ANCILLARY TESTS

Radiography and CT

- Evaluate component integrity, mineralization, etc.

SELECTED REFERENCES

1. Lin PT et al: Forensic considerations in a series of 14 deaths of patients with a left ventricular assist device. Acad Forensic Pathol. 9(3-4):200-11, 2019
2. Hanke JS et al: Five-year results of patients supported by HeartMate II: outcomes and adverse events. Eur J Cardiothorac Surg. 53(2):422-7, 2018
3. Sajgalik P et al: Current status of left ventricular assist device therapy. Mayo Clin Proc. 91(7):927-40, 2016
4. Kirklin JK et al: Sixth INTERMACS annual report: a 10,000-patient database. J Heart Lung Transplant. 33(6):555-64, 2014

Driveline From HeartMate II LVAD

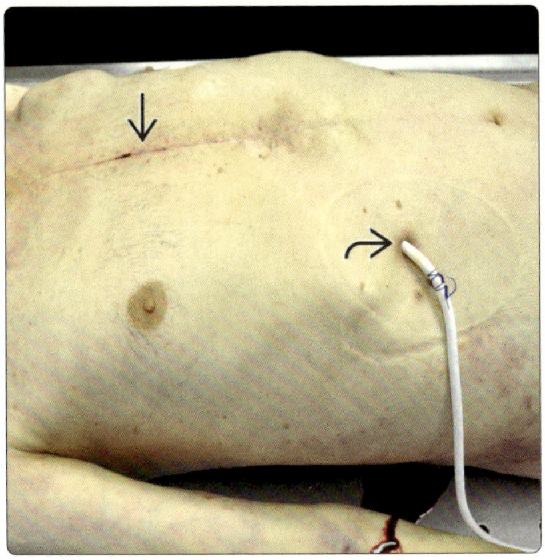

CardioWest Total Artificial Heart Without Atria

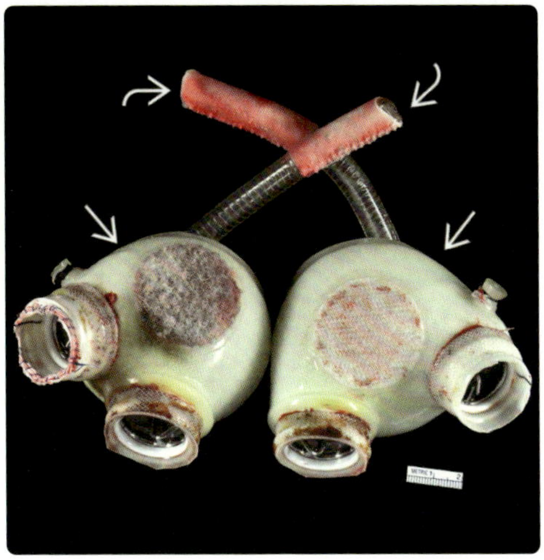

(Left) *Gross photograph shows HeartMate II LVAD is an intracorporeal device with nearly all components inside the chest (note thoracotomy scar →). Only the driveline → exits the body, which connects to an external driver console. This lowers the risk of infection and enables device portability.* **(Right)** *The CardioWest TAH is attached directly to the atria after surgical removal of the rest of the heart. Note the artificial ventricles → and drivelines →.*

HeartWare HVAD

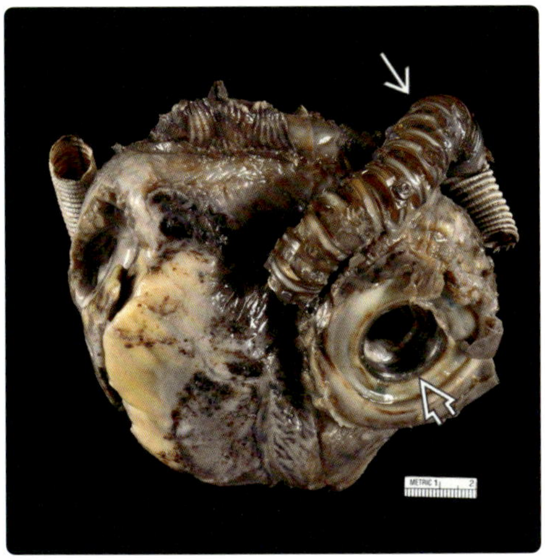

HeartWare HVAD Components

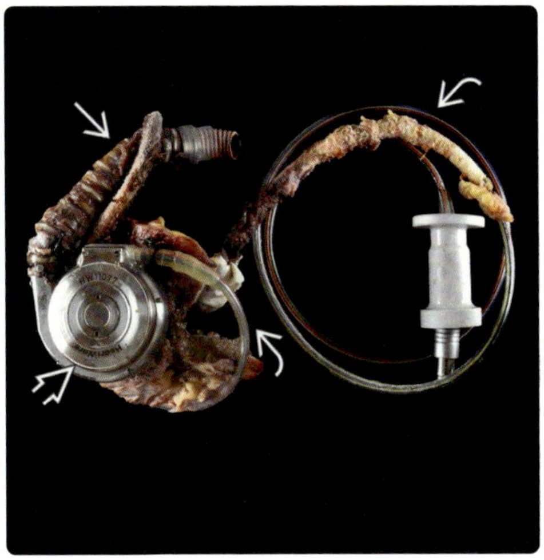

(Left) *Gross photograph shows the HeartWare HVAD is implantable within the pericardium with the pump → attached directly to the left ventricular apex and the outflow conduit → attached to the ascending aorta. The driveline is hidden under the specimen in this view.* **(Right)** *This gross photograph shows the heart has been largely removed from the HeartWare HVAD, revealing the device's components, including the pump →, outflow conduit →, and long, coiled driveline → with adherent subcutaneous tissue.*

HeartMate II LVAD Components

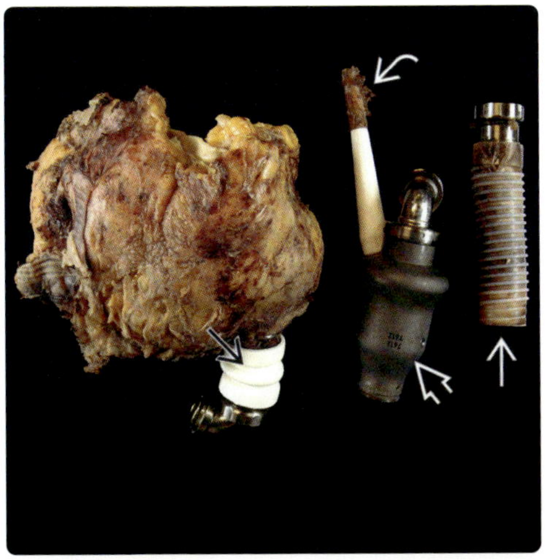

HeartMate II LVAD Pump Chamber

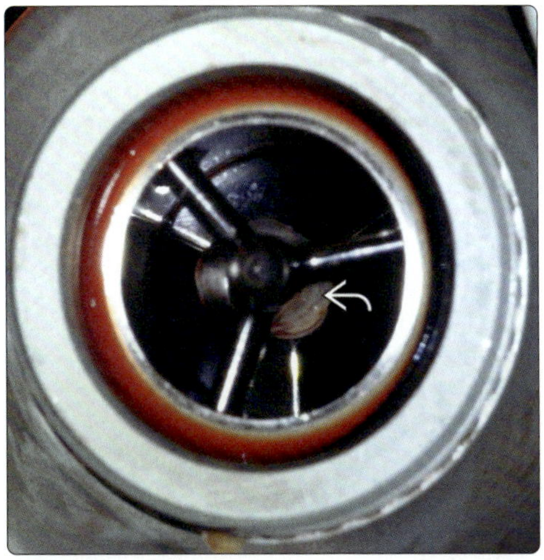

(Left) *Disassembly is essential for identifying thrombi, damage, and other device abnormalities. This gross photograph shows the inflow cannula →, pump →, outflow conduit →, and driveline → of a HeartMate II LVAD.* **(Right)** *This view into the pump chamber of a HeartMate II LVAD demonstrates old thrombus → surrounding the driveshaft above the impeller. Thrombus formation is an infrequent but important complication, and examination of VADs must include a careful search for thrombus.*

Heart Transplant

KEY FACTS

ETIOLOGY/PATHOGENESIS

- Cellular rejection (CR)
  - T-cell-mediated host response to allografted heart stimulated by "foreign" human leukocyte antigen (HLA) and other antigens expressed in graft tissue
- Antibody-mediated rejection (AMR)
  - Antibody-mediated host response to allografted heart with damage with complement activation
- Cardiac allograft vasculopathy (CAV)
  - Arterial narrowing due to concentric intima thickening by proliferating smooth muscle cells and fibroblasts

CLINICAL ISSUES

- Most rejection episodes occur within 6 months post transplant

MACROSCOPIC

- Rejection
  - May appear grossly normal
- CAV
  - Epicardial and intramyocardial artery involvement
- Complications
  - Malignancy (masses, lymphadenopathy)
  - Infection (pneumonia, abscess, meningitis, pyelonephritis)
  - Medication toxicity (cushingoid features, nephrosclerosis)

MICROSCOPIC

- CR
  - Perivascular/interstitial mononuclear inflammation
  - Myocyte damage in association with mononuclear inflammation
- AMR
  - Capillary endothelial cell swelling and injury
  - Positive staining for complement (C4d and C3d)
- CAV
  - Marked concentric intima thickening

Allograft Vasculopathy: Gross

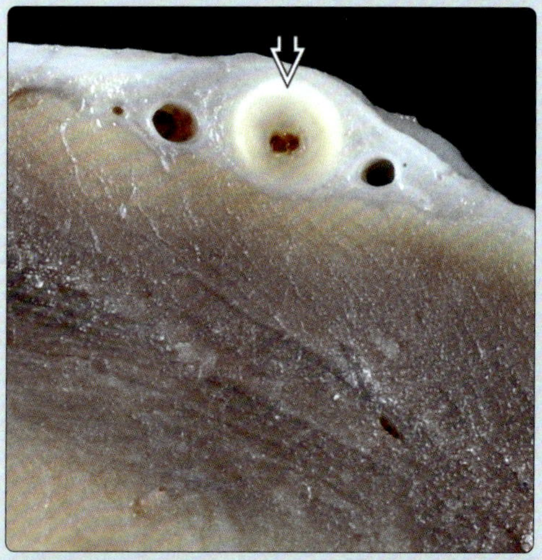

Acute Cellular Rejection

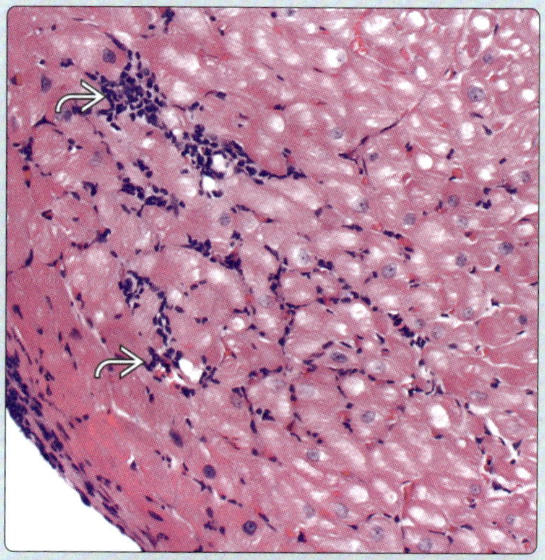

(Left) *Gross photograph of an autopsied heart from a patient with cardiac transplantation shows severe cardiac allograft vasculopathy with near-complete occlusion of the left anterior descending artery.* **(Right)** *H&E of an endomyocardial biopsy with obvious lymphoid infiltrate distorting the myocyte architecture and focally surrounding myocytes is shown. This process is diagnostic of cellular rejection.*

C3d Immunofluorescence

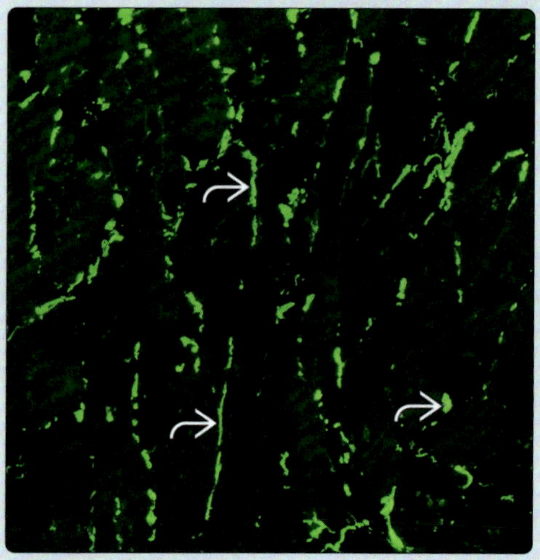

Deep Quilty Lesion

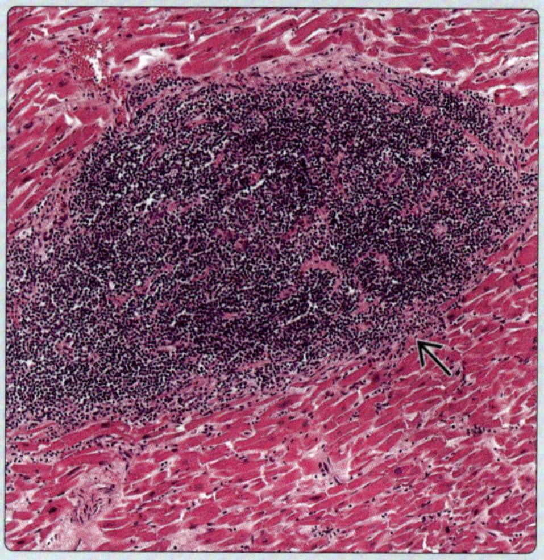

(Left) *Fluorescence photomicrograph shows positive capillary staining for C3d, one of the immunopathology criteria for antibody-mediated rejection.* **(Right)** *Photomicrograph shows a well-demarcated lymphoid aggregate deep in the myocardium. This most likely represents "deep" Quilty effect, a clinically insignificant and enigmatic finding in cardiac allografts.*

TERMINOLOGY

Synonyms

- Antibody-mediated rejection (AMR): Humoral rejection, vascular rejection
- Cardiac allograft vasculopathy (CAV): Transplant coronary artery disease, transplant vasculopathy, allograft arteriopathy, transplant arteriosclerosis

ETIOLOGY/PATHOGENESIS

Cellular Rejection

- T-cell-mediated host response to allografted heart stimulated by "foreign" human leukocyte antigen (HLA) and other antigens expressed in graft tissue
  - Class I antigens (HLA-A, -B, and -C) constitutively expressed on most heart cells, especially vascular endothelium
  - Class II antigens (HLA-DP, -DQ, and -DR) are constitutively expressed on vascular endothelium, resident macrophages
  - Presentation of antigen occurs to T cells directly or indirectly via antigen-presenting and endothelial cells
- T-cell antigen stimulation leads to graft injury
  - Activated T cells produce proinflammatory cytokines
  - Activated CD8(+) cytotoxic T cells participate in cytotoxic killing of graft myocytes
  - Activated T cells activate B cells and can stimulate donor-specific antibody production

Antibody-Mediated Rejection

- Antibody-mediated host response to allografted heart with damage from complement activation and antibody-dependent cellular cytotoxicity
  - Antibody binding to capillary antigen presented by endothelium activates endothelial signaling
  - Antibody binding initiates complement cascade
  - Complement split products and other chemoattractants lead to macrophage aggregation within injured vessels

Cardiac Allograft Vasculopathy

- Arterial narrowing due to concentric intima thickening by proliferating smooth muscle cells and fibroblasts, leading to chronic ischemia with secondary myocyte changes and interstitial fibrosis
- Proposed mechanisms include
  - Immunologic
    - Ongoing endothelial injury (such as with persistent or repetitive AMR)
    - Increased T-helper cell activity
    - HLA mismatch
  - Nonimmunologic
    - CMV infection
    - Coagulation cascade and fibrin deposition
    - Traditional atherosclerotic risk factors

CLINICAL ISSUES

Epidemiology

- Incidence
  - Most rejection episodes occur within 6 months post transplant
  - ~ 30% of recipients have some rejection during 1st year post transplant
  - Cellular and AMR can occur simultaneously
  - CAV incidence post transplant
    - 8% at 1 year
    - 20% at 3 years
    - 30% at 5 years
    - 50% at 10 years

Presentation

- Asymptomatic presentation is most common
- Symptoms occur only with moderate or severe ACR and include symptoms associated with heart failure
- Risk factors associated with cellular rejection (CR)
  - Noncompliance with immunosuppressive regimen
  - Diarrhea, vomiting interfering with medication absorption
  - Infections
  - Untoward effects/interference of other medications
  - Drastic changes in weight
- Risk factors associated with AMR
  - Young, female
  - Multiparity
  - Presensitization (panel-reactive antibody or single antigen bead)
  - Previous transplantation
  - Multiple transfusions

Treatment

- Options
  - CR
    - Mild rejection [International Society of Heart Lung Transplantation (ISHLT) 1R] may resolve spontaneously (~ 85%)
    - Pulse corticosteroids or modification of baseline calcineurin inhibitor dose
    - Antithymocyte globulin
  - AMR
    - Corticosteroids, augmented immunosuppressives
    - Rituximab, bortezomib
    - Plasmapheresis
  - CAV
    - Stents, mTOR inhibitors to stop progression

IMAGING

General Features

- Echocardiography
- Angiography

MACROSCOPIC

External Examination

- Median sternotomy
- Other scars
  - Coronary bypass grafting (harvest sites)
  - Ventricular assist device, driveline exit site
  - Chest tubes
- Congestive heart failure
  - Edema, ascites, hepatomegaly
- Sepsis/disseminated intravascular coagulation

- Petechiae, ecchymoses

Cardiac Allograft Vasculopathy

- Epicardial and intramyocardial artery involvement
- Vein involvement
- Subendocardial ischemic changes
- Interventions (e.g., stenting)

Complications

- Infection (pneumonia, urinary tract, abscess, meningitis, pyelonephritis)
- Malignancy (masses, metastases, lymphadenopathy, splenomegaly)
- Medication toxicity (cushingoid features, nephrosclerosis, adrenal atrophy)

Biopsy Sites

- Right ventricle apical trabeculations

MICROSCOPIC

Cellular Rejection

- Perivascular/interstitial mononuclear inflammation predominantly composed of activated lymphocytes and macrophages
- Myocyte damage in association with mononuclear inflammation
  - Damage is not myocyte necrosis but rather encroachment of inflammatory cells into myocyte borders, leading to architectural distortion
- In severe ACR, neutrophils &/or eosinophils may be present; such rejection is usually mixed with AMR
- Grading
  - ISHLT 2004 grading schema intended for biopsy but may be applied loosely (1R, 2R, 3R)
  - Alternatively, descriptive diagnosis of severity could be given (mild/moderate/severe; focal/diffuse, etc.)

Antibody-Mediated Rejection

- Histopathology
  - Capillary endothelial cell swelling and injury
  - Interstitial edema, hemorrhage
  - Adherence of macrophages to endothelium
  - Severe cases show edema, hemorrhage, karyorrhexis, vasculitis, and thrombi
  - Occasional neutrophils, eosinophils
- Immunopathology
  - Positive staining for complement (C4d and C3d)
  - CD68(+) intravascular macrophages

Cardiac Allograft Vasculopathy

- Epicardial coronary arteries
  - Marked concentric intima thickening
  - Smooth muscle cell proliferation
  - Intimal inflammatory cells
  - Variable lipid, foamy macrophages
- Intramyocardial arteries
  - Myointimal proliferative changes
  - Endothelialitis
  - Perivascular fibrosis
- Myocardium
  - Subendocardial sarcoplasmic vacuolization
  - Myocyte hypertrophy, interstitial fibrosis
  - Rare infarct-like changes

Other Conditions

- Posttransplant lymphoproliferative disorder
  - EBV(+) lymphoid proliferation
  - Polyclonal/polymorphous or monoclonal
- Infections
  - CMV, *Toxoplasma*, Chagas
- Recurrent amyloid

Quilty Effect

- Nodular subendocardial lymphoid aggregates
  - Well circumscribed, rounded
  - May extend or be seen deep to endocardium as well
- Prominent capillary vascularity within lymphoid aggregates
- B cells and follicular dendritic cells admixed in lymphoid aggregate

Biopsy Sites

- Fibrosis with entrapped myocytes and variable amount of mononuclear inflammation

"Harvesting" or Perioperative Ischemic Damage (for Fresh Transplants)

- Mixed infiltrate and coagulation necrosis secondary to perfusion-related damage to myocardium
- Resolves in initial weeks post transplant

ANCILLARY TESTS

Immunohistochemistry

- CD3, CD20; may be used to rule out posttransplant lymphoproliferative disorder and Quilty effect
- C4d to assess AMR (frozen tissue for immunofluorescence or else paraffin immunohistochemistry methods)
- CD68 to identify intravascular macrophages, which would support diagnosis of AMR

SELECTED REFERENCES

1. Gökler J et al: Indications, complications, and outcomes of cardiac surgery after heart transplantation: results from the Cash study. Front Cardiovasc Med. 10:879612, 2022
2. Berry GJ et al: The 2013 International Society for Heart and Lung Transplantation Working Formulation for the standardization of nomenclature in the pathologic diagnosis of antibody-mediated rejection in heart transplantation. J Heart Lung Transplant. 32(12):1147-62, 2013
3. Kittleson MM et al: Antibody-mediated rejection. Curr Opin Organ Transplant. 17(5):551-7, 2012
4. Kobashigawa J et al: Report from a consensus conference on antibody-mediated rejection in heart transplantation. J Heart Lung Transplant. 30(3):252-69, 2011
5. Lu WH et al: Diverse morphologic manifestations of cardiac allograft vasculopathy: a pathologic study of 64 allograft hearts. J Heart Lung Transplant. 30(9):1044-50, 2011
6. Tan CD et al: Update on cardiac transplantation pathology. Arch Pathol Lab Med. 131(8):1169-91, 2007
7. Marboe CC et al: Nodular endocardial infiltrates (Quilty lesions) cause significant variability in diagnosis of ISHLT grade 2 and 3A rejection in cardiac allograft recgripients. J Heart Lung Transplant. 24(7 Suppl):S219-26, 2005
8. Stewart S et al: Revision of the 1990 working formulation for the standardization of nomenclature in the diagnosis of heart rejection. J Heart Lung Transplant. 24(11):1710-20, 2005
9. Rowan RA et al: Pathologic changes in the long-term transplanted heart: a morphometric study of myocardial hypertrophy, vascularity, and fibrosis. Hum Pathol. 21(7):767-72, 1990

Acute Cellular Rejection: Perivascular Infiltrate

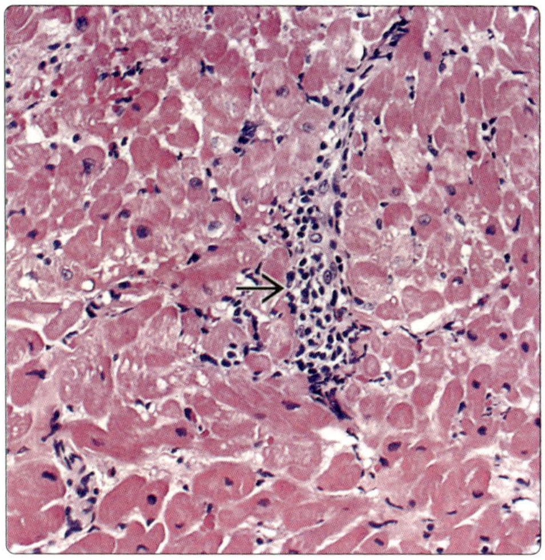

Acute Cellular Rejection: Autopsy

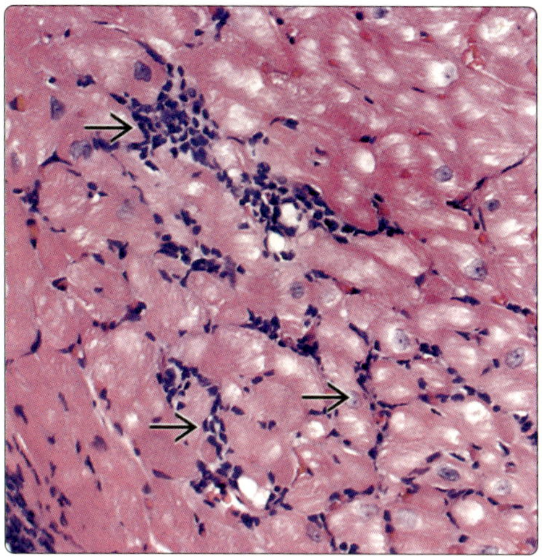

(Left) *Photomicrograph from a cardiac allograft at autopsy shows a small perivascular lymphocytic infiltrate* → *without obvious myocyte injury. This would be consistent with mild cellular rejection.* **(Right)** *A more diffuse lymphocytic infiltrate* → *is seen in this cardiac allograft at autopsy. There is still no obvious or definite myocyte injury, so it would be considered mild. The ISHLT grading system is intended for biopsies, and caution should be taken when applying this to autopsy.*

Severe Rejection

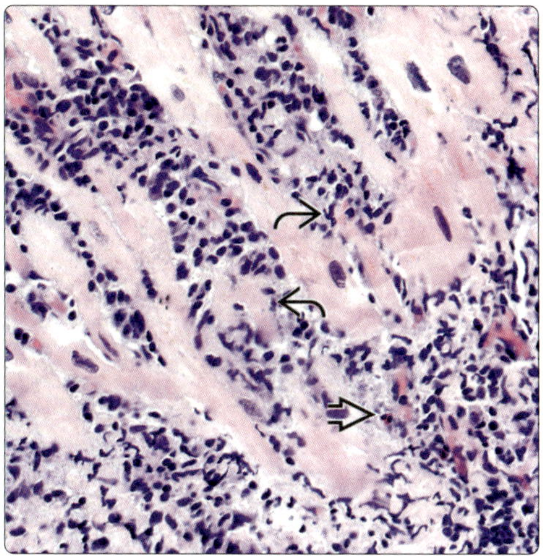

Severe Cellular Rejection

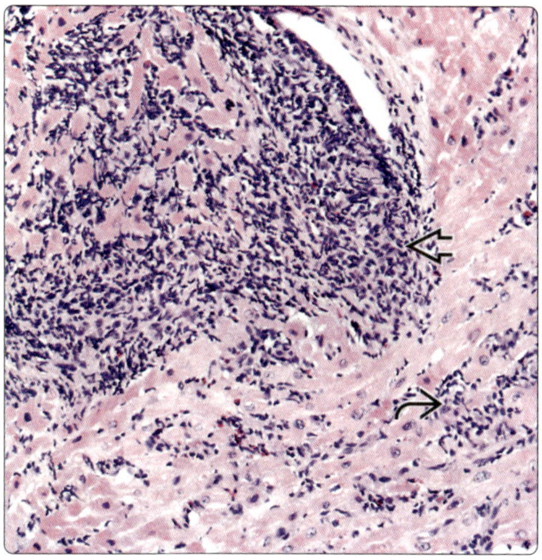

(Left) *Photomicrograph of a heart allograft at autopsy shows a lymphoid inflammatory infiltrate with rare eosinophils* →*, associated with multifocal myocyte injury* →*, consistent with more severe rejection. Clinical correlation would be needed to determine the role of rejection in the cause of death.* **(Right)** *This allograft heart at autopsy also showed marked perivascular infiltrate* → *with several foci of myocyte injury* →*, consistent with severe rejection.*

Multiple Quilty Lesions

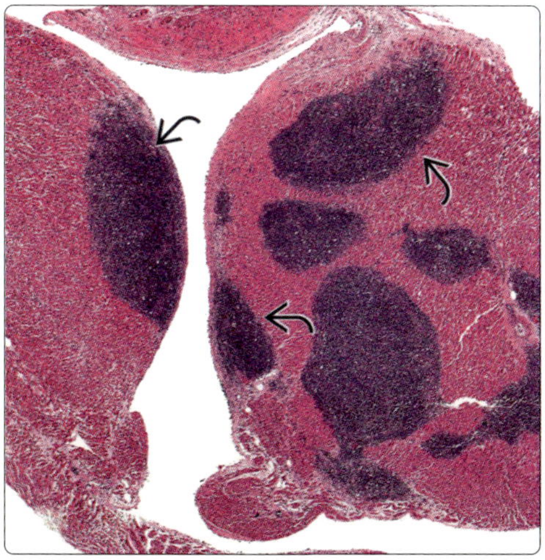

Quilty Effect

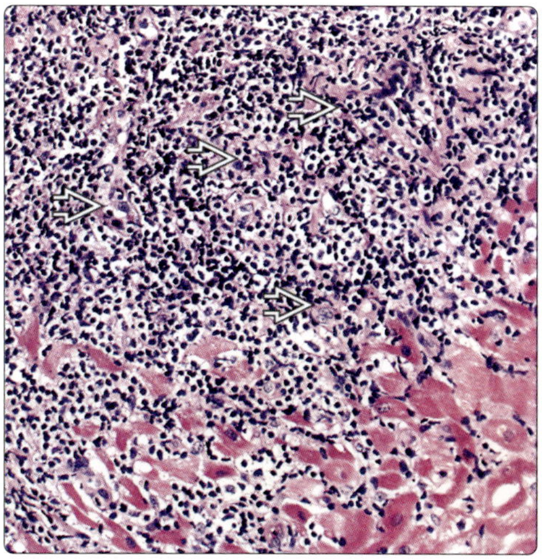

(Left) *Photomicrograph shows trabecular myocardium from the right ventricle of a transplant heart at autopsy. There are rounded lymphoid aggregates* → *without interstitial extension, consistent with Quilty effect.* **(Right)** *At higher magnification, Quilty effect shows proliferating capillaries* →*. This is helpful in the differential diagnosis with cellular rejection.*

Antibody-Mediated Rejection: Histologic Features

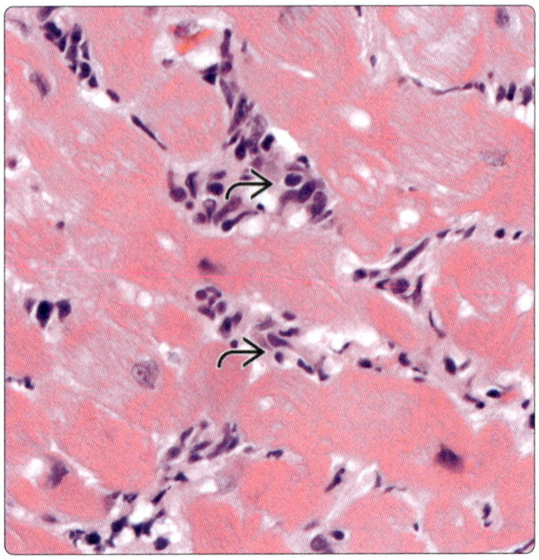

Interstitial Edema in Antibody-Mediated Rejection

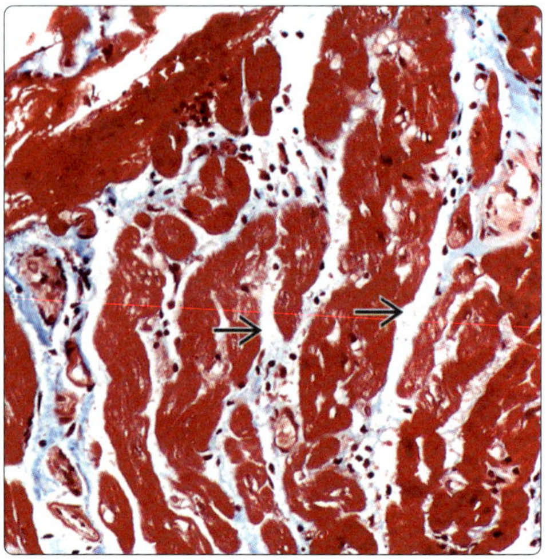

(Left) *High-power photomicrograph of cardiac transplant myocardium at autopsy shows prominent intravascular mononuclear cells, a hallmark of antibody-mediated rejection. Immunostaining for complement (C4d, C3d) &/or macrophages (CD68) should be performed to complete the diagnostic work-up.* **(Right)** *Trichrome stain shows another feature prominent in antibody-mediated rejection: Interstitial edema. The capillaries also show intravascular mononuclear cells.*

Vasculitis in Antibody-Mediated Rejection

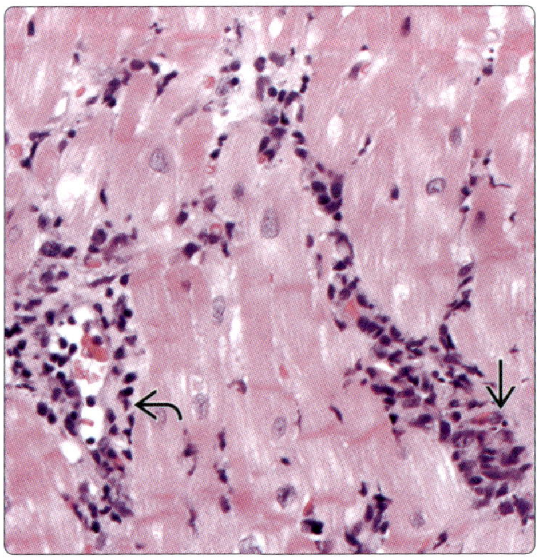

Severe Rejection: Overlapping Histology

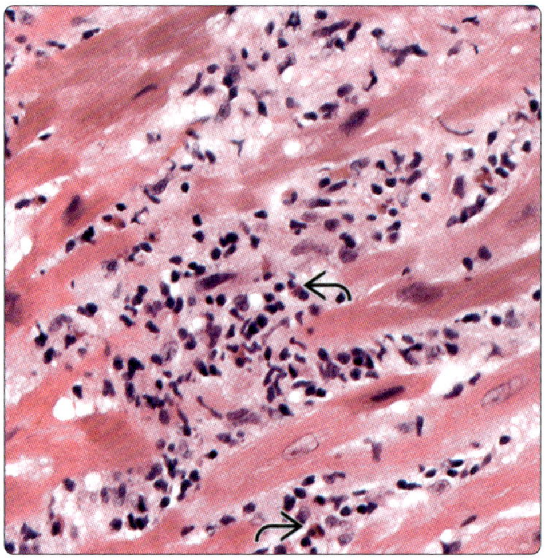

(Left) *High-magnification view of a transplant myocardium at autopsy shows more severe venular changes with transmural mononuclear inflammation and focal karyorrhectic debris. Complement stains were positive in this case.* **(Right)** *In severe rejection, it can be difficult to distinguish cellular rejection features from those of severe antibody-mediated rejection. Several eosinophils are seen in this case of severe rejection. Complement staining is helpful in cases like this.*

Immunofluorescence Staining for C4d

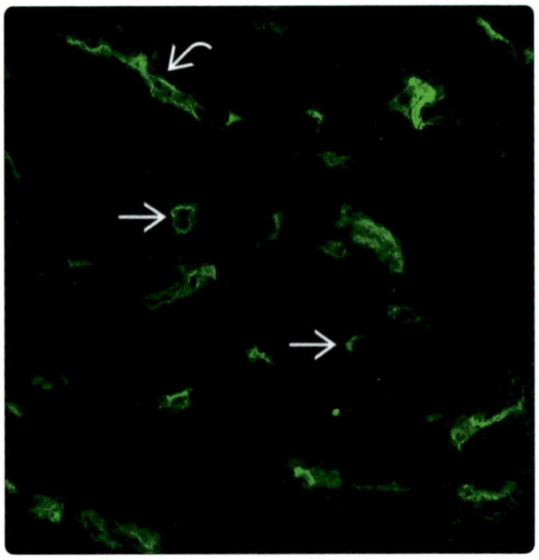

Immunoperoxidase Staining for C4d

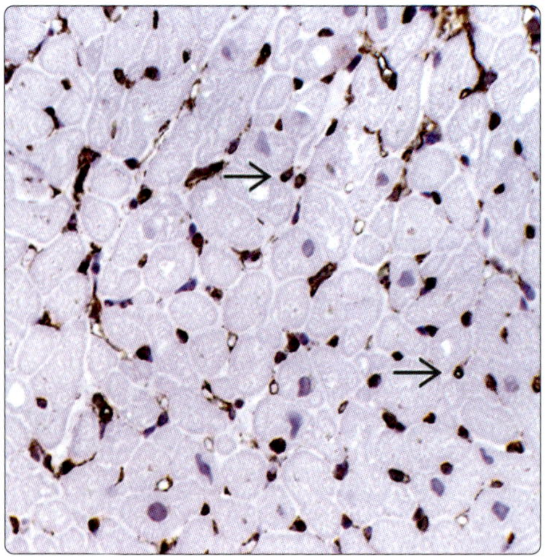

(Left) *Immunofluorescence staining of this cardiac allograft at autopsy is positive for C4d deposition. Capillaries are seen in cross section and longitudinal section.* **(Right)** *C4d staining can also be performed using immunohistochemistry techniques in paraffin sections at autopsy. The capillaries are strongly and diffusely positive. The staining is crisp, linear, and circumferential, all features that are helpful in excluding false-positive artifact staining.*

Cardiac Allograft Vasculopathy

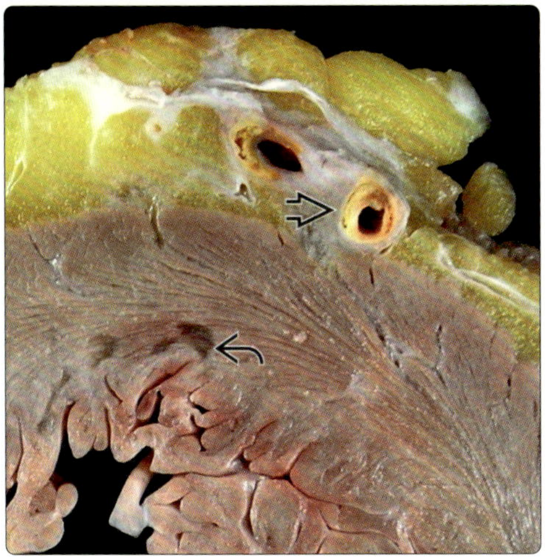

Cardiac Allograft Vasculopathy on Angiogram

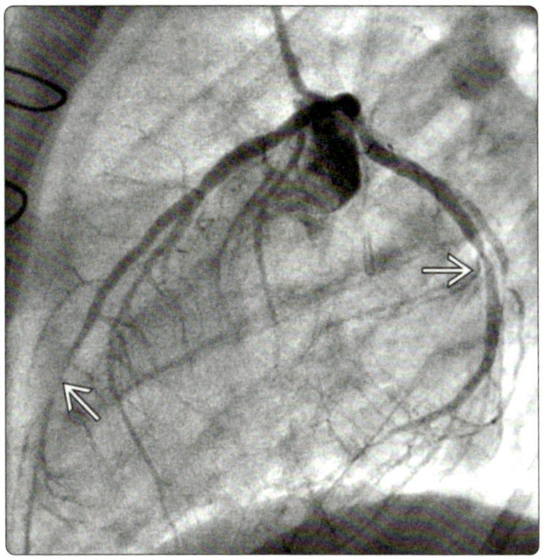

(Left) *Epicardial coronary artery from a transplanted heart at autopsy shows significant allograft vasculopathy ➡. There are also small, depressed, old subendocardial infarctions ➡ in the territory of this artery.* **(Right)** *Angiogram in a cardiac transplant patient shows areas of tapered narrowing ➡, consistent with graft vasculopathy. Since this is only a "luminogram," the degree of cross-sectional stenosis is likely to be greater than anticipated based on the angiogram.*

Allograft Vasculopathy

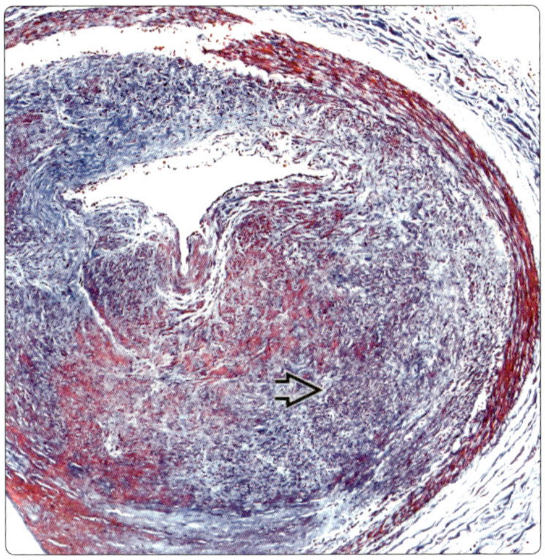

Cardiac Allograft Vasculopathy: Elastic Stain

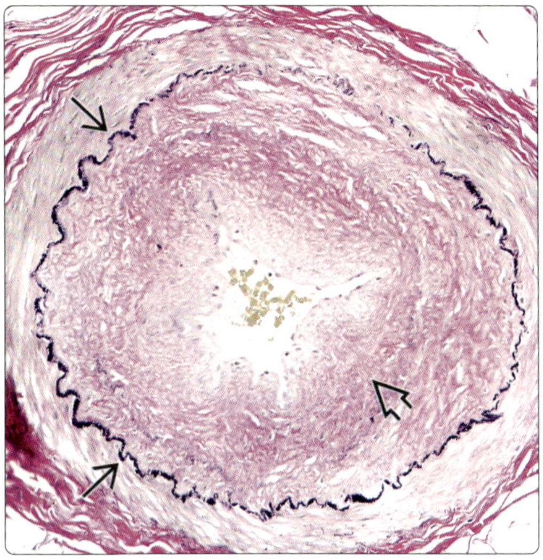

(Left) *Low-power photomicrograph of an epicardial coronary artery from an allograft heart at autopsy shows near-complete luminal occlusion. The intima has been expanded by smooth muscle cells and collagen ➡.* **(Right)** *Elastic stain highlights the internal elastic lamina ➡. The narrowing of this artery is due to an increase in collagen ➡ and proliferating vascular smooth muscle cells in the intimal layer (inside the internal elastic lamina).*

Vasculitis in Allograft Vasculopathy

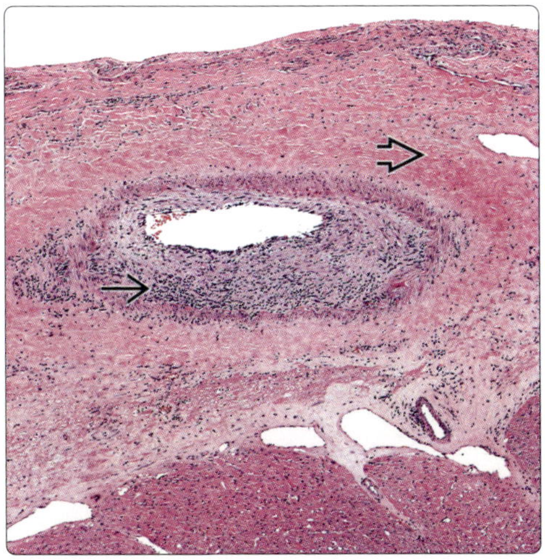

Subendocardial Ischemic Vacuolation

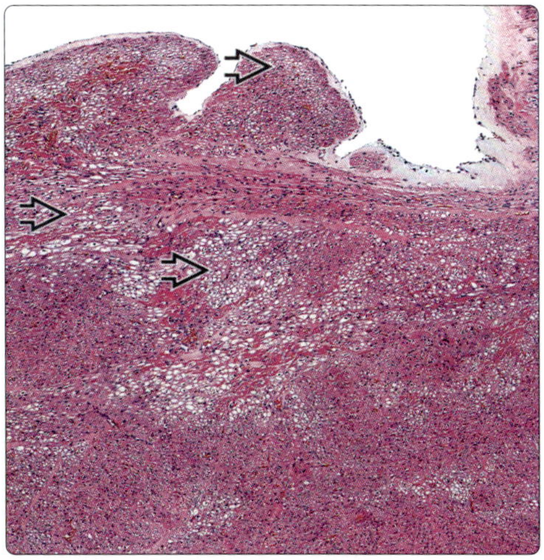

(Left) *Epicardial branch coronary artery from a transplanted heart at autopsy also shows inflammation, largely confined to the intima ➡. There is also an unusual amount of epicardial fibrosis ➡.* **(Right)** *Prominent subendocardial myocyte vacuolization change ➡ is seen in this allograft with cardiac allograft vasculopathy. This finding suggests ongoing chronic ischemia, leading to "hibernating" myocardium.*

Thoracic Aortic Aneurysm Repair

KEY FACTS

TERMINOLOGY

- Aneurysm: Localized pathologic dilatation of vessel wall at least 50% greater than normal; true aneurysm contains all layers of vessel wall

ETIOLOGY/PATHOGENESIS

- May be syndromic or nonsyndromic
- Syndromic: Marfan syndrome (fibrillin 1), vascular Ehlers-Danlos, Loeys-Dietz syndrome (types 1 and 2), familial thoracic aortic aneurysm (TAA) syndrome
- Nonsyndromic: 15% of patients with nonsyndromic TAA have positive family history
- 1.3% of general population has bicuspid aortic valve (BAV), and 14% of patients with TAA have BAV

CLINICAL ISSUES

- Usually silent until complications (dissection/rupture)
- Risk of rupture ↑ with ↑ size; > 6 cm has 30% risk of rupture/dissection
- Indications for repair: Size, growth rate, symptoms
- Endovascular repair: Fabric (polyester or PTFE)-covered metallic (nitinol, stainless steel) stent deployed across aneurysm to exclude it from aortic blood flow leading to aneurysm thrombosis and remodeling
- Open repair: Ascending and arch repair with coronary artery and branch vessel reimplantation ± aortic valve replacement

MICROSCOPIC

- Anastomotic sections: Adventitial granulation tissue and fibrosis with longer duration grafts, abscess if superimposed infection
- Aortic sections: Intramural hematoma (dissection), acute or chronic, medial degeneration, smooth muscle cell loss
- Heart with hypertrophy and areas of interstitial fibrosis in cases with aortic valve insufficiency, varying stages of acute and healing coagulative myocyte necrosis in cases with infarction

Histology of Aneurysm Wall

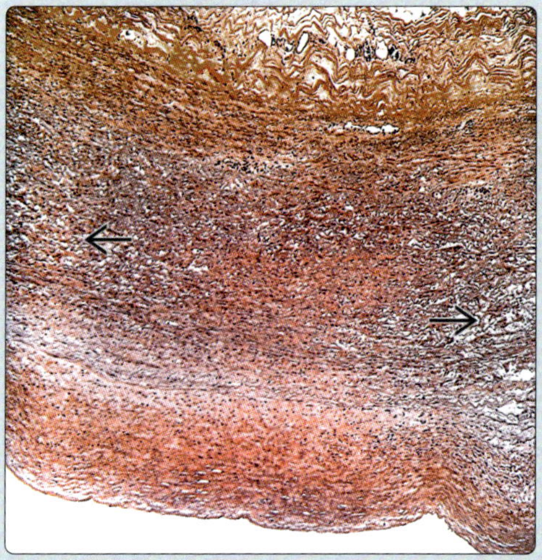

Ascending Aortic Aneurysm: In Situ View

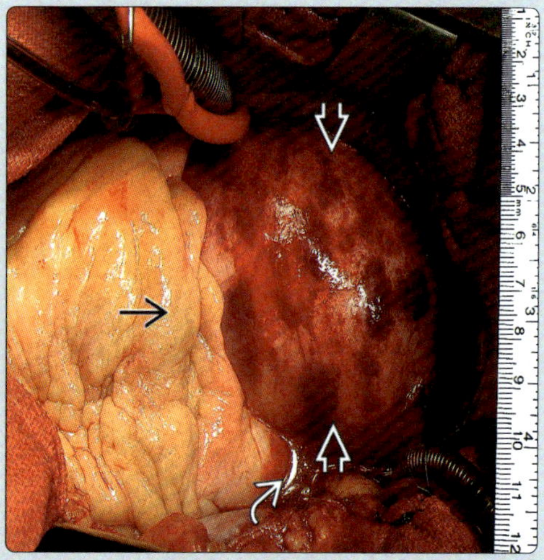

(Left) *Thoracic aneurysm wall shows degenerative changes in the media. The media demonstrates loss of staining of nuclei of smooth muscle cells and increase in proteoglycans* ⇒. **(Right)** *Ascending aortic aneurysm* ➡ *required repair due to its large size. The heart* ⇒ *and pulmonary artery* ➡ *are noted.*

Types of Thoracic Aneurysms

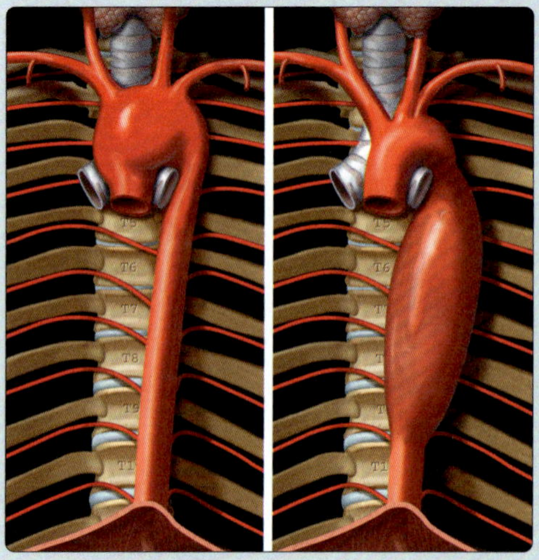

3D Sagittal Reconstruction

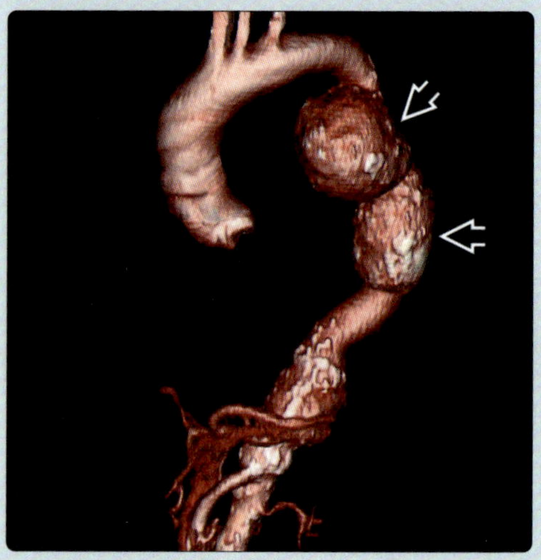

(Left) *Graphic shows types of aneurysms involving thoracic aorta. On the left, an ascending aneurysm is shown, and on the right, a descending thoracic aneurysm. Endograft repair is easier for the descending type.* **(Right)** *3D sagittal reconstruction of a complicated descending thoracic aortic aneurysm* ➡ *is shown.*

TERMINOLOGY

Abbreviations

- Thoracic aortic aneurysm (TAA) repair
- Thoracic endovascular aortic repair (TEVAR)
- Open thoracic aortic repair (OTAR)

Definitions

- Aneurysm: Localized pathologic dilatation of vessel wall at least 50% greater than normal
  - True aneurysm contains all layers of vessel wall
  - Aortic size ↑ with age (1-2 mm/year)
  - Normal ascending aorta generally < 3.5 cm; descending thoracic aorta generally < 2.5 cm

ETIOLOGY/PATHOGENESIS

Pathogenesis

- May be syndromic or nonsyndromic
- Syndromic: Marfan syndrome (fibrillin 1), vascular Ehlers-Danlos, Loeys-Dietz syndrome (types 1 and 2), familial TAA syndrome
- Nonsyndromic: 15% of patients with nonsyndromic TAA have positive family history
  - Genes associated with nonsyndromic TAA include *ACTA2*, *MYH11*, *TGFBR1*, and *TGFBR2*
    - These genes may be associated with TGF-β signaling, indicating similar pathogenesis to syndromic TAA
- Bicuspid aortic valve (BAV)
  - 1.3% of general population has BAV, and 14% of patients with TAA have BAV
  - Valve function may be stenotic, regurgitant, or normal, suggesting factors other than hemodynamics play role in formation of TAA with BAV

Infection

- Historically, syphilitic aortitis in tertiary syphilis was important cause of TAA; now rare
  - Proliferative endarteritis of vasa vasorum → ischemic injury to vascular media → aneurysmal dilatation

CLINICAL ISSUES

Epidemiology

- Incidence
  - TAA incidence is 10.4/100,000 person-years

Presentation

- Usually silent until complications (dissection/rupture)
  - Risk of rupture ↑ with ↑ size; > 6 cm has 30% risk of rupture/dissection
  - Rupture presents with acute pain, hypotension/shock
    - Pain location varies with site of aneurysm
      - Ascending: Anterior chest pain
      - Arch: Neck pain
      - Descending: Back pain between scapulae
  - Chronic pain seen with large aneurysms due to distention and compression of surrounding structures
  - Large aneurysms may present with superior vena cava (SVC) syndrome
    - 1st report of SVC syndrome was due to syphilitic ascending aortic aneurysm
    - Syndrome caused by partial to complete obstruction to blood flow in SVC ± thrombosis of vessel
    - Symptoms include dyspnea, facial swelling, facial congestion, cough, and arm swelling
- Postrepair complications
  - Shock, valvular insufficiency, stroke, embolic phenomena, ischemic myocardial, gastrointestinal and hepatic injury, acute tubular injury/necrosis, infection and ischemic spinal cord injury, thoracoabdominal or descending aortic aneurysm repair

Treatment

- Surgical approaches
  - Indications for repair
    - Size, growth rate, symptoms
  - Types of repair
    - Endovascular: Fabric (polyester or PTFE)-covered metallic (nitinol, stainless steel) stent deployed across aneurysm to exclude it from aortic blood flow leading to aneurysm thrombosis and remodeling
    - Most commonly used for descending thoracic aneurysms, ascending and aortic arch hybrid procedures (multiple grafts, combined endovascular and open procedures) used for ascending and arch repair
    - Open: Ascending and arch repair with coronary artery and branch vessel reimplantation ± aortic valve replacement (Bentall procedure: Ascending aortic aneurysm graft with aortic valve replacement and coronary artery reimplantation)

MACROSCOPIC

External Examination

- Pallor (hemorrhagic shock from rupture), petechiae (disseminated intravascular coagulation following rupture and hemorrhage), sternotomy incision (OTAR), groin incision (TEVAR)
- Facial congestion and swelling (SVC syndrome)
- Syndromic features
  - Marfan (thin, long limbs; arm span greater than height; long digits; pectus excavatum)
  - Loeys-Dietz (type 1 overlaps with Marfan with craniofacial anomalies bifid uvula, cleft palate hypertelorism), type 2 overlaps with Marfan and vascular Ehlers-Danlos (usually only bifid uvula, pectus, joint laxity and long digits, and bruising)
  - Vascular Ehlers-Danlos (bruising; velvety, translucent skin; small, lax joints)

Internal Examination

- In situ documentation of graft type, segment of aorta grafted (open or endovascular), length and patency of graft, patency of branch vessels, including coronary arteries in cases of ascending aneurysm, status of nongrafted aorta, presence of intramural hematoma (dissection in 15% of TAA)
  - Procure material for microbiologic culture studies if clinically indicated (suspected graft infection) immediately upon opening chest cavity
- Anastomotic integrity assessed by inspection and water infusion into aorta if concern for anastomotic integrity

Organ Examination

- Aorta and heart
  - Open aorta from distal aspect after inspecting graft and anastomoses and branch vessels
    - Section nongrafted aorta and anastomoses; Dacron graft material can be processed for histologic analysis
  - Ascending aorta: Inspect any coronary graft ostia or coronary buttons (reimplanted native coronary ostia)
    - Coronary reimplantation or bypass may be necessary in ascending aortic repair
    - Examine coronary arteries for evidence of dissection, surgical injury
  - Inspect aortic valve from aortic aspect
    - Native valve: Cusp number (check for BAV) and coaptation, surgical injury (suture, etc.), surgical repair (pledgeted sutures to resuspend valve cusps), vegetation
    - Bioprosthetic valve: May be part of ascending aorta replacement or separate; look for cusp integrity, thrombosis, surgical injury, vegetation
  - Heart
    - Size and weight: Dilated left ventricle with eccentric hypertrophy in aortic valve insufficiency, concentric hypertrophy with aortic stenosis and hypertension
    - Myocardial infarction (may be multifactorial): Operative stress, surgical injury, embolic, underlying coronary atherosclerosis
  - Respiratory
    - Cardiogenic pulmonary edema (congestive heart failure from aortic valve insufficiency, perioperative ischemic injury, etc.)
    - Noncardiogenic pulmonary edema (multifactorial): Operative stress, intercurrent sepsis, shock (hypovolemic from hemorrhage, or cardiogenic), aspiration
  - Gastrointestinal: Ischemic injury (shock)
  - Hepatobiliary
    - Congestion (congestive heart failure from aortic valve insufficiency), necrosis (shock liver)
    - Acute pancreatitis (uncommon complication of cardiopulmonary bypass)
  - Genitourinary: Acute tubular injury (operative stress, hypovolemic shock)
  - Central and peripheral nervous system
    - Spinal cord injury (ischemic) with descending aneurysm repair or arch repair with distal graft tunneled into descending aorta; examination of thoracic cord important in these cases
    - Appearance of central nervous system and spinal cord infarcts varies with duration from injury and presence or absence of hemorrhage

MICROSCOPIC

Histologic Features

- Heart and aorta
  - Anastomotic sections: Adventitial granulation tissue and fibrosis with longer duration grafts, abscess if superimposed infection
  - Aortic sections: Intramural hematoma (dissection), acute or chronic, medial degeneration, smooth muscle cell loss
  - If aneurysm from syphilitic aortitis (rare), intimal proliferation of adventitial vessels (vasa vasora), plasma cell-rich inflammation, and laminar necrosis of media due to ischemia
  - Heart with hypertrophy and areas of interstitial fibrosis in cases with aortic valve insufficiency, varying stages of acute and healing coagulative myocyte necrosis in cases with infarction
    - May see foreign material (suture, etc.) embolization related to surgery
- Respiratory system
  - Intraalveolar pale pink fluid (cardiogenic pulmonary edema); fibrin layering along alveolar septal walls ± evidence of organization (noncardiogenic pulmonary edema), intrabronchial and intraalveolar acute inflammation in pneumonia
    - With aspiration, may see intraairway or intraalveolar gastric content or aspirated squames from oral cavity and multinucleated giant cells with chronic aspiration
- Gastrointestinal system
  - Varying severity of ischemic injury with coagulative necrosis of mucosa to serosa (severe case), submucosal vascular thrombosis; may see atheroemboli or foreign material (suture) emboli related to operative intervention and catheterization
- Hepatobiliary system
  - Centrilobular hepatocyte necrosis and congestion; larger areas of necrosis affecting entire lobule and bridging from lobule to lobule in more severe shock
  - Coagulative necrosis of pancreatic parenchyma with fibrin thrombi in vessels in bypass-related acute pancreatitis
    - Usually seen in association with other shock changes, such as hepatic necrosis, intestinal ischemia, and acute tubular injury
- Genitourinary system
  - Loss of brush border of tubular epithelial cells with coagulative necrosis in more severe cases
- Central and peripheral nervous system
  - Cerebral and spinal cord infarct appearance varies with time from ischemic insult
    - 12 hours: Red neurons, vasogenic edema
    - 48 hours: Neutrophilic infiltrate begins to ↓ and phagocytes ↑ to become prominent cell type over ensuing weeks; reactive astrocytes appear at edge of infarct

DIFFERENTIAL DIAGNOSIS

Pseudoaneurysm

- Contained rupture of aorta
  - Contains hematoma surrounded by granulation tissue or fibrous tissue depending on age of pseudoaneurysm
  - Does not contain layers of vessel wall

SELECTED REFERENCES

1. Farinetti A et al: Changed pathophysiology of thoracic aorta after aortic arch repair. J Vasc Surg. 75(3):1122-3, 2022
2. Janko M et al: Thoracic endovascular aortic/aneurysm stent-graft repair (TEVAR) primer. J Card Surg. 37(7):2212-6, 2022
3. Ranney DN et al: Long-term results of endovascular repair for descending thoracic aortic aneurysms. J Vasc Surg. 67(2):363-8, 2018

Enhanced CT of Ascending Aortic Aneurysm

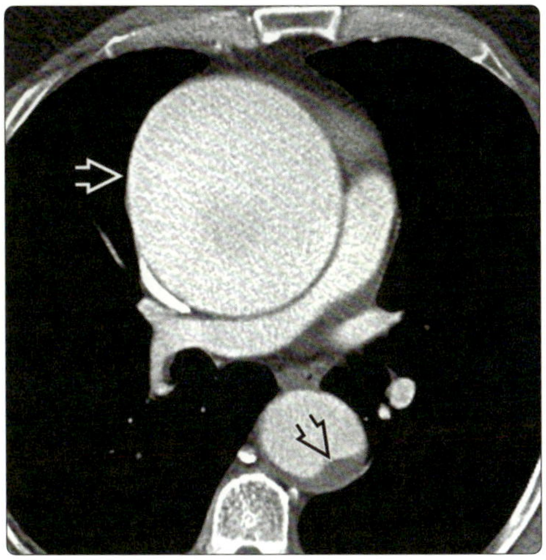

Ascending Aortic Aneurysm: In Situ View

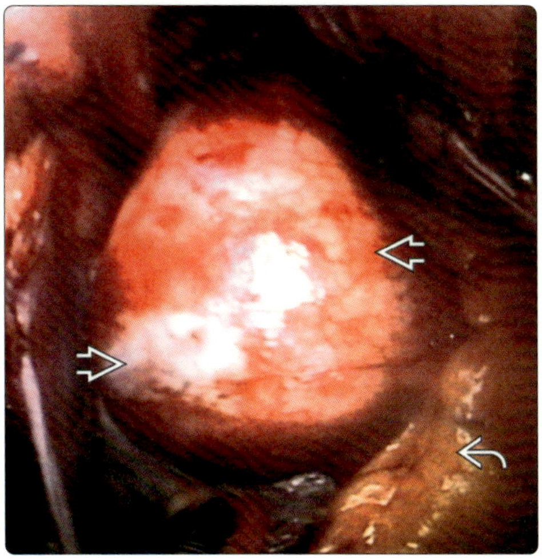

(Left) *Enhanced CT of the chest shows a large ascending aortic aneurysm ➡. There is atherosclerotic plaque in the descending aorta ➡, but the lumen is of normal caliber.* **(Right)** *In situ view shows a large ascending aortic aneurysm ➡ prior to repair. The heart ➡ is noted.*

Aortic Arch Aneurysm

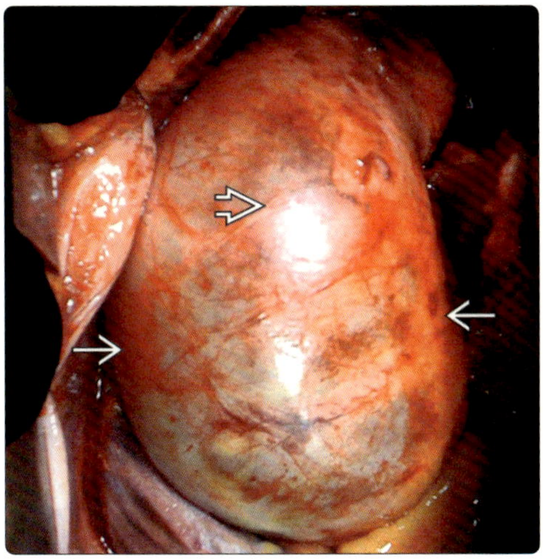

Aortic Arch Aneurysm Repair

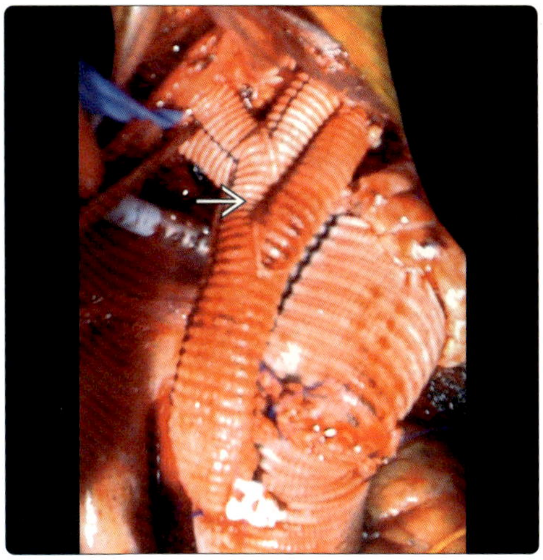

(Left) *Aortic arch is markedly dilated ➡, and the blue discoloration ➡ indicates an aortic dissection complicating this arch aneurysm.* **(Right)** *Aortic arch repair often includes repair of the arch vessels. Here, they are replaced with grafts ➡. If the ostia and the proximal arch vessels are intact, the vessel-bearing portion of the arch can also sometimes be resected and attached to the arch graft, similar to coronary buttons.*

Combined Aortic Aneurysm Repair and Coronary Bypass Grafting

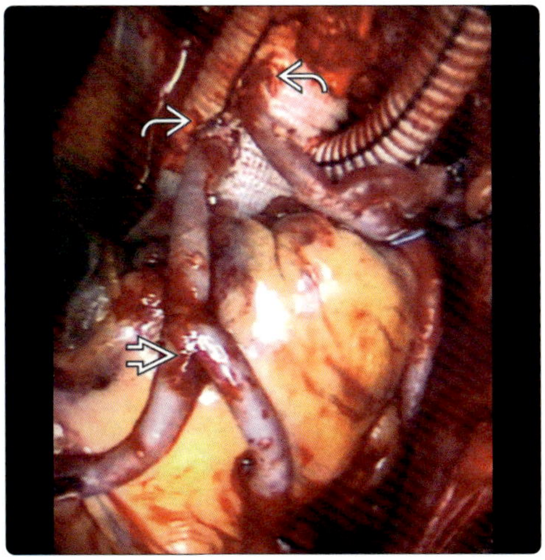

Aortic Root Replacement

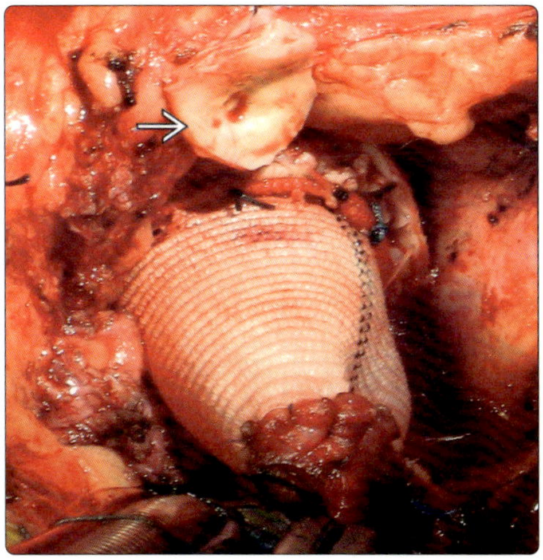

(Left) *Saphenous vein bypass grafts can be attached to ascending aortic grafts to perform a simultaneous coronary artery bypass procedure. In this case, 2 grafts are attached proximally ➡, and vein-to-vein Y grafts ➡ are used to bypass additional vessels.* **(Right)** *In this case of aortic root replacement, the coronary arteries are being reattached to the ascending graft as a coronary button ➡ that contains the coronary ostium and a portion of the surrounding aortic wall.*

(Left) *CT angiogram in a patient with Marfan syndrome and acute chest syndrome shows the classic tulip bulb appearance → due to annuloaortic ectasia. Other terms describing this appearance include onion bulb, pear-shaped, and Florence flask. (From DI: Cardiovascular.)* **(Right)** *Graphic compares a normal ascending aorta (left) with a well-defined sinotubular junction → and annuloaortic ectasia with sinotubular junction effacement (right), as seen in Marfan syndrome.*

CT Angiogram of Aortic Root Dilatation

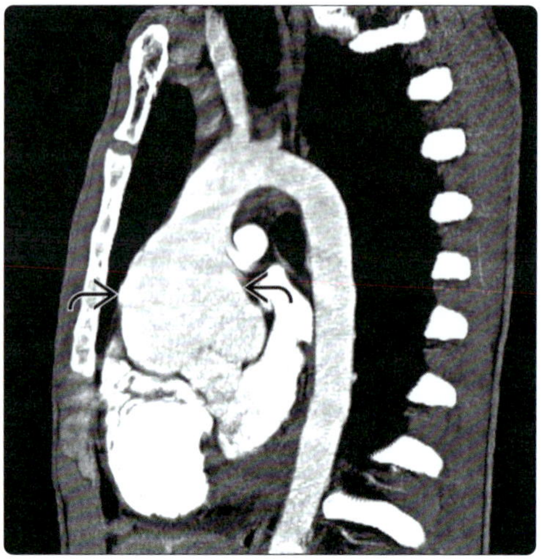

Aortic Root Changes in Marfan Syndrome

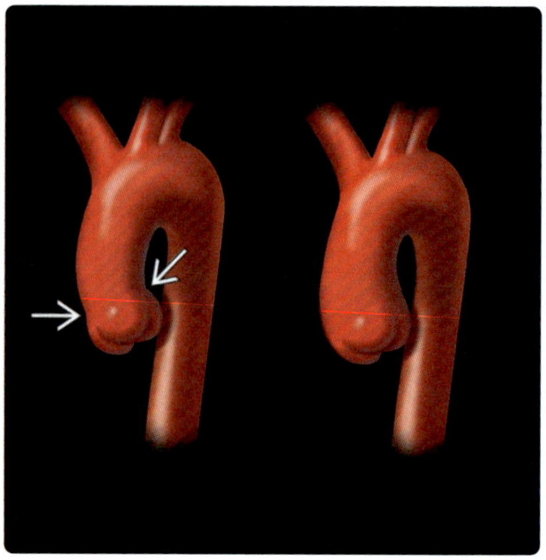

(Left) *This aortic root and ascending aortic aneurysm is being replaced with a valved conduit so the aortic valve, root, and ascending aorta are replaced simultaneously. In this photograph, the proximal suturing of the valve into the root is being performed. Multiple sutures → will anastomose the sewing ring of the valve → onto the root. (Courtesy J. Plate, MD and E. Pantin, MD.)* **(Right)** *The coronary buttons → have been anastomosed to the ascending aortic graft.*

Aortic Root and Ascending Aneurysm Replacement

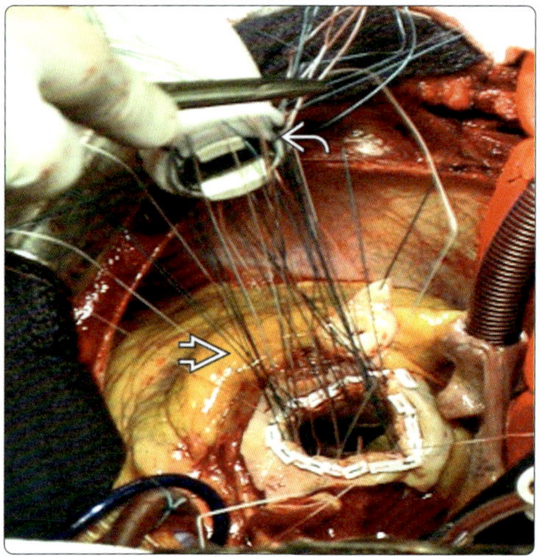

Ascending Aortic Graft

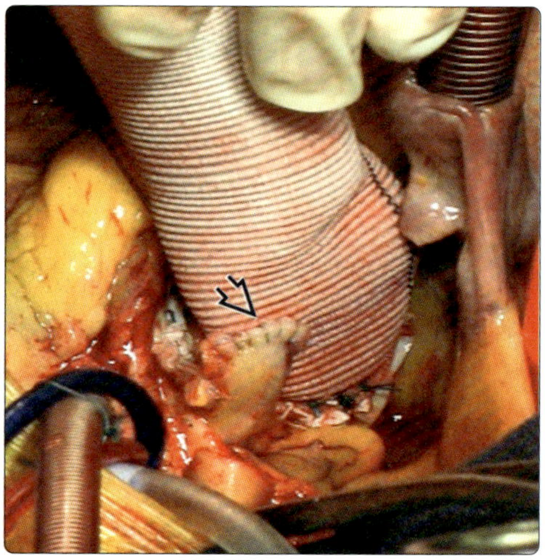

(Left) *This is the outflow view of an aortic valve that has been resuspended with 3 commissure pledgeted sutures →. There is excellent coaptation of the valve cusps after resuspension.* **(Right)** *Sagittal reconstructed CT shows a large descending thoracic aneurysm →. Descending aortic aneurysms are easier to repair with endografts than ascending aneurysms. (From DI: Chest.)*

Aortic Valve Repair

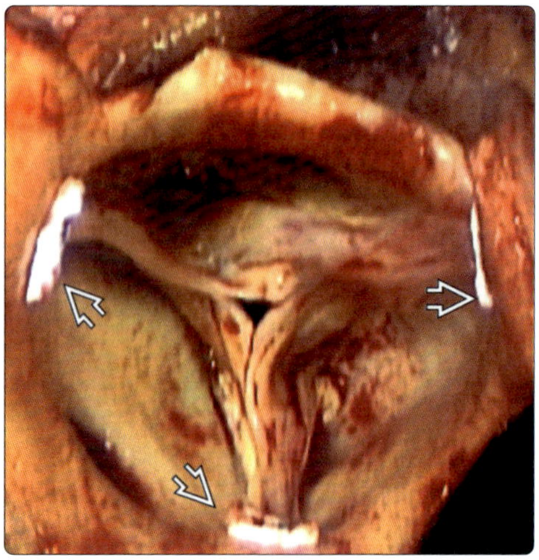

Descending Aortic Aneurysm

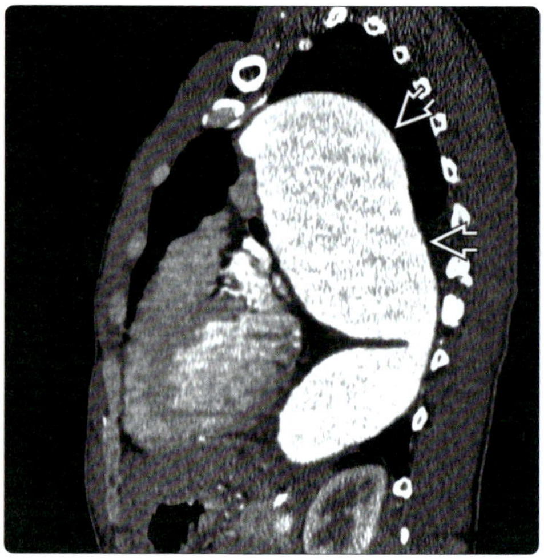

Thoracoabdominal Chronic Aortic Dissection

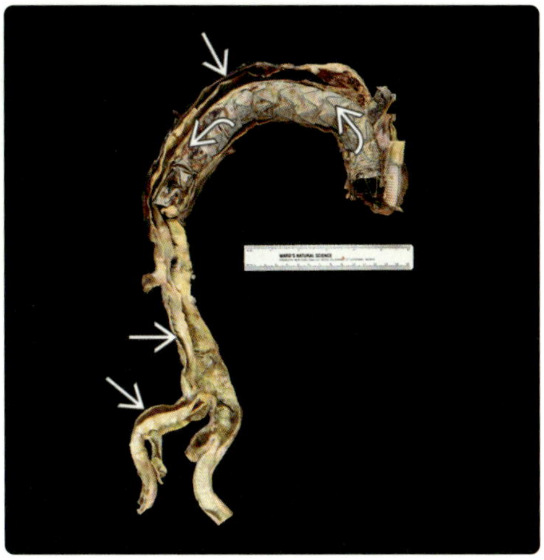

Aortic Arch Branched Graft and Endograft

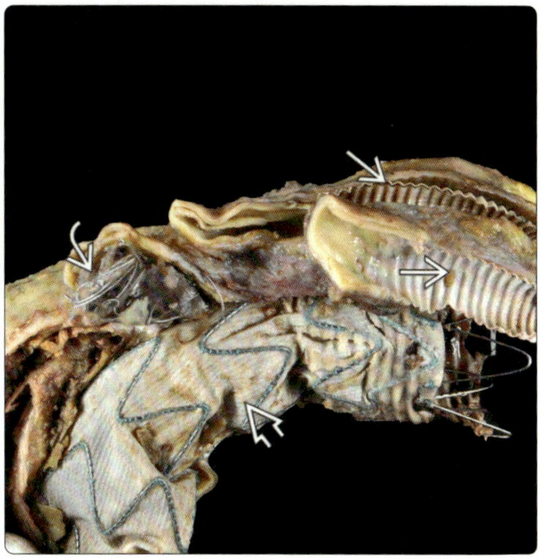

(Left) *Chronic aortic dissection ➡ extends the entire length of the aorta and into the iliac branch. Overlapping PTFE endografts ➡ have been placed in the ascending, arch, and descending thoracic aorta.* **(Right)** *Synthetic tube grafts to the aortic arch vessels ➡, an endograft with the arch itself ➡, and a endovascular coil ➡ are all seen in this image. The coiled arch branch was bypassed.*

Endograft Repair of Thoracic Aortic Aneurysm

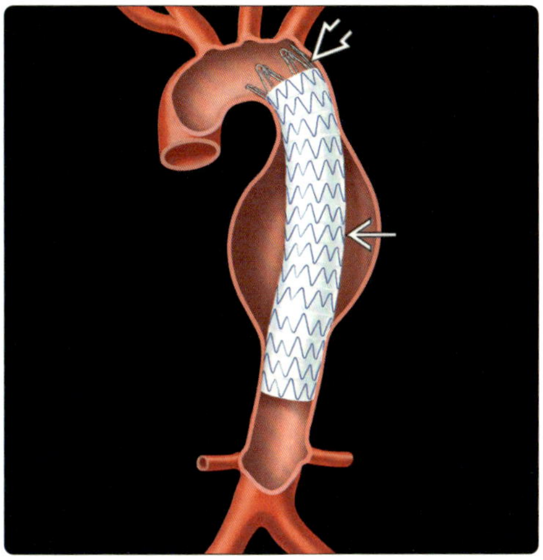

3D Reconstruction of Thoracoabdominal Aneurysm Endograft Repair

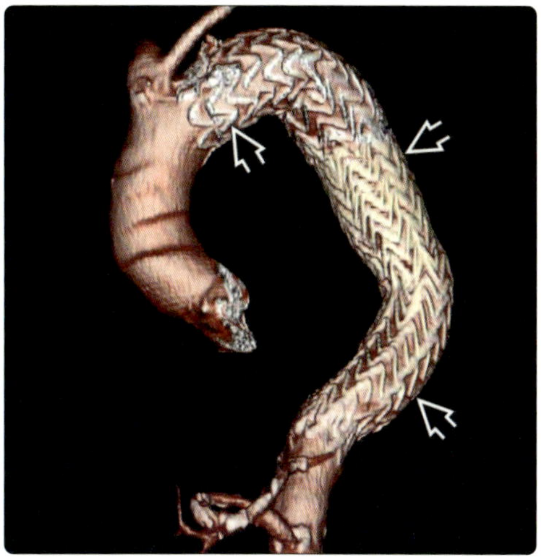

(Left) *Graphic shows a descending thoracic aneurysm repaired with an endograft. The endograft struts ➡ attach to the aortic wall. The body is composed of fabric-covered, self-expanding stents ➡.* **(Right)** *3D reconstruction shows a thoracoabdominal aneurysm after endograft repair ➡. The location of endografts should be determined by chart review, premortem imaging review, &/or postmortem/specimen imaging prior to aortic dissection to avoid iatrogenic injury to the graft. (From DI: Procedures.)*

Aortic Pseudoaneurysm

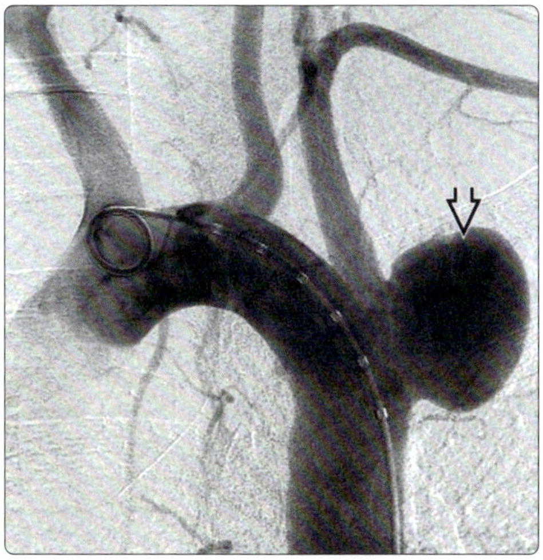

Aortic Pseudoaneurysm Endograft Repair

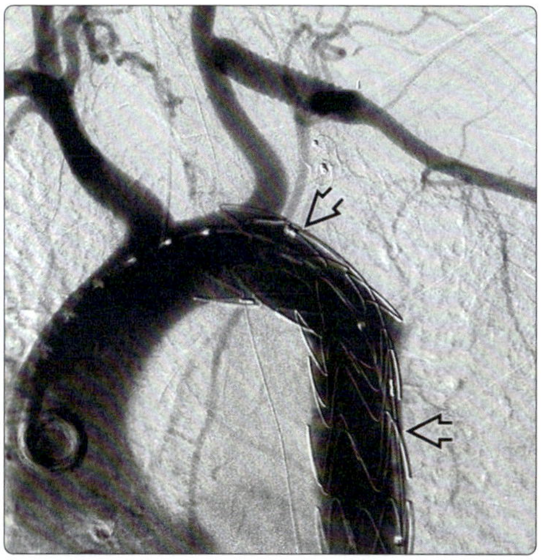

(Left) *Angiogram shows a large saccular aneurysm ➡. This is likely a pseudoaneurysm that represents a contained periaortic hematoma with retained communication to the aortic lumen.* **(Right)** *Angiogram in the same case after endograft repair ➡ is shown. The endograft excluded the pseudoaneurysm from the aortic blood flow. (From DI: Interventional Procedures.)*

Abdominal Aortic Aneurysm

KEY FACTS

TERMINOLOGY

- Aneurysm: Localized permanent pathologic dilatation of vessel wall with diameter at least 50% greater than normal

CLINICAL ISSUES

- Major risk factors
  - Nonmodifiable: ↑ age, male sex, family history
  - Modifiable: Hypertension, hyperlipidemia, smoking, obesity
- Clinical presentation usually due to complications of aneurysm/endografts
  - Rupture (abdominal pain/shock), emboli, compression (e.g., ureter azotemia), fistula (massive GI hemorrhage), infection (sepsis/shock), endoleaks
- Rupture risk ↑ with ↑ diameter; 4-5 cm: 1% per year; 5-6 cm: 11% per year; 6 cm: 25% per year: Repair usually at 5.5 cm
- M > F (4:1)

MACROSCOPIC

- Describe shape, length, position in relation to renal artery ostia (supra-/juxta-/infrarenal), and diameter
- Look for rupture if hemoperitoneum or retroperitoneal hematoma present
  - Most common site: Left lateral infrarenal

MICROSCOPIC

- Aneurysm: Atherosclerosis with marked degeneration of media; marked acute inflammation indicates possible infection (rare); malignancy related to stent (rare)
- Complications: Atheroemboli ± thrombosis/vasculitis, infarcts (kidney, intestine, brain, spleen)

TOP DIFFERENTIAL DIAGNOSES

- IgG4-related disease/inflammatory aortic aneurysm
  - Marked storiform adventitial fibrosis with extensive plasma cell infiltrate, composed of high percentage of IgG4(+) plasma cells

Saccular Abdominal Aortic Aneurysm

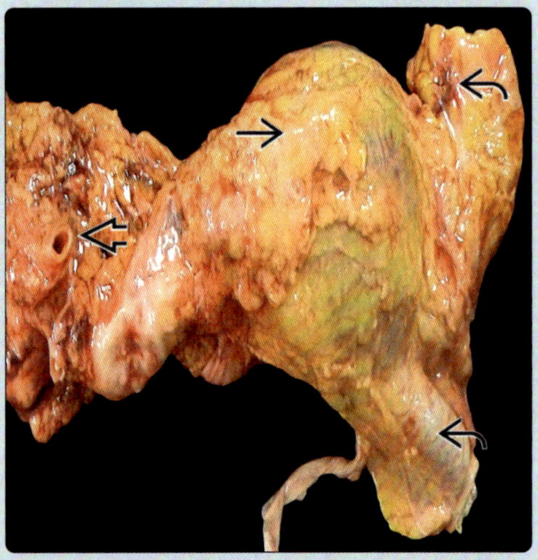

AAA With Left Renal Artery Obstruction

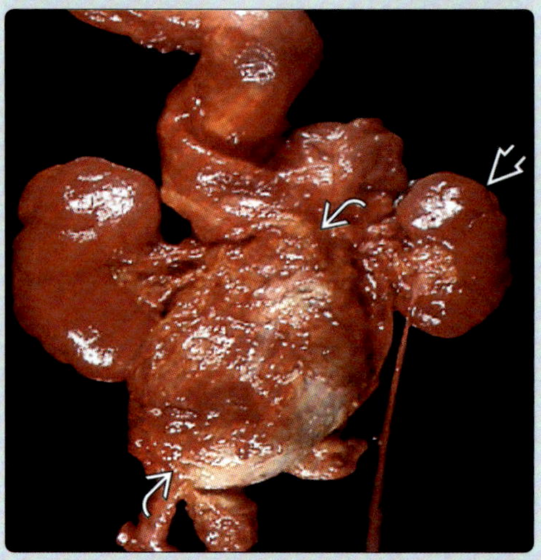

(Left) *This infrarenal, saccular abdominal aortic aneurysm (AAA) is distal to the superior mesenteric artery and renal arteries (not well visualized) and ends at the iliac vessels.* **(Right)** *Obstructive complications of AAA include major branch obstruction. This juxtarenal AAA is associated with obstruction of the left renal artery as denoted by the atrophic left kidney.*

Cloth-Covered Stent Within AAA

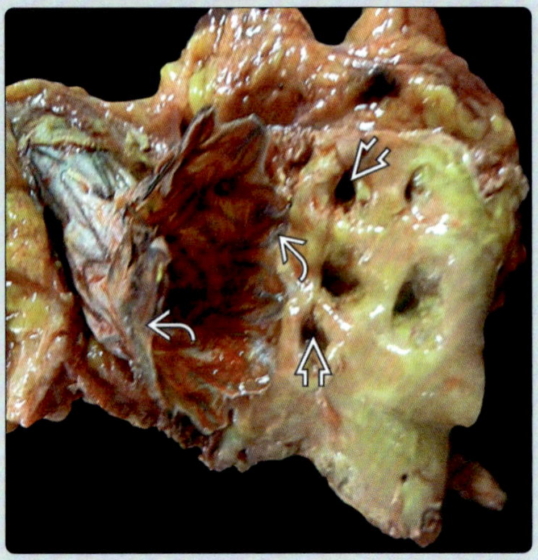

Histology of Aneurysm Wall

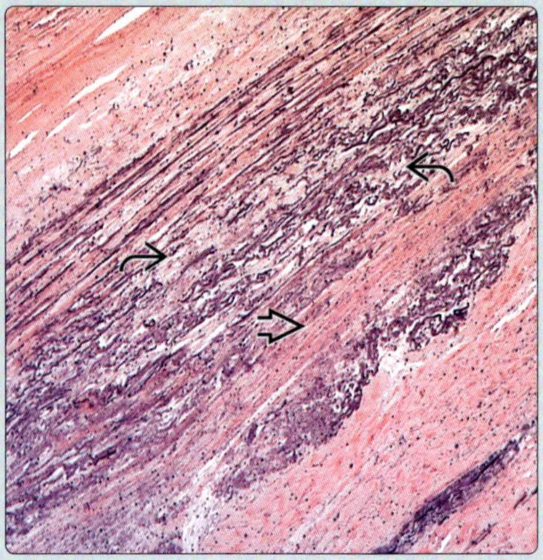

(Left) *This cloth-covered stent is attached proximally to the aorta beneath the renal artery ostia. This has become the primary mode of treatment for the majority of patients with AAA. Open repair is generally used for patients with complex anatomy or a coexisting process that prohibits endovascular aneurysm repair. (Courtesy J. Chiaffarano, MD.)* **(Right)** *Elastic stain of an aneurysm wall shows marked thinning and fragmentation of elastic lamellae and loss of elastic tissue.*

TERMINOLOGY

Abbreviations

- Abdominal aortic aneurysm (AAA)

Definitions

- Aneurysm: Localized permanent pathologic dilatation of vessel wall with diameter at least 50% greater than normal due to wall weakening
  - Abdominal aortic diameter < 3 cm
  - Normal diameter ↑ with age, varies with aortic location and body habitus

ETIOLOGY/PATHOGENESIS

Mechanisms of Aneurysm Development

- Proteolysis of structural components (elastic fibers) of vascular wall
- Loss of vascular smooth muscle cells by apoptosis and replacement by collagen
- Oxidative stress
- Chronic inflammatory response

CLINICAL ISSUES

Epidemiology

- Incidence
  - ~ 5-8% of male population age 65 years; 2% of female population of same age
    - True prevalence is hard to determine because AAA is usually asymptomatic
  - Mean annual incidence of new diagnoses of AAA in Western population ranges 0.4-0.67%
  - ↑ incidence of ruptured aneurysm, accounting for 1-2% of all deaths
- Sex
  - M > F (4:1)
- Major risk factors
  - Nonmodifiable
    - Older age
    - Male sex
    - Family history: ↑ prevalence among 1st-degree relatives
  - Modifiable
    - Hypertension
    - Hyperlipidemia
    - Smoking
    - Obesity

Presentation

- Usually due to complications of aneurysm/endografts
  - Rupture (abdominal pain/shock) most severe complication, associated with > 80% mortality
  - Emboli
  - Compression (e.g., ureter/azotemia)
  - Fistula (massive GI hemorrhage)
  - Infection (sepsis/shock)
  - Endoleaks

Laboratory Tests

- Hyperhomocysteinemia, hyperlipidemia, ↑ C-reactive protein (risk factor assessment)
- ↓ hemoglobin/hematocrit (normal if acute rupture, ↓ with slow leak), ↑ creatinine (acute tubular injury)
- Blood culture (infected aneurysm)

Treatment

- Surgical approaches
  - Aneurysm repair with endografts or open surgery is only option when aneurysm diameter > 5.5 cm to prevent rupture
- Medical treatment
  - Conservative management when diameter of AAA is maintained at 3-5 cm
    - Aneurysm growth monitored by ultrasound (most used methodology), MR, or CT
    - Control of risk factors: Statins, antiplatelet, antihypertensive, and antiinflammatory drugs
  - No medical treatment available to control aneurysm growth or prevent rupture

Prognosis

- Rupture risk ↑ with ↑ diameter; 4-5 cm: 1% per year: 5-6 cm: 11% per year; 6 cm: 25% per year
- Outcome in female patients with AAA is worse than in male patients: Rupture occurs at smaller AAA diameter; higher mortality rates post surgical repair are reported

Clinical Chart Review

- Risk factors for atherosclerosis/aneurysm, family history, clinical presentation suggestive of rupture/other complication
- History of intervention: Endovascular aneurysm repair ± endoleak
- Abdominal or aorta x-ray highlights endografts
  - Review recent imaging; history of endoleaks
- Other atherosclerotic complications (myocardial infarction, stroke)

MACROSCOPIC

External Examination

- Pallor &/or distended abdomen (rupture)
- Lower extremity changes related to aortic atherosclerotic disease/aneurysm
  - Loss of hair, thin skin, muscle atrophy, erythema, blue toe (embolic)
- Abdominal incision (aneurysm repair)
- Signs of risk factors for atherosclerosis
  - Xanthelasma (hypercholesterolemia)
  - Diagonal earlobe crease (Frank sign) (more sensitive in younger patients)

Internal Examination

- Hemoperitoneum or retroperitoneal hematoma

Organ Examination

- Aneurysm
  - Describe shape, length, position in relation to renal artery ostia (supra-/juxta-/infrarenal), and diameter
    - Fusiform: When dilatation of wall occurs in all directions of circumference
    - Saccular: When only part of circumference is dilated
  - Look for rupture if hemoperitoneum or retroperitoneal hematoma present

- Most common site: Left lateral infrarenal
- Endoleaks: Continued growth of aneurysm due to continued perfusion after endograft
  - Classification
    - Type I at graft anastomosis
    - Type II from branch vessels
    - Type III between stents/ruptured graft
    - Type IV through porous graft
    - Type V unknown
  - Clinical diagnosis but recent thrombus around stent supports diagnosis, and radiograph of stent can identify rupture of graft
- Aneurysm interior examination
  - Open aneurysm posteriorly; examine contents, relationship to/obstruction of branch vessels, presence of rupture
  - Describe stent appearance, location, adherence to underlying aortic wall, obstruction of ostia
  - Graft can be kept intact with sampling of aneurysm around graft
- Systemic atherosclerosis ± complications
  - Acute/chronic myocardial infarction, cerebral infarcts

MICROSCOPIC

Histologic Features

- Aneurysm
  - Atherosclerosis with marked degeneration of media
  - Variable degree of mononuclear inflammation (macrophages, lymphocytes, mast cells)
  - Marked acute inflammation indicates possible infection (rare)
  - Malignancy related to stent (rare)
- Rest of cardiovascular system
  - Coronary/carotid atherosclerosis acute plaque events (rupture, thrombosis)
  - Acute/chronic myocardial infarction, acute subendocardial ischemia (terminal shock)
- Other: Emboli/shock
  - Atheroemboli ± thrombosis/vasculitis
  - Infarcts (renal, intestine, spleen)
  - Acute tubular injury

ANCILLARY TESTS

Histochemistry

- Gram stain in cases of suspected infected aneurysms
- Elastic stain for evaluation of aneurysm wall

Immunohistochemistry

- IgG4/IgG to exclude IgG4 disease [percentage of IgG4(+) cells]

DIFFERENTIAL DIAGNOSIS

IgG4-Related Disease/Inflammatory Aortic Aneurysm

- Marked storiform adventitial fibrosis with extensive plasma cell infiltrate, composed of high percentage of IgG4 cells

Mycotic Aneurysm

- Weakening of aortic wall due to (usually bacterial) primary or secondary infection of existing atherosclerotic AAA

REPORTING

Aneurysm Incidental or Cause of Death

- Identify complications and risk factors for aneurysm

SELECTED REFERENCES

1. Liu B et al: Pathogenic mechanisms and the potential of drug therapies for aortic aneurysm. Am J Physiol Heart Circ Physiol. 318(3):H652-70, 2020
2. Blassova T et al: Inflammatory cell infiltrates, hypoxia, vascularization, pentraxin 3 and osteoprotegerin in abdominal aortic aneurysms - a quantitative histological study. PLoS One. 14(11):e0224818, 2019
3. Butcovan D et al: Sub-classification of non-inflammatory and inflammatory surgical aortic aneurysms and the association of histological characteristics with potential risk factors. Exp Ther Med. 18(4):3046-52, 2019
4. Kumar S et al: Role of noncoding RNAs in the pathogenesis of abdominal aortic aneurysm. Circ Res. 124(4):619-30, 2019
5. Pinard A et al: Genetics of thoracic and abdominal aortic diseases. Circ Res. 124(4):588-606, 2019
6. Prucha M et al: Abdominal aortic aneurysm as an IgG4-related disease. Clin Exp Immunol. 197(3):361-5, 2019
7. Quintana RA et al: Cellular mechanisms of aortic aneurysm formation. Circ Res. 124(4):607-18, 2019
8. Torres-Fonseca M et al: Pathophisiology of abdominal aortic aneurysm: biomarkers and novel therapeutic targets. Clin Investig Arterioscler. 31(4):166-77, 2019
9. van Laarhoven CJHCM et al: Polygenic susceptibility of aortic aneurysms associates to the diameter of the aneurysm sac: the Aneurysm-Express Biobank Cohort. Sci Rep. 9(1):19844, 2019
10. Das UN: Is aortic aneurysm preventable? J Transl Int Med. 5(2):72-8, 2017
11. Hourai R et al: IgG4-positive cell infiltration in various cardiovascular disorders - results from histopathological analysis of surgical samples. BMC Cardiovasc Disord. 17(1):52, 2017
12. Kumar Y et al: Abdominal aortic aneurysm: pictorial review of common appearances and complications. Ann Transl Med. 5(12):256, 2017
13. Meyermann K et al: Treatment of abdominal aortic pathology. Cardiol Clin. 35(3):431-9, 2017
14. Kent KC: Clinical practice: abdominal aortic aneurysms. N Engl J Med. 371(22):2101-8, 2014

Aorta Aneurysm Wall With Atherosclerosis

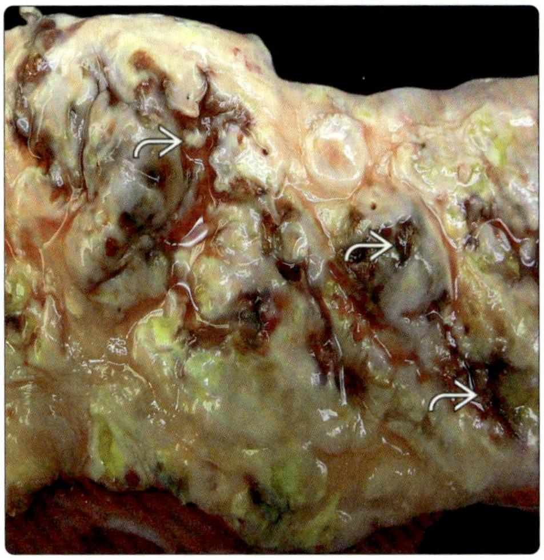

Histology of Aneurysm Wall

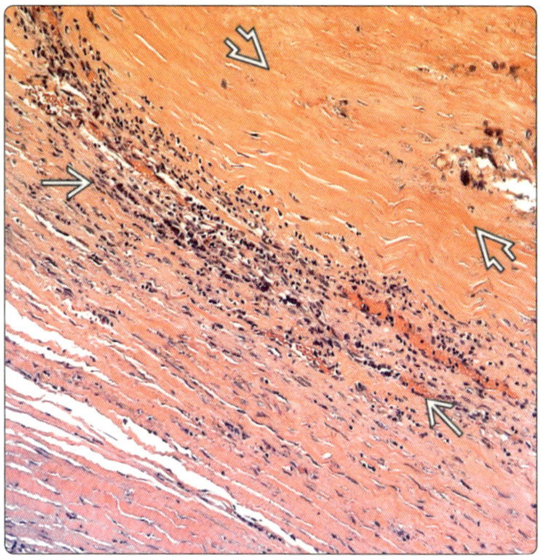

(Left) *This infrarenal aorta has a large atherosclerotic plaque burden and areas of plaque ulceration* ➢ *and aneurysm formation.* **(Right)** *Inflammation, including lymphocytes and occasional plasma cells, is common in aneurysm walls. There is marked destruction of the media* ➢*, and the inflammation is in the adventitial tissue* ➢*. Marked inflammation in a thick aneurysm wall with perianeurysmal adhesion would suggest inflammatory aortic aneurysm.*

Gross View of Endovascular Graft

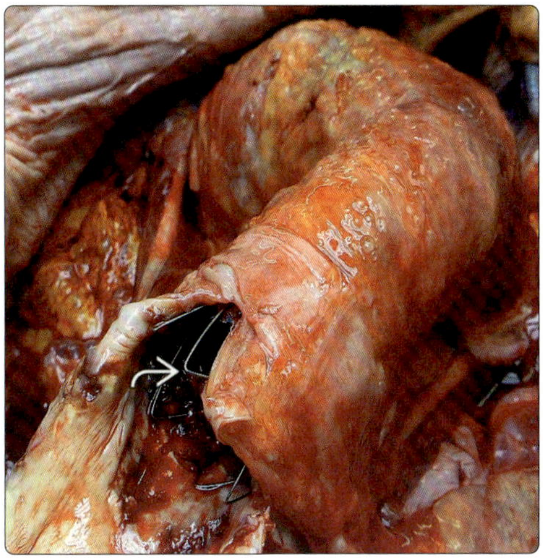

Ruptured AAA With Endovascular Stent

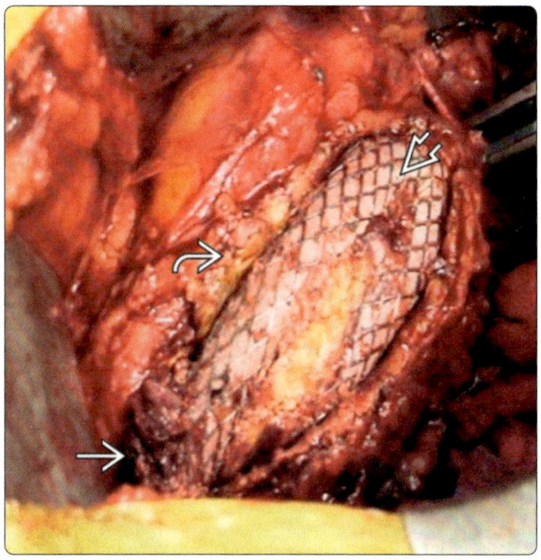

(Left) *Some endovascular grafts have a bare metal proximal portion* ➢ *in order to allow perfusion to major vessels, such as renal arteries, if the aneurysm is juxta- or suprarenal.* **(Right)** *This ruptured infrarenal aneurysm has an endovascular stent* ➢*. The aneurysm wall* ➢ *is thin, and there is hematoma* ➢ *around the distal aneurysm due to rupture. (Courtesy S. A. Rahimi, MD.)*

Aneurysm Wall With Overlying Thrombus

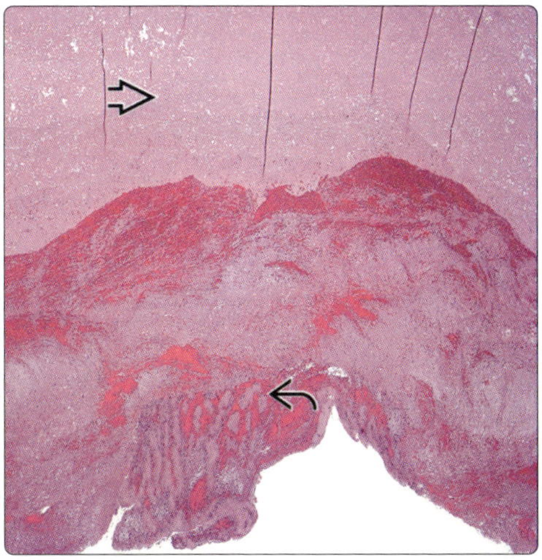

Cholesterol Emboli in Renal Artery Branch

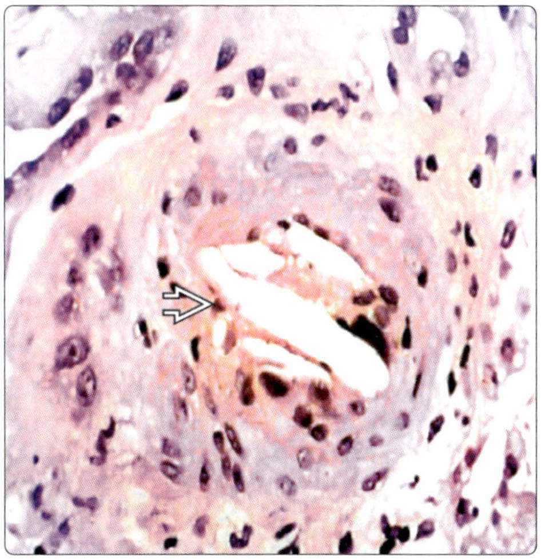

(Left) *Histologically, these thrombi show more recent thrombus along the luminal surface* ➢ *(layered RBCs, fibrin) and homogeneous older thrombus* ➢ *without cellular detail. Thrombus formation is a common finding in AAA and may contribute to aneurysm progression. (Courtesy E. Sadimin, MD.)* **(Right)** *Atheroembolic complications may be seen in atherosclerosis or aneurysmal disease. This renal artery is filled with cholesterol crystals* ➢*. The emboli arose from an AAA.*

KEY FACTS

ETIOLOGY/PATHOGENESIS

- Developmental aneurysms
  - Termed saccular, "berry," or congenital aneurysms (rarely appear at birth)
  - Lacks medial smooth muscle layer, precluding formation of internal elastic lamina
- Vertebrobasilar dolichoectasia (arteriopathy)
  - Focally dilated basilar artery; mostly in older men
  - Longstanding case may form fusiform aneurysm
- Vascular malformations
  - Arteriovenous malformation (AVM): No capillary bed; may cause seizures, prone to rupture
  - Cavernous angioma, prone to rupture
  - Capillary hemangioma
  - Telangiectasia (telangiectases)
  - Venous malformation, minor to extensive
  - Dural arteriovenous fistula or shunt; potential for major clinical hemorrhage
- *PIK3CA* mutations in sporadic cavernous AVM

CLINICAL ISSUES

- Subarachnoid or intraparenchymal hemorrhage, seizure disorder, fatal rupture
- Medical treatment (antiepileptics), open surgery, endovascular thrombosis-promoting procedures

MACROSCOPIC

- Aneurysm rupture often obscured by blood; multiple aneurysms common
- Common incidental finding (aneurysm, vascular malformation)

MICROSCOPIC

- Developmental aneurysmal wall characteristic
- Malformed vessels in AVM

Subarachnoid Hemorrhage: Sylvian Fissure

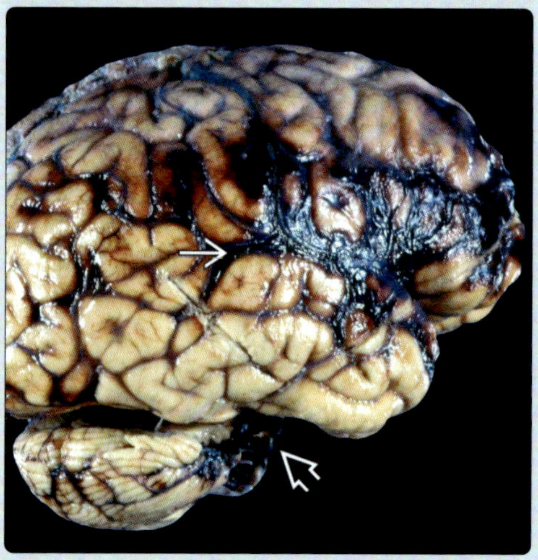

"Berry" Aneurysm of Circle of Willis

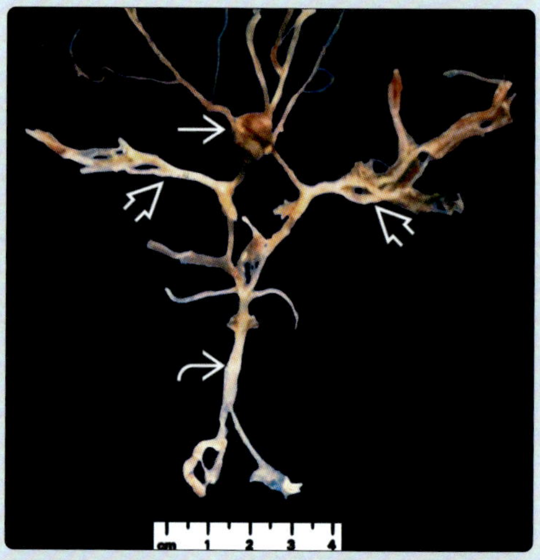

(Left) *Subarachnoid hemorrhage around the sylvian fissure ➡ suggests the location of the ruptured right middle cerebral artery aneurysm. Some subarachnoid blood has also settled over the brainstem ➡.* **(Right)** *A ruptured anterior communicating artery aneurysm ➡ is seen on the circle of Willis with arachnoidal tissue dissected away. The middle cerebral arteries ➡ and basilar artery ➡ are indicated.*

Arteriovenous Malformation: Cerebral Angiogram

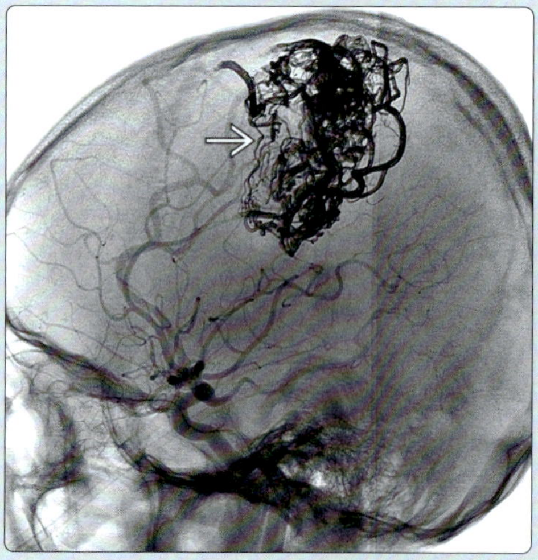

Arteriovenous Malformation: Post Onyx Embolization

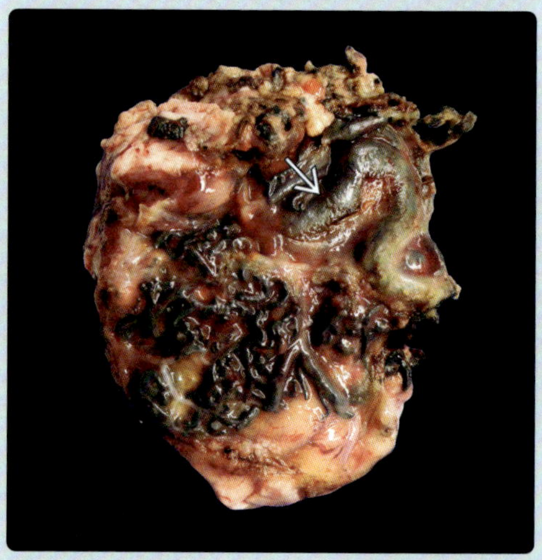

(Left) *Onyx injected into the feeding artery of a large frontoparietal arteriovenous malformation (AVM) ➡ has high attenuation, so that its distribution is clearly seen in this cerebral angiogram.* **(Right)** *Onyx, a viscous black polymer mixture, fills all vascular sizes in this cerebral AVM photographed in the surgical suite after excision. The dark, somewhat firm polymer is seen through the relatively thin (for size) abnormal vascular walls ➡. (Courtesy G. Gupta, MD.)*

ETIOLOGY/PATHOGENESIS

Developmental Aneurysms

- Saccular, "berry," or congenital (although rarely present at birth) aneurysms
- Lack medial smooth muscle layer, precluding formation of internal elastic lamina
  - Internal elastic lamina provides tensile strength
  - Systolic blood pressure enlarges wall over time into saccular aneurysm
- Usually at bifurcations (circle of Willis)
- Distal aneurysms (not at bifurcation) mostly cerebellar
- AVM-associated aneurysms (↑ hemodynamic instability): Alter prognosis, management

Acquired Aneurysms

- Vascular wall damage, repair
  - Trauma (pseudoaneurysm): Often near dural-free edge
  - Arteriovenous malformation (AVM)-associated acquired aneurysms
  - Spheroidal (early) or fusiform (late alteration)
- Intrinsic vascular wall weakness
  - Genetic predisposition
    - Vascular Ehlers-Danlos syndrome
    - Sickle cell anemia
- Vertebrobasilar dolichoectasia (arteriopathy)
  - Mostly older men; hypertension association
- Mycotic (infective) aneurysms
  - Usually secondary to bacterial endocarditis
  - Fungal infection (very rare)

Vascular Malformations

- Blood vessel hamartomas
  - Most cases sporadic
- Genetic background in some cases
  - Osler-Weber-Rendu disease
  - Sturge-Weber disease
  - *PIK3CA* mutations in sporadic cavernous AVM
- AVM
  - Arterial systolic pressure directly enters abnormal veins
  - Affected vessels leak → blood pigment, gliosis
  - Rupture not inevitable but may be fatal
- Cavernous angioma
  - Focally thin walls in large abnormal vessels may rupture
- Capillary hemangioma
  - Usually incidental finding
- Telangiectasia (telangiectases)
  - 4-12% of vascular malformations
- Venous malformation
  - Frequent; usually incidental finding
  - Low pressure; rupture infrequently
  - Vein of Galen aneurysmal malformation
    - Infrequent; may cause high-output cardiac failure
- Dural arteriovenous fistula or shunt
  - Direct connection between dural artery and brain/spinal cord blood vessels
    - Leak or sudden rupture into neural parenchyma
  - Foix-Alajouanine (venous congestive myelopathy)
    - Dural arterial reflux into spinal venous drainage

CLINICAL ISSUES

Presentation

- Developmental (saccular) aneurysms
  - Autopsy prevalence rate: 1-5%
  - Annual rupture rate: < 2%
    - Up to 80% do not rupture (incidental)
  - Can be incidental on imaging or autopsy
  - Subarachnoid hemorrhage (major presentation)
    - Headache, mental status change, neck stiffness, focal neurologic deficits, acute brain injury
  - Subdural hematoma (rare)
  - Distal embolization (rare)
- Acquired aneurysms
  - Infrequent, may be secondary to connective tissue disorder
  - Vertebrobasilar dolichoectasia
    - Stroke, central nerve or brainstem compression, cerebellar symptoms, hydrocephalus, fatal rupture
- AVM
  - Prevalence: 18/100,000 adults
    - Autopsy prevalence rate: 1-4%
    - Clinical imaging incidental rate: 0.05%
  - Lifetime bleeding risk: 17-90%
    - Depends on size, location (e.g., deep), venous drainage, associated aneurysm, previous bleed
  - Presentation with rupture
    - Hemorrhage (50%)
    - Seizure (25%)
    - Headache (25%)
  - Unruptured (present 2x as commonly as ruptured)
    - 1st hemorrhage fatality rate: 15-18%
    - 4-34% rerupture risk: ↑ for deep location
  - 3-16% associated developmental/acquired aneurysm
  - Worse prognosis if large or eloquent area [brainstem, thalamus, hypothalamus, motor or sensory (parietal, visual) cortex]
  - Better prognosis for small AVM (≤ 3 cm)
  - Angiographically occult AVM: < 3 cm or thrombosed
    - Annual bleeding risk: < 1%
- Cavernous angioma
  - Subarachnoid/intraparenchymal bleed with rupture
- Capillary hemangioma
  - Symptoms if size ↑ → tissue pressure
- Telangiectases and venous malformations
  - Commonly incidental
- Dural arteriovenous fistula or shunt
  - Leak or sudden rupture into neural parenchyma

Treatment

- Surgical approaches
  - AVM or cavernous angioma extent &/or vascular supply may limit or prevent surgical approach
- Aneurysm
  - Small (< 7-mm) aneurysms: Small rupture potential, traditionally observed but increasingly embolized
  - Surgical clipping (open): Larger aneurysms
  - Endovascular embolization (coils, stent-assisted coils, pipeline embolization mesh)
- AVM

- Staged multimodality for vessel obliteration
  - Stereotactic (focused) irradiation (radiosurgery)
  - Endovascular embolization (polymer, glue)
  - Excision; may follow radiation, embolization
- Observation: Active treatment ↑ harm if unruptured; case dependent
- Brainstem AVM: Single mode less harmful

Prognosis

- Developmental aneurysms
  - Subarachnoid hemorrhage
    - Mortality rate: 45%; most deaths in 1st week
    - Reduced mortality (13-35%) in experienced centers
    - Rebleed ↑ untreated or treated mortality rate
  - Morbidity/mortality factors
    - Acute brain injury: Vasospasm, hypoxia, infarcts
    - Rebleed risk: Older patient, size > 10 mm, blood pressure > 160 mm Hg, poor initial clinical status
    - Morbidity/mortality rate after endovascular coiling lower than after surgical clipping
    - Coil-packed ruptured aneurysm rebleed rate ~ 1% higher compared to clipping
    - Complications: Seizures, syndrome of inappropriate antidiuretic hormone secretion, hydrocephalus
  - Cause of death
    - Subarachnoid hemorrhage (acute brain injury)
    - Pneumonia, organ failure (cardiopulmonary)
    - Intracerebral hemorrhage (rare)
- AVM
  - Associated aneurysm(s) ↓ prognosis
    - Unruptured with associated aneurysm: 7% annual hemorrhage risk
  - Hemorrhage risk ↓ over time
  - Radiation ↑ rebleed risk for large AVM
  - Embolization alone ↑ hemorrhage risk for 1 year
  - Brainstem AVM prognosis favorable
  - Seizure risk same with drugs or surgery
  - Combined therapy compounds treatment-related risk
  - Cause of death
    - Intracerebral hemorrhage, herniation
    - Treatment complications, seizures
    - Operative complication

Pertinent Antemortem Data

- CBC, PT, aPTT
- CT, reconstructed CTA
- MR
- Conventional angiography
- Operative and radiation therapy report(s)

MACROSCOPIC

Aneurysm

- Incidental in some autopsies, usually circle of Willis
  - May be multiple, occasionally symmetrical
- Rupture with subarachnoid hemorrhage
  - Clip, coils, stent, mesh visible or palpable, if used
  - Blood often obscures aneurysm
    - Aneurysm usually at epicenter of hemorrhage
    - Dissect away blood and cerebral tissue as needed
    - May require multiple samples from hemorrhage to locate aneurysm microscopically
    - With no organ retention permitted, remove some blood and fix area(s) likely to contain aneurysm
    - Postmortem cerebral angiography for location (brain edema may interfere by vascular collapse)

Vascular Malformation

- Common incidental finding
  - Usually venous anomaly or telangiectasia
    - Occasionally, only old blood pigment or vague discoloration grossly
- Inoperable AVM or cavernous angioma
  - Often large; in brainstem, may be small
  - Often at least few vessels > 1 mm in diameter
  - Old blood pigment, firm surrounding gliosis
- Posttreatment lesion
  - Variable appearance
    - Residual vessels often grossly apparent
    - Embolized polymer in AVM, may migrate past malformed vessels

MICROSCOPIC

Histologic Features

- Aneurysm
  - Fraying, loss of internal elastic lamina
  - Collagenous tissue in sac wall, no smooth muscle
  - Rupture site, if seen, often in sac dome
- Dolichoectasia
  - Smooth muscle atrophy, frayed internal elastic lamina
- Vascular malformations
  - Back-to-back vessel walls in part or entirely
    - Wall thickness from capillary-like to very thick
  - AVM
    - No capillary bed; intervening parenchyma present
    - Old blood pigment, calcification/bone, gliosis
  - Cavernous angioma
    - Large, abnormal vessels, no intervening parenchyma
    - Old blood pigment, gliosis
  - Capillary hemangioma
    - Small, thin-walled vessels, little, if any, intervening parenchyma
  - Telangiectasia
    - Loosely clustered or scattered, very thin-walled, dilated branches
    - Wall: Endothelium, some pericytes
  - Venous malformation
    - Variable; very thin (focally endothelium and little adventitia) to very thick vessel walls
  - Dural arteriovenous fistula or shunt
    - Enlarged arterialized subarachnoid veins, thickened elastic laminae

SELECTED REFERENCES

1. Wang K et al: Exome-wide analysis of de novo and rare genetic variants in patients with brain arteriovenous malformation. Neurology. 98(16):e1670-8, 2022
2. Peyre M et al: Somatic PIK3CA mutations in sporadic cerebral cavernous malformations. N Engl J Med. 385(11):996-1004, 2021
3. McNulty ML et al: Management of unruptured intracranial aneurysms and arteriovenous malformations. Am J Ther. 18(1):64-9, 2011

Inferior Cerebellar Artery Aneurysm With Subarachnoid Hemorrhage

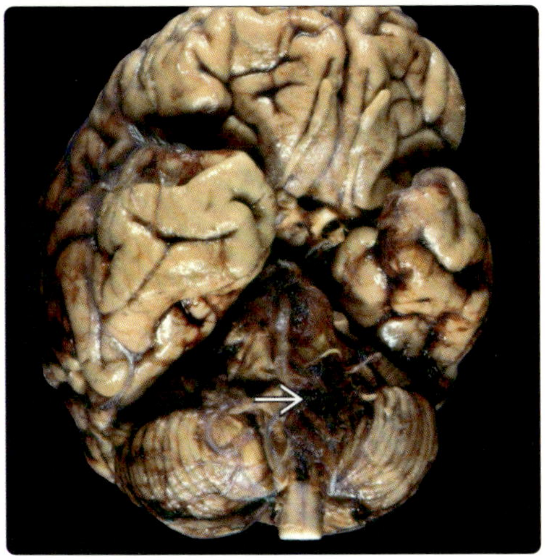

Basilar Artery Dolichoectasia

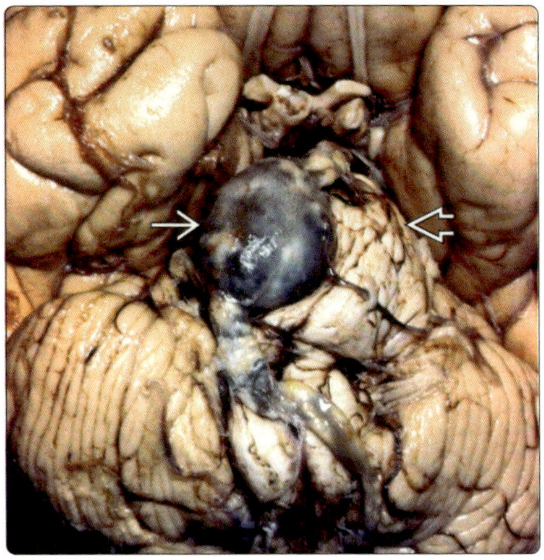

(Left) *Subarachnoid hemorrhage* ➡ *covers a ruptured distal aneurysm of the left posterior inferior cerebellar artery. An infarct in the medulla causes Wallenberg syndrome.* **(Right)** *Basilar artery dolichoectasia* ➡ *pushed the basis pontis laterally* ➡. *These spheroidal dilations become fusiform later. They can cause cardiorespiratory failure from pontine compression. Dolichoectasia ("long dilated") has hypertension, trauma, genetic, and AVM associations.*

Right Occipital Arteriovenous Malformation

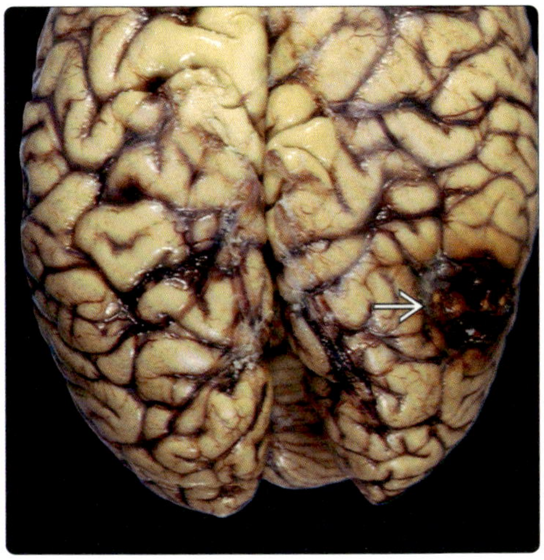

Right Frontal Arteriovenous Malformation

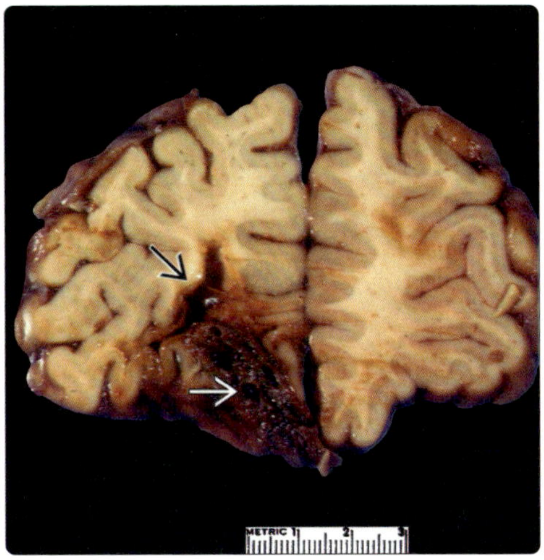

(Left) *A patient with a chronic seizure disorder had an AVM of the right occipital lobe* ➡. *No surgical procedure was performed, but a seizure was thought to have contributed to death.* **(Right)** *This patient with a chronic seizure disorder had a right medial frontal orbital AVM. Several abnormal vessels are large and easily seen* ➡. *Blood leakage and perhaps small ruptures resulted in a cavity in the white matter with blood-stained walls* ⇨.

Parietal Arteriovenous Malformation

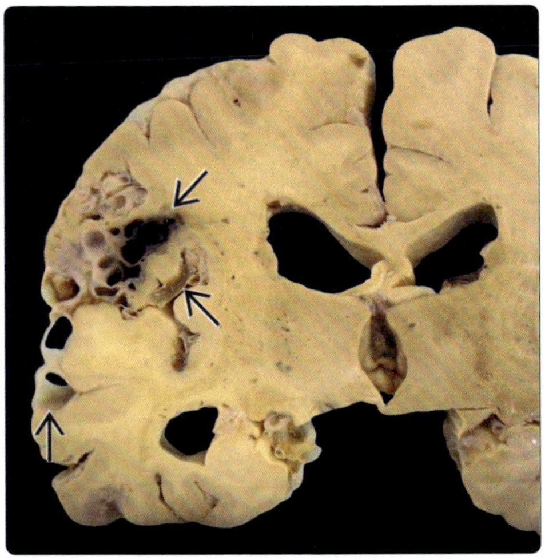

Basal Ganglia Vascular Malformation

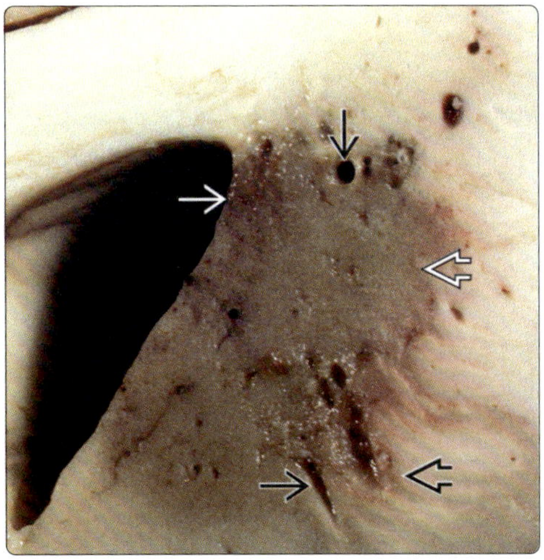

(Left) *Very wide-bore, back-to-back venous structures make up this extensive, inoperable cavernous angioma* ⇨ *that was present in several coronal cerebral sections and was the cause of death.* **(Right)** *Like many vascular malformations in the brain, this is a composite vascular malformation in the right corpus striatum, including the head of the caudate nucleus* ➡ *and the internal capsule* ⇨. *An area of telangiectasia* ➡ *is a classic punctate patch. Large venous channels* ⇨ *are in the same general vascular distribution.*

(Left) *A typical incidental venous malformation with a wide distribution is in the right occipital white matter with little cortical involvement.* **(Right)** *This is an incidental venous malformation involving the walls of the 4th ventricle. It provides an unusual view of the abnormal, low-flow venous structures that form such vascular hamartomas. Note the combination of small- and large-bore abnormal veins.*

Venous Malformation

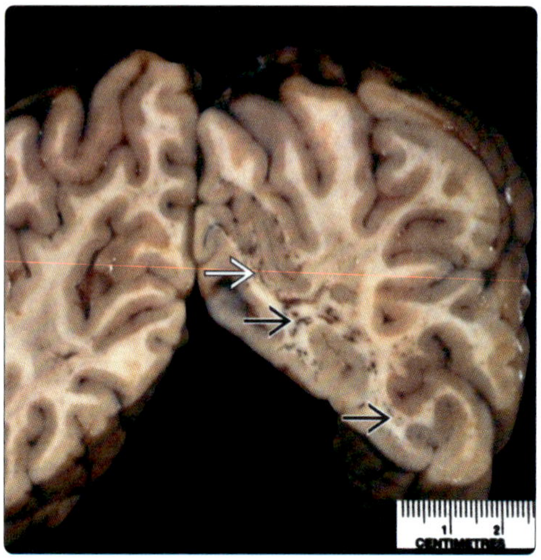

4th Ventricle Venous Malformation

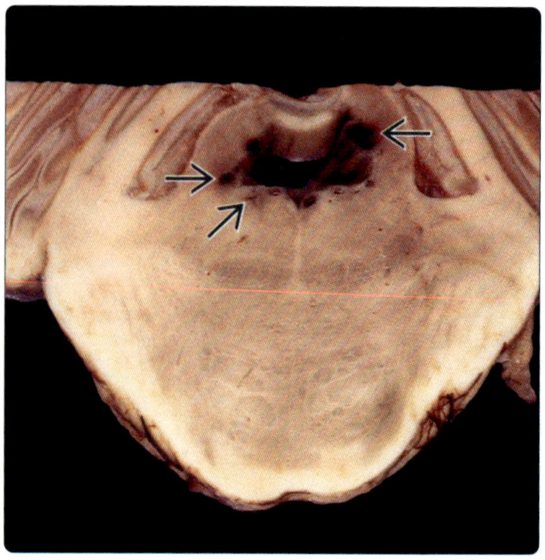

(Left) *A ruptured aneurysm of the anterior communicating artery was closed with 2 metal clips. The patient later died following further subarachnoid hemorrhage. At autopsy, the clips were removed to show crushed vascular tissue.* **(Right)** *Angiogram shows a dural arteriovenous fistula draining from the left transverse sinus to the basal ganglia. Most of these originate in association with a dural venous sinus. The patient presented with basal ganglia hemorrhage.*

Aneurysm Clips

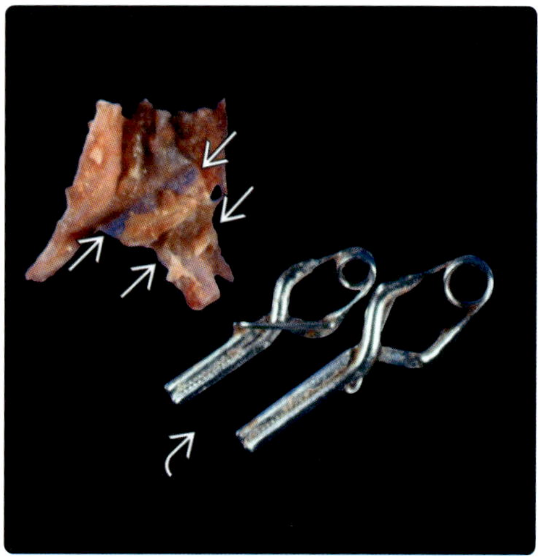

Dural Arteriovenous Fistula

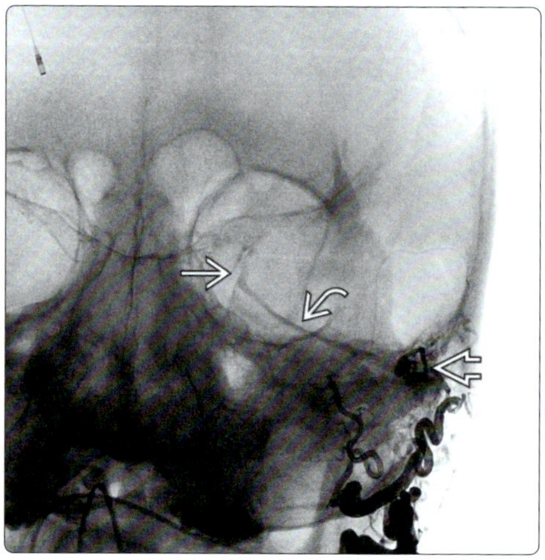

(Left) *Elastic stain of a middle cerebral artery shows a normal, wavy internal elastic lamina that ends at the aneurysmal neck. The aneurysmal wall is irregular and fibrotic. Subarachnoid blood surrounds the sac, which is intact in this field.* **(Right)** *The fibrous wall of a saccular aneurysm is seen, where the rupture site is filled by a delicate fibrin (and cellular) plug or fibrin net. The fibrin net is thought to be disrupted easily by blood flow, and this may be the cause of acute rebleeding prior to interventional therapy.*

Aneurysm Neck: Elastic Stain

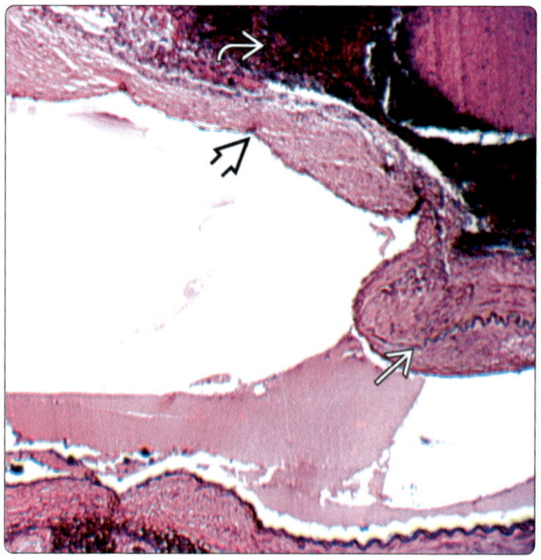

Ruptured Aneurysm

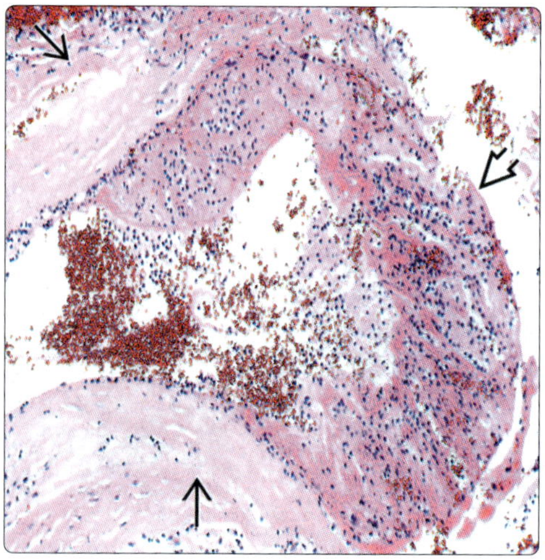

Infective or Mycotic Aneurysm

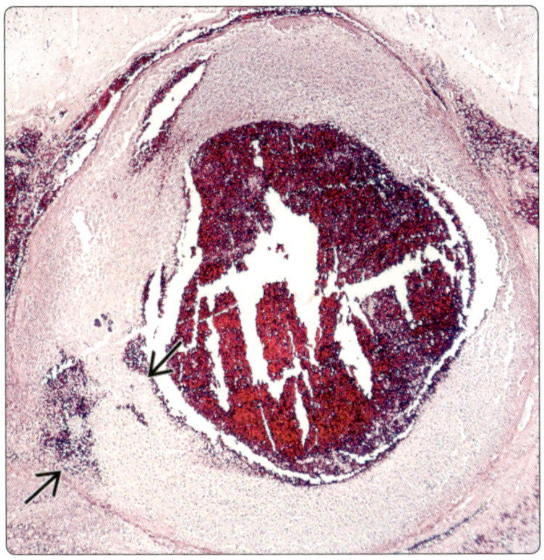

Onyx Embolization Material: Arteriovenous Malformation

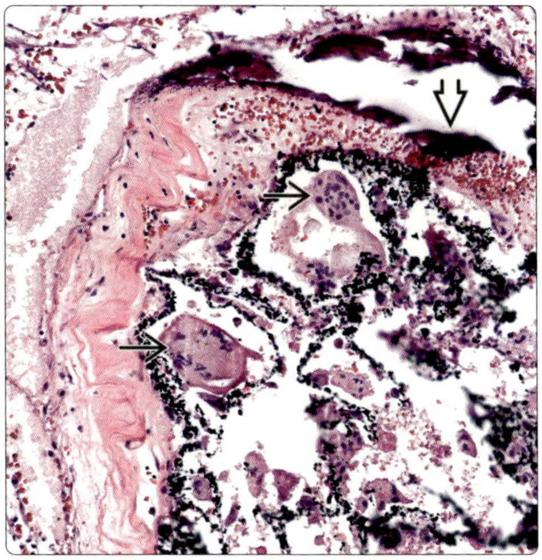

(Left) *This mycotic aneurysm, seen in cross section with H&E stain at low magnification, arose from a bacterial infection of the arterial wall. The wall is replaced by acute inflammatory cells and tissue debris* → *, predisposing to rupture.* **(Right)** *A dilated AVM channel has an irregular wall with focal calcification* → *. The lumen was embolized with Onyx polymer seen as discrete black particles that promote thrombosis. Foreign body giant cells* → *can respond to Onyx, as seen here.*

Abnormal Arteriovenous Malformation Aneurysm

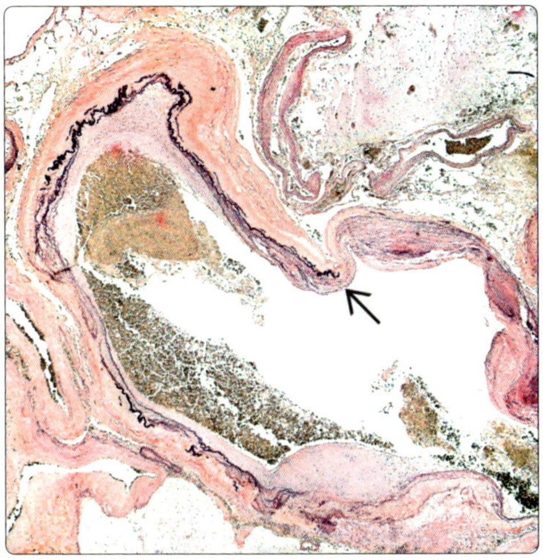

Cavernous Angioma

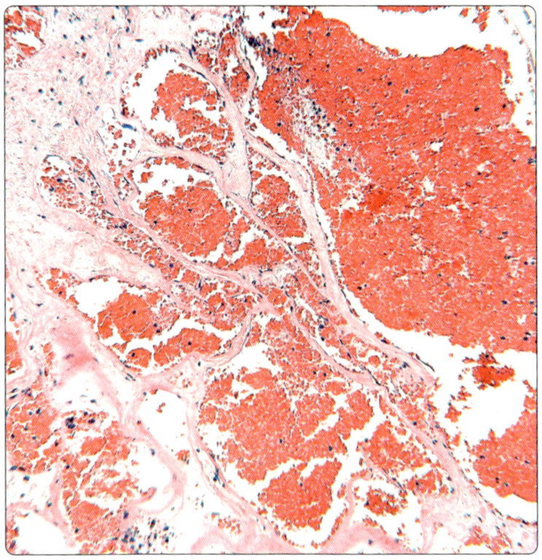

(Left) *Elastin stain (blue-black) at low magnification shows the reduplicated internal elastic lamina of an AVM artery ending* → *at the transition directly into a dilated, irregular vein. Systolic pressure acts directly on the venous wall.* **(Right)** *A cavernous angioma in the medulla, seen at medium magnification, has back-to-back dilated vessels with variable wall thickness without intervening parenchyma. Focal dystrophic ossification and old blood pigment were present.*

Cerebellar Telangiectatic Malformation

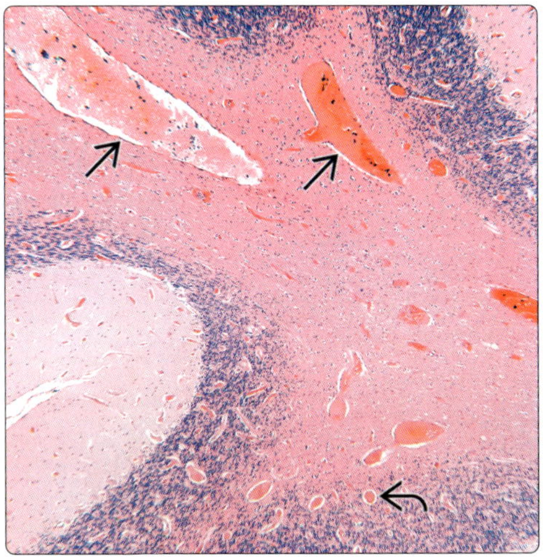

Capillary Hemangioma

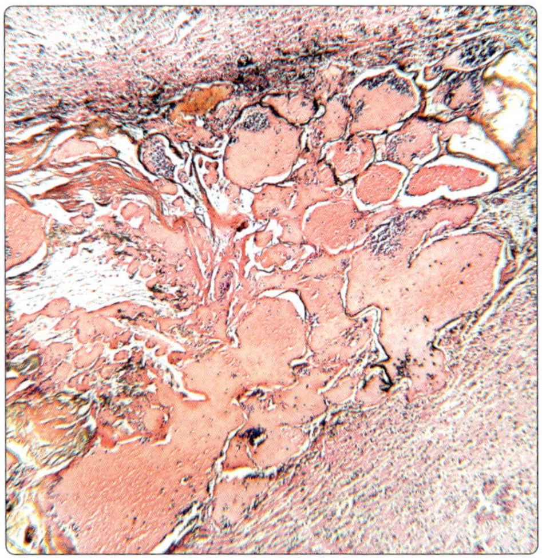

(Left) *An extensive incidental cerebellar telangiectatic malformation, seen in part at low magnification, is formed of many very thin-walled, dilated, small* → *and large vessels* → *with scant adventitia. The abnormal vascular tree has scattered branches.* **(Right)** *This small, incidental capillary hemangioma of back-to-back, dilated, thin-walled, capillary-like vessels in cerebral white matter is seen at low magnification. Capillary-like refers to the thin walls, not the wide lumina.*

INDEX

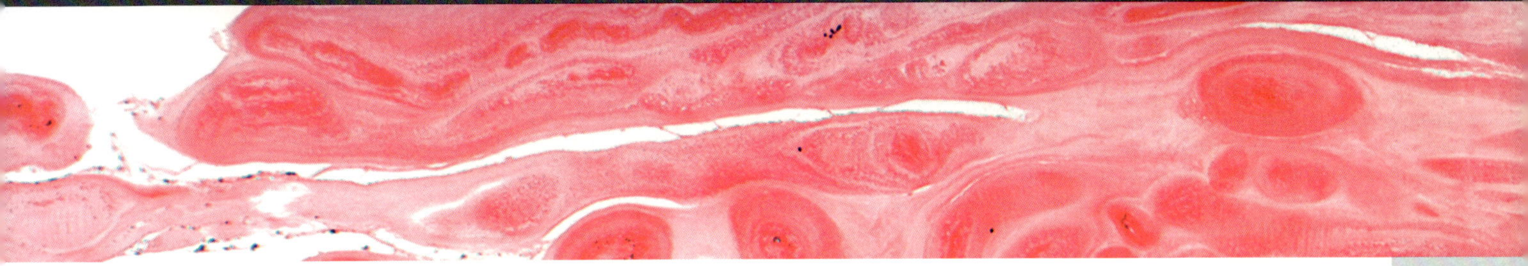

A

INDEX

INDEX

INDEX

B

INDEX

C

INDEX

INDEX

INDEX

INDEX

D

INDEX

E

INDEX

F

G

H

INDEX

INDEX

INDEX

INDEX

J

K

INDEX

L

M

INDEX

N

O

P

INDEX

INDEX

Q

R

S

INDEX

T

INDEX

U

INDEX

V

W

X